Get focused & study sma[illegible]

RELATED RESOU[illegible]

GET HELP WITH T[illegible] WHOLE NURSING PROCESS

Doenges & Moorhouse

APPLICATION OF NURSING PROCESS AND NURSING DIAGNOSIS

An Interactive Text for Diagnostic Reasoning

An interactive, workbook-style approach shows you how to develop the diagnostic reasoning and problem-solving skills you need to think like a nurse.

APPLY CARE PLANS TO THE NURSING PROCESS

Doenges, Moorhouse & Murr

NURSING CARE PLANS

Guidelines for Individualizing Client Care Across the Life Span

Turn to the all-in-one care planning resource. 167 care plans enhance your critical-thinking and analytical skills.

LEARN TO DEVELOP CONCEPT CARE MAPS

Schuster

CONCEPT MAPPING

A Critical Thinking Approach to Care Planning

Here's the clear, visual, and systematic model you need for mastering the whys and hows of concept mapping.

Check out our resources at **www.FADavis.com!**

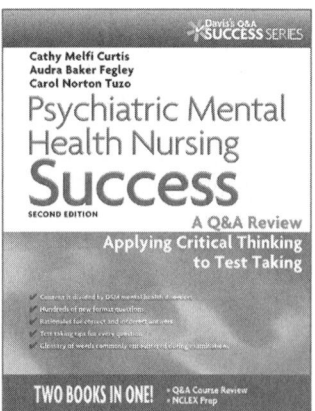

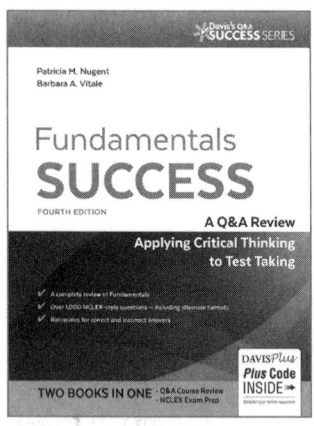

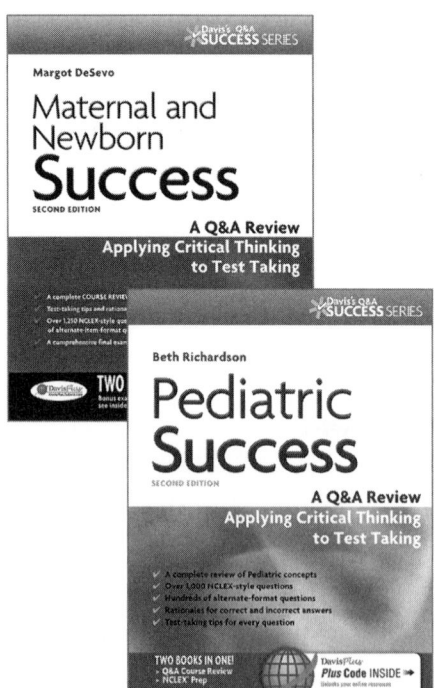

Nursing Diagnosis Manual

Planning, Individualizing, and Documenting Client Care

Marilynn E. Doenges, APN, BC—Retired
Clinical Specialist—Adult Psychiatric/Mental Health Nursing, Adjunct Faculty (Ret)
Beth-El College of Nursing and Health Sciences, CU–Springs
Colorado Springs, Colorado

Mary Frances Moorhouse, RN, MSN, CRRN
Nurse Consultant, TNT-RN Enterprises
Adjunct Nursing Faculty
Pikes Peak Community College
Colorado Springs, Colorado

Alice C. Murr, BSN, RN—Retired
Nurse Consultant
Parkville, Missouri

FIFTH EDITION

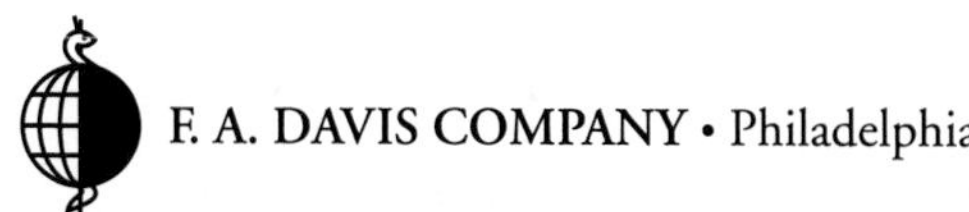

F. A. Davis Company
1915 Arch Street
Philadelphia, PA 19103
www.fadavis.com

Printed in the United States of America

Last digit indicates print number: 10 9 8 7 6 5 4

Acquisitions Editor: Megan Klim
Content Project Manager II: Amy M. Romano
Design and Illustrations Manager: Carolyn O'Brien

Library of Congress Cataloging-in-Publication Data

Names: Doenges, Marilynn E., 1922–, author. | Moorhouse, Mary Frances, 1947–, author. | Murr, Alice C., 1946–, author.
Title: Nursing diagnosis manual : planning, individualizing, and documenting client care / Marilynn E. Doenges, Mary Frances Moorhouse, Alice C. Murr.
Description: Fifth edition. | Philadelphia, PA : F.A. Davis Company, [2016] |
Includes bibliographical references and indexes.
Identifiers: LCCN 2015042538 | ISBN 9780803644748 | ISBN 0803644744
Subjects: | MESH: Nursing Diagnosis. | Nursing Records. | Patient Care Planning.
Classification: LCC RT48.6 | NLM WY 100.4 | DDC 616.07/5--dc23 LC record available at http://lccn.loc.gov/2015042538

To our spouses, children, parents, and friends, who much of the time have had to manage without us while we work and dream, as well as cope with our struggles and frustrations.

The Doenges families: the late Dean, Jim; Barbara and Bob Lanza; David, Monita, Matthew, and Tyler; and John, Holly, Nicole, and Kelsey; and the Daigle families: Nancy, Jim; Jennifer, Brandon, Annabelle, Will, and Henry Smith-Daigle; and Jonathan, Kim, and Mandalyn JoAn.

The Moorhouse family: the late Jan; sons Paul, Jason, and Thenderlyn Moorhouse; granddaughters Alexa and Tanner Plant; Mary Isabella Moorhouse; and the perfect great-grandchild, Quinton Russell Plant.

To my children: Kevin and Tammy Carroll and Darin and Ck Carroll; the best grandchildren ever: Chelsea-Jane and Joseph Bockerstette and Matthew, Joseph, Nathan, and Ben Carroll; and my perfect great-grandchildren: Maxwell Carroll Bockerstette and Eisley Jo Bockerstette. You are my joy. Mom/Grammy Murr.

To our FAD family, especially Megan Klim and Amy Romano, our production team who assisted us in meeting deadlines and completing this new edition, and Robert Allen for teaching old nurses new technology.

To the nurses we are writing for, who daily face the challenge of meeting the needs of clients in varied settings and are looking for a practical way to organize and document this care. We believe that nursing diagnosis and these guides will help.

And to NANDA-I and the international nurses who are facilitating the development and dissemination of nursing diagnoses—we continue to champion your efforts and the work of promoting standardized languages.

PREFACE

The American Nurses Association (ANA) *Social Policy Statement* of 1980 was the first to define nursing as the diagnosis and treatment of human responses to actual and potential health problems. This definition, when combined with the ANA *Scope and Standards of Practice,* has provided impetus and support for the use of nursing diagnosis. Defining *nursing* and its effect on client care supports the growing awareness that nursing care is a key factor in client survival and in the maintenance, rehabilitative, and preventive aspects of healthcare. Changes and new developments in healthcare delivery in the past decades have given rise to the need for a common framework of communication to ensure continuity of care for the client moving between multiple healthcare settings and providers.

This book is designed to aid the student nurse and the practitioner in identifying interventions commonly associated with specific nursing diagnoses as disseminated by NANDA International. These interventions are the activities needed to implement and document care provided to the individual client and can be used in varied settings from acute to community/home care.

Chapter 1 presents a brief discussion of the nursing process and introduces the concept of evidence-based practice. Standardized nursing languages (SNLs) are discussed in Chapter 2, with a focus on NANDA-I (nursing diagnoses), NIC (interventions), and NOC (outcomes). NANDA-I has 235 diagnosis labels with definitions, defining characteristics, and related or risk factors used to define a client need or problem. NIC is a comprehensive standardized language providing 554 direct and indirect intervention labels with definitions and a list of activities a nurse might choose to carry out each intervention. NOC language provides 490 outcome labels with definitions; a set of indicators describing specific client, caregiver, family, or community states related to the outcome; and a 5-point Likert-type measurement scale that can demonstrate client progress even when outcomes are not fully met. Chapter 3 addresses the assessment process using a nursing framework for data collection, such as the Diagnostic Divisions Assessment Tool.

A creative approach for developing and documenting the planning of care is demonstrated in Chapter 4. Mind or Concept Mapping is a technique or learning tool provided to assist you in achieving a holistic view of your client, enhance your critical-thinking skills, and facilitate the creative process of planning client care. For more in-depth information and inclusive plans of care related to specific medical/psychiatric/obstetrical and newborn conditions (with rationale and the application of the diagnoses), refer to the larger work also published by the F. A. Davis Company: *Nursing Care Plans: Guidelines for Individualizing Client Care Across the Life Span*, 9th ed. (Doenges, Moorhouse, & Murr, 2014). Psychiatric/mental health and maternal/newborn plans of care are available on the Davis Plus Web site.

Chapter 6 contains 850 disorders and health conditions reflecting all specialty areas with associated nursing diagnoses written as client problem/need statements to aid you in validating the assessment and diagnosis steps of the nursing process.

In Chapter 5, the heart of the book, all the nursing diagnoses are listed alphabetically for ease of reference and include the diagnoses accepted for use by NANDA-I 2015–2017. The alphabetization of diagnoses follows NANDA-I's own sequencing, whereby diagnoses are alphabetized first by their key term, which is capitalized. Subordinate terminology or descriptors of the diagnosis are presented in lowercase words and are alphabetized secondarily to the key term (for example, chronic Pain is alphabetized under P, following acute Pain). Each approved diagnosis includes its location in NANDA-I's Taxonomy II (see Appendix A), definition, and information divided into the NANDA-I categories of Related or Risk Factors and Defining Characteristics. Related/Risk Factors information reflects causative or contributing factors that can be useful for determining whether the diagnosis is applicable to a particular client.

Defining Characteristics (signs and symptoms or cues) are listed as subjective and/or objective and are used to confirm problem diagnoses, aid in formulating outcomes, and provide additional data for choosing appropriate interventions. We have not deleted or altered NANDA-I's listings; however, on occasion, we have added to their definitions and suggested additional criteria to provide clarification and direction. These additions are denoted with brackets [ ].

NANDA-I nursing diagnosis labels are designed to be multiaxial with seven axes or descriptors. An *axis* is defined as a dimension of the human response that is considered in the diagnostic process (see Appendix B). Sometimes an axis may be included in the diagnostic concept, such as ineffective community Coping, in which the unit of care (i.e., community) is named. Some are implicit, such as Activity Intolerance, in which the individual is the unit of care. At times, an axis may not be pertinent to a particular diagnosis and will not be a part of the nursing diagnosis label. For example, the time frame (e.g., acute, intermittent) or body part (e.g., cerebral, oral, skin) may not be relevant to each diagnostic situation.

Desired Outcomes/Evaluation Criteria are identified to assist you in formulating individual client outcomes and to support the evaluation process. Sample NOC linkages to the nursing diagnosis are provided.

Nursing priorities are used to group the suggested interventions, which are primarily directed to adult care, although interventions designated as across the lifespan do include pediatric and geriatric considerations and are designated by an icon. In general, the interventions can be used in multiple settings—acute care, rehabilitation, community clinics, home care, or private practice. Most interventions are independent or nursing originated; however, some interventions are collaborative orders (e.g., medical, psychiatric), and you will need to determine when this is necessary and take the appropriate action. Icons are also used to differentiate collaborative interventions, diagnostic studies, and medications, as well as transcultural considerations. All of these "specialized" interventions are presented with icons, rather than being broken out under separate headings, to maintain their sequence within the prioritization of all nursing interventions for the diagnosis. Additionally, in support of evidence-based practice, rationales are provided for the interventions and references for these rationales are cited.

The inclusion of Documentation Focus suggestions is to remind you of the importance and necessity of recording the steps of the nursing process.

As noted, with few exceptions, we have presented NANDA-I's recommendations as formulated. We support the belief that practicing nurses and researchers need to study, use, and evaluate the diagnoses as presented. Nurses can be creative as they use the standardized language, redefining and sharing information as the diagnoses are used with individual clients. As new nursing diagnoses are developed, it is important that the data they encompass are added to assessment tools and current databases. As part of the process by clinicians, educators, and researchers across practice specialties and academic settings to define, test, and refine nursing diagnosis, nurses are encouraged to share insights and ideas with NANDA-I at the following address: NANDA International, PO Box 157, Kaukauna, WI 54130–0157; e-mail: nanda.org.

Marilynn E. Doenges
Mary Frances Moorhouse
Alice C. Murr

CONTRIBUTORS

Diane Bligh, RN, MS, CNS
Associate Professor, Nursing
Front Range Community College
Westminster, Colorado

Caryn F. Demaree , RN, BSN, IBCLC
Lactation Specialist
Denver Health Medical Center
Denver, Colorado

Mary F. Johnston, RN, MSN
Retired Program Director, Nursing
Front Range Community College
Westminster, Colorado

Sheila Marquez, RN, BSN, PNP—Retired
Former Executive Director, Vice President/Chief Operating Officer
The Colorado SIDS Program, Inc.
Denver, Colorado

Susan Moberly, RNC, BSN, ICCE (Deceased)
Childbirth Educator
Obstetric Nursing and Lactation Consultant
Colorado Springs, Colorado

Alma Mueller, RN, MEd
Retired Chair and Professor of Nursing
Front Range Community College
Westminster, Colorado

Acknowledgment: A special thank you to our researchers who were so vital in locating evidence-based resources.

Mary Katherine Blackwell
Macon, Mississippi

Kathe L. Ellis
Colorado Springs, Colorado

REVIEWERS

Elizabeth Jean Hayes, RN, MS
Associate Professor
Purdue University North Central
Westville, Indiana

Janice Lowden-Stokley, MSN, RN
Associate Professor & Level III Coordinator
Adventist University of Health Sciences
Orlando, Florida

Mindy Thompson, RN, BSN
Nursing Instructor
Oklahoma State University Institute of Technology
Okmulgee, Oklahoma

CONTENTS

CHAPTER 1
The Nursing Process: The Foundation of Quality Client Care 1

CHAPTER 2
The Language of Nursing: NANDA, NIC, NOC, and Other Standardized Nursing Languages 9

CHAPTER 3
The Assessment Process: Developing the Client Database 13

CHAPTER 4
Concept or Mind Mapping to Create and Document the Plan of Care 24

CHAPTER 5
Nursing Diagnoses in Alphabetical Order 32

CHAPTER 6
Health Conditions and Client Concerns With Associated Nursing Diagnoses 943

APPENDIX A
NANDA-I's Taxonomy II 1065

APPENDIX B
Definitions of Taxonomy II Axes 1067

APPENDIX C
NANDA-I Nursing Diagnoses Organized According to Maslow's Hierarchy of Needs 1069

Index 1072

CHAPTER 1

The Nursing Process: The Foundation of Quality Client Care

Defining the Profession

In the world of healthcare, nursing has long struggled to establish itself as a profession. Dictionary terms describe nursing as "a calling requiring specialized knowledge and often long and intensive academic preparation; a principal calling, vocation, or employment; the whole body of persons engaged in a calling."[1] Throughout the history of nursing, unfavorable stereotypes (based on the view of nursing as subservient and dependent on the medical profession) have negatively affected the view of nursing as an independent entity. In its early developmental years, nursing did not seek or have the means to control its own practice. Florence Nightingale, in discussing the nature of nursing in 1859, observed that "nursing has been limited to signify little more than the administration of medicines and the application of poultices."[2] Although this attitude may persist to some degree, the nursing profession has defined what makes nursing unique and has identified a body of professional knowledge. As early as 1896, nurses in America banded together to seek standardization of educational programs and laws governing their practice. The task of nursing since that time has been to create descriptive terminology reflecting specific nursing functions and levels of competency.[3] Erickson, Tomlin, and Swain stated the belief that "nursing will thrive as a unique and valued profession when nurses present a theory and rationalistic model for their practice, correct misleading stereotypes, locate control with clients, and actively participate in processes for change."[4]

In the past several decades, more than a dozen prominent nursing scholars (e.g., Rogers, Parse, and Henderson) have developed conceptualizations to define the nature of nursing. Because much of nursing is nonphenomenological or nonobservable, the nature of nursing cannot be explained using the usual parameters of scientific investigation. Kikuchi proposes that conceptualizations about nursing are philosophic in nature and as such are still testable.[5] As nursing research continues the work of establishing the profession as independent in its own right, the value of nursing goals is being understood and the difference between nursing and other professions is being delineated. Nursing is now recognized as both a science and an art concerned with the physical, psychological, sociological, cultural, and spiritual concerns of the individual. The science of nursing is based on a broad theoretical framework; its art depends on the caring skills and abilities of the individual nurse. The importance of the nurse within the healthcare system is noted in many positive ways, and the profession of nursing is acknowledging the need for its practitioners to act professionally and be accountable for the care they provide.

Barely a century after Florence Nightingale noted that "the very elements of nursing are all but unknown," the American Nurses Association (ANA) developed its first Social Policy Statement in 1980, defining nursing as "the diagnosis and treatment of *human responses* to actual or potential health problems."[6] Human responses (defined as people's experiences with and responses to health, illness, and life events) are nursing's phenomena of concern. In 1995, this statement was revisited, updated, and titled "Nursing's Social Policy Statement." This policy statement acknowledged that since the release of the original statement, "nursing has been influenced by many social and professional changes, as well as by the science of caring."[7]

The statement delineated four essential features of today's contemporary nursing practice:

1. Attention to the full range of human experiences and responses to health and illness without restriction to a problem-focused orientation
2. Integration of objective data with knowledge gained from an understanding of the client's or group's subjective experience
3. Application of scientific knowledge to the processes of diagnosis and treatment
4. Provision of a caring relationship that facilitates health and healing[7]

Thus, nursing's role includes the promotion of health as well as the performance of activities that contribute to recovery from or adjustment to illness. This is reflected in ANA's 2003 Nursing's Social Policy Statement, which recognized nursing's full scope of care by defining nursing as "the protection, promotion, and optimization of health and abilities, prevention of illness and injury, alleviation of suffering through the diagnosis and treatment of human response, and advocacy in the care of individuals, families, communities, and populations."[8] Also, nurses support the right of clients to define their own health-related goals and to engage in care that reflects their personal values. Emphasis is placed on the mind-body-spirit connection with a holistic view of the individual as nurses facilitate the client's efforts in striving for growth and development.

In your readings, you will likely encounter other definitions of nursing. As your knowledge and experience develop, your definition of nursing may change to reflect your personal nursing philosophy, your focus on a particular care setting or population, or your specific role. For example, although the definition of nursing developed by Erickson, Tomlin, and Swain is more than 30 years old, it remains viable and timely because it incorporates the concepts noted previously with today's holistic approach to care. Their definition includes what nursing is, how it is accomplished, and the goals of nursing: "Nursing is the holistic helping of persons with their self-care activities in relation to their health. This is an interactive, interpersonal process that nurtures strengths to enable development, release, and channeling of resources for coping with one's circumstances and environment. The goal is to achieve a state of perceived optimum health and contentment."[4]

An understanding of human nature is certainly important in the development of a philosophy of nursing. Understanding that "needs motivate behavior" helps the nurse to determine the client's needs at a particular moment in time. Maslow's hierarchy of needs[9] provides a basis for understanding that unmet needs can interfere with an individual's holistic growth and may even result in physical or mental distress and illness. Other theorists have also studied how people are similar, providing the nurse with more information to help understand the client. For example, Erik Erikson's observations on the stages of psychological development suggest that the individual is a "work in progress" accomplishing age-specific maturational tasks throughout the lifespan. Piaget's cognitive stages address how thinking develops and how individuals adapt to and organize their environment intellectually.[4] However, in the end, the individual is the primary source of information about himself/herself. The nurse needs to listen with an open mind and empathic, unconditional acceptance to what the client is relating. Knowing how people are alike provides a basis to understanding human nature. However, each person is unique, and the nurse needs to look for the client's model of the world and how it relates to the client's own situation.

The nursing profession is further defined by fundamental philosophical beliefs that have been identified over time as essential to the practice of nursing. These values and assumptions offer guidance to the nurse and need to be kept in mind to enhance the quality of nursing care provided:

- The client is a human being who has worth and dignity.
- Humans manifest an essential unity of mind/body/spirit.[7]
- There are basic human needs that must be met (Maslow's hierarchy of needs).
- When these needs are not met, problems arise that may require intervention by another person until the individuals can resume responsibility for themselves.
- Human experience is contextually and culturally defined.[7]
- Health and illness are human experiences.[7]
- Clients have a right to quality health and nursing care delivered with interest, compassion, and competence with a focus on wellness and prevention.
- The presence of illness does not preclude health, nor does optimal health preclude illness.[7]
- The therapeutic nurse-client relationship is important in the nursing process and provision of individualized care.

Finally, the Code of Ethics for Nurses[10] addresses the need for nurses to respect human dignity, acknowledge the uniqueness of each client, and honor the client's right to privacy. The Code also calls on nurses to assume responsibility for individual nursing judgments and actions and for the delegation of nursing activities to others. Nurses are encouraged to maintain competence in nursing, contribute to the ongoing development of the profession, and participate in the implementation and improvement of standards. This last goal can be accomplished by using the results of nursing research to engage in evidence-based nursing practice.

The roots of evidence-based practice lie in the efforts of many in the past. Hippocrates described the symptoms and course of illnesses and related them to the seasons, geographical area, and types of people associated with each. These hypotheses founded the rational approach to the understanding of disease. As knowledge grew and the germ theory of disease was accepted, epidemiology began to count disease events, leading to the establishment of a central government agency to collect and record data. This led to the posing of questions in the form of testable hypotheses, the collection of data to support or refute hypotheses, and the development of statistical tools to summarize numerical data.[11] The work of Pasteur and Koch expanded the understanding of causal relationships between bacterial causes of many diseases, leading to reducing illness and mortality.

Florence Nightingale used statistics to measure health, identify causes of mortality, evaluate health services, and reform institutions. After the Crimean War, she began organizing committees, assembling data, and preparing reports and hearings on how administrative inadequacies affected clients' health. Her work resulted in British Army Hospital and government reforms in the interest of preventing death and disease. She became an honorary member of the American Statistical Association in 1874, and her papers were read at a National Social Science Congress in 1863 and at the nurses' congress of the Chicago World's Fair in 1893. The efforts of these pioneers laid the groundwork for the development of evidence-based practice.

Barnsteiner and Provost note that "the current definition [of evidence-based practice] is the integration of best research evidence with clinical expertise and patient values"[12]—that is, both research and nonresearch components are combined to create evidence-based practice. Quantitative research is invaluable in measuring the effectiveness of nursing interventions, while qualitative studies capture the preferences, attitudes, and values of healthcare consumers. However, the nurses' clinical judgment and individual client needs and perspectives must also be included. As nurses work to provide cost-effective care in the best setting for the client, "the most important [and challenging] requirement for practicing nurses in the 21st century will be to utilize [appropriate] evidence available to improve practice."[13]

Administering Nursing Care

Nursing leaders have identified a process that "combines the most desirable elements of the art of nursing with the most relevant elements of systems theory, using the scientific method."[14] This *nursing process* incorporates an interactive and interpersonal approach with a problem-solving and decision-making process that serves as a framework for the delivery of nursing care.[15–17]

The concept of a nursing process was first introduced in the 1950s as a three-step process of assessment, planning, and evaluation based on the scientific method of observing, measuring, gathering data, and analyzing the findings. Years of study, use, and refinement have led nurses to expand the nursing process to five distinct steps that provide an efficient method of organizing thought processes for clinical decision making, problem solving, and the delivery of higher-quality, individualized client care. The nursing process now consists of the following:

- *Assessment* or the systematic collection of data relating to clients;
- *Diagnosis or need identification* involving the analysis of collected data to identify the client's needs;
- *Planning,* which is a two-part process of identifying goals and the client's desired outcomes to address the assessed health and wellness needs along with the selection of appropriate nursing interventions to assist the client in attaining the outcomes;
- *Implementation* or putting the plan of care into action; and
- *Evaluation* by determining the client's progress toward attaining the identified outcomes and the

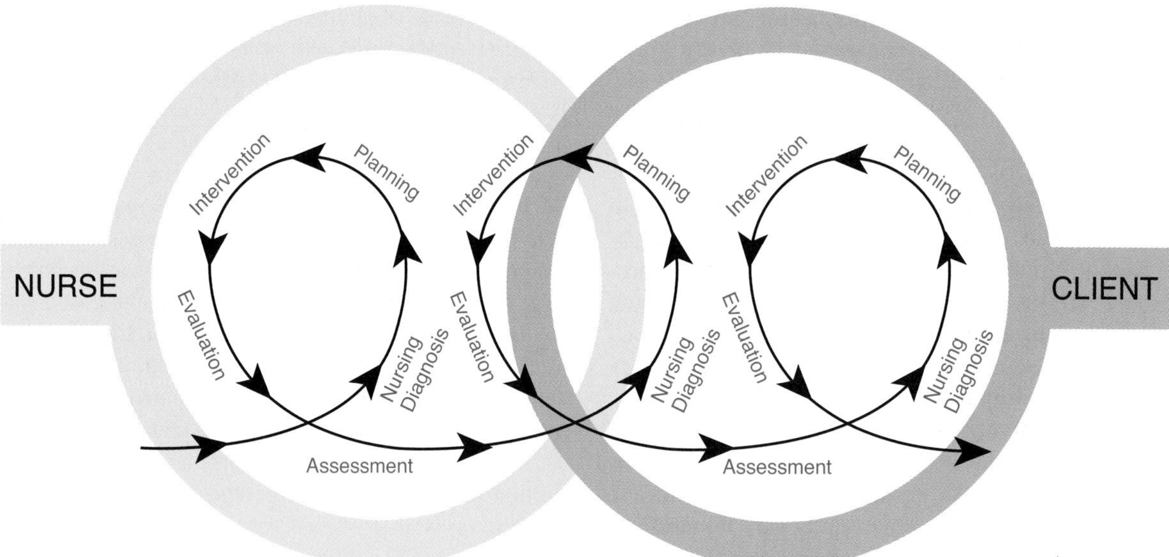

Figure 1.1 Diagram of the nursing process. The steps of the nursing process are interrelated, forming a continuous circle of thought and action that is both dynamic and cyclical.

client's response to and the effectiveness of the selected nursing interventions for the purpose of altering the plan as indicated.

Because these five steps are central to nursing actions in any setting, the nursing process is now included in the conceptual framework of nursing curricula and is accepted as part of the legal definition of nursing in the Nurse Practice Acts of most states.

When a client enters the healthcare system, whether as an inpatient, a clinic outpatient, or a homecare client, the nursing process steps are set into motion. The nurse collects data, identifies client needs (nursing diagnoses), establishes goals, creates measurable outcomes, and selects nursing interventions to assist the client in achieving these outcomes and goals. Finally, after the interventions have been implemented, the nurse evaluates the client's responses and the effectiveness of the plan of care in reaching the desired outcomes and goals to determine whether or not the needs or problems have been resolved and the client is ready to be discharged from the care setting. If the identified needs or problems remain unresolved, further assessment, additional nursing diagnoses, alteration of outcomes and goals, or changes of interventions are required.

Although we use the terms *assessment, diagnosis, planning, implementation,* and *evaluation* as separate, progressive steps, in reality they are interrelated. Together these steps form a continuous circle of thought and action that recycles throughout the client's contact with the healthcare system. Figure 1.1 depicts a model for visualizing this process. You can see that the nursing process uses the nursing diagnosis, which is the clinical judgment product of critical thinking. Based on this judgment, nursing interventions are selected and implemented. Figure 1.1 also shows how the progressive steps of the nursing process create an understandable model of both the products and the processes of critical thinking contained within the nursing process. The model graphically emphasizes both the dynamic and cyclic characteristics of the nursing process.

Application of the Nursing Process

The scientific method of problem solving introduced in the previous section is used almost instinctively by most people, without conscious awareness.

FOR EXAMPLE While studying for your semester finals, you snack on pepperoni pizza. After going to bed, you are awakened by a burning sensation in the center of your chest. You are young and in good health and note no other symptoms (assessment). You decide that your pain is the result of the spicy food you have eaten (diagnosis). You then determine that before you can return to sleep, you need to relieve the discomfort with an over-the-counter preparation (planning). You take a liquid antacid for your discomfort (implementation). Within a few minutes, you note the burning sensation is relieved, and you return to bed without further concern (evaluation).

As you see, this is a process you routinely use to solve problems in your life that can be readily applied to client-care situations. You need only to learn the new terms describing the nursing process rather than having to think about each step (assessment, diagnosis/need identification, planning, implementation, and evaluation) in an entirely new way.

To effectively use the nursing process, the nurse needs to possess and apply some basic abilities. Particularly important is a thorough knowledge of science and theory, not only as applied in nursing, but also in other related disciplines such as medicine and psychology. Creativity is needed in the application of nursing knowledge, as is adaptability in handling change and the many unexpected happenings that occur. As a nurse, you must make a commitment to practice your profession in the best possible way, trusting in yourself and your ability to do your job well and displaying the necessary leadership to organize and supervise as your position requires. In addition, intelligence, well-developed interpersonal skills, and competent technical skills are essential.

FOR EXAMPLE A diabetic client's irritable behavior could be the result of low serum glucose or the effects of excessive caffeine intake. However, it could also arise from a sense of helplessness regarding life events. A single behavior may have varied causes. It is important that your nursing assessment skills identify the underlying etiology to provide appropriate care.

The practice responsibilities presented in the definitions of nursing and the nursing process are explained in detail in the publication *Nursing: Scope & Standards of Practice*.[18] The standards provide workable guidelines to ensure that the practice of nursing can be carried out by each nurse. Table 1.1 presents an abbreviated description of the standards of clinical practice. With the ultimate goal of quality healthcare, the effective use of the nursing process will result in a viable nursing care system that is recognized and accepted as nursing's body of knowledge and that can be shared with other healthcare professionals.

TABLE 1.1 ANA Standards of Nursing Practice

Standards of Practice

Describe a competent level of nursing care as demonstrated by the nursing process that encompasses all significant actions taken by the nurse in providing care and forms the foundation of clinical decision making.

1. Assessment: The registered nurse (RN) collects comprehensive data pertinent to the healthcare consumer's health and/or situation.
2. Diagnosis: The RN analyzes the assessment data to determine the diagnoses or the issues.
3. Outcome Identification: The RN identifies expected outcomes for a plan individualized to the healthcare consumer or the situation.
4. Planning: The RN develops a plan that prescribes strategies and alternatives to attain expected outcomes.
5. Implementation: The RN implements the identified plan.
   a. Coordination of Care: The RN coordinates care delivery.
   b. Health Teaching and Health Promotion: The RN employs strategies to promote health and a safe environment.
   c. Consultation: The graduate-level specialty nurse or advanced-practice RN provides consultation to influence the identified plan, enhance the abilities of others, and effect change.
   d. Prescriptive Authority and Treatment: The advanced-practice RN uses prescriptive authority, procedures, referrals, treatments, and therapies in accordance with state and federal laws and regulations.
6. Evaluation: The RN evaluates progress toward attainment of outcomes.

(table continues on page 6)

TABLE 1.1 ANA Standards of Nursing Practice (continued)

Standards of Professional Performance
Describe roles expected of all professional nurses appropriate to their education, position, and practice setting.
7. Ethics: The RN integrates practices ethically.
8. Education: The RN attains knowledge and competence that reflect current nursing practice.
9. Evidence-Based Practice and Research: The RN integrates evidence and research findings into practice.
10. Quality of Practice: The RN contributes to quality nursing practice.
11. Communication: The RN communicates effectively in all areas of practice.
12. Leadership: The RN demonstrates leadership in the professional practice setting and the profession.
13. Collaboration: The RN collaborates with the healthcare consumer, her or his family, and others in the conduct of nursing practice.
14. Professional Practice Evaluation: The RN evaluates her or his own nursing practice in relation to professional practice standards and guidelines, relevant statutes, rules, and regulations.
15. Resource Utilization: The RN utilizes appropriate resources to plan and provide nursing services that are safe, effective, and financially responsible.
16. Environmental Health: The RN practices in an environmentally safe and healthy manner.

Source: American Nurses Association. (2010). *Nursing: Scope & Standards of Practice.* 2nd ed. Silver Spring, MD: Nursesbooks.org.

Advantages of Using the Nursing Process

There are many advantages to using the nursing process:

- The nursing process provides an organizing framework for meeting the individual needs of the client, the client's family/significant other(s), and the community.
- The steps of the nursing process focus the nurse's attention on the "individual" human responses of a client/family or group to a given health situation, resulting in a holistic plan of care addressing the specific needs of the client/family or group.
- The nursing process provides an organized, systematic method of problem solving (while still allowing for creative solutions) that may minimize dangerous errors or omissions in caregiving and avoid time-consuming repetition in care and documentation.
- The use of the nursing process promotes the active involvement of clients in their healthcare, enhancing consumer satisfaction. Such participation increases clients' sense of control over what is happening to them, stimulates problem solving, and promotes personal responsibility, all of which strengthen the client's commitment to achieving the identified goals.
- The use of the nursing process enables you as a nurse to have more control over your practice. This enhances the opportunity for you to use your knowledge, expertise, and intuition constructively and dynamically to increase the likelihood of a successful client outcome. This, in turn, promotes greater job satisfaction and your professional growth.
- The use of the nursing process provides a common language (nursing diagnosis) for practice, unifying the nursing profession. Using a system that clearly communicates the plan of care to coworkers and clients enhances continuity of care, promotes achievement of client goals, provides a vehicle for evaluation, and aids in the development of nursing standards. In addition, the structure of the process provides a format for documenting the client's response to all aspects of the planned care.
- The use of the nursing process provides a means of assessing nursing's economic contribution to client care. The nursing process supplies a vehicle for the quantitative and qualitative measurement of nursing care that meets the goal of cost-effectiveness and still promotes holistic care.

Summary

Nursing is continuing to evolve into a well-defined profession with a more clearly delineated definition and phenomena of concern. Fundamental philosophical beliefs and qualities have been identified that are important for the nurse to possess in order to provide quality care.

The nursing profession has developed a body of knowledge that contributes to the growth and well-being of the individual and the community, the prevention of illness, the maintenance and/or restoration of health, and the relief of pain and provision of support when a return to health is not possible. The nursing process is the basis of all nursing actions and is the essence of nursing, providing a flexible, orderly, and logical problem-solving approach for administering nursing care so that client (whether individual, community, or population) needs for such care are met comprehensively and effectively. It can be applied in any healthcare or educational setting, in any theoretical or conceptual framework, and within the context of any nursing philosophy.

Each step of the nursing process builds on and interacts with the other steps, ensuring an effective practice model. Inclusion of the standards of clinical nursing practice provides additional information to reinforce understanding and opportunities to apply knowledge.

Please note, the term *client* rather than *patient* is used in this book to reflect the philosophy that the individuals or groups you work with are legitimate members of the decision-making process with some degree of control over the planned regimen and are able, active participants in the planning and implementation of their care.[4]

Next, we introduce the language described in the nursing process. This includes NANDA International's classification of nursing diagnoses,[19] the Iowa Intervention and Outcome Projects: Nursing Interventions Classification (NIC),[20] and the Nursing Outcomes Classification (NOC).[21] NANDA-I, NIC, and NOC have combined their classification systems (NNN Alliance) to provide a comprehensive nursing language.

References

1. Merriam-Webster Online Dictionary. Retrieved May 7, 2003, from www.m-w.com/dictionary .htm.
2. Nightingale, F. (1859). *Notes on Nursing: What It Is and What It Is Not.* Facsimile edition. Philadelphia:: J. B. Lippincott, 1946.
3. Jacobi, E. M. (1976). Foreword. In Flanigan, L. (ed). *One Strong Voice: The Story of the American Nurses' Association.* Kansas City, MO: American Nurses Association.
4. Erickson, H. C., Tomlin, E. M., Swain, M. A. (1983). *Modeling and Role-Modeling: A Theory and Paradigm for Nursing.* Englewood Cliffs, NJ: Prentice Hall.
5. Kikuchi, J. F. (1999). Clarifying the nature of conceptualizations about nursing. *Canadian J Nurs Res,* 30(4), 115–128.
6. American Nurses Association. (1980). *Nursing: A Social Policy Statement.* Kansas City, MO: American Nurses Publishing.
7. American Nurses Association. (1995). *Nursing's Social Policy Statement.* Washington, DC: American Nurses Publishing.
8. Maslow, A. H. (1970). *Motivation and Personality.* 2d ed. New York, NY: Harper & Row.
9. American Nurses Association. (2003). *Nursing's Social Policy Statement.* Washington, DC: Nursesbooks.org.
10. Fowler, M. D. M. (ed.). (2008/reissue 2010). *Guide to the Code of Ethics for Nurses.* Washington, DC: Nursesbooks.org.
11. Stolley, P. D., Lasky, T. (1995). *Investigating Disease Patterns: The Science of Epidemiology.* (Scientific American Library, no. 57). New York, NY: WH Freeman.
12. Barnsteiner, J., Provost, S. (2002). How to implement evidence-based practice: Some tried and true pointers. *Reflect Nurs Leadersh,* 28(2), 18.
13. Amarsi, Y. (2002). Evidence-based nursing: Perspective from Pakistan. *Reflect Nurs Leadersh,* 28(2), 28.
14. Shore, L. S. (1988). *Nursing Diagnosis: What It Is and How to Do It, a Programmed Text.* Richmond, VA: Medical College of Virginia Hospitals.
15. Peplau, H. E. (1952). *Interpersonal Relations in Nursing: A Conceptual Frame of Reference for Psychodynamic Nursing.* New York, NY: Putnam.
16. King, L. (1971). *Toward a Theory for Nursing: General Concepts of Human Behavior.* New York, NY: Wiley.

17. Yura, H., Walsh, M. B. (1988). *The Nursing Process: Assessing, Planning, Implementing, Evaluating*. 5th ed. Norwalk, CT: Appleton & Lange.
18. American Nurses Association. (2010). *Nursing: Scope & Standards of Practice*. 2nd ed. Silver Spring, MD: Nursesbooks.org.
19. North American Nursing Diagnosis Association. (2001). *Nursing Diagnoses: Definitions & Classification*. Philadelphia, PA: NANDA.
20. Bulecheck, G. M., Butcher, H. K., Dochterman, J. M. (2008). *Nursing Interventions Classification (NIC)*. 5th ed. St. Louis, MO: Mosby.
21. Moorhead, S., Johnson, M., Maas, M., Swanson, E. (2008). *Nursing Outcomes Classification (NOC)*. 4th ed. St. Louis, MO: Mosby.

CHAPTER 2

The Language of Nursing: NANDA, NIC, NOC, and Other Standardized Nursing Languages

In this chapter, we look at the process and progress of describing the work of nursing because, as Lang has stated, "If we cannot name it, we cannot control it, practice it, teach it, finance it, or put it into public policy."[1] At first glance, nursing seems to be a simple task. However, over many years, the profession has struggled, in part as a result of changes in healthcare delivery and financing, the expansion of nursing's role, and the dawning of the computer age. Gordon reminds us that classification system development parallels knowledge development in a discipline.[2] As theory development and research have begun to define nursing, it has become necessary for nursing to find a common language to describe what nursing is, what nursing does, and how to codify it. Thus, the terms "classification systems" and "standardized language" have been embraced, and the work continues.

Changes in the healthcare system occur at an ever-increasing rate. One of these changes is the movement toward a paperless (computerized or electronic) client record. The use of electronic healthcare information systems is rapidly expanding, and the focus has shifted from its original uses—financial and personnel management functions—to the efficient documentation of the client encounter, whether a single office visit or a lengthy hospitalization. The move to electronic documentation is being fueled by changes in healthcare delivery and reimbursement as well as the growth of alternative healthcare settings (outpatient surgeries, home health, rehabilitation or subacute units, extended or long-term care facilities, etc.), all of which increase the need for a commonality of communication to ensure continuity of care for the client who moves from one setting or level of care to another.

These changes in the business and documentation of healthcare require the industry to generate data about its operations and outcomes. Evaluation and improvement of provided services are important to the delivery of cost-effective client care. Therefore, providers and consumers interested in outcomes of care benefit from accurate documentation of the care provided and the client's response. With the use of language or terminology that can be coded, healthcare information can be recorded in terms that are universal and easily entered into an electronic database and that can generate meaningful reporting data about its operation and outcomes. In short, standardized language is required.

A standardized language contains formalized terms that have definitions and guidelines for use. For example, if the impact of nursing care on financial and clinical outcomes is to be analyzed, coding of this information is essential. While it has been relatively easy to code medical procedures, nursing is more of an enigma because its work has not been so clearly defined.

Since the 1970s, nursing leaders have been working to define the profession of nursing and to develop a commonality of words describing practice (a framework of communication and documentation) so that nursing's contribution to healthcare is captured, is visible in healthcare databases, and is thereby recognized as essential. Therefore, the focus of the profession has been on the effort to classify tasks and to develop standardized nursing languages (SNLs) to better demonstrate what nursing is and what nursing does.

Around the world, nursing researchers continue their efforts to identify and label people's experiences with (and responses to) health, illness, and life processes as they relate to the scope of nursing practice. The use of universal nursing terminology directs our focus to the central content and process of nursing care by identifying, naming, and standardizing the "what" and "how" of the work of nursing—including both direct and indirect activities. This wider application for a standardized language has spurred its development.

A recognized pioneer in SNL is NANDA International's "nursing diagnosis."[3] Simply stated, a nursing diagnosis is defined as a clinical judgment about individual, family, or community responses to actual or potential health problems and life processes. Nursing diagnoses provide the basis for selecting nursing interventions to achieve outcomes for which the nurse is accountable.[4] NANDA-I nursing diagnoses currently include 235 labels with definitions, defining characteristics, and related or risk factors used to define a client need or problem. Once the client's need is defined, outcomes can be developed and nursing interventions chosen to achieve the desired outcomes.

The linkage of client problems or nursing diagnoses to specific nursing interventions and client outcomes has led to the development of several other SNLs, including Clinical Care Classification (originally Home Health Care Classification[5]),[6] Nursing Interventions Classification (NIC),[7] Nursing Outcomes Classification (NOC),[8] Omaha System-Community Health Classification System (OS),[9] Patient Care Data Set (now retired),[10] and Perioperative Nursing Data Set (PNDS).[11]

Whereas some of these languages (e.g., OS and PNDS) are designed for a specific client population, the NANDA-I, NIC, and NOC languages are comprehensively designed for use across systems and settings and at individual, family, and community or population levels.[12]

NIC is a comprehensive standardized language providing 554 direct and indirect intervention labels (Table 2.1) with definitions. A list of activities a nurse might choose to carry out for each intervention is also provided and can be modified as necessary to meet the specific needs of the client. These research-based interventions encompass a broad range of nursing practices, addressing both general practice and specialty areas, including direct care as well as support or administrative activities.

TABLE 2.1 Sample Nursing Interventions Classification Labels

Abuse Protection Support: Elder Acid-Base Monitoring Active Listening	Medication Administration: Intraspinal Mutual Goal Setting
Cardiac Care: Rehabilitation Code Management Community Health Development Complex Relationship Building Critical Path Development	Organ Procurement Ostomy Care
Dementia Management: Bathing Deposition/Testimony	Patient Rights Protection Peripherally Inserted Central (PIC) Catheter Care Phototherapy: Neonate Postmortem Care Preceptor: Student
Endotracheal Extubation	Relocation Stress Reduction
Forensic Data Collection	Sibling Support Staff Development
Gastrointestinal Intubation	Urinary Bladder Training
Infection Control: Intraoperative	Venous Access Device (VAD) Maintenance
Kangaroo Care	Wound Care

Source: Bulecheck, G., Butcher, H. K., Dochterman, J., Wagner, C. M. (2013). *Nursing Interventions Classifications (NIC)*. 6th ed. St. Louis, MO: Mosby.

TABLE 2.2 Sample Nursing Outcomes Classification Labels

Abusive Behavior Self-Restraint
Acceptance: Health Status

Blood Glucose Level
Breastfeeding Establishment: Infant

Comfortable Death
Community Health Status

Development: Late Adulthood

Falls Occurrence
Family Resiliency

Heedfulness of Affected Side

Immobility Consequences: Psycho-Cognitive
Information Processing

Kidney Function
Knowledge: Cancer Threat Reduction

Loneliness Severity

Mechanical Ventilation Weaning Response: Adult
Medication Response

Neurological Status: Spinal Sensory/Motor Function

Pain: Adverse Psychological Response
Parenting: Adolescent Physical Safety
Participation in Healthcare Decisions
Pre-Procedure Readiness

Quality of Life

Respiratory Status: Airway Patency
Risk Control: Tobacco Use

Safe Home Environment
Self-Care: Parenteral Medication
Student Health Status
Substance Addiction: Consequences
Swallowing Status: Pharyngeal Phase

Tissue Perfusion: Cardiac

Vision Compensation Behavior

Will to Live
Wound Healing: Secondary Intention

Source: Moorhead, S., Johnson, M., Maas, M. L., Swanson, E. (eds.). (2013). *Nursing Outcomes Classifications (NOC)*. 5th ed. St. Louis, MO: Mosby.

NOC is also a comprehensive standardized language providing 490 outcome labels (Table 2.2) with definitions; a set of indicators describing specific client, caregiver, family, or community states related to the outcome; and a five-point Likert-type scale that facilitates tracking clients across care settings and that can demonstrate client progress even when outcomes are not fully met. The outcomes are research based and are applicable in all care settings, clinical specialties, and across the lifespan.

In addition, NIC and NOC have been linked to the Omaha System problems, to resident assessment protocols used in extended/long-term care settings, and to NANDA-I. This last linkage created the NANDA, NIC, NOC (NNN) Taxonomy of Nursing Practice. The combination of NANDA-I nursing diagnoses, NOC outcomes, and NIC interventions in a common unifying structure provides a comprehensive nursing language recognized by the American Nurses Association (ANA) that is coded in the Systematized Nomenclature of Medicine (SNOMED), a multidisciplinary terminology supporting the electronic client record.

Having an SNL entered into international-coded terminology allows nurses to describe the care received by the client and to document the effects of that care on client outcomes, and it facilitates the comparison of nursing care across worldwide settings and diverse databases. In addition, it supports research by comparing client care delivered by nurses with that delivered by other providers, which is essential if nursing's contribution is to be recognized and nurses are to be reimbursed for the care they provide.

The current 12 versions of SNLs (consisting of two data element sets and 10 terminologies) recognized by the ANA have been submitted to the National Library of Medicine for inclusion in the Unified Medical Language System Metathesaurus. The Metathesaurus provides a uniform, integrated distribution format from over 100 biomedical vocabularies and classifications (the majority in English and some in multiple languages), and it links many different names for the same concepts, establishing new relationships among terms from different source vocabularies.

Indexing of the entire medical record supports disease management activities (including decision support systems), research, and analysis of outcomes for quality improvement for all healthcare disciplines. Coding also supports telehealth (the use of telecommunications technology to provide medical information and healthcare services over distance) and facilitates access to healthcare data across care settings and different computer systems.

So, to those who stated, "Nursing will thrive as a unique and valued profession when nurses present a theory and rationalistic model for their practice . . . and actively participate in processes for change,"[13] we answer, "We are actively participating in processes for change, and as a profession, we will continue to grow."

References

1. Clark, J., Lang, N. (1992). Nursing's next advance: An internal classification for nursing practice. *Int Nurs Rev*, 39, 109–111, 128.
2. Gordon, M. (1998). Nursing nomenclature and classification system development. *Online J Issues Nurs*. Retrieved from http://nursingworld.org/ojin/tpc7/tpc7_1.htm.
3. NANDA International. (2003). *Nursing Diagnoses: Definitions & Classifications 2003–2004*. Philadelphia, PA: NANDA International.
4. Carroll-Johnson, R. M. (ed). (1991). *Classification of Nursing Diagnoses: Proceedings of the Ninth Conference*. Philadelphia, PA: J. B. Lippincott.
5. Saba, V. K. (1994). *Home Health Care Classification (HHCC) of Nursing Diagnoses and Interventions*. (Revised). Washington, DC: Author.
6. Saba, V. K. (2007). *Clinical Care Classification (CCC) System Manual: A Guide to Nursing Documentation*. New York, NY: Springer.
7. McCloskey, J. C., Bulechek, G. M. (eds). (2004). *Nursing Interventions Classification (NIC)*. 4th ed. St. Louis, MO: Mosby.
8. Moorhead, S., Johnson, M., Maas, M. (eds). (2004). *Nursing Outcomes Classification (NOC)*. 3rd ed. St. Louis, MO: Mosby.
9. Martin, K. S., Scheet, N. J. (1992). *The Omaha System: Applications for Community Health Nursing*. Philadelphia, PA: W. B. Saunders.
10. Ozboldt, J. G. (1996). From minimum data to maximum impact: Using clinical data to strengthen patient care. *Adv Pract Nurs Q*, 1, 62–69.
11. Beyea, S. (2002). *Perioperative Nursing Data Set (PNDS)*. 2nd ed. Denver, CO: AORN.
12. Johnson, M., et al. (2001). *Nursing Diagnoses, Outcomes, and Interventions: NANDA, NOC, and NIC Linkages*. St. Louis, MO: Mosby.
13. Erickson, H. C., Tomlin, E. M., Swain, M. A. P. (1983). *Modeling and Role-Modeling*. Englewood Cliffs, NJ: Prentice Hall.

CHAPTER 3

The Assessment Process: Developing the Client Database

Nursing: Scope & Standards of Practice[1] addresses the assessment process. The standard stipulates that the data-collection process is systematic and ongoing, with the registered nurse collecting comprehensive data pertinent to the healthcare consumer's health and/or situation involving the healthcare consumer, family, and healthcare providers as appropriate, in holistic data collection. The priority of the data collection is based on the healthcare consumer's immediate condition or the anticipated needs of the healthcare consumer or situation. Data are collected using appropriate evidence-based assessment techniques, instruments, and tools with the relevant data documented in a retrievable format.

The Client Database

The assessment step of the nursing process is focused on eliciting a profile of the client that allows the nurse to identify client problems or needs and corresponding nursing diagnoses, to plan care, to implement interventions, and to evaluate outcomes. This profile, or *client database,* supplies a sense of the client's overall health status, providing a picture of the client's physical, psychosocial, emotional, sexual, cultural, spiritual/transpersonal, cognitive, age-related, and developmental levels; economic status; functional abilities; and lifestyle. It is a combination of data gathered from the history-taking interview (a method of obtaining SUBJECTIVE information by talking with the client or significant others and listening to their responses), from the physical examination (a "hands-on" means of obtaining OBJECTIVE information), and from the results of laboratory tests and diagnostic studies. To be more specific, subjective data are what the client/significant others perceive and report, and objective data are what the nurse observes and gathers from other sources.

Assessment involves three basic activities:

- Systematically gathering data
- Organizing or clustering the data collected
- Documenting the data in a retrievable format

Gathering Data—The Interview

Information in the client database is obtained primarily from the client (who is the most important or primary source) and then from family members/significant others (secondary sources), as appropriate, through conversation and by observation during a structured interview. Clearly, the interview involves more than simply exchanging and processing data. Nonverbal communication is as important as the client's choice of words in providing the data. The ability to collect data that are meaningful to the client's health concerns depends heavily on the nurse's knowledge base; on the choice and sequence of questions; and on the ability to give meaning to the client's responses, integrate the data gathered, and prioritize the resulting information. Insight into the nature and behavior of the client is essential as well.

The nurse's initial responsibility is to observe, collect, and record data without drawing conclusions or making judgments or assumptions. Self-awareness is a crucial factor in the interaction because perceptions, judgments, and assumptions can easily color the assessment findings unless they are recognized.

The quality of a history improves with experience with the interviewing process. Tips for obtaining a meaningful history include the following:

- Be a good listener.
- Listen carefully and attentively for whole thoughts and ideas, not merely isolated facts.
- Use the skills of active listening, silence, and acceptance to provide ample time for the person to respond. Be as objective as possible.
- Identify only the client's or significant others' contributions to the history.

The interview question is the major tool used to acquire information. How the question is phrased is a skill that is important in obtaining the desired results and in getting the information necessary to make accurate nursing diagnoses. *Note:* Some questioning strategies to avoid include closed-ended and leading questions, probing, and agreeing or disagreeing that imply that the client is "right" or "wrong." It is important to remember, too, that the client has the right to refuse to answer any question, no matter how reasonably phrased.

The following are nine effective data-collection questioning techniques:

1. Open-ended questions allow clients maximum freedom to respond in their own way, impose no limitations on how the question may be answered, and can produce considerable information.
2. Hypothetical questions pose a situation and ask the client how it might be handled.
3. Reflecting or "mirroring" responses is a useful technique in getting at underlying meanings that might not be verbalized clearly.
4. Focusing consists of eye contact (within cultural limits), body posture, and verbal responses.
5. Giving broad openings encourages the client to take the initiative in what is to be discussed.
6. Offering general leads encourages the client to continue.
7. Exploring pursues a topic in more depth.
8. Verbalizing the implied gives voice to what has been suggested.
9. Encouraging evaluation helps clients to consider the quality of their own experiences.

The client's medical diagnosis can provide a starting point for gathering data. Knowledge of the anatomy and physiology of the specific disease process and severity of the condition also helps in choosing and prioritizing precise portions of the assessment. For example, when examining a client with severe chest pain, it may be wise to evaluate the pain and the cardiovascular system in a focused assessment before addressing other areas, possibly at a later time. Likewise, the duration and length of any assessment depend on circumstances such as the client's condition and the situation's urgency.

The data collected about the client or significant others contain a vast amount of information, some of which may be repetitious. However, some of the data will be valuable for eliciting information that was not recalled or volunteered previously. Enough material needs to be noted in the history so that a complete picture is presented, and yet not so much that the information will not be read or used.

Gathering Data—The Physical Examination

The physical examination is performed to gather objective information and serves as a screening device. Four common methods used during the physical examination are inspection, palpation, percussion, and auscultation. These techniques incorporate the senses of sight, hearing, touch, and smell. For the data collected during the physical examination to be meaningful, it is vital to know the normal physical and emotional characteristics of humans well enough to be able to recognize deviations. To gain as much information as possible from the assessment procedure, the same format should be used each time a physical examination is performed to lessen the possibility of omissions.

Gathering Data—Laboratory Tests/Diagnostic Procedures

Laboratory and other diagnostic studies are a part of the information-gathering stage providing supportive evidence. These studies aid in the management, maintenance, and restoration of health. In reviewing and interpreting laboratory tests, it is important to remember that the origin of the test material does not always correlate to an organ or body system (e.g., a urine test to detect the presence of bilirubin and urobilinogen could indicate liver disease, biliary obstruction, or hemolytic disease). In some cases, the results of a test are *nonspecific* because they indicate only a disorder or abnormality and not the location of the cause of the problem (e.g., an elevated erythrocyte sedimentation rate suggests the presence but not the location of an inflammatory process).

In evaluating laboratory tests, it is advisable to consider which medications (e.g., heparin, promethazine) are being administered to the client, including over-the-counter and herbal supplements (e.g., vitamin E), because these have the potential to alter, blur, or falsify results, creating a misleading diagnostic picture.

Documenting and Clustering the Data

Data gathered during the interview and physical examination, as well as from other records/sources, are organized and recorded in a concise, systematic way and clustered into similar categories. Various formats have been used to accomplish this, including a review of body systems. This approach has been utilized by both medicine and nursing for many years but was initially developed to aid the physician in making medical diagnoses. Currently, nursing is developing and fine-tuning its own tools for recording and clustering data. Several nursing models available to guide data collection include Doenges and Moorhouse's Diagnostic Divisions (Table 3.1),[2,3] Gordon's Functional Health Patterns,[4] and Guzzetta's Clinical Assessment Tool.[5]

TABLE 3.1 General Assessment Tool

This is a suggested guideline/tool applicable in most care settings for creating a client database. It provides a nursing focus (Doenges & Moorhouse's Diagnostic Divisions of Nursing Diagnoses) that will facilitate planning client care. Although the sections are alphabetized here for ease of presentation, they can be prioritized or rearranged to meet individual needs. (Sample exerpts from psychiatric and obstetrical assessment tools are available on Davis Plus.)

Adult Medical/Surgical Assessment Tool

General Information

Name: ______ Age: ______ DOB: ______ Gender: ______ Race: ______
Admission Date: ______ Time: ______ From: ______
Reason for this visit/admission (primary concern): ______
Source of information: ______ Reliability (1–4, with 4 = very reliable): ______

Activity/Rest

Subjective (Reports)

Occupation: ______ Able to participate in usual activities/hobbies: ______ Leisure time/diversional activities: ______
Ambulatory: ______ Gait (describe): ______ Activity level (sedentary to very active; use scale if available): ______
Daily exercise (type): ______
Changes in muscle mass/tone/strength: ______
History of problems/limitations imposed by condition (e.g., immobility, transfer difficulties, weakness, breathlessness):
______
Feelings (e.g., exhaustion, restlessness, boredom, dissatisfaction): ______
Developmental factors (e.g., delayed/age appropriate): ______

(table continues on page 16)

TABLE 3.1 General Assessment Tool (continued)

Sleep: Hours: ______ Naps: ______ Aids: ______ Insomnia: ______ Related to: ______
Difficulty falling asleep: ______ Difficulty staying asleep: ______
Rested on awakening: ______ Excessive grogginess: ______ Bedtime rituals: ______
Relaxation techniques: ______ Sleeps on more than one pillow: ______
Use of oxygen (type): ______ When used: ______
Medications or herbals for/affecting sleep: ______

Objective (Exhibits)

Observed response to activity: Heart rate: ______ Rhythm (reg/irreg): ______ Blood pressure: ______ Respiratory rate: ______
Pulse oximetry: ______
Mental status (e.g., cognitive impairment, withdrawn/lethargic): ______
Neuromuscular assessment: Muscle mass/tone: ______ Posture (e.g., normal, stooped, curved spine): ______
Tremors (location): ______ ROM: ______
Strength: ______ Deformity: ______
Mobility aids (list): ______

Circulation

Subjective (Reports)

History of/treatment date: High blood pressure: ______ Brain injury: ______ Stroke: ______ Heart condition/surgery: ______ Rheumatic fever: ______ Palpitations: ______ Syncope: ______ Pain in legs: ______ Ankle/leg edema: ______ Blood clots: ______ Bleeding tendencies: ______ Spinal cord injury/dysreflexia episodes (describe): ______
Slow/delayed healing (describe): ______
Extremities: Numbness (location): ______ Tingling (location): ______
Cough (describe)/hemoptysis: ______
Change in frequency/amount of urine: ______
Medications/herbals: ______

Objective (Exhibits)

Color (e.g., pale, cyanotic, jaundiced, mottled, ruddy): Skin: ______ Mucous membranes: ______ Lips: ______ Nailbeds: ______
Conjunctiva: ______ Sclera: ______
Skin moisture (e.g., dry, diaphoretic): ______
BP (R & L): Lying: ______ Sitting: ______ Standing: ______ Pulse pressure: ______ Auscultatory gap: ______
Pulses (palpated 1–4 strength): Carotid: ______ Temporal: ______ Jugular: ______ Radial: ______ Femoral: ______ Popliteal: ______
Posttibial: ______ Dorsalis pedis: ______
Cardiac (palpation): Thrill: ______ Heaves: ______
Heart sounds (auscultation): Rate: ______ Rhythm: ______ Quality: ______ Friction rub: ______
Murmur (describe location/sounds): ______
Vascular bruit (location): ______ Jugular vein distention: ______
Breath sounds (describe location & sounds): ______
Extremities: Temperature: ______ Color: ______ Capillary refill (1–3 sec): ______ Edema (+1 to +4): ______
Varicosities (location): ______ Nail abnormalities: ______ Distribution/quality of hair: ______ Trophic skin changes: ______

Ego Integrity

Subjective (Reports)

Relationship status: ______
Expressed concerns (e.g., financial, relationships, recent or anticipated lifestyle/role changes, recent tour(s) of combat duty): ______
Stress factors: ______ Usual ways of handling stress: ______
Expression of feelings of: Anger: ______ Anxiety: ______ Fear: ______ Grief: ______ Helplessness: ______ Hopelessness: ______
Powerlessness: ______
Cultural factors/ethnic ties: ______
Religious affiliation: ______ Active/practicing: ______ Practices prayer/meditation: ______
Religious/spiritual concerns: ______ Desires clergy visit: ______
Expression of sense of connectedness/harmony with self and others: ______
Medications/herbals: ______

TABLE 3.1 continued

Objective (Exhibits)

Emotional status (check those that apply):
Calm: ____ Anxious: ____ Angry: ____ Withdrawn: ____ Fearful: ____ Irritable: ____ Restive: ____ Euphoric: ____
Observed body language: ____ Observed physiological responses (e.g., crying, change in voice quality/volume): ____
Changes in energy field: Temperature: ____ Color: ____ Distribution: ____ Movement: ____ Sounds: ____

Elimination

Subjective (Reports)

Usual bowel elimination pattern: ____ Character of stool (e.g., hard, soft, liquid): ____ Stool color (e.g., brown, black, yellow, clay colored, tarry): ____ Last BM/Character of stool: ____ Constipation (acute/chronic): ____ Diarrhea (acute/chronic): ____ Bowel incontinence: ____ History of bleeding: ____ Hemorrhoids/fistula: ____
Laxative use: ____ How often: ____ Enema/suppository: ____ How often: ____
Usual voiding pattern and character of urine: ____
Difficulty voiding: ____ Urgency: ____ Frequency: ____ Retention: ____ Bladder spasms: ____
Pain/burning: ____
Urinary incontinence (type & time of day usually occurs): ____
History of kidney/bladder disease or stones: ____
Diuretic use: ____ Other medications/herbals: ____

Objective (Exhibits)

Abdomen (auscultation): Bowel sounds (location/type): ____ Abdomen (palpation): Soft/firm: ____ Tenderness/pain (quadrant location): ____ Distention: ____ Palpable mass: ____ Size/girth: ____
Bladder palpable: ____ Residual (per scan): ____ Overflow voiding: ____
Rectal sphincter tone (describe): ____ Hemorrhoids/fistulas: ____
Stool in rectum: ____ Impaction: ____ Occult blood: (+ or –): ____
Presence/use of catheter or continence devices: ____ Ostomy appliances (describe appliance and location): ____

Food/Fluid

Subjective (Reports)

Usual diet (type): ____ Calorie/carbohydrate/protein/fat (g/day): ____ # of meals daily: ____ Snacks (# daily, time consumed, type): ____
Last meal consumed/content: ____
Food preferences: ____ Food allergies/intolerances: ____
Cultural or religious food preparation concerns/prohibitions: ____
Usual appetite: ____ Change in appetite: ____
Usual weight: ____ Unexpected/undesired weight loss or gain: ____
Nausea/vomiting: ____ Related to?____ Heartburn/indigestion: ____ Related to?____ Relieved by?____
Chewing/swallowing problems: ____ Gag/swallow reflex (present): ____
Facial injury/surgery: ____ Stroke/other neurologic deficit: ____
Teeth: Normal: ____ Dentures (full/partial): ____ Loose/absent teeth: ____ Sore mouth/gums: ____
Dental hygiene practices: ____ Professional dental care/frequency: ____
Diabetes/type: ____ Controlled with diet/pills/insulin: ____
Vitamin/food supplement use: ____ Medications/herbals: ____

Objective (Exhibits)

Current weight: ____ Height: ____ Body build: ____ Body fat %: ____
Skin turgor (e.g., firm, supple, dehydrated): ____ Mucous membranes (moist/dry): ____
Edema (describe): Generalized: ____ Dependent: ____ Feet/ankles: ____ Periorbital: ____ Abdominal/ascites: ____
Jugular vein distention: ____
Breath sounds (auscultation)/location: Normal: ____ Diminished: ____ Crackles: ____ Wheezes: ____
Condition of teeth/gums: ____ Appearance of tongue: ____ Mucous membranes: ____
Bowel sounds (quadrant location/type): ____ Hernia/masses: ____
Urine S/A or Chemstix: ____ Serum glucose (Glucometer): ____

(table continues on page 18)

TABLE 3.1 General Assessment Tool (continued)

Hygiene

Subjective (Reports)

Ability to carry out activities of daily living: Independent/dependent (levels 1–4, with 1 = *no assistance needed* to 4 = *completely dependent*):

Mobility: ______ Needs assistance (describe): ______ Assistance provided by: ______
Equipment/prosthetic devices required: ______
Feeding: ______ Needs assistance preparing/eating (describe): ______ Assistive devices: ______
Bathing: ______ Needs assistance setup/regulating water temperature/washing body parts (describe): ______
Preferred time of personal care/bath: ______
Dressing: ______ Needs assistance selecting clothing/dressing self (describe): ______
Toileting: ______ Needs assistance transferring/cleaning self (describe): ______

Objective (Exhibits)

General appearance: Manner of dress: ______ Grooming/personal habits: ______
Condition of hair/scalp: ______
Body odor: ______ Presence of vermin (e.g., lice, scabies): ______

Neurosensory

Subjective (Reports)

History of brain injury, trauma, stroke (residual effects): ______
Fainting spells/dizziness: ______ Headaches (location/type/frequency): ______
Tingling/numbness/weakness (location): ______
Seizures: ______ History/onset: ______ Type (e.g., generalized, partial): ______ Frequency: ______ Aura (describe): ______
Postictal state: ______ How controlled: ______
Vision loss/changes: ______ Glasses/contacts: ______ Last exam: ______ Glaucoma: ______ Cataract: ______ Eye surgery (type/date): ______
Hearing loss: ______ Sudden/gradual: ______ Hearing aids: ______ Last exam: ______
Sense of smell (changes): ______ Epistaxis: ______
Sense of taste (changes): ______
Other: ______

Objective (Exhibits)

Mental status (note duration of change):
Oriented: Time: ______ Place: ______ Person: ______ Situation: ______
Check all that apply: Alert: ______ Drowsy: ______ Lethargic: ______ Stuporous: ______ Comatose: ______
Cooperative: ______ Follows commands: ______ Agitated/restless: ______ Combative: ______
Delusions (describe): ______ Hallucinations (describe): ______
Affect (describe): ______ Speech: ______
Memory: Recent: ______ Remote: ______
Pupil shape: ______ Size/reaction: R/L: ______ Accommodation: ______
Facial droop: ______ Swallowing: ______
Hand grasp/release, R: ______ L: ______
Coordination: ______ Balance: ______ Walking: ______ Sitting: ______ Standing: ______
Deep tendon reflexes (present/absent/location): ______ Tremors: ______ Posturing: ______ Paralysis (L/R): ______

Pain/Discomfort

Subjective (Reports)

Primary focus: Location: ______ Intensity (use pain scale/pictures): ______
Quality (e.g., stabbing, aching, burning): ______ Radiation: ______
Frequency: ______ Duration: ______
Precipitating/aggravating factors: ______
How relieved: OTC/prescription: ______ Nonpharmaceuticals/therapies: ______
Associated symptoms (e.g., nausea, sleep problems, photosensitivity): ______
Effect on daily activities: ______ Relationships: ______ Job: ______ Enjoyment of life: ______
Additional pain focus/describe: ______
Cultural expectations regarding pain perception and expression: ______

TABLE 3.1 continued

Objective (Exhibits)

Facial grimacing: ______ Guarding affected area: ______ Posturing: ______ Behaviors: ______ Narrowed focus: ______
Emotional response (e.g., crying, withdrawal, anger): ______
Vital sign changes (acute pain): BP: ______ Pulse: ______ Respirations: ______

Respiration

Subjective (Reports)

Dyspnea/related to: ______ Precipitating factors: ______ Relieving factors: ______
Airway clearance (e.g., spontaneous/device): ______
Cough (e.g., hard, persistent, croupy): ______ Sputum color/character: ______ Requires suctioning: ______
History of/date: Bronchitis: ______ Emphysema: ______ Tuberculosis: ______ Recurrent pneumonia: ______ Exposure to noxious fumes/allergens, infectious agents/diseases, poisons: ______
Smoker: ______ packs/day: ______ # of pack years: ______ Cigar use: ______ Smokeless: ______
Use of respiratory aids: ______ Oxygen (type, frequency, rate): ______
Medications/herbals: ______

Objective (Exhibits)

Respirations (spontaneous/assisted): ______ Rate: ______ Depth: ______ Chest excursion (e.g., equal/symmetrical): ______ Use of accessory muscles: ______ Nasal flaring: ______ Fremitus: ______
Breath sounds (describe): ______ Egophony: ______
Skin/mucous membrane color (e.g., pale, cyanotic): ______ Clubbing of fingers: ______
Sputum characteristics: ______
Mentation (e.g., calm, anxious, restless): ______
Pulse oximetry: ______

Safety

Subjective (Reports)

Allergies/sensitivity (medications, foods, environment, iodine, latex): ______
Type of reaction: ______
Blood transfusion/number: ______ Date: ______ Reaction (describe): ______
Exposure to infectious diseases (e.g., measles, influenza, pink eye, whooping cough): ______
Exposure to pollution, toxins, poisons/pesticides, radiation (describe reactions): ______
Geographic areas lived in/recent travel: ______
Immunization history/date: Tetanus: ______ MMR: ______ Polio: ______ Hepatitis: ______ Pneumonia: ______ Influenza: ______ HPV: ______
Altered/suppressed immune system (list cause): ______
History of sexually transmitted infection (date/type): ______ Testing: ______
High-risk behaviors (specify): ______
Uses seat belt regularly: ______ Uses bike helmet: ______ Other safety devices: ______
Workplace safety/health issues (describe): ______ Occupation: ______ Currently working: ______ Rate working conditions (e.g., safety, noise, heating, water, ventilation): ______
History of injuries (e.g., fall, vehicle crash, blast, gunshot, electrical, chemical): ______ Fractures/dislocations: ______
Arthritis/unstable joints: ______ Joint replacement surgeries (type and date): ______ Back problems: ______
Skin problems (e.g., rashes, lesions, moles, breast lumps, enlarged nodes)/describe: ______
Delayed healing (describe): ______
Cognitive limitations (e.g., disorientation, confusion): ______
Sensory limitations (e.g., impaired vision/hearing, detecting heat/cold, taste, smell, touch): ______
Prosthesis (type and date received): ______ Ambulatory devices: ______
Violence (episodes or tendencies): ______

Objective (Exhibits)

Body temperature/method (e.g., oral, rectal, temporal, tympanic): ______
Skin integrity (mark location on diagram): Scars: ______ Rashes: ______ Lacerations: ______ Ulcerations: ______ Bruises: ______
Blisters: ______ Drainage: ______ Burns (degree/% of body surface): ______

(table continues on page 20)

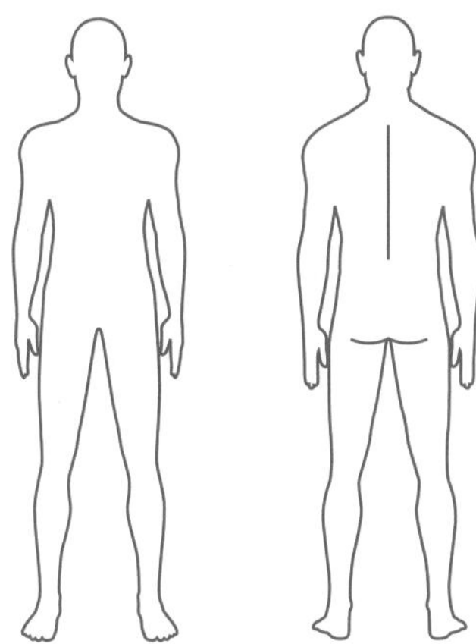

Musculoskeletal: General strength: ______ Muscle tone: ______ Gait: ______ ROM: ______ Paresthesia/paralysis: ______
Results of testing (e.g., cultures, immune function, TB, hepatitis): ______

Sexuality (Component of Social Interaction)

Subjective (Reports)

Sexually active: ______ Monogamous/committed relationship: ______ Use of condoms: ______
Birth control method: ______
Sexual concerns/difficulties: ______ Recent change in frequency/interest: ______ Pain/discomfort: ______

Objective (Exhibits)

Comfort level with subject matter: ______

Female: Subjective (Reports)

Menstruation: Age at menarche: ___ Length of cycle: ___ Duration: ___ Number of pads/tampons used/day: ___ Last menstrual period: ___ Bleeding between periods: ___ Menopausal: ___ Last period: ___ Hysterectomy (type/date): ___ Problems with: Hot flashes: ______ Night sweats: ______ Vaginal lubrication: ______ Vaginal discharge: ______
Gynecological/breast surgery (type and date): ______
Infertility concerns: ______ Type of therapy: ______
Pregnant now: ______ Para: ______ Gravida: ______ Due date: ______
Practices breast self-examination: ______ Last mammogram: ______ Last Pap smear: ______
Hormonal therapy: ______ Supplemental calcium: ______ Other medications/herbals: ______

Female: Objective (Exhibits)

Breast examination: ______
Genitalia: ______ Warts/lesions: ______ Vaginal bleeding/discharge: ______
Test results: ______ Pap: ______ Mammogram: ______ STI: ______

Male: Subjective (Reports)

Penis: Circumcised: ______ Lesions/discharge: ______ Vasectomy: ______
Prostate disorder/voiding difficulties: ______
Practice self-examination: Breast: ______ Testicles: ______
Last proctoscopic/prostate examination: ______ Last PSA: ______
Medications/herbals: ______

Male: Objective (Exhibits)

Genitalia: Penis: ______ Warts/lesions: ______ Bleeding/discharge: ______ Testicles (e.g., descended, lumps): ______
Prostate: ______
Breast examination: ______
Test results: ______ STI: ______ PSA: ______

TABLE 3.1 continued

Social Interactions

Subjective (Reports)

Relationship status: Single: ______ Married: ______ Living with partner: ______ Divorced: ______ Widowed: ______
Years in relationship: ______ Perception of relationship: ______ Concerns/stresses: ______
Role within family structure: ______ Number/age of children: ______
Individuals living in home: ______ Caregiver (to whom & how long): ______
Extended family/availability: ______ Other support person(s): ______
Perception of relationship with family members: ______
Ethnic/cultural affiliation: ______ Strength of ethnic identity: ______ Lives in ethnic community: ______
Feelings of (describe): Mistrust: ______ Rejection: ______ Unhappiness: ______ Loneliness/isolation: ______
Problems related to illness/condition: ______
Difficulties with communication (e.g., speech, another language, brain injury): ______
Use of communication aids (list): ______ Requires interpreter: ______
Genogram: (complete on separate form)

Objective (Exhibits)

Communication/speech: Clear: ______ Slurred: ______ Unintelligible: ______ Aphasic: ______
Unusual speech pattern/impairment: ______ Laryngectomy present: ______
Use of speech/communication aids: ______
Verbal/nonverbal communication with family/significant other(s): ______
Family interaction (behavioral) pattern: ______

Teaching/Learning

Subjective (Reports)

Communication: Dominant language (specify): ______ Second language: ______
Literate (reading/writing): ______
Education level: ______ Learning disabilities (specify): ______ Cognitive limitations: ______
Culture/ethnicity: ______ Where born: ______ If immigrant, how long in this country: ______
Health and illness beliefs/practices/customs: ______
Which family member makes healthcare decisions/is spokesperson for client: ______
Presence of Advance Directives: ______ Code status: ______ Durable Medical Power of Attorney: ______ Designee: ______
Health goals: ______
Current health problem: ______ Client understanding of problem: ______
Special healthcare concerns (e.g., impact of religious/cultural practices, healthcare decisions, family involvement): ______
Familial risk factors (indicate relationship): Diabetes: ______ Thyroid (specify): ______ Tuberculosis: ______ Heart disease: ______
Stroke: ______ High BP: ______
Epilepsy/seizures: ______ Kidney disease: ______ Cancer: ______ Mental illness/depression: ______ Other: ______
Prescribed medications (list each separately):
Drug: ______ Dose: ______ Times (circle last dose): ______
Take regularly: ______ Purpose: ______ Side effects/problems: ______
Nonprescription drugs/frequency:
OTC drugs: ______ Vitamins: ______ Herbals: ______ Street drugs: ______
Alcohol (amount/frequency): ______ Tobacco: ______ Smokeless tobacco: ______
Admitting diagnosis per provider: ______
Reason for hospitalization/visit per client: ______
History of current problem/concern: ______
Client expectations of this hospitalization/visit: ______
Will admission cause any lifestyle changes (describe): ______
Previous illnesses and/or hospitalizations/surgeries: ______
Evidence of failure to improve: ______
Last complete physical examination: ______

Discharge Plan Considerations

Projected length of stay (hours/days): ______ Anticipated date of discharge: ______
Date information obtained: ______ Source: ______

(table continues on page 22)

TABLE 3.1 General Assessment Tool (continued)

Resources available: Persons: ______ Financial: ______ Community supports: ______ Groups: ______
Areas that may require alteration/assistance: Food preparation: ___ Shopping: ___ Transportation: ___ Ambulation: ___
Self-care (specify): ______ Socialization: ______
Medication/IV therapy: ______ Treatments: ______ Wound care: ______ Supplies: ______
Homemaker/maintenance (specify): ______ Physical layout of home (specify): ______
Anticipated changes in living situation after discharge: ______ Living facility other than home (specify): ______
Referrals (date/source/services): Social services: ______ Rehabilitation: ______
Dietary: ______ Home care: ______ Resp/O_2: ______ Equipment: ______ Supplies: ______ Other: ______

The use of a nursing model as a framework for data collection (rather than a body systems approach [assessing the heart, moving on to the lungs, etc.] or the commonly known head-to-toe approach) has the advantage of focusing data collection on the nurse's phenomena of concern—the human responses to health, illness, and life processes.[6] This facilitates the identification and validation of *nursing* diagnosis labels to describe the data accurately.

Reviewing and Validating Findings

The nurse's initial responsibility is to observe, collect, and record data without drawing conclusions or making judgments or assumptions. Self-awareness is a crucial factor in this interaction because perceptions, judgments, and assumptions can easily color the assessment findings.

Validation is an ongoing process that occurs during the data-collection phase and upon its completion, which is when the data are reviewed and compared. The nurse should review the data to be sure that the recordings are factual, to identify errors of omission, and to compare the objective and subjective data for incongruencies or inconsistencies that require additional investigation or a more focused assessment. Data that are grossly abnormal are rechecked, and any temporary factors that may affect the data are identified and noted. Validation is particularly important when the data are conflicting, when the data sources may be unreliable, or when serious harm to the client could result from any inaccuracies. Validating the information reduces the possibility of drawing wrong inferences or conclusions that could result in inaccurate nursing diagnoses, incorrect outcomes, or inappropriate nursing actions. This can be done by sharing the assumptions with the individuals involved (e.g., client, significant other/family) and having them verify the accuracy of those conclusions. Sharing pertinent data with other healthcare professionals, such as the physician, dietitian, or physical therapist, can aid in collaborative planning of care. Data given in confidence should not be shared with other individuals (unless withholding that information would hinder appropriate evaluation or care of the client).

Summary

The assessment step of the nursing process emphasizes and should provide a holistic view of the client. The generalized assessment done during the overall data-gathering process creates a profile of the client. A focused, or more detailed, assessment may be warranted given the client's condition or emergent time constraints, or it may be done to obtain more information about a specific issue that needs expansion or clarification. Both types of assessments provide important data that complement each other. A successfully completed assessment creates a picture of clients' states of wellness, their response to health concerns or problems, and individual risk factors—this is the foundation for identifying appropriate nursing diagnoses, developing client outcomes, and choosing relevant interventions necessary for providing individualized care.

References

1. American Nurses Association. (2010). *Nursing: Scope & Standards of Practice*. 2nd ed. Silver Spring, MD: Nursesbooks.org.
2. Doenges, M. E., Moorhouse, M. F., Murr, A. C. (2010). *Nurse's Pocket Guide: Diagnoses, Interventions, and Rationales*. 12th ed. Philadelphia, PA: F. A. Davis.
3. Doenges, M. E., Moorhouse, M. F., Murr, A. C. (2010). *Nursing Care Plans: Guidelines for Individualizing Client Care Across the Lifespan*. 8th ed. Philadelphia, PA: F. A. Davis.
4. Gordon, M. (2008). *Assess Notes: Nursing Assessment and Diagnostic Reasoning*. Philadelphia, PA: F. A. Davis.
5. Guzzetta, C. E., et al. (1989). *Clinical Assessment Tools for Use With Nursing Diagnoses*. St. Louis, MO: Mosby.
6. American Nurses Association. (1995). *Nursing's Social Policy Statement*. Washington, DC: American Nurses Association.

CHAPTER 4

Concept or Mind Mapping to Create and Document the Plan of Care

The plan of care may be recorded on a single page or in a multiple-page format, with one page for each nursing diagnosis or client diagnostic statement. The format for documenting the plan of care is determined by agency policy. As a practicing professional, you might use a computer with a plan-of-care database, preprinted standardized care plan forms, or clinical pathways. Whichever form you use, the plan of care enables visualization of the nursing process and must reflect the basic nursing standards of care; personal client data; nonroutine care; and qualifiers for interventions and outcomes, such as time, frequency, and amount.

As students, you are asked to develop plans of care that often contain more detail than what you see in the hospital plans of care. This is to help you learn how to apply the nursing process and create individualized client care plans. However, even though much time and energy may be spent focusing on filling in the columns of traditional clinical care plan forms, some students never develop a holistic view of their clients and fail to visualize how each client need interacts with other identified needs. A new technique or *megacognitive* learning tool has been developed to assist you in visualizing the linkages and understanding the interrelationships among a client's health concerns, to enhance and evaluate your critical thinking skills, and to facilitate the creative process of planning client care.[1,2]

Concept or Mind Mapping Client Care

Have you ever asked yourself whether you are more right-brained or left-brained? Those who naturally use their left brains are more linear in their thinking. Right-brain thinkers see more in pictures and illustrations. It is best for nurses to use the whole brain (right and left) when thinking about providing the broad scope of nursing care to clients.

No More Columns!

Traditional nursing care plans are linear—that is, they are designed in columns. They speak almost exclusively to the left brain. The traditional nursing care plan is organized according to the nursing process, which guides us in problem-solving the nursing care we give. However, the linear nature of the traditional plan does not facilitate interconnecting data from one "row" to another or between parts in a column. Concept mapping allows us to show the interconnections among various client symptoms, interventions, and problems as they impact each other.

You can keep the parts that are great about traditional care plans (problem-solving and categorizing), but change the linear or columnar nature of the plan to a design that uses the whole brain—bringing left-brained, linear problem-solving together with the free-wheeling, interconnected, creative right brain. Joining concept mapping and care planning enables you to create a whole picture of a client with all the interconnections identified.

There are several diverse and innovative ways to mind map or to concept map nursing care plans.[3] The examples in this chapter use mind mapping and require placing the client at the center, with all ideas on one page (for a whole picture); the examples also use color coding and creative energy.[4,5] When doing a large mapped plan of care, a light poster board is often used so that all ideas fit on one page.

Components of a Concept Map

Tony Buzan developed the idea of mind mapping as a way to depict how ideas about a main subject are related. Mapping represents graphically the relationships and interrelationships of ideas and concepts.[6] It fosters and encourages critical thinking through brainstorming about a particular subject. Mueller, Johnston, and Bligh took the process of mind mapping and combined it with care planning to enhance nursing students' critical thinking and provision of holistic nursing care.[3] This process has also been referred to as concept mapping.

Instead of starting at the top of the page, concept mapping starts at the page's center. The main concept of our thinking goes in this center stage place.

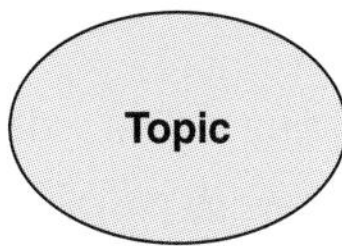

From that central thought, simply begin thinking of other main ideas that relate to the central topic. These ideas radiate out from the central idea likes spokes of a wheel (see subsequent discussion); however, they do not have to be added in a balanced manner; the "wheel" does not have to be round.

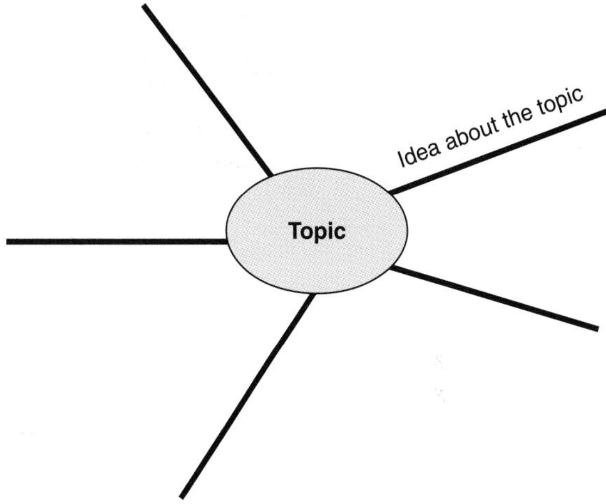

You will generate further ideas related to each spoke (see subsequent discussion); and your mind will race with even more ideas from those thoughts, which can be represented through pictures or words.

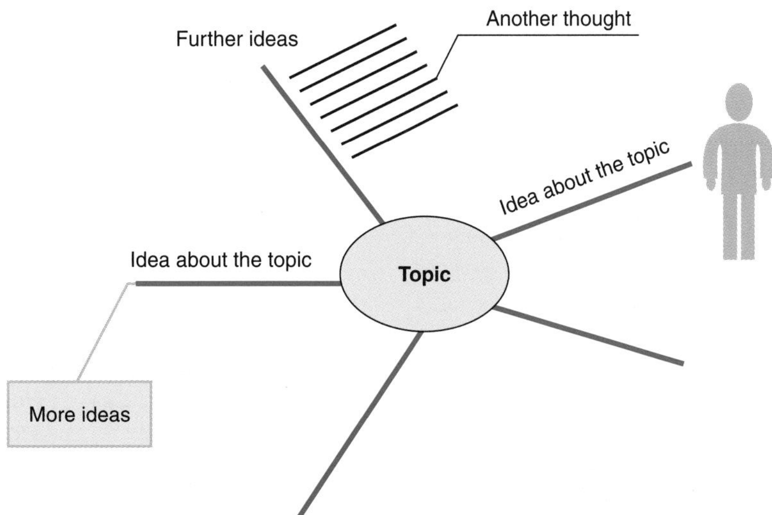

As you think of new ideas, write them down immediately. This may require going back and forth from one area of the page to another. Writing your concept map by hand allows you to move faster. Avoid using a computer to generate a map because it hinders the fast-paced process. You can group different concepts together by color coding or by placement on the page (see subsequent discussion).

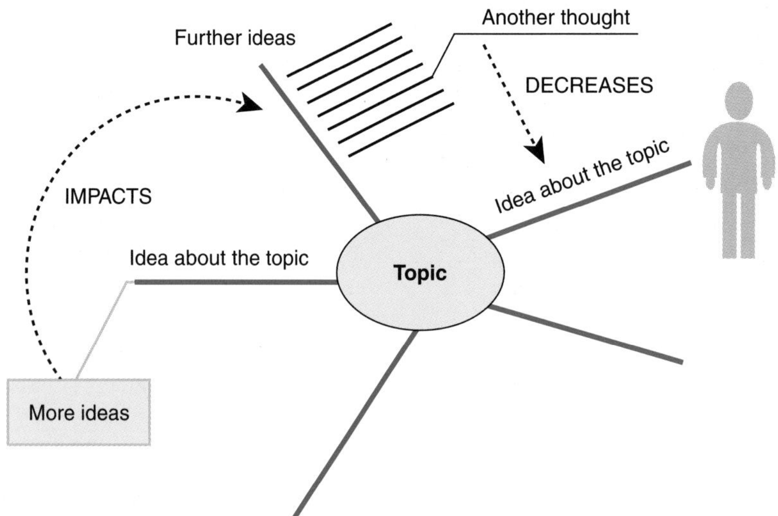

As you see connections and interconnections among groups of ideas, use arrows or lines to connect those concepts (refer to the dotted lines). You can also add defining phrases that explain how the interconnected thoughts relate to one another, as in the figure above.

Some left-brain thinkers find it very difficult to start their ideas in the middle of a page. If you are this type of thinker, try starting at the top of the page (see subsequent discussion), but you must still represent your ideas in illustration form, not in paragraphs.

Concept maps created by different people look different. They are unique to the mind's eye picture, so do not expect your map to be the same as someone else's.

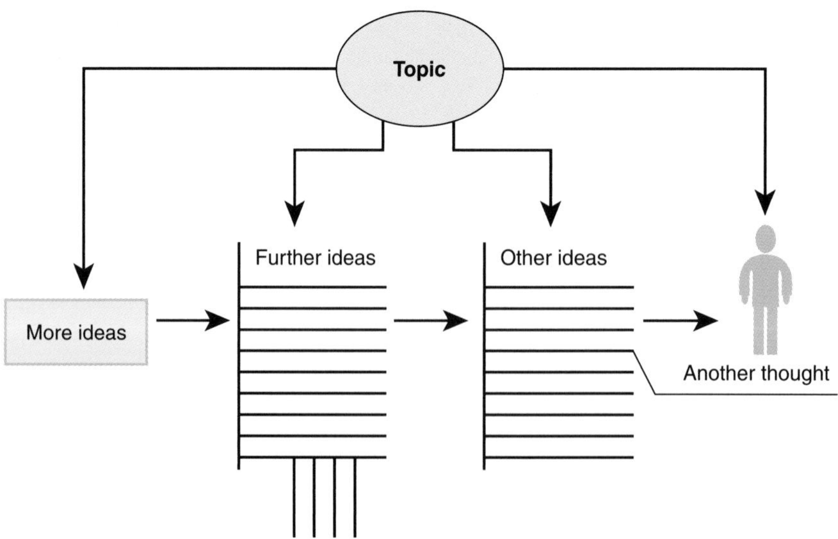

Concept Mapping a Plan of Care

Concept mapping is an exciting alternative format for illustrating a written plan of care. A mapped care plan will look very different from traditional plans of care, which are usually completed on linear forms.

To begin mapping a client plan of care, you must begin with the central topic—the client. Now you are thinking like a nurse. Create a shape that signifies "client" to you and place it at your map's center. If your hand just cannot start at the center, then put the shape at the top. This will help you remember that the client, not the medical diagnosis or condition, is the focus of your plan. All other pieces of the map will be connected in some manner to the client. Many different pieces of information about the client can be connected directly to the client. For example, each of the following pieces of critical client data could stem from the center:

- 78-year-old widower
- No family in the state
- Obese
- Medical diagnosis of recurrent community-acquired pneumonia

Now, you must do a bit of thinking about how you think. To create the rest of your map, ask yourself how *you* plan client care. For example, which of these items do you see first or think of first as the basis for your plan: the clustered assessment data, nursing diagnoses, or outcomes? Whichever piece you choose becomes your first layer of connections. Suppose when thinking about a plan of care for a female client with heart failure, you think first in terms of all the nursing diagnoses about that woman and her condition. Your map would start with the diagnoses featured as the first "branches," with each one listed separately in some way on the map.

Completing the map then becomes a matter of adding the rest of the pieces of the plan using the nursing process and your own way of thinking or planning as your guide. If you began your map using nursing diagnoses, you might think, "What signs and symptoms or data support these diagnoses?" Then, you would connect clusters of supporting data to the related nursing diagnosis. Or you might think, "What client outcomes am I trying to achieve when I address this nursing diagnosis?" In that case, you would next connect client outcomes (or NOC labels) to the nursing diagnoses.

To keep your map clear, as suggested previously, use different colors and maybe a different shape, spoke, or line for each piece of the care plan that you add. For example:

- Red for signs and symptoms (to signify danger)
- Yellow for nursing diagnoses (for "stop and think what this is")
- Green for nursing interventions or NIC labels (for "go")
- Blue (or some other color) for outcomes or NOC labels

When all the pieces of the nursing process are represented, each branch of the map is complete. There should be a nursing diagnosis (supported by subjective and objective assessment data), nursing interventions, desired client outcome(s), and any evaluation data, all connected in a manner that shows there is a relationship among them.

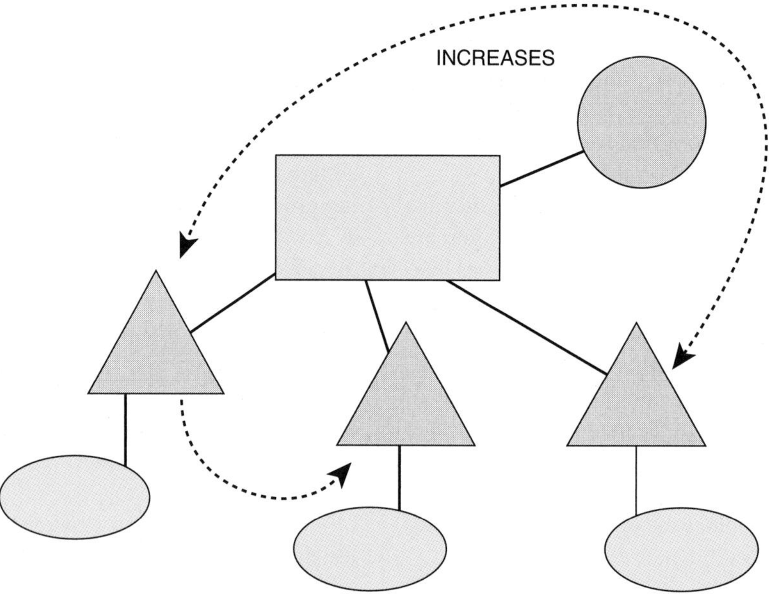

It is critical to understand that there is no preset order for the pieces because one cluster is not more or less important than another (or one is not "subsumed" under another). It is important, however, that those pieces within a branch be in the same order in each branch.

So, you might ask, how is this different from writing out information in a linear manner? What makes mapping so special? One of the things you may have discovered about caring for clients is that the care you deliver is very interconnected. Taking care of one problem often results in the simultaneous correction of another. For example, if you resolve a fluid volume problem in a client with heart failure, you will also positively impact the client's gas exchange and decrease his or her anxiety. These kinds of interconnections cannot be shown on linear plans of care, yet they are what practicing nurses see in their mind's eye all the time. These interconnections can be represented on a map with arrows or dotted or dashed lines that tie related ideas together. Then, defining phrases that explain the nature of the interconnection can be added to further clarify the relationship, as shown in Figure 4.1.

In addition to the pieces of the nursing process, other components of care can be illustrated on a map. Nurses have certain responsibilities when clients have diagnostic tests (such as an angiography or a bronchoscopy). These tests can be connected to the appropriate piece of your map, along with the correct nursing interventions related to those tests. Another item to be added is potential complications or collaborative problems.

Taking your clients' needs one step further: Try asking every client you have (medical, surgical, or otherwise), "What is the most important thing to you now in relation to why you are here?" Obtaining this information builds an alliance between you and your client, and together you can work toward that desired outcome. Add it to your map and see how your plan of care becomes more client centered (refer to Fig. 4.2).

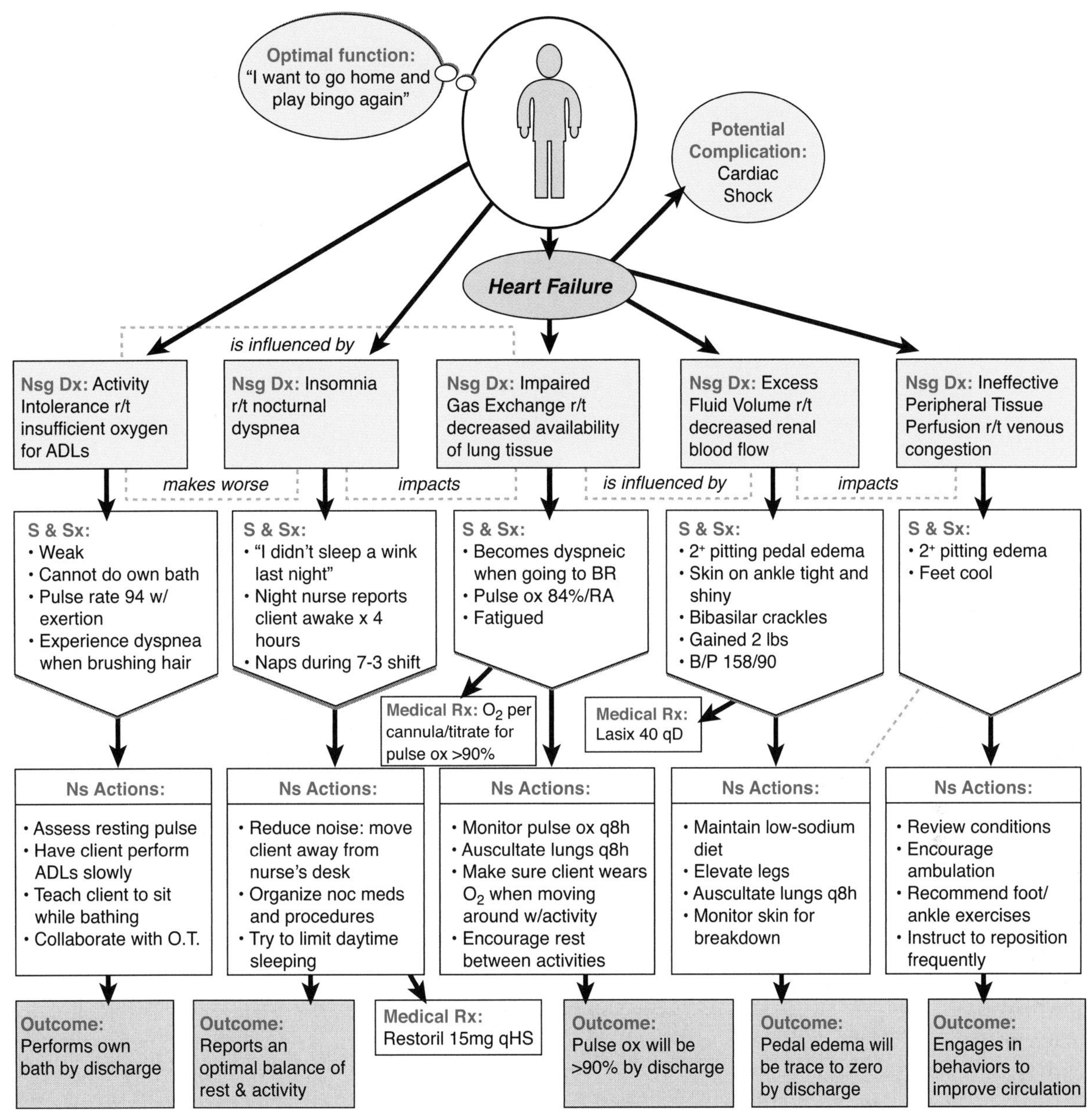

Figure 4.1 Concept map of a plan of care for a client with heart failure.

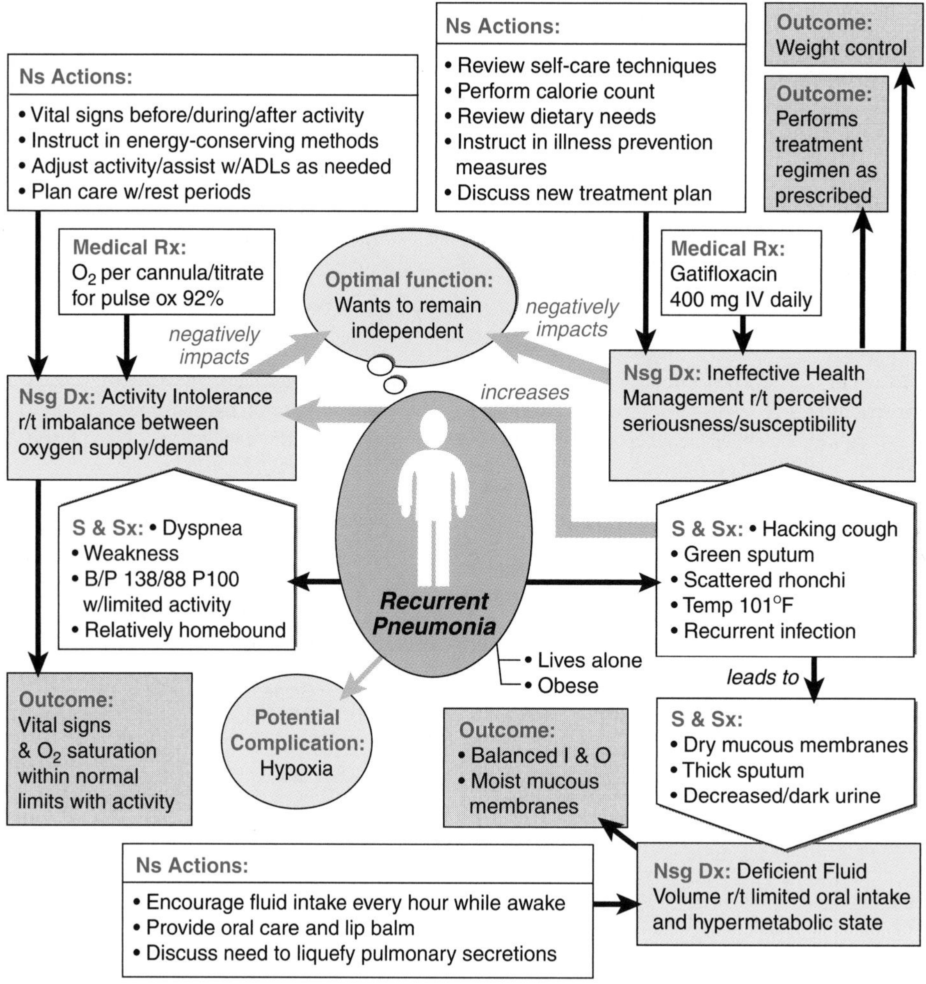

Figure 4.2 Concept map of a plan of care for a client with pneumonia.

Summary

Concept maps allow you to do something that is different and creative. They require you to think (and learn), make connections, and use colors and shapes. They help you to focus on the client, and having the map on one page helps you to understand the "whole picture" better. Concept maps also help you become better organized and develop your own unique approach to "thinking like a nurse" much sooner.

A student who had written many traditional plans of care in her previous nursing program wrote the following about concept-mapped care plans:

> *Concept mapping is painting a picture using colors of the rainbow on blank paper to tell the story of your client using "NANDA" nursing diagnoses and the*

nursing process. Previously, I was a student in prison (my mind) who hated the words "CARE PLAN," writing page after page in narrative form. It was laborious to do and boring to read. There was no life or heartbeat.

Concept mapping opened the prison doors, and my care plan took on human form with a VOICE, a beating HEART, and COLOR while still incorporating the nursing process and standardized nursing language. My mind now took on the professional thought process for which NANDA, NIC, and NOC were created to facilitate nursing; however, the magic was in concept mapping, which removed all my fears, and the client became a beautiful painting with a heartbeat.[3]

References

1. Gull, B., Bowman, J. (2006). Concept mapping: A strategy for teaching and evaluating critical thinking in nursing education. *Nurse Educ Pract*, 6(4), 199–206.
2. Hicks-Moore, S. (2005). Clinical concept maps in nursing education: An effective way to link theory and practice. *Nurse Educ Pract*, 5(6), 348–352.
3. Schuster, P. (2010). *Concept Mapping: A Critical-Thinking Approach to Care Planning*. Philadelphia: F. A. Davis.
4. Mueller, A., Johnston, M., Bligh, D. (2001). Mind-mapped care plans, a remarkable alternative to traditional nursing care plans. *Nurse Educ*, 26(2), 75–80.
5. Mueller, A., Johnston, M., Bligh, D. (2002). Viewpoint: Joining mind mapping and care planning to enhance student critical thinking and achieve holistic nursing care. *Int J Nurs Terminol Classif*, 13(1), 24–27.
6. Buzan, T. (1995). *The MindMap Book*. 2nd ed. London: BBC Books.

CHAPTER 5

Nursing Diagnoses in Alphabetical Order

Activity Intolerance [specify level]

Taxonomy II: Activity/Rest—Class 4 Cardiovascular/Pulmonary Responses (00092) [**Diagnostic Division:** Activity/Rest], Submitted 1982

DEFINITION: Insufficient physiological or psychological energy to endure or complete required or desired daily activities.

RELATED FACTORS

Generalized weakness
Sedentary lifestyle
Bedrest/immobility
Imbalance between oxygen supply and demand, [anemia]

DEFINING CHARACTERISTICS

Subjective

Reports fatigue, generalized weakness
Exertional discomfort, dyspnea

Objective

Abnormal heart rate or blood pressure response to activity
ECG change (e.g., arrhythmia, conduction abnormality, ischemia)

FUNCTIONAL LEVEL CLASSIFICATION (GORDON, 2014)[3]

Level I: Walk, regular pace, on level indefinitely; climb one flight or more but more short of breath than normally
Level II: Walk one city block [or] 500 ft on level; climb one flight slowly without stopping
Level III: Walk no more than 50 ft on level without stopping; unable to climb one flight of stairs without stopping

Information that appears in brackets has been added by the authors to clarify and enhance the use of the nursing diagnoses.

Level IV: Dyspnea and fatigue at rest
Sample Clinical Applications: Anemias, angina, aortic stenosis, bronchitis, emphysema, cancers, diabetes mellitus, dysmenorrhea, heart failure, HIV/AIDS, labor/preterm labor, leukemias, mitral stenosis, obesity, pain, pericarditis, peripheral vascular disease, rheumatic fever, thrombocytopenia, tuberculosis, uterine bleeding

DESIRED OUTCOMES/EVALUATION CRITERIA

Sample NOC linkages:
Activity Tolerance: Physiological response to energy-consuming movements with daily activities
Energy Conservation: Personal actions to manage energy for initiating and sustaining activity
Endurance: Capacity to sustain activity
Psychomotor Energy: Personal drive and energy to maintain activities of daily living, nutrition, and personal safety

Client Will (Include Specific Time Frame)
- Identify negative factors affecting activity tolerance and eliminate or reduce their effects when possible.
- Use identified techniques to enhance activity tolerance.
- Participate in necessary/desired activities.
- Report measurable increase in activity tolerance.
- Demonstrate a decrease in physiological signs of intolerance (e.g., pulse, respirations, and blood pressure remain within client's usual range).

ACTIONS/INTERVENTIONS

Sample NIC linkages:
Activity Therapy: Prescription of and assistance with specific physical, cognitive, social, and spiritual activities to increase the range, frequency, or duration of an individual's (or group's) activity
Energy Management: Regulating energy use to treat or prevent fatigue and optimize function
Exercise Promotion: Facilitation of regular physical activity to maintain or advance to a higher level of fitness and health

NURSING PRIORITY NO. 1 To identify causative/precipitating factors:

- Note presence of acute or chronic illness, such as heart failure, pulmonary disorders, hypothyroidism, diabetes mellitus, AIDS, anemias, cancers, acute and chronic pain, etc. *Many factors cause or contribute to fatigue, but the term "activity intolerance" implies that the client cannot endure or adapt to increased energy or oxygen demands caused by an activity.*[1,8,9]
- Assess cardiopulmonary response to physical activity by measuring vital signs, noting heart rate and regularity, respiratory rate and work of breathing, and blood pressure before, during, and after activity. Note progression or accelerating degree of fatigue. *Dramatic changes in heart rate and rhythm, changes in usual blood pressure, and progressively worsening fatigue result from imbalance of oxygen supply and demand. These changes are potentially greater in the frail, elderly population.*[1,3,10,11]
- Note treatment-related factors such as side effects and interactions of medications. *Can affect nature and degree of activity intolerance.*
- Determine if client is receiving medications such as vasodilators, diuretics, or beta blockers. *Orthostatic hypotension can occur with activity because of medication effects (vasodilation), fluid shifts (diuresis), or compromised cardiac pumping function.*[15]
- Note client reports of difficulty accomplishing tasks or desired activities. Evaluate current limitations or degree of deficit in light of usual status and what the client perceives causes, exacerbates, and helps the problem. *Provides comparative baseline, influences choice of interventions, and may reveal causes that the client is unaware of affecting energy, such as sleep deprivation, smoking, poor diet, depression, or lack of support.*[2,10,11]

- Ascertain ability to sit, stand, and move about as desired. Note degree of assistance necessary and/or use of assistive equipment. *Helps to differentiate between problems relating to movement and problems with oxygen supply and demand characterized by fatigue and weakness.*[2,8,9,11]
- Identify activity needs versus desires (e.g., client barely able to walk up stairs but states would like to play racquetball). *Assists caregiver in dealing with reality of situation as well as the feasibility of goals client wants to achieve when developing activity plan.*
- Assess emotional or psychological factors affecting the current situation. *Stress and/or depression may be exacerbating the effects of an illness, or depression may be the result of therapy and/or limitations.*

NURSING PRIORITY NO. 2 To assist client to deal with contributing factors and manage activities within individual limits:

- Monitor vital signs before and during activity, watching for changes in blood pressure, heart and respiratory rate, and postactivity vital sign response. *Vital signs may change during activity (including higher or lower pulse or blood pressure) and should return to baseline within 5 to 7 min after activity if response to activity is normal.*[1]
- Observe respiratory rate, noting breathing pattern, breath sounds, skin color, and mental status. *Pallor and/or cyanosis, presence of respiratory distress, or confusion may be indicative of need for oxygen during activities, especially if respiratory infection or compromise is present.*
- Plan care with rest periods between activities *to reduce fatigue.*
- Assist with self-care activities. Adjust activities or reduce intensity level, or discontinue activities that cause undesired physiological changes. *Prevents overexertion.*
- Increase exercise/activity levels gradually; encourage stopping to rest for 3 min during a 10-min walk, or sitting down instead of standing to brush hair. *Methods of conserving energy.*
- Encourage expression of feelings contributing to or resulting from condition. Provide positive atmosphere while acknowledging difficulty of the situation for the client. *Helps to minimize frustration, rechannel energy.*
- Involve client/significant others (SOs) in planning of activities as much as possible. *May give client opportunity to perform desired or essential activities during periods of peak energy.*
- Assist with activities and provide and monitor client's use of assistive devices. *Enables client to maintain mobility while protecting from injury.*
- Promote comfort measures and provide for relief of pain *to enhance client's ability and desire to participate in activities.*[9,11] (Refer to NDs acute Pain, chronic Pain.)
- Provide referral to collaborative disciplines, such as an exercise physiologist, psychological counseling/therapy, occupational/physical therapy, and recreation/leisure specialists. *May be needed to develop individually appropriate therapeutic regimens.*
- Prepare for/assist with and monitor effects of exercise-capacity testing. *May be performed to determine degree of oxygen desaturation and/or hypoxemia that occurs with exertion or to optimize titration of supplemental oxygen when used.*[5,8]
- Implement graded exercise or rehabilitation program under direct medical supervision. *Gradual increase in activity avoids excessive myocardial workload and associated oxygen demand and has been shown to exert positive health benefits, even in those with chronic diseases. One intervention review found that for people with mild to moderate systolic heart failure, there was neither a reduction nor an increase in the risk of death with exercise. However, following exercise training, there was a reduction in hospital admissions due to systolic heart failure.*[4]
- Administer supplemental oxygen, medications, prepare for surgery, and other treatments, as indicated. *Type of therapy or medication is dependent on the underlying condition and might include medications (e.g., antiarryhthmics, bronchodilators) or surgery (e.g., stents or coronary artery bypass graft) to improve myocardial perfusion and systemic circulation. Other treatments might include iron preparations or blood transfusion to treat severe anemia or use of oxygen and bronchodilators to improve respiratory function.*[6,7,12,14]

NURSING PRIORITY NO. 3 To promote wellness (Teaching/Discharge Considerations):

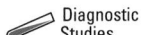

- Review expectations of client/SOs/providers and explore conflicts or differences. *Helps to establish goals and to reach agreement for the most effective plan.*
- Assist or direct client/SOs to plan for progressive increase of activity level, aiming for maximal activity within the client's ability. *Promotes improved or more normal activity level, stamina, and conditioning.*
- Instruct client/SOs in monitoring response to activity and in recognizing signs/symptoms that indicate need to alter activity level. *Assists in self-management of condition and in understanding of reportable problems. The 2008 Physical Guidelines for Americans summary of research studies confirms that "some physical activity is better than none" and that regular physical activity not only reduces the risk of many adverse outcomes, but also provides health benefits.* [8,9,13]
- Give client information that provides evidence of daily or weekly progress *to sustain motivation.*
- Assist client to learn and demonstrate appropriate safety measures, such as using assistive devices correctly, wearing glasses, and having a companion when walking *to prevent injuries.*
- Provide information about proper nutrition to meet metabolic and energy needs, obtaining or maintaining normal body weight. *Energy is improved when nutrients are sufficient to meet metabolic demands.*[1]
- Encourage client to use relaxation techniques, such as visualization or guided imagery, as appropriate. *Useful in maintaining positive attitude and enhancing sense of well-being.*
- Encourage participation in self-care, recreation, or social activities and hobbies appropriate for situation. (Refer to ND deficient Diversional Activity)
- Monitor laboratory values (such as for anemia) and pulse oximetry *to identify areas of concern that may require further assessment or intervention.*

DOCUMENTATION FOCUS

Assessment/Reassessment

- Level of activity as noted in Functional Level Classification.
- Causative or precipitating factors.
- Client reports of difficulty or change.

Planning

- Plan of care and who is involved in planning.
- Teaching plan.

Implementation/Evaluation

- Response to interventions, teaching, and actions performed.
- Modifications to plan of care.
- Attainment or progress toward desired outcome(s).

Discharge Planning

- Referrals to other resources.
- Long-term needs and who is responsible for actions.

References

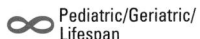

1. Newfield, S. A., Hinz, M. D., Scott-Tilley, D., et al. (2007). *Cox's Clinical Applications of Nursing Diagnosis: Adult, Child, Women's, Psychiatric, Gerontic, and Home Health Considerations.* 5th ed. Philadelphia, PA: F. A. Davis.
2. Stanley, M. (2005). In Blair, K. A., Beare, P. G. (eds). *Gerontological Nursing: Promoting Successful Aging with Older Adults.* 3rd ed. Philadelphia: F. A. Davis.
3. Gordon, M. (2014). *Manual of Nursing Diagnosis.* 13th ed. St. Louis, MO: Mosby.

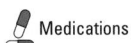

4. Taylor, R. S., Sagar, V. A., Davies, E. J., et al. (update 2014). Exercise-based rehabilitation for heart failure. *Cochrane Library*. Retrieved October 2015 from http://onlinelibrary.wiley.com/doi/10.1002/14651858.CD003331.pub4/full.
5. Foss, C. M., et al. (2001). Exercise testing for evaluation of hypoxemia and/or desaturation: Revision & update. *Resp Care*, 46(5), 514–522.
6. Gibbons, R. J., Chatterjee, K., Daley, J., et al. (1999). ACC/AHA/ACP-ASIM: Guidelines for the management of patients with chronic stable angina: A report of the American College of Cardiology/American Heart Association Task Force on Practice Guidelines. *J Am Coll Cardiol*, 99, 2829.
7. *Congestive Heart Failure in Adults*. (2002). Bloomington, MN: Institute for Clinical Systems Improvement.
8. Michael, K. M., Allen, J. K., Macko, R. E. (2006). Fatigue after stroke: Relationship to mobility, fitness, ambulatory activity, social support, and falls efficacy. *Rehabil Nurs*, 31(5), 210–217.
9. Graf, C. (2006). Functional decline in hospitalized older adults. *Am J Nurs*, 106(1), 58–67.
10. Winkelman, C., Chlan, L. (2009). Bed rest in health and critical illness: A body systems approach. *AACN Advanced Critical Care*, 20(3), 254–266.
11. Hurr, H. K., Park, S. M., Kim, S. S., et al. (2005). Activity intolerance and impaired physical mobility in elders. *Int J of Nursing Terminologies and Classifications*, 16(3–4), 47–53.
12. Exercise-induced bronchoconstriction and asthma: EPC Evidence Reports. (2010). *Agency for Healthcare Research and Quality*. Retrieved October 2015 from http://www.ahrq.gov/sites/default/files/wysiwyg/research/findings/evidence-based-reports/eibeia-evidence-report.pdf.
13. 2008 Physical Guidelines for Americans, Summary. (no date). *Office of Disease Prevention and Health Promotion*. Retrieved October 2015 from http://health.gov/paguidelines/guidelines/summary.aspx.
14. Koh, H. K., Tee, A., Lasserson, T. J., et al. (2007). Inhaled corticosteroids compared to placebo for prevention of exercise-induced bronchoconstriction. *Cochrane Library*. Retrieved October 2015 from http://onlinelibrary.wiley.com/doi/10.1002/14651858.CD002739.pub3/full.
15. Mussi, C., Ungar, A., Salvioli, G., et al. (2009). Orthostatic hypotension as cause of syncope in patients older than 65 years admitted to emergency departments for transient loss of consciousness. *J Gerentol A Biol Sci Med Sci*, 64(7), 801–806.

risk for Activity Intolerance

Taxonomy II: Activity/Rest—Class 4 Cardiovascular/Pulmonary Response (00094) [**Diagnostic Division:** Activity/Rest], Submitted 1982, revised 2013

DEFINITION: Vulnerable to experiencing insufficient physiological or psychological energy to endure or complete required or desired daily activities, which may compromise health.

RISK FACTORS

History of previous intolerance
Circulatory problem or respiratory condition, [dysrhythmias]
Physical deconditioning
Inexperience with an activity
NOTE: A risk diagnosis is not evidenced by signs and symptoms as the problem has not occurred; rather, nursing interventions are directed at prevention.
Sample Clinical Applications: Anemias, angina, aortic stenosis, bronchitis, emphysema, dysmenorrhea, heart failure, HIV/AIDS, labor/preterm labor, leukemias, mitral stenosis, obesity, pain, pericarditis, peripheral vascular disease, rheumatic fever, thrombocytopenia, tuberculosis, uterine bleeding

DESIRED OUTCOMES/EVALUATION CRITERIA

Sample NOC linkages:
Endurance: Capacity to sustain activity
Energy Conservation: Personal actions to manage energy for initiating and sustaining activity

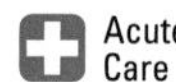

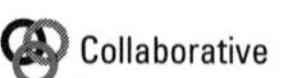

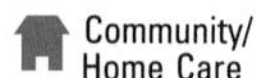

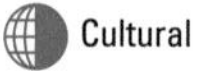

Psychomotor Energy: Personal drive and energy to maintain activities of daily living, nutrition, and personal safety

Client Will (Include Specific Time Frame)
- Verbalize understanding of potential loss of ability in relation to existing condition.
- Participate in conditioning or rehabilitation program to enhance ability to perform.
- Identify alternative ways to maintain desired activity level (e.g., if weather is bad, walking in a shopping mall could be an option).
- Identify conditions or symptoms that require medical reevaluation.

ACTIONS/INTERVENTIONS

Sample NIC linkages:
Energy Management: Regulating energy use to treat or prevent fatigue and optimize function
Exercise Promotion: Facilitation of regular physical activity to maintain or advance to a higher level of fitness and health

NURSING PRIORITY NO. 1 To assess factors affecting current situation:

- Note presence of medical diagnosis and/or therapeutic regimens (e.g., AIDS, chronic obstructive pulmonary disease, cancer, heart failure or other cardiac problems, anemia, multiple medications or treatment modalities, extensive surgical interventions, musculoskeletal trauma, neurological disorders). *These have potential for interfering with client's ability to perform at a desired level of activity. Note: Many factors cause or contribute to fatigue, but activity intolerance implies that the individual cannot endure or adapt to increased energy or oxygen demands caused by an activity.*[1]
- Ask client/significant other (SO) about usual level of energy *to identify potential problems and/or client's/SO's perception of client's energy and ability to perform needed or desired activities.*
- Identify factors (e.g., age, functional decline, painful conditions, breathing problems, client resistive to efforts; vision or hearing impairments, climate or weather; unsafe areas to exercise; need for mobility assistance) *that could block or affect desired level of activity.*
- Determine current activity level and physical condition with observation, exercise capacity testing, use of functional level classification system (e.g., Gordon's), as appropriate. *Provides baseline for comparison and opportunity to track changes.*

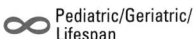

NURSING PRIORITY NO. 2 To develop/investigate alternative ways to remain active within the limits of the disabling condition/situation:

- Implement physical therapy or exercise program in conjunction with the client and other team members, such as a physical and/or occupational therapist, exercise or rehabilitation physiologist. *Collaborative program with short-term achievable goals enhances likelihood of success and may motivate client to adopt a lifestyle of physical exercise for enhancement of health.*[2]
- Promote or implement conditioning program and support inclusion in exercise or activity groups *to prevent or limit deterioration. Note, studies continue to support the positive effects of exercise training on exercise [activity] tolerance.*[6,7]
- Instruct client in proper performance of unfamiliar activities and/or alternate ways of doing familiar activities *to learn methods of conserving energy and promote safety in performing activities.*

NURSING PRIORITY NO. 3 To promote wellness (Teaching/Discharge Considerations):

- Discuss with client/SO relationship of illness or debilitating condition to inability to perform desired activity(ies). *Understanding these relationships can help with acceptance of limitations or reveal opportunity for changes of practical value.*[1,5]

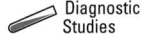

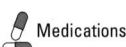

- Provide information regarding factors such as smoking when one has respiratory problems, weight management, lack of motivation or interest in exercise. *Education is essential to encourage modification of potential interferences to activity.*[3,4]
- Assist client/SO with planning for changes that may become necessary (e.g., shifting of family responsibilities, use of supplemental oxygen or medications to improve client's ability to participate in desired activities). *Anticipatory guidance facilitates adaptation if symptoms occur.*[3,4] (Refer to ND Activity Intolerance.)
- Identify and discuss symptoms for which client needs to seek medical assistance or evaluation, *providing for timely intervention.*[3]
- Refer to appropriate sources for assistance (e.g., smoking cessation, dietary counseling, psychological counseling) and/or assistive equipment, as needed, *to sustain or improve activity level and to promote client safety.*

DOCUMENTATION FOCUS

Assessment/Reassessment

- Identified and potential risk factors for individual.
- Current level of activity tolerance and blocks to activity.

Planning

- Treatment options, including physical therapy or exercise program, other assistive therapies and devices.
- Lifestyle changes that are planned, who is to be responsible for each action, monitoring methods.

Implementation/Evaluation

- Responses to interventions, teaching, and actions performed.
- Attainment or progress toward desired outcome(s).
- Modification of plan of care.

Discharge Planning

- Referrals for medical assistance and evaluation.

References

1. Cox, H. C., Sridaromont, K., King, M., et al. (2002). *Clinical Applications of Nursing Diagnosis: Adult, Child, Women's, Psychiatric, Gerontic, and Home Health Considerations.* 4th ed. Philadelphia, PA: F. A. Davis.
2. Stanley, M. (2004). In Blair, K. A., Beare, P. G. (eds). *Gerontological Nursing: Promoting Successful Aging in the Older Adult.* 3rd ed. Philadelphia, PA: F. A. Davis.
3. Pinkerman, C., Sander, P., Breeding, J. E., et al. (updated 2013). Heart failure in adults. *Institute for Clinical Systems Improvement.* Retrieved March 2015 from https://www.icsi.org/_asset/50qb52/HeartFailure.pdf.
4. Meleski, D. D. (2002). Families with chronically ill children. *Am J Nurs*, 102(5), 47–54.
5. Borroso, J., Hammill, B. G., Leserman, J., et al. (2010). Physiological and psychosocial factors that predict HIV-related fatigue. *AIDS Behav*, 14(6), 1415–1427.
6. Office of Disease Prevention and Health Promotion *2008 Physical Guidelines for Americans.* Retrieved March 2015 from http://www.health.gov/paguidelines/guidelines/summary.aspx.
7. Taylor, R. S., Briscoe, S., Lough, F., et al. (updated 2014). Exercise-based rehabilitation for heart failure. *Cochrane Database of Systematic Reviews.* Retrieved March 2015 from http://www.cochrane.org/CD003331/VASC_exercise-based-rehabilitation-for-heart-failure.

ineffective Activity Planning

Taxonomy II: Coping/Stress Tolerance—Class 2 Coping Responses (00199) [**Diagnostic Division:** Activity/Rest], Submitted 2008

DEFINITION: Inability to prepare for a set of actions fixed in time and under certain conditions.

RELATED FACTORS

Unrealistic perception of event [or] personal abilities
Insufficient social support
Insufficient information processing ability
Flight behavior when faced with proposed solution
Hedonism [motivated by pleasure and/or pain]

DEFINING CHARACTERISTICS

Subjective

Worried/excessive anxiety/fear about a task to be undertaken

Objective

Pattern of failure
Insufficient resources (e.g., financial, social, knowledge)
Absence of plan; insufficient organizational skills
Pattern of procrastination
Unmet goals for chosen activity

Sample Clinical Applications: Depression, bipolar disorder, learning disabilities or dyslexia, chronic conditions (e.g., fibromyalgia, fatigue syndrome)

DESIRED OUTCOMES/EVALUATION CRITERIA

Sample NOC linkages:

Motivation: Inner urge that moves or promotes an individual to positive action(s)
Support System Enhancement: Facilitation of support to patient by family, friends, and community

Client Will (Include Specific Time Frame)

- Acknowledge difficulty with follow-through of activity plan.
- Identify negative factors affecting ability to plan activities.
- Willingly prepare to develop own plan for activity.
- Report lessened anxiety and fear toward planning.
- Be aware of and make plan to deal with procrastination.

ACTIONS/INTERVENTIONS

Sample NIC linkages:

Self-Awareness Enhancement: Assisting a patient to explore and understand his/her thoughts, feelings, motivations, and behaviors
Values Clarification: Assisting another to clarify her/his own values in order to facilitate effective decision making

NURSING PRIORITY NO. 1 To identify causative/precipitating factors:

- Determine individual problems with planning and follow through with activity plan. *Identifies individual difficulties, such as anxiety regarding what kind of activity to choose, lack of resources, lack of confidence in own ability.*[1]

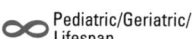

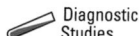

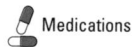

- Perform complete physical examination. *May have underlying problems, such as allergies, hypertension, asthma, that contribute to fatigue and difficulty undertaking task.*[2]
- Review medication regimen. *Side effects may contribute to fatigue, affecting client's desire to get involved in any activity.*[2]
- Assess mental status; use Beck's Depression scale as indicated. *Anxieties and depression can interfere with client's ability and desire to be active.*[5]
- Identify client's personal values and perception of self, including strengths and weaknesses. *Provides information that will be helpful in planning care and choosing goals for this individual.*[1]
- Determine client's need to be in control, fear of dependency on others (although may need assistance from others), belief he or she cannot do the task. *Indicative of external locus of control, where client sees others as having the control and ability.*[1]
- Identify cultural or religious issues that may affect how individual deals with issues of life. *Often person learns strict ideas in family of origin, such as rituals of Catholicism or the demands of prayers for Muslims, that affect how they see their ability to make choices or manage own life.*[1]
- Discuss awareness of procrastination, need for perfection, fear of failure. *Although client may not acknowledge it as a problem, this may be a factor in difficulty in planning for, choosing, and following through with activities that might be enjoyed.*[3,8,9]
- Assess client's ability to process information. *Low self-esteem, anxiety, and possibly difficulty with thinking ability may interfere with perception of the world.*[4]
- Discuss possibility that client is motivated by pleasure to avoid pain (hedonism). *Individual may seek activities that bring pleasure to avoid painful experiences and not realize he or she is using this to keep from completing tasks.*[4,7]
- Note availability and use of resources. *Client may have difficulty if family and friends are not supportive and other resources are not readily available.*[1]

NURSING PRIORITY NO. 2 To assist client to recognize and deal with individual factors and begin to plan appropriate activities:

- Encourage expression of feelings contributing to or resulting from situation. Maintain a positive atmosphere without being too cheerful. *Helps client to begin to be aware of frustration and redirect energy into productive actions.*[5]
- Discuss client's perception of self as worthless and not deserving of success and happiness. *This belief is common among individuals who struggle with feelings of low self-esteem/self-confidence. They believe that anything they do is bound to fail, and feelings of anxiety and worry contribute to failure. Procrastinating and postponing the task results in failure. Sometimes the underlying feelings are those of wanting to be perfect, and the task may not be perfect if it is finished.*[4,8]
- Gently confront ambivalent, angry, or depressed feelings. *Client may react negatively and withdraw if these feelings are not dealt with in a sensitive manner.*[1]
- Help client learn how to reframe negative thoughts about self into a positive view of what is happening. *Reframing turns a negative thought into something positive to change how it affects the individual.*[1]
- Involve client/significant others (SOs) in planning an activity. *Starting with one activity at a time and having the support of the family and nurse will help promote success.*[1]
- Direct client to break down desired activity into specific steps. *Makes activity more manageable, and as each step is accomplished, individual feels more confident about ability to finish the task.*[1]
- Encourage client to recognize procrastinating behaviors and make a decision to change. *Procrastination is a learned behavior, possibly in the family of origin, and serves many purposes for the individual. It can be changed but may require intensive therapy.*[3,8,9]
- Accompany client to activity of own choosing, encouraging participation together, if appropriate. *Support from caregiver may enable client to begin participating and gain confidence.*[1,9]
- Assist client to develop skills of relaxation, imagery or visualization, and mindfulness. *Using these techniques can help the client learn to overcome stress and be able to manage life's difficulties more effectively.*[2,6]

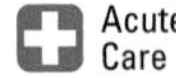

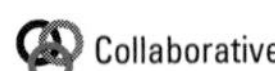

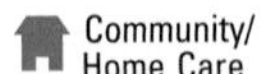

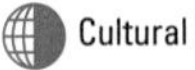

- Assist client to investigate the idea that seeking pleasure (hedonism) is interfering with motivation to accomplish goals. *Some philosophers believe that pleasure is the only good for a person, and the individual does not see other aspects of life, interfering with accomplishments.*[7]

NURSING PRIORITY NO. 3 To promote wellness (Teaching/Discharge Criteria):

- Assist client to identify life goals and priorities. *Often individual has not thought about the possibility of these ideas and, when asked to do this, begins to think he or she can accomplish some goals.*[1]
- Review treatment goals and expectations of client and SOs. *Helps to clarify what has been discussed and decisions that have been made and provides an opportunity to change goals as needed.*[1]
- Discuss progress in learning to relax and deal productively with anxieties and fears. *As client sees that progress is being made, feelings of worthwhileness will be enhanced and individual will be encouraged to continue working toward goals.*[2,3]
- Identify community resources such as social services, senior center, or classes *to provide support and options for activities and change.*
- Refer for cognitive therapy. *This structured therapy can help the individuals identify, evaluate, and modify underlying assumptions and dysfunctional beliefs they may have and begin the process of change. Learning to set own schedule with reminders can also help client to get tasks done in a timely manner.*[5]

DOCUMENTATION FOCUS

Assessment/Reassessment
- Specific problems exhibited by client.
- Causative or precipitating factors.
- Client reports of difficulty making and following through with plans.

Planning
- Plan of care and who is involved in planning.
- Teaching plan.

Implementation/Evaluation
- Response to interventions, teaching, and actions performed.
- Attainment or progress toward desired outcome(s).

Discharge Planning
- Referrals to other resources.
- Long-term needs and who is responsible for actions.

References

1. Schuyler, D. (2003). Cognitive therapy for depression. *Primary Psychiatry*, 10(5), 33–36.
2. Berczi, I. (1994). Stress and disease: The contributions of Hans Selye to neuroimmunology. In Berczi, I., Szélenyi, J. (eds). *Advances in Psychoneuroimmunology*. New York: Plenum Press, 1–15.
3. Marano, H. E. (2009). Ending procrastination. Retrieved January 2015 from http://www.psychologytoday.com/articles/200310/ending-procrastination.
4. Ellis, A. (1994). Showing people they are not worthless individuals. *Voices: The Art and Science of Psychotherapy*, 1(2), 74–77.
5. Beck, A. C., Beck, A. T. (1995). Cognitive therapy for depression. *Clin Psychol*, 48(3), 3–5.
6. Hopper, J. (2009; revised 2015). Mindfulness and kindness: Inner sources of freedom and happiness. Retrieved January 2015 from http://www.jimhopper.com/mindfulness/.
7. Moore, A. (2004; revised 2013). Hedonism. *The Stanford Encyclopedia of Philosophy*. Retrieved January 2015 http://plato.stanford.edu/entries/hedonism/.
8. California Polytechnic State University. (2012). Procrastination. Retrieved January 2015 from http://sas.calpoly.edu/asc/ssl/procrastination.html.
9. Gura, T. (2009). I'll do it tomorrow. *Scientific American Mind*, 19, 32–39.

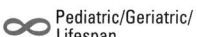

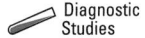

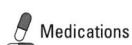

risk for ineffective Activity Planning

Taxonomy II: Coping/Stress Tolerance—Class 2 Coping Responses (0026) [**Diagnostic Division:** Activity/Rest], Submitted 2010; Revised 2013

DEFINITION: Vulnerable to an inability to prepare for a set of actions fixed in time and under certain conditions, which may compromise health.

RISK FACTORS

Unrealistic perception of events or personal abilities
Insufficient support systems
Insufficient information processing ability
Flight behavior when faced with proposed solution
Pattern of procrastination
Hedonism
Sample Clinical Applications: Depression, bipolar disorder, learning disabilities/dyslexia, chronic conditions (e.g., fibromyalgia, fatigue, multiple sclerosis).

DESIRED OUTCOMES/EVALUATION CRITERIA

Sample NOC linkages:
Motivation: Inner urge that motivates or prompts an individual to positive action(s)
Decision Making: Ability to make judgments and choose between two or more alternatives

Client Will (Include Specific Time Frame)
- Express awareness of negative factors or actions that can interfere with planning.
- Establish mindfulness and relaxation activities to lessen anxiety.
- Develop a plan, including the time frame, for a task to be completed.

ACTIONS/INTERVENTIONS

Sample NIC linkages:
Self-Responsibility Facilitation: Encouraging a patient to assume more responsibility for own behavior
Self-Modification Assistance: Reinforcement of self-directed change initiated by the patient to achieve personally important goals
Mutual Goal Setting: Collaborating with a patient to identify and prioritize care goals, then develop a plan for achieving those goals

NURSING PRIORITY NO. 1 To identify causative/precipitating factors related to risk:

- Determine circumstances of client's situation that may impact participating in selective activities. *Identifies areas for client to begin to change behavior.*
- Note client's ability to process information. *Compromised mental ability, low self-esteem, and anxiety can interfere with dealing with planning of activities of life.*[15]
- Review health history and medications. *Underlying physical problems, such as fatigue or medication side effects, can affect ability to engage in tasks.*[3,11,18]
- Evaluate mental status, using Beck's Depression scale or other inventories as indicated. *Depression, anxiety, and/or mental illness can potentially interfere with client's ability to plan desired activities.*[16]
- Discuss religious/cultural and personal values and perception of self, including view of strengths and weaknesses. *These factors affect every aspect of client's life, including how he/she views ability to make choices or manage life.*[9,15]

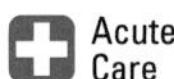

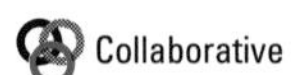

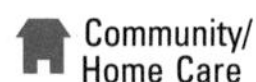

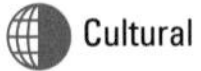

- Ascertain need for control, fear of dependency on others, or belief they will not be able to do the task. *Although client may need assistance, he/she may have external locus of control and see others as having control and the ability to do things the client is not able to do.*[17]
- Investigate client's awareness of procrastination, need for perfection, or fear of failure. *These issues may be interfering with client's choosing to manage planning of life activities.*[8]
- Discuss issue of avoiding pain by seeking pleasure (hedonism). *People sometimes avoid pain by choosing activities that provide pleasure but don't get needed tasks accomplished.*[7,8,9]
- Note availability and use of resources and support. *Lack of resources or insufficient support limit client's ability to engage in activities.*

NURSING PRIORITY NO. 2 To assist client to recognize and deal with risk factors that interfere with appropriate activities:

- Encourage recognition of feelings associated with issues that prevent client from planning desired activities. *Awareness of frustration and/or anxiety will help client redirect energy into productive activities.*[5,10]
- Help client to reframe negative thoughts about self into a positive view of what he/she is able to achieve. *The belief that individuals are worthless and not deserving of success and happiness is prevalent among many people who are anxious, leading to the belief that anything tried is doomed to failure.*[2,5,6,14]
- Encourage client to recognize procrastinating behaviors and make a decision to change. *Often this learned behavior comes from the family of origin. A decision to change may require therapy to change the ingrained habit.*[5,11,13]
- Develop a plan with the client to deal with activities in small steps. *Learning to do this will help client to feel more organized and successful in completing the desired task.*[4,5,12]
- Encourage client to engage in activity of choice with a friend, family member. *Support may encourage client to pursue activity and be successful at completion.*[1]
- Investigate with the client the possibility that seeking pleasure (hedonism) may interfere with achieving life goals. *Individual may believe that pleasure is the only good and avoid tasks or activities viewed as not fun or pleasurable thereby interfering with accomplishments.*[7]

NURSING PRIORITY NO. 3 To promote wellness (Teaching/Discharge Criteria):

- Identify life goals and priorities. *If the individual has never thought about setting goals, he or she may begin to think about the possibility of being successful.*[12]
- Discuss use of relaxation techniques and mindfulness to deal with anxieties and stressors. *Enables client to deal with life's difficulties more effectively, helping client to view self as worthwhile and encouraging continued work toward goals.*[3,6]
- Identify community resources, such as social services, senior center, or classes. *Provides an opportunity to be involved in different activities and be successful in trying new activities.*
- Refer for cognitive therapy as indicated. *May help client to deal with basic assumptions and dysfunctional beliefs in order to become successful.*[5,13]

DOCUMENTATION FOCUS

Assessment/Reassessment

- Individual risk factors identified.
- Client concerns or difficulty making and following through with plan.

Planning

- Plan of care and who is involved in planning.
- Teaching plan.

Implementation/Evaluation

- Response to interventions, teaching, and actions performed.
- Attainment or progress toward outcomes.
- Client's plan for the future.

Discharge Planning

- Referrals to other resources.
- Long-term need and who is responsible for actions.

References

1. Davis, J. L. (2005, reviewed 2009). Coping with Anxiety. Retrieved January 2015 from http://www.webmd.com/anxiety-panic/guide/coping-with-anxiety.
2. Blanicka, P. (2002). Reframing: The essence of mediation. Retrieved January 2015 from http://www.mediate.com/articles//blanciak.cfm.
3. Stress relievers: Top 10 picks to tame stress. (2013). Mayo Clinic Staff. Retrieved January 2015 from http://www.mayoclinic.com/health/stress-relievers/MY01373.
4. Marano, H. E. (2003, revised 2009). Ending procrastination. *Psychology Today*. Retrieved January 2015 from http://www.psychologytoday.com/articles/200310/ending-procrastination.
5. Butler, A. C., Beck, A. T. (1995). Cognitive therapy for depression. *Clin Psychol*, 48(3), 3–5.
6. Hopper, J. (revised 2015). Mindfulness and kindness: Inner sources of freedom and happiness. Retrieved January 2015 from http://www.jimhopper.com/mindfulness/.
7. Moore, A. (2004). Hedonism. *The Stanford Encyclopedia of Philosophy*. Retrieved November 2012 from http://plato.stanford.edu/entries/hedonism/.
8. Gura, T. (2009). I'll do it tomorrow. *Scientific American Mind*, December/January, 32–39.
9. The Arizona Direct Care Curriculum Project. (2011). Activity Planning. Principles of Caregiving: Aging and Physical Disabilities, Chapter 7. Retrieved January 2015 from http://www.azdirectcare.org/uploads/APDChap7-ActivityPlanningJan11.pdf.
10. Reblin, M., Uchino, B. N. (2008). Social and emotional support and its implication for health. *Curr Opin Psychiatry*, 21(2), 201–205.
11. Marano, H. E. (2003, revised 2010). Procrastination: Ten things to know. *Psychology Today*. Retrieved January 2015 from http://www.psychologytoday.com/articles/200308/procrastination-ten-things-know.
12. No author listed. (1996–2015). Personal goal setting—Planning to live your life your way. MindTools. Retrieved January 2015 from http://www.mindtools.com/page6.html.
13. Pucci, A. R. (2010). *The Client's Guide to Cognitive-Behavioral Therapy*. Weirton, WV: National Association of Cognitive-Behavioral Therapists.
14. Townsend, M. T. (2010). *Essentials of Psychiatric Mental Health Nursing: Concepts of Care in Evidence-Based Practice*. 5th ed. Philadelphia, PA: F. A. Davis, 143–146.
15. Das, J. P., Naglieri, J. A., Murphy, D. B. (1995). Individual differences in cognitive processes of planning: A personality variable? The Psychological Record. Digital book. Retrieved January 2015 from http://www.thefreelibrary.com/Individual+differences+in+cognitive+processes+of+planning%3A+a...-a017150075.
16. Beck Institute for Cognitive Behavior Therapy. (No date listed). Professional Tools & Resources: Patient assessment tools. Retrieved January 2015 from http://www.beckinstitute.org/beck-inventory-and-scales/.
17. No author. Stress, definition of stress, stressor, What is stress? What is eustress? Retrieved November 2012 from http://www.morgancc.edu/abm/curric/SG/Cert9/ABM_153/U4/Stress,%20Definition%20of%20Stress,%20Stressor,%20What%20is%20Stress,%20Eustress.PDF.
18. Scott, E. (2012). Top 10 Things to Know about the Effects of Stress. About.com. Retrieved November 2012 from http://stress.about.com/od/understandingstress/tp/effects_stress.htm.

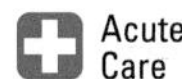

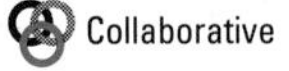

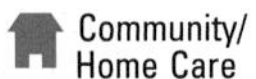

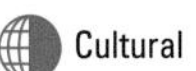

decreased intracranial Adaptive Capacity

Taxonomy II: Coping/Stress Tolerance—Class 3 Neurobehavioral Stress (00049) [**Diagnostic Division:** Circulation], Submitted 1994

DEFINITION: Intracranial fluid dynamic mechanisms that normally compensate for increases in intracranial volume are compromised, resulting in repeated disproportionate increases in intracranial pressure (ICP) in response to a variety of noxious and non-noxious stimuli.

RELATED FACTORS

Brain injuries (e.g., cerebrovascular impairment, neurological illness, trauma, tumor)
Sustained increase in intracranial pressure (ICP) of 10 to 15 mmHg
Decreased cerebral perfusion pressure ≥50 to 60 mmHg
Systemic hypotension with intracranial hypertension

DEFINING CHARACTERISTICS

Objective

Repeated increase in ICP of ≥10 mmHg for ≥5 min following external stimuli
Disproportionate increase in ICP following stimulus
Elevated P_2 ICP waveform
Volume-pressure response test variation (volume: pressure ratio 2, pressure-volume index <10)
Baseline ICP ≥10 mmHg
Wide-amplitude ICP waveform

Sample Clinical Applications: Traumatic brain injury (TBI), cerebral edema, stroke, cranial tumors/hematomas, hydrocephalus

DESIRED OUTCOMES/EVALUATION CRITERIA

Sample NOC linkages:

Tissue Perfusion: Cerebral: Adequacy of blood flow through the cerebral vasculature to maintain brain function

Neurological Status: Ability of the peripheral and central nervous system to receive, process, and respond to internal and external stimuli

Client Will (Include Specific Time Frame)

- Demonstrate stable ICP as evidenced by normalization of pressure waveforms and response to stimuli.
- Display improved neurological signs.

ACTIONS/INTERVENTIONS

Sample NIC linkages:

Cerebral Edema Management: Limitation of secondary cerebral injury resulting from swelling of brain tissue

Cerebral Perfusion Promotion: Promotion of adequate perfusion and limitation of complications for a patient experiencing or at risk for inadequate cerebral perfusion

ICP Monitoring: Measurement and interpretation of patient data to regulate ICP

NURSING PRIORITY NO. 1 To assess causative/contributing factors:

- Determine factors related to individual situation (e.g., trauma such as fall, motor vehicle crash, gunshot wound, infection such as meningitis or encephalitis; brain tumor) and potential for increased ICP.

Deterioration in neurological signs/symptoms or failure to improve after initial insult may reflect decreased adaptive capacity.

- Review results of diagnostic imaging (e.g., cerebral computed tomography [CT] scans) *to note location, type, and severity of intracranial injury. CT scan is sensitive to acute hemorrhage or skull fractures and aids in evaluating mass effect and midline shift, obliteration of the basal cisterns, or evidence of herniation.*[6]
- Monitor for change in ICP (e.g., worsening neurological signs or variations in ICP monitor waveform and pressure) and corresponding event (e.g., coughing, suctioning, position change, noise such as monitor alarms, family visit). *ICP monitoring may be done in a critically ill client with a Glasgow Coma Scale (GCS) score of 8 or less. The ICP offers data that supplement the neurological examination and can be crucial in a client whose examination findings are affected by sedatives, paralytics, or other factors. Elevated pressure can be caused by the injury, environmental stimuli, or treatment modalities. Note: More advanced technologies are being used in some neurotrauma intensive care units to monitor electroencephalograph and bispectral index readings at the bedside to evaluate brain function while the client is in induced coma sedation with agents such as pentobarbital or propofol (Diprivan).*[2,3,6,14]

NURSING PRIORITY NO. 2 To note degree of impairment:

- Evaluate level of consciousness using GCS. *GCS remains the gold standard for objectively assessing individuals with TBIs. It assesses eye opening (e.g., awake, opens only to painful movement, keeps eyes closed), position or movement (e.g., spontaneous, purposeful, posturing), pupils (size, shape, equality, light reactivity), and consciousness or mental status (e.g., comatose, responds to pain, awake or confused). Low numbers (e.g., <8) are typically seen in clients with severe head injury and impaired cerebral perfusion requiring critical care interventions.*[2,3,6,9]
- Note purposeful and nonpurposeful motor response (e.g., posturing), comparing right and left sides. *Posturing and abnormal flexion of extremities usually indicate diffuse cortical damage. Absence of spontaneous movement on one side indicates damage to the motor tracts in the opposite cerebral hemisphere.*[1]
- Test for presence or absence of reflexes (e.g., blink, cough, gag, Babinski's reflex) and nuchal rigidity. *Helps identify location of injury (e.g., loss of blink reflex suggests damage to the pons and medulla, absence of cough and gag reflexes reflects damage to medulla, presence of Babinski's reflex indicates injury along pyramidal pathways in the brain).*[1]
- Monitor vital signs and cardiac rhythm before, during, and after activity. *Helps determine parameters for "safe" activity. Mean arterial blood pressure should be maintained above 90 mmHg to maintain cerebral perfusion pressure (CCP) greater than 70 mmHg, which reflects adequate blood supply to the brain. Fever in brain injury can be associated with injury to the hypothalamus or bleeding, systemic infection (e.g., pneumonia), or drugs. Hyperthermia exacerbates cerebral ischemia. Irregular respiration patterns can suggest location of cerebral insult. Cardiac dysrhythmias can be due to brainstem injury and stimulation of the sympathetic nervous system. Bradycardia may occur with high ICP.*[2,3,6]
- Monitor pulse oximetry or arterial blood gases, particularly pH, CO_2, and PaO_2. *A $PaCO_2$ level of 30 to 35 mmHg maintains cerebral blood flow and adequate cerebral oxygenation, while a PaO_2 of less than 65 mmHg may cause cerebral vascular dilation and further tissue damage.*[2,3,12]
- Monitor urine output and serum sodium. *Posttraumatic neuroendocrine dysfunction can result in a hyponatremic or hypernatremic state. When hyponatremia exists, cerebral edema or syndrome of inappropriate antidiuretic hormone can occur, requiring correction with fluid restriction and hypertonic IV solution. Hypernatremia can occur because of injury to the hypothalamus or pituitary stalk, causing diabetes insipidus, resulting in huge urine losses, or can be the result of excessive diuresis due to use of mannitol or furosemide administered to reduce cerebral edema.*[3]

NURSING PRIORITY NO. 3 To minimize/correct causative factors/maximize perfusion:

- Perform periodic assessments of the client's level of consciousness and/or neurological status, blood pressure, breath sounds, temperature, amount of respiratory secretions, central venous pressure, heart rate and rhythm, fluid balance, nutritional status, and serial laboratory values, as with any critically ill client.

- Perform interventions specific to client with increased ICP:
  - Elevate head of bed as individually appropriate. *Optimal head of bed position is determined by both ICP and coronary perfusion pressure measurements—that is, which degree of elevation lowers ICP while maintaining adequate cerebral blood flow. Studies show that in most cases, an elevation of 30 degrees significantly decreases ICP while maintaining cerebral blood flow.*[6,7]
  - Maintain head and neck in neutral position, supporting with small towel rolls or pillows *to maximize venous return. Note: Lateral and rotational neck flexion has been shown to be the most consistent trigger of sustained increases in ICP.*[3,4]
  - Avoid causing hip flexion of 90 degrees or more. *Hip flexion may trap venous blood in the intra-abdominal space, increasing abdominal and intrathoracic pressure and reducing venous outflow from the head, increasing cerebral pressure.*[5]
  - Limit or prevent activities such as coughing, vomiting, and straining at stool and avoid or restrict use of restraints. *These factors often increase intrathoracic/abdominal pressures or agitation and markedly increase ICP.*[1]
  - Suction with caution and only when needed. Pass catheter just beyond end of endotracheal tube without touching tracheal wall or carina. Administer lidocaine intratracheally if indicated *to reduce cough reflex. Note: Studies have noted significant increase in ICP and decrease in CCP in ventilated clients with brain injury, especially if they are not well sedated.*[3,15]
  - Hyperoxygenate before suctioning as appropriate *to minimize hypoxia. Note: Studies show that in most clients, hyperventilation is not necessary; however, therapeutic hyperventilation ($PaCO_2$ of 30 to 35 mm) may be used for a short period of time in acute neurological deterioration to reduce intracranial hypertension while other methods of ICP control are initiated.*[3,7,8,11]
- Investigate increased restlessness *to determine causative factors and initiate corrective measures as indicated:*
  - Decrease extraneous stimuli and provide comfort measures (e.g., quiet environment, soft voice, tapes of familiar voices played through earphones, back massage, gentle touch as tolerated) *to reduce central nervous system stimulation and promote relaxation.*[4]
  - Limit painful procedures (e.g., venipunctures, redundant neurological evaluations) to those that are absolutely necessary *in order to minimize preventable elevations in ICP.*[3]
  - Provide rest periods between care activities and limit duration of procedures. Lower lighting and noise levels and schedule and limit activities *to provide a restful environment and limit spikes in ICP associated with noxious stimuli.*[3]
  - Encourage family/significant others to talk to client. *Familiar voices appear to have a relaxing effect on many comatose individuals (thereby reducing ICP).*[1]
- Administer and restrict fluid intake as necessary, and administer IV fluids via pump or control device *to maintain intravascular volume sufficient to maintain cerebral perfusion while preventing inadvertent vascular overload, cerebral edema, and increased ICP.*[6]
- Weigh as indicated. Calculate fluid balance every shift/daily *to determine fluid needs, maintain hydration, and prevent fluid overload.*[1]
- Monitor and manage body temperature. Regulate environmental temperature and bed linens and use cooling blanket as indicated *to decrease metabolic and oxygen needs when fever is present or when therapeutic hypothermia therapy is used. Lowering the body temperature has been shown to lower ICP and improve outcomes for recovery.*[3,6,13]
- Provide appropriate safety measures/initiate treatment for seizures *to prevent injury and increase of ICP or hypoxia.*
- Administer supplemental oxygen as indicated *to prevent cerebral ischemia.*
- Administer medications (e.g., antihypertensives, diuretics, analgesics, sedatives, antipyretics, vasopressors, antiseizure drugs, neuromuscular blocking agents, corticosteroids) as appropriate *to maintain cerebral homeostasis and manage symptoms associated with neurological injury. Note: Controversy continues concerning the use of steroids in the setting of TBI. One 2004 study showed a significantly increased risk of death in clients treated with steroids after TBI.*[12]

- Administer enteral or parenteral nutrition *to achieve positive nitrogen balance, reducing effects of post–brain injury metabolic and catabolic states, which can lead to complications such as immunosuppression, infection, poor wound healing, loss of body mass, and multiple organ dysfunction. Studies have shown that parenteral nutritional support can be given to these clients without worsening cerebral edema.*[10]
- Prepare client for surgery as indicated (e.g., evacuation of hematoma or space-occupying lesion) *to reduce ICP and enhance circulation.*

NURSING PRIORITY NO. 4 To promote wellness (Teaching/Discharge Considerations):

- Discuss with caregivers specific situations (e.g., if client choking or experiencing pain, needing to be repositioned, constipated, blocked urinary flow) and review appropriate interventions *to prevent or limit episodic increases in ICP.*
- Identify signs/symptoms suggesting increased ICP (in client at risk without an ICP monitor), such as restlessness and deterioration in neurological responses. Review appropriate interventions.

DOCUMENTATION FOCUS

Assessment/Reassessment

- Neurological findings, noting right and left sides separately (e.g., pupils, motor response, reflexes, restlessness, nuchal rigidity); GCS.
- Response to activities and events (e.g., changes in pressure waveforms or vital signs).
- Presence and characteristics of seizure activity.

Planning

- Plan of care and who is involved in planning.
- Teaching plan.

Implementation/Evaluation

- Response to interventions and actions performed.
- Attainment or progress toward desired outcome(s).
- Modifications to plan of care.

Discharge Planning

- Future needs, plan for meeting them, and determining who is responsible for actions.
- Referrals as identified.

References

1. Doenges, M. E., Moorhouse, M. F., Murr, A. C. (2010). Craniocerebral trauma (acute rehabilitative phase). *Nursing Care Plans: Guidelines for Individualizing Client Care Across the Life Span.* 8th ed. Philadelphia, PA: F. A. Davis.
2. Brain Trauma Foundation Team (2007). Indications for intracranial monitoring: Guidelines for the management of severe traumatic brain injury. *J Neurotrauma*, 24: Suppl 1, S37–S44.
3. McNett, M. M., Gianakis, A. (2011). Nursing interventions for critically ill traumatic brain injury patients. *J Neurosci Nurs*, 42(2), 71–77.
4. Mitchell, P. H., Habermann, B. (1999). Rethinking physiological stability: Touch and intracranial pressure. *Biol Res Nurs*, 1(1), 12–19.
5. Vos, H. R. (1993). Making headway with intracranial hypertension. *Am J Nurs*, 93(2), 28–35.
6. Rangel-Castilla, L., Gasco, J., Hanbali, F., et al. (2011). Closed head trauma. Retrieved January 2012 from http://emedicine.medscape.com/article/251834-overview.
7. Reddy, L. (2006). Heads up on cerebral bleeds. *Nursing*, 3(5), 4–9. Suppl, ED Insider.
8. Zink, E. K., McQuillan, K. (2005). Managing traumatic brain injury. *Nursing*, 35(9), 36–43.
9. Teasdale, G., Jennett, B. (1974). Assessment of coma and impaired consciousness: A practical scale. *Lancet*, 2(7872), 81–84.
10. Brain Trauma Foundation Team: Guidelines for the management of severe traumatic brain injury (2007). Nutrition. *Lancet*, 24:Supp 1, S77–S78.

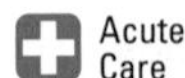

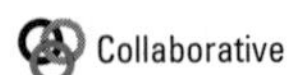

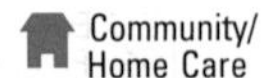

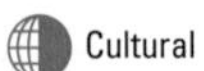

11. Rangel-Castillo, L., Roberstson, C. S. (2006). Management of intracranial hypertension. *Crit Care Clin*, 22(4), 713–732.
12. Roberts, I., Yates, D., Sandercock, P., et al. (2004). Effect of intravenous corticosteroids on death within 14 days in 10,008 adults with clinically significant head injury (MRC CRASH trial): Randomized placebo-controlled trial. *Lancet*, 364, 1321–1328.
13. Sahuquillo, J., Vilalta, A. (2007). Cooling the injured brain: How does moderate hypothermia influence the pathophysiology of traumatic brain injury? *Curr Pharm Des*, 13, 2310–2322.
14. Littlejohns, L., Bader, M. (2009). *Monitoring Technologies in Critically Ill Neuroscience Patients.* Boston: Jones and Bartlett.
15. Gemma, M., Tommasino, C., Cerri, M., et al. (2002). Intracranial effects of endotracheal suctioning in the acute phase of head injury. *J Neurosurg Anesth*, 14(1), 50–54.

ineffective Airway Clearance

Taxonomy II: Safety/Protection—Class 2 Physical Injury (00031) [**Diagnostic Division:** Respiration], Submitted 1980; Revised 1996, 1998

DEFINITION: Inability to clear secretions or obstructions from the respiratory tract to maintain a clear airway.

RELATED FACTORS

Environmental

Smoking; exposure to smoke; secondhand smoke

Obstructed airway

Retained secretions; exudate in the alveoli; excessive mucus; airway spasm; foreign body in airway; presence of artificial airway

Chronic obstructive pulmonary disease [COPD]; hyperplasia of the bronchial walls

Physiological

Asthma; allergic airways

Neuromuscular dysfunction

Infection

DEFINING CHARACTERISTICS

Subjective

Dyspnea

Objective

Diminished breath sounds; adventitious breath sounds [rales, crackles, rhonchi, wheezes]

Ineffective or absence of cough; excessive sputum

Alteration in respiratory rate or pattern

Difficulty vocalizing

Wide-eyed look; restlessness

Orthopnea

Cyanosis

Sample Clinical Applications: COPD, pneumonia, influenza, acute respiratory distress syndrome (ARDS), cancer of lung, cancer of head and neck, congestive heart failure (CHF), cystic fibrosis, neuromuscular diseases such as cerebral palsy; spinal cord injury, inhalation injuries

(continues on page 50)

ineffective Airway Clearance (continued)

DESIRED OUTCOMES/EVALUATION CRITERIA

Sample NOC linkages:

Respiratory Status: Airway Patency: Open, clear tracheobronchial passages for air exchange
Aspiration Prevention: Personal actions to prevent the passage of fluid and solid particles into the lung
Cognition: Ability to execute complex mental processes

Client Will (Include Specific Time Frame)

- Maintain airway patency.
- Expectorate or clear secretions readily.
- Demonstrate absence or reduction of congestion with breath sounds clear, respirations noiseless, and improved oxygen exchange (e.g., absence of cyanosis, arterial blood gas [ABG] results within client norms).
- Verbalize understanding of cause(s) and therapeutic management regimen.
- Demonstrate behaviors to improve or maintain clear airway.
- Identify potential complications and how to initiate appropriate preventive or corrective actions.

ACTIONS/INTERVENTIONS

Sample NIC linkages:

Airway Management: Facilitation of patency of air passages
Respiratory Monitoring: Collection and analysis of patient data to ensure airway patency and adequate gas exchange
Cough Enhancement: Promotion of deep inhalation by the patient with subsequent generation of high intrathoracic pressures and compression of underlying lung parenchyma for the forceful expulsion of air

NURSING PRIORITY NO. 1 To maintain adequate, patent airway:

- Identify client populations at risk. *Persons with impaired ciliary function (e.g., cystic fibrosis, lung transplant recipients); those with excessive or abnormal mucus production (e.g., asthma, emphysema, pneumonia, dehydration, bronchiectasis, mechanical ventilation); those with impaired cough function (e.g., neuromuscular diseases, such as muscular dystrophy, multiple sclerosis and other neuromotor conditions, such as cerebral palsy, spinal cord injury); those with swallowing abnormalities (e.g., poststroke, seizures, head/neck cancer, coma/sedation, tracheostomy, facial burns/trauma/surgery); those who are immobile (e.g., sedated individual, frail elderly, developmentally delayed, institutionalized client with multiple high-risk conditions); and infants/children (e.g., feeding intolerance, abdominal distention, emotional stressors that may compromise airway) are all at risk for problems with maintenance of open airways.*[1,2]
- Assess level of consciousness/cognition and ability to protect own airway. *This information is essential for identifying potential for airway problems, providing baseline level of care needed, and influencing choice of interventions.*
- Evaluate respiratory rate/depth and breath sounds. *Tachypnea is usually present to some degree and may be pronounced during respiratory stress. Respirations may be shallow. Some degree of bronchospasm is present with obstruction in airways and may/may not be manifested in adventitious breath sounds, such as scattered moist crackles (bronchitis), faint sounds with expiratory wheezes (emphysema), or absent breath sounds (severe asthma).*[2]
- Position head appropriate for age and condition/disorder. *Repositioning head may, at times, be all that is needed to open or maintain open airway in at-rest or compromised individual, such as one with sleep apnea.*
- ∞ Insert oral airway, using correct size for adult or child, when indicated. Have appropriate emergency equipment at bedside (such as tracheostomy equipment, ambu-bag, suction apparatus) *to restore or maintain an effective airway.*[3,4]
- Evaluate amount and type of secretions being produced. *Excessive and/or sticky mucus can completely obstruct or make it difficult to maintain effective airways, especially if client has impaired cough function, is very young or elderly, is developmentally delayed, has restrictive or obstructive lung disease, or is mechanically ventilated.*[2,5]

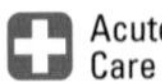

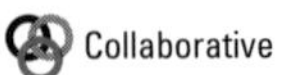

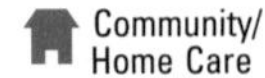

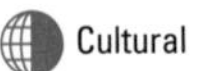

- Note ability to, and effectiveness of, cough. *Cough function may be absent, weak, or ineffective in diseases and conditions such as extremes in age (e.g., premature infant or elderly), cerebral palsy, muscular dystrophy, spinal cord injury, brain injury, postsurgery, and/or mechanical ventilation due to mechanisms affecting muscles of throat, chest, and lungs.*[5,6]
- Suction (nasal, tracheal, oral), when indicated, using correct-size catheter and suction timing for child or adult *to clear airway when secretions are blocking airways, client is unable to clear airway by coughing, cough is ineffective, infant is unable to take oral feedings because of secretions, or ventilated client is showing desaturation of oxygen by oximetry or ABGs.*[2,5,7]
- Assist with or prepare for appropriate testing (e.g., pulmonary function test or sleep studies) *to identify causative or precipitating factors.*
- Assist with procedures (e.g., bronchoscopy, tracheostomy) *to clear or maintain open airway.*
- Keep environment free of smoke, dust, and feather pillows according to individual situation. *Remove precipitators of allergic types of respiratory reactions that can trigger/exacerbate acute episode.*[3]

NURSING PRIORITY NO. 2 To mobilize secretions:

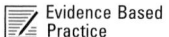

- Elevate head of the bed or change position, as needed. *Elevation or upright position facilitates respiratory function by use of gravity; however, the client in severe distress will seek position of comfort.*[3]
- Position appropriately (e.g., head of bed elevated, client on side, rather than supine) and discourage use of oil-based products around nose *to prevent vomiting with aspiration into lungs.* (Refer to NDs risk for Aspiration, impaired Swallowing.)
- Exercise diligence in providing oral hygiene, removing substances, and keeping oral mucosa hydrated. *Airways can be obstructed by substances such as blood or thickened secretions. These can be managed by strict attention to good oral hygiene, especially in the client who is unable to provide that for self. Note: Instances of inspissated (thickened, dense, dehydrated) secretions as the cause of death have been reported.*[2]
- Encourage and instruct in deep-breathing and directed-coughing exercises; teach (presurgically) and reinforce (postsurgically) breathing and coughing while splinting incision *to maximize cough effort, lung expansion, and drainage and to reduce impairment associated with pain.*
- Mobilize client as soon as possible. *Reduces risk or effects of atelectasis, enhancing lung expansion and drainage of different lung segments.*[5]
- Administer analgesics, as indicated. *Analgesics may be needed to improve cough effort when pain is inhibiting. Note: Overmedication, especially with opioids, can depress respirations and cough effort.*
- Administer medications (e.g., expectorants, anti-inflammatory agents, bronchodilators, mucolytic agents), as indicated, *to relax smooth respiratory musculature, reduce airway edema, and mobilize secretions.*[8]
- Increase fluid intake to at least 2,000 mL/day within cardiac tolerance (may require IV in acutely ill, hospitalized client). Encourage or provide warm versus cold liquids, as appropriate. *Warm hydration can help liquefy viscous secretions and improve secretion clearance. Note: Individuals with compromised cardiac function may develop symptoms of CHF (crackles, edema, weight gain).*[4,5]
- Provide ultrasonic nebulizer or room humidifier, as needed, *to deliver supplemental humidification, helping to reduce viscosity of secretions.*
- Assist with use of respiratory devices and treatments (e.g., intermittent positive-pressure breathing [IPPB], incentive spirometer [IS], positive expiratory pressure mask, mechanical ventilation, airway clearance vest/oscillatory airway device [flutter], assisted and directed cough techniques). *Various therapies/modalities may be required to maintain adequate airways and improve respiratory function and gas exchange depending on the cause for airway impairment. For example, an evidence-based review supports the notion that in cervical spinal cord individuals, cough can be made more effective by using manual assistance or positive-pressure insufflation devices. However, in clients with COPD, these same devices can be detrimental, causing decreased peak expiratory flow.* (Refer to NDs ineffective Breathing Pattern, impaired Gas Exchange, impaired spontaneous Ventilation.)[3,12]
- Perform or assist client in learning airway clearance techniques, particularly when airway congestion is a chronic or long-term condition. *Numerous techniques may be used, including (but not limited to) postural*

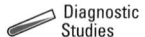

drainage and percussion, flutter devices, high-frequency chest compression with an inflatable vest, intrapulmonary percussive ventilation administered by a percussinator, and active cycle breathing, as indicated. Many of these techniques are the result of research in treatments of cystic fibrosis and muscular dystrophy as well as other chronic lung diseases. NOTE: Studies show that while these modalities yield short-term improvements in airway clearance, more studies are needed to measure long-term and clinically important endpoints like quality of life or rates of exacerbations.[1,12]

NURSING PRIORITY NO. 3 To assess changes, note complications:

- Auscultate breath sounds, noting changes in air movement *to ascertain current status and effects of treatments to clear airways.*
- Monitor vital signs, noting blood pressure or pulse changes. Observe for increased respiratory rate, restlessness or anxiety, and use of accessory muscles for breathing, *suggesting advancing respiratory distress.*
- Monitor and document serial chest radiographs, ABGs, pulse oximetry readings. *Identifies baseline status, influences interventions, and monitors progress of condition and/or treatment response.*
- Evaluate changes in sleep pattern, noting insomnia or daytime somnolence. *May be evidence of nighttime airway incompetence or sleep apnea.* (Refer to NDs Insomnia, Sleep Deprivation)
- Document response to drug therapy and/or development of adverse reactions or side effects with antimicrobial agents, steroids, expectorants, and bronchodilators. *Pharmacological therapy is used to prevent and control symptoms, reduce severity of exacerbations, and improve health status. The choice of medications depends on availability of the medication, the client's decision making about medication regimen, and response to any given medication.*[10]
- Observe for signs/symptoms of infection (e.g., increased dyspnea, onset of fever, increase in sputum volume, change in color or character) *to identify infectious process and promote timely intervention.*[10]
- Obtain sputum specimen, preferably before antimicrobial therapy is initiated, *to verify appropriateness of therapy. Note: The presence of purulent sputum during an exacerbation of symptoms is a sufficient indication for starting antibiotic therapy, but a sputum culture and antibiogram (antibiotic sensitivity) may be done if the illness is not responding to the initial antibiotic.*[10]

NURSING PRIORITY NO. 4 To promote wellness (Teaching/Discharge Considerations):

- Assess client's/caregiver's knowledge of contributing causes, treatment plan, specific medications, and therapeutic procedures *to determine educational needs.*
- Provide information about the necessity of raising and expectorating secretions versus swallowing them *to note changes in color and amount in the event that medical intervention may be needed to prevent or treat infection.*
- Identify signs/symptoms to be reported to primary care provider. *Prompt evaluation and intervention are required to prevent/treat infection.*
- Demonstrate or assist client/significant other (SO) in performing specific airway clearance techniques (e.g., forced expiratory breathing [also called "huffing"] or respiratory muscle strength training, use of vest, chest percussion), if indicated.[11]
- Review breathing exercises, effective coughing techniques, and use of adjunct devices (e.g., IPPB or IS) in preoperative teaching *to facilitate postoperative recovery and reduce risk of pneumonia.*
- Instruct client/SO/caregiver in use of inhalers and other respiratory drugs. Include expected effects and information regarding possible side effects and interactions of respiratory drugs with other medications, over-the-counter medications, and herbals. Discuss symptoms requiring medical follow-up. *Client is often taking multiple medications that have similar side effects and potential for interactions. It is important to understand the difference between nuisance side effects (e.g., fast heartbeat after albuterol inhaler) and adverse effects (e.g., chest pain, hallucinations, or uncontrolled cardiac arrhythmia).*[9]
- Encourage and provide opportunities for rest; limit activities to level of respiratory tolerance. *Prevents or diminishes fatigue associated with underlying condition or efforts to clear airways.*
- Urge reduction or cessation of smoking. *Smoking is known to increase production of mucus and to paralyze (or cause loss of) cilia needed to move secretions to clear airway and improve lung function.*[10]

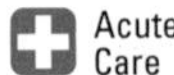

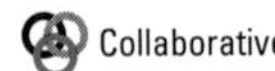

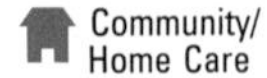

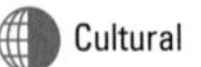

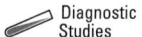

- Refer to appropriate support groups (e.g., smoking-cessation clinic, COPD exercise group, weight reduction, American Lung Association, Cystic Fibrosis Foundation, Muscular Dystrophy Association).
- Instruct in use of nocturnal positive pressure airflow for treatment of sleep apnea. (Refer to NDs Insomnia, Sleep Deprivation.)

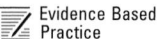

DOCUMENTATION FOCUS

Assessment/Reassessment

- Related factors for individual client.
- Breath sounds, presence and character of secretions, use of accessory muscles for breathing.
- Character of cough and sputum.

Planning

- Plan of care and who is involved in planning.
- Teaching plan.

Implementation/Evaluation

- Client's response to interventions, teaching, and actions performed.
- Attainment or progress toward desired outcome(s).
- Modifications to plan of care.

Discharge Planning

- Long-term needs and who is responsible for actions to be taken.
- Specific referrals made.

References

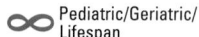

1. Clinical policy bulletin: Chest physiotherapy and airway clearance devices. (1995, updated 2010). *Aetna's Clinical Policy Bulletin.* Retrieved January 2011 from http://www.aetna.com/cpb/medical/data/1_99/0067.html.
2. Prahlow, J. A., Prahlow, T. J., Rakow, R. J. (2009). Case study: Asphyxia caused by inspissated oral and nasopharyngeal secretions. *Am J Nurs,* 109(6), 38–43.
3. McCool, F. D., Rosen, M. J. (2006). Nonpharmacologic airway clearance therapies: ACCP evidence-based clinical practice guidelines. *Chest,* 129 (Supp), 250S–259S.
4. Cox, H. C., et al. (2002). *Clinical Applications of Nursing Diagnosis: Adult, Child, Psychiatric, Gerontic, and Home Health Considerations.* 4th ed. Philadelphia, PA: F. A. Davis, 244–249.
5. Fink, J. B., Hunt, G. E. (eds). (1999). *Clinical Practice in Respiratory Care.* Baltimore, MD: Lippincott, Williams & Wilkins.
6. Blair, K. A. (1999). The aging pulmonary system. In Stanley, M., Beare, P. G. (eds). *Gerontological Nursing.* 2nd ed. Philadelphia, PA: F. A. Davis.
7. American Association for Respiratory Care. (1996). Suctioning of the patient in the home. Clinical practice guidelines. *Respir Care,* 44(1), 99–104.
8. Deglin, J. H., Vallerand, A. H., Sanoski, C. A. (2011). Bronchodilators: Pharmacologic Profile G56. *Davis's Drug Guide for Nurses.* 12th ed. Philadelphia, PA: F. A. Davis.
9. Yngsdal-Krenz, R. (Spring 1999). Airway clearance techniques. Center Focus, newsletter of the University of Wisconsin, Madison.
10. Global strategy for the diagnosis, management, and prevention of chronic obstructive pulmonary disease. Global Initiative for Chronic Obstructive Lung Disease, revised 2011. Retrieved October 2015 from http://www.goldcopd.org/uploads/users/files/GOLD_Report_2011_Feb21.pdf.
11. AHRQ Evidence Report Summaries. Treatment of disease following spinal cord injury: Summary. (2001). Retrieved October 2015 from http://www.ncbi.nlm.nih.gov/books/NBK11884/.
12. Samsa, G. P., Govert, J., Matchar, D. B., et al. (2002). Use of data from randomized trial designs in evidence reports: An application to treatment of pulmonary disease following spinal cord injury. *J Rehabil Res Dev,* 39, 41–52.

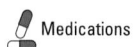

risk for Allergy Response

Taxonomy II: Safety/Protection—Class 5 Defensive Processes (00217) [**Diagnostic Division:** Safety], Submitted 1988; revised 2013

DEFINITION: Vulnerable to an exaggerated immune response or reaction to substances, which may compromise health.

RISK FACTORS

Allergy to insect sting
Exposure to allergen (e.g., pharmaceutical agent)
Exposure to environmental allergen (e.g., dander, dust, mold, pollen)
Exposure to toxic chemical
Food allergy (e.g., avocado, banana, shellfish, mushroom, tropical fruit)
Repeated exposure to allergen-producing environmental substance
Sample Clinical Applications: Asthma, conjunctivitis; eczema and other allergic skin rashes; food allergies and intolerances; hay fever; hives; insect stings

DESIRED OUTCOMES/EVALUATION CRITERIA

Sample NOC linkages:
Allergic Response: Localized: Severity of localized hypersensitive immune response to a specific environmental (exogenous) antigen
Allergic Response: Systemic: Severity of systemic hypersensitive immune response to a specific environmental (exogenous) antigen
Risk Control: Personal actions to prevent, eliminate, or reduce modifiable health threats

Client Will (Include Specific Time Frame)
- Be free of signs of hypersensitive response
- Verbalize understanding of individual risks and responsibilities in avoiding exposure
- Identify signs/symptoms requiring prompt response

ACTIONS/INTERVENTIONS

Sample NIC linkages:
Allergy Management: Identification, treatment, and prevention of allergic responses to food, medications, insect bites, contrast material, blood, and other substances

NURSING PRIORITY NO. 1 To identify causative/precipitating factors related to risk:

- Question client regarding known allergies upon admission to healthcare facility. *Basic safety information to help healthcare providers prevent/prepare for safe environment for client while providing care.*
- Ascertain type of allergy and usual symptoms if client reports history of allergies (e.g., seasonal rhinitis ["hay-fever"], allergic dermatitis, conjunctivitis, environmental asthma, environmental substances [e.g., mold, dust, pet dander], insect sting reactions, food intolerance, immunodeficiency such as Addison's disease, drug or transfusion reaction. *Allergies can manifest as local reactions (as may occur in skin rashes) or be systemic. Responses are many and variable. Client/caregiver may be aware of some allergies, but not all of them. It is also possible that client is having a first time allergic reaction to a substance and not know what substance caused the reaction.*[5]

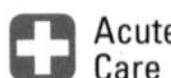

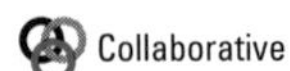

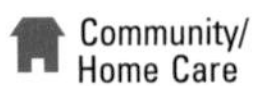

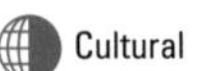

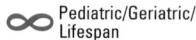

- Obtain written list of drug allergies upon first contact with client. *Helps prevent adverse drug events (ADEs) while client in facility care and aids in differentiating side effects from allergic responses. May also help improve client's understanding of reportable symptoms.*[1]
- Discuss possibility of latex allergy when entering facility care, especially when procedures are anticipated (e.g., laboratory, emergency department, operating room, wound care management, one-day surgery, dental) *so that proper precautions can be taken by healthcare providers. Note: The most severe reactions tend to occur with latex proteins contacting internal tissues during invasive procedures and when they touch mucous membranes of the mouth, vagina, urethra, or rectum.*[2] (Refer to ND Latex Allergy Response for related interventions.)
- Note client's age. *Although allergies can occur at any time in client's lifespan, there are some that can start early in life. These include food allergies (e.g., peanuts) and respiratory ailments (e.g., asthma). Note: In 2013 8.3% of children in the United States currently had asthma.*[3]
- Perform challenge or patch test, if appropriate, *to identify specific allergens in client with known type IV hypersensitivity. Note: Emergency department diagnosis and management depend on the history and physical examination.*
- Note response to radioallergosorbent test (RAST) or enzyme-linked latex-specific IgE (ELISA), where available. *Performed to measure the quantity of IgE antibodies in serum after exposure to specific antigens and has generally replaced skin tests and provocation tests, which are inconvenient, often painful, and/or hazardous to the client. Note: These tests are useful in nonemergent evaluations.*[34]

NURSING PRIORITY NO. 2 To take measures to avoid exposure and reduce/limit allergic response:

- Discuss client's current symptoms, noting reports of rash, hives, itching; teary eyes, localized swelling (e.g., of lips) or diarrhea, nausea, and feeling of faintness. Try to ascertain if client/care provider associates these symptoms with certain food, substances, or environmental factors. *May help isolate cause for a reaction. Baseline for determining where the client is along a continuum of symptoms so that appropriate treatments can be initiated.*[4]
- Provide allergen-free environment (e.g., clean, dust-free room, use of air filters to reduce mold and pollens in air, etc.) *to reduce client exposure to allergens.*
- Collaborate with all healthcare providers to administer medications and perform procedures with client's allergies in mind. Perform challenge or patch test, if appropriate.
- Encourage client to wear medical ID bracelet/necklace *to alert providers to condition if client is unresponsive or unable to relay information for any reason.*
- Refer to physician/allergy specialists as indicated *for interventions related to specific allergy conditions.*

NURSING PRIORITY NO. 3 To promote wellness (Teaching/Discharge Criteria):

- Instruct in/review with client and care provider(s) ways to prevent or limit client exposures. *May need or desire information regarding ways to reduce allergens at home, school, or work; may desire information regarding potential exposures when traveling, or how to manage food allergies when eating in restaurants.*[5]
- Instruct in signs of reaction and emergency treatment needs. *Allergic reactions range from skin irritation to anaphylaxis. Reaction may be gradual but progressive, affecting multiple body systems, or may be sudden, requiring lifesaving treatment. Allergy can result in chronic illness, disability, career loss, hardship, and death.*
- Emphasize the critical importance of taking immediate action for moderate to severe hypersensitivity reactions *to limit life-threatening symptoms.*
- Demonstrate equipment and injection procedure, and recommend client carry auto-injectable epinephrine *to provide timely emergency treatment, as needed.*
- Emphasize necessity of informing all new care providers of allergies *to reduce preventable exposures.*
- Provide audiovisual resources and assistance numbers for emergencies. *When allergy is suspected or the potential for allergy exists, protection must begin with identification and removal of possible sources.*

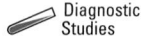

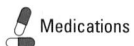

DOCUMENTATION FOCUS

Assessment/Reassessment

- Individual risk factors identified.
- Client concerns or difficulty making and following through with plan.

Planning

- Plan of care and who is involved in planning.
- Teaching plan.

Implementation/Evaluation

- Response to interventions, teaching, and actions performed.
- Attainment or progress toward outcomes.

Discharge Planning

- Referrals to other resources.
- Long-term need and who is responsible for actions.

References

1. Vallente, S., Murray, L. P. (2011). Creative strategies to improve patient safety: Allergies and adverse drug reactions. *J Nurses Staff Dev*, 27(1), E1–E5.
2. Mecurio, J. (2011). Creating a latex-safe perioperative environment. *OR Nurse*, 5(6), 18–25.
3. Centers for Disease Control and Prevention (CDC). (2013). Asthma Surveillance. Retrieved March 2015 http://www.cdc.gov/asthma/asthmadata.htm.
4. No author listed. (update 2014). Article for Lab Tests Online. Various pages. Retrieved March 2015 from http://labtestsonline.org/understanding/analytes/allergy/tab/test.
5. Asthma and Allergy Foundation of America. (No date). Allergy overview: Various pages. Retrieved March 2015 from http://www.asthmapact.org/.

Anxiety [specify level: mild, moderate, severe, panic]

Taxonomy II: Coping/Stress Tolerance—Class 2 Coping Responses (00146) [**Diagnostic Division:** Ego Integrity], Submitted 1973; Revised 1982, 1998

DEFINITION: Vague uneasy feeling of discomfort or dread accompanied by an autonomic response (the source is often nonspecific or unknown to the individual); a feeling of apprehension caused by anticipation of danger. It is an alerting sign that warns of impending danger and enables the individual to take measures to deal with that threat.

RELATED FACTORS

Conflict about life goals; value conflict
Situational or maturational crisis
Stressors
Family history of anxiety; heredity
Interpersonal transmission or contagion
Threat to current status
Threat of death [perceived or actual]
Major change (e.g., health status; role function or status; environment; economic status)
Unmet needs
Exposure to toxins
Substance abuse

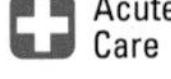

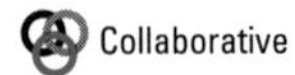

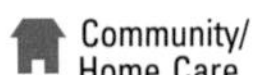

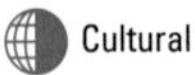

DEFINING CHARACTERISTICS

Subjective

Behavioral: Worried about change in life event; insomnia
Affective: Regretful; rattled; distress; apprehensiveness; uncertain; fear; feeling of inadequacy; worried; helplessness
Cognitive: Fear; awareness of physiological symptoms
Physiological: Shakiness
Sympathetic: Dry mouth; heart palpitations; weakness; anorexia; diarrhea
Parasympathetic: Tingling in extremities; nausea; abdominal pain; diarrhea; urinary frequency, hesitancy, urgency; faintness; fatigue; alteration in sleep pattern

Objective

Behavioral: Poor eye contact; glancing about; scanning behavior; hypervigilance; extraneous movement; fidgeting; restlessness; decrease in productivity
Affective: Increase in wariness; self-focus; irritability; jitteriness; overexcitement; anguish
Cognitive: Preoccupation; alteration in attention, concentration; forgetfulness; diminished ability to learn or problem solve; rumination; tendency to blame others; blocking of thoughts; confusion; decrease in perceptual field
Physiological: Voice quivering; trembling; hand tremors; increase in tension; facial tension; increase in perspiration
Sympathetic: Cardiovascular excitation; facial flushing; superficial vasoconstriction; increase in heart or respiratory rate; increase in blood pressure; alteration in respiratory pattern; pupil dilation; twitching; brisk reflexes
Parasympathetic: Decrease in blood pressure or heart rate
Sample Clinical Applications: Major life changes or events, hospital admissions, surgery, cancer, hyperthyroidism, drug intoxication or abuse, mental health disorders

DESIRED OUTCOMES/EVALUATION CRITERIA

Sample NOC linkages:

Anxiety Level: Severity of manifested apprehension, tension, or uneasiness arising from an unidentifiable source
Anxiety Self-Control: Personal actions to eliminate or reduce feelings of apprehension, tension, or uneasiness from an unidentifiable source
Coping: Personal actions to manage stressors that tax an individual's resources

Client Will (Include Specific Time Frame)

- Verbalize awareness of feelings of anxiety.
- Appear relaxed and report anxiety is reduced to a manageable level.
- Identify healthy ways to deal with and express anxiety.
- Demonstrate problem-solving skills.
- Use resources and support systems effectively.

ACTIONS/INTERVENTIONS

Sample NIC linkages:

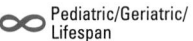

Anxiety Reduction: Minimizing apprehension, dread, foreboding, or uneasiness related to an unidentified source or anticipated danger
Calming Technique: Reducing anxiety in patient experiencing acute distress
Dementia Management: Provision of a modified environment for the patient who is experiencing a chronic confusional state

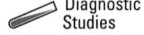

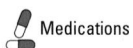

NURSING PRIORITY NO. 1 To assess level of anxiety:

- Review familial and physiological factors, such as genetic depressive factors and psychiatric illness, active medical conditions (e.g., thyroid problems, metabolic imbalances, cardiopulmonary disease, anemia, dysrhythmias), and recent or ongoing stressors (e.g., family member illness or death, spousal conflict or abuse, loss of job). *These factors can cause or exacerbate anxiety and anxiety disorders.*[6,12,13]
- Determine current prescribed medication regimen and recent drug history of prescribed or over-the-counter (OTC) medications (e.g., steroids, thyroid preparations, weight-loss pills, caffeine). *Can heighten feelings or sense of anxiety.*[12,13]
- Identify client's perception of the threat represented by the situation. *Distorted perceptions of the situation may magnify feelings. Understanding client's point of view promotes a more accurate plan of care.*[1]
- Note cultural factors that may influence anxiety. *Individual responses are influenced by the cultural values and beliefs and culturally learned patterns of family of origin.*[3]
- Monitor physical responses (e.g., palpitations, rapid pulse, repetitive movements, pacing). *Changes in vital signs may suggest degree of anxiety client is experiencing or reflect the impact of physiological factors such as endocrine imbalances and medication effect.*[6]
- Observe behavior indicative of anxiety, *which can be a clue to the client's level of anxiety:*

  Mild

  Alert, more aware of environment, attention focused on environment and immediate events.
  Restless, irritable, wakeful, reports of insomnia.
  Motivated to deal with existing problems in this state.

  Moderate

  Perception narrower, concentration increased, able to ignore distractions in dealing with problem(s).
  Voice quivers or changes pitch.
  Trembling, increased pulse or respirations.

  Severe

  Range of perception is reduced, anxiety interferes with effective functioning.
  Preoccupied with feelings of discomfort or sense of impending doom.
  Increased pulse or respirations with reports of dizziness, tingling sensations, headache, etc.

  Panic

  Ability to concentrate is disrupted, behavior is disintegrated, client distorts the situation and does not have realistic perceptions of what is happening.
  May be experiencing terror or confusion or be unable to speak or move (paralyzed with fear).
- Note own feelings of anxiety or uneasiness. *Feelings of anxiety are circular, and those in contact with the client may find themselves feeling more anxious.*[2]
- Note use of drugs (including alcohol and other drugs), insomnia or excessive sleeping, and limited or avoidance of interactions with others, *which may be behavioral indicators of use of drugs to deal with problems or may indicate withdrawal from drugs or substances.*[4]
- Review results of diagnostic tests (e.g., drug screens, cardiac testing, complete blood count, chemistry panel), *which can point to physiological sources of anxiety.*
- Review coping skills used in past. *Can determine those that might be helpful in current circumstances.*[5]

NURSING PRIORITY NO. 2 To assist client to identify feelings and begin to deal with problems:

- Establish a therapeutic relationship, conveying empathy and unconditional positive regard. *Enables client to become comfortable and to begin looking at feelings and dealing with situation.*[2]
- Be available to client for listening and talking. *Establishes rapport, promotes expression of feelings, and helps client/significant other look at realities of the illness or treatment without confronting issues they are not ready to deal with.*[2]

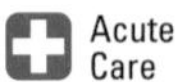
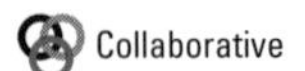
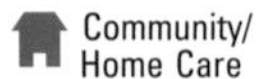
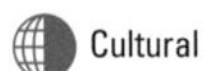

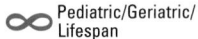

- Encourage client to acknowledge and to express feelings—for example, crying (sadness), laughing (fear, denial), or swearing (fear, anger)—using active-listening, reflection techniques. *Often, acknowledging feelings enables client to accept and deal more appropriately with situation, thus relieving anxiety.*[7]
- Assist client to develop self-awareness of verbal and nonverbal behaviors. *Becoming aware helps client to control these behaviors and begin to deal with issues that are causing anxiety.*[8]
- Clarify meaning of feelings or actions by providing feedback and checking meaning with the client. *Validates meaning and ensures accuracy of communication.*[9]
- Acknowledge anxiety or fear. Do not deny or reassure client that everything will be all right. *Validates reality of feelings. False reassurances may be interpreted as lack of understanding or dishonesty, further isolating client.*[2]
- Be aware of defense mechanisms being used (e.g., denial, regression). *Use of defense mechanisms may be a helpful coping mechanism initially. However, continued use of such mechanisms diverts the energy that the client needs for healing, thus delaying the client from focusing and dealing with the actual problem.*[5]
- Identify coping skills the individual is using currently, such as anger, daydreaming, forgetfulness, eating, smoking, or lack of problem solving. *These may be useful for the moment but may eventually interfere with resolution of current situation.*[5]
- Provide accurate information about the situation. *Helps client to identify what is reality based and provides opportunity for client to feel reassured.*[10]
- ∞ Respond truthfully, avoid bribing, and provide physical contact (e.g., hugging, rocking) when client is a child. *Soothes fears and provides assurance. Children need to recognize that their feelings are not different from others'.*[4]

NURSING PRIORITY NO. 3 To provide measures to comfort and aid client to handle problematic situations:

- Provide comfort measures (e.g., calm or quiet environment, soft music, warm bath, back rub, Therapeutic Touch). *Aids in meeting basic human need, decreasing sense of isolation, and assisting client to feel less anxious. Therapeutic Touch requires the nurse to have specific knowledge and experience to use the hands to correct energy field disturbances by redirecting human energies to help or heal.*[2,10]
- ∞ Modify procedures as necessary (e.g., substitute oral for intramuscular medications, combine blood draws or use fingerstick method). *Limits degree of stress and avoids overwhelming child or anxious adult.*[1]
- ∞ Manage environmental factors, such as harsh lighting, high traffic flow, excessive noise. *May be confusing or stressful to older individuals. Managing these factors can lessen anxiety, especially when client is in strange and unusual circumstances.*[1]
- Discuss the use of music and accommodate client's preferences. *Promotes calming atmosphere, helping to alleviate anxiety.*[2]
- Accept client as is. *The client may need to be where he or she is at this point in time, such as in denial after receiving the diagnosis of a terminal illness.*[2]
- Allow the behavior to belong to the client; do not respond personally. *Reacting personally can escalate the situation, promoting a nontherapeutic situation and increasing anxiety.*
- Assist client to use anxiety for coping with the situation if helpful. *Moderate anxiety heightens awareness and can help client to focus on dealing with problems.*[8]
- Encourage awareness of negative self-talk and discuss replacing with positive statements, such as using "can" instead of "can't," etc. *Negative self-talk promotes feelings of anxiety and self-doubt. Becoming aware and replacing these thoughts can enhance sense of self-worth and reduce anxiety.*[8]

PANIC STATE

- Stay with client, maintaining a calm, confident manner. *Presence communicates caring and helps client to regain control and sense of calm.*
- Speak in brief statements using simple words. *Client is not able to comprehend complex information at this time.*

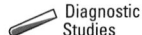

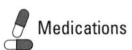

- Provide for nonthreatening, consistent environment or atmosphere. Minimize stimuli and monitor visitors and interactions with others. *Lessens effect of transmission of anxious feelings.*
- Set limits on inappropriate behavior and help client to develop acceptable ways of dealing with anxiety.
- Provide safe controls and environment until client regains control. *Behavior may result in damage or injury that client will regret when control is regained, diminishing sense of self-worth.*
- Gradually increase activities and involvement with others as anxiety is decreased. *Promotes sense of normalcy, helps control feelings of anxiety.*
- Use cognitive therapy to focus on and correct faulty catastrophic interpretations of physical symptoms. *For example, thoughts of dying increase anxiety and feelings of panic. Controlling these thoughts allows client to look at situation more realistically and begin to deal appropriately with what is happening.*
- Administer anti-anxiety agents or sedatives, as ordered. *Appropriate medication can be helpful in enabling the client to regain control.*

NURSING PRIORITY NO. 4 To promote wellness (Teaching/Discharge Considerations):

- Assist client to identify and deal with precipitating factors and learn new methods of coping with disabling anxiety. *Lessens possibility of repeat episodes.*[8]
- Review happenings, thoughts, and feelings preceding the anxiety attack. *Identifies factors that led to onset of attack, promoting opportunity to prevent recurrences.*[1]
- Identify actions and activities the client has previously used to cope successfully when feeling nervous or anxious. *Realizing that individual already has coping skills that can be applied in current and future situations can empower client.*[1]
- List helpful resources and people, including available hotline or crisis managers. *Provides ongoing and timely support.*[1]
- Encourage client to develop a regular exercise or activity program. *May be helpful in reducing level of anxiety by relieving tension and has been shown to raise endorphin levels to enhance sense of well-being.*[1]
- Assist in developing skills (e.g., awareness of negative thoughts, saying "Stop" and substituting a positive thought). *Eliminating negative self-talk can lead to feelings of positive self-esteem. (Note: Mild phobias seem to respond better to behavioral therapy.)*[9]
- Review such strategies as role-playing, use of visualizations to practice anticipated events, and prayer or meditation. *These activities can help the client practice behaviors in a safe and supportive environment, enabling individual to manage anxiety-provoking situations.*[9]
- Review medication regimen and possible interactions, especially with OTC drugs, alcohol, and herbal products. *Enhances understanding of reason for medication and can avoid untoward or harmful reactions from incompatible drugs.*[11]
- Discuss appropriate drug substitutions or changes in dosage or time of dose. *Ensures proper dosage and avoids untoward side effects. This is especially important in the elderly, who are particularly susceptible to multidrug complications.*[11]
- Refer to physician for drug management program or alteration of prescription regimen. *Drugs that often cause symptoms of anxiety include aminophylline, anticholinergics, dopamine, levodopa, salicylates, and steroids. Monitoring provides opportunity to correct possible undesirable effects of these drugs.*[11]
- Refer to individual and/or group therapy, as appropriate. *May be useful to help client deal with chronic anxiety states.*[1]

DOCUMENTATION FOCUS

Assessment/Reassessment

- Level of anxiety and precipitating or aggravating factors.
- Description of feelings (expressed and displayed).
- Awareness or ability to recognize and express feelings.
- Related substance use, if present.

Planning
- Treatment plan and individual responsibility for specific activities.
- Teaching plan.

Implementation/Evaluation
- Client involvement and response to interventions, teaching, and actions performed.
- Attainment or progress toward desired outcome(s).
- Modifications to plan of care.

Discharge Planning
- Referrals and follow-up plan.
- Specific referrals made.

References

1. Andrews, G., Creamer, M., Crino, R., et al. (2002). *The Treatment of Anxiety Disorders: Clinician Guides and Patient Manuals*. 2nd ed. Cambridge, UK: Cambridge University Press.
2. Brantley, P. J., Mehan, D. J., Ames, S. C., et al. (1999). Minor stressors and generalized anxiety disorder among low-income patients attending primary care clinics. *J Nerv Ment Dis*, 87, 435–440.
3. Lipson, J. G., Dibble, S. L., Minarik, P. A. (1996). *Culture & Nursing Care: A Pocket Guide. School of Nursing*. San Francisco, CA: UCSF Nursing Press.
4. National Institute of Mental Health. (2005). *Anxiety Disorders*. Retrieved January 2012 from http://www.nimh.nih.gov/health/publications/anxiety-disorders/complete-index.shtml.
5. Wittchen, H. U., Hoyer, J. (2001). Generalized anxiety disorder: Nature and course. *J Clin Psychiatry*, 62(supplement 11), S15–S19.
6. Kunert, P. K. (2002). Stress and adaptation. In Porth, C. M. (ed). *Pathophysiology: Concepts of Altered Health States*. Philadelphia, PA: Lippincott.
7. Moller, M. D., Murphy, M. F. (1998). *Recovering from Psychosis: A Wellness Approach*. Nine Mile Falls, WA: Psychiatric Rehabilitation Nurses Inc.
8. Bohrer, G. J. (2002). Anxiety, emotional and physical discomfort. *NurseWeek*, 3(1), 21–22. (Mountain West edition).
9. Burns, D. D. (1999). *Feeling Good: The New Mood Therapy*. New York: Avon.
10. Hutchison, C. P. (1999). Healing touch: An energetic approach. *Am J Nurs*, 99(4), 43–48.
11. Hayes, P. E., Dommisse, C. S. (1987). Current concepts in clinical therapeutics: Anxiety disorders, part 1. *Clin Pharm*, 6(21), 140–147.
12. Murphy, K. (2005). Anxiety: When is it too much? *Nursing Made Incredibly Easy!*, 3(5), 22–31.
13. Yeats, W. R., Bernstein, B. E., Bessman, E., et al. (updated 2012). *Anxiety Disorders*. Retrieved January 2012 from http://emedicine.medscape.com/article/286227-overview.

risk for Aspiration

Taxonomy II: Safety/Protection—Class 2 Physical Injury (00039) [**Diagnostic Division:** Respiration], Submitted 1988; Revised 2013

DEFINITION: Vulnerable to entry of gastrointestinal secretions, oropharyngeal secretions, solids or fluids into the tracheobronchial passages, which may compromise health.

RISK FACTORS

Barrier to elevating upper body; facial surgery or trauma; neck surgery or trauma; oral surgery or trauma; wired jaw

Decrease in gastrointestinal motility; delayed gastric emptying; incompetent lower esophageal sphincter; increase in gastric residual; increase in intragastric pressure

Decrease in level of consciousness; depressed gag reflex; impaired ability to swallow; ineffective cough

(continues on page 62)

risk for Aspiration (continued)
Presence or oral/nasal tube (e.g., tracheal, feeding); enteral feedings
Treatment regimen
NOTE: A risk diagnosis is not evidenced by signs and symptoms, as the problem has not occurred; rather, nursing interventions are directed at prevention.
Sample Clinical Applications: Facial, jaw, neck surgery; vomiting, bulimia nervosa, presence of nasogastric tube, enteral feedings; brain injury, spinal cord injury

DESIRED OUTCOMES/EVALUATION CRITERIA

Sample NOC linkages:
Aspiration Prevention: Personal actions to prevent the passage of fluid and solid particles into the lungs
Neurological Status: Ability of the peripheral and central nervous system to receive, process, and respond to internal and external stimuli
Respiratory Status: Airway Patency: Open, clear tracheobronchial passages for air exchange

Client/Caregiver Will (Include Specific Time Frame)
- Experience no aspiration as evidenced by noiseless respirations; clear breath sounds; clear, odorless secretions.
- Identify causative or risk factors.
- Demonstrate techniques to prevent and/or correct aspiration.

ACTIONS/INTERVENTIONS

Sample NIC linkages:
Aspiration Precautions: Prevention or minimization of risk factors in the patient at risk for aspiration
Artificial Airway Management: Maintenance of endotracheal and tracheostomy tubes and prevention of complications associated with their use
Postanesthesia Care: Monitoring and management of the patient who has recently undergone general or regional anesthesia

NURSING PRIORITY NO. 1 To assess causative/contributing factors:

- Identify at-risk client according to condition/disease process as listed in Risk Factors *to determine when more active observation and/or interventions may be required.*
- ∞ Assess for age-related risk factors potentiating risk of aspiration (e.g., premature infant, elderly infirm). *Aspiration pneumonia is more common in extremely young or old individuals, and it commonly occurs in those with chronically impaired airway defense mechanisms, including gag reflex, coughing, ciliary movement, and immune mechanisms that aid in removing material from the lower airways.*[4,13]
- Note level of consciousness or awareness of surroundings and cognitive impairment. *Aspiration is common in comatose clients owing to inability to cough or swallow adequately and/or presence of artificial airway, mechanical ventilation, and tube feedings.*[1,13]
- Evaluate neuromuscular dysfunction, if present, noting muscle groups involved, degree of impairment, and whether acute or of a progressive nature (e.g., stroke, cerebral palsy, Parkinson's disease, progressive supranuclear palsy, similar disabling brain diseases; Guillain-Barré syndrome, amyotrophic lateral sclerosis, psychiatric client following electric shock therapy). *May result in temporary or chronic, progressive impairment of protective muscle functions.*[7,11]
- Assess client's ability to swallow and cough; note quality of voice. *Although aspiration during swallowing is best detected by procedures such as video fluoroscopy, clinical observations are important. Sudden respiratory symptoms (such as severe coughing and cyanosis or wet phlegmy voice quality) are indicative of potential aspiration. Also individuals with impaired or absent cough reflexes (such as may occur after a stroke, in Parkinson's disease, or during sedation) are at high risk for "silent" aspiration.*[4,9]

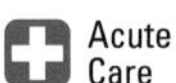
Acute Care
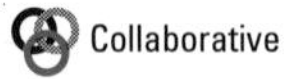
Collaborative
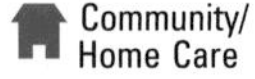
Community/ Home Care
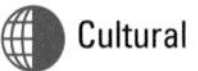
Cultural

- Observe for neck and facial edema; e.g., client with head or neck surgery or a tracheal or bronchial injury (upper torso burns, inhalation or chemical injury). *Problems with swallowing and maintenance of airways can be expected in this client, and the potential is high for aspiration and aspiration pneumonia.*
- Assess amount and consistency of respiratory secretions and rate and depth of respirations. *Helps differentiate the potential cause for risk of aspiration. The major pathophysiological dysfunction is the inability of the epiglottis and true vocal cords to move to close the trachea (e.g., changes in the structures themselves or because messages to the brain are absent, decreased, or impaired). Problems with coughing (clearing airways) and swallowing (pooling of saliva, liquids) increase risk of aspiration and respiratory complications.*[2–4]
- Auscultate lung sounds periodically (especially in client who is coughing frequently or not coughing at all; client with artificial airways, endotracheal and tracheostomy tubes; ventilator client being tube-fed, immediately following extubation), and observe chest radiographs *to determine decreased breath sounds, rales, or dullness to percussion that could indicate presence of aspirated food or secretions and "silent aspiration" leading to aspiration pneumonia. Note: Aspiration is the most common route of entry for both community- and hospital-acquired pneumonia.*[5]
- Evaluate for/note presence of gastrointenstinal (GI) pathology and motility disorders. *Nausea with vomiting (associated with metabolic disorders, following surgery, or with certain medications) and gastroesophageal reflux disease can cause inhalation of gastric contents.*[3,6]
- Note administration of enteral feedings, which may be initiated when oral nutrition is not possible, such as in head injury, stroke, or other neurological disorders, head and neck surgery, esophageal obstruction, and discontinuous GI tract. *Potential exists for regurgitation and aspiration with the use of small or larger bore nasogastric feeding tubes, even with proper tube placement, necessitating the need for clients at high risk for aspiration associated with nasogastroenteral feedings to be evaluated for enteral feedings into the jejunum.*[7]
- Ascertain lifestyle habits (e.g., chronic use of alcohol and drugs, alcohol intoxication, tobacco, other central nervous system–suppressant drugs). *Can affect awareness as well as impair gag and swallow mechanisms.*[5]
- Assist with and review diagnostic studies (e.g., video-fluoroscopy, fiber-optic endoscopy) *that may be done to assess for presence and degree of impairment. Note: One recent retrospective study of 2,000 clients evaluated by video-fluoroscopy revealed that of those who aspirated, 55% had no protective cough reflex (silent aspiration).*[9,11]

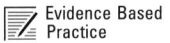

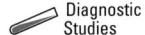

NURSING PRIORITY NO. 2 To assist in correcting factors that can lead to aspiration:

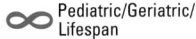

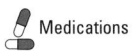

- Place client in proper position for age and condition or disease affecting airways. *Adult and child should be upright for meals to decrease likelihood of drainage into trachea and to reduce reflux and improve gastric emptying.*[2,4] *Prone position may provide shorter gastric emptying time and decreased incidence of regurgitation and subsequent aspiration in premature infants.*[8]
- Encourage client to cough, as able, to clear secretions. *May simply need to be reminded or encouraged to cough (such as might occur in elderly person with delayed gag reflex or in postoperative, sedated client).*[2]
- Provide close monitoring for use of oxygen masks in clients at risk for vomiting. Refrain from using oxygen mask for comatose individuals.
- Keep wire cutters or scissors with client at all times when jaws are wired or banded *to facilitate clearing airway in emergencies.*
- Assist with oral care, postural drainage, and other respiratory therapies *to remove or mobilize thickened secretions that may interfere with swallowing and block airway.*[6]
- In client requiring suctioning to manage secretions:[6,9,10,]
  Maintain operational suction equipment at bedside or chairside.
  Suction (oral cavity, nose, and endotracheal/tracheostomy tube) as needed, using correct size of catheter and timing for adult or child *to clear secretions in client with more frequent or congested-sounding cough; presence of coarse rhonchi and expiratory wheezing (audible with or without auscultation); visible secretions; increased peak pressures during volume-cycled ventilation; indication from client that suctioning is necessary; suspected aspiration of gastric or upper airway secretions; or otherwise unexplained increases in shortness of breath, respiratory rate, or heart rate.*

Avoid triggering gag mechanism when performing suction or mouth care.

Avoid keeping client supine or flat when on mechanical ventilation (especially when also receiving enteral feedings). *Supine positioning and enteral feeding have been shown to be independent risk factors for the development of aspiration pneumonia.*

- For a verified swallowing problem:[3–5,11]

Provide a rest period prior to feeding time. *Rested person may have less difficulty with swallowing.*

Elevate client to highest or best possible position for eating and drinking.

Feed slowly and instruct client to take small bites and to chew thoroughly.

Vary placement of food in client's mouth according to type of deficit (e.g., place food in right side of mouth if facial weakness present on left side). Use semisolid or soft foods that stick together and form a bolus (e.g., casseroles, puddings, stews), *which aids swallowing effort by improving client's ability to manipulate food with the tongue.*

Avoid pureed foods and mucus-producing foods (milk).

Determine food and liquid viscosity best tolerated by client. Add thickening agent to liquids, as appropriate. *Some individuals may swallow thickened liquids better than thin liquids.*

Offer very warm or very cold liquids *to activate temperature receptors in the mouth that help to stimulate swallowing.*

Avoid washing solids down with liquids *to prevent bolus of food pushing down too rapidly, increasing risk of aspiration.*

- Provide oral medications in elixir form or crushed, if appropriate. Have client self-medicate when possible. Time medications to coincide with meals when possible.
- Refer to physician and/or speech language pathologist, as appropriate, *for medical and surgical interventions or for specific exercises to strengthen muscles and techniques to enhance swallowing.*
- When feeding tube is in place:[4,12,13]

Note radiograph and/or measurement of aspirate pH following placement of feeding tube *to verify correct position.*

Ask client about feeling of fullness and/or measure residuals just prior to feeding and several hours after feeding, when appropriate, *to prevent overfeeding.*

Elevate head of bed 30 degrees during and for at least 30 minutes after bolus feedings.

- Determine best position for infant/child (e.g., with the head of bed elevated 30 degrees and infant propped on right side after feeding). *Upper airway patency is facilitated by upright position, and turning to right side decreases likelihood of drainage into trachea.*
- Provide oral medications in elixir form or crushed, if appropriate.
- Minimize use of sedatives/hypnotics when possible. *Agents can impair coughing and swallowing.*

NURSING PRIORITY NO. 3 To promote wellness (Teaching/Discharge Considerations):

- Review individual risk or potentiating factors with client/care provider.
- Provide information about the effects of aspiration on the lungs. *Note: Severe coughing and cyanosis associated with eating or drinking and voice change after swallowing indicate onset of respiratory symptoms associated with aspiration and require intervention for actual presence of aspiration.*[4,12]
- Instruct in safety concerns when feeding orally or tube feeding. (Refer to ND impaired Swallowing.)
- Train client to suction self or train family members in suction techniques (especially if client has constant or copious oral secretions) *to enhance safety/self-sufficiency.*
- Instruct individual/family member to avoid or limit activities after eating that increase intra-abdominal pressure (straining, strenuous exercise, tight or constrictive clothing). *May slow digestion or increase risk of regurgitation.*

DOCUMENTATION FOCUS

Assessment/Reassessment

- Assessment findings and conditions that could lead to problems of aspiration.
- Verification of tube placement, observations of physical findings.

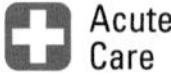

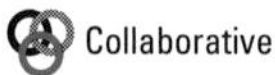

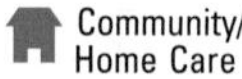

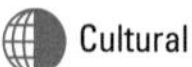

Planning
- Interventions to prevent aspiration or reduce risk factors and who is involved in the planning.
- Teaching plan.

Implementation/Evaluation
- Client's responses to interventions, teaching, and actions performed.
- Foods and fluids client handles with ease or difficulty.
- Amount and frequency of intake.
- Attainment or progress toward desired outcome(s).
- Modifications to plan of care.

Discharge Planning
- Long-term needs and who is responsible for actions to be taken.

References

1. Swaminathan, A., Stearns, D. A., Varkey, S. B. (updated 2014). Aspiration pneumonia. Retrieved March 2015 from http://emedicine.medscape.com/article/296198-overview.
2. Cox, H. C., et al. (2002). *Clinical Applications of Nursing Diagnosis: Adult, Child, Women's, Psychiatric, Gerontic, and Home Health Considerations*. 4th ed. Philadelphia, PA: F. A. Davis.
3. American Medical Directors Association. Altered nutritional status in the long term care setting. (2010). Retrieved March 2015 from http://www.guideline.gov/content.aspx?id=15590.
4. Metheny, N. A., Boltz, M., Greenberg, S. A. (2008). Preventing aspiration in older adults with dysphagia. *Am J Nurs*, 108(2), 45–46.
5. Galvan, T. J. (2001). Dysphagia: Going down and staying down. *Am J Nurs*, 101(1), 37.
6. Prahlow, J. A., Prahlow, T. J., Rakow, R. J. (2009). Case study: Asphyxia caused by inspissated oral and nasopharyngeal secretions. *Am J Nurs*, 109(38), 43.
7. Goodwin, R. S. (1996). Prevention of aspiration pneumonia: A research-based protocol. *Dimens Crit Care Nurs*, 15(2), 58–71.
8. Apnea of Prematurity. Clinical Practice Guideline. (February 1999). National Association of Neonatal Nurses.
9. Garon, B. R., Sierzant, T., Ormiston, C. (2009). Silent aspiration: Results of 2,000 video fluoroscopic evaluations. *J Neurosci Nurs*, 41(4), 178–185.
10. American Association for Respiratory Care. (2010). AARC Clinical Practice Guidelines: Endotracheal suctioning of mechanically ventilated patients with artificial airways 2010. *Respir Care*, 55(6), 758–764.
11. Bowman, A., Breiner, J. E., Dorschug, K. C., et al. (2005). Implementation of an evidence-based feeding protocol and aspiration risk reduction algorithm. *Crit Care Nurs Q*, 28(4), 324–333.
12. Smith Hammond, C. A., Goldstein, L. B. (2006). Cough and aspiration of food and liquids due to oral-pharyngeal dysphagia: ACCP evidence-based clinical practice guidelines, EBP compendium. *Chest*, 129(1 Suppl), 154S–168S.
13. McClave, S. A., Lukan, J. K., Lowen, J. K., et al. (2005). Poor validity of residual volumes as a marker for risk of aspiration in critically ill patients. *Crit Care Med*, 33(2), 324–330.

risk for impaired Attachment

Taxonomy II: Role Relationships—Class 2 Family Relationships (00058) [**Diagnostic Division:** Social Interaction], Submitted as Risk for Impaired Parent/Infant/Child Attachment 1994; Revised 2008, 2013

DEFINITION: Vulnerable to disruption of the interactive process between parent/significant other and child that fosters the development of a protective and nurturing reciprocal relationship.

RISK FACTORS

Inability of parent to meet personal needs

Anxiety; [parents who themselves experienced impaired attachment]

(continues on page 66)

risk for impaired Attachment (continued)

Prematurity; child's illness prevents effective initiation of parental contact
Disorganized infant behavior; parental conflict resulting from disorganized infant behavior
Parent-child separation; physical barrier (e.g., infant in isolette); insufficient privacy
Substance abuse
[Difficult pregnancy and/or birth]
[Uncertainty of paternity; conception as a result of rape/sexual abuse]
NOTE: A risk diagnosis is not evidenced by signs and symptoms, as the problem has not occurred; rather, nursing interventions are directed at prevention.

Sample Clinical Applications: Prematurity, genetic or congenital conditions, autism, attention deficit disorder, developmental delay (parent or child), substance abuse (parent), bipolar disorder (parent)

DESIRED OUTCOMES/EVALUATION CRITERIA

Sample NOC linkages:

Parent-Infant Attachment: Parent and infant behaviors that demonstrate an enduring affectionate bond

Parenting Performance: Parental actions to provide a child a nurturing and constructive physical, emotional, and social environment

Child Development: [specify age group]: Milestones of physical, cognitive, and psychosocial progression by [specify] months/years of age

Parent Will (Include Specific Time Frame)

- Identify and prioritize family strengths and needs.
- Exhibit nurturing and protective behaviors toward child.
- Identify and use resources to meet needs of family members.
- Demonstrate techniques to enhance behavioral organization of the infant/child.
- Engage in mutually satisfying interactions with child.

ACTIONS/INTERVENTIONS

Sample NIC linkages:

Attachment Promotion: Facilitation of the development of the parent-infant relationship

Parenting Promotion: Providing parenting information, support, and coordination of comprehensive services to high-risk families

Environmental Management: Attachment Process: Manipulation of the patient's surroundings to facilitate the development of the parent-infant relationship

NURSING PRIORITY NO. 1 To identify causative/contributing factors:

- Interview parents, noting their perception of situation and individual concerns. *Identifies problem areas and strengths to formulate appropriate plans to change situation that is currently creating problems for the parents.*[8]
- Assess parent/child interactions. *Identifies relationships, communication skills, and feelings about one another. The way in which a parent responds to a child and how the child responds to the parent largely determines how the child develops. Identifying the way in which the family responds to one another is crucial in determining the need for and type of interventions required.*[8]
- Ascertain availability and use of resources to include extended family, support groups, and finances. *Lack of support from or presence of extended family, lack of involvement in groups (e.g., church) or specific resources (e.g., La Leche League), and financial stresses can affect family negatively, interfering with ability to deal effectively with parenting responsibilities. Parents need support from both inside and outside the family.*[9,12]

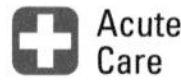

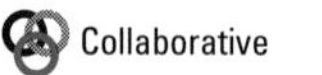

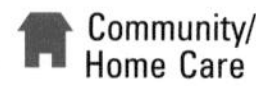

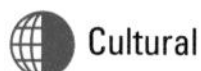

- Determine emotional and behavioral problems of the child. *Attachment-disordered children are unable to give and receive love and affection, defy parental rules and authority, and are physically and emotionally abusive, creating ongoing stress and turmoil in the family and in future relationships.*[12]
- Evaluate parents' ability to provide protective environment and to participate in reciprocal relationship. *Parents may be immature, may be substance abusers, or may be mentally ill and unable or unwilling to assume the task of parenting. The ways in which the parent responds to the child are critical to the child's development, and interventions need to be directed at helping the parents to deal with their own issues and learn positive parenting skills.*[1,7]
- Note attachment behaviors between parent and child(ren), recognizing cultural background. *For example, lack of eye contact and touching may indicate bonding problems. Behaviors such as eye-to-eye contact, use of en face position, and talking to the infant in a high-pitched voice are indicative of attachment behaviors in American culture but may not be appropriate in another culture. Failure to bond effectively is thought to affect subsequent parent-child interaction.*[4,5]
- Assess parenting skill level, considering intellectual, emotional, and physical strengths and limitations. *Identifies areas of need for further education, skill training, and factors that might interfere with ability to assimilate new information.*[1,2]

NURSING PRIORITY NO. 2 To enhance behavioral organization of infant/child:

- Identify infant's strengths and vulnerabilities. *Each child is born with his or her own temperament that affects interactions with caregivers, and when these are known, actions can be taken to assist parents/caregivers to parent appropriately.*[2,7,11]
- Educate parents regarding child growth and development, addressing parental perceptions. *Parents often have misconceptions about the abilities of their children, and providing correct information clarifies expectations and is more realistic.*[6]
- Assist parents in modifying the environment. *The environment can be changed to provide appropriate stimulation (e.g., to diminish stimulation before bedtime, to simplify when the environment is too complex to handle, to provide life space where the child can play unrestricted, resulting in freedom for the child to meet his or her needs).*[2,7] (Refer to ND readiness for enhanced organized Infant Behavior.)
- Model caregiving techniques that best support behavioral organization, such as attachment parenting. *Recognizing that the child deserves to have his or her needs taken seriously and responding to those needs in a loving fashion promotes trust, and children learn to model their behavior after what they have seen the parents do.*[9,11]
- Respond consistently with nurturance to infant/child. *Babies come wired with an ability to signal their needs by crying, and when parents respond to these signals, they develop a sensitivity that in turn develops parental intuition, providing infants with gratification of their needs and trust in their environment.*[10]

NURSING PRIORITY NO. 3 To enhance best functioning of parents:

- Develop a therapeutic nurse-client relationship. Provide a consistently warm, nurturant, and nonjudgmental environment. *Parents are often surprised to find that a tiny infant can cause so many changes in their lives and need help to adjust to this new experience. The warm, caring relationship of the nurse can help with this adjustment and provide the information and empathy they need at this time.*[1]
- Assist parents in identifying and prioritizing family strengths and needs. *Promotes positive attitude by looking at what they already do well and using those skills to address needs.*[2]
- Support and guide parents in process of assessing resources. *Outside support is important at this time, and making sure that parents receive the help they need will help them in this adjustment period.*[12]
- Involve parents in activities with the infant/child that they can accomplish successfully. *Activities such as Baby Gymboree and baby yoga enable the parents to get to know their child and themselves, enhancing their confidence and self-concept.*[12]

- Recognize and provide positive feedback for nurturant and protective parenting behaviors. *Using "I" messages to let parents know their behaviors are effective reinforces continuation of desired behaviors and promotes feelings of confidence in their abilities.*[2,12]

NURSING PRIORITY NO. 4 To support parent/child attachment during separation:

- Provide parents with telephone contact as appropriate. *Knowing there is someone they can call if they have problems provides a sense of security.*[3]
- Establish a routine time for daily phone calls or initiate calls as indicated when child is hospitalized. *Provides sense of consistency and control; allows for planning of other activities so parents can maintain contact and get information on a regular basis.*[1]
- Minimize number of professionals on team with whom parents must have contact. *Parents begin to know the individuals they are dealing with on a regular basis, fostering trust in these relationships and providing opportunities for modeling and learning.*[3]
- Invite parents to use resources, such as the Ronald McDonald House, or provide a listing of a variety of local accommodations and restaurants. *When child is hospitalized out of town, parents need to have a place to stay so they can have ready access to the hospital and be able to rest and refresh from time to time.*[3]
- Arrange for parents to receive photos and progress reports from the child. *Provides information and comfort as the child progresses, allowing the parents to continue to have hope for a positive resolution.*[3]
- Suggest parents provide a photo and/or audiotape of themselves for the child. *Provides a connection during the separation, sustaining attachment between parent and child.*[1]
- Consider use of a contract with parents. *Clearly communicating expectations of both family and staff serves as a reminder of what each person has committed to and serves as a tool to evaluate whether expectations are being maintained.*[3]
- Suggest parents keep a journal of infant/child progress. *Serves as a reminder of the progress that is being made, especially when they become discouraged and believe infant/child is "never" going to be better.*[3]
- Provide "homelike" environment for situations requiring supervision of visits. *An environment that is comfortable supports the family as they work toward resolving conflicts and promotes a sense of hopefulness, enabling them to experience success when family is involved with a legal situation.*[12]

NURSING PRIORITY NO. 5 To promote wellness (Teaching/Discharge Considerations):

- Refer to addiction counseling or treatment, individual counseling, or family therapies as indicated. *May need additional assistance when situation is complicated by drug abuse (including alcohol), mental illness, disruptions in caregiving, or parents who are burned out with caring for child with attachment or other difficulties.*[12,13]
- Identify services for transportation, financial resources, housing, etc. *Assistance with these needs can help families focus on therapeutic regimen and on issues of parenting to improve family dynamics.*[9]
- Develop support systems appropriate to situation (e.g., extended family, friends, social worker). *Depending on individual situation, support from extended family, friends, social worker, or therapist can assist family to deal with attachment disorders.*[10]
- Explore community resources (e.g., church affiliations, volunteer groups, day/respite care). *Church affiliations, volunteer groups, day or respite care can help parents who are overwhelmed with care of a child with attachment or other disorder.*[12]

DOCUMENTATION FOCUS

Assessment/Reassessment

- Identified behaviors of both parents and child.
- Specific risk factors, individual perceptions and concerns.
- Interactions between parent and child.

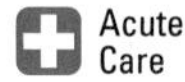

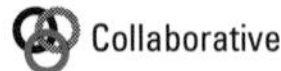

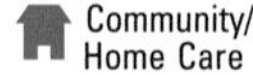

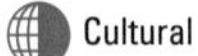

Planning

- Plan of care and who is involved in planning.
- Teaching plan.

Implementation/Evaluation

- Parents'/child's responses to interventions, teaching, and actions performed.
- Attainment or progress toward desired outcomes.
- Modifications to plan of care.

Discharge Planning

- Long-term needs and who is responsible.
- Plan for home visits to support parents and to ensure infant/child safety and well-being.
- Specific referrals made.

References

1. Linwood, A. S. (no date). Parent-child relationships. Encyclopedia of Children's Health. Retrieved March 2015 from http://www.healthofchildren.com/P/Parent-Child-Relationships.html.
2. Gordon, T. How children really react to control. Retrieved March 2015 from http://www.naturalchild.org/guest/thomas_gordon.html.
3. Melnyk, B. M. (2000). Intervention studies involving parents of hospitalized young children: An analysis of the past and future recommendations. *J Ped Nurs*, 15(1), 4–13.
4. Lipson, J. G., Dibble, S. L., Minarik, P. A. (1996). *Culture & Nursing Care. A Pocket Guide*. San Francisco, CA: UCSF Nursing Press.
5. Martin, J. (1993). The gentle truth about infant bonding. *Parenting*, (December).
6. Dowshen, S. (updated 2013). Your child's growth. Retrieved March 2015 from http://kidshealth.org/parent/growth/growing/childs_growth.html#.
7. New, M. (updated 2012). Developing your child's self-esteem. Retrieved March 2015 from http://kidshealth.org/parent/emotions/feelings/self_esteem.html#.
8. Gordon, T. What every parent should know. Retrieved March 2015 from http://www.gordontraining.com/artman2/uploads/1/What_Every_Parent_Should_Know_1.pdf.
9. Henningsen, M. (1996). *Attachment Disorder: Theory, Parenting and Therapy*. Evergreen, CO: Evergreen Family Counseling Center.
10. Sears, W. (1999). *Attachment Parenting: A Style That Works. Nighttime Parenting: How to Get Your Baby and Child to Sleep.* (La Leche International Book, revised edition). New York: Plume.
11. Benaroch, R. (reviewer) (2014). What is attachment parenting? WebMD Health and Parenting. Retrieved March 2015 from http://www.webmd.com/parenting/what-is-attachment-parenting.
12. Adventures in parenting. (2001). U.S. Department of Health and Human Services. Retrieved March 2015 from https://www.nichd.nih.gov/publications/pubs/adv_in_parenting/documents/adventures_in_parenting_rev.pdf.
13. DrugFacts: Treatment approaches for drug addiction. (2009). National Institute of Drug Abuse. Retrieved March 2015 from http://www.drugabuse.gov/publications/drugfacts/treatment-approaches-drug-addiction.

Autonomic Dysreflexia

Taxonomy II: Coping/Stress Tolerance—Class 3 Neurobehavioral Stress (00009) [**Diagnostic Division:** Circulation], Submitted 1988

DEFINITION: Life-threatening, uninhibited sympathetic response of the nervous system to a noxious stimulus after a spinal cord injury (SCI) at T7 or above.

RELATED FACTORS

Bladder or bowel distention; [catheter insertion, constipation, obstruction; irrigation]
Skin irritation
Insufficient [client] or caregiver knowledge
[Sexual excitation; menstruation; pregnancy; labor and delivery]
[Environmental temperature extremes]

DEFINING CHARACTERISTICS

Subjective

Headache (a diffuse pain in different portions of the head and not confined to any nerve distribution area)
Paresthesia, chilling, blurred vision, chest pain, metallic taste in mouth, nasal congestion

Objective

Paroxysmal hypertension [sudden periodic elevated blood pressure with systolic pressure >140 mmHg and diastolic >90 mmHg]
Bradycardia or tachycardia
Diaphoresis (above the injury), red splotches on skin (above the injury), pallor (below the injury)
Horner's syndrome [contraction of the pupil, partial ptosis of the eyelid, enophthalmos, and sometimes loss of sweating over the affected side of the face]; conjunctival congestion
Pilomotor reflex
Sample Clinical Applications: Spinal cord injury

DESIRED OUTCOMES/EVALUATION CRITERIA

Sample NOC linkages:
Neurological Status: Autonomic: Ability of the autonomic nervous system to coordinate visceral and homeostatic function
Knowledge: Disease Process: Extent of understanding conveyed about a specific disease process
Neurological Status: Autonomic: Ability of the autonomic nervous system to coordinate visceral and homeostatic function

Client/Caregiver Will (Include Specific Time Frame)

- Identify specific precipitating factors.
- Recognize signs and symptoms of syndrome.
- Demonstrate corrective techniques.

Client Will
Experience no episodes of dysreflexia or seek medical intervention in a timely manner.

ACTIONS/INTERVENTIONS

Sample NIC linkages:
Dysreflexia Management: Prevention and elimination of stimuli that cause hyperactive reflexes and inappropriate autonomic responses in a patient with a cervical or high thoracic cord lesion

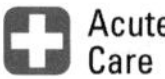

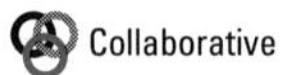

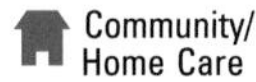

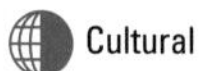

Urinary Elimination Management [or] Bowel Management: Maintenance of an optimum urinary elimination pattern/establishment and maintenance of a regular pattern of bowel elimination
Anxiety Reduction: Minimizing apprehension, dread, foreboding, or uneasiness related to an unidentified source or anticipated danger

NURSING PRIORITY NO. 1 To assess for precipitating factors:

- Note phase and specifics of injury. *Autonomic dysreflexia (AD) occurs in about 29% of persons with complete tetraplegia (quadraplegia). AD does not occur in the acute phase of SPI. However, some studies have identified factors that may point toward a client's likelihood of developing AD, and perhaps early in recovery. These include higher level of injury (cervical versus thoracic involvement) and more complete lesions.*[1–3,6–11]
- Assess for bladder distention, presence of bladder spasms or stones, or acute urinary tract infection. *The most common stimulus for AD is bladder irritation or overstretch associated with urinary retention or infection, blocked catheter, overfilled collection bag, or noncompliance with intermittent catheterization.*
- Evaluate for bowel distention, fecal impaction, or problems with bowel management program. *Bowel irritation or overstretch is associated with constipation or impaction; digital stimulation, suppository, or enema use during bowel program; hemorrhoids or fissures; and/or infection of gastrointestinal tract, such as might occur with ulcers or appendicitis.*
- Observe skin and tissue pressure areas, especially following prolonged sitting. *Skin and tissue irritants include direct pressure (e.g., object in chair or shoe, leg straps, abdominal support, orthotics), wounds (e.g., bruise, abrasion, lacerations, pressure ulcer), ingrown toenail, tight clothing, or sunburn or other burn.*
- Inquire about sexual activity and/or determine if reproductive issues are involved. *Overstimulation or vibration, sexual intercourse and ejaculation, scrotal compression, menstrual cramps, and/or pregnancy (especially labor and delivery) are known precipitants.*
- Inform client/care providers of additional precipitators during course of care. *Client is prone to physical conditions or treatments (e.g., intolerance to temperature extremes; deep vein thrombosis; kidney stones; fractures or other trauma; surgical, dental, diagnostic procedures), any of which can precipitate AD.*
- Note environmental temperature for extremes/drafts, *which can precipitate episode.*

NURSING PRIORITY NO. 2 To provide for early detection and immediate intervention:

- Investigate associated complaints/syndrome of symptoms (e.g., severe pounding headache, [blood pressure may be >200/100 mmHg], chest pain, irregular heart rate or dysrhythmias, blurred vision, nausea, facial flushing, metallic taste, severe anxiety; minimal symptoms or expressed complaints in presence of significantly elevated blood pressure—silent AD]). *Body's reaction to misinterpreted sensations from below the injury site, resulting in an autonomic reflex, can cause blood vessels to constrict and increase blood pressure. This is a potentially life-threatening condition, requiring immediate and correct action.*[1–3,6,7]
- Note onset of crying, irritability, or somnolence in infant or child *who may present with nonspecific symptoms and may not be able to verbalize discomfort.*[1]
- Locate and attempt to eliminate causative stimulus, moving in a stepwise fashion: *Cause can be anything that would normally cause pain or discomfort below level of injury.*[1–7]
  - Assess for bladder distention: *Note: The two most common inciting stimuli are bladder and bowel distention, respectively, commonly a blocked urinary catheter.*[3]
  - Empty bladder by voiding or catheterization, applying local anesthetic ointment (if indicated/per facility procedure *to prevent exacerbation of AD by procedure*).
  - Ascertain that urine is free-flowing if Foley or suprapubic catheter is in place, empty drainage bag, straighten tubing if kinked, and lower drainage bag if it is higher than bladder.
  - Irrigate gently or change catheter, if it is not draining freely.
- Note color, character, and odor of urine; obtain specimen for culture as indicated *(acute urinary infection can cause AD).*[3]

- Check for distended bowel *(if urinary problem is not causing AD):* Note: Fecal impaction is the second most common cause of AD.[6]
  - Perform digital stimulation, checking for constipation or impacted stool. (If symptoms first appear while performing digital stimulation, stop procedure.)
  - Apply local anesthetic ointment to rectum; remove impaction after symptoms subside *to remove causative problem without causing additional symptoms.*
- Check for skin pressure or irritation *(if bowel problem is not causing AD):*
  - Perform a pressure release if sitting.
  - Check for tight clothing, straps, and belts.
  - Note whether pressure sore has developed or changed.
  - Observe for bruising and signs of infection.
  - Check for ingrown toenail, other injury to skin or tissue (e.g., burns, sunburn), or fractured bones.
- Check for other possible causes *(if skin pressure is not causing AD):*
  - Menstrual cramps, sexual activity, or labor and delivery.
  - Abdominal conditions (e.g., colitis, ulcer).
  - Environmental temperature extremes.
- Take steps to reduce blood pressure, thereby *reducing potential for stroke (primary concern):*[1–7]
  - Elevate head of bed immediately or place in sitting position with legs hanging down. *Lowers blood pressure by pooling of blood in legs and decreases intracranial pressure caused by vasodilation in the brain, thus reducing headache.*[3]
  - Loosen any clothing or restrictive devices. *Lowers blood pressure by pooling of blood in abdomen and lower extremities.*
  - Monitor vital signs frequently during acute episode. *Blood pressure may fluctuate quickly due to impaired autonomic regulation.* Continue to monitor blood pressure at intervals during procedures to remove cause of AD and after acute episodic symptoms subside *to evaluate effectiveness of interventions and antihypertensives.*
- Administer medications, as indicated. *If an episode is particularly severe, or persists after removal of suspected cause, antihypertensive medications with rapid onset and short duration (e.g., nifedipine, nitrates, mecamylamine diazoxide, phenoxybenzamine) may be used to block excessive autonomic nerve transmission, normalize heart rate, and reduce hypertension.*[1,4,6]
- Know contraindications and cautions associated with antihypertensive medications; adjust dosage of antihypertensive medications carefully for child, elderly person, individual with known heart disease, male client using sildenafil for sexual activity, and pregnant woman. *Prevents complications, including unknown reactions in a child or systemic hypotension or seizure activity.*[6] *Note: Use of nitrate-containing medications is an absolute contraindication to sildenafil use because of the possibility of a fatal response.*[1,3]

NURSING PRIORITY NO. 3 To promote wellness (Teaching/Discharge Considerations):

- Discuss with client/caregivers warning signs of AD, as listed previously. Be aware of client's communication abilities. *AD can occur at any age from infant to very old, and the individual may not be able to verbalize a pounding headache, which is often the first symptom during onset of AD.*[1,8]
- Ascertain that client/caregivers understand ways to avoid onset or treat syndrome as noted previously. Provide information card and instruct and periodically reinforce teaching, as needed, regarding:[1,2,5–8]
  - Maintaining indwelling catheter by keeping tubing free of kinks, keeping bag empty and situated below bladder level, and checking daily for deposits (bladder grit) inside catheter.
  - Performing intermittent catheterization as often as necessary *to prevent overfilling or distention.*
  - Monitoring for adequate spontaneous voiding, noting frequency and amount.
  - Maintaining a regular and effective bowel evacuation program.
  - Performing routine skin assessments.

Acute Care 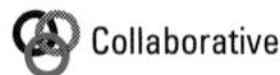 Collaborative 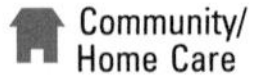 Community/ Home Care 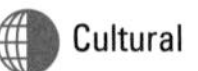 Cultural

Monitoring all systems for signs of infection and reporting promptly *for timely medical treatment.* Scheduling routine medical evaluations.

- Instruct family member/caregiver in client's "normal" blood pressure range and proper blood pressure monitoring and plan for monitoring hypertension during acute episodes. *A spinal cord–injured client's (both adult and child) baseline blood pressure is lower than that of a noninjured person. Blood pressure 20 to 40 mmHg higher than reference range may be a sign of AD.*[6]
- Review proper use and administration of medications, when used. *Client may have medication(s) both for emergent situations and/or prevention of AD, and if so, he or she should receive medication instructions, as well as symptoms to report for immediate or emergent care, when blood pressure is not responsive.*[1,8]
- Refer for or advise treatment of sexual and reproductive concerns, as indicated. *Client requires information and monitoring regarding sexual issues that can precipitate AD, including vibration to achieve orgasm, use of erectile dysfunction medication, and labor and delivery.*[3,9]
- Recommend wearing medical alert bracelet or necklace and carrying information card about signs/symptoms of AD and usual methods of treatment. *Provides vital information in emergency.*
- Assist client/family in identifying emergency referrals (e.g., physician, rehabilitation nurse/home-care supervisor). Place telephone number(s) in prominent place or program numbers into client's/caregiver's cell phone.

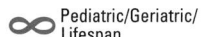

DOCUMENTATION FOCUS

Assessment/Reassessment

- Individual findings, noting previous episodes, precipitating factors, and individual signs/symptoms.

Planning

- Plan of care and who is involved in planning.
- Teaching plan.

Implementation/Evaluation

- Client's responses to interventions and actions performed, understanding of teaching.
- Attainment or progress toward desired outcome(s).
- Modifications to plan of care.

Discharge Planning

- Long-term needs and who is responsible for actions to be taken.

References

1. Consortium for Spinal Cord Medicine/Paralyzed Veterans of America. (2001). *Acute Management of Autonomic Dysreflexia: Individuals with Spinal Cord Injury Presenting to Health-Care Facilities: Clinical Practice Guidelines.* 2nd ed. Retrieved March 2015 from http://www.guideline.gov/content.aspx?id=2964.
2. Acuff, M. (2005). Autonomic dysreflexia: What it is, what it does, and what to do if you experience it. *The Missouri Model Spinal Cord Injury System.* Columbia, MO: University of Missouri-Columbia, School of Health Professions.
3. Saulino, M. F. (updated 2014). Rehabilitation of persons with spinal cord injuries. Retrieved March 2015 from http://emedicine.medscape.com/article/1265209/overview.
4. Deglan, J. H., Vallerand, A. H. (2011). *Davis's Drug Guide for Nurses.* 12th ed. Philadelphia, PA: F. A. Davis.
5. No author listed. (2009). Other complications of spinal cord injury: Autonomic dysreflexia (hyperreflexia) treatment. RehabTeamSite. Retrieved March 2015 from http://calder.med.miami.edu/pointis/automatic.html.
6. Consortium for Spinal Cord Medicine. (1997). Autonomic dysreflexia: What you should know. Retrieved March 2015 from http://www.scicpg.org/cpg_cons_pdf/ADC.pdf.
7. Stephenson, R. O., Berliner, J. (updated 2014). Autonomic dysreflexia in spinal cord injury. Retrieved January 2011 from http://emedicine.medscape.com/article/322809-overview.

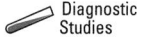

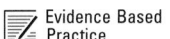

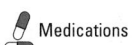

8. Cody, T., Zieroff, V. (2009). Autonomic dysreflexia. Northeast Rehabilitation Health Network. Retrieved March 2015 from http://www.sci-info-pages.com/ad.html.
9. Ducharme, S. (2000). Sexuality and spinal cord injury. *Paraplegia News*. Retrieved March 2015 from www.stanleyducharme.com/resources/sex_spinalcord_injury.htm.
10. Krassioukov, A. V., Furlan, J. C., Fehlings, M. G. (2003). Autonomic dysreflexia in acute spinal cord injury: An under-recognized clinical entity. *J Neurotrauma*, 20(8), 707–716.
11. Widerstrom-Noga, E., Cruz-Almeida, Y., Krassioukov, A. (2004). Is there a relationship between chronic pain and autonomic dysreflexia in persons with cervical spinal cord injury? *J Neurotrauma*, 21(2), 195–204.

risk for Autonomic Dysreflexia

Taxonomy II: Coping/Stress Tolerance—Class 3 Neurobehavioral Stress (00010) [**Diagnostic Division:** Circulation], Submitted 1988; Revised 2000, 2013

DEFINITION: Vulnerable to life-threatening, uninhibited response of the sympathetic nervous system post-spinal shock, in an individual with a spinal cord injury or lesion at T6 or above (has been demonstrated in clients with injuries at T7 and T8), which may compromise health.

RISK FACTORS

Cardiopulmonary Stimuli
Deep vein thromobis; pulmonary emboli

Gastrointestinal Stimuli
Bowel distention, constipation; difficult passage of feces; fecal impaction
Digital stimulation; enemas; suppositories
Gastrointestinal system pathology; esphogeal reflux disease; gallstones; hemorrhoids

Musculoskeletal-Integumentary Stimuli
Cutaneous stimulation (e.g., pressure ulcer, ingrown toenail, dressing, burns, rash); sunburn; wounds
Pressure over bony prominences/genitalia; range-of-motion exercises; spasm
Fracture; heterotrophic bone

Neurological Stimuli
Painful or irritating stimuli below the level of injury

Regulatory Stimuli
Temperature fluctuations; extremes of environmental temperatures

Reproductive Stimuli
Sexual intercourse; ejaculation; [vibrator overstimulation]
Menstruation; pregnancy; labor and delivery; ovarian cyst

Situational Stimuli
Constrictive clothing (e.g., straps, stockings, shoes)
Pharmaceutical agent [e.g., decongestants, sympathomimetics, vasoconstrictors]; substance withdrawal (e.g., narcotic/opiate)
Positioning; surgical [or diagnostic] procedure

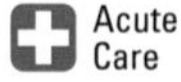

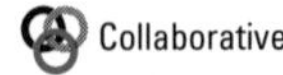

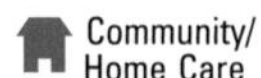

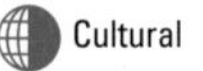

Urological Stimuli
Bladder distention or spasm
Detrusor sphincter dyssynergia
Urinary catheterization; instrumentation; surgery
Urinary tract infection; cystitis; urethritis; epididymitis; renal calculi
NOTE: A risk diagnosis is not evidenced by signs and symptoms as the problem has not occurred; rather, nursing interventions are directed at prevention.
Sample Clinical Applications: Spinal cord injury

DESIRED OUTCOMES/EVALUATION CRITERIA

Sample NOC linkages:
Risk Control: Personal actions to prevent, eliminate, or reduce modifiable health threats
Knowledge: Disease Process: Extent of understanding conveyed about a specific disease process
Caregiver Home Care Readiness: Extent of preparedness of a caregiver to assume responsibility for the healthcare of a family member in the home

Client/Caregiver Will (Include Specific Time Frame)
- Identify risk factors present.
- Demonstrate preventive or corrective techniques.
- Client will be free of episodes of dysreflexia.

ACTIONS/INTERVENTIONS

Sample NIC linkages:
Dysreflexia Management: Prevention and elimination of stimuli that cause hyperactive reflexes and inappropriate autonomic responses in a patient with a cervical or high thoracic cord lesion
Surveillance: Purposeful and ongoing acquisition, interpretation, and synthesis of patient data for clinical decision making
Medication Management: Facilitation of safe and effective use of prescription and over-the-counter drugs

NURSING PRIORITY NO. 1 To assess risk factors present:

- Monitor for potential precipitating factors, including urological (e.g., bladder distention, acute urinary tract infection, kidney stones), gastrointestinal (e.g., bowel overdistention, hemorrhoids, digital stimulation), cutaneous (e.g., pressure ulcers, extreme external temperatures, dressing changes), reproductive (e.g., sexual activity, menstruation, pregnancy/delivery), and miscellaneous (e.g., pulmonary emboli, drug reaction, deep vein thrombosis). (Refer to ND Autonomic Dysreflexia for a more complete listing of precipitating factors, if indicated.[1,2,6,7])

NURSING PRIORITY NO. 2 To prevent occurrence:

- Monitor vital signs routinely, noting changes in blood pressure, heart rate, and temperature, especially during times of physical stress *to identify trends and intervene in a timely manner.*[1,2] *Note: The baseline blood pressure in spinal cord–injured clients (adult and child) is lower than in the general population; therefore, an elevation of 20 to 40 mm Hg above baseline may be indicative of autonomic dysreflexia (AD).*[6,7]
- Instruct all caregivers in regularly timed elimination and safe bowel and bladder or catheter care, as well as in interventions for long-term prevention of skin stress or breakdown (e.g., appropriate padding for skin and tissues, proper positioning with frequent pressure-relief actions, routine foot and toenail care) *to reduce risk of AD episode. Note: The two most common inciting stimuli are bladder and bowel distention, respectively; commonly a blocked urinary catheter.*[1,3,5,7]

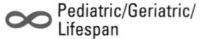

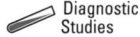

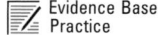

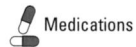

- Instruct client/caregivers in additional preventive interventions (e.g., temperature control; preventing pressure ulcers, blisters, ingrown toenails; checking frequently for tight clothes or leg straps; sunburn and other burn prevention).[1,4–7]
- Administer antihypertensive medications, as indicated. *At-risk client may be placed on routine "maintenance dose," such as when noxious stimuli cannot be removed (e.g., presence of chronic sacral pressure ulcer, fracture, acute postoperative pain).*[1]
- Refer to ND Autonomic Dysreflexia.

NURSING PRIORITY NO. 3 To promote wellness (Teaching/Discharge Considerations):

- Review warning signs of AD with client/caregiver (e.g., sudden, severe pounding headache; flushed, red face; increased blood pressure/acute hypertension; nasal congestion; anxiety; blurred vision; metallic taste in mouth; sweating and/or flushing above the level of SCI; goose bumps; bradycardia, cardiac irregularities). *AD can develop rapidly (in minutes), thus requiring quick intervention.*
- Be aware of client's communication abilities. *AD can occur at any age, from infant to very old, and the individual may not be able to verbalize a pounding headache, which is often the first symptom during onset of AD.*[1]
- Ascertain that client/caregiver understands ways to avoid onset of syndrome. Provide information card and instruct and periodically reinforce teaching, as needed, regarding the following:[1–7]
  - Keeping indwelling catheter free of kinks, keeping bag empty and situated below bladder level, and checking daily for deposits (bladder grit) inside catheter,
  - Catheterizing as often as necessary *to prevent overfilling,*
  - Monitoring voiding patterns for adequate frequency and amount,
  - Performing regular bowel evacuation program,
  - Performing routine skin assessments, and
  - Monitoring all systems for signs/symptoms of infection and reporting promptly *for timely medical treatment.*
- Instruct family member/caregiver in proper blood pressure monitoring.
- Review use and administration of medications, when used. *Some clients are on medications routinely, and if so, they should receive instructions for routine administration, as well as symptoms to report for immediate or emergent care, when blood pressure is not responsive.*[1,6]
- Emphasize importance of regularly scheduled medical evaluations *to monitor status and identify developing problems.*
- Recommend wearing a medical alert bracelet or necklace with information card about signs/symptoms of AD and usual methods of treatment. *Provides vital information in emergencies.*
- Assist client/family in identifying emergency referrals (e.g., physician, rehabilitation nurse, or home-care supervisor). Place telephone number(s) in prominent place or program into client's/caregiver's cell phone.

DOCUMENTATION FOCUS

Assessment/Reassessment

- Individual risk factors.
- Previous episodes, precipitating factors, and individual signs/symptoms.

Planning

- Plan of care and who is involved in planning.
- Teaching plan.

Implementation/Evaluation

- Client's responses to interventions and actions performed, understanding of teaching.
- Attainment or progress toward desired outcome(s).
- Modifications to plan of care.

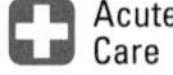

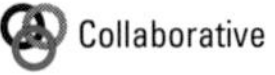

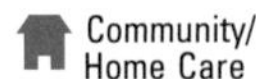

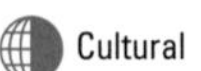

Discharge Planning

- Long-term needs and who is responsible for actions to be taken.

References

1. Consortium for Spinal Cord Medicine. (2001). *Acute Management of Autonomic Dysreflexia: Individuals with Spinal Cord Injury Presenting to Health-Care Facilities: Clinical Practice Guidelines.* 2nd ed. Retrieved March 2015 from http://www.guideline.gov/content.aspx?id=2964.
2. Acuff, M. (2005). Autonomic Dysreflexia: What It Is, What It Does, and What to Do if You Experience It. *The Missouri Model Spinal Cord Injury System.* Columbia, MO: University of Missouri-Columbia, School of Health Professions.
3. Saulino, M. F. Rehabilitation of persons with spinal cord injuries. Retrieved March 2015 from http://emedicine.medscape.com/article/1265209/overview.
4. No author listed. (Updated 2009). Other complications of spinal cord injury: Autonomic dysreflexia (hyperreflexia) treatment. RehabTeam. Retrieved March 2015 from http://calder.med.miami.edu/pointis/symptoms.html.
5. National Spinal Cord Injury Association. (Updated 2011). SCI complications resource: Autonomic dysreflexia. Retrieved March 2015 http://www.spinalcord.org/news.
6. Stephenson, R. O. (updated 2014). Autonomic dysreflexia in spinal cord injury. Retrieved March 2015 from http://emedicine.medscape.com/article/322809-overview.
7. No author listed. (2009). Autonomic dysreflexia. Article for Northeast Rehabilitation Health Network. Retrieved March 2015 from http://www.sci-info-pages.com/ad.html.

disorganized infant Behavior

Taxonomy II: Coping/Stress Tolerance—Class 3 Neurobehavioral Stress (00116) [**Diagnostic Division:** Neurosensory], Submitted 1994; 1998

DEFINITION: Disintegrated physiological and neurobehavioral responses of infant to the environment.

RELATED FACTORS

Prenatal

Congenital or genetic disorders; exposure to teratogen

Postnatal

Feeding intolerance; malnutrition
Impaired motor functioning; oral impairment
Invasive procedure; pain

Individual

Low postconceptual age; prematurity; immature neurological functioning
Illness [hypoxia or birth asphyxia]

Environmental

Inadequate physical environment; insufficient containment within environment
Insufficient sensory stimulation, overstimulation, or deprivation

Caregiver

Cue misreading; insufficient knowledge of behavioral cues
Environmental overstimulation

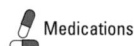

(continues on page 78)

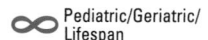

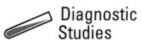

disorganized infant Behavior (continued)

DEFINING CHARACTERISTICS

Objective

Attention-interaction system: Impaired response to sensory stimuli (e.g., difficult to soothe, unable to sustain alert status)

Motor system:

Alteration in primitive reflexes; exaggerated startle response; jitteriness

Finger splay; fisting; hands to face; hyperextension of extremities

Impaired motor tone; tremor, twitching; uncoordinated movements

Physiological:

Abnormal skin color (e.g., pale, dusky, cyanosis)

Arrhythmia; bradycardia; tachycardia

Feeding intolerances

"Time-out signals" (e.g., gaze, grasp, hiccough, cough, sneeze, sigh, slack jaw, open mouth, tongue thrust)

Regulatory problems: Inability to inhibit startle reflex; irritability

State-organization system:

Active-awake (e.g., fussy, worried gaze); quiet-awake (e.g., staring, gaze aversion)

Diffuse alpha EEG activity with eyes closed; state-oscillation

Irritable crying

Sample Clinical Applications: Prematurity, congenital or genetic disorders, meconium aspiration, respiratory distress syndrome, small for gestational age

DESIRED OUTCOMES/EVALUATION CRITERIA

Sample NOC linkages:

Neurological Status: Ability of the peripheral and central nervous system to receive, process, and respond to internal and external stimuli

Preterm Infant Organization: Extrauterine integration of physiological and behavioral function by the infant born 24 to 37 (term) weeks gestation

Infant Will (Include Specific Time Frame)

- Exhibit organized behaviors that allow the achievement of optimal potential for growth and development as evidenced by modulation of physiological, motor, state, and attentional-interactive functioning.

Sample NOC linkages:

Child Development [specify age 1, 2 months]: Milestones of physical, cognitive, and psychosocial progression by [specify] months of age

Parent/Caregiver Will

- Recognize individual infant cues.
- Identify appropriate responses (including environmental modifications) to infant's cues.
- Verbalize readiness to assume caregiving independently.

ACTIONS/INTERVENTIONS

Sample NIC linkages:

Environmental Management: Manipulation of the patient's surroundings for therapeutic benefit, sensory appeal, and psychological well-being

Developmental Enhancement: Infant: Facilitating optimal physical, cognitive, social, and emotional growth of child under 1 year of age

Newborn Care: Management of neonate during the transition to extrauterine life and subsequent period of stabilization

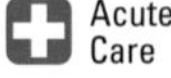
Acute Care

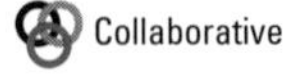
Collaborative

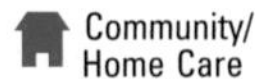
Community/ Home Care

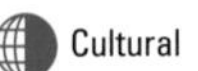
Cultural

NURSING PRIORITY NO. 1 To assess causative/contributing factors:

- Determine infant's chronological and developmental age; note length of gestation. *These factors (prematurity, infant maturity, and stages of development) help to determine plan of care.*[1,2]
- Observe for cues suggesting presence of situations that may result in pain or discomfort. *Some behavior that appears to be disorganized may be caused by a pain source that, once identified, may be alleviated.*[1]
- Determine adequacy of physiological support. *Identifies areas of additional need.*[1]
- Evaluate level and appropriateness of environmental stimuli. *Infant behavior is affected by a wide range of stimuli. Careful assessment narrows focus of concerns.*[2]
- Ascertain parents' understanding of infant's needs and abilities. *Identifies knowledge base and areas of learning needed.*[2–4]
- Listen to parents' concerns about their capabilities to meet infant's needs. *Active listening can reassure parents, pinpoint areas to be addressed, and provide an opportunity to correct misconceptions.*[2,3]

NURSING PRIORITY NO. 2 To assist parents in providing coregulation to the infant:

- Provide a calm, nurturant, physical, and emotional environment. *Provides optimal infant comfort. Models behavior for parent(s) and optimizes learning.*[2,3]
- Encourage parents to hold infant, including skin-to-skin contact as appropriate. *Touch enhances parent-infant bonding and provides means of calming.*[3] *Research suggests skin-to-skin contact or kangaroo care may have a positive effect on infant development by enhancing neurophysiological organization and an indirect effect by improving parental mood, perceptions, and interactive behavior.*[6]
- Model gentle handling of baby and appropriate responses to infant behavior. *Provides cues to parent.*[3]
- Support and encourage parents to be with infant and participate actively in all aspects of care. *Situation may seem overwhelming to new parents. Emotional and physical support enhances coping. Parents who are able to help in the care of their infant express lower levels of helplessness and powerlessness.*[1,2]
- Encourage parents to refrain from social interaction during feedings as appropriate. *Infant may have difficulty/lack necessary energy to manage feeding and social stimulation simultaneously.*[5]
- Provide positive feedback for progressive parental involvement in caregiving process. *Transfer of care from staff to parents progresses along a continuum as parents' confidence level increases and they are able to take on more complex care activities.*[7]
- Discuss infant growth and development, pointing out current status and progressive expectations as appropriate. *Augments parent knowledge of coregulation.*[2]
- Incorporate the parents' observations and suggestions into plan of care. *Demonstrates valuing of parents' input and encourages continued involvement.*[2,4]

NURSING PRIORITY NO. 3 To deliver care within the infant's stress threshold:

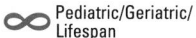

- Provide a consistent caregiver. *Facilitates recognition of infant cues or changes in behavior. Communication is optimized if family is familiar with caregiver.*[2]
- Identify infant's individual self-regulatory behaviors (e.g., sucking, mouthing; grasp, hand-to-mouth, face behaviors; foot clasp, brace; limb flexion, trunk tuck; boundary seeking).
- Support hands to mouth and face; offer pacifier or nonnutritive sucking at the breast with gavage feedings. *Provides opportunities for infant to self-regulate.*[2,5]
- Avoid aversive oral stimulation, such as routine oral suctioning; suction endotracheal tube only when clinically indicated. *Maximizes infant comfort, preventing undue/noxious stimulation.*[1,2]
- Use Oxyhood large enough to cover the infant's chest so arms will be inside the hood. *Allows for hand-to-mouth self-calming activities during this therapy.*[2]
- Provide opportunities for infant to grasp. *Helps with development of motor function skills and can have a calming effect.*[2,5]

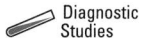

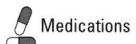

- Provide boundaries or containment during all activities. Use swaddling, nesting, bunting, and caregiver's hands as indicated. *Enhances infant's feelings of security and safeness. Avoids startle reflex and accompanying distress.*[2,3]
- Allow adequate time and opportunities to hold infant. Handle infant very gently; move infant smoothly, slowly, and keep contained, avoiding sudden or abrupt movements. *Provides comfort to infant and models behavior to parent(s).*[3]
- Maintain normal alignment, position infant with limbs softly flexed and shoulders and hips adducted slightly. Use appropriate-sized diapers. *Avoids unnecessary discomfort.*[2]
- Evaluate chest for adequate expansion, placing rolls under trunk if prone position is indicated. *Provides for ease of respirations.*[2]
- Avoid restraints, including at IV sites. If an IV board is necessary, secure to limb positioned in normal alignment. *Optimizes comfort and movement.*[1,2]
- Provide a pressure-eliminating mattress, water bed, or gel pillow for infant who does not tolerate frequent position changes. *Minimizes tissue pressure and risk of tissue injury.*[2]
- Visually assess color, respirations, activity, and invasive lines without disturbing infant. Assess with "hands on" every 4 hr as indicated and prn. *Allows for undisturbed rest and quiet periods.*[2,3]
- Group care activities, schedule time for rest, and organize sleep and wake states to maximize tolerance of infant. Defer routine care when infant is in quiet sleep. *Gives infant a sense of routine and also provides for undisturbed rest and longer periods of quiet.*[2,3,5]
- Provide care with baby in side-lying position. Begin by talking softly to the baby and then placing hands in a containing hold on baby, allowing baby to prepare. Proceed with least invasive manipulations first. *Gradual build from comforting touch, to nursing care, to invasive interventions decreases overall stress of infant. Shortens perception of "being bothered" time and facilitates a more rapid calming phase.*[3]
- Respond promptly to infant's agitation or restlessness. Provide "time-out" when infant shows early cues of overstimulation. Comfort and support the infant after stressful interventions. *Decreases stress for both infant and family. Facilitates calming phase.*[3]
- Remain at infant's bedside for several minutes after procedures and caregiving to monitor infant's response and provide necessary support. *Allows for more rapid intervention(s) if infant becomes overstressed.*[3]
- Administer analgesics as individually appropriate. *Maintains optimal comfort.*[1–4]

NURSING PRIORITY NO. 4 To modify the environment to provide appropriate stimulation:

- Introduce stimulation as a single mode and assess individual tolerance.

LIGHT/VISION

- Reduce lighting perceived by infant; introduce diurnal lighting (and activity) when infant achieves physiological stability. (Daylight levels of 20 to 30 candles and nightlight levels of less than 10 candles are suggested.) Change light levels gradually to allow infant time to adjust. *Lowering light levels reduces visual stimulation and provides a comforting environment. Diurnal lighting allows the stable infant to begin perception of day and night cycles and to establish circadian rhythms.*[1]
- Protect the infant's eyes from bright illumination during examinations and procedures, as well as from indirect sources, such as neighboring phototherapy treatments. *Prevents retinal damage and reduces visual stressors.*[2]
- Deliver phototherapy (when required) with Biliblanket devices if available. *Alleviates need for eye patches to protect vision.*[2]
- Provide a caregiver's face (preferably a parent's) as visual stimulus when infant shows readiness (awake, attentive). *Begins process of visual recognition.*[1]
- Evaluate/readjust placement of pictures, stuffed animal, etc., within infant's immediate environment. *Promotes state maintenance and smooth transition, allowing infant to look away easily when visual stimuli become stressful.*[5]

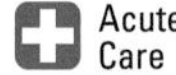

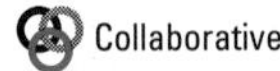

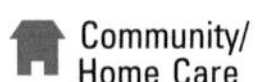

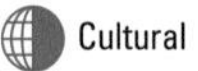

SOUND

- Identify sources of noise in environment and eliminate/reduce *to minimize auditory stimulus, reduce startle response in infant, and provide a comforting environment:*[2]
  Speak in a low voice.
  Reduce volume on alarms and telephones to safe but not excessive volume.
  Pad metal trash can lids.
  Open paper packages such as IV tubing and suction catheters slowly and at a distance from bedside.
  Conduct rounds or report away from bedside.
  Place soft, thick fabric such as blanket rolls and toys near infant's head *to absorb sound.*
  Keep all incubator portholes closed, closing with two hands *to avoid loud snap with closure and associated startle response.*
- Refrain from playing musical toys or tape players inside incubator. *Even very soft sounds echo in an enclosed space. What an adult may find soothing is likely to overstimulate an infant.*[2,3]
- Avoid placing items on top of incubator; if necessary to do so, pad surface well. *Contact with the external parts of the incubator causes reverberation inside the chamber.*
- Conduct regular decibel (dB) checks of interior noise level in incubator (recommended not to exceed 60 dB). *Verifies that decibel levels are within acceptable range.*[2]
- Provide auditory stimulation to console and support infant before and through handling or to reinforce restfulness. *Provides modeling of behavior for family and increased comfort for infant.*[3]

OLFACTORY

- Be cautious in exposing infant to strong odors (e.g., alcohol, Betadine, perfumes). *Olfactory capability of the infant is very sensitive.*[1]
- Place a cloth or gauze pad scented with milk near the infant's face during gavage feeding. *Enhances association of milk with act of feeding and gastric fullness.*[2]
- Invite parents to leave near infant a handkerchief that they have scented by wearing close to their body. *Strengthens infant recognition of parents.*[2]

VESTIBULAR

- Move and handle the infant slowly and gently. Do not restrict spontaneous movement. *Maintains comfort while encouraging motor function skill.*[2]
- Provide vestibular stimulation *to console, stabilize breathing/heart rate, or enhance growth.* Use a water bed (with or without oscillation); a motorized, moving bed or cradle; or rocking in the arms of a caregiver.

GUSTATORY

- Dip pacifier in milk and offer to infant for sucking and tasting during gavage feeding. *Further enhances feeding recognition with touch and taste cues.*[2]

TACTILE

- Maintain skin integrity and monitor closely. Limit frequency of invasive procedures. *Decreases chance of infections. Decreases infant discomfort.*[1]
- Minimize use of chemicals on skin (e.g., alcohol, povidone-iodine, solvents) and remove afterward with warm water. *Chemical compounds remove the natural protective mechanisms of skin, and infants are often very sensitive to integumentary injury.*[1]
- Limit use of tape and adhesives directly on skin. Use DuoDerm under tape. *Helps prevent dermal injury and allergic reactions.*[1]
- Touch infant with a firm, containing touch; avoid light stroking. Provide a sheepskin or soft linen. *Note: Tactile experience is the primary sensory mode of the infant. Light stroking can cause tickle sensations that are irritating rather than pleasurable. Firm touch is reassuring.*[2]

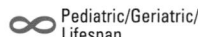

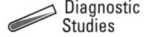

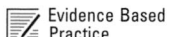

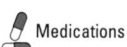

- Encourage frequent parental holding of infant (including skin-to-skin). Supplement activity with extended family, staff, volunteers. *For family members, touch enhances bonding. If family is not readily available, infant needs regular skin-to-skin contact from caregivers for comfort and reassurance.*[3]

NURSING PRIORITY NO. 5 To promote wellness (Teaching/Discharge Considerations):

- Evaluate home environment to identify appropriate modifications. *Helps the family identify needs and begin to mentally prepare for infant homecoming.*[3]
- Identify community resources (e.g., early stimulation program, qualified childcare facilities or respite care, visiting nurse, home-care support, specialty organizations). *Begins process of resource utilization.*[2–4]
- Determine sources for equipment and therapy needs. *Facilitates transition to at-home care.*[3]
- Refer to support or therapy groups as indicated. *Provides role models, facilitates adjustment to new roles and responsibilities, and enhances coping.*[2,3]
- Provide contact number, as appropriate (e.g., primary nurse). *Supports adjustment to home setting and enhances problem solving.*[3]
- Refer to additional NDs such as risk for impaired Attachment, risk for caregiver Role Strain, compromised/disabled/readiness for enhanced family Coping, risk for delayed Development.

DOCUMENTATION FOCUS

Assessment/Reassessment

- Findings, including infant's cues of stress, self-regulation, and readiness for stimulation; chronological and developmental age.
- Parent's concerns, level of knowledge.

Planning

- Plan of care and who is involved in the planning.
- Teaching plan.

Implementation/Evaluation

- Infant's responses to interventions and actions performed.
- Parents' participation and response to interactions and teaching.
- Attainment or progress toward desired outcome(s).
- Modifications of plan of care.

Discharge Planning

- Long-term needs and who is responsible for actions to be taken.
- Specific referrals made.

References

1. Greene, M. F., Creasy, R., Resnik, R., et al. (2008). *Creasy & Resnik's Maternal-Fetal Medicine.* 6th ed. Philadelphia: W. B. Saunders.
2. London, M. L., Ladewig, P. W., Ball, J. W., et al. (2006). *Maternal & Child Nursing Care.* 2nd ed. Upper Saddle River, NJ: Prentice Hall.
3. Ladewig, P., London, M. L., Davidson, M. W. (2009). *Contemporary Maternal-Newborn Nursing Care.* 7th ed. Upper Saddle River, NJ: Prentice Hall.
4. Lowdermilk, D., Perry, S. (2009). *Maternity & Women's Health Care.* 7th ed. St. Louis, MO: Mosby.
5. LaRossa, M. M. (No date). Understanding preterm infant behavior in the NICU. Retrieved March 2015 from http://www.pediatrics.emory.edu/divisions/neonatology/dpc/nicubeh.html.
6. Feldman, R., Eidelman, A. I., Sirota, L., et al. (2002). Comparison of skin-to-skin (kangaroo) and traditional care: Parenting outcomes and preterm infant development. *Pediatrics,* 110(1), 16–26.
7. Scharer, K., Brooks, G. (1994). Mothers of chronically ill neonates and primary nurses in the NICU: Transfer of care. *Neonatal Network,* 13(5), 37–46.

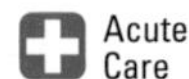

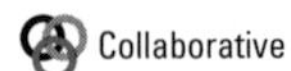

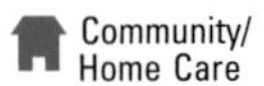

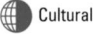

readiness for enhanced organized infant Behavior

Taxonomy II: Coping/Stress Tolerance—Class 3 Neurobehavioral Stress (00117) [**Diagnostic Division:** Neurosensory], Submitted 1994; Revised 2013

DEFINITION: A pattern of modulation of the physiological and behavioral systems of functioning (i.e., autonomic, motor, state-organization, self-regulatory, and attentional-interactional systems) in an infant, which can be improved.

DEFINING CHARACTERISTICS

Objective

Parent expresses desire to enhance cue recognition
Parent expresses desire to enhance recognition of infant's self-regulatory behaviors

Sample Clinical Applications: Prematurity, congenital or genetic disorders, meconium aspiration, respiratory distress syndrome, small for gestational age

DESIRED OUTCOMES/EVALUATION CRITERIA

Sample NOC linkages:

Preterm Infant Organization: Extrauterine integration of physiologic and behavioral function by the infant born 24 to 37 (term) weeks gestation

Neurological Status: Ability of the peripheral and central nervous system to receive, process, and respond to internal and external stimuli

Infant Will (Include Specific Time Frame)

- Modulate physiological and behavioral systems of functioning.
- Achieve higher levels of integration in response to environmental stimuli.

Sample NOC linkages:

Child Development: [specify age group 1 or 2 months]: Milestones of physical, cognitive, and psychosocial progression by [specify] months of age

Knowledge: Infant Care: Extent of understanding conveyed about caring for a baby from birth to first birthday

Parent/Caregiver Will (Include Specific Time Frame)

- Identify cues reflecting infant's stress threshold and current status.
- Develop or modify responses (including environment) to promote infant adaptation and development.

ACTIONS/INTERVENTIONS

Sample NIC linkages:

Developmental Enhancement: Infant: Facilitating optimal physical, cognitive, social, and emotional growth of child under 1 year of age

Environmental Management: Manipulation of the patient's surroundings for therapeutic benefit, sensory appeal, and psychological well-being

NURSING PRIORITY NO. 1 To assess infant status and parental skill level:

- Determine infant's chronological and developmental age; note length of gestation. *These factors (prematurity, infant maturity, and stages of development) help to determine plan of care.*[1,2,5]

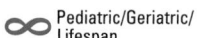

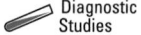

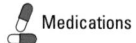

- Identify infant's individual self-regulatory behaviors: suck, mouth; grasp, hand-to-mouth, face behaviors; foot clasp, brace; limb flexion, trunk tuck; boundary seeking. *Assessing the infant's own regulatory coping tools alerts family and caregiver when infant is entering a stress cycle and helps determine if the infant needs assistance coping. This knowledge also helps in development of a care plan if situation warrants.*[1,2,4]
- Observe for cues suggesting presence of situations that may result in pain/discomfort. *Some behavior that appears to be disorganized may be caused by a pain source that, once identified, may be alleviated.*[1]
- Evaluate level and appropriateness of environmental stimuli. *Infant behavior is affected by a wide range of stimuli. Careful assessment narrows focus of concerns.*[2]
- Ascertain parents' understanding of infant's needs and abilities. *Identifies knowledge base and areas of additional learning need.*[2–4]
- Listen, or active-listen, to parents' perceptions of their capabilities to promote infant's development. *When parents feel their thoughts and concerns are heard, they will feel reassured that they will be able to handle the situation.*[2,3]

NURSING PRIORITY NO. 2 To assist parents to enhance infant's integration:

- Provide positive feedback for parental involvement in caregiving process. Transfer of care from staff to parents progresses along a continuum as parents' confidence level increases and they are able to take on more responsibility.[7]
- Discuss use of skin-to-skin contact (kangaroo care [KC]) as appropriate. *Research suggests KC may have a positive effect on infant development by enhancing neurophysiological organization and an indirect effect by improving parental mood, perceptions, and interactive behavior.*[6]
- Review infant growth and development, pointing out current status and progressive expectations. *Increases parental knowledge base and level of confidence.*[2–4]
- Identify cues reflecting infant stress. *Attention to cues allows for early intervention in case of problem development.*[2–4]
- Discuss possible modifications of environmental stimuli, handling, activity schedule, sleep, and pain control needs based on infant's behavioral cues. *Stimulation that is properly timed and appropriate in complexity and intensity allows the infant to maintain a stable balance of his/her subsystems and enhances development.*[5]
- Discuss parents' perceptions of needs and provide recommendations for modifications of environmental stimuli, activity schedule, sleep, and pain control needs. *While care provided is satisfactory, some modifications may enhance infant's integration and development.*[1,4]
- Incorporate parents' observations and suggestions into plan of care. *Demonstrates value of and regard for parents' input and enhances sense of ability to deal with situation.*[2,4]

NURSING PRIORITY NO. 3 To promote wellness (Teaching/Learning Considerations):

- Identify community resources (e.g., visiting nurse, home-care support, childcare). *Begins process of resource utilization.*[2–4]
- Refer to support group or individual role model *to facilitate ongoing adjustment to new roles and responsibilities and problem solving.*[2,3]
- Refer to additional NDs, for example, readiness for enhanced family Coping.

DOCUMENTATION FOCUS

Assessment/Reassessment

- Findings, including infant's self-regulation and readiness for stimulation; chronological and developmental age.
- Parents' concerns, level of knowledge.

Planning

- Plan of care and who is involved in the planning.
- Teaching plan.

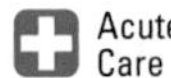

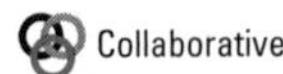

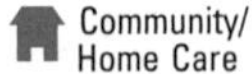

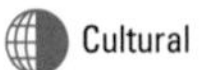

Implementation/Evaluation

- Infant's responses to interventions and actions performed.
- Parents' participation and response to interactions/teaching.
- Attainment or progress toward desired outcome(s).
- Modifications of plan of care.

Discharge Planning

- Long-term needs and who is responsible for actions to be taken.
- Specific referrals made.

References

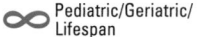

1. Greene, M. F., Creasy, R., Resnik, R., et al. (2008). *Creasy & Resnik's Maternal-Fetal Medicine*. 6th ed. Philadelphia, PA: W. B. Saunders.
2. London, M., Ladewig, P., Ball, J., et al. (2006). *Maternal & Child Nursing Care*. 2nd ed. Upper Saddle River, NJ: Prentice Hall.
3. Ladewig, P., London, M. L., Davidson, M. W. (2009). *Contemporary Maternal-Newborn Nursing Care*. 7th ed. Upper Saddle River, NJ: Prentice Hall.
4. Lowdermilk, D., Perry, S. (2009). *Maternity & Women's Health Care*. 7th ed. St. Louis, MO: Mosby.
5. LaRossa, M. M. Understanding preterm infant behavior in the NICU. Retrieved April 2012 from http://www.pediatrics.emory.edu/divisions/neonatology/dpc/nicubeh.html.
6. Feldman, R., Eidelman, A. I., Sirota, L., et al. (2002). Comparison of skin-to-skin (kangaroo) and traditional care: Parenting outcomes and preterm infant development. *Pediatrics*, 110(1), 16–26.
7. Scharer, K., Brooks, G. (1994). Mothers of chronically ill neonates and primary nurses in the NICU: Transfer of care. *Neonatal Network*, 13(5), 37–46.

risk for disorganized infant Behavior

Taxonomy II: Coping/Stress Tolerance—Class 3 Neurobehavioral Stress (00115) [**Diagnostic Division:** Neurosensory], Submitted 1994; revised 2013

DEFINITION: Vulnerable to alteration in integration and modulation of the physiological and behavioral systems of functioning (i.e., autonomic, motor, state-organization, self-regulatory, and attentional-interactional systems), which may compromise health.

RISK FACTORS

Impaired motor functioning; oral impairment

Insufficient containment within environment; parent expresses desire to enhance environmental conditions

Prematurity; [hypoxia and/or birth asphyxia]

Procedure or invasive procedure; pain

NOTE: A risk diagnosis is not evidenced by signs and symptoms, as the problem has not occurred; rather, nursing interventions are directed at prevention.

Sample Clinical Applications: Prematurity, congenital or genetic disorders, meconium aspiration, respiratory distress syndrome, small for gestational age

DESIRED OUTCOMES/EVALUATION CRITERIA

Sample NOC linkages:

Preterm Infant Organization: Extrauterine integration of physiologic and behavioral function by the infant born 24 to 37 (term) weeks gestation

Neurological Status: Ability of the peripheral and central nervous system to receive, process, and respond to internal and external stimuli

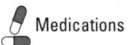

(continues on page 86)

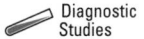

risk for disorganized infant Behavior (continued)

Infant Will (Include specific time frame)
- Exhibit organized behaviors that allow the achievement of optimal potential for growth and development as evidenced by modulation of physiological, motor, state, and attentional-interactive functioning.

Sample NOC linkages:

Child Development: [specify age group 1 or 2 months]: Milestones of physical, cognitive, and psychosocial progression by [specify] months of age

Knowledge: Infant Care: Extent of understanding conveyed about caring for a baby from birth to first birthday

Parent/Caregiver Will (Include specific time frame)
- Identify cues reflecting infant's stress threshold and current status.
- Develop or modify responses (including environment) to promote infant adaptation and development.

ACTIONS/INTERVENTIONS AND DOCUMENTATION FOCUS

Refer to ND disorganized infant Behavior for Actions/Interventions and Documentation Focus.

risk for Bleeding

Taxonomy II: Safety/Protection—Class 2 Physical Injury (00206) [**Diagnostic Division:** Circulation], Submitted 2008; Revised 2013

DEFINITION: Vulnerable to decrease in blood volume that may compromise health.

RISK FACTORS

Aneurysm; disseminated intravascular coagulapathy; inherent coagulopathy (e.g., thrombocytopenia)
Gastrointestinal condition (e.g., ulcer, polyps, varices); impaired liver function (e.g., cirrhosis, hepatitis)
History of falls; trauma
Insufficient knowledge of bleeding precautions
Pregnancy complication (e.g., premature rupture of membranes, placenta previa/abruption, multiple gestation; postpartum complications (e.g., uterine atony, retained placenta
Treatment regimen [e.g., surgery, medications, administration of platelet-deficient blood products, chemotherapy]; circumcision

Note: A risk diagnosis is not evidenced by signs and symptoms, as the problem has not occurred; rather, nursing interventions are directed at prevention.

Sample Clinical Applications: Trauma, brain injury, femur fracture, aortic aneurysm, esophageal varices, pancreatitis, sickle cell anemia, surgery; use of anticoagulants

DESIRED OUTCOMES/EVALUATION CRITERIA

Sample NOC linkages:

Blood Loss Severity: Severity of internal/external hemorrhage

Blood Coagulation: Extent to which blood clots within normal period of time

Risk Control: Personal actions to prevent, eliminate, or reduce modifiable health threats

Client Will (Include Specific Time Frame)
- Be free of signs of active bleeding, such as hemoptysis, hematuria, or hematemesis, or excessive blood loss as evidenced by stable vital signs, skin and mucous membranes free of pallor, usual mentation, and urinary output.

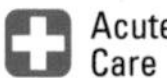
Acute Care
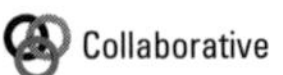
Collaborative
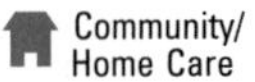
Community/ Home Care
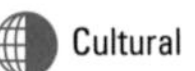
Cultural

- Display laboratory results for clotting times and factors within normal range for individual.
- Identify individual risks and engage in appropriate behaviors or lifestyle changes to prevent or reduce frequency of bleeding episodes.

ACTIONS/INTERVENTIONS

Sample NIC linkages:

Bleeding Precautions: Reduction of stimuli that may induce bleeding or hemorrhage in at-risk patients

Bleeding Reduction [specify]: Limitation of the loss of blood volume during an episode of bleeding

NURSING PRIORITY NO. 1 To assess risk factors:

- Assess client risk. Note possible medical diagnoses or disease processes that may lead to bleeding as listed in Risk Factors, such as known or suspected major trauma, coagulopathies, gastric ulcers, liver disorders, pregnancy-related complications, malignancies, gram-negative sepsis, etc.
- Note type of injury(ies) present when client presents with trauma. *The pattern and extent of injury and bleeding may or may not be readily determined. For example, unbroken skin can hide a significant injury where a large amount of blood is lost within soft tissues or a crush injury resulting in interruption of the integrity of the pelvic ring can cause life-threatening bleeding from three sources (arterial, venous, and bone edge).*[1,10,11]
- Determine presence of hereditary factors, such as hereditary hemorrhagic telangiectasia, hemophilia, or other factor deficiencies; thrombocytopenia. *Hereditary bleeding or clotting disorders predispose client to bleeding complications, either spontaneous bleeding, such as nosebleeds and acute and chronic digestive tract bleeding,*[2] *or failure to clot in a timely manner.*[1]
- Obtain detailed history if a familial bleeding disorder is suspected. *Specialized testing may be needed and/or referral to hematologist.*[1]
- Note client's gender. *While bleeding disorders are common in both men and women, women are affected more due to the increased risk of blood loss related to menstrual cycle and child delivery procedures.*[1,3]
- Note pregnancy-related factors, as indicated. *Many factors can occur, including overdistention of the uterus—pregnant with multiples, prolonged or rapid labor, lacerations occurring during vaginal delivery, or retained placenta that can place mother at risk for postpartum bleeding.*
- Evaluate client's medication regimen. *Use of medications, such as NSAIDs, anticoagulants, corticosteroids, and certain herbals (e.g., gingko biloba), predispose client to bleeding.*[4]

NURSING PRIORITY NO. 2 To evaluate for potential bleeding:

- Monitor perineum and fundal height in postpartum client and wounds, dressings, and tubes in client with trauma, surgery, or other invasive procedures *to identify active blood loss. Note: Hemorrhage may occur because of inability to achieve hemostasis in the setting of injury or may result from the development of a coagulopathy.*[2] *Excessive bleeding may be defined by the individual client's physician or the facility's written policy—such as saturating two perineal pads/hr or more than 200 mL/chest tube drainage in 4 hr.*[5]
- Evaluate and mark boundaries of soft tissues in enclosed structures such as a leg or abdomen *to document expanding bruise or hematomas. Helps in identifying bleeding that may be occurring in a closed space, which renders client susceptible to complications, such as compartment syndrome or hypovolemia; permits earlier intervention.*
- Assess vital signs, including blood pressure, pulse (may be elevated initially), and respirations. Measure blood pressure lying, sitting, and standing as indicated *to evaluate for orthostatic hypotension. Note: Vital signs do not reflect the quantity of hemorrhage accurately! Fit, young patients may lose 40% of their blood volume before the systolic blood pressure drops below 100 mmHg, whereas the elderly may become hypotensive with volume loss of as little as 10%.* Monitor invasive hemodynamic parameters when present (e.g., central venous pressure) *to determine if intravascular fluid deficit exists. Note: Client could lose up to 2 liters of blood into chest, abdomen, or pelvis before hypotension signals the presence of a problem.*[6] *The American*

College of Surgeons Advanced Trauma Life Support lists four classes of hemorrhage, with class I involving up to 15% blood volume loss and little change in vital signs and class IV involving blood loss greater than 40% of circulating volume and requiring aggressive resuscitation to prevent death.[7]

- Hematest all secretions and excretions for occult blood *to more accurately determine possible source of bleeding when blood loss is occurring and urgency of the situation.*
- Note client report of pain in specific areas and whether pain is increasing, diffuse, or localized. *Can help identify bleeding into tissues, organs, or body cavities.*
- Assess skin color and moisture, urinary output, and level of consciousness or mentation. *Changes in these signs may be indicative of blood loss affecting systemic circulation or local organ function such as kidneys or brain.*
- Review laboratory data (e.g., complete blood count, including hemoglobin [Hb], platelet numbers, and function; and other coagulation factors, which may be known by number—factor I, factor II, etc., or by name—prothrombin time, partial thromboplastin time, fibrinogen, etc.) *to evaluate bleeding risk. An abrupt drop in Hb of 2 g/dL can indicate active bleeding.*[8] *Note: When one or more of these factors are missing, produced in too small a quantity, or not functioning correctly, excessive bleeding can occur. Loss of factors may be due to acute blood loss, transfusion of factor-deficient blood, presence of inherited bleeding disorders, drugs that alter factors (e.g., warfarin, steroids, contraceptives, NSAIDs), or medical conditions affecting organs, such as cirrhosis of the liver.*[9]
- Prepare client for, or assist with, diagnostic studies, such as x-rays, computed tomography or magnetic resonance imaging scans, ultrasound, or colonoscopy, *to determine presence of injuries or disorders that could cause internal bleeding (e.g., ectopic pregnancy, damaged spleen following vehicle crash, epidural hemorrhage 2 days after a fall, reports of rectal bleeding).*

NURSING PRIORITY NO. 3 To prevent bleeding/correct potential causes of excessive blood loss:

- Apply direct pressure and ice to bleeding site, insert nasal packing, or perform fundal massage as appropriate.
- Restrict activity and encourage bedrest or chairrest until bleeding abates.
- Maintain patency of vascular access *for fluid administration or blood replacement as indicated.*
- Assist with treatment of underlying conditions causing or contributing to blood loss, such as medical treatment of systemic infections or balloon tamponade of esophageal varices prior to sclerotherapy; proton pump inhibitor medications or antibiotics for gastric ulcer; and surgery for internal abdominal trauma or retained placenta. *Treatment of underlying conditions may prevent or halt bleeding complications.*
- Provide special intervention for an at-risk client (e.g., individual with bone marrow suppression, chemotherapy, uremia) *to prevent bleeding associated with tissue injury:*

  Monitor closely for overt bleeding.

  Observe for diffuse oozing from tubes, wounds, and orifices with no observable clotting *to identify excessive bleeding and/or possible coagulopathy. Note: Client with certain conditions, such as obstetric complications, gram-negative sepsis, or massive trauma, may be predisposed to develop consumptive coagulopathy or disseminated intravascular coagulation, a potentially lethal phenomenon characterized by simultaneous clotting and continual bleeding.*[2]

  Maintain pressure or pressure dressings as indicated for a longer period of time. *May be required to stop bleeding, such as pressure dressings over arterial puncture site or surgical dressings.*

  Hematest secretions and excretions for occult blood *for early identification of internal bleeding.*

  Protect client from trauma such as falls, accidental or intentional blows, or lacerations *that could cause bleeding.*

  Use soft toothbrush or toothettes for oral care *to reduce risk of injury to oral mucosa.*
- Collaborate in evaluating need for replacing blood loss or specific components and be prepared for emergency interventions. *Institution or physician may have specific guidelines for transfusion, such as platelet count less than 20,000/mcL or Hg less than 7 g/dL, in addition to the client's clinical status.*
- Be prepared to administer hemostatic agents, such as desmopressin, *which promotes clotting and may stop bleeding by increasing coagulation factor VIII and the von Willebrand factor,* or medications to prevent

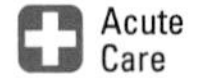
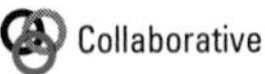
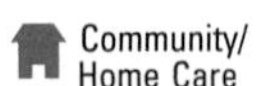
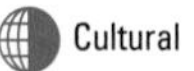

bleeding, such as proton pump inhibitors *to reduce the risk of gastrointestinal bleeding and need for replacement transfusion.*

NURSING PRIORITY NO. 4 To promote wellness (Teaching/Discharge Considerations):

- Provide information to client/family about hereditary or familial problems that predispose to bleeding complications.
- Instruct at-risk client and family regarding:

Specific signs of bleeding requiring healthcare provider notification, such as active bright bleeding anywhere, prolonged epistaxis or trauma in client with known factor bleeding tendencies, black tarry stools, weakness, vertigo, syncope, etc.

The need to inform healthcare providers when taking aspirin and other anticoagulants (e.g., Coumadin, Plavix), especially when elective surgery or other invasive procedure is planned. *These agents will most likely be withheld for a period of time prior to elective procedures to reduce potential for excessive blood loss.*

Importance of periodic review of client's medication regimen *to identify medications that might cause or exacerbate bleeding problems. Note: Some prescriptions, over-the-counter medications, and herbals (e.g., vitamin E, ginkgo, ginger, garlic, fish oils) promote bleeding.*[5]

Necessity of regular medical and laboratory follow-up when on anticoagulants, such as Coumadin (warfarin), *to determine needed dosage changes or client management issues requiring monitoring and/or modification.*

Dietary measures to improve blood clotting, such as foods rich in vitamin K.

The need to avoid alcohol in diagnosed liver disorders or seek treatment for alcoholism in presence of alcoholic varices.

Techniques for postpartum client to check her own fundus and perform fundal massage as indicated and to contact physician for postdischarge bleeding that is bright red or dark red with large clots. *May prevent blood loss complications, especially if client is discharged early from hospital.*

DOCUMENTATION FOCUS

Assessment/Reassessment

- Individual factors that may potentiate blood loss—type of injuries, obstetrical complications, etc.
- Baseline vital signs, mentation, urinary output, and subsequent assessments.
- Results of laboratory tests or diagnostic procedures.

Planning

- Plan of care and who is involved in the planning.
- Teaching plan.

Implementation/Evaluation

- Responses to interventions, teaching, and actions performed.
- Attainment or progress toward desired outcome(s).
- Modifications to plan of care.

Discharge Planning

- Long-term needs, identifying who is responsible for actions to be taken.
- Community resources or support for chronic problems.
- Specific referrals made.

References

1. Lambing, A. (2007). Bleeding disorders: Patient history key to diagnosis. *Nurs Pract*, 32(12), 16–24.
2. Ragsdale, J. A. (2007). Hereditary hemorrhagic telangiectasia from epistaxis to life-threatening GI bleeding. *Gastroenterol Nurs*, 30(4), 293–299.
3. Sommers, M. S., Johnson, S. A., Beery, T. A. (2007). *Diseases and Disorders: A Nursing Therapeutics Manual*. 3rd ed. Philadelphia: F. A. Davis.
4. Ayers, D. M., Montgomery, M. (2009). Putting a stop to dysfunctional uterine bleeding. *Nursing*, 39(1), 44–50.
5. Beattie, S. (2007). Bedside emergency: Hemorrhage. *RN*, 70(8), 30–34.
6. Dutton, R. P. (2007). Current concepts in hemorrhagic shock. *Anesthesiol Clin North Am*, 25(1), 23–34.
7. Cabañas, J. G., Manning, J. E., Cairns, C. B. (2011). Fluid and blood resuscitation. *Tintinalli's Emergency Medicine: A Comprehensive Study Guide*. 7th ed. New York: McGraw-Hill.
8. Spahn, D. R., Cerny, V., Coats, T. J., et al. (2006). Management of bleeding following major trauma: A European guideline. *Crit Care*, 11(1), 414.
9. Leeuwen, A. M., Kranpitz, T. R., Smith, L. (2006). *Davis Comprehensive Handbook of Diagnostic Tests with Nursing Implications*. 2nd ed. Philadelphia: F. A. Davis.
10. Smeltzer, M. D. (2010). Making a point about open fractures. *Nursing*, 40(2), 24–30.
11. Bodden, J. (2009). Treatment options in the hemodynamically unstable patient with a pelvic fracture. *Orthop Nurs*, 28(3), 109–114.

risk for unstable Blood Glucose Level

Taxonomy II: Nutrition—Class 4 Metabolism (00179) [**Diagnostic Division:** Food/Fluid], Submitted 2006; Revised 2013

DEFINITION: Vulnerable to variation in blood glucose/sugar levels from the normal range, which may compromise health.

RISK FACTORS

Does not accept diagnosis; insufficient knowledge of diabetes management

Insufficient diabetes management or nonadherence to diabetes management plan; inadequate blood glucose monitoring; ineffective medication management

Insufficient dietary intake; excessive weight gain or loss; rapid growth period; pregnancy

Compromised physical health status

Average daily physical activity is less than recommended for gender and age

Excessive stress; alteration in mental status

Delay in cognitive development

Note: A risk diagnosis is not evidenced by signs and symptoms, as the problem has not occurred; rather, nursing interventions are directed at prevention.

Sample Clinical Applications: Diabetes mellitus, diabetic ketoacidosis, hypoglycemia, gestational diabetes, corticosteroid use, total parenteral nutrition (TPN)

DESIRED OUTCOMES/EVALUATION CRITERIA

Sample **NOC** linkages:

Knowledge: Diabetes Management: Extent of understanding conveyed about diabetes mellitus, its treatment, and the prevention of complications

Diabetes Self-Management: Personal actions to manage diabetes mellitus, its treatment, and prevention of disease progression

Blood Glucose Level: Extent to which glucose levels in plasma and urine are maintained in normal range

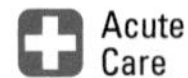

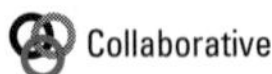

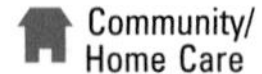

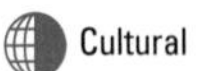

Client/caregiver Will (Include Specific Time Frame)

- Acknowledge factors that may lead to unstable glucose.
- Verbalize understanding of body and energy needs.
- Verbalize plan for modifying factors to prevent or minimize shifts in glucose level.
- Maintain glucose in satisfactory range.

ACTIONS/INTERVENTIONS

Sample NIC linkages:

Hyperglycemia Management: Preventing and treating above-normal blood glucose levels

Teaching: Disease Process: Assisting the patient to understand information related to a specific disease process

Teaching: Prescribed Medication: Preparing a patient to safely take prescribed medications and monitor for their effects

NURSING PRIORITY NO. 1 To assess risk/contributing factors:

- Determine individual factors as listed in Risk Factors. *Client or family history of diabetes, known diabetic with poor glucose control, eating disorders (e.g., morbid obesity), poor exercise habits, and failure to recognize changes in glucose needs or control due to adolescent growth spurts or pregnancy can result in problems with glucose stability.*
- Ascertain client's/significant other (SO)'s knowledge and understanding of condition and treatment needs.
- Identify individual perceptions and expectations of treatment regimen.
- Note influence of cultural, ethnic origin, socioeconomic, or religious factors impacting diabetes recognition and care, including how person with diabetes is viewed by family and community; the seeking and receiving of health care, management of factors such as dietary practices, weight, blood pressure, and lipids; and expectations of outcomes. *These factors influence client's ability to manage condition and must be considered when planning care. Numerous U.S. studies in recent years have shown that diabetes and its complications disproportionately affect African Americans and Hispanics, with few individuals receiving treatment for hyperlipidemia or albuminuria, and that there are differences in the control of glucose and hypertension. Disparities have also been found in A_1C levels between Hispanic and non-Hispanic white adults. Some ethnic groups use folk medicine and popular remedies such as bitter food and herbs to reduce blood sugar; others may practice fasting or prayer. However, because food patterns are learned in family context and have highly symbolic associations, food choices and preparation may be the most difficult aspects of diabetes management.*[11–13]
- Determine client's awareness and ability to be responsible for dealing with situation. *Age, developmental level, and current health status affect client's ability to provide for own safety.*
- Assess client family/SO(s) support of client. *Client may need assistance with lifestyle changes (e.g., food preparation, consumption, timing of intake and/or exercise, administration of medications).*
- Note availability and use of resources.

NURSING PRIORITY NO. 2 To assist client to develop preventative strategies to avoid glucose instability:

- Ascertain whether client and SO(s) are certain they are obtaining accurate readings on glucose-monitoring device and are adept at using device. *In addition to checking blood glucose more frequently when it is unstable, it is wise to ascertain that equipment is functioning properly and being used correctly. All available devices will provide accurate readings if properly used and maintained and routinely calibrated. However, there are many other factors that may affect the accuracy of numbers, such as size of blood drop with fingersticking, forgetting a bolus from insulin pump, and injecting insulin into lumpy subcutaneous site. Note: Although expensive and not widely used yet, recent technology advances include a real-time continuous blood glucose monitoring system that is a tool for detecting blood glucose trends, as well as a warning system for extreme highs and lows.*[1,15]

- Provide information on balancing food intake, antidiabetic agents, and energy expenditure.
- Review medical necessity for regularly scheduled lab screening and monitoring tests for diabetes. *Screening tests may include fasting plasma glucose or oral glucose tolerance tests. In the known or sick diabetic, tests can include fasting, daily (or numerous times in a day) finger-stick glucose levels. Also, in diabetics, regular testing of hemoglobin (Hgb)A_1C and the estimated average glucose help determine glucose control over time (few months). Recent guidelines state that "HgbA_1C level less than 7% is a reasonable goal for many, but not all patients and should be based on individualized assessment of risk for complications."* [2,3,14]
- Discuss home glucose monitoring according to individual parameters (e.g., six times per day for normal day and more frequently during times of stress) *to identify and manage glucose fluctuations.*[2]
- Identify common situations that could contribute to client's glucose instability on daily, occasional, or crisis basis. *Multiple factors can be in play at any time, such as missing meals, an adolescent growth spurt, or infection or other illness.*
- Review client's diet, especially carbohydrate intake. *Glucose balance is determined by the amount of carbohydrates consumed, which should be determined in needed grams/day.*[4]
- Encourage client to read labels and choose carbohydrates described as having a low glycemic index (GI) and foods with adequate protein, higher fiber, and low fat content. *These foods produce a slower rise in blood glucose and more stable release of insulin. Note: For most people with diabetes, the first tool for managing blood glucose is some form of carbohydrate counting. Because the type of carbohydrate also affects glucose, using the GI may be helpful in "fine-tuning" blood glucose management.*[5]
- Discuss how client's antidiabetic medication(s) work. *Drugs and combinations of drugs work in varying ways with different blood glucose control and side effects. Understanding drug actions can help client avoid or reduce risk of potential for hypoglycemic reactions.*[6]

For client receiving insulin:

- Emphasize importance of checking expiration dates of medication, inspecting insulin for cloudiness if it is normally clear, and monitoring proper storage and preparation (when mixing is required). *Affects insulin absorbability and effectiveness.*[1]
- Review type(s) of insulin used (e.g., rapid, short, intermediate, long-acting, combinations, premixed) and delivery method (e.g., subcutaneous, intramuscular injection; prefilled pen; pump). Note time when short-acting and long-acting insulins are administered. Remind client that only short-acting insulin is used in pump. *Affects timing of effects and provides clues to potential timing of glucose instability.*[1,7]
- Check injection sites periodically. *Insulin absorption can vary from day to day in healthy sites and is less absorbable in lumpy sites.*[7]
- Ascertain that all injections are being given. *Children, teenagers, and elderly clients may forget injections or be unable to self-inject; they may need reminders and supervision.*[1]

NURSING PRIORITY NO. 3 To promote wellness (Teaching/Discharge Considerations):

- Review individual risk factors and provide information *to assist client in efforts to avoid complications, such as caused by chronic hyperglycemia and acute hypoglycemia. Note: Hyperglycemia is most commonly caused by alterations in nutrition needs, inactivity, or inadequate use of antidiabetic medications. Hypoglycemia is the most common complication of antidiabetic therapy, stress, and exercise.*[1,8–10]
- Emphasize consequences of actions and choices—both immediate and long term.
- Engage client/family/caregiver in formulating a plan *to manage blood glucose level, incorporating lifestyle, age, developmental level, physical and psychological ability to manage condition.*
- Consult with dietitian about specific dietary needs based on individual situation (e.g., growth spurt, pregnancy, change in activity level following injury).
- Encourage client to develop a system for self-monitoring *to provide a sense of control and enable client to follow own progress and assist with making choices.*

- Refer to appropriate community resources, diabetic educator, and/or support groups as needed *for lifestyle modification, medical management, referral for insulin pump or glucose monitor, financial assistance for supplies, etc.*

DOCUMENTATION FOCUS

Assessment/Reassessment

- Findings related to individual situation, risk factors, current caloric intake, and dietary pattern; prescription medication use; monitoring of condition.
- Client's/caregiver's understanding of individual risks and potential complications.
- Results of laboratory tests and finger-stick testing.

Planning

- Plan of care and who is involved in planning.
- Teaching plan.

Implementation/Evaluation

- Individual responses to interventions, teaching, and actions performed.
- Specific actions and changes that are made.
- Attainment or progress toward desired outcomes.
- Modifications to plan of care.

Discharge Planning

- Long-term plans for ongoing needs, monitoring and management of condition, and who is responsible for actions to be taken.
- Sources for equipment and supplies.
- Specific referrals made.

References

1. Ambler, G. R. (2010). Monitoring diabetes control (Chapter 7). In Cameron, F. J. (ed). *Caring for Diabetes in Children and Adolescents.* 3rd ed. Homebush, NSW: Blue Star Print Group.
2. Gardner, B. M. (2002). Current approaches to type 2 diabetes mellitus. Retrieved March 2015 from www.medscape.com/viewarticle/444348.
3. Buse, J. B. (2003). Normal A1c but unstable blood glucose. Retrieved March 2015 from http://www.medscape.com/viewarticle/463024.
4. Moshang, J. (2005). The growing problem of type 2 diabetes. *LPN*, 1(3), 26–34.
5. American Diabetes Association. (updated 2014). Glycemic index and diabetes. Retrieved March 2015 from http://www.diabetes.org/food-and-fitness/food/what-can-i-eat/understanding-carbohydrates/glycemic-index-and-diabetes.html.
6. Griffin, R. M. (2011). New type 2 diabetes treatment options. Retrieved March 2015 from http://diabetes.webmd.com/features/new-treatments.
7. Mathur, R. (2011). Insulin therapy for diabetes: Past, present and future. Retrieved March 2015 from hhttp://www.medicinenet.com/script/main/art.asp?articlekey=11441.
8. Iscoe, K. E., Campbell, J. E., Jamnik, V., et al. (2006). Efficacy of continuous real-time blood glucose monitoring during and after prolonged high-intensity cycling exercise: Spinning with a continuous glucose monitoring system. *Diabetes Technol Ther*, 8(6), 627–635.
9. McLeod, M. E. (2006). Interventions for clients with diabetes mellitus. In Ignativicius, D. D., Workman, M. L. (eds). *Medical-Surgical Nursing: Critical Thinking for Collaborative Care.* 5th ed. Philadelphia: Elsevier Saunders.
10. Asp, A. A. (2005). Diabetes mellitus. In Copstead, L. C., Banasik, J. L. (eds). *Pathophysiology.* 3rd ed. Philadelphia: Elsevier Saunders.
11. Bonds, D. E., Zaccaro, D. J., Karter, A. J., et al. (2004). Ethnic and racial differences in diabetes care: The insulin resistance atherosclerosis study. *Diabetes Care*, 26(4), 1040–1046.
12. Kirk, J. K., Passmore, L. V., Bell, R. A., et al. (2008). Disparities in A_1C levels between Hispanic and non-Hispanic white adults with diabetes: A meta-analysis. *Diabetes Care*, 31(2), 240–246.

13. Tripp-Reimer, T., Choi, E., Kelley, L. S., et al. (2001). Cultural barriers to care: Inverting the problem. *Diabetes Spectrum*, 14(1), 13–22.
14. Quaseem, A., Vijan, S., Snow, J. T., et al. (2007). Glycemic control and type 2 diabetes mellitis: The optimal hemoblogin A_1 C targets: A guidance statement from the American College of Physicians. *Ann Intern Med*, 147(6), 417–422.
15. Ramchandani, N., Saadon, Y., Jornsay, D. (2010). Diabetes under control: Real-time glucose monitoring. *Am J Nurs*, 110(4), 60–63.

disturbed Body Image

Taxonomy II: Self-Perception—Class 3 Body Image (00118) [**Diagnostic Division:** Ego Integrity], Submitted 1973; Revised 1998

DEFINITION: Confusion in [and/or dissatisfaction with] mental picture of one's physical self.

RELATED FACTORS

Illness; trauma; injury; surgical procedure; treatment regimen
Alteration in body function (due to anomaly, disease, medication, pregnancy, radiation, surgery, trauma, etc.)
Cultural or spiritual incongruences
Alteration in self-perception, cognitive functioning
Impaired psychosocial functioning
Developmental transition
[Significance of body part or functioning with regard to age, gender, developmental level, or basic human needs]

DEFINING CHARACTERISTICS

Subjective

Alteration in view of one's body (e.g., appearance, structure, function)
Perceptions that reflect an altered view of one's body appearance
Fear of reaction by others
Focus on past strength, function, or appearance
Negative feeling about body
Preoccupation with change or loss
Refusal to verify actual change
Emphasis on remaining strengths
Personalization of body part/loss by name
Depersonalization of body part/loss by use of impersonal pronouns

Objective

Behavior of: acknowledging one's body, monitoring one's body
Nonverbal response to actual or perceived change in body (e.g., appearance, structure, function)
Alteration in body structure or function; absence of body part
Avoids looking at or touching one's body
Trauma to nonfunctioning part
Change in ability to estimate spatial relationship of body to environment
Extension of body boundary (e.g., includes external object)
Hiding or overexposure of body part

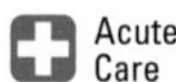

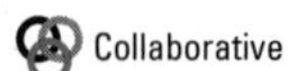

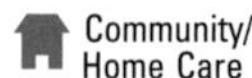

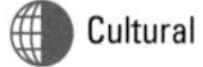

Change in lifestyle, social involvement
Heightened achievement
[Aggression; low frustration tolerance level]
Sample Clinical Applications: Eating disorders (anorexia/bulimia nervosa), traumatic injuries, amputation, ostomies, aging process, arthritis, pregnancy, chronic renal failure, renal dialysis, burns

DESIRED OUTCOMES/EVALUATION CRITERIA

Sample NOC linkages:
Body Image: Positive perception of own appearance and body functions
Self-Esteem: Personal judgment of self-worth
Adaptation to Physical Disability: Adaptive response to a significant functional challenge due to a physical disability

Client Will (Include Specific Time Frames)

- Verbalize acceptance of self in situation (e.g., chronic progressive disease, amputee, decreased independence, weight as is, effects of therapeutic regimen).
- Verbalize relief of anxiety and adaptation to altered body image.
- Verbalize understanding of body changes.
- Recognize and incorporate body image change into self-concept in accurate manner without negating self-esteem.
- Seek information and actively pursue growth.
- Acknowledge self as an individual who has responsibility for self.
- Use adaptive devices or prosthesis appropriately.

ACTIONS/INTERVENTIONS

Sample NIC linkages:
Body Image Enhancement: Improving a patient's conscious and unconscious perceptions and attitudes toward his or her body
Developmental Enhancement: Adolescent: Facilitating optimal physical, cognitive, social, and emotional growth of individuals during the transition from childhood to adulthood
Self-Esteem Enhancement: Assisting a patient to increase his or her personal judgment of self-worth

NURSING PRIORITY NO. 1 To assess causative/contributing factors:

- Discuss pathophysiology present or situation affecting the individual and refer to additional NDs, as appropriate. For example, when alteration in body image is related to neurological deficit (e.g., stroke), refer to ND Unilateral Neglect; for presence of severe, ongoing pain, refer to ND chronic Pain; or for loss of sexual desire/ability, refer to ND Sexual Dysfunction.
- Determine whether condition is permanent with no hope for resolution. (May be associated with other NDs such as Self-Esteem [specify] or risk for impaired Attachment when child is affected.) *Identifies appropriate interventions based on reality of situation and need to plan for long- or short-term prognosis. Note: There is always something that can be done to enhance acceptance, and it is important to hold out the possibility of living a good life with the disability.*[1]
- Assess the mental and physical influence of illness or condition on the client's emotional state (e.g., diseases of the endocrine system, use of steroid therapy). *Some diseases can have a profound effect on one's emotions and need to be considered in the evaluation and treatment of the individual's behavior and reaction to the current situation.*[1,9]
- Evaluate level of client's knowledge of and anxiety related to situation. Observe emotional changes. *Provides information about starting point for providing information about illness. Emotional changes may indicate level of anxiety and need for intervention to lower anxiety before learning can take place.*[1]

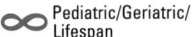

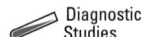

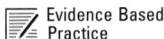

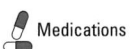

- Recognize behavior indicative of overt preoccupation with body and its processes. *May interfere with ability to engage in therapy and indicate need to provide interventions to deal with concern before beginning therapy.*[2,3]
- Assume all individuals are sensitive to changes in appearance, but avoid stereotyping. *Not all individuals react to body changes in the same way, and it is important to determine how this person is reacting to changes.*[2,3]
- Have client describe self, noting what is positive and what is negative. Be aware of how client believes others see self. *Identifies self-image and whether there is a discrepancy between own view and how client believes others see him or her, which may have an effect on how client perceives changes that have occurred.*[3,4]
- ∞ Discuss meaning of loss or change to client. *A small (seemingly trivial) loss may have a big impact (such as the use of a urinary catheter or enema for bowel continence). A change in function (such as immobility) may be more difficult for some to deal with than a change in appearance. Permanent facial scarring of child may be difficult for parents to accept.*[1]
- ∞ Use developmentally appropriate communication techniques for determining exact expression of body image in child (e.g., puppet play or constructive dialogue for toddler). *Developmental capacity must guide interaction to gain accurate information.*[4]
- Note signs of grieving or indicators of severe or prolonged depression. *May require evaluation of need for counseling or medications.*[3]
- Determine ethnic background and cultural or religious perceptions and considerations. *Understanding how these factors affect the individual in this situation and how they may influence how individual deals with what has happened is necessary to develop appropriate interventions.*[5]
- Identify social aspects of illness or disease. *Sexually transmitted infections, sterility, or chronic conditions (e.g., vitiligo, multiple sclerosis) may affect how client views self and functions in social settings and how others view the client.*[2,8]
- Observe interaction of client with significant others (SOs). *Distortions in body image may be unconsciously reinforced by family members, or secondary gain issues may interfere with progress.*[2,8]

NURSING PRIORITY NO. 2. To determine coping abilities and skills:

- Assess client's current level of adaptation and progress. *Client may have already adapted somewhat, and information provides starting point for developing plan of care.*[2]
- Listen to client's comments and note responses to the situation. *Different situations are upsetting to different people, depending on individual coping skills, severity of the perceived changes in body image, and past experiences with similar illnesses/conditions.*[2–4,8]
- Note withdrawn behavior and the use of denial. *May be normal response to situation or may be indicative of mental illness (e.g., depression, schizophrenia).*[6] (Refer to ND ineffective Denial.)
- Note dependence on prescription medications or use of addictive substances/alcohol. *May reflect dysfunctional coping as client turns to use of these substances to avoid dealing with changes that are occurring to body or ability to function in his or her accustomed manner.*[6]
- Identify previously used coping strategies and effectiveness. *Familiar coping strategies can be used to begin adaptation to current situation.*[2]
- Determine individual/family/community resources. *Can provide efficient assistance and support to enable the client to adapt to changing circumstances.*[4]

NURSING PRIORITY NO. 3 To assist client and SO(s) to deal with/accept issues of self-concept related to body image:

- Establish a therapeutic nurse-client relationship. *Conveys an attitude of caring and develops a sense of trust in which client can discuss concerns and find answers to issues confronting him or her in new situation.*[4,8]
- Visit client frequently and acknowledge the individual as someone who is worthwhile. *Provides opportunities for listening to concerns and questions to promote dealing positively with individual situation and change in body image.*[1]

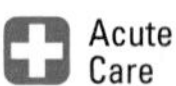
Acute Care
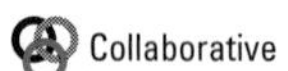
Collaborative
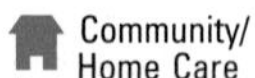
Community/ Home Care
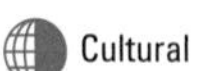
Cultural

- Assist in correcting underlying problems when possible. *Promotes optimal healing and adaptation to individual situation (i.e., amputation, presence of colostomy, mastectomy, impotence).*[1]
- Provide assistance with self-care needs or measures, as necessary, while promoting individual abilities and independence. *Client needs support to achieve the goal of independence and positive return to managing own life.*[4]
- Work with client's self-concept without moral judgments regarding client's efforts or progress (e.g., "You should be progressing faster; you're weak, lazy, not trying hard enough"). *Such statements diminish self-esteem and are counterproductive to progress. Positive reinforcement encourages client to continue efforts and strive for improvement.*[2,8]
- Discuss concerns about fear of mutilation, prognosis, and rejection when client is facing surgery or potentially poor outcome of procedure or illness. *Addresses realities and provides emotional support to enable client to be ready to deal with whatever the outcome may be.*[1]
- Acknowledge and accept feelings of dependency, grief, and hostility. *Conveys a message of understanding.*[1]
- Encourage verbalization of anticipated conflicts *to enhance handling of potential situations. Provides an opportunity to imagine and practice how different situations can be dealt with, thus promoting confidence.*[4]
- Encourage client and SO(s) to communicate feelings to each other and discuss situation openly. *Enhances relationship, improving sense of self-worth and sense of support.*[2]
- Alert staff to be cognizant of own facial expressions and other nonverbal behaviors. *Important to convey acceptance and not revulsion, especially when the client's appearance is affected. Clients are very sensitive to reactions of those around them, and negative reactions will affect self-esteem and may retard adaptation to situation.*[1]
- Encourage family members to treat client normally and not as an invalid. *Helps client return to own routine and begin to gain confidence in ability to manage own life.*[1]
- Encourage client to look at and touch affected body part *to begin to incorporate changes into body image. Acceptance will enhance self-esteem and enable client to move forward in a positive manner.*[1,7]
- Allow client to use denial without participating (e.g., client may at first refuse to look at a colostomy; the nurse says, "I am going to change your colostomy now" and proceeds with the task). *Provides individual time to adapt to situation.*[4,9]
- Set limits on maladaptive behavior; assist client to identify positive behaviors. *Self-esteem will be damaged if client is allowed to continue behaviors that are destructive or not helpful, and adaptation to new image will be delayed.*[4,10]
- Provide accurate information, as desired or requested. Reinforce previously given information. *Accurate knowledge helps client make better decisions for the future.*[4]
- Discuss the availability of prosthetics, reconstructive surgery, and physical and occupational therapy or other referrals, as dictated by individual situation. *Provides hope that situation is not impossible and the future does not look so bleak.*[1,7,8]
- Help client to select and creatively use clothing or makeup *to minimize body changes and enhance appearance.*[1]
- Discuss reasons for infectious isolation and procedures when used, and make time to sit down and talk or listen to client while in the room. *Promotes understanding and decreases sense of isolation and loneliness.*[1]

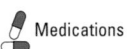

NURSING PRIORITY NO. 4 To promote wellness (Teaching/Discharge Considerations):

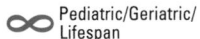

- Begin counseling or other therapies (e.g., biofeedback or relaxation techniques) as soon as possible. *Provides early and ongoing sources of support to promote rehabilitation in a timely manner.*[1]
- Provide information at client's level of acceptance and in small segments. *Allows for easier assimilation.*[1,2,7]
- Clarify misconceptions and reinforce explanations given by other health team members. *Ensures client is hearing factual information to make the best decisions for own situation.*[1,2,7]
- Include client in decision-making process and problem-solving activities. *Promotes adherence to decisions and plans that are made.*[1]

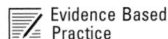

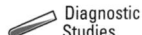

- Assist client to incorporate therapeutic regimen into activities of daily living (e.g., specific exercises, housework activities). *Promotes continuation of program by helping client see that progress can be made within own daily activities.*[1]
- Identify and plan for alterations to home and work environment or activities when necessary. *Accommodates individual needs and supports independence.*[1,9]
- Assist client in learning strategies for dealing with feelings and venting emotions. *Helps individual move toward healing and optimal recuperation.*[1,2]
- Offer positive reinforcement for efforts made (e.g., wearing makeup, using prosthetic device). *Client needs to hear that what he or she is doing is helping.*[1,9]
- Refer to appropriate support groups. *May need additional help to adjust to new situation and life changes.*[1]

DOCUMENTATION FOCUS

Assessment/Reassessment

- Observations, presence of maladaptive behaviors, emotional changes, stage of grieving, level of independence.
- Physical wounds, dressings; use of life support–type machine (e.g., ventilator, dialysis machine).
- Meaning of loss or change to client.
- Support systems available (e.g., SOs, friends, groups).

Planning

- Plan of care and who is involved in planning.
- Teaching plan.

Implementation/Evaluation

- Client's response to interventions, teaching, and actions performed.
- Attainment or progress toward desired outcome(s).
- Modifications of plan of care.

Discharge Planning

- Long-term needs and who is responsible for actions.
- Specific referrals made (e.g., rehabilitation center, community resources).

References

1. Tagkalakis, P., Demiri, E. (2009). A fear avoidance model in facial burn body image disturbance. *Ann Burns Fire Disasters*, 22(4), 203–207.
2. No author listed. (2009). Body image. Women's Health. Retrieved April 2015 from http://www.womenshealth.gov/body-image/.
3. Kilic, E., Taycan, O., Belli, A. K., et al. (2007). The effect of permanent ostomy on body image, self-esteem, marital adjustment, and sexual functioning. *Turk Psikiyatri Derg*, 18(4), 302–310.
4. Gerber, R. (2010). Beauty and body image in the media. Media Awareness Network. Retrieved April 2015 from http://www.media-awareness.ca/english/issues/stereotyping/women_and_girls/women_beauty.cfm?RenderForPrint=1.
5. George, J. B., Franko, D. L. (2010). Cultural issues in eating pathology and body image among children and adolescents. *J Pediatr Psychol*, 35(3), 231–242.
6. Pimenta, A. M., Sanchez-Villegas, A., Bes-Rastrolo, M., et al. (2009). Relationship between body image disturbance and incidence of depression: The SUN prospective cohort. *BMC Public Health*, 9(1), 1471–2458.
7. Aacovou, I. (2005). The role of the nurse in the rehabilitation of patients with radical changes in body image due to burn injuries. *Ann Burns Fire Disasters*, 18(2), 89–94.
8. Breakey, J. W. (1997). Body image: The inner mirror. *J Prosthet Orthot*, 9(3), 107–112.
9. Kater, K. (updated 2012). Healthy Bodies curriculum. Retrieved April 2015 from http://bodyimagehealth.org/resources/.
10. Reasoner, R. (2010). The true meaning of self-esteem. National Association for Self-Esteem. Retrieved April 2015 from http://www.self-esteem-nase.org/what.php.

risk for imbalanced Body Temperature

Taxonomy II: Safety/Protection—Class 6 Thermoregulation (00005) [**Diagnostic Division:** Safety], Submitted 1986; Revised 2000, 2013

DEFINITION: Vulnerable to failure to maintain body temperature within normal parameters, which may compromise health.

RISK FACTORS

Acute brain injury; sepsis
Alteration in metabolic rate; condition affecting temperature regulation; increase in oxygen demand; inefficient nonshivering thermogenesis
Decreased sweat response; dehydration
Extremes of age or weight; increased body surface area to weight ratio; insufficient supply of subcutaneous fat
Extremes of environmental temperature; improper clothing for environmental temperature;
Inactivity; vigorous activity
Pharmaceutical agent; sedation
Note: A risk diagnosis is not evidenced by signs and symptoms, as the problem has not occurred; rather, nursing interventions are directed at prevention.
Sample Clinical Applications: Any infectious process, surgical procedures, brain injuries, hypo/hyperthyroidism, prematurity

DESIRED OUTCOMES/EVALUATION CRITERIA

Sample NOC linkages:
Thermoregulation: Balance among heat production, heat gain, and heat loss
Thermoregulation: Newborn: Balance among heat production, heat gain, and heat loss during the first 28 days of life
Post-Procedure Recovery: Extent to which an individual returns to baseline function following a procedure(s) requiring anesthesia or sedation

Client Will (Include Specific Time Frame)
- Maintain body temperature within normal range.
- Verbalize understanding of individual risk factors and appropriate interventions.
- Demonstrate behaviors for monitoring and maintaining appropriate body temperature.

ACTIONS/INTERVENTIONS

Sample NIC linkages:
Risk Identification: Analysis of risk factors, determination of health risks, and prioritization of risk reduction strategies for an individual or group
Temperature Regulation: Attaining or maintaining body temperature within a normal range
Temperature Regulation: Intraoperative: Attaining or maintaining desired intraoperative body temperature

NURSING PRIORITY NO. 1 To identify causative/risk factors present:

- Note presence of condition that can affect body's heat production and heat dissipation (e.g., spinal cord injury; burns or skin diseases; endocrine disorders; neurological disorders, such as Parkinson's disease; kidney disease; being significantly overweight or underweight).[3,4,7]

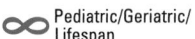

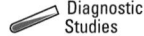

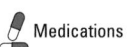

- Determine if present illness or condition has resulted from exposure to environmental factors, surgery, infection, or trauma. *Helps to determine the scope of interventions that may be needed (e.g., simple addition of warm blankets after surgery or hypothermia therapy following brain trauma).*[1,8]
- Monitor laboratory values (e.g., tests indicative of infection, thyroid or other endocrine tests, drug screens) *to identify potential internal causes of temperature imbalances.*
- Note client's age (e.g., premature neonate, young child, or aging individual), *as it can directly impact ability to maintain or regulate body temperature and respond to changes in environment.*[5,7]
- Assess nutritional status *to determine metabolism effect on body temperature and to identify foods or nutrient deficits that affect metabolism.*

NURSING PRIORITY NO. 2 To prevent occurrence of temperature alteration:

- Monitor temperature regularly, measuring core body temperature whenever needed to observe this vital sign. Exercise care in selecting appropriate thermometer for client's age and clinical condition, and observe for inconsistencies in readings obtained with various instruments. Observe temperature reading for trends, and avoid basing therapeutic decisions solely on thermometer readings. *Traditionally, temperature measurements have been taken orally (good in alert, oriented adults), rectally (accurate, but not always easy to obtain), or axillary (readings may be lower than core temperature), with each site offering advantages and disadvantages in terms of accuracy and safety. Newer technologies allow temperatures to be instantly measured. Tympanic temperature measurement is a noninvasive way to measure core temperature, as blood is supplied to the tympanic membrane by the carotid artery.*[3] *In adult intensive-care patients, both oral and temporal artery measurements have been found to be accurate and precise.*[9] *Note: Research shows that many factors affect the accuracy and precision of various temperature measurement methods; for example, oral measurements can be changed by incorrect positioning of the probe or by drinking hot/cold liquids, and ear-based measurements can be affected by excessive ear wax or taking temperature in the ear that has been against a pillow.*[2]
- Maintain comfortable ambient environment *to reduce effect on body-temperature alterations:*[1,4,6,7]
  Provide environmental heating or cooling measures, as needed, such as space heater or air conditioner or fans.
  Ascertain that cooling and warming equipment and supplies are available during or following procedures and surgery.
- Dress or discuss with client/caregivers appropriate dressing for client's condition:[6–8]
  Wear layers of clothing that can be removed or added as needed. Wear hat and gloves in cold weather; wear light, loose protective clothing in hot weather; and wear water-resistant outer gear *to protect from changes in weather or wet weather chill.*
  Cover infant's head with knit cap, use layers of lightweight blankets, and provide for skin-to skin contact with mother. Place newborn infant under a radiant warmer. Teach parents to dress infant appropriately for weather and home environment. *Newborns/infants, especially very low weight neonates, can have temperature instability with heat loss greatest through head and by evaporation and convection.*[5]
  Limit clothing or remove blanket from premature infant placed in incubator *to prevent overheating in climate-controlled environment.*
- Maintain adequate fluid intake. Offer cool or warm liquids, as appropriate. *Hydration assists in maintaining normal body temperature.*[1,4,7,8]
- Restore and maintain core temperature within client's normal range. (If temperature is below or above normal range, or parameters defined by physician, refer to NDs Hypothermia or Hyperthermia for additional interventions.)
- Recommend lifestyle changes, such as cessation of substance use, normalization of body weight, nutritious meals, or regular exercise *to maximize metabolism and general health.*[1]
- Refer at-risk persons to appropriate community resources (e.g., home care, social services, Foster Adult Care, housing agencies) *to provide assistance to meet individual needs.*[1]

NURSING PRIORITY NO. 3 To promote wellness (Teaching/Discharge Considerations):

- Review potential problem or individual risk factors with client/significant other(s).
- Discuss effects of age and gender with client/caregiver, as appropriate. *Older or debilitated persons, infants, and young children typically feel more comfortable in higher ambient temperatures. Women notice feeling cool quicker than men, which may be related to body size or to differences in metabolism and the rate that blood flows to extremities to regulate body temperature.*[6,7]
- Instruct in measures to protect from identified risk factors. *Provides understanding for ways in managing lifestyle and environment (e.g., adding or removing clothing, adding or removing heat sources, evaluating home or shelter for ability to manage heat and cold, addressing nutritional and hydration status) and enhances self-care abilities.*[6]
- Review client's medications for possible thermoregulatory side effects (e.g., diuretics, certain sedatives and antipsychotic agents, some heart and blood pressure medications, anesthesia).[1,7,8]
- Discuss with client using sympathomimetics (e.g., cocaine, methamphetamines) the effects of drug on body temperature regulation.[1,7,8]
- Identify ways to prevent accidental thermoregulation problems. *For example, hypothermia can result from overzealous cooling to reduce fever or maintaining too warm an environment when client has lost the ability to perspire can lead to hyperthermia.*

DOCUMENTATION FOCUS

Assessment/Reassessment

- Identified individual causative or risk factors.
- Record of core temperature, initially and prn.
- Results of diagnostic studies and laboratory tests.

Planning

- Plan of care and who is involved in planning.
- Teaching plan, including best ambient temperature and ways to prevent hypothermia or hyperthermia.

Implementation/Evaluation

- Response to interventions, teaching, and actions performed.
- Attainment or progress toward desired outcome(s).
- Modifications to plan of care.

Discharge Planning

- Long-term needs and who is responsible for actions.
- Specific referrals made.

References

1. Doenges, M. E., Moorhouse, M. F., Murr, A. C. (2010). Surgical intervention. *Nursing Care Plans: Nursing Care Plans Across the Life Span.* 8th ed. Philadelphia: F. A. Davis.
2. Bridges, E., Thomas, K. (2009). Noninvasive measurement of body temperature in critically ill patients. *Crit Care Nurse*, 29(3), 94–97.
3. Sund-Lavander, M., Grodzinsky, E., Lloyd, D., et al. (2004). Errors in body temperature measurement in febrile intensive care patients. *Int J Nurs Pract*, 10(5), 216–223.
4. American Academy of Pediatrics: Section on Anesthesiology. (1999). Guidelines for the pediatric perioperative anesthesia environment. *Pediatrics*, 103(2), 512–515.

5. Knobel, R., Holditch-Davis, D. (2007). Thermoregulation and heat loss prevention after birth and during neonatal intensive care unit stabilization of extremely low birth weight infants. *J Obstet Gynecol Neonatal Nurs*, 36(3), 280–287.
6. Beattie, S. (2006). In from the cold. *RN*, 69(11), 22–27.
7. Knies, R. C. (No date). Geriatric thermoregulation. Emergency Nursing World! Retrieved March 2015 from http://enw.org/Research-GeriTherm.htm.
8. Helman, R. S., Habal, R. (updated 2014). Heatstroke. Retrieved March 2014 from http://emedicine.medscape.com/article/166320-overview.
9. Moore, K. (2008). Hypothermia in trauma. *J Trauma Nurs*, 15(2), 62–64.

ineffective Breastfeeding

Taxonomy II: Nutrition—Class 1 Ingestion (00104) [**Diagnostic Division:** Food/Fluid], Submitted 1988; Revised 2010, 2013

DEFINITION: Difficulty providing milk to an infant or young child directly from the breasts, which may compromise nutritional status of the infant/child.

RELATED FACTORS

Insufficient parental knowledge regarding importance of breastfeeding or breastfeeding techniques
Insufficient opportunity for suckling at the breast; inadequate milk supply; delayed lactogenesis II
Prematurity [late preterm (35 to 37 weeks)]; poor infant sucking reflex
Oropharyngeal defect [e.g., cleft palate/lip, ankyloglossia (tongue tied)]
Supplemental feedings with artificial nipple; pacifier use
Maternal anxiety or ambivalence, fatigue, pain, obesity
Previous history of breastfeeding failure
Interrupted breastfeeding; short maternity leave
Maternal breast anomaly; previous breast surgery

DEFINING CHARACTERISTICS

Subjective

Sore nipples persisting beyond the first week of breastfeeding
Insufficient emptying of each breast per feeding
Perceived inadequate milk supply

Objective

Insufficient opportunity for suckling at the breast
Infant inability to latch on to maternal breast correctly; unsustained suckling at the breast
Infant arching or crying at the breast; resisting latching on to breast
Infant crying within the first hour after breastfeeding; fussing within 1 hour of breastfeeding; unresponsive to other comfort measures
Insufficient signs of oxytocin release
Inadequate infant stooling
Insufficient infant weight gain; sustained infant weight loss

Sample Clinical Applications: Prematurity, cleft lip/palate, ankyloglossia, Down Syndrome, child abuse or neglect, failure to thrive, diseases/infections of the breast

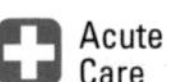

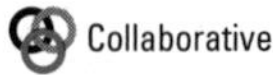

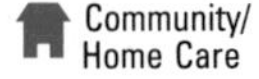

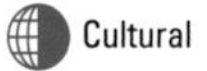

DESIRED OUTCOMES/EVALUATION CRITERIA

Sample NOC linkages:

Knowledge: Breastfeeding: Extent of understanding conveyed about lactation and nourishment of infant through breastfeeding

Breastfeeding Establishment: Maternal [or] Infant: Maternal establishment of proper attachment of an infant to and sucking from the breast for nourishment during the first 3 weeks of breastfeeding/infant attachment to and sucking from the mother's breast for nourishment during the first 3 weeks of breastfeeding

Breastfeeding Maintenance: Continuation of breastfeeding from establishment to weaning for nourishment of an infant/toddler

Client Will (Include Specific Time Frame)

- Verbalize understanding of causative or contributing factors.
- Demonstrate techniques to enhance breastfeeding experience.
- Assume responsibility for effective breastfeeding.
- Achieve mutually satisfactory breastfeeding regimen with infant content after feedings, gaining weight appropriately, and output within normal range.

ACTIONS/INTERVENTIONS

Sample NIC linkages:

Breastfeeding Assistance: Preparing a new mother to breastfeed her infant

Lactation Counseling: Use of an interactive helping process to assist in maintenance of successful breastfeeding

Support Group: Use of a group environment to provide emotional support and health-related information for members

NURSING PRIORITY NO. 1 To identify maternal causative/contributing factors:

- Assess client knowledge about breastfeeding and extent of instruction previously received. *Provides baseline information for identifying needs and developing plan of care.*[1,7]
- Encourage discussion of current and previous breastfeeding experience(s). *Identifies current needs and problems encountered to develop a plan of care.*[5]
- Note previous unsatisfactory experience (including self or others). *Often unsolved problems and stories told by others may cause doubt about chance for success.*[1]
- Perform physical assessment, noting appearance of breasts and nipples, marked asymmetry of breasts, obvious inverted or flat nipples, and minimal or no breast enlargement during pregnancy. *Identifies existing problems that may interfere with successful breastfeeding experience and provides opportunity to correct them when possible.*[1,7]
- Determine whether lactation failure is primary (i.e., maternal prolactin deficiency/serum prolactin levels, inadequate mammary gland tissue, breast surgery that has damaged the nipple, areola enervation, pituitary disorders) or secondary (i.e., sore nipples, severe engorgement, plugged milk ducts, mastitis, inhibition of letdown reflex, maternal/infant separation with disruption of feedings). *Primary failure may be irremediable, and alternate plans may need to be made. Secondary failure can be remedied so breastfeeding efforts can be successful.*[5] *Note: Overweight women and obese women are 2.5 times and 3.6 times, respectively, less successful in initiating breastfeeding than the general population.*[9]
- Note history of pregnancy, labor, and delivery (vaginal or cesarean section); other recent or current surgery; preexisting medical problems (e.g., diabetes mellitus, seizure disorder, cardiac diseases, presence of disabilities); or if client is adoptive mother. *While some conditions may preclude breastfeeding and alternate plans need to be made, others will need specific plans for monitoring and treatment to ensure successful breastfeeding.*[5]

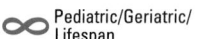

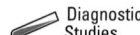

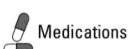

- Identify maternal support systems and presence and response of significant other (SO), extended family, and friends. *Infant's father and maternal grandmother (in addition to caring healthcare providers) are important factors in whether breastfeeding is successful.*[8] *Having sufficient support enhances opportunity for a successful breastfeeding experience. Negative attitudes and comments interfere with efforts and may cause client to abandon attempt to breastfeed.*[5]
- Ascertain mother's age, number of children at home, and need to return to work or school. *These factors may have a detrimental effect on desire to breastfeed. Immaturity may influence mother to avoid breastfeeding, believing that it will be inconvenient, or may cause her to be insensitive to the infant's needs. The stress of the responsibility of other children or the need to return to work can affect the ability to manage effective breastfeeding; mother will need support and information to be successful.*[6]
- Determine maternal feelings (e.g., fear, anxiety, ambivalence, depression). *Indicators of underlying emotional state that may suggest need for intervention and referral.*[1]
- Ascertain cultural expectations or conflicts about breastfeeding and beliefs and practices regarding lactation, letdown techniques, and maternal food preferences. *Understanding impact of culture and idiosyncrasies of specific feeding practices is important to determine the effect on infant feeding. The practice may be different but not inferior. For example, in some cultures, colostrum is not offered to the newborn. Intervention is only necessary if the practice/belief is harmful to the infant.*[1,3,8]
- Note incorrect myths or misunderstandings, especially in teenage mothers *who are more likely to have limited knowledge and more concerns about body image issues.*[8]

NURSING PRIORITY NO. 2 To assess infant causative/contributing factors:

- Determine suckling problems or infant anomaly (e.g., cleft lip/palate). *These factors indicate need for interventions directed at correcting individual situation. Conditions such as cleft palate need evaluation for correction and individualized instruction in holding infant upright and using special nipple or feeding device, such as a Haberman feeder.*[1,2] *Note: One study indicated that about one-half of mothers in the study were unable to breastfeed infants with cleft lip and/or palate.*[14]
- Note prematurity. *Degree of prematurity will dictate type of interventions needed to deal with situation. Infant may be put to breast if sufficiently developed or mother may pump breast and the breast milk given via gavage. If infant breastfeeds, mother should pump afterwards because the premature infant's suck cannot empty breast.* [2]
- Encourage mother to keep a log of intake and output. Review feeding schedule to note increased demand for feeding (at least eight times/day, taking both breasts at each feeding for more than 15 min on each side) or use of supplements with artificial nipple. *Provides opportunity to evaluate infant's growth, determine whether sufficient nourishment is provided, and make adjustments as needed.*[2]
- Evaluate baby latching and note observable signs of inadequate infant intake. *Inadequate latching, baby latching onto mother's nipples with sustained suckling but minimal audible swallowing noted, infant arching and crying at the breasts with resistance to latching on, decreased urinary output/frequency of stools, and inadequate weight gain all indicate need for evaluation and intervention.*[1,7]
- Determine whether baby is content after feeding or exhibits fussiness and crying within the first hour after breastfeeding. *Suggests unsatisfactory breastfeeding process.*[1]
- Note any correlation between maternal ingestion of certain foods and "colicky" response of infant. *Some foods may seem to result in reaction by the infant, and identification and elimination may correct the problem.*[2]

NURSING PRIORITY NO. 3 To assist mother to develop skills of successful breastfeeding:

- Provide emotional support to mother. Use one-to-one instruction with each feeding during hospital stay/clinic visit. *New mothers say they would like more support, encouragement, and practical information, especially when they are discharged early. Contact during each feeding provides the opportunity to develop nurse-client*

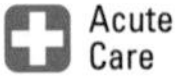

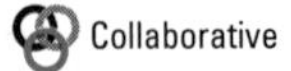

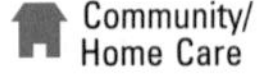

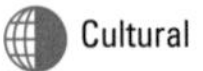

relationship in which these goals can be attained.[1] *Note: Adoptive mothers choosing to breastfeed will require more supportive instruction from a lactation consultant to assist with induced lactation techniques.*[8]

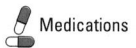

- Encourage skin-to-skin or kangaroo care, especially for the premature infant. *Studies show that early skin-to-skin mother-infant contact is correlated with exclusive breastfeeding while in the hospital.*[16,21]
- Inform mother how to assess and correct a latch if needed. Demonstrate asymmetric latch by aiming infant's lower lip as far from base of the nipple as possible and then bringing infant's chin and lower jaw in contact with breast while mouth is wide open and before upper lip touches breast. *This position allows infant to use both tongue and jaw more effectively to obtain milk from the breast.*[17,21]
- Discuss early infant feeding cues (e.g., rooting, lip smacking, sucking fingers or hand) versus the late cue of crying. *New mothers may not be aware that these behaviors indicate hunger and may not respond appropriately. Early recognition of infant hunger promotes timely and more rewarding feeding experience for infant and mother.*[1,8]
- Recommend avoidance or overuse of supplemental bottle feedings and pacifiers (unless specifically indicated). *These can lessen infant's desire to breastfeed. The shape of the mouth and lips and the sucking mechanism are different for breast and bottle, and the infant may be confused by the difference, causing interference in the breastfeeding process and increasing risk of early weaning. Note: Adoptive mothers may not develop a full breast milk supply, necessitating supplemental feedings.*[1,8]
- Restrict use of nipple shields (i.e., only temporarily to help draw the nipple out) and then place baby directly on nipple. *These have been found to contribute to lactation failures. Shields prevent the infant's mouth from coming into contact with the mother's nipple, which is necessary for continued release of prolactin (promoting milk production) and can interfere with or prevent establishment of adequate milk supply. However, temporary use of shield may be beneficial in the presence of severe nipple cracking. Hand pumps can also help draw a flat nipple out before latching.*[6]
- Discuss and demonstrate breastfeeding aids (e.g., infant sling, nursing footstool, or pillows) and suggest using a variety of nursing positions *to find the most comfortable ones for mother and infant. Positions particularly helpful for "plus-sized" women or those with large breasts include the "football" hold, with infant's head to mother's breast and body curved around behind her, or lying down to nurse.*[10]
- Encourage frequent rest periods, sharing household and child-care duties. *The new mother may feel overwhelmed with taking care of infant and carrying out other household duties; having assistance can limit fatigue and facilitate relaxation at feeding times.*[6] *Note: Research suggests a correlation between psychological stress and development of breast disease (e.g., breast pain, milk stasis, mastitis) leading to early weaning.*[19]
- Suggest abstinence or restriction of tobacco, caffeine, alcohol, drugs, and excess sugar, as appropriate. *May affect milk production/letdown reflex and can be passed on to the infant.*[1]
- Promote early management of breastfeeding problems. *Dealing with problems in a timely manner will promote successful breastfeeding.*[1,7]

For example:

Engorgement: Wear supportive bra; apply heat or cool applications to the breasts and massage from chest wall down to nipple; soothe "fussy baby" before latching on the breast and properly position baby on breast/nipple; alternate the side on which baby starts nursing; nurse round the clock or pump with piston-type electric breast pump with bilateral collection chambers at least 8 to 12 times/day; and avoid using bottle, pacifier, or supplements.[13]

Sore nipples: Wear 100% cotton fabrics, do not use soap/alcohol/drying agents on nipples, and avoid use of nipple shields or nursing pads that contain plastic; cleanse and pat dry with a clean cloth; apply thin layer of highly purified anhydrous (HPA) lanolin on nipple. *Note:* This cream is edible and does not need to be removed before breastfeeding.[12,18] Administer a mild pain reliever as appropriate. Infant should latch on least sore side or begin with hand expression to establish letdown reflex, properly position infant on breast and nipple, and use a variety of nursing positions. Break suction after breastfeeding is complete.

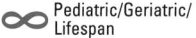

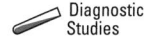

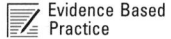

Clogged ducts: Use larger bra or extender to avoid pressure on site; use moist or dry heat and gently massage from above plug down to nipple; nurse infant, hand express, or pump after massage; and nurse more often on affected side.

Inhibited letdown: Use relaxation techniques before nursing (e.g., maintain quiet atmosphere, massage, apply heat to breasts, have beverage available, assume position of comfort, place infant on mother's chest, skin-to skin). Encourage mother to relax and enjoy her baby.

Mastitis: Promote bedrest (with infant) for several days; administer antibiotics; provide warm, moist heat before and during nursing; and empty breasts completely, continuing to nurse baby at least 8 to 12 times/ day, or pumping breasts for 24 hours, and then resuming breastfeeding as appropriate.

- Demonstrate use of hand expression, hand pump, and electric piston-type breast pump with bilateral collection chamber when necessary to maintain or increase milk supply. *Note: Studies indicate that mothers taught hands-on pumping increased the mean daily volume of milk by 48%.*[20] *The need to use a pump to store milk for feedings while the mother is away (i.e., going back to work or simply to allow time away from the infant) demands some degree of proficiency in the use of the pump.*[1]

NURSING PRIORITY NO. 4 To condition infant to breastfeed:

- Scent breast pad with breast milk and leave in bed with infant along with mother's photograph when separated from mother for medical purposes (e.g., prematurity).
- Increase skin-to-skin contact (kangaroo care).
- Provide practice times at breast for infant to "lick and learn."
- Express small amounts of milk into baby's mouth.
- Have mother pump breast after feeding to enhance milk production.
- Use supplemental nutrition system cautiously when necessary.
- Identify special interventions for feeding in presence of cleft lip/palate.

These measures promote optimal interaction between mother and infant and provide adequate nourishment for the infant, enhancing successful breastfeeding.[1,21]

NURSING PRIORITY NO. 5 To promote wellness (Teaching/Discharge Considerations):

- Schedule follow-up visits with healthcare provider 24 to 48 hours after hospital discharge and 2 weeks after birth. *Provides opportunity to evaluate milk intake and breastfeeding process, adequacy of home situation, and answer mother's questions.*[2]
- Recommend monitoring number of infant's wet and soiled diapers. *Stools should be yellow in color and infant should have at least six wet diapers a day to determine that infant is receiving sufficient intake.*[6]
- Weigh infant at least every third day initially as indicated and record. *Provides record of appropriate weight gain verifying adequacy of nutritional intake or indicates need for evaluation of insufficient weight gain.*[1] *Note: Most infants lose 5% to 7% of their birth weight in the first few days of life.*[12]
- Educate father/SO about benefits of breastfeeding and how to manage common lactation challenges. *Enlisting support of father/SO is associated with higher ratio of successful breastfeeding at 6 months.*[11]
- Discuss with spouse/SO mother's need for rest, relaxation, and time together with spouse and with other children as appropriate. *Promotes understanding of mother's needs and cooperation with incorporation of new member into family. Spouse and children feel included when they have time alone with mother and are more willing to allow mother time with infant and for herself.*[4]
- Instruct in use of relaxation techniques. *Facilitates release of oxytocin improving milk removal.*[21]
- Promote peer and cultural group counseling for teen mothers. *Provides positive role model that teen can relate to and feel comfortable with discussing concerns and feelings.*[8]
- Discuss importance of adequate nutrition and fluid intake, prenatal vitamins, or other vitamin or mineral supplements, such as vitamin C, as indicated. *During lactation, there is an increased need for energy, and supplementation of protein, minerals, and vitamins is necessary to provide nourishment for the infant and to*

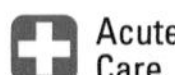
Acute Care
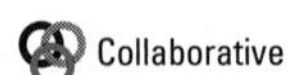
Collaborative
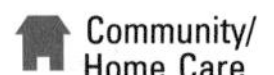
Community/ Home Care
 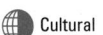
Cultural

protect mother's stores, along with extra fluid intake. Alternating different types of fluid, water, juices, decaffeinated tea, and milk can help mother promote sufficient intake. Beer and wine are not recommended for increasing lactation.[4]

- Address specific problems (e.g., suckling problems, prematurity, anomalies). *Individualized planning can enhance mother's understanding and ability to manage situation.*[1,7]
- Discuss timing of introduction of solid foods and importance of delaying until infant is at least 4 months, preferably 6 months old. *American Academy of Pediatrics and the World Health Organization recommend delaying solids until at least 6 months. If supplementation is necessary, infant can be finger fed, spoon fed, cup fed, or syringe fed.*[10,15]
- Inform mother that the return of menses varies in nursing mothers and usually averages 3 to 36 weeks with ovulation returning in 17 to 28 weeks. *Return of menstruation does not affect breastfeeding, and breastfeeding is not a reliable method of birth control.*[1]
- Refer to support groups (e.g., La Leche League, parenting support groups, stress reduction, or other community resources as indicated). *Provides information and visible support for ensuring an effective outcome.*[5]
- Provide bibliotherapy and appropriate Web sites for further information. *Additional resources to assist mother and family learn and apply new skills.*[1]

DOCUMENTATION FOCUS

Assessment/Reassessment

- Identified assessment factors, both maternal and infant (e.g., is engorgement present, is infant demonstrating adequate weight gain without supplementation).

Planning

- Plan of care, specific interventions, and who is involved in planning.
- Teaching plan.

Implementation/Evaluation

- Mother's/infant's responses to interventions, teaching, and actions performed.
- Changes in infant's weight and output.
- Attainment or progress toward desired outcome(s).
- Modifications to plan of care.

Discharge Planning

- Referrals that have been made and mother's choice of participation.

References

1. Ladewig, P., London, M., Davidson, M. (2009). *Contemporary Maternal-Newborn Nursing Care.* 7th ed. Upper Saddle River, NJ: Prentice Hall.
2. Riodan, J., Auerbach, K. (2010). *Breastfeeding and Human Lactation.* 4th ed. Boston: Jones & Bartlett.
3. Purnell, L. D. (2011). *Guide to Culturally Competent Health Care.* 2nd ed. Philadelphia: F. A. Davis.
4. Lowdermilk, D. L., Cashion, M. C., Perry, S. E. (2011). *Maternity & Women's Health Care.* 10th ed. St. Louis, MO: Mosby.
5. Doenges, M., Moorhouse, M. (1999). *Maternal/Newborn Plans of Care: Guidelines for Individualizing Care.* 3rd ed. Philadelphia: F. A. Davis.
6. Phillips, C. R. (1996). *Family-Centered Maternity and Newborn Care.* 4th ed. St. Louis, MO: Mosby.
7. London, M. L., Ladewig, P. W., Ball, J. W., et al. (2010). *Maternal and Child Nursing Care.* 3rd ed. Upper Saddle River, NJ: Prentice Hall.
8. American Academy of Family Physicians. Breastfeeding (Position paper). Retrieved October 2015 from www.aafp.org/about/policies/all/breastfeeding-support.html.
9. Oddy, W. H., Jianghong, L., Landsborough, L., et al. (2006). The association of maternal overweight and obesity with breastfeeding duration. *J Pediatr,* 149(2), 185–191.
10. American Academy of Pediatrics. (Revised 2013). Ten steps to support parents' choice to breastfeed their baby. Retrieved October 2015 from www.aap.org/breastfeeding/files/pdf/tenstepsposter.pdf.

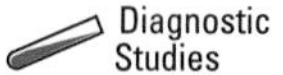
Diagnostic Studies
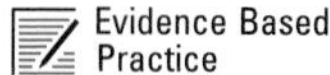
Evidence Based Practice
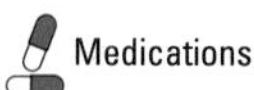
Medications

Pediatric/Geriatric/Lifespan

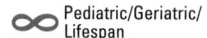

11. Pisacane, A., Continisio, G. I., Aldinucci, M., et al. (2005). A controlled trial of the father's role in breast-feeding promotion. *Pediatrics*, 116(4), e494–e498.
12. Lawrence, R. A., Lawrence, R. M. (2005). *Breast-feeding: A Guide for the Medical Profession.* 6th ed. St. Louis, MO: Mosby.
13. Morbacher, N., Kendall-Tackett, K. (2010). *Breast-feeding Made Simple: Seven Natural Laws for Nursing Mothers.* 2nd ed. Oakland, CA.: New Harbinger.
14. Trenouth, M. J., Campbell, A. N. (1996). Questionnaire evaluation of feeding methods for cleft lip and palate neonates. *Int J Pediatr Dent*, 6(4), 241–244.
15. No author listed. Up to what age can a baby stay well nourished by just being breastfed? World Health Organization. Retrieved October 2015 from http://www.who.int/features/qa/21/en/.
16. Bramson, L., Lee, J. W., Moore, E., et al. (2010). Effect of early skin-to-skin mother-infant contact during the first three hours following birth on exclusive breast-feeding during the maternity hospital stay. *J Hum Lact*, 26(2), 130–137.
17. Neifert, M. (2009). *Great Expectations: The Essential Guide to Breastfeeding.* New York: Sterling.
18. Abou-Dakn, M., Fluhr, J. W., Gensch, M., et al. (2011). Positive effect of HPA lanolin versus expressed breastmilk on painful and damaged nipples during lactation. *Skin Pharmacol Physiol*, 24(11), 27–35.
19. Abou-Dakn, M., Schafer-Graf, U., Wockel, A. (2009). Psychological stress and breast disease during lactation. *Breastfeed Rev*, 17(3), 19–26.
20. Morton, J., Hall, J. Y., Wong, R. J., et al. (2009). Combining hand techniques with electric pumping increases milk production in mothers of preterm infants. *J Perinatol*, 29(11), 757–764.
21. The Academy of Breastfeeding Medicine Protocol Committee. (2011). Protocol #9: Use of galactogogues in initiating or augmenting maternal milk supply. *Breastfeeding Med*, 6(1), 41–49.

interrupted Breastfeeding

Taxonomy II: Nutrition—Class 1 Ingestion (00105) [**Diagnostic Division:** Food/Fluid], Submitted 1992; Revised 2013

DEFINITION: Break in the continuity of providing milk to an infant or young child directly from the breasts, which may compromise breastfeeding success and/or nutritional status of the infant/child.

RELATED FACTORS

Maternal/infant illness
Prematurity
Maternal-infant separation; maternal employment; hospitalization of child
Contraindications to breastfeeding (e.g., pharmaceutical agents)
Need to abruptly wean infant

DEFINING CHARACTERISTICS

Subjective
Nonexclusive breastfeeding
Sample Clinical Applications: Prematurity, postpartum depression, conditions requiring hospitalization of infant or mother, occasionally maternal medication or drug use

DESIRED OUTCOMES/EVALUATION CRITERIA

Sample NOC linkages:
Knowledge: Breastfeeding: Extent of understanding conveyed about lactation and nourishment of infant through breastfeeding

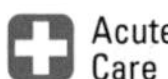

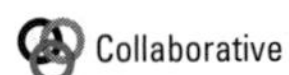

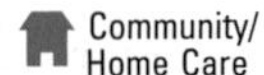

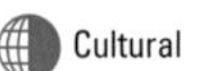

Breastfeeding Maintenance: Continuation of breastfeeding from establishment to weaning for nourishment of an infant/toddler
Parent-Infant Attachment: Parent and infant behaviors that demonstrate an enduring affectionate bond

Client Will (Include Specific Time Frame)
- Identify and demonstrate techniques to sustain lactation until breastfeeding is re-initiated.
- Achieve mutually satisfactory feeding regimen with infant content after feedings and gaining weight appropriately.
- Achieve weaning and cessation of lactation, if desired or necessary.

ACTIONS/INTERVENTIONS

Sample NIC linkages:
Lactation Counseling: Use of an interactive helping process to assist in maintenance of successful breastfeeding
Coping Enhancement: Assisting a patient to adapt to perceived stressors, changes, or threats that interfere with meeting life demands and roles
Bottle Feeding: Preparation and administration of fluids to an infant via a bottle

NURSING PRIORITY NO. 1 To identify causative/contributing factors:

- Assess client knowledge and perceptions about breastfeeding and extent of instruction that has been given. *Provides baseline information to develop plan of care for individual situation.*[1,8]
- Note myths or misunderstandings, especially in some cultures, and in teenage mothers, *who are more likely to have limited knowledge and concerns about body image issues.*[9]
- Encourage discussion of current and previous breastfeeding experience(s). *Useful for determining efforts needed to continue breastfeeding, if desired, while circumstances interrupting process are resolved, if possible.*[2]
- Ascertain cultural expectations or conflicts. *The dominant culture in America has sexualized women's breasts, and mother may be embarrassed by breastfeeding or father/partner may not want mother to breastfeed. Mother may believe her independence will be curtailed by breastfeeding. Studies have shown that in the United States, breastfeeding rates vary, not only by race and ethnicity, but also by geographic location. For example, the rate of breastfeeding among African American mothers in the Southeast has lagged behind other areas in the country.*[1,3,19]
- Determine support systems available to mother/family. *Infant's father and maternal grandmother (in addition to caring healthcare providers) are important factors in whether breastfeeding is successful and sustained.*[9]
- Identify factors necessitating interruption or, occasionally, cessation of breastfeeding (e.g., maternal illness, drug use) or desire or need to wean infant. *In general, infants with chronic diseases benefit from breastfeeding, and only a few maternal infections (e.g., HIV, active/untreated tuberculosis for initial 2 weeks of multidrug therapy, active herpes simplex of the breasts, development of chickenpox within 5 days prior to delivery or 2 days after delivery) are hazardous to breastfeeding infants. In addition, use of antiretroviral medications, chemotherapy agents, or maternal substance abuse usually requires weaning of infant. Exposure to radiation therapy requires interruption of breastfeeding for length of time radioactivity is known to be present in breast milk and is therefore dependent on agent used. Note: Mother can "pump and dump" her breastmilk to maintain supply and continue to breastfeed after her condition has resolved (e.g., chicken pox).*[1,8–11,18]
- Determine maternal responsibilities, routines, and scheduled activities. *Caretaking of siblings, employment in or out of the home, and work or school schedules of family members may affect ability to visit hospitalized infant when this is the reason for mother/infant separation.*[6,7]

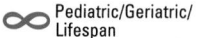

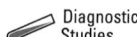

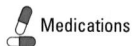

NURSING PRIORITY NO. 2 To assist mother to maintain breastfeeding, as desired:

- Provide information, as needed, regarding need or decision to interrupt breastfeeding.
- Give emotional support to mother and support her decision regarding cessation or continuation of breastfeeding. *Many women are ambivalent about breastfeeding, and providing information about the pros and cons of both breastfeeding and bottle-feeding, along with support for the mother's/couple's decision, will promote a positive experience.*[1,8]
- Promote peer counseling for teen mothers. *Provides positive role model teen can relate to and feel comfortable with discussing concerns and feelings.*[9]
- Educate father/significant other (SO) about the benefits of breastfeeding and how to manage common lactation challenges. *Enlisting support of father/SO is associated with higher ratio of successful breastfeeding at 6 months.*[12]
- Discuss and demonstrate use of breastfeeding aids (e.g., infant sling, nursing footstool or pillows, hand expression, manual and/or electric piston-type breast pump). *Enhances comfort and relaxation for breastfeeding. When circumstances dictate that mother and infant are separated for a time, whether due to illness, prematurity, or returning to work or school, the milk supply can be maintained by use of the pump. Storing the milk for future use enables the infant to continue to receive the value of breast milk. Learning the correct technique is important for successful use of the pump.*[1,4,13,15]
- Review techniques for storage and use of expressed breast milk. *Provides safety and optimal nutrition, promoting continuation of the breastfeeding process.*[1]
- Determine if a routine visiting schedule or advance warning can be provided. *When infant remains in the hospital or when working mother continues to nurse, it helps to make preparations so that infant will be hungry and ready to feed when the mother arrives. A sleepy baby can be gently played with to arouse him or her; clothing can be loosened or diaper changed, exposing infant to room air; or if infant is hungry and upset, a calm voice and gentle rocking can calm the infant and prepare him or her to nurse.*[1]
- Provide privacy and calm surroundings when mother breastfeeds in hospital or work setting. *Note: Federal law 2010 requires an employer to provide a place and reasonable break time for an employee to express her breast milk for her baby for 1 year after birth.*[20]
- Problem-solve return-to-work or school issues or periodic infant care requiring bottle or supplemental feeding.[14,15]
- Recommend using expressed breast milk instead of formula or at least partial breastfeeding for as long as mother and child are satisfied. *Prevents temporary interruption in breastfeeding, decreasing the risk of premature weaning.*[13,15]

NURSING PRIORITY NO. 3 To promote successful infant feeding:

- Recommend or provide for infant sucking on a regular basis, especially if gavage feedings are part of the therapeutic regimen. *Reinforces that feeding time is pleasurable and enhances digestion.*[1]
- Explain anticipated changes in feeding needs and frequency. *Growth spurts require increased intake or more feedings by infant.*[13]
- Discuss proper use and choice of supplemental nutrition and alternate feeding methods (e.g., bottle or syringe, finger feeding, cup feeding, or supplemental nursing system feeding). *If infant is not receiving sufficient nourishment, whether by mother's choice to reduce number of feedings (e.g., returning to work) or necessity (e.g., specific maternal illness, medication use), other means for supplementing intake must be taken, and mother needs to be given information regarding method chosen.*[1]
- Review safety precautions when bottle-feeding is necessary/chosen. *Identifying importance of proper flow of formula from nipple, frequency of burping, holding bottle instead of propping, techniques of formula preparation, and sterilization techniques are necessary for successful bottle-feeding.*[1]

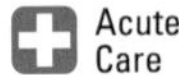

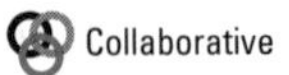

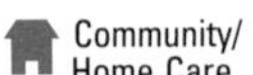

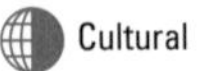

NURSING PRIORITY NO. 4 To promote wellness (Teaching/Discharge Considerations):

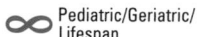

- Encourage mother to obtain adequate rest, maintain fluid and nutritional intake, continue to take her prenatal vitamins, and schedule breast pumping every 3 hours while awake, as indicated. *Sustains adequate milk production and enhances breastfeeding process when mother and infant are separated for any reason.*[1,8]
- Suggest abstinence or restriction of tobacco, caffeine, alcohol, drugs, and excess sugar, as appropriate, when breastfeeding is re-initiated. *These substances may affect milk production/letdown reflex and can be passed on to the infant.*[1]
- Identify other means of nurturing and strengthening infant attachment, such as skin-to-skin or kangaroo care. *Activities that provide comfort, consolation, and play activities help mother become comfortable with handling the infant, thus enhancing relationship.*[7,15]
- Refer to support groups (e.g., La Leche League, Lact-Aid) or community resources (e.g., public health nurse; lactation specialist; Women, Infants, and Children [WIC] program; and electric pump rental programs). *Additional support may provide assistance, supplies, and education to promote a successful outcome. WIC and other federal programs support breastfeeding through education and enhanced nutritional intake.*[5,15]
- Promote use of bibliotherapy and appropriate Web sites. *Provides additional sources of information.*[5]
- Discuss timing of introduction of solid foods and importance of delaying until infant is at least 4 months, preferably 6 months old if possible. *American Academy of Pediatrics and the World Health Organization recommend delaying solids until at least 6 months. If supplementation is necessary, infant can be finger fed, spoon fed, cup fed, or syringe fed.*[13,21]

NURSING PRIORITY NO. 5 To assist mother in weaning process, when desired:

- Discuss reducing frequency of daily feedings or breast pumping by once every 2 to 3 days. *Preferred method of weaning, if circumstance permits, to reduce problems associated with engorgement.*[16,17]
- Encourage wearing a snug, well-fitting bra, but refrain from binding breasts, *because of increased risk of clogged milk ducts and inflammation.*[15,16]
- Recommend expressing some milk from breasts regularly each day over a 1- to 3-week period, if necessary, *to reduce discomfort associated with engorgement until milk production decreases.*[16,17]
- Suggest holding infant differently during bottle-feeding or interactions or having another family member give infant's bottle feeding *to prevent infant rooting for mother's breast and limit stimulation of her nipples.*
- Discuss use of ibuprofen or acetaminophen *for discomfort during weaning process.*[8]
- Suggest use of ice packs to breast tissue (not nipples) for 15 to 20 min at least four times a day *to help reduce swelling during sudden weaning.*[17]

DOCUMENTATION FOCUS

Assessment/Reassessment

- Baseline findings maternal/infant factors, including mother's milk supply, infant nourishment.
- Reason for interruption or cessation of breastfeeding.
- Number of wet and soiled diapers daily, log of intake and output, as appropriate, and periodic weight.

Planning

- Method of feeding chosen.
- Plan of care and who is involved in planning.
- Teaching plan.

Implementation/Evaluation

- Maternal response to interventions, teaching, and actions performed.
- Infant's response to feeding and method.
- Whether infant appears satisfied or still seems to be hungry.

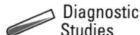

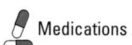

- Attainment or progress toward desired outcome(s).
- Modifications to plan of care.

Discharge Planning

- Referrals, plan for follow-up, and who is responsible.
- Specific referrals made.

References

1. Ladewig, P., London, M., Davidson, M. (2009). *Contemporary Maternal-Newborn Nursing Care.* 7th ed. Upper Saddle River, NJ: Prentice Hall.
2. Riodan, J., Auerbach, K. (2010). *Breastfeeding and Human Lactation.* 4th ed. Boston: Jones & Bartlett.
3. Purnell, L. D. (2011). *Guide to Culturally Competent Health Care.* 2nd ed. Philadelphia: F. A. Davis.
4. Lowdermilk, D. L., Cashion, M. C., Perry, S. (2011). *Maternal and Woman's Health Care.* 10th ed. St. Louis, MO: Mosby.
5. Doenges, M., Moorhouse, M. (1999). *Maternal/Newborn Plans of Care: Guidelines for Individualizing Care.* 3rd ed. Philadelphia: F. A. Davis.
6. Phillips, C. R. (2003). *Family-Centered Maternity and Newborn Care.* Maynard, MA: Jones & Bartlett Learning.
7. Cox, H., et al. (2007). *Clinical Applications of Nursing Diagnosis: Adult, Child, Women's, Psychiatric, Gerontic and Home Health Considerations.* 5th ed. Philadelphia: F. A. Davis.
8. London, M., Ladewig, P. A., Ball, J. W., et al. (2010). *Maternal and Child Nursing Care.* 3rd ed. Upper Saddle River, NJ: Prentice Hall.
9. American Academy of Family Physicians. Breastfeeding (Position paper). Retrieved October 2015 from www.aafp.org/about/policies/all/breastfeeding-support.html.
10. Centers for Disease Control and Prevention. (2015). When should a mother avoid breastfeeding? Retrieved October 2015 from http://www.cdc.gov/breastfeeding/disease/.
11. United States National Library of Medicine. (no date listed). Toxnet: Drugs and Lactation Database. (LactMed). Retrieved October 2015 from http://toxnet.nlm.nih.gov/newtoxnet/lactmed.htm.
12. Pisacane, A., Continisio, G. I., Aldinucci, N., et al. (2005). A controlled trial of the father's role in breastfeeding promotion. *Pediatrics*, 116(4), e494–e498.
13. American Academy of Pediatrics. (Revised July 2013). Ten steps to support parents' choice to breastfeed their baby. Retrieved October 2015 from www2.aap.org/breastfeeding/files/tenstepsposter.pdf.
14. U.S. Department of Health and Human Services, Office on Women's Health. (Update 2012). *Common breastfeeding challenges.* Retrieved October 2015 from http://www.womenshealth.gov/breastfeeding/common-challenges/.
15. Smith, A. (updated 2015). Breast infections and plugged ducts. *Breastfeeding Basics.* Retrieved October 2015 from http://www.breastfeedingbasics.com/articles/breast-infections-and-plugged-ducts.
16. Children's Hospitals and Clinics of Minnesota Patient/Family Education Resources. (reviewed 2015). *Breastfeeding: Weaning.* Retrieved October 2015 from http://www.childrensmn.org/educationmaterials/childrensmn/article/15846/breastfeeding-weaning/.
17. Smith, A. Breastfeeding Basics: Weaning. Retrieved November 2015 from www.breastfeeding-basics.com/articles/weaning-your-baby.
18. Hale, T. W. (2010). *Medications and Mothers' Milk: A Manual of Lactational Pharmacology.* 14th ed. Amarillo, TX: Pharmasoft Medical Pub.
19. Wozniki, K. (2010). Breastfeeding rates vary by race, region. Retrieved October 2015 from WebMD Health News. http://www.medicinenet.com/script/main/art.asp?articlekey=114787.
20. U.S. Department of Labor. (revised 2013). Fact Sheet #73. Retrieved October 2015 from http://www.dol.gov/whd/regs/compliance/whdfs73.htm.
21. World Health Organization. Up to what age can a baby stay well nourished by just being breastfed? Retrieved October 2015 from http://www.who.int/features/qa/21/en/index.html.

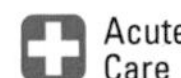

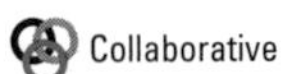

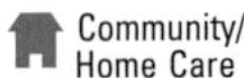

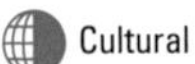

readiness for enhanced Breastfeeding

Taxonomy II: Nutrition—Class 1 Ingestion (00106) [**Diagnostic Division:** Food/Fluid], Submitted 1990; Revised 2010, 2013

DEFINITION: A pattern of providing milk to an infant or young child directly from the breasts, which may be strengthened.

DEFINING CHARACTERISTICS

Subjective

Mother expresses desire to enhance ability to exclusively breastfeed
Mother expresses desire to provide breast milk for child's nutritional needs

Sample Clinical Applications: Wellness diagnosis associated with pre-/postnatal client

DESIRED OUTCOMES/EVALUATION CRITERIA

Sample NOC linkages:

Breastfeeding Establishment: Infant: Infant attachment to and sucking from the mother's breast for nourishment during the first 3 weeks
Breastfeeding Establishment: Maternal: Maternal establishment of proper attachment of an infant to and sucking from the breast for nourishment during the first 3 weeks of breastfeeding
Breastfeeding Maintenance: Continuation of breastfeeding from establishment to weaning for nourishment of an infant/toddler

Client Will (Include Specific Time Frame)

- Verbalize understanding of breastfeeding techniques, good latch, and lactogenesis.
- Demonstrate effective techniques for breastfeeding.
- Demonstrate family involvement and support.
- Attend classes, read appropriate materials, or access resources as necessary.
- Verbalize understanding of the benefits of human milk.

ACTIONS/INTERVENTIONS

Sample NIC linkages:

Lactation Counseling: Use of an interactive helping process to assist in maintenance of successful breastfeeding
Anticipatory Guidance: Preparation of patient for an anticipated developmental and/or situational crisis
Teaching: Infant Nutrition (specify age): Instruction on nutrition and feeding practices during the first year of life

NURSING PRIORITY NO. 1 To determine individual learning needs:

- Assess mother's desires/plan for feeding infant. *Provides information for developing plan of care.*[1]
- Assess mother's knowledge and previous experience with breastfeeding. *Provides information for developing plan of care. Accurate knowledge and previous experience can lead to a positive breastfeeding experience.*[1]
- Note cultural and societal influences regarding infant feeding (breastfeeding/bottle-feeding), lactation process, letdown techniques, and maternal food preferences. *In Western cultures, the breast has taken on a sexual connotation, and some mothers may be embarrassed to breastfeed. While breastfeeding may be accepted, in some cultures, certain beliefs may affect specific feeding practices (e.g., in Mexican American, Navajo,*

Filipino, and Vietnamese cultures, colostrum is often not offered to the newborn; breastfeeding sometimes begins only after the milk flow is established).[3]

- Note myths or misunderstandings, especially in teenage mothers *who are more likely to have limited knowledge and concerns about body image issues.*[6]
- Monitor effectiveness of current breastfeeding efforts. *Determining the actions client is taking provides information about measures that may enhance efforts to be successful in endeavor.*[1]
- Determine support systems available to mother/family. *Presence of adequate support can provide encouragement to mother who may be feeling nervous and unsure about new role.*[1,6]

NURSING PRIORITY NO. 2 To promote effective breastfeeding behaviors:

- Initiate breastfeeding within first hour after birth. *The time of the first feeding is determined by the infant's physiological and behavioral cues. Throughout the first 2 hours after birth, the infant is usually alert and ready to nurse. Early feedings are of great benefit to mother and infant because oxytocin release is stimulated, helping to expel the placenta and prevent excessive maternal blood loss; the infant receives the immunological protection of colostrum; peristalsis is stimulated; lactation is accelerated; and maternal-infant bonding is enhanced.*[2]
- Encourage skin-to-skin contact. Place infant on mother's stomach, skin-to-skin after delivery. *Many full-term infants are alert and capable of latching onto mother's breast without assistance.*[9] *Studies show that early skin-to-skin mother-infant contact is correlated with exclusive breastfeeding while in the hospital.*[10]
- Demonstrate asymmetric latch aiming infant's lower lip as far from base of the nipple as possible, then bringing infant's chin and lower jaw in contact with breast while mouth is wide open and before upper lip touches breast. *This position allows infant to use both tongue and jaw more effectively to obtain milk from the breast.*[9]
- Demonstrate how to support and position infant and use of aids (e.g., infant sling, nursing footstool, or pillows). *The mother should be made as comfortable as possible and given specific instructions for positioning self and baby depending on the type of birth (e.g., cesarean section or vaginal).*[1,5]
- Observe mother's return demonstration/teach back. *Provides practice and the opportunity to correct misunderstandings and add additional information to promote optimal experience for breastfeeding.*[1]
- Keep infant with mother for unrestricted breastfeeding duration and frequency. *Rooming-in offers opportunity for spontaneous encounters for the family to practice handling skills and increase confidence in own ability. It also encourages feeding in response to cues from the baby and increases bonding.*[1]
- Discuss early infant feeding cues (e.g., rooting, lip smacking, sucking fingers or hand) versus the late cue of crying. *Early recognition of infant hunger promotes timely and more rewarding feeding experience for infant and mother.* NOTE: For healthy infants, discourage use of pacifiers and artificial nipples in first month of life *to avoid "nipple confusion" and to establish mother's milk supply.*[6]
- Encourage mother to follow a well-balanced diet containing an extra 500 calories/day, continue her prenatal vitamins, and drink at least 2,000 to 3,000 mL of fluid/day. *There is an increased need for maternal energy, protein, minerals, and vitamins, as well as increased fluid intake, during lactation to restore what the mother loses in secreting milk to provide adequate nutrients for the nourishment of the infant and to protect the mother's own stores.*[4]
- Provide information, as needed, in support of breastfeeding. *Having adequate information about the nutritional, psychological, immunological advantages, contraindications, and disadvantages of breastfeeding helps the parents to make a decision that is best for the family. Many mothers indicate that if they had had adequate information, they would have chosen to breastfeed.*[1]
- Promote peer counseling for teen mothers. *Provides positive role model teen can relate to and feel comfortable with discussing concerns and feelings.*[6]

NURSING PRIORITY NO. 3 To enhance optimum wellness (Teaching/Discharge Considerations):

- Provide for follow-up contact or home visit 48 hours after discharge; repeat visit as necessary. *Provides opportunity to assess adequacy of home situation and breastfeeding efforts as well as support and assistance with problem solving, if needed.*[1]

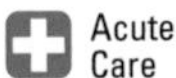

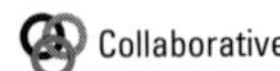

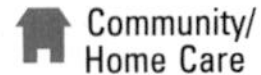

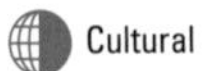

- Recommend monitoring number of infant's wet diapers (at least six wet diapers in 24 hours suggests adequate hydration) and soiled diapers (breastfed baby's stool will be yellow in color). *Often mothers who are breastfeeding worry about whether infant is getting adequate nutrition because they cannot measure the amount of milk being received, and having this information can allay these fears.*[1]
- Encourage mother and other family members to express feelings and concerns, and active-listen *to determine nature of concerns. Identifying the concerns of the parents promotes problem solving and alleviation of worries and fears. When individuals do not express these concerns, they can become frustrated, which can interfere with successful breastfeeding.*[1]
- Educate father/significant other (SO) about benefits of breastfeeding and how to manage common lactation challenges. *Enlisting support of father/SO is associated with higher ratio of successful breastfeeding at 6 months.*[8]
- Review techniques for expression and storage of breast milk to help sustain breastfeeding activity. *Having this information enables the mother to successfully manage continuation of breastfeeding while engaging in activities outside the home for specified periods of time.*[1]
- Explain changes in feeding needs and frequency. *Growth spurts require increased intake or more feedings by infant.*[5]
- Review normal nursing behaviors of older breastfeeding infants/toddlers.[5]
- Discuss importance of delaying introduction of solid foods until infant is at least 4 months, preferably 6 months old. *Note:* American Academy of Pediatrics and the World Health Organization recommend delaying solids until at least 6 months.[5,11]
- Recommend avoidance of specific medications or substances (e.g., estrogen-containing contraceptives, bromocriptine, nicotine, alcohol) *known to decrease milk supply. Note: Small amounts of alcohol have not been shown to be detrimental.*[6,7]
- Emphasize importance of client notifying healthcare providers, dentists, and pharmacists of breastfeeding status.
- Problem solve return-to-work issues or periodic infant care requiring bottle or supplemental feeding. *Enables mothers who need or desire to return to work (for economic or personal reasons) or who simply want to attend activities without the infant to deal with these issues, thus allowing more freedom while maintaining adequate breastfeeding.*[1]
- Recommend using expressed breast milk instead of formula or at least partial breastfeeding for as long as mother and child are satisfied.[6]
- Refer to support groups, such as La Leche League, as indicated. Provide mother with phone number of support person or group, prior to leaving hospital. *While the father or SO is the most important support person in Western society, family support systems may be lacking information about other support systems/groups.*[1]
- Refer to ND ineffective Breastfeeding for more specific information, as appropriate.

DOCUMENTATION FOCUS

Assessment/Reassessment

- Identified assessment factors (maternal and infant).
- Number of daily wet and soiled diapers and periodic weight.

Planning

- Plan of care, specific interventions, and who is involved in the planning.
- Teaching plan.

Implementation/Evaluation

- Mother's response to interventions, teaching plan, and actions performed.
- Effectiveness of infant's efforts to feed.
- Attainment or progress toward desired outcome(s).
- Modifications to plan of care.

Discharge Planning

- Long-term needs, referrals made, and who is responsible for follow-up actions.

References

1. Ladewig, P., London, M., Davidson, M. (2009). *Contemporary Maternal-Newborn Nursing Care.* 7th ed. Upper Saddle River, NJ: Prentice Hall.
2. Riodan, J., Auerbach, K. (2010). *Breastfeeding and Human Lactation.* 4th ed. Boston: Jones & Bartlett.
3. Purnell, L. D. (2011). *Guide to Culturally Competent Health Care.* 2nd ed. Philadelphia: F. A. Davis.
4. Lowdermilk, D., Cashion, M., Perry, S. (2012). *Maternity & Women's Health Care.* 10th ed. St. Louis, MO: Elsevier-Mosby.
5. American Academy of Pediatrics. Ten steps to support parents' choice to breastfeed their baby. Retrieved October 2015 from www2.aap.org/breastfeeding/files/pdf/tenstepsposter.pdf.
6. American Academy of Family Physicians. (2011). Breastfeeding (position paper). Retrieved October 2015 from www.aafp.org/about/policies/all/breastfeeding-support.html.
7. Callen, J., Pinelli, J. (2005). A review of the literature examining the benefits and challenges, incidence and duration, and barriers to breastfeeding in preterm infants. *Adv Neonatal Care*, 5(2), 72–88.
8. Pisacane, A., Continisio, G. I., Aldinucci, M., et al. (2005). A controlled trial of the father's role in breastfeeding promotion. *Pediatrics*, 116(4), e494–e498.
9. Neifert, M. (2009). *Great Expectations: The Essential Guide to Breastfeeding.* New York: Sterling.
10. Bramson, L., Lee, J. W., Montgomery, S., et al. (2010). Effect of early skin-to-skin mother-infant contact during the first three hours following birth on exclusive breast-feeding during the maternity hospital stay. *J Hum Lact*, 26(2), 130–137.
11. World Health Organization. Up to what age can a baby stay well nourished by just being breastfed? Retrieved October 2015 from http://www.who.int/features/qa/21/en/index.html.

insufficient Breast Milk

Taxonomy II: Nutrition—Class 1 Ingestion (00216) [**Diagnostic Division:** Food/Fluid], Submitted 2010

DEFINITION: Low production of maternal breast milk.

RELATED FACTORS

Mother

Insufficient fluid volume [e.g., dehydration, hemorrhage]

Smoking; alcohol consumption

Malnutrition

Treatment regimen [e.g., medication side effects—contraceptives, diuretics]

Pregnancy

Infant

Ineffective latching on to breast, sucking reflex

Insufficient opportunity for suckling at the breast or suckling time at breast

Rejection of breast

DEFINING CHARACTERISTICS

Objective

Mother

Expressed breast milk less than prescribed volume

Delay in milk production

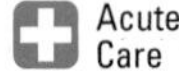

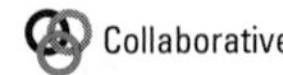

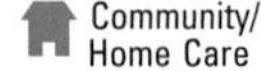

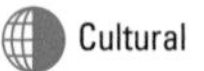

Absence of milk production with nipple stimulation

Infant

Frequently seeks to suckle at breast; prolonged breastfeeding time

Suckling time at breast appears unsatisfactory; frequent crying

Refuses to suckle at breast

Voids small amounts of concentrated urine; constipation

Weight gain is 500 g in a month

Sample Clinical Applications: Conditions resulting in dehydration, such as fluid volume depletion, hemorrhage; malnutrition; premature infant with inability to suck vigorously, or mother not pumping to promote supply; adolescent mother; use/abuse of substances and/or certain medications.

DESIRED OUTCOMES/EVALUATION CRITERIA

Sample NOC linkages:

Knowledge: Breastfeeding: Extent of understanding conveyed about lactation and nourishment of an infant through breastfeeding

Breastfeeding Establishment: Maternal: Maternal establishment of proper attachment of an infant to and sucking from the breast for nourishment during the first three weeks of breastfeeding

Breastfeeding Maintenance: Continuation of breastfeeding from establishment to weaning for nourishment of infant/toddler

Client Will [Include Specific Time Frame]

- Develop plan to correct/change contributing factors.
- Engage in techniques to enhance milk production.
- Achieve mutually satisfactory breastfeeding pattern with infant content after feedings and gaining weight appropriately.

ACTIONS/INTERVENTIONS

Sample NIC linkages:

Breastfeeding Assistance: Preparing a new mother to breastfeed her infant

Lactation Counseling: Use of an interactive helping process to assist in maintenance of successful breastfeeding

NURSING PRIORITY NO. 1 To identify maternal causative or contributing factors:

- Assess mother's knowledge about breastfeeding and extent of instruction that has been provided. Determine previous breastfeeding experience. *Lack of knowledge, unresolved problems, or stories told by others may cause client to doubt abilities and chances for success.*[8,13]
- Identify cultural expectations and conflicts about breastfeeding and beliefs or practices regarding lactation, letdown techniques, and maternal food preferences. *Understanding the impact of culture and idiosyncrasies of specific feeding practices is important to determine the effect on infant breastfeeding success.*[8,11,14]
- Note incorrect myths/misunderstandings, especially in teenage mothers. *Adolescents are more likely to have limited knowledge, difficulty managing time demands of school/work, concerns about body image issues, and feel overwhelmed.*[8,14]
- Identify maternal support systems and presence/response of significant others (SOs)/extended family. *Negative attitudes and comments interfere with efforts and may cause client to prematurely abandon attempt to breastfeed.*[14]
- Determine use of supplemental feedings for infant. *Unless medically indicated, routine supplementation increases risk for decrease in mother's milk supply.*[14]

- Perform physical examination, noting appearance of breasts and nipples, marked asymmetry of breasts, obvious inverted or flat nipples, minimal or no breast enlargement during pregnancy. *Inadequate mammary gland tissue, breast surgery that has damaged the nipple, areola enervation results in irremediable primary lactation failure.*[9,13]
- Assess for other causes of primary lactation failure. *Maternal prolactin deficiency/serum prolactin levels, pituitary or thyroid disorders, and anemia may be corrected with medication.*[4,9]
- Review lifestyle for common causes of secondary lactation failure. *Smoking, caffeine/alcohol use, birth control pills containing estrogen, medications (e.g., antihistamines, decongestants, diuretics), stress, and fatigue are known to inhibit milk production.*[1,4,9]
- Determine desire/motivation to breastfeed. *Increasing milk supply can be intense, requiring commitment to therapeutic regimen and possible lifestyle changes.*

NURSING PRIORITY NO. 2 To identify infant causative or contributing factors:

- Observe infant at breast to evaluate latching-on skill and presence of suck/swallow difficulties. *Poor latching-on, lack of audible swallowing/gulp are associated with inadequate intake. The infant gets substantial amounts of milk when drinking with an open—pause—close type of suck. Note: Open—pause—close is one suck; the pause is not a pause between sucks.*[3]
- Observe signs of inadequate infant intake. *Infant arching and crying at the breast with resistance to latching-on, decreased urinary output/frequency of stools, and inadequate weight gain indicate need for further evaluation and intervention.*[11,13]
- Review feeding schedule—frequency, length of feeding, and taking one or both breasts at each feeding. *Provides information regarding whether sufficient nutrition is being provided.*[10]

NURSING PRIORITY NO. 3 To increase mother's milk supply:

- Instruct on how to differentiate between perceived and actual insufficient milk supply. *Normal breastfeeding frequencies, suckling times, and amounts vary not only between mothers, but also based on infant's needs/moods. Milk production is likely to be a reflection of the infant's appetite rather than the mother's ability to produce milk.*[4,5]
- Provide emotional support to mother. Use one-to-one instruction with each feeding during hospital stay, clinic, or home visit. *Increases likelihood of continuation of breastfeeding efforts and achievement of goals.*[11,14]
- Refer adoptive mothers choosing to breastfeed to a lactation consultant. *Adoptive mothers choosing to breastfeed will require more supportive instruction from a professional consultant to assist with induced lactation techniques.*[14]
- Inform mother how to assess and correct a latch if needed. Demonstrate asymmetric latch, aiming infant's lower lip as far from base of the nipple as possible and then bringing infant's chin and lower jaw in contact with breast while mouth is wide open and before upper lip touches breast. *Correct latching-on is the most effective way to stimulate milk supply.*[2,9]
- Encourage unrestricted frequency and duration of breastfeeding. *Provides stimulation of breast tissue and may increase milk supply naturally.*[9]
- Recommend reducing or stopping supplemental feedings if used. *Gradual tapering off of supplementation can increase frequency/duration of infant's breastfeeding stimulating maternal milk production.*[9,14]
- Demonstrate breast massage technique. *Improves oxytocin release and milk removal to increase milk supply naturally.*[9,14] *Also, gently massaging breast while infant feeds from it can improve the release of higher-calorie-hindmilk from the milk glands.*[1,9]
- Use breast pump 8 to 12 times a day. *Expressing with a hospital-grade, double (automatic) pump is ideal for stimulation/reestablishing milk supply.*[1,9]
- Recommend mother adjust the electric pump to her maximum comfortable vacuum. *Enhances milk flow rate and milk yield and minimizes occurrence of tissue damage.*[9]

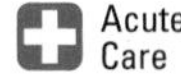

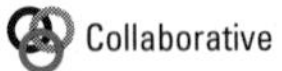

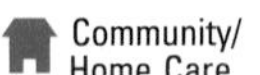

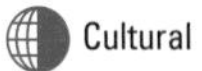

- Suggest using a breast pump or hand expression after infant finishes breastfeeding. *Continued breast stimulation cues the mother's body that more milk is needed, increasing supply.*[7]
- Encourage use of relaxation techniques during hand or mechanical expression. Facilitates oxytocin release to improve milk removal.[9]
- Monitor increased filling of breasts in response to nursing and/or pumping *to help evaluate effectiveness of interventions.*
- Discuss appropriate/safe use of herbal supplements. *Herbs such as sage, parsley, oregano, peppermint, jasmine, and yarrow may have a negative effect on milk supply if taken in large quantities. A number of herbs have been used for centuries to stimulate milk production, with fenugreek (*Trigonella foenum-graecum*) being the most commonly recommended herbal galactogogue to facilitate lactation.*[4,9]
- Discuss possible use of prescribed medications (galactogogues) to increase milk production. *Domperidone (Motilium) is approved by the American Academy of Pediatrics for use in breastfeeding mothers and has fewer side effects. Metoclopramide (Reglan) has been shown to increase milk supply anywhere from 72% to 110% depending on how many weeks postpartum a mother is.*[1,6,9]

NURSING PRIORITY NO. 4 To promote optimal success and satisfaction of breastfeeding process for mother and infant:

- Encourage frequent rest periods, sharing household and child care tasks. *Having assistance can limit fatigue (known to impact milk production) and facilitate relaxation at feeding time.*[12]
- Discuss with spouse/SO mother's requirement for rest, relaxation, and time together with family members. *Enhances understanding of mother's needs, and family members feel included and more willing to support breastfeeding activity/treatment plan.*[11]
- Arrange dietary consult to review nutritional needs and vitamin/mineral supplements, such as vitamin C, as indicated. *During lactation, there is an increased need for energy requiring supplementation of protein, vitamins, and minerals to provide nourishment for the infant.*[11]
- Stress importance of adequate fluid intake. *Alternating types of fluids (e.g., water, juice, decaffeinated tea/coffee, milk) enhances intake promoting milk production. Note: Beer and wine are not recommended for increasing lactation.*[11]
- Encourage peer counseling for teen mothers. *Provides positive role model that teen can relate to and feel comfortable with discussing concerns and feelings.*[14]
- Recommend monitoring number of infant's wet and soiled diapers. *Stools should be yellow in color and infant should have at least six wet diapers a day to determine that infant is receiving sufficient intake.*[12]
- Weigh infant every 3 days, or as directed by primary provider/lactation consultant, and record. *Monitors weight gain verifying adequacy of intake or need for additional interventions.*[11]
- Identify products/programs for cessation of smoking. *Smoking can interfere with the release of oxytocin, which stimulates the letdown reflex, and can negatively affect milk production.*[4,9,11]
- Refer to support groups (e.g., La Leche League International, parenting support groups, stress management class, or other community resources, as indicated). *Provides information and ongoing support increasing likelihood of successful breastfeeding.*[9]

DOCUMENTATION FOCUS

Assessment/Reassessment

- Identified maternal assessment factors—hydration level, medication use, lifestyle choices.
- Cultural factors, support systems.
- Findings of breast examination.
- Infant assessment factors—latching-on technique, hydration level/number of wet diapers, weight gain/loss.
- Use of supplemental feedings.

Planning

- Plan of care, specific interventions, and who is involved in planning.
- Individual teaching plan.

Implementation/Evaluation

- Mother's/infant's responses to interventions, teaching, and actions performed.
- Change in infant's weight.
- Attainment or progress toward desired outcomes.
- Modification to plan of care.

Discharge Planning

- Specific referrals made.

References

1. Nagin, M. J. (updated 2015). Relactation—How to increase your milk supply. Retrieved October 2015 from http://breastfeeding.about.com/od/lactation/a/relactation.htm.
2. Murray, D. (updated 2015). 6 Ways to naturally increase your breast milk supply. Retrieved October 2015 from http://breastfeeding.about.com/od/milksupplyproblems/a/Increasing-Your-Milk-Supply-Naturally.htm.
3. Iannelli, V. (updated 2014). Breastfeeding your child effectively—Breastfeeding and breast compression. Retrieved October 2015 from http://pediatrics.about.com/od/breastfeeding/a/compression.htm.
4. Murray, D. (updated 2014). Things that can decrease your milk supply. Retrieved October 2015 from http://breastfeeding.about.com/od/breastfeedingwork/a/compression.htm.
5. Daly, S. E. J., Hartmann, P. E. (1995). Infant demand and milk supply, part 1: Infant demand and milk production in lactating women. *J Hum Lact*, 11(1), 21–26.
6. Kent, J. C., Prime, D. K., Garbin, C. F. (2012). Principles for maintaining or increasing breast milk production. *J Obstet Gynecol Neonatal Nurs*, 41(1), 114–121.
7. Morton, J., Hall, J. Y., Wong, R. J., et al. (2009). Combining hand techniques with electric pumping increases milk production in mothers of preterm infants. *J Perinatol*, 29(11), 757–764.
8. Wambach, K. A., Cohen, S. M. (2009). Breast feeding experiences of urban adolescent mothers. *J Pediatr Nurs*, 24(4), 244–254.
9. The Academy of Breastfeeding Medicine Protocol Committee. (2011). Protocol #9: Use of galactogogues in initiating or augmenting maternal milk supply. *Breastfeeding Med*, 6(1), 41–49.
10. Smith, A. (2013). Increasing Your Milk Supply. Retrieved October 2015 from http://www.breastfeedingbasics.com/article/increasing-your-milk-supply.
11. Ladewig, P., London, M., Davidson, M. (2009). *Contemporary Maternal-Newborn Nursing Care*. 7th ed. Upper Saddle River, NJ: Prentice Hall.
12. Riodan, J., Auerbach, K. (2010). *Breastfeeding and Human Lactation*. 4th ed. Boston: Jones & Bartlett.
13. Lowdermilk, D. L., Cashion, M. C., Perry, S. E. (2011). *Maternity & Women's Health Care*. 10th ed. St. Louis, MO: Mosby.
14. Phillips, C. R. (1996). *Family-Centered Maternity and Newborn Care*. 4th ed. St. Louis, MO: Mosby.

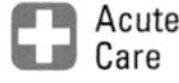

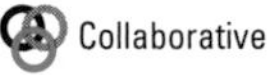

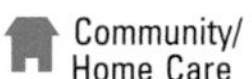

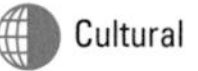

ineffective Breathing Pattern

Taxonomy II: Activity/Rest—Class 4 Cardiovascular/Pulmonary Responses (00032) [**Diagnostic Division:** Respiration], Submitted 1980; Revised 1996, 1998, 2010

DEFINITION: Inspiration and/or expiration that does not provide adequate ventilation.

RELATED FACTORS

Neuromuscular impairment; spinal cord injury (SCI); neurological impairment (e.g., positive EEG, head trauma, seizure disorders) or immaturity
Musculoskeletal impairment; bony or chest wall deformity
Anxiety; [panic attacks]
Pain
Fatigue; [deconditioning]; respiratory muscle fatigue
Body position that inhibits lung expansion; obesity
Hyperventilation; hypoventilation syndrome; [alteration of client's normal O_2:CO_2 ratio (e.g., lung diseases, pulmonary hypertension, airway obstruction, O_2 therapy in chronic obstructive pulmonary disease—COPD)]

DEFINING CHARACTERISTICS

Subjective

Dyspnea; [feeling breathless]
Orthopnea

Objective

Bradypnea; tachypnea
Abnormal breathing pattern (e.g., rate, rhythm, depth)
Prolonged expiration phases; pursed-lip breathing
Decrease in minute ventilation or vital capacity
Decrease in inspiratory or expiratory pressure
Use of accessory muscles to breathe; use of three-point position
Altered chest excursion; [paradoxical breathing patterns]
Nasal flaring; [grunting]
Increase in anterior-posterior diameter
Sample Clinical Applications: COPD, emphysema, asthma, pneumonia, chest trauma or surgery, SCI, Guillain-Barré syndrome, traumatic brain injury, cystic fibrosis, drug or alcohol toxicity

DESIRED OUTCOMES/EVALUATION CRITERIA

Sample NOC linkages:
Respiratory Status: Ventilation: Movement of air in and out of the lungs
Fatigue Level: Severity of observed or reported prolonged fatigue
Anxiety Level: Severity of manifested apprehension, tension, or uneasiness arising from an unidentifiable source

Client Will (Include Specific Time Frame)

- Establish a normal, effective respiratory pattern.
- Be free of cyanosis and other signs/symptoms of hypoxia with arterial blood gases (ABGs) within client's normal/acceptable range.
- Verbalize awareness of causative factors and initiate needed lifestyle changes.
- Demonstrate appropriate coping behaviors.

(continues on page 122)

ineffective Breathing Pattern (continued)
ACTIONS/INTERVENTIONS

Sample NIC linkages:
Ventilation Assistance: Promotion of an optimal spontaneous breathing pattern that maximizes oxygen and carbon dioxide exchange in the lungs
Airway Management: Facilitation of patency of air passages
Respiratory Monitoring: Collection and analysis of patient data to ensure airway patency and adequate gas exchange

NURSING PRIORITY NO. 1 To identify etiology/precipitating factors:

- Identify age and ethnic group of client who may be at increased risk. *Respiratory ailments in general are increased in infants and children with neuromuscular disorders, the frail elderly, and persons living in highly polluted environments.*[1,2] *Studies have linked air pollution to heart disease, asthma, and other diseases. Communities that live in areas, such as close to freeways or high traffic areas, with high levels of air toxins are especially vulnerable.*[3,4] *People most at risk for infectious pneumonias include the very young and frail elderly; those suffering from chronic respiratory or circulatory problems; and those with compromised immune systems from congenital deficiencies, AIDS, cancers, and cancer therapies.*[2,5]
- Ascertain if client has history of underlying respiratory disorder or if this is a new condition with potential for breathing problems or exacerbation of preexisting problems (e.g., asthma, other acute upper respiratory infection, lung cancer, neuromuscular disorders, heart disease, sepsis, burns, acute chest or brain trauma). *Important in pointing to cause for current breathing problems.*[6]
- Assess for pregnancy, other abdominal distention, and muscle guarding. *Distended abdomen and muscle tension can impede diaphragmatic excursion and reduce lung expansion.*
- Note current symptoms and how they relate to past history. *Assessing current illness, including history of (1) onset and duration of symptoms; (2) how they are similar to or different from past symptoms; (3) precipitating, relieving, and exacerbating factors; and (4) exposures (e.g., environmental toxins, alcohol or other drugs, source of infection) may help in selecting the correct diagnosis.*
- Note emotional state. *Gasping, crying, anxiety, irritability, struggling, look of fear, report of tingling lips or fingers, withdrawal, and self-focus are responses often associated with respiratory distress. Emotional changes can accompany a condition or precipitate or aggravate ineffective breathing patterns.*[5–9]
- Evaluate client's respiratory status:

  Note rate and depth of respirations, counting for 1 full minute, if rate is irregular. *Rate may be faster or slower than usual. In infants and younger children, rate increases dramatically relative to anxiety, crying, fever, or disease. Depth may be difficult to evaluate but is usually described as shallow, normal, or deep.*[5,7,8]

  Note client's reports and perceptions of breathing ease. *Client may report a range of symptoms (e.g., air hunger, shortness of breath with speaking, activity, or at rest) and demonstrate a wide range of signs (e.g., tachypnea, gasping, wheezing, coughing).*

  Observe characteristics of breathing pattern. *May note use of accessory muscles for breathing, sternal retractions (infants and young children), nasal flaring, or pursed-lip breathing. Client may change position in effort to breathe easier. Irregular patterns may be pathological (e.g., prolonged expiration, periods of apnea, obvious agonal breathing) with pronounced alterations in conditions such as severe asthma attack, brainstem damage, or impending respiratory failure.*[5–7]

  Auscultate and percuss chest, describing presence, absence, and character of breath sounds. *Air should be moving freely through air passages (differs from ineffective airway clearance), but ventilatory effort may be insufficient to bring in enough oxygen or to exchange sufficient amounts of carbon dioxide, such as might*

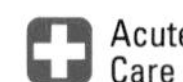
Acute Care
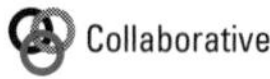
Collaborative
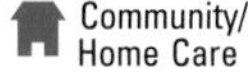
Community/ Home Care
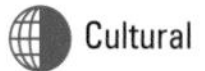
Cultural

occur in asthma or congenital heart disease. Abnormal breath sounds are indicative of numerous problems (e.g., obstruction by foreign object, hypoventilation such as might occur with chest or spinal cord injuries, atelectasis, or presence of secretions, improper endotracheal [ET] tube placement, collapsed lung) and must be evaluated and reported for further intervention.[5,8,9]

Observe chest size, shape, and symmetry of movement. *Changes in movement of chest wall (such as might occur with chest trauma, chest wall deformities) can impair breathing patterns.*

Note color of skin and mucous membranes. *If pallor, duskiness, and/or cyanosis are present, supplemental oxygen and/or other interventions may be required.* (Refer to ND impaired Gas Exchange.)

Note presence and character of cough. *Cough function may be weak or ineffective in conditions such as extremes in age (e.g., premature infant or elderly); in diseases (e.g., cerebral palsy, muscular dystrophy, SCI, brain injury); after surgery; and/or in mechanical ventilation due to mechanisms affecting muscles of throat, chest, and lungs. Cough that is persistent and constant can interfere with breathing (such as can occur with asthma, acute bronchitis, cystic fibrosis, croup, whooping cough).*[1,6–10] (Refer to ND ineffective Airway Clearance.)

- Assess client's awareness and cognition. *Affects ability to manage own airway and cooperate with interventions such as controlling breathing and managing secretions.*[2,8,9]
- Assist with and monitor results of diagnostic testing (e.g., pulmonary or cardiac function studies, neuromuscular evaluation, sleep studies) *to diagnose presence and severity of lung diseases and degree of respiratory compromise.*
- Review chest radiographs and laboratory data (e.g., ABGs, pulse oximetry at rest and activity *to determine degree of oxygenation, CO_2 retention)* and pulmonary function studies (such as spirometry) *to determine effectiveness of inhalation and exhalation.*[9]

NURSING PRIORITY NO. 2 To provide for relief of causative factors, promoting ease of breathing:[6–11]

- Assist in treatment of underlying conditions, administering medications and therapies as ordered.
- Suction airway to clear secretions as needed. (Refer to ND ineffective Airway Clearance for additional interventions.)
- Maintain emergency equipment in readily accessible location and include age- and size-appropriate airway, ET, and tracheostomy tubes (e.g., infant, child, adolescent, adult).
- Administer oxygen (by cannula, mask, mechanical ventilation) at lowest concentration needed (per ABGs, pulse oximetry) *for underlying pulmonary condition and current respiratory problem.*[11–13] (Refer to ND impaired Gas Exchange for additional interventions.)
- Elevate head of bed or have client sit up in chair; support with pillows *to prevent slumping and promote rest,* or place in position of comfort, as appropriate, *to promote maximal inspiration.*
- Reposition client frequently *to enhance respiratory effort and ventilation of all lung segments, especially if immobility is a factor.*
- Encourage early ambulation using assistive devices, as individually indicated. Involve client in program of exercise training *to prevent onset or reduce severity of respiratory complications and to improve respiratory muscle strength.*[11]
- Direct client in breathing efforts as needed. Encourage slower and deeper respirations and use of the pursed-lip technique, *to assist client in "taking control" of the situation, especially when condition is associated with anxiety and air hunger.*
- Coach client in effective coughing techniques. Place in appropriate position for clearing airways. Splint rib cage and surgical incisions as appropriate. Medicate for pain, as indicated. *Promotes breathing that is more effective and airway management when client is guarding, as might occur with chest, rib cage, or abdominal injuries or surgeries.* (Refer to NDs acute Pain; chronic Pain for additional interventions.)
- Provide and assist with use of respiratory therapy adjuncts.
- Maintain calm attitude while working with client/significant others (SOs). Provide quiet environment, instruct and reinforce client in the use of relaxation techniques, and administer anti-anxiety medications as indicated *to*

reduce intensity of anxiety and deal with fear that may be present. (Refer to NDs Fear; Anxiety for additional interventions.)

- Avoid overfeeding, such as might occur with young infant or client on tube feedings. *Abdominal distention can interfere with breathing as well as increase the risk of aspiration.*
- Ascertain that client possesses and properly operates continuous positive airway pressure machine *when obstructive sleep apnea is causing breathing problems.*
- Maintain emergency equipment in readily accessible location and include age/size-appropriate ET/tracheostomy tubes (e.g., infant, child, adolescent, adult) *when ventilatory support might be needed.*
- Assist with bronchoscopy or chest tube insertion as indicated.

NURSING PRIORITY NO. 3 To promote wellness (Teaching/Discharge Considerations):

- Review with client/SO the type of respiratory condition, treatments, rehabilitation measures, and quality-of-life issues. *Many conditions with impaired breathing are associated with chronic conditions that require lifetime management by client and healthcare providers.*
- Instruct and reinforce breathing retraining. *Education may include many measures, such as conscious control of respiratory rate, effective use of accessory muscles, breathing exercises (diaphragmatic, abdominal breathing, inspiratory resistive, pursed-lip), and assistive devices such as rocking bed.*[6]
- Discuss relationship of smoking to respiratory function. Stress importance of smoking cessation and a smoke-free environment.
- Encourage client/SO(s) to develop a plan for smoking cessation. Provide appropriate referrals.
- Encourage self-assessment and symptom management:[6–11]
  Use of equipment to identify respiratory decompensation, such as peak flow meter.
  Appropriate use of oxygen (dosage, route, safety factors).
  Medication regimen, including actions, side effects, and potential interactions of medications, over-the-counter drugs, vitamins, and herbal supplements.
  Home treatments such as metered-dose inhalers, compressor, nebulizer, and chest physiotherapies.
  Dietary patterns and needs; access to foods and nutrients supportive of health and breathing.
  Management of personal environment, including stress reduction, rest and sleep, social events, travel, and recreation issues.
  Avoidance of known irritants, allergens, and sick persons.
  Immunizations against influenza and pneumonia.
  Early intervention when respiratory symptoms occur and what symptoms require reporting to medical providers or seeking emergency care.
- Discuss benefits of exercise for endurance, muscle strengthening, and flexibility training *to improve general health and respiratory muscle function.*
- Refer to physical therapy and pulmonary rehabilitation programs and resources as indicated.[11,12]
- Review energy conservation techniques (e.g., sitting instead of standing to wash dishes, pacing activities, taking short rest periods between activities) *to limit fatigue and improve endurance.*
- Review environmental factors (e.g., exposure to dust, high pollen counts, severe weather, perfumes, animal dander, household chemicals, fumes, secondhand smoke; insufficient home support for safe care) *that may require avoidance/modification of lifestyle or environment to limit impact on client's breathing.*[12–14]
- Reinforce instruction in proper use and safety concerns for home oxygen therapy and/or use of respirator or diaphragmatic stimulator, rocking bed, or apnea monitor, when used. *Protects client's safety, especially when used in the very young or fragile elderly or when a cognitive or neuromuscular impairment is present.*
- Discuss impact of respiratory condition on occupational performance, as well as work environment issues that affect client.
- Provide referrals as indicated by individual situation. *May include a wide variety of services and providers, including support groups, a comprehensive rehabilitation program, occupational nurse, oxygen and durable medical equipment companies for supplies, home health services, occupational and physical therapy,*

transportation, assisted or alternate living facilities, local and national Lung Association chapters, and Web sites for educational materials.

DOCUMENTATION FOCUS

Assessment/Reassessment

- Relevant history of problem.
- Respiratory pattern, breath sounds, use of accessory muscles.
- Laboratory values.
- Use of respiratory supports, ventilator settings, etc.

Planning

- Plan of care, specific interventions, and who is involved in the planning.
- Teaching plan.

Implementation/Evaluation

- Response to interventions, teaching, actions performed, and treatment regimen.
- Mastery of skills, level of independence.
- Attainment or progress toward desired outcome(s).
- Modifications to plan of care.

Discharge Planning

- Long-term needs, including appropriate referrals and action taken, available resources.
- Specific referrals provided.

References

1. Bradley, J. S., et al. (2011). The management of Community-Acquired Pneumonia in Infants and Children Older Than 3 Months of Age. Retrieved October 2015 from http://www.idsociety.org/uploadedFiles/IDSA/Guidelines-Patient_Care/PDF_Library/2011%20CAP%20in%20Children.pdf.
2. Stanley, M., Blair, K. A., Beare, P. G. (2005). *Gerontological Nursing: Promoting Successful Aging with Older Adults.* 3rd ed. Philadelphia: F. A. Davis.
3. American Lung Association. State of lung disease in diverse communities 2010. Retrieved October 2015 from http://www.action.lung.org/site/DocServer/state-of-lung-disease-in-diverse-communities-2010.pdf?docID=8744.
4. Purnell, L. D. (2011). *A Guide to Culturally Competent Health Care.* 2nd ed. Philadelphia: F. A. Davis.
5. Williams, M. E. (2009). The basic geriatric respiratory examination. Retrieved October 2015 from http://www.medscape.com/viewarticle/712242.
6. Rabe, K. F., Hurd, S., Anzueto, A., et al. (2007). Global strategy for the diagnosis, management, and prevention of chronic obstructive pulmonary disease. *Am J Respir Crit Care Med*, 176, 532–555.
7. Engel, J. (2002). *Mosby's Pocket Guide to Pediatric Assessment.* 4th ed. St. Louis, MO: Mosby.
8. Cox, H. C., Sridaromont, K., King, M., et al. (2002). *Clinical Applications of Nursing Diagnosis: Adult, Child, Women's, Gerontic, and Home Health Considerations.* 4th ed. Philadelphia: F. A. Davis, 256–261.
9. Doenges, M. E., Moorhouse, M. F., Murr, A. C. (2010). *Nurse's Pocket Guide: Diagnoses, Prioritized Interventions and Rationales.* 12th ed. Philadelphia: F. A. Davis, 151–155.
10. Irwin, R. S. (2006). Introduction to the diagnosis and management of cough: ACCP evidence-based clinical practice guidelines. *Chest*, 129(1 Suppl), 255–275.
11. Ries, A. L., Bauldoff, G. S., Carlin, B. W., et al. (1997, revised 2007). Pulmonary rehabilitation: Joint ACCP/AACVPR evidence-based clinical practice guidelines. Retrieved October 2015 from http://journal.publications.chestnet.org/article.aspx?articleid=1209436.
12. Bauldoff, G. S., Diaz, P. T. (2006). Improving outcomes for COPD patients. *Nurs Pract*, 31(8), 26–43.
13. Pruitt, B. (2006). Weaning patients from mechanical ventilation. *Nursing*, 36(9), 36–41.
14. Garyi, J. P. (update 2015). Exercise-induced asthma. Retrieved October 2015 from http://emedicine.medscape.com/article/1938228-overview.

decreased Cardiac Output

Taxonomy II: Activity/Rest—Class 4 Cardiovascular/Pulmonary Responses (00029) [**Diagnostic Division:** Circulation], Submitted 1979; Revised 1996, 2000

DEFINITION: Inadequate blood pumped by the heart to meet the metabolic demands of the body. [Note: In a hypermetabolic state, although cardiac output may be within normal range, it may still be inadequate to meet the needs of the body's tissues. Cardiac output and tissue perfusion are interrelated, although there are differences. When cardiac output is decreased, tissue perfusion problems will develop; however, tissue perfusion problems can exist without decreased cardiac output.]

RELATED FACTORS

Alteration in heart rate or rhythm
Altered afterload [e.g., systemic vascular resistance]
Altered contractility [e.g., ventricular-septal rupture, ventricular aneurysm, papillary muscle rupture, valvular disease]
Altered preload [e.g., decreased venous return]
Altered stroke volume

DEFINING CHARACTERISTICS

Subjective

Altered Heart Rate/Rhythm: Heart palpitations
Altered Preload: Fatigue
Altered Afterload: Dyspnea; [feeling breathless]
Altered Contractility: Orthopnea; paroxysmal nocturnal dyspnea [PND]
Behavioral/Emotional: Anxiety

Objective

Altered Heart Rate/Rhythm: Bradycardia; tachycardia; ECG [electrocardiogram] changes (e.g., arrhythmia, conduction abnormality, ischemia)
Altered Preload: Jugular vein distention; edema; weight gain; increase or decrease in central venous pressure (CVP); increase or decrease in pulmonary artery wedge pressure (PAWP); heart murmur
Altered Afterload: Clammy skin; abnormal skin color (e.g., pale, dusky, cyanosis); prolonged capillary refill; decreased peripheral pulses; alterations in blood pressure readings; increase or decrease in systemic vascular resistance; increase or decrease in pulmonary vascular resistance; oliguria
Altered Contractility: Adventitious breath sounds; cough; decreased cardiac index; decrease in ejection fraction; decrease in stroke volume index (SVI) or left ventricular stroke work index (LVSWI); presence of S_3 or S_4 sounds [gallop rhythm]
Behavioral/Emotional: Restlessness
Sample Clinical Applications: Myocardial infarction (MI), congestive heart failure, valvular heart disease, dysrhythmias, cardiomyopathy, cardiac contusions/trauma, pericarditis, ventricular aneurysm

DESIRED OUTCOMES/EVALUATION CRITERIA

Sample NOC linkages:

Cardiac Pump Effectiveness: Adequacy of blood volume ejected from the left ventricle to support systemic perfusion pressure
Circulation Status: Unobstructed, unidirectional blood flow at an appropriate pressure through large vessels of the systemic and pulmonary circuits
Energy Conservation: Personal actions to manage energy for initiating and sustaining activity

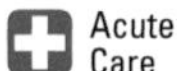

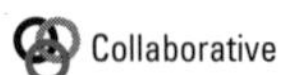

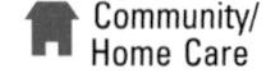

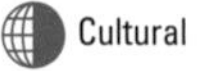

Client Will (Include Specific Time Frame)

- Display hemodynamic stability (e.g., blood pressure, cardiac output, urinary output, peripheral pulses).
- Report or demonstrate decreased episodes of dyspnea, angina, and dysrhythmias.
- Demonstrate an increase in activity tolerance.
- Verbalize knowledge of the disease process, individual risk factors, and treatment plan.
- Participate in activities that reduce the workload of the heart (e.g., stress management or therapeutic medication regimen program, weight reduction, balanced activity/rest plan, proper use of supplemental oxygen, cessation of smoking).
- Identify signs of cardiac decompensation, alter activities, and seek help appropriately.

ACTIONS/INTERVENTIONS

Sample NIC linkages:

Hemodynamic Regulation: Optimization of heart rate, preload, afterload, and contractility

Cardiac Care: Limitation of complications resulting from an imbalance between myocardial oxygen supply and demand for a patient with symptoms of impaired cardiac function

Circulatory Care: Mechanical Assist Devices: Temporary support of the circulation through the use of mechanical devices or pumps

NURSING PRIORITY NO. 1 To identify causative/contributing factors:

- Review clients at risk as noted in Related Factors and Defining Characteristics. *In addition to individuals obviously at risk with known cardiac problems, there is a potential for cardiac output problems in persons with trauma; hemorrhage; alcohol and other drug intoxication, withdrawal, chronic use, or overdose; pregnant women with hypertensive states; individuals with chronic renal failure; individuals with brainstem trauma or spinal cord injury at T8 or above.*
- Note age, gender and ethnic-related cardiovascular considerations, e.g., *in infants, failure to thrive with poor ability to suck and feed can be an indication of heart problems.*[1] *Contractile force is naturally decreased in the elderly with reduced ability to increase cardiac output in response to increased demand. Also, arteries are stiffer, veins are more dilated, and heart valves are less competent, often resulting in systemic hypertension and blood pooling.*[3] *The prevalence of heart failure is 2.7% of the population between 45 and 55 years and increases to a rate of 7.8% for persons older than 65 years.*[4] *When in the supine position, pregnant women incur decreased vascular return during the second and third trimesters, potentially compromising cardiac output.*[2] *Generally, higher-risk populations include African Americans, Hispanics, Native Americans, and recent immigrants from developing nations, Russia, and the former Soviet republics. The higher prevalence of heart failure in African Americans, Hispanics, and Native Americans is directly related to the higher incidence and prevalence of hypertension and diabetes.*[4,5]
- Review diagnostic studies, including, but not limited to, chest radiograph, cardiac stress testing, ECG, echocardiogram, cardiac output and ventricular ejection studies, and heart scan or catheterization. *For example, ECG may show previous or evolving MI, left ventricular hypertrophy, and valvular stenosis. Doppler flow echocardiogram showing an ejection fraction (EF) less than 40% is indicative of systolic dysfunction, but many clients with clinical diagnosis of heart failure have a normal EF. Although cardiac output can be high in certain types of heart failure, a client with severe heart failure (HF) will have decreased cardiac output (less than 4 L/m) owing either to an increased hemodynamic burden or to a reduction in oxygen delivery to the myocardium, resulting in impaired contraction. Additional cardiac studies (e.g., radionuclide scans or catheterization) may be indicated to assess left ventricular function, valvular function, and coronary circulation. Chest radiography may show enlarged heart, pulmonary infiltrates.*[6–8,12,13]
- Review laboratory data, including, but not limited to, complete blood count, electrolytes, arterial blood gases (ABGs), and cardiac biomarkers (e.g., creatine kinase and its subclasses, troponins, myoglobin, and LDH); lactate; brain natriuretic peptide; kidney, thyroid, and liver function studies; and cultures (e.g., blood,

wound, secretions), bleeding, and coagulation studies *to identify imbalances, disease processes, and effects of interventions.*[6,12]

NURSING PRIORITY NO. 2 To assess degree of debilitation:

- Assess for signs of poor ventricular function or impending cardiac failure and shock:[2,3,7–12]

  Client reports or demonstrates extreme fatigue, intolerance for activity, sudden or progressive weight gain, swelling of extremities, and progressive shortness of breath.

  Client reports chest pain. *May indicate evolving heart attack; can also accompany congestive heart failure. Chest pain may be atypical in women experiencing an MI and is often atypical in the elderly owing to altered pain perception.*

  Mental status changes. *Confusion, agitation, decreased cognition, and coma may occur due to decreased brain perfusion.*

  Changes in heart rate or rhythm: Tachycardia at rest, bradycardia, atrial fibrillation, or multiple dysrhythmias may be noted. *Heart irritability is common, reflecting conduction defects and/or ischemia.*

  Heart sounds may be distant, with irregular rhythms; murmurs—systolic *(valvular stenosis and shunting)* and diastolic *(aortic or pulmonary insufficiency)* or gallop rhythm (S_3, S_4) noted *when heart failure is present and ventricles are stiff.*

  Peripheral pulses may be weak and thready, *reflecting hypotension, vasoconstriction, shunting, and venous congestion.*

  ∞ Changes in skin color, moisture, temperature, and capillary refill time. *Pallor or cyanosis; cool, moist skin; and slow capillary refill time may be present because of peripheral vasoconstriction and decreased oxygen saturation. Note: Children with chronic heart failure and adults with chronic obstructive pulmonary disease often show clubbing of fingertips.*

  Blood pressure changes. *Hypertension may be chronic or blood pressure elevated initially in client with impending cardiogenic, hypovolemic, or septic shock. Later, as cardiac output decreases, profound hypotension can be present, often with narrowed pulse pressure.*

  Breath sounds may reveal bilateral crackles and wheezing *associated with congestion. Respiratory distress and failure often occur as shock progresses.*

  Edema with neck vein distention is often present, and pitting edema is noted in extremities and dependent portions of body *because of impaired venous return.* Other veins in trunk and extremities can be prominent *owing to venous congestion.*

  ∞ Urinary output may be decreased or absent, *reflecting poor perfusion of kidneys. Note: Output less than 30 mL/hr (adult) or less than 10 mL/hr (child) indicates inadequate renal perfusion.*

NURSING PRIORITY NO. 3 To minimize/correct causative factors, maximize cardiac output:

Acute/severe phase[7–10,12,15]

- Keep client on bedrest or chairrest in position of comfort. *Decreases oxygen consumption and demand, reducing myocardial workload and risk of decomposition. Note: In congestive state, client may be placed in semi-Fowler's or high Fowler's position to reduce preload and ventricular filling. A supine position may be needed to increase venous return and promote diuresis. May raise legs 20 to 30 degrees in shock situation (Trendelenburg position); however, current data to support the use of the Trendelenburg position during shock are limited and do not reveal any beneficial or sustained changes in systolic blood pressure or cardiac output.*[18]
- Administer supplemental oxygen, as indicated (by cannula, mask, endotracheal or tracheostomy tube with mechanical ventilation), *to improve cardiac function by increasing available oxygen and reducing oxygen consumption. Note: A critically ill client may be on ventilator to support cardiopulmonary function.*[12]
- Monitor vital signs frequently *to evaluate response to treatments and activities.* Perform periodic hemodynamic measurements, as indicated (e.g., arterial, CVP, PAWP, left atrial pressure; cardiac output and

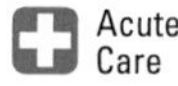
Acute Care
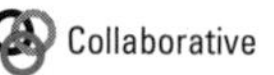
Collaborative
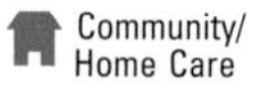
Community/Home Care
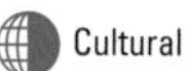
Cultural

cardiac index, oxygen saturation). *These measurements (via central line monitoring) are commonly used in the critically ill to provide continuous, accurate assessment of cardiac function and response to inotropic and vasoactive medications that affect cardiac contractility and systemic circulation (preload and afterload). Note: A multicenter research study evaluating the clinical effectiveness of clinical management guided by a pulmonary artery catheter in adult intensive care patients (*N = *1,041) found no clear evidence that management guided by a pulmonary catheter was either beneficial or harmful.*[15,17]

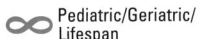

- Monitor cardiac rhythm continuously *to note changes and evaluate effectiveness of medications and devices (e.g., implanted pacemaker/defibrillator).*
- Administer or restrict fluids, as indicated. *Replacement of blood and large amounts of IV fluids may be needed if low output state is due to hypovolemia.* Use infusion pumps for IVs *to monitor IV rates closely to prevent bolus or exacerbation of fluid overload.*
- Assess hourly or periodic urinary output and daily weight, noting 24-hr total fluid balance *to evaluate kidney function and effects of interventions, as well as to allow for timely alterations in therapeutic regimen.*
- Administer medications as indicated (e.g., inotropic drugs *to maintain systemic perfusion and preserve end-organ performance,* antiarrhythmics *to improve cardiac output;* diuretics *to reduce congestion by improving urinary output;* vasopressors and/or dilators as indicated *to manage systemic effects of vasoconstriction and low cardiac output;* pain medications and anti-anxiety agents *to reduce oxygen demand and myocardial workload;* anticoagulants *to improve blood flow and prevent thromboemboli). Note: Studies show that some antiarrhythmics have negative inotropic effects, and some, particularly the class I and class III drugs, have proarrhythmic effects. Amiodarone (Cordarone) and dofetilide (Tikosyn) are two antiarrhythmic agents found to have neutral effects on mortality in clinical trials of patients with HF.*[7]
- Note reports of anorexia or nausea and limit or withhold oral intake as indicated. *Symptoms may be systemic reaction to low cardiac output, visceral congestion, or reaction to medications or pain.*
- Assist with preparations for and monitor response to support procedures or devices as indicated (e.g., cardioversion, pacemaker, angioplasty and stent placement, coronary artery bypass graft or valve replacement, intra-aortic balloon pump, left ventricular assist device [LVAD]). *Any number of interventions may be required to correct a condition causing heart failure or to support a failing heart during recovery from myocardial infarction, while awaiting transplantation, or for long-term management of chronic heart failure. Note: The application of LVAD during reperfusion procedures causes reduction of the left ventricular preload, increases regional myocardial blood flow and lactate extraction, and improves general cardiac function.*[7]
- Promote rest periods in bed or chair with upper body elevated, as indicated, *to reduce catecholamine-induced stress response and cardiac workload:*[11,15]
  Decrease stimuli, providing quiet environment.
  Schedule activities and assessments *to maximize sleep periods.*
  Assist with or perform self-care activities for client.
  Avoid the use of restraints whenever possible, especially if client is confused.
- Use sedation and analgesics, as indicated, with caution *to achieve desired rest state without compromising hemodynamic responses.*

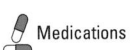

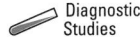

Postacute/Chronic Phase[6,7,11]

- Provide for adequate rest, positioning client for maximum comfort.
- Encourage changing positions slowly, dangling legs before standing *to reduce risk of orthostatic hypotension.*
- Increase activity levels gradually as permitted by individual condition, noting vital sign response to activity.
- Administer medications, as appropriate, and monitor cardiac responses.
- Encourage relaxation techniques *to reduce anxiety and muscle tension.*
- Refer for nutritional needs assessment and management *to provide for supportive nutrition while meeting diet restrictions (e.g., IV nutrition or total parenteral nutrition, sodium-restricted or other type of diet with frequent small feedings).*
- Monitor intake/output and calculate 24-hr fluid balance. Provide or restrict fluids, as indicated, *to maximize cardiac output and improve tissue perfusion.*[15]

NURSING PRIORITY NO. 4 To enhance safety/prevent complications :[2,14,15]

- Wash hands before and after client contact, maintain aseptic technique during invasive procedures, and provide site care, as indicated, *to prevent hospital-acquired infection.* (Refer to ND risk for Infection for additional interventions.)
- Provide antipyretics and fever control actions as indicated. Adjust ambient environmental temperature *to maintain body temperature in near-normal range.*
- Maintain patency of invasive intravascular monitoring and infusion lines and tape connections *to prevent exsanguination or air embolus.*
- Minimize activities that can elicit Valsalva response (e.g., rectal straining, vomiting, spasmodic coughing with suctioning, prolonged breath-holding during pushing stage of labor) and encourage client to breathe deeply in and out during activities that increase risk of Valsalva effect. *Valsalva response to breath-holding causes increased intrathoracic pressure, reducing cardiac output and blood pressure.*[14]
- Avoid prolonged sitting position for all clients and supine position for sleep or exercise for gravid clients (second and third trimesters) *to maximize vascular return.*[2,15]
- Elevate legs when in sitting position and edematous extremities when at rest. Apply antiembolic hose or sequential compression devices when indicated, being sure they are individually fitted and appropriately applied. *Limits venous stasis, improves venous return, and reduces risk of thrombophlebitis.* (Refer to ND ineffective peripheral Tissue Perfusion for additional interventions.)
- Provide skin care, a special bed or mattress (e.g., air, water, gel, foam), and assist with frequent position changes *to prevent the development of pressure ulcers.*
- Provide psychological support *to reduce anxiety and its adverse effects on cardiac function:*
  Maintain calm attitude and limit stressful stimuli.
  Provide and encourage use of relaxation techniques, such as massage therapy, soothing music, or quiet activities.
  Promote visits from family/significant others *to provide positive social interaction.*
  Provide information about testing procedures and client participation.
  Explain limitations imposed by condition and dietary and fluid restrictions.
  Share information about positive signs of improvement.

NURSING PRIORITY NO. 5 To promote wellness (Teaching/Discharge Considerations) :[11,16]

- Provide information to clients/caregivers on individual condition, therapies, and expected outcomes. Use various forms of teaching according to client needs, desires, and learning style.
- Direct client and/or caregivers to resources for emergency assistance, financial help, durable medical supplies, and psychosocial support and respite, especially when client has impaired functional capabilities or requires supporting equipment (e.g., pacemaker, LVAD, or 24-hr oxygen).
- Emphasize importance of regular medical follow-up care *to monitor client's condition and response to treatment and provide the most effective care.*
- Educate client/caregivers about drug regimen, including indications, dose and dosing schedules, potential adverse side effects, or drug/drug interactions. *Client is often on multiple medications, which can be difficult to manage, thus increasing potential that medications can be missed or incorrectly used.*
- Emphasize reporting of adverse and nuisance side effects of medications *so that adjustments can be made in dosing or another class of medication considered.*
- Discuss significant signs/symptoms that need to be reported to healthcare provider, such as *unrelieved or increased chest pain, dyspnea, fever, swelling of ankles, and sudden unexplained cough—these are all "danger signs" that require immediate evaluation and possible change of usual therapies.*
- Provide instruction for home monitoring of weight, pulse, and blood pressure, as appropriate, *to detect change and allow for timely intervention.*
- Recommend annual flu shot, and pneumonia vaccination (when needed).

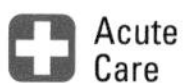

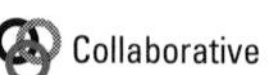

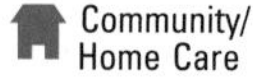

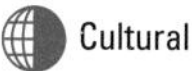

- Discuss individual's particular risk factors (e.g., smoking, stress, obesity, recent MI) and specific resources for assistance (e.g., written information sheets, direction to helpful Web sites, formalized rehabilitation programs, home interventions) for management of identified factors for:
  Smoking cessation
  Stress management techniques
  Energy conservation techniques
  Nutrition education regarding specific needs (e.g., to improve general health status, reduce or gain weight, lower cholesterol levels, manage sodium)
  Exercise and activity plan
- Refer to NDs Activity Intolerance, deficient Diversional Activity, ineffective Coping, ineffective Breathing Pattern, compromised family Coping, deficient/excess Fluid Volume, imbalanced Nutrition: less than body requirements, Overweight, acute/chronic Pain, risk for decreased cardiac Tissue Perfusion, ineffective peripheral Tissue Perfusion, Sexual Dysfunction, as indicated.

DOCUMENTATION FOCUS

Assessment/Reassessment

- Baseline and subsequent findings and individual hemodynamic parameters, heart and breath sounds, ECG pattern, presence and strength of peripheral pulses, skin and tissue status, renal output, and mentation.

Planning

- Plan of care and who is involved in planning.
- Teaching plan.

Implementation/Evaluation

- Client's responses to interventions, teaching, and actions performed.
- Status and disposition at discharge.
- Attainment or progress toward desired outcome(s).
- Modifications to plan of care.

Discharge Planning

- Discharge considerations and who will be responsible for carrying out individual actions.
- Long-term needs.
- Specific referrals made.

References

1. Newfield, S. A., Hinz, M. D., Tilley, D. S., et al. (2007). *Cox's Clinical Applications of Nursing Diagnosis: Adult, Child, Women's Psychiatric, Gerontic, and Home Health Considerations*. 5th ed. Philadelphia: F. A. Davis.
2. Ladewig, P., London, M., Davidson, M., et al. (2001). *Contemporary Maternal-Newborn Nursing Care*. 5th ed. Upper Saddle River, NJ: Prentice Hall.
3. Stanley, M., Beare, P. G. (1999). *Gerontological Nursing: A Health Promotion/Protection Approach*. 2nd ed. Philadelphia: F. A. Davis.
4. National Heart, Lung, and Blood Institute. (2012). Disease statistics data points for graphics. NHLBI Fact Book. Retrieved December 2014 from http://www.nhlbi.nih.gov/about/documents/factbook/2012/chapter4data#gr29.
5. Purnell, L. D. (2008). *Guide to Culturally Competent Health Care*. 2nd ed. Philadelphia: F. A. Davis.
6. Dumitru, I., Baker, M. M. (2014). Heart failure. Retrieved December 2014 from http://emedicine.medscape.com/article/163062-workup.
7. 2013 ACCF/AHA guideline for the management of heart failure. (2013). *American College of Cardiology Foundation/American Heart Association Task Force on Practice Guidelines*. Retrieved December 2014 from http://content.onlinejacc.org/article.aspx?articleid=1695825.
8. Department of Veterans Affairs, Veterans Health Administration. (2003). *The pharmacologic management of chronic heart failure*. Washington, DC: Department of Veterans Affairs, Veterans Health Administration.

9. Bond, A. E., Nelson, K., Germany, C. L., et al. (2003). The left ventricular assist device. *Am J Nurs*, 103(1), 33–40.
10. Gawlinski, A., McAtee, M. E. (2002). Biventricular pacing: New treatment for patients with heart failure: Important nursing implications. *Am J Nurs Suppl Critical Care Update*, 102(5), 4–7.
11. American Heart Association, the Council on Clinical Cardiology, the Councils on Cardiovascular Nursing, et al. Core components of cardiac rehabilitation secondary prevention programs: 2007 update. (2007). *Circulation*, 115, 2675–2682.
12. Ren, X., Lenneman, A., Ooi, H. H. (Updated 2014). Cardiogenic shock. Retrieved December 2014 from http://emedicine.medscape.com/article/152191-overview.
13. Olade, R. B. (Updated 2014). Cardiac catheterization of the left heart. Retrieved December 2014 from http://emedicine.medscape.com/article/1819224-overview.
14. Hiner, B. C. (2005). Valsalva maneuver. *Clin Med Res*, 3(2), 55.
15. Cheever, K. H. (2005). An overview of pulmonary arterial hypertension: Risks, pathogenesis, clinical manifestations, and management. *J Cardiovasc Nurs*, 20(2), 108–116.
16. Purgason, K. (2006). Broken hearts: Differentiating stress-induced cardiomyopathy from acute myocardial infarction in the patient presenting with acute coronary syndrome. *Dimens Crit Care Nurs*, 25(6), 247–253.
17. Harvey, S. (2005). Assessment of the clinical effectiveness of the pulmonary catheters in the management of patients in intensive care; (PAC-Man): A randomised controlled trial. *Lancet*, 366(9484), 472–477.
18. Bridges, N., Jarquin-Valdivia, A. A. (2005). Use of the Trendelenburg position as the resuscitation position: To T or not to T? *Am J Crit Care*, 13(5), 464–468.

risk for decreased Cardiac Output

Taxonomy II: Activity/Rest—Class 4 Cardiovascular/Pulmonary Responses (00240) [**Diagnostic Division:** Circulation], Submitted 2013

DEFINITION: Vulnerable to inadequate blood pumped by the heart to meet the metabolic demands of the body, which may compromise health.

RISK FACTORS

Alteration in heart rate or rhythm
Altered afterload
Altered contractility
Altered preload
Altered stroke volume

DESIRED OUTCOMES/EVALUATION CRITERIA

Sample NOC linkages:

Cardiac Pump Effectiveness: Adequacy of blood volume ejected from the left ventricle to support systemic perfusion pressure

Circulation Status: Unobstructed, unidirectional blood flow at an appropriate pressure through large vessels of the systemic and pulmonary circuits

Energy Conservation: Personal actions to manage energy for initiating and sustaining activity

Client Will (Include Specific Time Frame)

- Display hemodynamic stability (e.g., blood pressure, cardiac output, urinary output, peripheral pulses).
- Verbalize knowledge of the disease process and individual risk factors.
- Participate in activities that reduce risk factors (e.g., stress management or therapeutic medication regimen program, weight reduction, balanced activity/rest plan, proper use of supplemental oxygen, cessation of smoking).

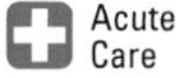

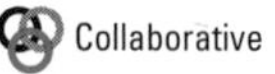

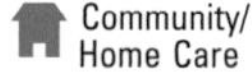

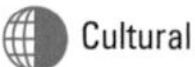

ACTIONS/INTERVENTIONS

Sample NIC linkages:

Cardiac Risk Management: Prevention of an acute episode of impaired cardiac function by minimizing contributing events and risk factors

Hemodynamic Regulation: Optimization of heart rate, preload, afterload, and contractility

NURSING PRIORITY NO. 1 To identify client at risk:

- Identify client at risk: *In addition to an individual obviously at risk because of known cardiac problems, there is a potential for cardiac output issues in others (e.g., person with traumatic injuries and hemorrhage; brainstem trauma; spinal cord injury at T8 or above; alcohol and other drug intoxication, substance withdrawal or overdose; pregnant woman with hypertensive states; individual with chronic renal failure).*
- Note age, gender, and ethnic-related cardiovascular considerations. For example, *in infants, failure to thrive with poor ability to suck and feed can be indications of heart problems;*[1] *contractile force is naturally decreased in the elderly with reduced ability to increase cardiac output in response to increased demand;*[2] *when in the supine position, pregnant women incur decreased vascular return during the second and third trimesters, potentially compromising cardiac output;*[3] *and generally, higher-risk populations include African Americans, Hispanics, Native Americans, and recent immigrants from developing nations, Russia, and the former Soviet republics.*[4,5]
- Assess for signs of poor ventricular function or impending cardiac failure:[2,6,7,9,10]

  Note reports of extreme fatigue, intolerance for activity, sudden or progressive weight gain, swelling of extremities, and progressive shortness of breath.

  Evaluate reports of chest pain. *May indicate evolving heart attack; can also accompany congestive heart failure.*

  Observe for mental status changes. *Confusion, agitation, and altered cognition may occur due to decreased brain perfusion.*

  Note changes in heart rate or rhythm: *Heart irritability is common, reflecting conduction defects and/or ischemia.*

  Assess heart sounds. *May become distant, with irregular rhythms; murmurs.*

  Palpate peripheral pulses, *which may become weak and thready.*

  Observe skin, noting color, moisture, temperature, and capillary refill time. *Pallor or cyanosis; cool, moist skin; and slow capillary refill time can occur with peripheral vasoconstriction and decreased oxygen saturation.*

  Evaluate blood pressure changes. *Client may have chronic hypertension. Blood pressure can be elevated initially, followed by hypotension in client with impending cardiogenic, hypovolemic, or septic shock.*

  Auscultate breath sounds. *Bilateral crackles and wheezing can occur associated with congestion.*

  Check for dependent or generalized edema with neck vein distention, *which can occur because of impaired venous return.*

  Observe for changes in urinary output, *which may be decreased or be caused by dehydration, hypovolemia, or poor perfusion of kidneys.*
- Review laboratory data, including, but not limited to, complete blood count, electrolytes, arterial blood gases, cardiac biomarkers (e.g., creatine kinase and its subclasses, troponins, myoglobin, LDH); lactate; brain natriuretic peptide; kidney, thyroid, and liver function studies; cultures (e.g., blood, wound, secretions); bleeding and coagulation studies, *to identify client at risk and promote early intervention, if indicated.*[6,7]
- Refer to ND decreased Cardiac Output for additional assessments and interventions as indicated.

NURSING PRIORITY NO. 2 To minimize risk factors, maximize cardiac output:[6–8,10]

- Provide for adequate rest.
- Increase activity levels gradually as permitted by individual condition, noting vital sign response to activity.

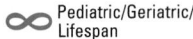

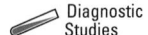

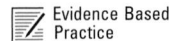

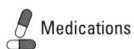

- Administer medications, as appropriate, and monitor cardiac responses.
- Encourage relaxation techniques *to reduce anxiety and muscle tension.*
- Elevate legs when in sitting position and edematous extremities when at rest. Apply antiembolic hose or sequential compression devices when indicated, ensuring they are individually fitted and appropriately applied. *Limits venous stasis, improves venous return, and reduces risk of thrombophlebitis.*
- Avoid prolonged sitting position for all clients and supine position for sleep or exercise for gravid clients (second and third trimesters) *to maximize vascular return.*[2,3]

NURSING PRIORITY NO. 3 To promote wellness (Teaching/Discharge Considerations):[6–8]

- Discuss individual's particular risk factors (e.g., smoking, stress, obesity, recent MI) and specific resources for assistance (e.g., written information sheets, direction to helpful Web sites, formalized rehabilitation programs, home interventions) for management of identified risk factors.
- Provide information to clients/caregivers on individual condition, therapies, and expected outcomes.
- Educate client/caregivers about drug regimen, including indications, dose and dosing schedules, potential adverse side effects, or drug/drug interactions.
- Provide instruction for home monitoring of weight, pulse, and blood pressure, as appropriate.
- Discuss significant signs/symptoms that need to be reported to healthcare provider, such as unrelieved or increased chest pain, dyspnea, fever, swelling of ankles, and sudden unexplained cough.
- Emphasize importance of regular medical follow-up care *to monitor client's condition and provide early intervention when indicated to prevent complications.*

DOCUMENTATION FOCUS

Assessment/Reassessment

- Baseline and subsequent findings and individual hemodynamic parameters, heart and breath sounds, ECG pattern, presence and strength of peripheral pulses, skin and tissue status, renal output, and mentation.

Planning

- Plan of care and who is involved in planning.
- Teaching plan.

Implementation/Evaluation

- Client's responses to interventions, teaching, and actions performed.
- Status and disposition at discharge.
- Attainment or progress toward desired outcome(s).
- Modifications to plan of care.

Discharge Planning

- Discharge considerations and who will be responsible for carrying out individual actions.
- Long-term needs.
- Specific referrals made.

References

1. Newfield, S. A., Hinz, M. D., Tilley, D. S., et al. (2007). *Cox's Clinical Applications of Nursing Diagnosis: Adult, Child, Women's Psychiatric, Gerontic, and Home Health Considerations.* 5th ed. Philadelphia: F. A. Davis.
2. Stanley, M., Beare, P. G. (1999). *Gerontological Nursing: A Health Promotion/Protection Approach.* 2nd ed. Philadelphia: F. A. Davis.
3. Ladewig, P., London, M., Davidson, M., et al. (2001). *Contemporary Maternal-Newborn Nursing Care.* 5th ed. Upper Saddle River, NJ: Prentice Hall.
4. National Heart, Lung, and Blood Institute. (2012). Disease statistics data points for graphics. NHLBI Fact Book. Retrieved December 2014 from http://www.nhlbi.nih.gov/about/documents/factbook/2012/chapter4data#gr29.

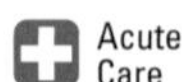

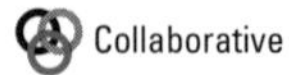

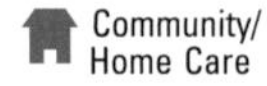

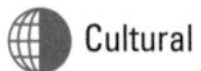

5. Purnell, L. D. (2008). *Guide to Culturally Competent Health Care*. 2nd ed. Philadelphia: F. A. Davis.
6. Dumitru, I., Baker, M. M. (2014). Heart failure. Retrieved December 2014 from http://emedicine.medscape.com/article/163062-workup.
7. American College of Cardiology Foundation/American Heart Association Task Force on Practice Guidelines. (2013). 2013 ACCF/AHA guideline for the management of heart failure. Retrieved December 2014 from http://content.onlinejacc.org/article.aspx?articleid=1695825.
8. American Heart Association, the Council on Clinical Cardiology, the Councils on Cardiovascular Nursing, et al. Core components of cardiac rehabilitation secondary prevention programs: 2007 update. (2007). *Circulation*, 115, 2675–2682.
9. Ren, X., Lenneman, A., Ooi, H. H. (Updated 2014). Cardiogenic shock. Retrieved December 2014 from http://emedicine.medscape.com/article/152191-overview.
10. Cheever, K. H. (2005). An overview of pulmonary arterial hypertension: Risks, pathogenesis, clinical manifestations, and management. *J Cardiovasc Nurs*, 20(2), 108–116.

risk for impaired Cardiovascular Function

Taxonomy II: Activity/Rest—Class 4 Cardiovascular/Pulmonary Response (00239) [**Diagnostic Division:** Circulation], Submitted 2013

DEFINITION: Vulnerable to internal or external causes, which damage one or more vital organs and the circulatory system itself.

RISK FACTORS

Age ≤65
Diabetes mellitus
Hypertension, dyslipidemia
Family history of cardiovascular disease; history of cardiovascular disease
Insufficient knowledge of modifiable risk factors; obesity; sedentary lifestyle; smoking
Pharmaceutical agent
Note: A risk diagnosis is not evidenced by signs and symptoms as the problem has not occurred; rather, nursing interventions are directed at prevention

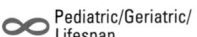

Sample Clinical Applications: Angina, coronary artery disease, hypertension, diabetes, cardiac surgery, bariatric surgery, substance abuse

DESIRED OUTCOMES/EVALUATION CRITERIA

Sample NOC linkages:

Circulation Status: Unobstructed, unidirectional blood flow at an appropriate pressure through large vessels of the systemic and pulmonary circuits

Cardiac Pump Effectiveness: Adequacy of blood volume ejected from the left ventricle to support systemic perfusion pressure

Tissue Perfusion: Adequacy of the blood flow through body organs to function at the cellular level

Client Will (Include Specific Time Frame)

- Be free of cardiovascular symptoms, such as hypertension, chest pain, activity intolerance, altered mental status, changes in heart rate or rhythm, syncope, decreased skin temperature, and diminished peripheral pulses.
- Verbalize knowledge of the disease process, individual risk factors, and treatment plan.
- Participate in activities that promote cardiovascular health (e.g., stress management, therapeutic medication regimen program, weight reduction, balanced activity/rest plan, cessation of smoking).

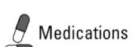

(continues on page 136)

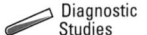

risk for impaired Cardiovascular Function (continued)
ACTIONS/INTERVENTIONS

Sample NIC linkages:
Cardiac Risk Management: Prevention of an acute episode of impaired cardiac function by minimizing contributing events and risk factors
Circulatory Care: Arterial Insufficiency: Promotion of arterial circulation

NURSING PRIORITY NO. 1 To identify client at risk:

- Note client's age and gender and family history when assessing risk for cardiovascular disease (CVD). *Risks that can't be controlled include increasing age, gender, and heredity. The American Heart Association states that "risk for heart disorders increases with age, and men are still considered at higher risk for myocardial infarction and experience them earlier in life. The majority of both sexes who die of coronary heart disease are 65 and older."*[1] *A family's history of CVD helps identify a client's risk. For example, if a first-degree blood relative has had coronary heart disease or stroke before the age of 55 years (for a male relative) or 65 years (for a female relative), the risk increases. Risk for stroke is similar for men and women.*[2]
- Review with client past history of conditions associated with cardiovascular impairment, such as heart attack, stroke, diabetes, and peripheral vascular conditions, *to help assess current risk for recurrence.*
- Determine if client has condition known as "metabolic syndrome" (i.e., large waistline, high triglcyeride level, low HDL cholesterol level [or is on medications to lower triglycerides or cholesterol]; is hypertensive and has high fasting blood glucose or A1C). *Metabolic risk factors are strongly associated with increased risk for heart disease and stroke, especially when combined with other risk factors such as smoking, a sedentary lifestyle, and obesity.*[3,4,21]
- Inquire about client's current and past history of smoking. *Smoking is associated with vasoconstriction, which causes decreased blood flow and reduced oxygenation of organs, which can impair cardiovascular function.*[5] *Smoking is a major cause of CVD and causes one of every three deaths from CVD, according to the 2014 Surgeon General's report on smoking and health.*[6] *Not only has cigarette smoking been determined to play a critical role in the development of premature coronary heart disease, but it has also been found to act synergistically with other conventional risk factors, greatly increasing the baseline risk associated with each risk factor individually.*[7]
- Note client's weight and dietary habits *to determine if obesity or poor nutrition are risk factors. Note: Studies have shown that overweight and obesity predispose to or are associated with numerous cardiac complications such as coronary heart disease, heart failure, and sudden death because of their impact on the cardiovascular system.*[8]

NURSING PRIORITY NO. 2 To determine changes in cardiovascular status:

- Investigate reports of chest pain, headache, or pain in extremities *to identify potential problem with cardiovascular perfusion.*
- Measure client's blood pressure at each medical provider visit *to identify high blood pressure (risk factor) or unknown or uncontrolled hypertension. Note: A 2003–2010 analysis report by the Centers of Disease Control of hypertension in the United States revealed that "overall prevalence of hypertension among adults aged ≥18 years was 30.4% or an estimated 66.9 million. Among those with hypertension, an estimated 35.8 million (53.5%) did not have their hypertension controlled. Among these, an estimated 14.1 million (39.4%) were not aware of their hypertension."*[9,10]
- Investigate reports of difficulty breathing; note respiratory rate outside of acceptable parameters, *which can be indicative of oxygen exchange problems with potential for cardiac and/or systemic vascular dysfunction.*[5]

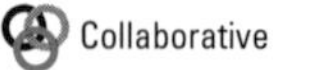

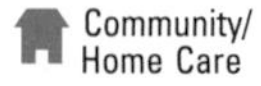

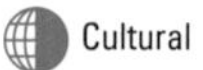

- Review diagnostic studies, including, but not limited to electrocardiogram, echocardiogram, body mass scan or other nutrition screen, and screening heart scan *to determine if cardiovascular concerns are developing.*
- Review laboratory data, including, but not limited to, lipid studies (e.g., cholesterol, triglycerides), electrolytes, fasting blood glucose, glucose tolerance, insulin resistance, and A1C; cardiac biomarkers; and kidney, thyroid, and liver function studies *to identify imbalances or disease processes and to take preventive measures when needed. Note: Familial hypercholesterolemia (FH) is an inherited disorder that is thought to lead to aggressive and premature-onset cardiovascular disease. FH is being studied by a multiagency-funded study in West Virginia that "screens 5th graders for high cholesterol and other factors that can lead to early onset of heart disease and additional health risks. The screenings identify children who may have familial hypercholesterolemia, genetic conditions that predispose them to early cardiac problems. Since 1998, the program has screened 100,000 fifth graders and secured treatment for many children and family members identified as having a genetic predisposition to developing early-onset heart disease."*[11] *Note: It has long been known that an association exits between diabetes mellitus and increased cardiovascular risk. The Australian Diabetes, Obesity and Lifestyle Study (2007) of 10,428 participants studied the relationship between milder elevations of blood glucose and mortality. This study investigated whether impaired fasting glucose and impaired glucose tolerance also increase the risk of all-cause and CVD mortality. They found a "strong association between abnormal glucose metabolism and mortality, and it suggests that this condition contributes to a large number of cardiovascular deaths in the general population."*[12]
- Assess for restlessness; fatigue; changes in level of consciousness; increased capillary refill time; diminished peripheral pulses; and pale, cool skin. *Signs and symptoms of inadequate systemic perfusion, which can cause or affect cardiovascular function.*[13]
- Assess heart sounds and pulses. *Helps identify conditions associated with inadequate myocardial or systemic tissue perfusion, dehydration, immobility, electrolyte, or acid-base imbalances.*[13]
- Investigate reports of difficulty breathing; note respiratory rate outside of acceptable parameters, *which can be indicative of oxygen exchange problems with potential for cardiopulmonary dysfunction.*[15]
- Assess for extremity discoloration, changes in pulses, temperature or color, and client report of discomfort/pain. *These signs and symptoms are associated with systemic or peripheral vascular conditions.*[14,16]

NURSING PRIORITY NO. 3 To promote cardiovascular health (Teaching/Discharge Considerations):

- Discuss the risk factors (e.g., family history, obesity, age, smoking, hypertension, diabetes, clotting disorders) and potential outcomes of atherosclerosis (e.g., systemic and cardiac disease conditions). *Information necessary for client to make informed decisions concerning risk factors and to commit to lifestyle changes necessary to prevent onset of complications or manage symptoms when condition is present.*[2,7]
- Review difference between modifiable and nonmodifiable risk factors *to assist client/significant others (SOs) in understanding those areas in which he/she can take action or make healthy choices:*
  - Recommend maintenance of normal weight or weight loss if client is obese *to decrease risk associated with overweight and obesity.*[8]
  - Encourage smoking cessation, when indicated, offering information about stop-smoking aids and programs. *Smoking causes vasoconstriction compromising systemic and peripheral perfusion. Smoking cessation is important in the medical management of many contributors to heart attack and stroke. These include atherosclerosis (fatty buildups in arteries), thrombosis (blood clots), artery spasm (e.g., coronary, carotid, cerebral), and cardiac dysrhythmias.*[17]
  - Encourage client to engage in regular exercise *to enhance circulation and promote healthy blood pressure and general well-being.*[18]
  - Review medications on regular basis *to manage those that affect cardiac function or those given to prevent blood pressure or thromboembolic problems.*
  - Discuss drug use where indicated (including cocaine, methamphetamines, alcohol) *to educate client regarding effect of drug on cardiovascular system.*[19,20]

Encourage client in high-risk categories (e.g., strong family history, diabetic, prior history of cardiac event) to have regular medical examinations *to provide timely intervention, when needed.*

- Refer to educational or community resources, as indicated. *Client/SO(s) may benefit from instruction and support provided by agencies to engage in healthier heart activities (e.g., weight loss, smoking cessation, exercise).*
- Instruct in blood pressure monitoring at home if indicated; advise purchase of home monitoring equipment; refer to community resources as indicated. *Facilitates management of hypertension, which is a major risk factor for damage to blood vessels or organ function.*[14]

DOCUMENTATION FOCUS

Assessment/Reassessment

- Individual findings, noting specific risk factors including diet, exercise, and smoking.
- Vital signs, pulse oximetry, cardiac rhythm, presence of dysrhythmias.
- Status of organ function (e.g., mentation, breath sounds, kidney output).

Planning

- Plan of care and who is involved in planning.
- Teaching plan.

Implementation/Evaluation

- Response to interventions, teaching, and actions performed.
- Attainment or progress toward desired outcome(s).
- Modifications to plan of care.

Discharge Planning

- Long-term needs and who is responsible for actions to be taken.
- Available resources, specific referrals made.

References

1. Bingaman, M. (2013). AHA scientific position on risk factors of coronary heart disease. American Heart Association (Summary by ehow contributor Bingaman). Retrieved February 2015 from http://www.ehow.com/about_5171788_uncontrollable-risk-factors-heart-disease.html.
2. World Health Organization, World Heart Federation, and World Stroke Organization. (2015). Cardiovascular disease risk factors. Retrieved February 2015 from http://www.world-heart-federation.org/press/fact-sheets/cardiovascular-disease-risk-factors/.
3. National Heart, Lung, and Blood Institute. (2011). What is metabolic syndrome? Retrieved February 2015 from http://www.nhlbi.nih.gov/health/health-topics/topics/ms.
4. Alberti, K. G., Zimmett, P., Shaw, J. (2006). Metabolic syndrome—a new world-wide definition. A Consensus Statement from the International Diabetes Federation. *Diabet Med*, 23(5), 469–480.
5. Jubran, A. (1999). Pulse oximetry. *Crit Care*, 3(2), R11–R17.
6. No author listed. (2014). Smoking and cardiovascular disease. Centers for Disease Control and Prevention: 2014 Surgeon General's Report: The Health Consequences of Smoking—50 Years of Progress. Retrieved February 2015 from http://www.cdc.gov/tobacco/data_statistics/sgr/50th-anniversary/index.htm#fact-sheets.
7. Keil, U., Liese, A. D., Hense, H. W., et al. (1998). Classical risk factors and their impact on incident non-fatal and fatal myocardial infarction and all-cause mortality in southern Germany: Results from the MONICA Augsburg cohort study 1984–1992 Monitoring Trends and Determinants in Cardiovascular Diseases. *Eur Heart*, 19, 1197–1207.
8. Poirier, P., Eckel, R. H. (2002). Obesity and cardiovascular diseases. *Curr Atheroscler Rep*, 4, 448–453.
9. No author listed. (2012). Vital signs: Awareness and treatment of uncontrolled hypertension among adults—United States, 2003–2010. Centers for Disease Control and Prevention: Morbidity and Mortality Weekly Report. Retrieved February 2015 from http://www.cdc.gov/mmwr/preview/mmwrhtml/mm6135a3.htm.
10. No author listed. (Updated 2015). About FH. The FH Foundation. Retrieved February 2015 from http://thefhfoundation.org/about-fh/what-is-fh/.

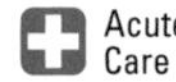

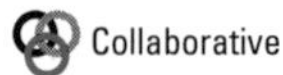

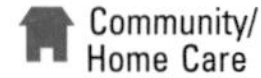

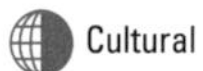

11. AHRQ Innovations Exchange. (2010, updated 2014). Statewide screening of fifth graders leads to identification and treatment of those with genetic predisposition to early-onset heart disease. Agency for Healthcare Research and Quality. Retrieved February 2015 from https://innovations.ahrq.gov/profiles/statewide-screening-fifth-graders-leads-identification-and-treatment-those-genetic.
12. Healy, G. N., Wijndaele, K., Dunstan, D. W., (2008). Objectively measured sedentary time, physical activity, and metabolic risk: The Australian Diabetes, Obesity and Lifestyle Study. *Diabet Care*, 2(3), 369–371.
13. Breitenbach, J. E. (2007). Putting an end to perfusion confusion. *Nursing Made Incredibly Easy!*, 5(3), 50–60.
14. Bartley, M. K. (2006). Keep venous thromboembolism at bay. *Nursing*, 10(3), 36–41.
15. The Task Force for the Diagnosis and Management of Acute Pulmonary Embolism of the European Society of Cardiology Endorsed by the European Respiratory Society. (2014). 2014 ESC Guidelines on the diagnosis and management of acute pulmonary embolism. Retrieved February 2015 from http://eurheartj.oxfordjournals.org/content/early/2014/08/28/eurheartj.ehu283.
16. Eberhardt, R. T., Raffetto, J. D. (2005). Chronic venous insufficiency. *Circulation*, 111(18), 2398–2409.
17. Centers for Disease Control and Prevention. (2014). Health effects of cigarette smoking. Retrieved February 2015 from http://www.cdc.gov/tobacco/data_statistics/fact_sheets/health_effects/effects_cig_smoking/.
18. Frost, K. L., Topp, R. (2006). A physical activity Rx for the hypertensive patient. *Nurs Pract*, 31(4), 29–37.
19. Aslibekyan, S., Levitan, E. B., Mittleman, M. A. (2008). Prevalent cocaine use and myocardial infarction. *Am J Cardiol*, 102(8), 966–969.
20. Richards, J. R., Derlet, R. W., Albertson, T. E. (Updated 2014). Methamphetamine toxicity. Retrieved February 2015 from http://emedicine.medscape.com/article/820918-overview.
21. Barr, E. L., Zimmett, P. Z., Welborn, T. A., et al. (2007). Epidemiology: Risk of cardiovascular and all-cause mortality in individuals with diabetes mellitus, impaired fasting glucose, and impaired glucose tolerance. *Circulation*, 116(2), 151–157.

ineffective Childbearing Process

Taxonomy II: Sexuality—Class 3 Reproduction (00221) [**Diagnostic Division:** Sexuality], Submitted 2010

DEFINITION: Pregnancy and childbirth process and care of the newborn* that does not match the environmental context, norms, and expectations.

RELATED

Insufficient knowledge of childbearing process; unrealistic birth plan
Unplanned/unwanted pregnancy
Inconsistent prenatal health visits; insufficient prenatal care
Inadequate maternal nutrition
Substance abuse
Insufficient parental role model or cognitive readiness for parenting
Low maternal confidence
Maternal powerlessness, psychological distress; insufficient support systems
Unsafe environment; domestic violence

(continues on page 140)

*The original Japanese term for "childbearing" (*shussan ikujikoudou*), which encompasses both childbirth and rearing of the neonate. It is one of the main concepts of Japanese midwifery.

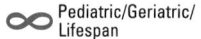

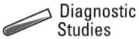

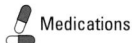

ineffective Childbearing Process (continued)

DEFINING CHARACTERISTICS

Subjective

During Pregnancy

Inadequate prenatal lifestyle (e.g., nutrition, elimination, sleep, exercise, personal hygiene)

Ineffective management of unpleasant symptoms in pregnancy

Unrealistic birth plan

During Labor and Delivery

Inadequate lifestyle for stage of labor (e.g., nutrition, elimination, sleep, exercise, personal hygiene)

*After Birth**

Inadequate postpartum lifestyle (e.g., nutrition, elimination, sleep, exercise, personal hygiene)

Objective

During Pregnancy

Inadequate prenatal care

Insufficient access of support system

Inadequate preparation of the home environment

Inadequate preparation of newborn care items; insufficient respect for unborn baby

During Labor and Delivery

Inappropriate response to onset of labor; decrease in proactivity during labor and delivery

Insufficient attachment behavior

Insufficient access of support system

*After Birth**

Insufficient attachment behavior

Inappropriate baby feeding techniques; inadequate baby care techniques

Unsafe environment for an infant

Inappropriate breast care

Insufficient access of support system

Sample Clinical Applications: First, second, and third trimester of pregnancy; labor and delivery, postpartum, newborn

DESIRED OUTCOMES/EVALUATION CRITERIA

Sample NOC linkages:

Prenatal Health Behavior: Personal actions to promote a healthy pregnancy and a healthy newborn

Maternal Status: Antepartum/Intrapartum/Postpartum [specify]: Extent to which maternal well-being is within normal limits from conception to the onset of labor/from onset of labor to delivery/from delivery of placenta to completion of involution

Knowledge: Infant Care: Extent of understanding conveyed about caring for a baby from birth to first birthday

Client Will (Include Specific Time Frame)

- Demonstrate healthy pregnancy free of preventable complications.
- Engage in activities to prepare for birth process and care of newborn.
- Experience complication-free labor and childbirth.
- Verbalize understanding of care requirements to promote health of self and infant.

ACTIONS/INTERVENTIONS

Sample NIC linkages:

Childbirth Preparation: Providing information and support to facilitate childbirth and to enhance the ability of an individual to develop and perform the parental role

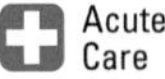

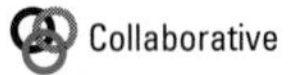

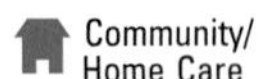

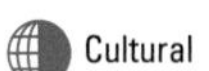

Prenatal Care: Monitoring and management of patient during pregnancy to prevent complications of pregnancy and promote a healthy outcome for both mother and infant
Attachment Promotion: Facilitation of the development of the parent-infant relationship

NURSING PRIORITY NO. 1 To determine causative factors and individual needs:

DURING PREGNANCY

- Determine maternal health/nutritional status, usual pregravid weight, and dietary pattern. *Research studies have found a positive correlation between pregravid maternal obesity and increased perinatal morbidity rates (e.g., hypertension and gestational diabetes) associated with preterm births and macrosomia.*[16]
- Note use of alcohol/other drugs, nicotine. *Maternal pregnancy complications and negative effects on the developing fetus are increased with the use of tobacco, alcohol, and illicit drugs. Smoking negatively affects placental circulation, even smoking fewer than 10 cigarettes/day is associated with an increased risk of fetal death, damage in utero, abruptio placenta, placenta previa, and low birth weights.*[4,8,13–15,20] *Note: Prescription medications may also be dangerous to the fetus, requiring a risk/benefit analysis for therapeutic choices and appropriate dosage.*[12]
- Evaluate current knowledge regarding physiological and psychological changes associated with pregnancy. *Provides information to assist in identifying needs and creating individual plan of care.*[2,3]
- Identify involvement/response of child's father to pregnancy. *Helps clarify whether or not father is likely to be supportive or has the potential of posing a threat to the safety and well-being of mother/fetus.*[19]
- Determine individual family stressors, economic situation/financial needs, and availability/use of resources *to identify necessary referrals. Impact of pregnancy on family with limited resources can create added stress and result in limited prenatal care and preparation for newborn.*[1,2]
- Verify environmental well-being and safety of client/family. *Women experiencing intimate partner violence both prior to and/or during pregnancy are at higher risk for multiple poor maternal and infant health outcomes.*[18,19]
- Determine cultural expectations/beliefs about childbearing, self-care, and so on. Identify who provides support/instruction within the client's culture (e.g., grandmother/other family member, cuerandero/doula, other cultural healer). Work with support person(s) as desired by client, using an interpreter as needed. *Helps ensure quality and continuity of care because support person(s) can reinforce information provided.*[1,2,4]
- Ascertain client's commitments to work, family, and self; roles/responsibilities within family unit; and use of supportive resources. *Helps in setting realistic priorities to assist client in making adjustments, such as changing work hours, shifting of household chores, curtailing some outside commitments.*[12,17] *Note: Initially even if the pregnancy is planned, the expectant mother may feel ambivalence toward the pregnancy because of personal or professional goals, financial concerns, and/or possible role changes.*[1,2]
- Determine client's/couple's perception of fetus as a separate entity and extent of preparations being made for this infant. *Absence of activities such as choosing a name or nicknaming the baby in utero and home preparations indicate lack of completion of psychological tasks of pregnancy. Note: Cultural or familial beliefs may limit visible preparations out of concern that bad outcome might result.*[2]

DURING LABOR AND DELIVERY

- Ascertain client's understanding and expectations of the labor process and who will participate/provide support.
- Determine presence/appropriateness of birth plan developed by client/couple and any associated cultural expectations/preferences. *Identifies areas to address to ensure that choices made are amenable to the specific care setting, reflect reality of client/fetal status, and accommodate individual wishes. Note: Some cultures or personal values may limit male involvement in the delivery process, necessitating the identification of other support person(s).*[1,6,10]

AFTER BIRTH

- Determine plan for discharge after delivery and home care support/needs. *Important to facilitate discharge and ensure client/infant needs will be met.*[3]

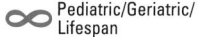

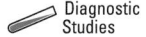

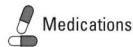

- Appraise level of parent's understanding of physiological needs and adaptation to extrauterine life associated with maintenance of body temperature, nutrition, respiratory needs, and bowel and bladder functioning. *Identifies areas of concern/need requiring development of teaching plan and/or demonstration of care activities.*[3,12]
- Assess mother's strengths and needs, noting age, relationship status, and reactions of family members. *Identifies potential risk factors that influence the client's/couple's ability to assume role of parenthood. For example, an adolescent still formulating goals and identity may have difficulty accepting the infant as a person. The single parent who lacks support systems may have difficulty assuming sole responsibility for parenting.*[1,6]
- Ascertain nature of emotional and physical parenting that client/couple received during their childhood. *Parenting role is learned, and individuals use their own parents as role models. Those who experienced a negative upbringing or poor parenting may require additional support to meet the challenges of effective parenting.*

NURSING PRIORITY NO. 2 To promote optimal maternal well-being:

DURING PREGNANCY

- Emphasize importance of maternal well-being including discussion of nutrition, regular moderate exercise, comfort measures, rest, and sexual activity. *Fetal well-being is directly related to maternal health, especially during the first trimester, when developing organ systems are most vulnerable to injury from environmental or hereditary factors:*
  - Review nutrition requirements and optimal prenatal weight gain to support maternal-fetal needs. *Dietary focus should be on balanced nutrients and calories to produce appropriate weight gain and to supply vitamins and minerals for healthy fetus. Inadequate prenatal weight gain and/or below normal prepregnancy weight increases the risk of intrauterine growth retardation in the fetus and delivery of a low-birth-weight infant.*[8,12]
  - Encourage moderate exercise such as walking, or non-weight-bearing activities (e.g., swimming, bicycling) in accordance with client's physical condition and cultural beliefs. *Nonendurance antepartal exercise tends to shorten labor, increases likelihood of a spontaneous vaginal delivery, and decreases need for oxytocin augmentation.*[4,5] *In some cultures, inactivity may be viewed as a protection for the mother.*[1,6]
  - Recommend a consistent sleep and rest schedule (e.g., 1- to 2-hour daytime nap and 8 hours of sleep each night) in a dark, comfortable room. *Provides rest to meet metabolic needs associated with growth of maternal and fetal tissues.*[12]
- Provide necessary referrals (e.g., dietitian, social services, supplemental nutrition assistance programs including the Women, Infants, and Children program) as indicated. *May need additional assistance with nutritional choices and may have budget or financial constraints. Supplemental federal/state food programs help promote optimal maternal, fetal, and infant nutrition.*[12]
- Encourage participation in a smoking-cessation program and alcohol/drug abstinence as appropriate. *Reduces risk of premature birth, stillbirth, low birth weight, congenital defects, drug withdrawal of newborn, and fetal alcohol syndrome.*[14]
- Explain psychological reactions, including ambivalence, introspection, stress reactions, and emotional lability, as being characteristic of pregnancy. *Helps client/couple understand mood swings and may provide opportunity for partner to offer support and affection at these times.*[4] *Note: However, the stressors associated with pregnancy may lead to abuse/exacerbate existing abusive behavior.*[18,19]
- Discuss personal situation and options, providing information about resources available to client. *Partner may be upset about an unplanned pregnancy, financial concern regarding supporting the child, or even jealousy that attention is shifting to the unborn child, creating safety issues for client/family.*[19]
- Identify reportable potential danger signals of pregnancy, such as bleeding, cramping, acute abdominal pain, backache, edema, visual disturbances, headaches, and pelvic pressure. *Helps client distinguish normal from abnormal findings, thus assisting her in seeking timely, appropriate healthcare.*[12] (Refer to ND risk for disturbed Maternal-Fetal Dyad for additional interventions.)

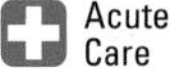

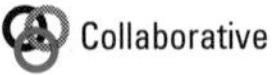

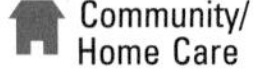

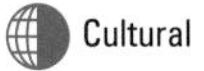

DURING LABOR AND DELIVERY

- Monitor labor progress and maternal and fetal well-being per protocol. Provide continuous intrapartal professional support/doula. *Fear of abandonment can intensify as labor progresses. The client may experience increased anxiety and/or loss of control when left unattended. Doulas can provide client with emotional, physical, and informational support as an adjunct to primary nurse.*[2,8]
- Identify client's support person/coach and ascertain that the individual is providing support the client requires. *Coach may be client's husband/significant other (SO) or doula, and he or she needs to include physical and emotional support for the mother and aid in initiation of bonding with the neonate.*[4]

AFTER BIRTH

- Promote sleep and rest. *Reduces metabolic rate and allows energy and oxygen to be used for healing process.*[12]
- Ascertain client's perception of labor and delivery, length of labor, and client's fatigue level. *There is a correlation between length of labor and the ability of some clients to assume responsibility for self-care/infant care tasks and activities.*
- Assess client's readiness for learning. Assist client in identifying needs. *The postpartum period provides an opportunity to foster maternal growth, maturation, and competence. However, the client needs time to move from "taking-in" to a "taking-hold" phase, in which her receptiveness and readiness is heightened and she is emotionally and physically ready for learning new information to facilitate mastery of her new role.*[4]
- Provide information about self-care, including perineal care and hygiene; physiological changes, including normal progression of lochial flow; need for sleep and rest; importance of progressive postpartum exercise program; and role changes. *Helps prevent infection, fosters healing and recuperation, and contributes to positive adaptation to physical and emotional changes, enhancing feelings of general well-being.*[12]
- Review nipple and breast care, special dietary needs for lactating mother, factors that facilitate or interfere with successful breastfeeding, use of breast pump and appropriate suppliers, and proper storage of expressed milk. *Prevents nipple cracking and soreness enhancing comfort, facilitates role of breastfeeding mother, and helps ensure adequate milk supply.*[8]
- Discuss normal psychological changes and needs associated with the postpartal period. *Client's emotional state may be somewhat labile at this time and often is influenced by physical well-being. Anticipating such changes may reduce the stress associated with this transition period that necessitates learning new roles and taking on new responsibilities.*[4,8,12]
- Discuss sexuality needs and plans for contraception. Provide information about available methods, including advantages/disadvantages. *Client/couple may need clarification regarding available contraception methods and the fact that pregnancy could occur even prior to the 4- to 6-week postpartum visit.*[8]
- Reinforce importance of postpartum examination by healthcare provider and interim follow-up as appropriate. *Follow-up visit is necessary to evaluate recovery of reproductive organs, healing of episiotomy/laceration-repair, general well-being, and adaptation to life changes.*[12]

NURSING PRIORITY NO. 3 To promote appropriate participation in childbearing process:

DURING PREGNANCY

- Develop nurse-client relationship, maintaining an open attitude toward beliefs of client/couple. *Acceptance is important to developing and maintaining relationship and supporting independence.*[2]
- Explain office visit routine and rationale for ongoing screening and close monitoring (e.g., urine testing, blood pressure monitoring, weight, fetal growth). Emphasize importance of keeping regular appointments. *Reinforces relationship between health assessment and positive outcomes for mother and baby.*[12]
- Suggest father/siblings attend office visits and listen to fetal heart tones as appropriate. *Promotes a sense of involvement and helps make baby a reality for family members.*

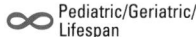

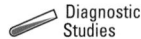

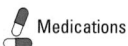

- Provide anticipatory guidance regarding health habits/lifestyle and employment concerns:
  Review physical changes to be expected during each trimester. *Questions will continue to arise as new changes occur, regardless of whether changes are anticipated or unexpected, and knowledge of normal variations can be reassuring. Also prepares client/couple for managing common discomforts associated with pregnancy.*[4,12]
  Discuss signs/symptoms requiring evaluation by primary provider during prenatal period (e.g., excessive vomiting, fever, unresolved illness of any kind, decreased fetal movement). *Allows for timely intervention.*[12]
  Identify anticipatory adaptations for SO/family necessitated by pregnancy. *Family members will need to be flexible in adjusting own roles and responsibilities in order to assist client to meet her needs related to the demands of pregnancy, both expected and unplanned, such as prolonged nausea, fatigue, and emotional lability.*[12]
  Provide information about potential teratogens, such as alcohol, nicotine, illicit drugs, the STORCH group of viruses (syphilis, toxoplasmosis, other, rubella, cytomegalovirus, herpes simplex), and HIV. *Helps client make informed decisions/choices about behaviors/environment that can promote healthy offspring. Note: Research supports the attribution of a wide range of negative effects in the neonate from alcohol and recreational drug use and smoking.*[4,8,13–15]
- Provide information about need for additional laboratory studies and diagnostic tests or procedure(s). Review risks and potential side effects. *Aids in making informed decisions and choosing treatment options.*[8,12]
- Discuss signs of labor onset; how to distinguish between false and true labor, when to notify healthcare provider, and when to leave for birth center/hospital as appropriate; and stages of labor and delivery. *Helps ensure timely arrival and enhances coping with labor/delivery process.*[12]
- Determine anticipated infant feeding plan. Discuss physiology and benefits of breastfeeding. *Breastfeeding provides a protective effect against respiratory illnesses, ear infections, gastrointestinal diseases, and allergies, including asthma, eczema, and atopic dermatitis.*[9]
- Encourage attendance at prenatal and childbirth classes. Provide information about father/sibling or grandparent participation in classes and delivery if client desires. *Knowledge gained helps reduce fear of unknown and increases confidence that client/couple can manage the preparation for the birth of their child. Helps family members to realize they are an integral part of the pregnancy and delivery.*[11,12]

DURING LABOR AND DELIVERY

- Support use of positive coping mechanisms. *Enhances feelings of competence and fosters self-esteem.*[12]
- Demonstrate behaviors and techniques (e.g., breathing, focused imagery, music, other distractions; aromatherapy; abdominal effleurage, back or leg rubs, sacral pressure, repositioning, back rest; oral care, linen changes, shower/tub use) that partner can use to assist with pain control and relaxation. *Enhances feeling of well-being. May block pain impulses within the cerebral cortex through conditioned responses and cutaneous stimulation, facilitating progression of normal labor.*[4]
- Discuss available analgesics, appropriate timing, usual responses and side effects (client and fetal), and duration of analgesia effect in light of current situation. *Allows client to make informed choices about means of pain control and can allay client's fears and anxieties about medication use. Note: If conservative measures are not effective and increasing muscle tension impedes progress of labor, judicious use of medication can enhance relaxation, shorten labor, limit fatigue, and prevent complications.*[4]
- Honor client's decision about the use or nonuse of medication in a nonjudgmental manner. Continue encouragement for efforts and use of relaxation techniques. *Enhances client's sense of control and may prevent or reduce need for medication. Note: Continued support may be needed to help reduce feelings of failure in the client/couple who may have anticipated an unmedicated birth and did not follow through with that plan.*[12]

AFTER BIRTH

- Monitor and document the client's/couple's interactions with infant. *Presence of bonding acquaintance behaviors (e.g., making eye contact, using high-pitched voice and en face [face-to-face] position as culturally appropriate, calling infant by name, holding infant closely) are indicators of beginning the attachment process.*[2,12]

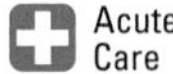

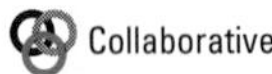

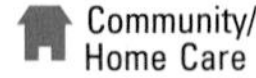

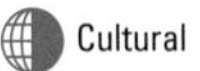

- Initiate early breast or oral feeding according to facility protocol and client preference. *Initiating feeding for breastfed infants usually occurs in the delivery room; otherwise, 5 to 15 mL of sterile water may be offered in the nursery to assess effectiveness of sucking, swallowing, gag reflexes, and patency of esophagus. If aspirated, sterile water is easily absorbed by pulmonary tissues.*[7,9]
- Provide for unlimited participation of father and siblings. Ascertain whether siblings attended orientation program. *Facilitates family development and ongoing process of acquaintance/attachment and helps family members feel more comfortable caring for newborn.*

NURSING PRIORITY NO. 4 To promote optimal well-being of newborn (Teaching/Discharge Considerations):

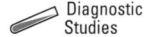

- Provide information about newborn interactional capabilities, states of consciousness, and means of stimulating cognitive development. *Helps parents recognize and respond to infant cues during interactional process and fosters optimal interaction, attachment behaviors, and cognitive development in infant. The state of consciousness can be divided into the sleep and the wake states, involving separate predictable behavioral characteristics.*[12]
- Note father's/partner's response to birth and to parenting role. *Client's ability to adapt positively to parenting may be strongly influenced by partner's reaction.*
- Discuss normal variations and characteristics of infant, such as caput succedaneum, cephalohematoma, pseudomenstruation, breast enlargement, physiological jaundice, and milia. *Helps parents recognize normal variations and may reduce anxiety.*[4,12]
- Demonstrate/supervise infant care activities related to feeding and holding; bathing, diapering, and clothing; care of umbilical cord stump; and care of circumcised male infant. *Promotes understanding of principles and techniques of newborn care, fosters parents' skills as caregivers, and enhances self-confidence.*[3,12]
- Note frequency, amount, and length of feeding. Encourage demand feedings instead of scheduled feedings. Note frequency, amount, and appearance of regurgitation. *Hunger and length of time between feedings vary from feeding to feeding, and excessive regurgitation increases replacement needs.*[7,9]
- Evaluate neonate and maternal satisfaction following feedings. *Provides opportunity to answer client questions, offer encouragement for efforts, identify needs, and problem solve situations.*[7,9]
- Discuss physiological needs and adaptation to extrauterine life, including maintenance of body temperature, nutritional requirements, respiratory needs, and bowel and bladder functioning. *Enhances parents' ability to provide for neonates' well-being.*[3,12]
- Emphasize newborn's need for follow-up laboratory tests, regular evaluations by healthcare provider, and timely immunizations. *Ongoing evaluation is important for monitoring growth and achievement of development milestones. Immunizations are necessary to protect the infant from childhood diseases and associated serious complications.*[12]
- Identify manifestations of illness and infection and when to contact healthcare provider. Demonstrate proper technique for taking temperature, administering oral medication, or providing other care activities for infant as required. *Early recognition of illness and prompt use of healthcare facilitate timely treatment and positive outcomes.*[12]
- Provide oral and written/pictorial information and reliable Web sites about infant care and development, feeding, and safety issues. Offer appropriate resources in client's dominant language reflecting cultural beliefs. *Maximizes learning, providing opportunity to review information as needed to engage in new caretaking role, identify necessary supplies/safety needs, and prepare for feeding method of choice.*[8,12]
- Refer breastfeeding client to lactation consultant/support group (e.g., La Leche League, Lact-Aid) as appropriate. *Provides ongoing support to promote a successful breastfeeding outcome.*[7,9]
- Discuss available community support groups/parenting class as indicated. *Increases parents' knowledge of child rearing and child development and provides a supportive atmosphere while parents incorporate new roles.*

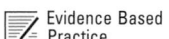

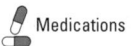

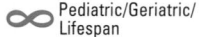

DOCUMENTATION FOCUS

Assessment/Reassessment

- Assessment findings, general health, previous pregnancy experience, any safety concerns.
- Knowledge of pre/postpartum needs and newborn care.
- Cultural beliefs and expectations.
- Specific birth plan and individuals to be involved in delivery.
- Arrangement for postpartum period and preparation for newborn.

Planning

- Plan of care and who is involved in planning.
- Individual teaching plans for pregnancy, labor/delivery, postpartum self-care, and infant care.

Implementation/Evaluation

- Response to interventions, teaching, and actions performed.
- Attainment or progress toward desired outcomes.
- Modifications to plan of care.

Discharge Planning

- Long-term needs and who is responsible for actions to be taken.
- Available resources, specific referrals made.

References

1. Lauderdale, J. In Andrews, M. M., Boyle, J. S. (eds.). (2007). Transcultural perspectives in childbearing. *Transcultural Concepts in Nursing Care.* 5th ed. Philadelphia: Wolters Kluwer Health, Lippincott Williams & Wilkins.
2. Purnell, L. D., Paulanka, B. J. (2008). *Transcultural Health Care: Culturally Competent Approach.* 3rd ed. Philadelphia: F. A. Davis.
3. Bastable, S. B. (2005). *Essentials of Patient Education.* Sudbury, MA: Jones and Bartlett.
4. Editorial Staff. (2008). Complications and high-risk conditions of the prenatal period. *Straight A's in Maternal-Neonatal Nursing.* 2nd ed. Philadelphia: Wolters Kluwer, Lippincott Williams & Wilkins.
5. American College of Obstetricians and Gynecologists, Committee on Obstetric Practice. (2002). Exercise during pregnancy and the postpartum period. ACOG Committee Opinion 267. *Obst Gynecol,* 99(1), 171–173.
6. Editorial Staff. (2007). Cultural childbearing practices. *Lippincott Manual of Nursing Practice Pocket Guides: Maternal-Neonatal Nursing.* Philadelphia: Lippincott Williams & Wilkins.
7. Meek, J. Y. (ed). (2002). *The American Academy of Pediatrics New Mothers Guide to Breastfeeding.* New York: Bantam.
8. Holloway, B., Moredich, C., Aduddell, K. (2006). *OB/Peds Women's Health Notes: Nurses' Clinical Pocket Guide.* Philadelphia: F. A. Davis.
9. American Academy of Pediatrics. (2005). Breastfeeding and the use of human milk. *Pediatrics,* 115(2), 496–506.
10. Murry, M., Huelsmann, G. (2009). *Labor and Delivery Nursing: Guide to Evidence-Based Practice.* New York: Springer.
11. Mayo Clinic Staff. (Updated 2014). Childbirth education: Get ready for labor and delivery. Retrieved March 2015 from http://www.mayoclinic.org/healthy-living/pregnancy-week-by-week/in-depth/pregnancy/art-20044568.
12. Ricci, S. S., Kyle, T. (2008). *Maternity and Pediatric Nursing.* Philadelphia: Lippincott Williams & Wilkins.
13. Surgeon General. (2005). Surgeon General's advisory on alcohol use in pregnancy. Retrieved March 2015 from www.surgeongeneral.gov/pressreleases/sg02222005.html.
14. March of Dimes. (2008). Street drugs and pregnancy. Retrieved March 2015 from http://www.marchofdimes.org/pregnancy/illicit-drug-use-during-pregnancy.aspx#.
15. Acharya, K. S., Groutegut, C. A. (Updated 2015). Psychosocial and environmental pregnancy risks. Retrieved March 2015 from http://emedicine.medscape.com/article/259346-overview.
16. Ehrenberg, H. M. (2009). Maternal obesity, uterine activity, and the risk of spontaneous preterm birth. *Obstet Gynecol,* 113(1), 48–52.

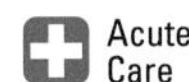

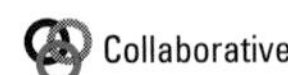

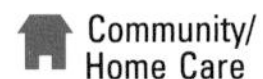

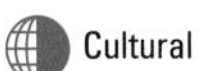

17. March of Dimes. (Updated 2014). Being pregnant at work. Retrieved March 2015 from www.marchofdimes.com/pnhec/159_11488.asp.
18. Silverman, J. G., Decker, M. R., Reed, E., et al. (2006). Intimate partner violence victimization prior to and during pregnancy among women residing in 26 U.S. states: Associations with maternal and neonatal health. *Am J Obstet Gynecol*, 195(1), 140–148.
19. March of Dimes. (2008). Abuse during pregnancy. Retrieved March 2015 from http://www.marchofdimes.org/pregnancy/abuse-during-pregnancy.aspx.
20. Shankaran, S., Lester, B. M., Das, A., et al. (2007). Impact of maternal substance use during pregnancy on childhood outcome. *Semin Fetal Neonatal Med*, 12(2), 143–150.

readiness for enhanced Childbearing Process

Taxonomy II: Sexuality—Class 3 Reproduction (00208) [**Diagnostic Division:** Sexuality], Submitted 2008; Revised 2013

DEFINITION: A pattern of preparing for and maintaining a healthy pregnancy, childbirth process, and care of newborn for ensuring well-being, which can be strengthened.

DEFINING CHARACTERISTICS

During Pregnancy

Subjective

Expresses desire to enhance prenatal lifestyle (e.g., nutrition, elimination, sleep, exercise, personal hygiene)
Expresses desire to enhance knowledge of childbearing process
Expresses desire to enhance management of unpleasant pregnancy symptoms
Expresses desire to enhance preparation for newborn

During Labor and Delivery

Subjective

Expresses desire to enhance lifestyle appropriate for stage of labor (e.g., nutrition, elimination, sleep, exercise, personal hygiene)
Expresses desire to enhance proactivity during labor and delivery

*After Birth**

Subjective

Expresses desire to enhance attachment behavior, baby care/feeding techniques, environmental safety for the baby
Expresses desire to enhance postpartum lifestyle (e.g., nutrition, elimination, sleep, exercise, personal hygiene), breast care
Expresses desire to enhance use of support system

Sample Clinical Applications: First, second, and third trimesters of pregnancy; labor and delivery; postpartum; newborn

(continues on page 148)

*The original Japanese term for "childbearing" (*shussan ikujikoudou*), which encompasses both childbirth and rearing of the neonate. It is one of the main concepts of Japanese midwifery.

readiness for enhanced Childbearing Process (continued)

DESIRED OUTCOMES/EVALUATION CRITERIA

Sample NOC linkages:

Knowledge: Pregnancy: Extent of understanding conveyed about promotion of a healthy pregnancy and prevention of complications

Knowledge: Labor & Delivery: Extent of understanding conveyed about labor and vaginal delivery

Knowledge: Infant Care: Extent of understanding conveyed about caring for a baby from birth to first birthday

Client Will (Include Specific Time Frame)

- Demonstrate healthy pregnancy free of preventable complications.
- Engage in activities to prepare for birth process and care of newborn.
- Experience complication-free labor and childbirth.
- Display culturally appropriate bonding behaviors.
- Verbalize understanding of care requirements to promote health of self and infant.

ACTIONS/INTERVENTIONS

Sample NIC linkages:

Childbirth Preparation: Providing information and support to facilitate childbirth and to enhance the ability of an individual to develop and perform the parental role

Postpartal Care: Monitoring and management of the patient who has recently given birth

Parent Education: Infant: Instruction on nurturing and physical care needed during the first year of life

NURSING PRIORITY NO. 1 To determine individual needs:

DURING PREGNANCY

- Evaluate current knowledge and cultural beliefs regarding normal physiological and psychological changes of pregnancy, as well as beliefs about activities, self-care, and so on. *Provides information to assist in identifying needs and creating individual plan of care.*[2,3]
- Determine degree of motivation for learning. *Client may have difficulty learning unless the need for it is clear.*[3]
- Identify who provides support/instruction within the client's culture (e.g., grandmother, other family member, curandero or doula, other cultural healer). Work with support person(s) when possible, using interpreter as needed. *Helps ensure quality and continuity of care because support person(s) may be more successful than the healthcare provider in communicating information.*[1,2,4]
- Determine client's commitments to work, family, community, and self; roles and responsibilities within family unit; and use of supportive resources. *Helps in setting realistic priorities to assist client in making adjustments, such as changing work hours, shifting of household chores and responsibilities, prioritizing and curtailing some outside commitments, etc.*[12,17]
- Evaluate the client's/couple's response to pregnancy, individual and family stressors, and cultural implications of pregnancy and childbirth. *The client's/couple's ability to adapt positively depends on support systems, cultural beliefs, resources, and effective coping mechanisms developed in dealing with past stressors. Initially, even if the pregnancy is planned, the expectant mother may feel ambivalent toward the pregnancy because of personal or professional goals, financial concerns, and possible role changes that a child will necessitate.*[1,2]
- Determine client's/couple's perception of fetus as a separate entity and extent of preparations being made for this infant. *Activities such as choosing a name or nicknaming the baby in utero and home preparations indicate completion of psychological tasks of pregnancy. Note: Cultural or familial beliefs may limit visible preparations out of concern that bad outcome may result.*[2]
- Assess economic situation and financial needs. Note use of available resources. *Impact of pregnancy on family with limited resources can create added stress and result in limited prenatal care and preparation for newborn.*

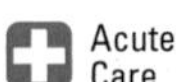

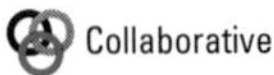

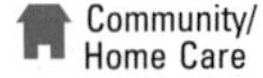

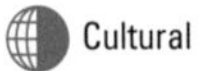

- Determine usual pregravid weight and dietary patterns. *Research studies have found a positive correlation between pregravid maternal obesity and increased perinatal morbidity rates (e.g., hypertension and gestational diabetes) associated with preterm births and macrosomia.*[16]

DURING LABOR AND DELIVERY

- Ascertain client's understanding and expectations of the labor process. *The client's/couple's coping skills are most challenged during the active and transition phases as contractions become increasingly intense. Lack of knowledge, misconceptions, or unrealistic expectations can have a negative impact on coping abilities.*
- Review birth plan developed by client/partner. Note cultural expectations/preferences. *Verifies that choices made are amenable to the specific care setting, accommodate individual wishes, and reflect client/fetal status. Note: Some cultures or personal values may limit male involvement in the delivery process, necessitating the identification of other support person(s).*[1,6,10]

AFTER BIRTH

- Determine plan for discharge after delivery and home care support and needs. *Early planning can facilitate discharge and help ensure that client/infant needs will be met.*[3]
- Ascertain client's perception of labor and delivery, length of labor, and client's fatigue level. *There is a correlation between length of labor and the ability of some clients to assume responsibility for self-care/infant care tasks and activities.*
- Assess mother's strengths and needs, noting age, marital status or relationship, presence and reaction of siblings and other family, available sources of support, and cultural background. *Identifies potential risk factors and sources of support, which influence the client's/couple's ability to assume role of parenthood. For example, the adolescent may still be formulating goals and an identity. She may have difficulty accepting the infant as a person and coping with full-time parenting responsibility. The single parent who lacks support systems may have difficulty assuming sole responsibility for parenting. Cultures in which the extended family members live together may provide more emotional and physical support, facilitating adoption of the new role.*[1,6]
- Appraise level of parents' understanding of infant's physiological needs and adaptation to extrauterine life associated with maintenance of body temperature, nutrition, respiratory needs, and bowel and bladder functioning. *Identifies areas of concern/need, which could require additional information and/or demonstration of care activities.*[3,12]
- Evaluate nature of emotional and physical parenting that client/couple received during their childhood. *Parenting role is learned, and individuals use their own parents as role models. Those who experienced a negative upbringing or poor parenting may require additional support to meet the challenges of effective parenting.*
- Note father's/partner's response to birth and to parenting role. *Client's ability to adapt positively to parenting may be strongly influenced by the father's/partner's reaction.*
- Assess client's readiness and motivation for learning. Assist client/couple in identifying needs. *The postpartal period provides an opportunity to foster maternal growth, maturation, and competence. However, the client needs time to move from a "taking-in" to a "taking-hold" phase, in which her receptiveness and readiness is heightened and she is emotionally and physically ready for learning new information to facilitate mastery of her new role.*[4]

NURSING PRIORITY NO. 2 To promote maximum participation in childbearing process:

DURING PREGNANCY

- Maintain open attitude toward beliefs of client/couple. *Acceptance is important to developing and maintaining relationship and supporting independence.*[2]
- Explain office visit routine and rationale for ongoing screening and close monitoring (e.g., urine testing, blood pressure monitoring, weight, fetal growth). Emphasize importance of keeping regular appointments. *Reinforces relationship between health assessment and positive outcome for mother/baby.*[12]

- Suggest father/siblings attend prenatal office visits and listen to fetal heart tones as appropriate. *Promotes a sense of involvement and helps make baby a reality for family members.*
- Provide information about need for additional laboratory studies and diagnostic tests or procedure(s). Review risks and potential side effects. *Aids in making informed decisions.*[8,12]
- Discuss any medications that may be needed to control or treat medical conditions. *Helpful in choosing treatment options because need must be weighed against possible harmful effects on the fetus.*[12]
- Provide anticipatory guidance, including discussion of nutrition, regular moderate exercise, comfort measures, rest, employment, breast care, sexual activity, and health habits and lifestyle. *Information encourages acceptance of responsibility and promotes self-care:*

  Review nutrition requirements and optimal prenatal weight gain to support maternal-fetal needs. *Dietary focus should be on balanced nutrients and calories to produce appropriate weight gain and to supply adequate vitamins and minerals for healthy fetus. Inadequate prenatal weight gain and/or below normal prepregnancy weight increases the risk of intrauterine growth restriction in the fetus and delivery of a low-birth-weight infant.*[8,12]

  Encourage moderate exercise such as walking or non-weight-bearing activities (e.g., swimming, bicycling) in accordance with client's physical condition and cultural beliefs. *Nonendurance, antepartal exercise regimens tend to shorten labor, increase likelihood of a spontaneous vaginal delivery, and decrease need for oxytocin augmentation.*[4,5] *In some cultures, inactivity may be viewed as a protection for mother/child.*[1,6]

  Recommend a consistent sleep and rest schedule (e.g., 1- to 2-hour daytime nap and 8 hours of sleep each night) in a dark, cool room. *Provides rest to meet metabolic needs associated with growth of maternal/fetal tissues.*[12]

  Identify anticipatory adaptations for significant other (SO)/family necessitated by pregnancy. *Family members will need to be flexible in adjusting own roles and responsibilities in order to assist client to meet her needs related to the demands of pregnancy, both expected and unplanned, such as prolonged nausea, fatigue, and emotional lability.*[12]

  Provide or reinforce information about potential teratogens, such as alcohol, nicotine, illicit drugs, the STORCH group of viruses (**s**yphilis, **t**oxoplasmosis, **o**ther, **r**ubella, **c**ytomegalovirus, **h**erpes simplex), and HIV. *Helps client make informed decisions and choices about behaviors and environment that can promote healthy offspring. Note: Research supports the fact that alcohol and recreational drug use can lead to a wide range of negative effects in the neonate. Smoking negatively affects placental circulation; even smoking fewer than 10 cigarettes per day is associated with an increased risk of fetal death, damage in utero, abruptio placentae, placenta previa, and low birth weight.*[4,8,13–15]

- Use various methods for learning, including pictures, to discuss fetal development. *Visualization enhances reality of child and strengthens learning process.*[4]
- Discuss signs of labor onset; how to distinguish between false and true labor, when to notify healthcare provider, and when to leave for hospital or birth center; and stages of labor and delivery. *Helps client to recognize onset of labor, to ensure timely arrival, and to cope with labor and delivery process.*[12]
- Review signs/symptoms requiring evaluation by primary provider during prenatal period (e.g., excessive vomiting, fever, unresolved illness of any kind, decreased fetal movement). *Allows for timely intervention.*[12]

DURING LABOR AND DELIVERY

- Identify client's support person/coach and ascertain that the individual is providing support that client requires. *Coach may be client's husband/SO or doula, and support can take the form of physical and emotional support for the mother and aid in initiation of bonding with the neonate.*[4]
- Demonstrate or review behaviors and techniques (e.g., breathing, focused imagery, music, other distraction; aromatherapy; abdominal effleurage, back and leg rubs, sacral pressure, repositioning, back rest; oral and perineal care, linen changes; shower or hot tub use) partner can use to assist with pain control and relaxation. *Enhances feeling of well-being. May block pain impulses within the cerebral cortex through conditioned responses and cutaneous stimulation, facilitating progression of normal labor.*[4]
- Discuss available analgesics, usual responses and side effects (client and fetal), and duration of analgesic effect in light of current situation. *Allows client to make informed choice about means of pain control and can*

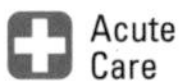

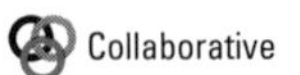

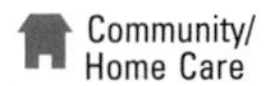

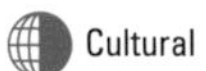

allay client's fears or anxieties about medication use. Note: If conservative measures are not effective and increasing muscle tension impedes progress of labor, judicious use of medication can enhance relaxation, shorten labor, limit fatigue, and prevent complications.[4]

- Support client's decision about the use or nonuse of medication in a nonjudgmental manner. Continue encouragement for efforts and use of relaxation techniques. *Enhances client sense of control and may prevent or decrease need for medication. Note: Continued support may be needed to help reduce feelings of failure in the client/couple who may have anticipated an unmedicated birth and did not follow through with that plan.*[12]

AFTER BIRTH

- Initiate early breastfeeding or oral feeding according to hospital protocol. *Initial feeding for breastfed infants usually occurs in the delivery room. Otherwise, 5 to 15 mL of sterile water may be offered in the nursery to assess effectiveness of sucking, swallowing, gag reflexes, and patency of esophagus. If aspirated, sterile water is easily absorbed by pulmonary tissues.*[7,9]
- Note frequency and amount and length of feedings. Encourage demand feedings instead of "scheduled" feedings. *Hunger and length of time between feedings vary from feeding to feeding.*[7,9] Note frequency, amount, and appearance of regurgitation. *Excessive regurgitation increases feeding needs.*
- Evaluate neonate/maternal satisfaction following feedings. *Provides opportunity to answer client questions, offer encouragement for efforts, identify needs, and problem solve solutions.*[7,9]
- Demonstrate and supervise infant care activities related to feeding and holding; bathing, diapering, and clothing; care of circumcised male infant; and care of umbilical cord stump. Provide written and pictorial information for parents to refer to after discharge. *Promotes understanding of principles and techniques of newborn care and fosters parents' skills as caregivers.*[3,12]
- Provide information about newborn interactional capabilities, states of consciousness, and means of stimulating cognitive development. *Helps parents recognize and respond to infant cues during interactional process and fosters optimal interaction, attachment behaviors, and cognitive development in infant. The state of consciousness can be divided into the sleep and the wake states, involving separate and predictable behavioral characteristics.*[12]
- Promote sleep and rest. *Reduces metabolic rate and allows nutrition and oxygen to be used for healing process rather than for energy needs.*[12]
- Provide for unlimited participation for father and siblings. Ascertain whether siblings attended an orientation program. *Facilitates family development and ongoing process of acquaintance and attachment. Helps family members feel comfortable caring for newborn.*
- Monitor and document the client's/couple's interactions with infant. Note presence of bonding (acquaintance) behaviors (e.g., making eye contact, using high-pitched voice and en face [face-to-face] position as culturally appropriate, calling infant by name, holding infant closely).[2,12]

NURSING PRIORITY NO. 3 To enhance optimal well-being:

DURING PREGNANCY

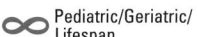

- Emphasize importance of maternal well-being. *Fetal well-being is directly related to maternal well-being, especially during the first trimester, when developing organ systems are most vulnerable to injury from environmental or hereditary factors.*
- Review physical changes to be expected during each trimester. *Questions will continue to arise as new changes occur, regardless of whether changes are expected or unexpected, and knowledge of "what's normal" can be reassuring. Also prepares client/couple for managing common discomforts associated with pregnancy.*[4,12]
- Explain psychological reactions, including ambivalence, introspection, stress reactions, and emotional lability, as being characteristic of pregnancy. *Helps client/couple understand mood swings and may provide opportunities for partner to offer support/affection at these times.*[4]
- Provide necessary referrals (e.g., dietitian, social services, Supplemental Nutrition Assistance Program (SNAP) or the Women, Infants, and Children [WIC] food program) as indicated. *May need additional*

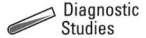

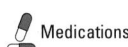

assistance with nutritional choices and may have budget or financial constraints. Supplemental federally funded food program helps promote optimal maternal, fetal, and infant nutrition.[12]

- Identify reportable danger signals of pregnancy, such as bleeding, cramping, acute abdominal pain, backache, edema, visual disturbance, headaches, and pelvic pressure. *Helps client to distinguish normal from abnormal findings, thus assisting her in seeking timely, appropriate healthcare.*[12]
- Encourage attendance at prenatal and childbirth classes. Provide information about father/sibling or grandparent participation in classes and delivery as client desires. *Knowledge gained helps reduce fear of unknown and increases confidence that couple can manage the preparation for the birth of their child. Helps family members to realize they are an integral part of the pregnancy and delivery.*[11,12]
- Provide list of appropriate reading materials for client, couple, and siblings regarding adjusting to newborn. *Information helps individual realistically analyze changes in family structure, roles, and behaviors.*[3]

DURING LABOR AND DELIVERY

- Monitor labor progress and maternal and fetal well-being per protocol. Provide continuous intrapartal professional support or a doula. *Fear of abandonment can intensify as labor progresses. The client may experience increased anxiety and/or loss of control when left unattended. Doulas can provide client with emotional, physical, and informational support as an adjunct to primary nurse.*[2,8]
- Reinforce use of positive coping mechanisms. *Enhances feelings of competence and fosters self-esteem.*[12]

AFTER BIRTH

- Provide information about self-care, including perineal care and hygiene; physiological changes, including normal progression of lochial discharge; needs for sleep and rest; importance of progressive postpartal exercise program; and role changes. *Helps prevent infection, fosters healing and recuperation, and contributes to positive adaptation to physical and emotional changes enhancing feelings of general well-being.*[12]
- Review normal psychological changes and needs associated with the postpartal period. *Client's emotional state may be somewhat labile at this time and often is influenced by physical well-being. Anticipating such changes may reduce the stress associated with this transition period that necessitates learning new roles and taking on new responsibilities.*[4,8,12]
- Discuss sexuality needs and plans for contraception. Provide information about available methods, including advantages and disadvantages. *Couple may need clarification regarding available contraceptive methods and the fact that pregnancy could occur even prior to the 4- to 6-week postpartum visit.*[8]
- Reinforce importance of postpartal examination by healthcare provider and interim follow-up as appropriate. *Follow-up visit is necessary to evaluate recovery of reproductive organs, healing of episiotomy or laceration repair, general well-being, and adaptation to life changes.*[12]
- Provide oral and written information about infant care and development, feeding, and safety issues. Offer appropriate references. Elicit cultural beliefs. *Helps prepare for new caretaking role, acquiring necessary items of furniture, clothing, and supplies; helps prepare for breastfeeding and/or bottle feeding.*[8,12]
- Discuss physiology and benefits of breastfeeding, nipple and breast care, special dietary needs, factors that facilitate or interfere with successful breastfeeding, and use of breast pump and appropriate suppliers. *Helps ensure adequate milk supply, prevents nipple cracking and soreness, facilitates comfort, and establishes role of breastfeeding mother.*[8]
- Refer client to support groups (e.g., La Leche League International, Lact-Aid) or a lactation consultant. *Provides ongoing help to promote a successful breastfeeding outcome.*[7,9]
- Identify available community resources as indicated (e.g., WIC program). *WIC and other federal programs support well-being through client education and enhanced nutritional intake for infant.*[12]
- Discuss normal variations and characteristics of infant, such as caput succedaneum, cephalohematoma, pseudomenstruation, breast enlargement, physiologic jaundice, and milia. *Helps parents to recognize normal variations and may reduce anxiety.*[4,12]
- Emphasize newborn's need for follow-up evaluation by healthcare provider and timely immunizations. *Ongoing evaluation is important for monitoring growth and development. Immunizations are necessary to protect the infant from childhood diseases with associated serious complications.*[12]

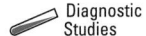

- Identify manifestations of illness and infection and when a healthcare provider should be contacted. Demonstrate proper technique for taking temperature, administering oral medications, or providing other care activities as required. *Early recognition of illness and prompt use of healthcare facilitate treatment and positive outcome.*[12]
- Refer client/couple to community postpartal parent groups. *Increases parents' knowledge of child rearing and child development and provides supportive atmosphere while parents incorporate new roles.*

DOCUMENTATION FOCUS

Assessment/Reassessment

- Assessment findings, general health, previous pregnancy experience.
- Cultural beliefs and expectations.
- Specific birth plan and individuals to be involved in delivery.
- Arrangements for postpartal recovery period.
- Response to newborn.

Planning

- Plan of care and who is involved in planning.
- Teaching plan.

Implementation/Evaluation

- Response to interventions, teaching, and actions performed.
- Attainment or progress toward desired outcome(s).
- Modifications to plan of care.

Discharge Planning

- Long-term needs and who is responsible for actions to be taken.
- Available resources, specific referrals made.

References

1. Lauderdale, J. (2007). Transcultural perspectives in childbearing. In Andrews, M. M., Boyle, J. S. (eds). *Transcultural Concepts in Nursing Care*. 5th ed. Philadelphia: Wolters Kluwer Health, Lippincott Williams & Wilkins.
2. Purnell, L. D., Paulanka, B. J. (2008). *Transcultural Health Care: Culturally Competent Approach*. 3rd ed. Philadelphia: F. A. Davis.
3. Bastable, S. B. (2005). *Essentials of Patient Education*. Sudbury, MA: Jones and Bartlett.
4. Editorial Staff. (2008). Complications and high-risk conditions of the prenatal period. *Straight A's in Maternal-Neonatal Nursing*. 2nd ed. Philadelphia: Wolters Kluwer, Lippincott Williams & Wilkins.
5. American College of Obstetricians and Gynecologists, Committee on Obstetric Practice. (2002). Exercise during pregnancy and the postpartum period. ACOG Committee Opinion 267. *Obstet Gynecol*, 99(1), 171–173.
6. Editorial Staff. (2007). Cultural childbearing practices. *Lippincott Manual of Nursing Practice Pocket Guides: Maternal-Neonatal Nursing*. Philadelphia: Lippincott Williams & Wilkins.
7. Meek, J. (ed.) (2002). *The American Academy of Pediatrics New Mothers Guide to Breastfeeding*. New York: Bantam.
8. Holloway, B., Moredich, C., Aduddell, K. (2006). *OB Peds Women's Health Notes: Nurses Clinical Pocket Guide*. Philadelphia: F. A. Davis.
9. American Academy of Family Physicians. Breastfeeding, family physicians supporting (Position paper). Retrieved October 2015 from http://www.aafp.org/policies/all/breastfeeding-support.html.
10. Murry, M., Huelsmann, G. (2008). *Labor and Delivery Nursing: Guide to Evidence-Based Practice*. New York: Springer.
11. Mayo Clinic Staff. (update 2014). Childbirth classes: Get ready for labor and delivery. Retrieved October 2015 from http://www.mayoclinic.org/healthy-lifestyle/pregnancy-week-by-week/in-depth/pregnancy/art-20044568.
12. Ricci, S. S., Kyle, T. (2008). *Maternity and Pediatric Nursing*. Philadelphia: Lippincott Williams & Wilkins.
13. Surgeon General. (2005, revised 2007). Surgeon General's advisory on alcohol use in pregnancy. Retrieved October 2015 http://www.cdc.gov/mmwr/preview/mmwrhtml/mm5409a6.htm.

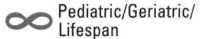

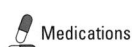

14. March of Dimes. (update 2013). Street drugs and pregnancy. Retrieved October 2015 from http://www.marchofdimes.org/pregnancy/street-drugs-and-pregnancy.aspx.
15. Acharya, K. S., Grotegut, C. A. (2015). Psychosocial and environmental pregnancy risks. Retrieved October 2015 from http://emedicine.medscape.com/article/259346-overview.
16. Ehrenberg, H. M. (2009). Maternal obesity, uterine activity, and the risk of spontaneous preterm birth. *Obstet Gynecol*, 113(1), 48–52.
17. March of Dimes. (update 2014). Being pregnant at work. Retrieved October 2015 from http://www.marchofdimes.org/pregnancy/being-pregnant-at-work.aspx.

risk for ineffective Childbearing Process

Taxonomy II: Sexuality—Class 3 Reproduction (00227) [**Diagnostic Division:** Sexuality], Submitted 2010; Revised 2013

DEFINITION: Vulnerable to not matching environmental context, norms and expectations of pregnancy, childbirth process, and the care of the newborn.

RISK FACTORS

Insufficient knowledge of childbearing process; unrealistic birth plan
Unplanned/unwanted pregnancy
Inconsistent prenatal health visits; insufficient prenatal care
Inadequate maternal nutrition
Substance abuse
Insufficient support system
Low maternal confidence
Maternal powerlessness/psychological distress
Domestic violence
Insufficient parental role model/cognitive readiness for parenting
Note: A risk diagnosis is not evidenced by signs and symptoms, as the problem has not occurred; rather, nursing interventions are directed at prevention.
Sample Clinical Applications: First, second, and third trimester of pregnancy; labor and delivery, postpartum, newborn

DESIRED OUTCOMES/EVALUATION CRITERIA

Sample NOC linkages:
Prenatal Health Behavior: Personal actions to promote a healthy pregnancy and a healthy newborn
Maternal Status: Antepartum/Intrapartum/Postpartum [specify]: Extent to which maternal well-being is within normal limits from conception to the onset of labor/from onset of labor to delivery/from delivery of placenta to completion of involution
Knowledge: Infant Care: Extent of understanding conveyed about caring for a baby from birth to first birthday

Client Will (Include Specific Time Frame)
- Acknowledge and address individual risk factors.
- Demonstrate healthy pregnancy free of preventable complications.
- Engage in activities to prepare for birth process and care of newborn.

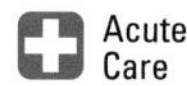

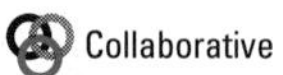

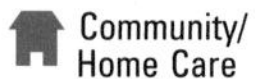

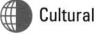

- Experience complication-free labor and childbirth.
- Verbalize understanding of care requirements to promote health of self and infant.

Refer to ND ineffective Childbearing Process *for Interventions and Documentation Focus*

impaired Comfort

Taxonomy II: Comfort—Class 1 Physical Comfort/Class 2 Environmental Comfort/Class 3 Social Comfort (00214) [**Diagnostic Division:** Pain/Discomfort], Submitted 2008; Revised 2010

DEFINITION: Perceived lack of ease, relief and transcendence in physical, psychospiritual, environmental, cultural, and/or social dimensions.

RELATED FACTORS

Illness-related symptoms; treatment regimen
Insufficient environmental or situational control
Insufficient privacy
Noxious environmental stimuli
Insufficient resources (e.g., financial, social, knowledge)

DEFINING CHARACTERISTICS

Subjective

Distressing symptoms; feeling of hunger, discomfort; itching; feeling cold, hot
Alteration in sleep pattern, inability to relax
Anxiety, fear; uneasy in situation

Objective

Restlessness; irritability; sighing; moaning; crying
Sample Clinical Applications: Presence of chronic physical or psychological conditions

DESIRED OUTCOMES/EVALUATION CRITERIA

Sample NOC linkages:

Symptom Control: Personal actions to minimize perceived adverse changes in physical and emotional functioning
Comfort Status: Overall physical, psychospiritual, sociocultural, and environmental ease and safety of an individual
Quality of Life: Extent of positive perception of current life circumstances

Client Will (Include Specific Time Frame)

Engage in behaviors or lifestyle changes to increase level of ease.
Verbalize sense of comfort and contentment.
Participate in desirable and realistic health-seeking behaviors.

(continues on page 156)

impaired Comfort (continued)
ACTIONS/INTERVENTIONS

Sample NIC linkages:
Environmental Management: Comfort: Manipulation of the patient's surroundings for promotion of optimal comfort
Relaxation Therapy: Use of techniques to encourage and elicit relaxation for the purpose of decreasing undesirable signs and symptoms such as pain, muscle tension, or anxiety
Self-Awareness Enhancement: Assisting a patient to explore and understand his/her thoughts, feelings, motivations, and behaviors

NURSING PRIORITY NO. 1 To assess etiology/precipitating contributory factors:

- Determine the type of discomfort client is experiencing, such as physical pain; feeling of discontent; lack of ease with self, environment, or sociocultural settings; or inability to rise above one's problems or pain (lack of transcendence). Have client rate total comfort using a 0–10 scale, with 10 being as comfortable as possible, or a "general comfort" questionnaire using a Likert-type scale. *A comfort scale is similar to a pain rating scale and can help client identify focus of discomfort (e.g., physical, emotional, social, etc.).*[1,5,10]
- Note cultural or religious beliefs and values that impact perceptions and expectations of comfort.
- Ascertain locus of control. *Presence of external locus of control may hamper efforts to achieve sense of peace or contentment.*
- Discuss concerns with client and active-listen to identify underlying issues (e.g., physical and/or emotional stressors; external factors such as environmental surroundings, social interactions) that could impact client's ability to control own well-being. *Helps to determine client's specific needs and ability to change own situation.*
- Establish context(s) in which lack of comfort is realized: physical—pertaining to bodily sensations; psychospiritual—pertaining to internal awareness of self and meaning in one's life, relationship to a higher order or being; environmental—pertaining to external surroundings, conditions, and influences; sociocultural—pertaining to interpersonal, family, and societal relationships.[1]

PHYSICAL

- Determine how client is managing pain and pain components. *Lack of control may be related to other issues or emotions such as fear, loneliness, anxiety, noxious stimuli, and anger.*[1]
- Ascertain what has been tried or is required for comfort or rest (e.g., head of bed up or down, music on or off, white noise, rocking motion, certain person or thing; ability to express and/or manage conflicts).[2]

PSYCHOSPIRITUAL

- Determine how psychological and spiritual indicators overlap (e.g., meaningfulness, faith, identity, self-esteem) for client.[1]
- Ascertain if client/significant other (SO) desires support regarding spiritual enrichment, including prayer, meditation, or access to spiritual counselor of choice.[3]

ENVIRONMENTAL

- Determine that client's environment respects privacy and provides natural lighting and readily accessible view to outdoors—*an aspect that can be manipulated to enhance comfort.*[1,3]

SOCIOCULTURAL

- Ascertain meaning of comfort in context of interpersonal, family, and cultural values and societal relationships.[4,10]
- Validate client/SO understanding of client's situation and ongoing methods of managing condition, as appropriate and/or desired by client. *Considers client/family needs in this area and shows appreciation for their desires.*[4]

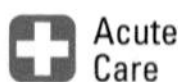

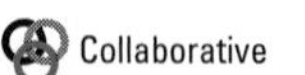

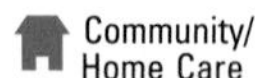

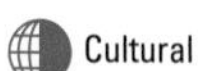

NURSING PRIORITY NO. 2 To assist client to alleviate discomfort:

- Review knowledge base and note coping skills that have been used previously to change behavior and promote well-being. *Brings these to client's awareness and promotes use in current situation.*[8]
- Acknowledge client's strengths in present situation and build on those strengths in planning for future.

PHYSICAL

- Collaborate in treating and managing medical conditions involving oxygenation, elimination, mobility, cognitive abilities, electrolyte balance, thermoregulation, and hydration, *to promote physical stability.*[2,5,6]
- Work with client to prevent pain, nausea, itching, thirst, and other physical discomforts.
- Review medications or treatment regimen *to determine possible changes or options to reduce side effects.*
- Suggest parent be present during procedures *to comfort child.*
- Provide age-appropriate comfort measures (e.g., back rub, change of position, cuddling, use of heat or cold) *to provide nonpharmacological pain management.*
- Discuss interventions and activities to promote ease, such as Therapeutic Touch, massage, healing touch, biofeedback, self-hypnosis, guided imagery, breathing exercises, play therapy, and humor, *to promote relaxation and refocus attention. Note: Studies show that client must be comfortable with touch in order to receive the full benefit of massage.*[9]
- Assist client to use and modify medication regimen *to make best use of pharmacological pain or symptom management.*
- Assist client/SO(s) to develop plan for activity and exercise within individual ability emphasizing necessity of allowing sufficient time to finish activities.
- Maintain open and flexible visitation with client's desired persons.
- Encourage and plan care to allow individually adequate rest periods *to prevent fatigue.* Schedule activities for periods when client has the most energy *to maximize participation.*
- Discuss routines to promote restful sleep.

PSYCHOSPIRITUAL

- Interact with client in therapeutic manner. *The nurse could be the most important comfort intervention for meeting client's needs. For example, assuring client that nausea can be treated successfully with both pharmacologic and nonpharmacologic methods may be more effective than simply administering antiemetic without reassurance and comforting presence.*[7]
- Encourage verbalization of feelings and make time for listening and interacting.
- Identify ways (e.g., meditation, sharing oneself with others, being out in nature or garden, other spiritual activities) to achieve connectedness or harmony with self, others, nature, and/or a higher power.
- Establish realistic activity goals with client. *Enhances commitment to promoting optimal outcomes.*
- Involve client/SO(s) in schedule planning and decisions about timing and spacing of treatments *to promote relaxation and reduce sense of boredom.*
- Encourage client to do whatever possible (e.g., self-care, sit up in chair, walk). *Enhances self-esteem and independence.*
- Use distraction with music, chatting, texting with family/friends, watching TV or videos, or playing computer games *to limit dwelling on negatives and to transcend unpleasant sensations and situations.*
- Encourage client to make use of beneficial coping behaviors and develop assertiveness skills, prioritizing goals and activities. *Promotes sense of control and improves self-esteem.*
- Offer or identify opportunities for client to participate in experiences that enhance control and independence.

ENVIRONMENTAL

- Provide quiet environment and calm activities.
- Provide for periodic changes in the personal surroundings when client is confined. Use the individual's input in creating the changes (e.g., seasonal bulletin boards, color changes, rearranging furniture, pictures).

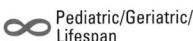

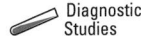

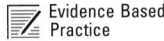

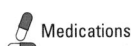

- Suggest activities, such as bird feeders or baths for bird-watching, a garden in a window box or terrarium, or a fishbowl or aquarium, *to stimulate observation as well as involvement and participation in an activity.*

SOCIOCULTURAL

- Encourage age-appropriate diversional activities (e.g., TV, radio, computer games, playtime, socialization or outings with others).
- Avoid overstimulation or understimulation (cognitive and sensory).
- Make appropriate referrals to available support groups, hobby clubs, and service organizations.

NURSING PRIORITY NO. 3 To promote wellness (Teaching/Discharge Considerations):

- Provide information about condition, health risk factors, or concerns in desired format (e.g., pictures, TV programs, articles, handouts, audio/visual materials; classes, group discussions, Internet Web sites, other databases) as appropriate. *Use of multiple modalities enhances acquisition and retention of information and gives client choices for accessing and applying information.*

PHYSICAL

- Promote overall health measures (e.g., nutrition, adequate fluid intake, appropriate vitamin or iron supplementation).
- Discuss potential complications and possible need for medical follow-up or alternative therapies. *Timely recognition and intervention can promote wellness.*
- Assist client/SO(s) to identify and acquire necessary equipment (e.g., lifts, commode chair, safety grab bars, personal hygiene supplies) to meet individual needs.

PSYCHOSPIRITUAL

- Collaborate with others when client expresses interest in lessons, counseling, coaching, and/or mentoring *to meet or enhance emotional and spiritual comfort.*
- Encourage client's contributions toward meeting realistic goals.
- Recommend client take time to be introspective in the search for contentment or transcendence.

ENVIRONMENTAL

- Create a compassionate supportive and therapeutic environment incorporating client's cultural, age, and developmental factors.
- Correct environmental hazards that could influence safety and negatively affect comfort.
- Arrange for home visit and evaluation as needed.
- Discuss long-term plan for taking care of environmental needs.

SOCIOCULTURAL

- Advocate for growth-promoting environment in conflict situations and consider issues from client/family and cultural perspective.
- Identify resources or referrals (e.g., knowledge and skills, financial resources and assistance; personal or psychological support group; social activities).

DOCUMENTATION FOCUS

Assessment/Reassessment

- Individual findings, including client's description of current status or situation, and factors impacting sense of comfort.
- Pertinent cultural or religious beliefs and values.
- Medication use and nonpharmacological measures.

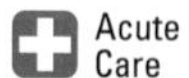

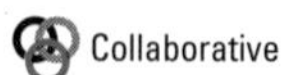

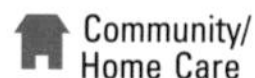

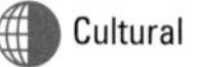

Planning
- Plan of care, specific interventions, and who is involved in planning.
- Teaching plan.

Implementation/Evaluation
- Responses to interventions, teaching, and actions performed.
- Attainment or progress toward desired outcome(s).
- Modifications to plan of care.

Discharge Planning
- Long-term needs and who is responsible for actions to be taken.
- Specific referrals made.

References

1. Kolcaba, K. Y., Fisher, E. M. (1996). A holistic perspective on comfort care as an advance directive. *Crit Care Nurs Q*, 18(4), 66–67.
2. Kolcaba, K., DiMarco, M. A. (2005). Comfort theory and its application to pediatric nursing. *Pediatr Nurs*, 31(3), 187–194.
3. Barclay, L., Lie, D. (2007). New guidelines issued for family support in patient-centered ICU. *CME/CE for Medscape*. Retrieved October 2015 from http://www.medscape.org/viewarticle/551738.
4. Malinowski, A., Stamler, L. L. (2002). Comfort: Exploration of the concept in nursing. *J Adv Nurs*, 39(6), 599–606.
5. Kolcaba, K. (2003). *Comfort Theory and Practice: A Vision for Holistic Health and Research*. New York: Springer.
6. Kaplow, R. (2003). AACN synergy model for patient care: A framework to optimize outcomes. *Crit Care Nurse Suppl*(February), 27–30.
7. Wilson, L., Kolcaba, K. (2004). Practical application of comfort theory in the perianesthesia setting. *J Perianesth Nurs*, 19(3), 164–173.
8. Townsend, M. C. (2005). *Psychiatric Mental Health Nursing Concepts of Care*. 5th ed. Philadelphia: F. A. Davis.
9. Andrade, C., Clifford, P. (2001). *Outcome Based Massage*. 2nd ed. Philadelphia: Lippincott Williams & Wilkins.
10. Kolcaba, K. (2003). *Comfort Theory and Practice*. New York: Springer.

readiness for enhanced Comfort

Taxonomy II: Comfort—Class 1 Physical Comfort/Class 2 Environmental Comfort/Class 3 Social Comfort (00183)
[**Diagnostic Division:** Pain/Discomfort], Submitted 2006; Revised 2013

DEFINITION: A pattern of ease, relief, and transcendence in physical, psychospiritual, environmental, or social dimensions, which can be strengthened.

DEFINING CHARACTERISTICS

Subjective
Expresses desire to enhance comfort or feeling of contentment
Expresses desire to enhance relaxation
Expresses desire to enhance resolution of complaints
Sample Clinical Applications: Presence of chronic physical or psychological conditions, or any individual seeking improved quality of life

(continues on page 160)

readiness for enhanced Comfort (continued)

DESIRED OUTCOMES/EVALUATION CRITERIA

Sample NOC linkages:

Comfort Status: Overall physical, psychospiritual, sociocultural, and environmental ease and safety of an individual

Personal Well-Being: Extent of positive perception of one's health status

Quality of Life: Extent of positive perception of current life circumstances

Client Will (Include Specific Time Frame)

- Verbalize sense of comfort or contentment.
- Demonstrate behaviors of optimal level of ease.
- Participate in desirable and realistic health-seeking behaviors.

ACTIONS/INTERVENTIONS

Sample NIC linkages:

Self-Modification Assistance: Reinforcement of self-directed change initiated by the patient to achieve personally important goals

Relaxation Therapy: Use of techniques to encourage and elicit relaxation for the purpose of decreasing undesirable signs and symptoms such as pain, muscle tension, or anxiety

Self-Awareness Enhancement: Exploration and understanding of patient's thoughts, feelings, motivations, and behaviors

NURSING PRIORITY NO. 1 To determine current level of comfort/motivation for growth:

- Determine the type of comfort client is experiencing: (1) relief—as from pain, (2) ease—a state of calm or contentment, or (3) transcendence—a state in which one rises above one's problems or pain.[1]
- Note cultural or religious beliefs and values that impact perceptions of comfort.
- Ascertain motivation and expectations for improvement. *Motivation to improve and high expectations can encourage client to make changes that will improve his or her life. However, presence of external locus of control or unrealistic expectations may hamper efforts.*
- Discuss concerns with client and active-listen to identify underlying issues (e.g., physical or emotional stressors; external factors such as environmental surroundings, social interactions) that could impact client's ability to control own well-being. *Helps to determine client's level of satisfaction with current situation and readiness for change.*
- Establish context(s) in which comfort is realized: (1) physical—pertaining to bodily sensations; (2) psychospiritual—pertaining to internal awareness of self and meaning in one's life; relationship to a higher order or being; (3) environmental—pertaining to external surroundings, conditions, and influences; or (4) sociocultural—pertaining to interpersonal, family, and societal relationships.[1]

PHYSICAL

- Verify that client is managing pain and pain components effectively. *Success in this arena usually addresses other issues or emotions (e.g., fear, loneliness, anxiety, noxious stimuli, anger).*[1]
- Ascertain what is used or required for comfort or rest (e.g., head of bed up or down, music on or off, white noise, rocking motion, certain person or thing, ability to express and/or manage conflicts).[2]

PSYCHOSPIRITUAL

- Determine how psychological and spiritual indicators overlap (e.g., meaningfulness, faith, identity, self-esteem) for client in enhancing comfort.[1]

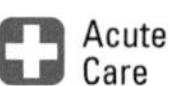

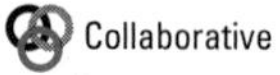

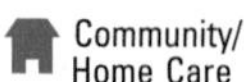

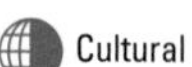

- Ascertain that client/significant other (SO) has received desired support regarding spiritual enrichment, including prayer, meditation, or access to spiritual counselor of choice.[3]

ENVIRONMENTAL
- Determine that client's environment respects privacy and provides natural lighting and readily accessible view to outdoors—*an aspect that can be manipulated to enhance comfort.*[1,3]

SOCIOCULTURAL
- Ascertain meaning of comfort in context of interpersonal, family, and cultural values and societal relationships.[4]
- Validate client/SO understanding of client's situation and ongoing methods of managing condition, as appropriate or desired by client. *Considers client/family needs in this area and shows appreciation for their desires.*[4]

NURSING PRIORITY NO. 2 To assist client in developing plan to improve comfort:
- Review knowledge base and note coping skills that have been used previously to change behavior and promote well-being. *Brings these to client's awareness and promotes use in current situation.*[8]
- Acknowledge client's strengths in present situation that can be used to build on in planning for future.

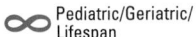

PHYSICAL
- Collaborate in treating or managing medical conditions involving oxygenation, elimination, mobility, cognitive abilities, electrolyte balance, thermoregulation, and hydration *to promote physical stability.*[2,5,6]
- Work with client to prevent pain, nausea, itching, thirst, and other physical discomforts.
- Suggest parent be present during procedures *to comfort child.*
- Suggest age-appropriate comfort measures (e.g., back rub, change of position, cuddling, use of heat or cold) *to provide nonpharmacological pain management.*
- Participate in interventions and age-appropriate activities, such as Therapeutic Touch, biofeedback, self-hypnosis, guided imagery, breathing exercises, play therapy, and humor, *that promote ease and relaxation and can refocus attention.*
- Assist client to use or modify medication regimen *to make best use of pharmacological pain management.*
- Assist client/SO(s) to develop or modify plan for activity and exercise within individual ability, emphasizing necessity of allowing sufficient time to finish activities.
- Maintain open and flexible visitation with client's desired persons.
- Encourage and plan care to allow individually adequate rest periods *to prevent fatigue.* Encourage client to schedule activities for periods when he/she has the most energy *to maximize effectiveness.*
- Discuss routines to promote restful sleep.

PSYCHOSPIRITUAL
- Interact with client in therapeutic manner. *The nurse could be the most important comfort intervention for meeting client's needs. For example, assuring client that nausea can be treated successfully with both pharmacological and nonpharmacological methods may be more effective than simply administering an antiemetic without reassurance and comforting presence.*[7]
- Encourage verbalization of feelings and make time for active-listening and interacting.
- Identify ways (e.g., meditation, sharing oneself with others, being out in nature or garden, other spiritual activities) to achieve connectedness or harmony with self, others, nature, or a higher power.
- Establish realistic activity goals with client. *Enhances commitment to promoting optimal outcomes.*
- Involve client/SO(s) in schedule planning and decisions about timing and spacing of treatments *to promote relaxation and desire for involvement in plan.*
- Encourage client to do whatever possible (e.g., self-care, sit up in chair, walk). *Enhances self-esteem and independence.*

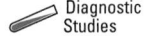

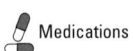

- Use distraction with music, chatting or texting with family/friends, watching TV, and playing video or computer games *to limit dwelling on negatives and to transcend unpleasant sensations and situations.*
- Encourage client to make use of beneficial coping behaviors and assertiveness skills, prioritizing goals and activities. *Promotes sense of control and improves self-esteem.*
- Offer and identify opportunities for client to participate in experiences that enhance control and independence.

ENVIRONMENTAL

- Provide quiet environment and calm activities.
- Provide for periodic changes in the personal surroundings when client is confined. Use the individual's input in creating the changes (e.g., seasonal bulletin boards, color changes, rearranging furniture, pictures).
- Suggest activities, such as bird-watching, planting a garden in a window box or terrarium, or populating a fishbowl or aquarium, *to stimulate observation as well as involvement and participation in activity.*

SOCIOCULTURAL

- Encourage age-appropriate diversional activities (e.g., TV, radio, playtime, socialization or outings with others).
- Avoid overstimulation or understimulation (cognitive and sensory).
- Make appropriate referrals to available support groups, hobby clubs, or service organizations.

NURSING PRIORITY NO. 3 To promote optimum wellness (Teaching/Discharge Considerations):

- Provide information about condition, health risk factors, or concerns in desired format (e.g., pictures, TV programs, articles, handouts, audio/visual materials, classes, group discussions, Web sites, other databases), as appropriate. *Use of multiple modalities enhances acquisition and retention of information and gives client choices for accessing and applying information.*

PHYSICAL

- Promote overall health measures (e.g., nutrition, adequate fluid intake, appropriate vitamin and iron supplementation).
- Discuss potential complications and possible need for medical follow-up or alternative therapies. *Timely recognition and intervention can promote wellness.*
- Assist client/SO(s) to identify and acquire necessary equipment (e.g., lifts, commode chair, safety grab bars, personal hygiene supplies) to meet individual needs.

PSYCHOSPIRITUAL

- Collaborate with others when client expresses interest in lessons, counseling, coaching, or mentoring to meet or enhance emotional and spiritual comfort.
- Promote client's contributions toward meeting realistic goals.
- Encourage client to take time to be introspective in the search for contentment or transcendence.

ENVIRONMENTAL

- Promote a compassionate, supportive, and therapeutic environment that incorporates client's cultural, age, and developmental factors.
- Review environmental hazards that could influence safety or negatively affect comfort.
- Arrange for home visit and evaluation, as needed.
- Discuss long-term plan for taking care of environmental needs.

SOCIOCULTURAL

- Advocate for growth-promoting environment in conflict situations and consider issues from client/family and cultural perspective.
- Support client/SO access to resources (e.g., knowledge and skills, financial resources or assistance, personal or psychological support, social systems).

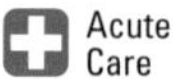

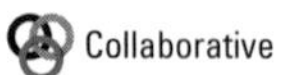

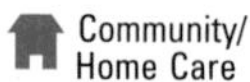

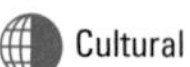

DOCUMENTATION FOCUS

Assessment/Reassessment

- Individual findings, including client's description of current status or situation.
- Motivation and expectations for change.
- Pertinent cultural or religious beliefs and values.
- Medication use and nonpharmacological measures.

Planning

- Plan of care, specific interventions, and who is involved in planning.
- Teaching plan.

Implementation/Evaluation

- Responses to interventions, teaching, and actions performed.
- Attainment or progress toward desired outcome(s).
- Modifications to plan of care.

Discharge Planning

- Long-term needs and who is responsible for actions to be taken.
- Specific referrals made.

References

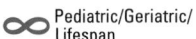

1. Kolcaba, K. Y., Fisher, E. M. (1996). A holistic perspective on comfort care as an advance directive. *Crit Care Nurs Q*, 18(4), 66–67.
2. Kolcaba, K., DiMarco, M. A. (2005). Comfort theory and its application to pediatric nursing. *Pediatr Nurse*, 31(3), 187–194.
3. Barclay, L., Lie, D. (2007). New guidelines issued for family support in patient-centered ICU. Retrieved October 2015 from http://www.medscape.org/viewarticle/551738.
4. Malinowski, A., Stamler, L. L. (2002). Comfort: Exploration of the concept in nursing. *J Adv Nurs*, 39(6), 599–606.
5. Kolcaba, K. (2003). *Comfort Theory and Practice: A Vision for Holistic Health and Research*. New York: Springer.
6. Kaplow, R. (2003). AACN synergy model for patient care: A framework to optimize outcomes. *Crit Care Nurse Suppl (Feb)*, 27–30.
7. Wilson, L., Kolcaba, K. (2004). Practical application of comfort theory in the perianesthesia setting. *J Perianesth Nurs*, 19(3), 164–173.
8. Townsend, M. C. (2005). *Psychiatric Mental Health Nursing Concepts of Care*. 5th ed. Philadelphia: F. A. Davis.

impaired verbal Communication

Taxonomy II: Perception/Cognition—Class 5 Communication (00051) [**Diagnostic Division:** Social Interaction], Submitted 1983; Revised 1996, 1998

DEFINITION: Decreased, delayed, or absent ability to receive, process, transmit, and/or use a system of symbols.

RELATED FACTORS

Alteration in development
Physical barrier (e.g., tracheostomy, intubation); oropharyngeal defect
Physiological conditions (e.g., decreased circulation to brain, weakened musculoskeletal system); central nervous system impairment

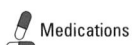

(continues on page 164)

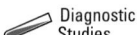

impaired verbal Communication (continued)

Vulnerability; emotional disturbance; psychotic disorder
Environmental barrier
Cultural incongruence
Insufficient information
Treatment regimen
Alteration in self-concept; low self-esteem
Alteration in perception
Absence of significant others

DEFINING CHARACTERISTICS

Objective

Inability to speak language of caregiver
Difficulty speaking/verbalizing; stuttering; slurred speech
Does not speak; refusal to speak; inability to speak
Difficulty forming sentences or words (e.g., aphonia, dyslalia, dysarthria)
Difficulty expressing thoughts verbally (e.g., aphasia, dysphasia, apraxia, dyslexia)
Inappropriate verbalization [e.g., incessant, loose association of ideas; flight of ideas]
Difficulty comprehending or maintaining communication
Absence of eye contact; difficulty in selective attending; partial or total visual deficit
Inability to, or difficulty in, use of facial or body expressions
Dyspnea
Disorientation to person, space, time
[Inability to modulate speech; message inappropriate to content]
[Use of nonverbal cues (e.g., pleading eyes, gestures, turning away)]

Sample Clinical Applications: Brain injury or stroke, facial trauma, head or neck cancer, radical neck surgery, laryngectomy, cleft lip/palate, dementia, Tourette's syndrome, autism, schizophrenia

DESIRED OUTCOMES/EVALUATION CRITERIA

Sample NOC linkages:

Communication: Reception, interpretation, and expression of spoken, written, and nonverbal messages
Communication: Expressive: Expression of meaningful verbal or nonverbal messages
Information Processing: Ability to acquire, organize, and use information

Client Will (Include Specific Time Frame)

- Verbalize or indicate an understanding of the communication difficulty and plans for ways of handling.
- Establish method of communication in which needs can be expressed.
- Participate in therapeutic communication (e.g., using silence, acceptance, restating, reflecting, active-listening, and "I" messages).
- Demonstrate congruent verbal and nonverbal communication.
- Use resources appropriately.

ACTIONS/INTERVENTIONS

Sample NIC linkages:

Communication Enhancement: Speech Deficit: Assistance in accepting and learning alternative methods for living with impaired speech

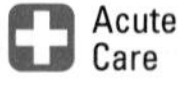
Acute Care
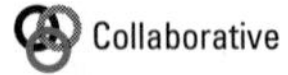
Collaborative
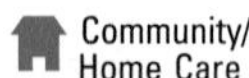
Community/ Home Care
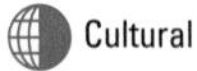
Cultural

Communication Enhancement: Hearing Deficit: Assistance in accepting and learning alternative methods for living with diminished hearing
Active Listening: Attending closely to and attaching significance to a patient's verbal and nonverbal messages

NURSING PRIORITY NO. 1 To assess causative/contributing factors:

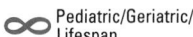

- Identify physiological or neurological conditions impacting speech, such as severe shortness of breath, cleft palate, facial trauma, neuromuscular weakness, stroke, brain tumors or infections, dementia, brain trauma, and deafness or hard of hearing.
- Review results of diagnostic studies (e.g., speech, language, and hearing evaluations, neurological testing or brain function studies—such as electroencephalogram, computed tomography scan, psychological evaluations) *to assess and delineate underlying conditions affecting verbal communication.*
- Note new onset or diagnosis of deficits that will progress or permanently affect speech.
- Note presence of physical barriers, including tracheostomy/intubation and wired jaws, or problem resulting in failure of voice production or "problem voice" *(pitch, loudness, or quality calls attention to voice rather than what speaker is saying, as might occur with electronic voice box or "talking valves" when tracheostomy in place).*[7,8]
- Determine age and developmental considerations when performing verbal examination, noting: (1) child too young for language or has developmental delays affecting speech and language skills or comprehension; (2) autism or other mental impairments; and (3) older client doesn't or isn't able to speak, verbalizes with difficulty, or has difficulty hearing or comprehending language or concepts. (The verbal examination should be adapted to the patient's communication skills and should use clear and concrete language, structure, reassurance, and support.)[1–3]
- Obtain history of hearing and speech-related pathophysiology or trauma (e.g., cleft lip/palate, traumatic brain injury, shaken baby syndrome, frequent ear infections affecting hearing, sensorineural changes associated with aging).
- Identify dominant language spoken. *Knowing the client's primary language and fluency in other languages is important to communication. For example, while some individuals may seem to be fluent in conversational English, they may still have limited understanding, especially the language of health professionals, and have difficulty answering questions, describing symptoms, or following directions.*[3,6,16]
- Ascertain whether client is recent immigrant, country of origin, and what cultural, ethnic group client identifies as own *(e.g., recent immigrant may identify with home country and its people, beliefs, and healthcare practices).*[6]
- Determine cultural factors affecting communication, such as beliefs concerning touch, eye contact, and verbal communications. *Certain cultures may prohibit client from speaking directly to healthcare provider; some cultures may interpret direct eye contact as disrespectful, impolite, an invasion of privacy, or aggressive.*[4] *Silence and tone of voice has various meanings, and slang words can cause confusion or misunderstandings.*[5]
- Identify environmental barriers, such as recent or chronic exposure to hazardous noise in home, job, recreation, or healthcare setting (e.g., rock music, jackhammer, snowmobile, lawn mower, truck traffic or busy highway, heavy equipment, medical equipment). *Noise not only affects hearing, but also increases blood pressure and breathing rate, can have negative cardiovascular effects, disturbs digestion, increases fatigue, causes irritability, and reduces attention to tasks.*[9]
- Investigate client reports of problems such as constantly raising voice to be heard, can't hear someone 2 feet away, conversation in room sounds muffled or dull, too much energy required to listen, or pain or ringing in ears after exposure to noise.[9]
- Determine if client with communication impairment has a speech or language problem or both. *When a speech problem is present, the language code can be correct, but words might be garbled, person may stutter, or*

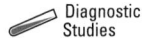

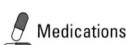

there may be problems with voice. Language and speech problems can exist together or by themselves. Language is a code made up of rules (e.g., what words mean, how to make new words, how to combine words, what combinations work in what situations). When a person cannot understand the language code, there is a receptive problem.[10]

- Determine presence of psychological or emotional barriers, such as history or presence of psychiatric conditions (e.g., bipolar disorder, schizoid or affective behavior); high level of anxiety, frustration, or fear; and presence of angry, hostile behavior. Note effect on speech and communication.[1,4]
- Identify information barriers, such as lack of knowledge or misunderstanding of terms related to client's medical conditions, procedures, treatments, and equipment.[4]
- Assess level of understanding in a sensitive manner. *Individual may be reluctant to say he or she doesn't understand or may be embarrassed to ask for help. Head nodding and smiles do not always mean comprehension.*[16]

NURSING PRIORITY NO. 2 To assist client to establish a means of communication to express needs, wants, ideas, and questions:

- Ascertain that you have client's attention before communicating.
- Establish rapport with client, initiate eye contact, shake hands, address by preferred name, meet family members present, ask simple questions, smile, and engage in brief social conversation if appropriate. *Helps establish a trusting relationship with client/family, demonstrating caring about the client as a person.*[2–4,18]
- Advise other care providers of client's communication deficits (e.g., deafness, aphasia, mechanical ventilation strategies) and needed means of communication (e.g., writing pad, signing, yes/no responses, gestures, picture board) *to minimize client's frustration and promote understanding.*[19]
- Provide and encourage use of glasses, hearing aids, dentures, and electronic speech devices as needed *to maximize sensory perception and improve speech patterns.*[2,4]
- Maintain a calm, unhurried manner and sit at client's eye level if possible. Provide sufficient time for client to respond. *Sitting down conveys that nurse has time and interest in communicating.*
- Pay attention to speaker. Be an active listener.
- ∞ Begin conversation with elderly individual with casual and familiar topics (e.g., weather, happenings with family members) *to convey interest and stimulate conversation and reminiscence.*[2,14]
- Reduce environmental distractions and background noise (e.g., close the door, turn down the radio or television).[14,20,21]
- Refrain from shouting when directing speech to a confused, deaf, or hearing-impaired client. Speak slowly and clearly, pitching voice low *to increase likelihood of being understood.*[2,15,20,21]
- Be honest and let the speaker know when you have difficulty understanding. Repeat part of message that you do understand *so speaker does not have to repeat entire message.*[11]
- Clarify type and special features of aphasia, when present. *Aphasia is a temporary, permanent, or progressive impairment of language affecting production or comprehension of speech and the ability to read or write. Some people with aphasia have problems primarily with expressive language (what is said), while others have problems with receptive language (what is understood). Aphasia can also be global (person understands almost nothing that is said and says little or nothing).*[4,11]
- Note diagnosis of apraxia (impairment in carrying out purposeful movements affecting rhythm and timing of speech), dysarthria (language code can be correct but the right body parts do not move at the right time to produce the right message), or dementia (defect is in decline in mental functions, including memory, attention, intellect, and personality) *to help clarify individual needs, appropriate interventions.*[11,12]
- Determine meaning of words used by the client and congruency of communication and nonverbal messages.
- Evaluate the meaning of words that are used/needed to describe aspects of healthcare (e.g., pain) and ascertain how to communicate important concepts.[5]
- Observe body language, eye movements, and behavioral clues. *For example, client may react with tears, grimacing, stiff posture, turning away, or angry outbursts when pain present.*[13]

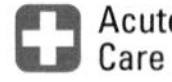

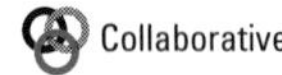

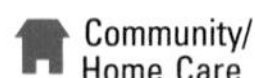

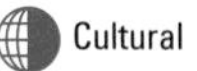

- Use confrontation skills, when appropriate, within an established nurse-client relationship *to clarify discrepancies between verbal and nonverbal cues.*[4,15]
- Point to objects or demonstrate desired actions when client has difficulty with language. *Speaker's own body language can be used to assist client's understanding.*
- Validate meaning of nonverbal communication; do not make assumptions *because they may be wrong.* Be honest; if you do not understand, seek assistance from others.[18]
- Work with confused, brain-injured, mentally disabled, or sensory-deprived client *to correctly interpret his or her environment.* Establish understanding and convey to others meaning of symbolic speech *to reduce frustration.* Teach basic signs such as "eat," "toilet," "more," and "finished" *to communicate basic needs.*[4,15]
- Provide reality orientation by responding with simple, straightforward, honest statements. Associate words with objects using repetition and redundancy *to improve communication patterns.*[2,4,15]
- Assess psychological response to communication impairment and willingness to find alternative means of communication.
- Identify family member who can speak for client and who is the family decision maker regarding healthcare decisions.[5,16]
- Note SO's/parents'/caregiver's speech patterns and interactive manner of communicating with client, including gestures.[20]
- Obtain interpreter with language or signing abilities and preferably with medical knowledge when needed. *Federal law mandates that interpretation services be made available. A trained, professional interpreter who translates precisely and possesses a basic understanding of medical terminology and healthcare ethics is preferred (over a family member) to enhance client and provider interactions.*[6,17]
- Evaluate ability to read and write, as well as musculoskeletal status, including manual dexterity (e.g., ability to hold a pen and write), and the need or desire for pictures or written communications and instructions as part of treatment plan.
- Plan for and provide alternative methods of communication:[2–4,17,22]

  Provide pad and pencil or a slate board *when client is able to write but cannot speak.*

  Use letter or picture board *when client can't write and picture concepts are understandable to both parties Note: Studies show that visual aids may improve the accuracy of medication assessment and may be especially beneficial for clients with communication barriers.*[22]

  Establish hand or eye signals *when client can understand language but cannot speak or has physical barrier to writing.*

  Remove isolation mask *when client is deaf and reads lips.*

  Obtain or provide access to typewriter or computer *if communication impairment is long-standing or client is used to this method.*
- Consider form of communication when placing IV. *IV positioned in hand or wrist may limit ability to write or sign.*
- Answer call bell promptly. Anticipate needs and avoid leaving client alone with no way to summon assistance. *Reduces fear, conveys caring to client, and protects nurse from problems associated with failure to provide due care.*[4]
- Refer for appropriate therapies and support services. *Client and family may have multiple needs (e.g., sources for further examinations and rehabilitation services, local community or national support groups and services for disabled, financial assistance with obtaining necessary aids for improving communication).*[4]

NURSING PRIORITY NO. 3 To promote wellness (Teaching/Discharge Considerations):

- Encourage family presence and use of touch. Involve them in plan of care as much as possible. *Enhances participation and commitment to plan, assists in normalizing family role patterns, and provides support and encouragement when learning new patterns of communicating.*[4]
- Review information about condition, prognosis, and treatment with client/SOs, reinforcing that loss of speech does not imply loss of intelligence.

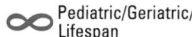

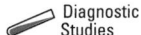

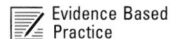

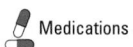

- Teach client and family the needed techniques for communication, whether it be speech or language techniques or alternate modes of communicating. Encourage family to involve client in family activities using enhanced communication techniques. *Reduces stress of difficult situation and promotes earlier return to more normal life patterns.*[4]
- Assess family for possible role changes resulting from client's impairment. Discuss methods of dealing with impairment.
- Use and assist client/SO(s) to learn therapeutic communication skills of acknowledgment, active-listening, and "I" messages. *Improves general communication skills, emphasizes acceptance, and conveys respect.*
- Discuss ways to provide environmental stimuli as appropriate *to maintain contact with reality or reduce environmental stimuli or noise. Unwanted sound affects physical health, increases fatigue, reduces attention to tasks, and makes speech communication more difficult.*[9,14]
- Refer to appropriate resources (e.g., speech or language therapist, support groups [e.g., stroke club], individual/family and/or psychiatric counseling) *to address long-term needs and enhance coping skills.*
- Refer to NDs ineffective Coping, disabled family Coping, Anxiety, Fear for additional interventions.

DOCUMENTATION FOCUS

Assessment/Reassessment

- Assessment findings, pertinent history information (i.e., physical, psychological, or cultural concerns).
- Meaning of nonverbal cues, level of anxiety client exhibits.

Planning

- Plan of care and specific interventions (e.g., type of alternative communication, translator).
- Teaching plan.

Implementation/Evaluation

- Response to interventions, teaching, and actions performed.
- Attainment or progress toward desired outcomes.
- Modifications to plan of care.

Discharge Planning

- Discharge needs, referrals made, additional resources available.

References

1. Szymanski, L., King, B. (1999). Practice parameters for the assessment and treatment of children, adolescents, and adults with mental retardation and comorbid mental disorders. American Academy of Child and Adolescent Psychiatry Working Group on Quality Issues. *J Am Acad Child Adolesc Psychiatry*, 38(12 suppl), 5S–31S.
2. Stanley, M., Beare, P. G. (1999). *Gerontological Nursing: A Health Promotion Approach.* 2nd ed. Philadelphia: F. A. Davis.
3. Newfield, S. A., Hinz, M. D., Tilley, D. S., et al. (2007). *Cox's Clinical Applications of Nursing Diagnosis: Adult, Child, Women's, Psychiatric, Gerontic, and Home Health Considerations.* 5th ed. Philadelphia: F. A. Davis.
4. Doenges, M. E., Moorhouse, M. F., Murr, A. C. (2010). *Nurse's Pocket Guide: Diagnoses, Interventions, and Rationales.* 12th ed. Philadelphia: F. A. Davis, 193–198.
5. Purnell, L. D. (2009). *Guide to Culturally Competent Health Care.* 2nd ed. Philadelphia: F. A. Davis.
6. Enslein, J., Tripp-Reimer, T., Kelley, L. S., et al. (2002). Evidence-based protocol: Interpreter facilitation for individuals with limited English proficiency. *J Gerontol Nurs*, 28(7), 5–13.
7. American Speech-Language-Hearing Association. Voice disorders. Retrieved October 2015 from http://www.asha.org/public/speech/disorders/voice.htm.
8. American Speech-Language-Hearing Association. Speech for patients with tracheostomies or ventilators (information sheet). Retrieved October 2015 from http://www.asha.org/public/speech/disorders/tracheostomies.htm.
9. American Speech-Language-Hearing Association. Noise (information sheet). Retrieved October 2015 from http://www.asha.org/uploadedFiles/AIS-Noise.pdf#search=%22Noise%22.

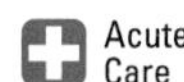

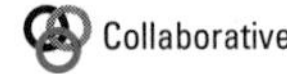

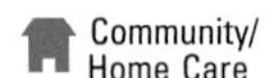

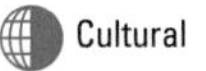

10. American Speech-Language-Hearing Association. What is language? What is speech? Retrieved October 2015 from http://www.asha.org/public/speech/development/language_speech/.
11. National Aphasia Association. (No date). More aphasia facts. Retrieved July 2011 from http://www.aphasia.org/Aphasia%20Facts/aphasia_facts.html.
12. National Aphasia Association. (No date). Understanding primary progressive aphasia. Retrieved July 2011 from http://www.aphasia.org/Aphasia%20Facts/understanding_primary_progressive_aphasia.html.
13. Hahn, J. (1999). Cueing in to patient language. *Reflections*, 25(1), 8–11.
14. Smith, K. (2001). I can hear you, but I can't understand you. Retrieved October 2015 from http://audioconsult.com/2011/08/i-can-year-you-%E2%80%A6-but-i-can%E2%80%99t-understand-you%E2%80%A6/.
15. Sendlebach, S., Guthrie, P. F. (2009). Acute confusion/delirium. *J Gerontological Nurs*, 35(11), 11–18.
16. Purnell, L. D. (2009). *Transcultural Health Care: A Culturally Competent Approach*. 3rd ed. Philadelphia: F. A. Davis.
17. Harquez-Rebello, M. C., Tornel-Costa, M. C. (1997). Design of a non-verbal method of communication using cartoons. *Rev Neurol*, 25(148), 2027–2045.
18. No author listed. (2005). Understanding transcultural nursing. *Nursing*, 35(1), 14–23.
19. Kirshner, D. (2015). Aphasia. Retrieved July 2011 from http://emedicine.medscape.com/article/1135944-overview.
20. Wallhagen, M. I., Pettengill, E., Whiteside, M. (2006). Sensory impairment in older adults part 1: Hearing loss. *Am J Nurs*, 106(10), 40–49.
21. Sommer, K. D., Sommer, N. W. (2002). When your patient is hearing impaired. *RN*, 65(12), 28–32.
22. Schillinger, D., Matchtinger, E. L., Wang, F., et al. (2006). Language, literacy, and communication regarding medication in an anticoagulation clinic: A comparison of verbal vs. visual assessment. *J Health Commun*, 11(7), 651–654.

readiness for enhanced Communication

Taxonomy II: Perception/Cognition—Class 5 Communication (00157) [**Diagnostic Division:** Teaching/Learning], Submitted 2002; Revised 2013

DEFINITION: A pattern of exchanging information and ideas with others, which can be strengthened.

DEFINING CHARACTERISTICS

Subjective

Expresses desire to enhance communication

Sample Clinical Applications: Brain injury or stroke, head or neck cancer, facial trauma, cleft lip/palate, Tourette's syndrome, autism, foreign-born individual communicating in second language

DESIRED OUTCOMES/EVALUATION CRITERIA

Sample NOC linkages:

Communication: Reception, interpretation, and expression of spoken, written, and nonverbal messages
Communication: Expressive: Expression of meaningful verbal and/or nonverbal messages
Information Processing: Ability to acquire, organize, and use information

Client/SO/Caregiver Will (Include Specific Time Frame)

- Verbalize or indicate an understanding of the communication process.
- Identify ways to improve communication.

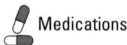

(continues on page 170)

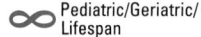

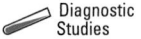

readiness for enhanced Communication (continued)
ACTIONS/INTERVENTIONS

Sample NIC linkages:
Communication Enhancement: Speech Deficit: Assistance in accepting and learning alternative methods for living with impaired speech
Communication Enhancement: Hearing Deficit: Assistance in accepting and learning alternative methods for living with diminished hearing
Active Listening: Attending closely to and attaching significance to a patient's verbal and nonverbal messages

NURSING PRIORITY NO. 1 To assess how client is managing communication and potential difficulties:

- Ascertain circumstances that result in client's desire to improve communication. *Many factors are involved in communication, and identifying specific needs and expectations helps in developing realistic goals and determining likelihood of success.*
- Ascertain motivation and expectations for change. *Motivation to improve and high expectations can encourage client to make changes that will improve his or her life. However, presence of external locus of control or unrealistic expectations may hamper efforts.*
- Evaluate mental status. *Disorientation, acute or chronic confusion, or psychotic conditions may be affecting speech and the communication of thoughts, needs, and desires.*
- Determine client's developmental level of speech and language comprehension. *Provides baseline information for developing plan for improvement.*
- Determine ability to read and write preferred language. *Evaluating grasp of language as well as musculoskeletal status, including manual dexterity (e.g., ability to hold a pen and write), provides information about nature of client's situation. Educational plan can address language skills. Neuromuscular deficits require individual physical or occupational therapeutic program to improve.*
- Determine country of origin, dominant language, whether client is recent immigrant, and what cultural or ethnic group client identifies as own. *Recent immigrant may identify with home country and its people, language, beliefs, and healthcare practices, thus affecting desire to learn language skills and ability to improve interactions in new country.*[1]
- Ascertain if interpreter is needed or desired. *Law mandates that interpretation services be made available. A trained, professional interpreter who translates precisely and possesses a basic understanding of medical terminology and healthcare ethics is preferred over a family member to enhance client and provider interaction and sharing of information.*[1]
- Determine comfort level in expression of feelings and concepts in nonproficient language. *Concern about language skills can impact perception of own ability to communicate effectively.*
- Note any physical challenges to effective communication (e.g., hearing impairment, talking tracheostomy apparatus, wired jaws) or physiological or neurological conditions (e.g., severe shortness of breath, neuromuscular weakness, stroke, brain trauma, deafness, cleft palate, facial trauma). *Client may be dealing with speech or language comprehension or have voice production problems (pitch, loudness, quality) that call attention to voice rather than what speaker is saying. These barriers may need to be addressed to enable client to improve communication skills.*[2,3]
- Clarify meaning of words used by the client to describe important aspects of life and health or well-being (e.g., pain, sorrow, anxiety). *Words can easily be misinterpreted when sender and receiver have different ideas about their meanings. This can affect the way both client and caregivers communicate important concepts. Restating what one has heard can clarify whether an expressed statement has been understood or misinterpreted.*[4]
- Determine presence of emotional lability or frequency of unstable behaviors. *Emotional or psychiatric issues can affect communication and interfere with understanding.*

Acute Care 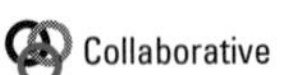 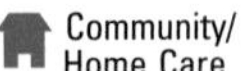 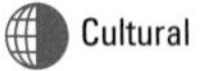

- Evaluate congruency of verbal and nonverbal messages. *Communication is enhanced when verbal and nonverbal messages are congruent.*[5]
- Determine lack of knowledge or misunderstanding of terms related to client's specific situation. *Indicators of need for additional information; clarification to help client improve ability to communicate.*
- Evaluate need or desire for pictures or written communications and instructions as part of treatment plan. *Alternative methods of communication can help client feel understood and promote feelings of satisfaction with interaction.*

NURSING PRIORITY NO. 2 To improve client's ability to communicate thoughts, needs, and ideas:

- Maintain a calm, unhurried manner. Provide sufficient time for client to respond. *An atmosphere in which client is free to speak without fear of criticism provides the opportunity to explore all the issues involved in making decisions to improve communication skills.*[10]
- Pay attention to speaker. Be an active listener. *The use of active-listening communicates acceptance and respect for the client, establishing trust and promoting openness and honest expression. It communicates a belief that the client is a capable and competent person.*
- Sit down and maintain eye contact, preferably at the client's level, and spend time with the client. *Conveys message that the nurse has time and interest in communicating.*[10]
- Encourage client to express feelings and clarify meaning of nonverbal clues. *Client may be reluctant to share dissatisfaction with events.*
- Help client identify and learn to avoid use of nontherapeutic communication. *These barriers are recognized as detriments to open communication, and learning to avoid them maximizes the effectiveness of communication between client and others.*
- Obtain interpreter with language or signing abilities as needed. *May be needed to enhance understanding of words and language concepts to ascertain that interpretation of communication is accurate.*[6,10]
- Encourage use of pad and pencil, slate board, or letter or picture board when interacting or to interface in new situations, as indicated. *When client has physical impairments that interfere with spoken communication, alternative means can provide concepts that are understandable to both parties.*[4,10]
- Obtain or provide access to voice-enabled computer. *Use of these devices may be more helpful when communication challenges are long-standing or when client is used to using them.*[1]
- Respect client's cultural communication needs. *Different cultures can dictate beliefs of what is normal or abnormal (i.e., in some cultures, eye-to-eye contact is considered disrespectful, impolite, or an invasion of privacy; silence and tone of voice have various meanings, and slang words can cause confusion).*[4]
- Provide or encourage use of glasses, hearing aids, dentures, or electronic speech devices, as needed. *These devices maximize sensory perception and can improve understanding and enhance speech patterns.*[7]
- Reduce distractions and background noises (e.g., close the door, turn down the radio or television). *A distracting environment can interfere with communication, limiting attention to tasks, and makes speech and communication more difficult. Reducing noise can help both parties hear clearly, improving understanding.*[8]
- Associate words with objects using repetition and redundancy, point to objects, or demonstrate desired actions. *Speaker's own body language can be used to enhance client's understanding when neurological conditions result in difficulty understanding language.*[9]
- Use confrontation skills carefully, when appropriate, and within an established nurse-client relationship. *Can be used to clarify discrepancies between verbal and nonverbal cues, enabling client to look at areas that may require change.*[10]

NURSING PRIORITY NO. 3 To promote optimum communication:

- Discuss with family/significant other (SO) and other caregivers effective ways in which the client communicates. *Identifying positive aspects of current communication skills enables family members to learn and move forward in desire to enhance ways of interacting.*[10]

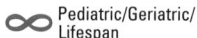

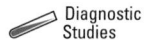

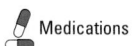

- Encourage client and family to familiarize themselves with and use new or developing communication technologies. *Enhances family relationships and promotes self-esteem for all members, as they are able to communicate regardless of problems (e.g., progressive neurological disorder) that could interfere with ability to interact.*[10]
- Reinforce client's/SO's learning and use of therapeutic communication skills of acknowledgment, active-listening, and "I" messages. *Improves general communication skills, emphasizes acceptance, and conveys respect, enabling family relationships to improve.*
- Refer to appropriate resources (e.g., speech therapist, language classes, individual/family or psychiatric counseling). *May need further assistance to overcome challenges as family reaches toward desired goal of enhanced communication.*

DOCUMENTATION FOCUS

Assessment/Reassessment

- Assessment findings, pertinent history information (i.e., physical, psychological, or cultural concerns).
- Meaning of nonverbal cues, level of anxiety client exhibits.
- Motivation and expectations for change.

Planning

- Plan of care and specific interventions (e.g., type of alternative communication, translator).
- Teaching plan.

Implementation/Evaluation

- Progress toward desired outcome(s).
- Modifications to plan of care.

Discharge Planning

- Discharge needs, referrals made, additional resources available.

References

1. Enslein, J., Tripp-Reimer, T., Kelley, L. S., et al. (2002). Evidence-based protocol: Interpreter facilitation for persons with limited English proficiency. *J Gerontol Nurs*, 28(7), 5–13.
2. American Speech-Language-Hearing Association. Voice disorders. Retrieved October 2015 from http://www.asha.org/public/speech/disorders/voice.
3. American Speech-Language-Hearing Association. Speech for patients with tracheostomies or ventilators. Retrieved October 2015 from http://www.asha.org/public/speech/disorders/tracheostomies.htm.
4. Purnell, L. (2009). *Guide to Culturally Competent Health Care.* 2nd ed. Philadelphia: F. A. Davis.
5. Hahn, J. (1999). Cueing in to client language. *Reflections*, 25(1), 8–11.
6. American Speech-Language-Hearing Association. What is language? What is speech? Retrieved October 2015 from http://www.asha.org/public/speech/development/language_speech.
7. Stanley, M., Beare, P. G. (1999). *Gerontological Nursing: A Health Promotion Approach.* 2nd ed. Philadelphia: F. A. Davis.
8. American Speech-Language-Hearing Association. Noise (information sheet). Retrieved October 2015 from http://www.asha.org/uploadedFiles/AIS-Noise.pdf#search=%22Noise%22.
9. Sendlebach, S., Guthrie, P. F. (2009). Acute confusion/delirium. *J Gerontol Nurs*, 35(11), 11–18.
10. Newfield, S. A., Hinz, M. D., Tilley, D. S., et al. (2005). *Cox's Clinical Applications of Nursing Diagnosis: Adult, Child, Women's, Psychiatric, Gerontic, and Home Health Considerations.* 5th ed. Philadelphia: F. A. Davis.

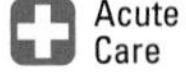

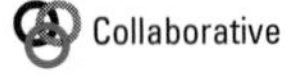

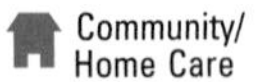

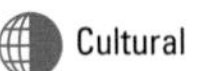

acute Confusion

Taxonomy II: Perception/Cognition—Class 4 Cognition (00128) [**Diagnostic Division:** Neurosensory], Submitted 1994; Revised 2006

DEFINITION: Abrupt onset of reversible disturbances of consciousness, attention, cognition, and perception that develop over a short period of time.

RELATED FACTORS

Age ≥60 years
Alteration in sleep-wake cycle
Delirium [including mania/other psychiatric disorder]; dementia
Substance abuse
[Endocrine or metabolic crisis, liver or renal failure; hypoxemia, hypercarbia; shock]

DEFINING CHARACTERISTICS

Subjective

Hallucinations [visual or auditory]
[Exaggerated emotional responses]

Objective

Agitation; restlessness
Alteration in cognitive functioning, or level of consciousness
Alteration in psychomotor functioning
Misperception
Inability to initiate goal-directed or purposeful behavior
Inability to follow through with goal-directed or purposeful behavior

Sample Clinical Applications: Brain injury or stroke, respiratory conditions with hypoxia, medication adverse reactions, drug or alcohol intoxication, hyperthermia, infectious processes, malnutrition, eating disorders, fluid and electrolyte imbalances, chemical exposure

DESIRED OUTCOMES/EVALUATION CRITERIA

Sample NOC linkages:

Acute Confusion Level: Severity of disturbance in consciousness and cognition that develops over a short period of time
Information Processing: Ability to acquire, organize, and use information
Distorted Thought Self-Control: Self-restraint of disruption in perception, thought processes, and thought content

Client/Caregiver Will (Include Specific Time Frame)

- Regain and maintain usual reality orientation and level of consciousness.
- Verbalize understanding of causative factors when known.
- Initiate lifestyle or behavior changes to prevent or minimize recurrence of problem.

ACTIONS/INTERVENTIONS

Sample NIC linkages:

Delirium Management: Provision of a safe and therapeutic environment for the patient who is experiencing an acute confusional state

(continues on page 174)

acute Confusion (continued)
Reality Orientation: Promotions of patient's awareness of personal identity, time, and environment
Delusion Management: Promoting the comfort, safety, and reality orientation of a patient experiencing false, fixed beliefs that have little or no basis in reality

NURSING PRIORITY NO. 1 To assess causative/contributing factors:

- Identify factors present, such as recent surgery or trauma; use of large numbers of medications (polypharmacy); intoxication with/withdrawal from a substance (e.g., prescription and over-the-counter [OTC] drugs; alcohol, illicit drugs); history or current seizure activity, episodes of fever, pain, presence of acute infection (especially occult urinary tract infection in elderly client); traumatic events; person with dementia experiencing sudden change in environment, unfamiliar surroundings or people). *Acute confusion is a symptom associated with numerous causes (e.g., hypoxia; metabolic/endocrine/neurological conditions, toxins; electrolyte abnormalities; systemic or central nervous system infections; nutritional deficiencies, acute psychiatric disorders). Note: Delirium due to physical illness is more frequent among the very young and the elderly. Delirium due to drug and alcohol intoxication or withdrawal is more common in persons aged mid-teens to late 30s. Studies show that age greater than 60 is the client-related factor that has been associated with the greatest neuropsychological changes after cardiac surgery.*[2,11,12,15]
- Assess mental status. *Typical symptoms of delirium include anxiety, disorientation, tremors, hallucinations, delusions, and incoherence. Onset is usually sudden, developing over a few hours or days, and resolving over varying periods of time.*[2,15]
- Evaluate vital signs. *Signs of poor tissue perfusion (i.e., hypotension, tachycardia, tachypnea, or fever) may identify underlying cardiovascular or infectious cause for mental status changes. Note: Clients with delirium frequently display elevated blood pressure because of adrenergic overload in the sympathetic nervous system. Heart rate can be either elevated or decreased.*[11]
- Determine current medications and drug use (especially anti-anxiety agents, barbiturates, certain antipsychotic agents; methyldopa, disulfiram, cocaine, alcohol, amphetamines, hallucinogens, opiates). *Use, misuse, overdose, and withdrawal of many drugs are associated with high risk of confusion and delirium.*[1,11]
- Investigate possibility of alcohol or illicit drug intoxication or withdrawal or prescription or OTC medication toxicity, side effects, or interactions. *Noncompliance with regimen, sudden discontinuation or overuse of substances, and certain drug combinations increase risk of toxic reactions and adverse reactions or interactions.*[1,2,12]
- Evaluate for exacerbation of psychiatric conditions (e.g., mood disorder, dissociative disorders, dementia). *Identification of the presence of mental illness provides opportunity for correct treatment and medication.*[10,11]
- Assess diet and nutritional status to identify possible deficiencies of essential nutrients and vitamins. *Failure to eat (forgetfulness or lack of food) can lead to deficiencies (e.g., vitamin B_{12}, folate, thiamine, iron) that could affect mental status.*[2,11]
- Evaluate sleep and rest status, noting deprivation or oversleeping. *Discomfort, worry, and lack of sleep and rest can cause or exacerbate confusion.* (Refer to ND Insomnia, disturbed Sleep Pattern as appropriate.)
- Monitor laboratory values (e.g., complete blood count, blood cultures; oxygen saturation and in some cases, arterial blood gases with carbon monoxide; blood urea nitrogen and creatinine levels; electrolytes; thyroid function studies; liver function studies, ammonia levels; serum glucose; urinalysis for infection and drug analysis; specific drug toxicologies, drug levels [including peak and trough, as appropriate]).[1–7,11]
- Review results of diagnostic studies (e.g., delirium assessment tools, such as the Confusion Assessment Method, delirium index, Mini Mental State Examination, etc; brain scans or imaging studies, electroencephalogram, lumbar puncture and cerebrospinal fluid studies). *Mental status instruments are helpful because they directly test the client's cognitive performance. However, performance is strongly affected by age, educational level, ethnicity, and language, and they may be difficult for the acutely ill client to perform.*[5,11]

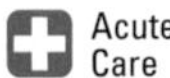
Acute Care
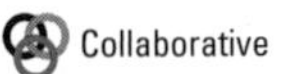
Collaborative
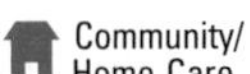
Community/ Home Care
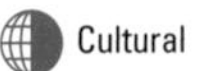
Cultural

NURSING PRIORITY NO. 2 To determine degree of impairment:

- Talk with client/significant others (SOs) to determine client's physical, functional, cognitive, and behavioral baseline; observed changes; and onset and precipitator of changes *to understand and clarify the current situation.*[1]
- Collaborate with medical and psychiatric providers *to evaluate extent of impairment in orientation, attention span, ability to follow directions, send and receive communication, and appropriateness of response.*[1]
- Note occurrence and timing of agitation, hallucinations, and violent behaviors *(e.g., delirium may occur as early as 1 or 2 days after last drink in an alcoholic; "Sundowners syndrome" may occur in intensive care unit, with client oriented during daylight hours but confused during night).*[1,3]
- Determine threat to safety of client/others. *Delirium can cause client to become verbally and physically aggressive, resulting in behavior threatening to safety of self and others.*

NURSING PRIORITY NO. 3 To maximize level of function, prevent further deterioration:

- Assist with treatment of underlying problem. *Interventions to establish and maintain normal fluid and electrolyte balance and oxygenation, treat infectious process or pain, detoxify from alcohol and other drugs, and provide psychological interventions can resolve or diminish confusion.*[1–7,9,11,12,14]
- Monitor and adjust medication regimen and note response. Determine which medications can be changed or eliminated when polypharmacy, side effects, or adverse reactions are determined to be associated with current condition.
- Implement helpful communication measures:[1–7,9,11,14]
  Use short, simple sentences. Speak slowly and clearly.
  Call client by name and identify yourself at each contact.
  Tell client what you want done, not what to do.
  Orient client to surroundings, staff, and necessary activities as often as needed.
  Acknowledge client's fears and feelings. *Confusion can be very frightening, especially when client knows thinking is not normal.*
  Listen to what client says and try to identify message and emotion or need being communicated.
  Limit choices and decisions until client is able to make them.
  Give simple directions. Allow sufficient time for client to respond, communicate, and make decisions.
  Present reality concisely and briefly and avoid challenging illogical thinking. *Defensive reactions may result.*
  Refer to ND impaired verbal Communication for additional interventions.
- Manage environment, using the following measures:[1–7,9,11,14]
  Provide undisturbed rest periods. Eliminate extraneous noise and stimuli. *Preventing overstimulation can help client relax and can result in reduced level of confusion.*[10]
  Provide calm and comfortable environment with good lighting. Encourage client to use vision or hearing aids, when needed, *to reduce disorientation and discomfort from sensory overload or deprivation.*
  Observe client on regular basis, informing client of this schedule.
  Provide adequate supervision (may need one-to-one during severe episode), remove harmful objects from environment, provide siderails and seizure precautions, place call bell and position needed items within reach, clear traffic paths, and ambulate with devices *to meet client's safety needs and reduce risk of falls.*
  Provide clear feedback on appropriate and inappropriate behavior.
  Remove client from situation; provide time-out or seclusion, as indicated, *for protection of client/others.*
  Encourage family/SO(s) to participate in reorientation and provide ongoing normal life input (e.g., current news and family happenings). Provide normal levels of essential sensory and tactile stimulation—include personal items and pictures. *Client may respond positively to well-known person and familiar items.*
- Note behavior that may be indicative of potential for violence and take appropriate actions to prevent injury to client/caregiver. (Refer to ND risk for self-/other-directed Violence.)

- Administer medication cautiously to control restlessness, agitation, and hallucinations. *Depending on the cause of acute delirium, medications could include sedatives, neuroleptics, and antidotes. Sedation with conventional antipsychotic agents (e.g., haloperidol, lorazepam, droperidol) may be used, although many other agents may be tried, including electrolytes, glucose, vitamins, antibiotics, etc. (Note: Sedation should be avoided if it will interfere with, or cloud the results of, serial neurological examinations.*[2,5–7,11])
- Assist with treatment of alcohol or drug intoxication and/or withdrawal, as indicated.[11,12,14]
- Avoid or limit use of restraints. *May worsen agitation and increase likelihood of untoward complications including injury or death.*[5,12]
- Mobilize elderly client (especially after orthopedic injury) as soon as possible. *Older person with low level of activity prior to crisis is at particular risk for acute confusion and may fare better when out of bed.*[4,14]
- Establish and maintain elimination patterns. *Disruption of elimination may be a cause for confusion, or changes in elimination may also be a symptom of acute confusion.*[5]
- Consult with psychiatric clinical nurse specialist or psychiatrist for additional interventions related to disruptive behaviors, psychosis, and unresolved symptoms.
- Refer to ND [disturbed Sensory Perception (Specify)] for additional interventions.

NURSING PRIORITY NO. 4 To promote wellness (Teaching/Discharge Considerations):

- Explain reason for confusion, if known. *Acute confusion usually subsides over time as client recovers from underlying cause or adjusts to situation, but it can be frightening to client/SO. Information about cause and treatment to improve condition may be helpful in managing sense of fear and powerlessness.*[13,14]
- Educate SO/caregivers to monitor client at home for sudden change in cognition and behavior. *An acute change is a classic presentation of delirium and should be considered a medical emergency. Early intervention can often prevent long-term complications.*[8]
- Discuss need for ongoing medical review of client's medications to limit possibility of misuse and/or potential for dangerous side effects or interactions. *Medications are frequent precipitants of acute confusion, especially in very young or old.*[8,9]
- Emphasize importance of keeping vision and hearing aids in good repair and readily available *to improve client's interpretation of environmental stimuli and communication.*
- Provide appropriate referrals. *Additional assistance may be required for client with confusion (e.g., cognitive retraining, substance abuse support groups, medication monitoring program, Meals on Wheels, home health, and adult day care).*[1]

DOCUMENTATION FOCUS

Assessment/Reassessment

- Nature, duration, frequency of problem.
- Current and previous level of function, effect on independence and lifestyle (including safety concerns).

Planning

- Plan of care and who is involved in planning.
- Teaching plan.

Implementation/Evaluation

- Response to interventions and actions performed.
- Attainment or progress toward desired outcomes.
- Modifications to plan of care.

Discharge Planning

- Long-term needs and who is responsible for actions to be taken.
- Available resources and specific referrals.

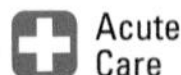

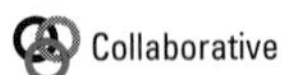

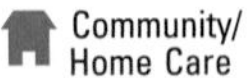

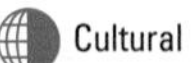

References

1. Doenges, M. E., Moorhouse, M. F., Murr, A. C. (2010). *Nurse's Pocket Guide: Diagnoses, Prioritized Interventions and Rationales.* 12th ed. Philadelphia: F. A. Davis, 211–215.
2. Alagiakrishnan, K. (2014). Delerium. Retrieved March 2015 from http://emedicine.medscape.com/article/288890-overview.
3. Stanley, M., Bear, P. G. (1999). *Gerontological Nursing: A Health Promotion/Protection Approach.* 2nd ed. Philadelphia: F. A. Davis, 342–349.
4. Matthiesen, V., Sivertsen, L., Foreman, M. D., et al. (1994). Acute confusion: Nursing intervention in older patients. *Orthop Nurs*, 13(2), 21–27.
5. Sendelbach, S., Guthrie, P. F. (2009). Acute confusion/delirium. *J Gerontol Nurs*, 35(11), 11–18.
6. American Psychiatric Association. Practice guideline for the treatment of patients with delirium. (1999). *Am J Psychiatry*, 156(5 Suppl), 1–20.
7. Alexopoulas, G. S. (2007). Treatment of dementia and agitation: A guide for families and caregiver. *J Psychiatric Pract*, 13(3), 12–20.
8. Ackley, B. J., Ladwig, G. B. (2002). *Nursing Diagnosis Handbook: A Guide to Planning Care.* 5th ed. St. Louis, MO: Mosby.
9. Cox, H. C., Sridaromont, K., King, M., et al. (2002). *Clinical Applications of Nursing Diagnosis: Adult, Child, Women's, Psychiatric, Gerontic, and Home Health Considerations.* 4th ed. Philadelphia: F. A. Davis.
10. Doenges, M. E., Townsend, M. C., Moorhouse, M. F. (1999). *Psychiatric Care Plans Guidelines for Individualizing Care.* 3rd ed. Philadelphia: F. A. Davis.
11. Gerstein, P. S. (Updated 2013). Delirium, dementia, and amnesia in emergency medicine. Retrieved March 2015 from http://emedicine.medscape.com/article/793247-overview.
12. Jennings-Ingle, S. (2007). The sobering facts about alcohol withdrawal syndrome. *Nursing Made Incredibly Easy!*, 5(1), 50–60.
13. McCaffrey, R., Rozzano, L. (2006). The effect of music on pain and acute confusion in older adults undergoing hip and knee surgery. *Holist Nurs Pract*, 20(5), 218–224.
14. Naylor, M. D., Stephens, C., Bowles, K. H., et al. (2005). Cognitively impaired older adults. *Am J Nurs*, 105(2), 52–61.
15. Bryson, G. L., Wynand, A. (2006). Evidence-based clinical update: General anesthesia and the risk of delirium and postoperative cognitive dysfunction. *Can J Anaesth*, 53(7), 669–677.

chronic Confusion

Taxonomy II: Perception/Cognition—Class 4 Cognition (00129) [**Diagnostic Division:** Neurosensory], Submitted 1994

DEFINITION: Irreversible, long-standing, and/or progressive deterioration of intellect and personality characterized by decreased ability to interpret environmental stimuli and decreased capacity for intellectual thought processes and manifested by disturbances of memory, orientation, and behavior.

RELATED FACTORS

Alzheimer's disease
Korsakoff's psychosis
Multi-infarct dementia
Cerebral vascular attack
Brain injury (e.g., cerebrovascular impairment, neurological illness, trauma, tumor)

DEFINING CHARACTERISTICS

Objective

Alteration in interpretation or response to stimuli
Progressive alteration in cognitive functioning; chronic cognitive impairment; organic brain disorder
Normal level of consciousness

(continues on page 178)

chronic Confusion (continued)
Impaired social functioning
Alteration in short-term or long-term memory
Alteration in personality
Sample Clinical Applications: Brain injury or stroke, dementia/Alzheimer's disease, medication adverse reactions, drug or alcohol abuse, malnutrition, eating disorders, chemical exposure

DESIRED OUTCOME/EVALUATION CRITERIA

Sample NOC linkages:
Physical Injury Severity: Severity of injuries from accidents and trauma
Cognitive Orientation: Ability to identify person, place, and time accurately

Client Will (Include Specific Time Frame)
- Remain safe and free from harm.
- Maintain usual level of orientation.

Sample NOC linkages:
Knowledge: Disease Process: Extent of understanding conveyed about a specific disease process

Family/Significant Other (SO) Will (Include Specific Time Frame)
- Verbalize understanding of disease process and prognosis and client's needs.
- Identify and participate in interventions to deal effectively with situation.
- Provide for maximal independence while meeting safety needs of client.

ACTIONS/INTERVENTIONS

Sample NIC linkages:
Dementia Management: Provision of a modified environment for the patient who is experiencing a chronic confusional state
Calming Technique: Reducing anxiety in patient experiencing acute distress
Surveillance: Purposeful and ongoing acquisition, interpretation, and synthesis of patient data for clinical decision making

NURSING PRIORITY NO. 1 To assess degree of impairment:

- Determine the underlying cause for chronic confusion, as noted in Related Factors. *Helps to sort out possible causes and likelihood for improvement, as well as helping to identify potentially useful interventions and therapies.*[1]
- Review and evaluate responses on diagnostic examinations (e.g., cognitive, functional capacity, behavior, memory impairments, reality orientation, attention span, quality of life). *A combination of tests (e.g., Confusion Assessment Method, Mini-Mental State Examination, Montreal Cognitive Assessment, Alzheimer's Disease Assessment Scale, Brief Dementia Severity Rating Scale, Neuropsychiatric Inventory, Functional Assessment Questionnaire, Clinical Global Impression of Change) is often needed to complete an evaluation of client's overall condition relating to chronic or irreversible condition. Note: Studies show that while a single screening test may identify cognitive decline and functional impairment, many tests serve different clinical and research functions. Therefore, clinical testing will continue to evolve.*[2,3,7]
- Talk with SO(s) regarding baseline behaviors, length of time since onset or progression of problem, their perception of prognosis, and other pertinent information and concerns for client. *The client's SO/primary caregiver is an invaluable and essential source of information, regarding history and current situation, as both cognitive and behavioral symptoms tend to change over time and are often variable from day to day. If history reveals a gradual and insidious decline over months to years and if memory loss is a prominent part of the*

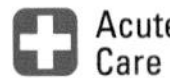 Acute Care 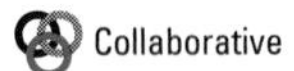 Collaborative 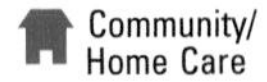 Community/Home Care 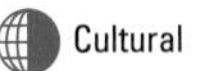 Cultural

confusion, dementia is likely. Conditions that permanently damage brain structure and tissue (e.g., vascular, traumatic, infectious or demyelinating conditions) can lead to dementia in person of any age.[1–4,8,9]

- Obtain information regarding recent changes or disruptions in client's health or routine. *Decline in physical health or disruption in daily living situation (e.g., hospitalization, change in medications, or moving to new home) can exacerbate agitation or bring on acute confusion.* (Refer to ND acute Confusion.)
- Evaluate client's response to primary care providers as well as receptiveness to interventions. *Awareness of these dynamics is helpful for evaluation of ongoing needs for both client and caregiver as client becomes increasingly dependent on caregivers or resistant to interventions.*
- Determine client and caregiver anxiety level in relation to situation. Note behavior that may be indicative of potential for violence. *The diagnosis of irreversible condition, the organic brain changes, and the day-to-day problems of living with it causes great stress and can potentiate violence.*[4]

NURSING PRIORITY NO. 2 To limit effects of deterioration/maximize level of function:

- Monitor for treatable conditions (e.g., depression, infections, malnutrition, electrolyte imbalances, and adverse medication reactions) *that may contribute to or exacerbate distress, discomfort, and agitation.*[1–6]
- Implement behavioral and environmental management interventions to promote orientation, provide opportunity for client interaction using current cognitive skills, and preserve client's dignity and safety:[6,9,11,12]

  Ascertain interventions previously used or tried and evaluate effectiveness.

  Provide calm environment and minimize relocations; eliminate extraneous noise and stimuli *that may increase client's level of agitation or confusion.*

  Introduce yourself at each contact, if needed. Call client by preferred name.

  Use touch judiciously. Tell client what is being done before touching *to reduce sense of surprise or negative reaction.*

  Be supportive and sensitive to fears, misperceived threats, and frustration with expressing what is wanted.

  Be open and honest when discussing client's disease, abilities, and prognosis.

  Maintain continuity of caregivers and care routines as much as possible.

  Use positive statements, offer guided choices between two options.

  Avoid speaking in loud voice, crowding, restraining, shaming, demanding, or condescending actions toward client.

  Set limits on acting-out behavior *for safety of client/others.*

  Remove from stressors and agitation triggers or danger, move client to quieter place, and offer privacy.

  Simplify client's tasks and routines *to accommodate fluctuating abilities and to reduce agitation associated with multiple options or demands.*

  Provide for or assist with daily care activities, including bathing, dressing, grooming, toileting, and exercise. *Client may "forget" how to perform activities of daily living.*

  Monitor and assist with meeting nutritional needs and feeding and fluid intake and monitor weight. Provide finger food if client has problems with eating utensils or is unable to sit to eat.

  Assist with toileting and perineal care, as needed. Provide incontinence supplies.

  Allow adequate rest between stimulating events.

  Use lighting and visual aids *to reduce confusion.*

  Encourage family/SO(s) to provide ongoing orientation/input to include current news and family happenings.

  Maintain reality-oriented relationship and environment (e.g., clocks, calendars, personal items, seasonal decorations).

  Encourage participation in resocialization groups *to help restore or maintain client's independence and dignity.*

  Allow client to reminisce or exist in own reality if not detrimental to well-being.

  Avoid challenging illogical thinking *because defensive reactions may result.*

  Provide appropriate safety measures. *Client who is confused needs close supervision. Safety measures (such as use of identification bracelet and alarms on unlocked exits, lockup of toxic substances and medication, supervision of outdoor activities and wandering, removal of car or car keys, lowered temperature on hot water tank) can prevent injuries.*[4]

- Avoid use of restraints as much as possible. Investigate use of alternatives (such as bed nets, electronic bed pads, chair alarms, laptop trays), when required. *Although restraints can prevent falls, they can increase client's agitation and distress, resulting in injury or even death.*[7,9,10]
- Administer medications (e.g., antidepressants, anxiolytics, antipsychotics), as ordered, at lowest possible therapeutic dose. Monitor for expected and/or adverse responses, side effects, and interactions. *May be used to manage symptoms of psychosis and aggressive behaviors but need to be used cautiously.*[5]
- Implement complementary therapies (e.g., music or dance therapy; animal-assisted therapy; massage, Therapeutic Touch [if touch is tolerated], aromatherapy, bright light treatment) as ordered or desired. Monitor client's response to each modality and modify as indicated. *Use of alternative therapies tailored to the client's preferences, skills, and abilities can be calming and provide relaxation and can be carried out by a wide range of health and social care providers and volunteers.*[11]
- Refer to NDs acute Confusion, impaired Memory, impaired verbal Communication for additional interventions.

NURSING PRIORITY NO. 3 To assist SO(s) to develop coping strategies:

- Determine family dynamics, cultural values, resources, availability, and willingness to participate in meeting client's needs. Evaluate SO's attention to own needs, including health status, grieving process, and respite. *Primary caregiver and other members of family will suffer from the stress that accompanies caregiving and will require ongoing information and support.*
- Discuss caregiver burden when appropriate. Provide educational materials and list of available resources, help lines, Web sites, and so forth, as desired, *to assist SO(s) in dealing and coping with long-term care issues.*[5,7,9] (Refer to NDs caregiver Role Strain, risk for caregiver Role Strain.)
- Involve SO(s) in care and discharge planning. Maintain frequent interactions with SOs *in order to relay information, to change care strategies, try different responses, or implement other problem-solving solutions.*[6]
- Identify appropriate community resources (e.g., Alzheimer's Disease and Related Disorders Association, stroke or other brain injury support groups, senior support groups, specialist day services, home care, respite care; adult placement and short-term residential care; clergy, social services, occupational and physical therapists; assistive technology and telecare; attorney services for advance directives, durable power of attorney) *to provide support for client and SOs and assist with problem solving.*[5,11]

NURSING PRIORITY NO. 4 To promote optimal functioning and safety (Teaching/Discharge Considerations):

- Discuss how client's condition may progress, ongoing age-appropriate treatment needs, and appropriate follow-up. *Intermittent evaluations are needed to determine client's general health, any deterioration in cognitive function, or required adjustment in medication regimen to help the client maintain the highest possible level of functioning.*[6]
- Review medications with SO/caregiver(s), including dosage, route, action, expected and reportable side effects, and potential drug interactions *to prevent or limit complications associated with multiple psychiatric and central nervous system medications.*[5]
- Develop plan of care with family to meet client's and SO's individual needs. *The individual plan is dependent on cultural and belief patterns as well as family resources (personal, emotional, financial).*[6]
- Instruct SO/caregivers to share information about client's condition, functional status, and medications whenever encountering new providers. *Clients often have multiple doctors, each of whom may prescribe medications with potential for adverse effects and overmedication.*
- Provide appropriate referrals (e.g., Meals on Wheels, adult day care, home-care agency, nursing home placement, respite care for family member). *May need additional assistance to maintain the client in the home setting or make arrangements for placement if necessary.*[6]

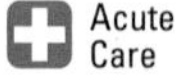
Acute Care
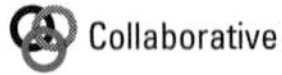
Collaborative
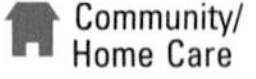
Community/ Home Care
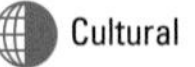
Cultural

DOCUMENTATION FOCUS

Assessment/Reassessment
- Individual findings, including current level of function, recent changes, and rate of anticipated changes.
- Client/caregiver response to situation.
- Results of diagnostic testing.

Planning
- Plan of care and who is involved in planning.
- Teaching Plan

Implementation/Evaluation
- Response to interventions and actions performed.
- Attainment or progress toward desired outcomes.
- Modifications to plan of care.

Discharge Planning
- Long-term needs and who is responsible for actions to be taken.
- Available resources, specific referrals made.

References

1. Bostwick, J. M. (2000). The many faces of confusion: Timing and collateral history often holds the key to diagnosis. *Postgrad Med*, 108(6), 60–72.
2. Alzheimer's Disease and Related Disorders Association. (Updated 2015). Disease tests for Alzheimer's disease and dementia. Retrieved April 2015 from http://www.alz.org/alzheimers_disease_steps_to_diagnosis.asp.
3. Vayda, E. P., Patterson, M. B., Whitehouse, P. J. (2010). The future of dementia: A case of hardening of the categories. *Am J Geriatr Psych*, 18(9), 755–758.
4. Alexopoulas, G. S., Jeste, D. V., Chug, H., et al. (2005). Treatment of dementia and agitation: A guideline for families and caregivers: Expert Consensus Guideline Series. *A Postgraduate Medicine Special Report*, January; 23(1), 18–22.
5. Sommers, M. S., Johnson, S. A., Beery, T. A. (2007). Alzheimer's disease. *Diseases and Disorders: A Nursing Therapeutics Manual*. 3rd ed. Philadelphia: F. A. Davis.
6. Kovach, C. R., Wilson, S. A. (2004). Dementia in older adults. In Stanley, M., et al. (eds). *Gerontological Nursing: Promoting Successful Aging with Older Adults*. 3rd ed. Philadelphia: F. A. Davis.
7. Boissonneault, G. (2010). MCI and dementia: Diagnosis and treatment. *JAAPA*, January; 23(1), 18–22.
8. Borbasi, S., Jones, J., Lockwood, C., et al. (2006). Health professionals' perspective of providing care to people with dementia in the acute setting: Toward better practice. *Geriatr Nurs*, 27(5), 300–308.
9. Kirshner, H. S. (2010). Confusional states and acute memory disorders. Retrieved July 2011 from http://emedicine.medscape.com/article/1135767-overview#showall.
10. Evans, L. K., Cotter, V. T. (2007). Avoiding restraints in patients with dementia: Understanding, prevention, and management are the keys. *Am J Nurs*, 108(3), 40–49.
11. National Collaborating Centre for Mental Health, Social Care Institute for Excellence, National Institute for Health and Clinical Excellence. (2006). Dementia: Supporting people with dementia and their carers in health and social care; National Clinical Guideline. Retrieved October 2015 from http://www.guideline.co.uk/central_nervous_system_nice_dementia#.ViUkpv9dHIU.
12. Alzheimer's Disease and Related Disorders Association. (2015). Treatments for Alzheimer's disease. Retrieved April 2015 from http://www.alz.org/alzheimers_disease_treatments_for_behavior.asp.

risk for acute Confusion

Taxonomy II: Perception/Cognition—Class 4 Cognition (00173) [**Diagnostic Division:** Neurosensory], Submitted 2006; Revised 2013

DEFINITION: Vulnerable to reversible disturbances of consciousness, attention, cognition, and perception that develop over a short period of time, which may compromise health.

RISK FACTORS

Age ≥60 years; male gender
Alteration in cognitive functioning; dementia
Alteration in sleep-wake cycle; sensory deprivation
Dehydration; malnutrition
History of cerebral vascular accident
History of metabolic functioning (e.g., azotemia, decreased hemoglobin, electrolyte imbalance, increase in blood urea nitrogen/creatinine)
Impaired mobility; inappropriate use of restraints; pain
Pharmaceutical agent
Substance abuse
Infection; urinary retention
Note: A risk diagnosis is not evidenced by signs and symptoms, as the problem has not occurred; rather, nursing interventions are directed at prevention.
Sample Clinical Applications: Brain injury or stroke, respiratory conditions with hypoxia, medication adverse reactions.

DESIRED OUTCOMES/EVALUATION CRITERIA

Sample NOC linkages:
Cognition: Ability to execute complex mental processes
Information Processing: Ability to acquire, organize, and use information
Risk Control: Personal actions to prevent, eliminate, or reduce modifiable health threats

Client/Caregiver Will (Include Specific Time Frame)
- Maintain usual level of consciousness and cognition.
- Verbalize understanding of individual cause and risk factor(s).
- Engage in activities or interventions to prevent or reduce risk of confusion.

ACTIONS/INTERVENTIONS

Sample NIC linkages:
Reality Orientation: Promotions of patient's awareness of personal identity, time, and environment
Teaching: Disease Process: Assisting the patient to understand information related to a specific disease process
Surveillance: Purposeful and ongoing acquisition, interpretation, and synthesis of patient data for clinical decision making

NURSING PRIORITY NO. 1 To assess causative/contributing factors:

- ∞ Identify risk factors present, such as recent trauma or fall; use of large numbers of medications (polypharmacy); intoxication with/withdrawal from a substance (e.g., prescription and over-the-counter [OTC] drugs;

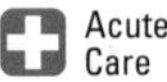

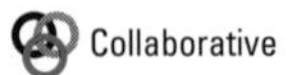

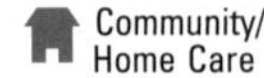

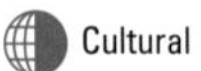

alcohol, illicit drugs); history or current seizures; episodes of fever, pain, or acute infection; exposure to toxic substances; traumatic events in client/significant other (SO) life; person with dementia experiencing sudden change in environment/unfamiliar surroundings or people; and exacerbation of psychiatric conditions (e.g., mood disorder, dissociative disorders). *Individuals are at risk of developing confusion associated with numerous causes (e.g., hypoxia, abnormal metabolic conditions, ingestion of toxins or medications, electrolyte abnormalities, sepsis/systemic infections, nutritional deficiencies, endocrine disorders, central nervous system infections, other neurological pathology, acute psychiatric disorders). Note: Delirium due to physical illness is more frequent among the very young and the elderly. Delirium due to drug and alcohol intoxication or withdrawal is more common in persons aged mid-teens to late 30s.*[2–5]

- Evaluate vital signs for indicators of poor tissue perfusion (i.e., hypotension, tachycardia, tachypnea). *May identify underlying cardiovascular or infectious cause for mental status changes.*
- Assess mental status. *Typical symptoms of delirium include anxiety, disorientation, tremors, hallucinations, delusions, and incoherence. Onset is usually sudden, developing over a few hours or days, and resolving over varying periods of time.*[2,6]
- Determine current medication regimen/drug use—especially anti-anxiety agents, barbiturates, certain antipsychotic agents, methyldopa, disulfiram, cocaine, alcohol, amphetamines, hallucinogens, and opiates, *which are associated with high risk of confusion, disorientation, and delirium;* and OTC medications, such as Benadryl and Tylenol PM, *which can cause an exaggerated response (including "Sundowners syndrome") in elderly individuals.* Note schedule of use (e.g., cimetidine + antacid, digoxin + diuretics). *Combinations can increase risk of adverse reactions/interactions, thus affecting mental status.*[2–5]
- Determine client's mobility and functional level. *Conditions or situations that limit client's mobility and independence potentiate prospect of acute confusional state.*
- Ascertain life events (e.g., death of spouse/other family member, absence of known care provider, move from lifelong home, catastrophic natural disaster) *that can affect client's perceptions, attention, and concentration.*[3]
- Assess diet and nutritional status *to identify possible deficiencies of essential nutrients and vitamins that could affect mental status.*[2,5]
- Evaluate sleep and rest status, noting deprivation or oversleeping. *Discomfort, worry, and lack of sleep and rest can cause or exacerbate confusion.* (Refer to NDs Insomnia, Sleep Deprivation, as appropriate.)
- Monitor laboratory values (e.g., complete blood count, blood cultures; oxygen saturation and, in some cases, arterial blood gases with carbon monoxide; BUN and Cr levels; electrolytes; thyroid function studies; liver function studies, ammonia levels; serum glucose; urinalysis for infection and drug analysis; specific drug toxicologies and drug levels [including peak and trough, as appropriate]) *to identify imbalances that have potential for causing confusion.*[1,2,5]

NURSING PRIORITY NO. 2 To reduce/correct existing risk factors:

- Assist with treatment of underlying problem (e.g., drug intoxication or substance abuse, infectious processes, hypoxemia, biochemical imbalances, nutritional deficits, pain management) *to reduce potential for confusion.*[1,2,5]
- Monitor and adjust medication regimen and note response. *May identify medications that can be changed or eliminated in client prone to adverse or exaggerated responses to medications (including confusion).*[1,2,5]
- Provide normal levels of essential sensory and tactile stimulation—include personal items and pictures, desired music, activities, and contacts. Encourage family/SO(s) to participate in orientation by providing ongoing input (e.g., current news and family happenings).[1,2]
- Maintain calm environment and eliminate extraneous noise and stimuli *to prevent overstimulation.*
- Provide adequate supervision: remove harmful objects from environment, provide siderails and seizure precautions, place call bell and position needed items within reach, clear traffic paths, and ambulate with devices *to meet client's safety needs and reduce risk of falls.*
- Encourage client to use vision or hearing aids and other adaptive equipment when needed *to assist client in interpretation of environment and communication.*

- Avoid or limit use of restraints. *Can cause agitation and increase likelihood of untoward complications.*[4,7]
- Promote early ambulation and recreational activities *to enhance well-being and reduce effects of prolonged bedrest or inactivity.*[1]
- Establish and maintain elimination patterns. *Disruption of elimination may be a cause for confusion or precipitate delerium.*[7]

NURSING PRIORITY NO. 3 To promote wellness (Teaching/Discharge Considerations):

- Assist with treatment of underlying medical conditions and/or management of risk factors *to reduce or limit potential for conditions associated with confusion.*[1,2,5]
- Discuss need for ongoing medical review of client's medications *to limit possibility of misuse or potential for dangerous side effects or interactions.*[1]
- Review ways to maximize sleep (e.g., preferred bedtime rituals; comfortable room temperature, bedding, and pillows; eliminate or reduce extraneous noise or stimuli and interruptions) *to prevent confusional state caused by sleep deprivation.*[1]
- Provide appropriate referrals (e.g., medication monitoring program, nutritionist, substance abuse treatment, support groups, home health and adult day care).[1,2]

DOCUMENTATION FOCUS

Assessment/Reassessment

- Existing conditions and risk factors for individual.
- Current level of function, effect on independence and ability to meet own needs, including food and fluid intake and medication use.

Planning

- Plan of care and who is involved in planning.
- Teaching plan.

Implementation/Evaluation

- Response to interventions and actions performed.
- Attainment or progress toward desired outcomes.
- Modifications to plan of care.

Discharge Planning

- Long-term needs and who is responsible for actions to be taken.
- Available resources and specific referrals.

References

1. Acute confusion. In Doenges, M. E., Moorhouse, M. F., Murr, A. C. (eds). (2010). *Nurse's Pocket Guide: Diagnoses, Prioritized Interventions and Rationales*. 12th ed. Philadelphia: F. A. Davis, 211–215.
2. Alagiakrishnan, K. (2014). Delerium. Retrieved March 2015 from http://emedicine.medscape.com/article/288890-overview.
3. Naylor, M. D., Stephens, C., Bowles, K. H., et al. (2005). Cognitively impaired older adults. *Am J Nurs*, 105(2), 52–61.
4. Jennings-Ingle, S. (2007). The sobering facts about alcohol withdrawal syndrome. *Nursing Made Incredibly Easy!*, 5(1), 50–60.
5. American Medical Directors Association. (2008). Delirium and acute problematic behavior in the long-term-care setting. *Agency for Healthcare Research and Quality Guideline*. Retrieved March 2015 from http://www.guideline.gov/content.aspx?id=12379.
6. Bryson, G. L., Wynand, A. (2006). Evidence-based clinical update: General anesthesia and the risk of delirium and postoperative cognitive dysfunction. *Can J Anaesth*, 53(7), 669–677.
7. Sendelbach, S., Guthrie, P. F. (2009). Acute confusion/delirium. *J Gerontol Nurs*, 35(11), 11–18.

Constipation

Taxonomy II: Elimination and Exchange—Class 2 Gastrointestinal Function (00011) [**Diagnostic Division:** Elimination], Submitted 1975; Revised 1998

DEFINITION: Decrease in normal frequency of defecation accompanied by difficult or incomplete passage of stool and/or passage of excessively hard, dry stool.

Author note: After reviewing current research and all NDs involving constipation it appears that chronic functional Constipation is actually the more commonly occurring form. To this end the assessment and interventions here reflect only what is presented in the Related Factors and Defining Characteristics. More in depth assessment and interventions will be found in chronic functional Constipation.

RELATED FACTORS

Functional
Abdominal muscle weakness
Average daily physical activity is less than recommended for gender and age
Habitually ignores urge to defecate; irregular defecation habits; inadequate toileting habits
Recent environmental change

Mechanical
Electrolyte imbalance
Hemorrhoids; pregnancy; obesity
Neurological impairment (e.g., positive EEG, head trauma, seizure disorders); Hirschsprung's disease; tumor
Prostate enlargement; postsurgical bowel obstruction; [colostomy]
Rectal abscess, ulcer; rectal prolapse; rectal anal fissure or stricture; rectocele

Pharmacological
Pharmaceutical agent; laxative abuse

Physiological
Eating habit change (e.g., foods, eating times); insufficient dietary habits; insufficient fiber or fluid intake; dehydration
Inadequate dentition or oral hygiene
Decrease in gastrointestinal motility

Psychological
Emotional disturbance; depression; confusion

DEFINING CHARACTERISTICS

Subjective
Abdominal pain; pain with defecation
Change in bowel pattern; decrease in frequency or volume of stool; hard, formed stool; inability to defecate
Increase in abdominal pressure; feeling of rectal fullness or pressure; straining with defecation
Indigestion; vomiting; headache; fatigue

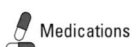

Objective
Hard, formed stool
Straining with defecation

(continues on page 186)

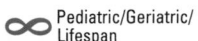

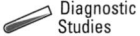

Constipation (continued)
Hypoactive or hyperactive bowel sounds; borborygmi
Distended abdomen; abdominal tenderness with/without palpable muscle resistance; palpable abdominal or rectal mass
Percussed abdominal dullness
Presence of soft pastelike stool in rectum; liquid stool; bright red blood with stool
Severe flatus; anorexia
Atypical presentations in older adults (e.g., changes in mental status, urinary incontinence, unexplained falls, elevated body temperature)
Sample Clinical Applications: Abdominal or pelvic surgeries; hemorrhoids, anal lesions, irritable bowel syndrome, diverticulitis, spinal cord injury (SCI), multiple sclerosis (MS), and other neurological conditions; hypothyroidism, iron deficiency anemia; uremia, kidney dialysis; Alzheimer's disease/other dementias or psychiatric conditions

DESIRED OUTCOMES/EVALUATION CRITERIA

Sample NOC linkages:
Bowel Elimination: Formation and evacuation of stool
Nutritional Status: Nutrient Intake: Nutrient intake to meet metabolic needs
Self-Care: Non-Parenteral Medications: Ability to administer oral and topical medications to meet therapeutic goals independently with or without assistive device

Client Will (Include Specific Time Frame)
- Establish or regain normal pattern of bowel functioning.
- Verbalize understanding of etiology and appropriate interventions or solutions for individual situation.
- Demonstrate behaviors or lifestyle changes to prevent recurrence of problem.
- Participate in bowel program, as indicated.

ACTIONS/INTERVENTIONS

Sample NIC linkages:
Constipation/Impaction Management: Prevention and alleviation of constipation/impaction
Bowel Management: Establishment and maintenance of a regular pattern of bowel elimination
Ostomy Care: Maintenance of elimination through a stoma and care of surrounding tissue

NURSING PRIORITY NO. 1 To identify causative/contributing factors:

- Review medical/surgical history as indicated in Related Factors above *to identify conditions commonly associated with constipation.* (Refer to ND chronic functional Constipation).
- ∞ Note client's age. *Constipation is more likely to occur in individuals older than 65 years of age, but can occur in any age from infant to elderly. A bottle-fed infant is more prone to constipation than a breastfed infant, especially when formula contains iron. Toddlers are at risk because of developmental factors (e.g., too young, too interested in other things, rigid schedule during potty training), and children and adolescents are at risk because of unwillingness to take breaks from play, poor eating and fluid intake habits, and withholding because of perceived lack of privacy. Many older adults experience constipation as a result of duller nerve sensations, immobility, dehydration, and electrolyte imbalances; incomplete emptying of the bowel; or failing to attend to signals to defecate.*[1–4,7]
- Review daily dietary regimen, noting if diet is deficient in fiber. *Imbalanced nutrition influences the amount and consistency of feces.*

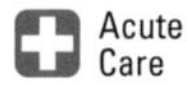
Acute Care
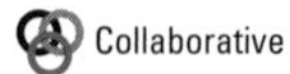
Collaborative
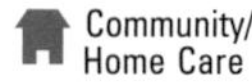
Community/ Home Care
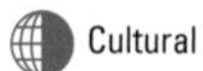
Cultural

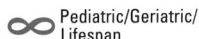

- Assess general oral and dental health. *Dental problems can impact dietary intake (e.g., loss of teeth or other oral conditions can force individuals to eat soft foods or liquids mostly lacking in fiber).*[3]
- Determine fluid intake *to note deficits.*
- Evaluate medication or drug usage *for agents that could slow passage of stool and cause or exacerbate constipation.*
- Note energy and activity level and exercise pattern. *Lack of physical activity or regular exercise is often a factor in constipation.*
- Identify areas of life changes or stressors. *Factors such as pregnancy, travel, traumas, changes in personal relationships, occupational factors, or financial concerns can cause or exacerbate constipation.*[5]
- Determine access to bathroom, privacy, and ability to perform self-care activities.
- Investigate reports of pain with defecation. *Hemorrhoids, rectal fissures or prolapse, skin breakdown, or other abnormal findings may be hindering passage of stool or causing client to hold stool.*[1,4–6]
- Discuss laxative and enema use. Note signs or reports of laxative abuse or overuse of stimulant laxatives. *This is most common among older adults preoccupied with having daily bowel movement.*[4,5,7]
- Auscultate abdomen for presence, location, and characteristics of bowel sounds *reflecting bowel activity.*
- Palpate abdomen for hardness, distension, and masses *indicating possible obstruction or retention of stool.*
- Perform digital rectal examination, as indicated, *to evaluate rectal tone and detect tenderness, blood, or detect fecal impaction.*
- Assist with medical work-up (e.g., x-rays, abdominal imaging, colonoscopy, proctosigmoidoscopy, anorectal function tests; colonic transit studies, stool sample tests) *for identification of possible causative factors.* Refer to ND: chronic functional Constipation for further assessments and interventions regarding dietary issues in constipation.

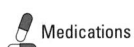

NURSING PRIORITY NO. 2 To determine usual pattern of elimination:

- Discuss customary elimination habits (e.g., normal urge time [client unable to eliminate unless in own home, passing hard stool after prolonged effort, anal pain or bleeding]). Determine what feature the client finds most distressing. *Helps to identify and clarify client's perception of problem. For example, constipation has been defined as not only infrequent stools, but also straining with bowel movements, hard stools, unproductive urges, and feeling of incomplete evacuation.*[6]
- Note factors that usually stimulate bowel activity and any interferences present. *Client may describe having to sit in a particular position or needing to apply perineal pressure or digital stimulation to start stool. Interferences can include not wanting to use a particular facility or not wanting to interrupt play or an activity.*[6]

NURSING PRIORITY NO. 3 To assess current pattern of elimination:

- Note color, odor, consistency, amount, and frequency of stool following each bowel movement during assessment phase. *Provides a baseline for comparison, promoting recognition of changes. If usual number of weekly bowel movements is decreased to three or less, stool is hard and formed, or client is straining, constipation is likely present.*[2]
- Ascertain duration of current problem and client's degree of concern. *Long-standing condition that client has "lived with" may not cause undue concern, while acute postsurgical constipation can cause great distress. Client's response may/may not be congruent with the severity of condition.*
- Note pharmacological agents client has used (e.g., fiber pills, laxatives, suppositories, enemas) *to determine effectiveness of current regimen and whether laxative use is appropriate and helpful.*

NURSING PRIORITY NO. 4 To facilitate return to usual/acceptable pattern of elimination:

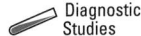

- Promote lifestyle changes.[1–8]

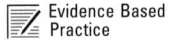

Limit foods with little or no fiber or diet high in fats (e.g., ice cream, cheese, meats, fast foods, processed foods). Note: Clients with descending or sigmoid colostomy must avoid constipation. Some may find it helpful to create their own dietary bulk laxative by combining unprocessed millers bran, applesauce, and prune juice.

Promote adequate fluid intake, including water, high-fiber fruit and vegetable juices, fruit/vegetable smoothies, and popsicles. Suggest drinking warm, stimulating fluids (e.g., decaffeinated coffee, hot water, tea) *to avoid dehydration; promote moist, soft feces; and facilitate passage of stool.*

Encourage daily activity and exercise within limits of individual ability *to stimulate contractions of the intestines.*

Encourage client to not ignore urge. Provide privacy and routinely scheduled time for defecation (bathroom or commode preferable to bedpan) *to promote psychological readiness and comfort.*

- Provide sitz bath before stools *to relax sphincter* and after stools *for cleansing and soothing effect to rectal area.*[4]
- Review client's current medication regime with physician *to determine if drugs contributing to constipation can be discontinued or changed.*
- Administer stool softeners *(to provide moisture to stool),* mild stimulants *(to cause rhythmic contractions of the bowel),* lubricants *(to enable stool to more easily pass),* saline or hyperosmolar laxatives, or bulk-forming agents *(to draw water into colon)* as ordered or routinely, when appropriate (e.g., for client receiving opiates, decreased level of activity/immobility).[1–3,5–8]
- Apply lubricant/anesthetic ointment to anus, if needed.
- Establish bowel program to include predictable interval timing for colostomy irrigation or toileting, use of particular position for defecation, abdominal massage, colostomy irrigation, biofeedback for pelvic floor dysfunction, and medications as indicated *to provide predictable and effective elimination and reduce evacuation problems when long-term or permanent bowel dysfunction is present.*

NURSING PRIORITY NO. 5 To promote wellness (Teaching/Discharge Considerations):[1,6]

- Discuss client's particular anatomy and physiology of bowel and acceptable variations in elimination.
- Provide information and resources to client/significant other about relationship of diet, fluid, exercise, and healthy elimination.
- Provide social and emotional support *to help client manage actual or potential disabilities associated with long-term bowel management.* Discuss rationale for and encourage continuation of successful interventions.
- Encourage client to maintain elimination diary, if appropriate, *to facilitate monitoring of long-term problem and choice of interventions.*
- Work to implement bowel management program that is easily replicated in home and community settings.
- Identify specific actions to be taken if problem does not resolve *to promote timely intervention, thereby enhancing client's independence.*

DOCUMENTATION FOCUS

Assessment/Reassessment

- Usual and current bowel pattern, duration of the problem, and interventions used.
- Characteristics of stool.
- Individual contributing factors.

Planning

- Plan of care, specific interventions or changes in lifestyle necessary to correct individual situation, and who is involved in planning.
- Teaching plan.

Implementation/Evaluation

- Responses to interventions, teaching, and actions performed.
- Change in bowel pattern, character of stool.
- Attainment or progress toward desired outcomes.
- Modifications to plan of care.

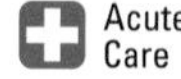

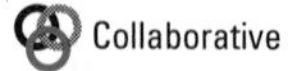

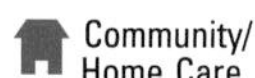

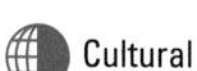

Discharge Planning

- Individual long-term needs, noting who is responsible for actions to be taken.
- Recommendations for follow-up care.
- Specific referrals made.

References

1. McKay, S. L., Fravel, M., Scanlon, C. (2012). Evidence-based practice: Management of constipation. *J Gerontol Nurs*, 38(7), 9–15.
2. Ferry, R. J. (Updated 2014). Constipation in children. Retrieved August 2014 from http://www.emedicinehealth.com/constipation_in_children/page3_em.htm.
3. Stanley, M. (1999). The aging gastrointestinal system, with nutritional considerations. In Stanley, M., Beare, P. G. (eds). *Gerontological Nursing: A Health Promotion/Protection Approach.* 7th ed. Philadelphia: F. A. Davis, 180–181.
4. Watson, L. (2010). Childhood constipation. *Community Pract*, 83(7), 40–42.
5. National Digestive Diseases Information Clearinghouse. (Updated 2014). Constipation. Retrieved July 2014 from http://digestive.hiddk.hih.gove/ddiseases/pubs/constipation/.
6. Locke, G. R., Pemberton, J. H., Phillips, S. F. (2000). American Gastroenterological Association: Medical position statement: Guidelines on constipation. *Gastroenterology*, 119(6), 1761–1778.
7. Basson, M. D. (Updated 2014). Constipation in adults. Retrieved July 2014 from http://emedicine.medscape.com/article/184704-overview.
8. CancerConnect.com staff. (2015). Living with a colostomy. Retrieved March 2015 from http://news.cancerconnect.com/colon-cancertipsliving-with-a-colostomy/.

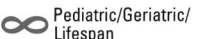

chronic functional Constipation

Taxonomy II: Elimination and Exchange—Class 2 Gastrointestinal Function (00235) [**Diagnostic Division:** Elimination], Submitted 2013

DEFINITION: Infrequent or difficult evacuation of feces, which has been present for at least 3 of the prior 12 months.

RELATED FACTORS

Anal fissure/stricture; hemorrhoids; proctitis
Insufficient dietary/fluid intake; dehydration; low fiber diet; low calorie intake; diet disproportionately high in protein and fat; failure to thrive
Inflammatory bowel disease; chronic intestinal pseudo-obstruction; ischemic stenosis; postinflammatory stenosis; surgical stenosis; colorectal cancer; extra intestinal mass; Hirschprung's disease
Sedentary lifestyle; impaired mobility; Parkinson's disease; slow colon transit time
Spinal cord injury; paraplegia; multiple sclerosis; autonomic neuropathy; myotonic dystrophy; cerebral vascular accident
Pharmaceutical agent; polypharmacy
Pregnancy; perineal damage; pelvic floor dysfunction
Hypercalcemia; hypothyroidism; panhypopituitarism
Diabetes mellitus; chronic renal insufficiency; scleroderma; dermatomyositis
Depression; dementia; habitually ignores urge to defecate

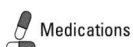

(continues on page 190)

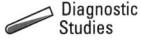

chronic functional Constipation (continued)

DEFINING CHARACTERISTICS

Subjective

Pain with defecation
Prolonged straining
[Feeling as though stool is still in rectum after bowel movement]
[Feeling as though something is blocking stool from passing]
[Using fingers to help with stool passage]

Objective

ADULT: Presence of 2 of the following symptoms on Rome III classification system:
Lumpy or hard stools; or straining; or sensation of incomplete evacuation; or sensation of anorectal obstructions; or manual maneuvers to facilitate defecations (digital manipulation, pelvic floor support) in 25% of defecations; 3 evacuations per week
CHILD 4 years: Presence of 2 criteria on Roman III Pediatric classification system for 1 month:
2 defecations per week; 1 episode of fecal incontinence per week; stool retentive posturing; painful or hard bowel movements; presence of large fecal mass in the rectum; large diameter stools that may obstruct the toilet
CHILD 4 years: Presence of 2 criteria on roman III Pediatric classification system for 2 months:
2 defecations per week; 1 episode of fecal incontinence per week; stool retentive posturing; painful or hard bowel movements; presence of large fecal mass in the rectum; large diameter stools that may obstruct the toilet
Abdominal distention
Palpable abdominal mass
Type 1 or 2 Bristol Stool Chart
Fecal impaction
Fecal incontinence (in children)
Leakage of stool with digital stimulation
Positive fecal occult blood
Prolonged straining Type 1 or 2 Bristol Stool Chart
Type 1 or 2 Bristol Stool Chart: after "Prolonged straining"
Sample Clinical Applications: Abdominal surgeries, hemorrhoids, anal lesions, irritable bowel syndrome, diverticulitis, spinal cord injury (SCI), multiple sclerosis (MS), hypothyroidism, iron deficiency, scleroderma, Alzheimer's disease/dementia

DESIRED OUTCOMES/EVALUATION CRITERIA

Sample NOC linkages:

Bowel Elimination: Formation and evacuation of stool
Gastrointestinal Function: Ability of the gastrointestinal tract to ingest and digest food products, absorb nutrients, and eliminate waste

Client Will (Include Specific Time Frame)

- Establish or regain normal pattern of bowel functioning.
- Document that bowel function has improved, noting an increase in frequency of stools and/or decrease in straining at stool.
- Verbalize understanding of etiology and appropriate interventions or solutions for individual situation.

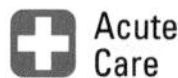

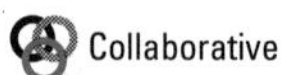

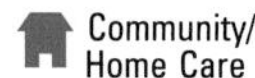

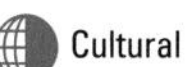

ACTIONS/INTERVENTIONS

Sample NIC linkages:
Constipation/Impaction Management: Prevention and alleviation of constipation/impaction
Bowel Management: Establishment and maintenance of a regular pattern of bowel elimination
Medication Management: Facilitation of safe and effective use of prescription and over-the-counter drugs

NURSING PRIORITY NO. 1 To identify causative/contributing factors:

- Review medical/surgical history *to identify conditions commonly associated with functional constipation. Causes may be classified as primary and secondary. Primary causes are related to problems inherent to the intestine; subdivided into normal-transit constipation, slow-transit constipation, and anorectal dysfunction. Secondary causes include gastrointestinal disorders (e.g., intestinal tumors, stenosis; idiopathic megacolon; rectocele, rectal prolapse, anal fissure; irritable bowel syndrome), metabolic and endocrine disorders (e.g., hyper/hypocalcemia, diabetes, hyperparathyroidism, chronic renal insufficiency), neurological conditions (e.g., Parkinson's disease, stroke, dementia syndromes, multiple sclerosis, spinal cord injuries), psychogenic disorders (e.g., anxiety, depression), dehydration, and the use of a variety of medications (e.g., opioids, anti-inflammatories, calcium channel blockers, calcium and iron supplements, anticholinergics, antipsychotics, antihistamines).*[1,2,14] *Note: Functional constipation can also be associated with symptoms arising in the mid or lower gastrointestinal tract that are not otherwise attributable to anatomic or biochemical defects. There is increasing evidence that a considerable number of individuals with constipation also have a disorder of the process of rectal evacuation.*[4,11,14]
- Note client's age, gender, and general health status. *Constipation is more likely to occur in individuals older than 65 years of age, but it may occur in client of any age with chronic or debilitating conditions. Approximately 95% of childhood constipation is functional in nature without any obvious cause. Children with anorectal malformations and Hirschsprung's disease have abnormal peristaltic waves in the colon, which result either in stagnant stool or an overactive colon.*[2,6–8,10] *Note: Prevalence estimates by gender support a female-to-male ratio of 2.2:1.*[14]
- Evaluate current medications or drug usage *for agents that could slow passage of stool and cause or exacerbate constipation (e.g., opioids, anti-inflammatories, calcium channel blockers, calcium and iron supplements, anticholinergics, antidepressants, antipsychotics, antihistamines, anticonvulsants, diuretics, chemotherapy, contrast media, steroids).*[1–3]
- Note interventions client has tried *to relieve current situation (e.g., fiber pills, laxatives, suppositories, enemas)* and document success or lack of effectiveness.
- Assist with medical work-up (e.g., lower GI series x-rays, abdominal imaging [e.g., defecography], colonoscopy, sigmoidoscopy; anorectal function tests [e.g., anal manometry, blood expulsion tests]; colonic transit studies) *for identification of possible causative factors and to show how well food moves through the colon.*[8,9,12]

NURSING PRIORITY NO. 2 To assess current pattern of elimination:[10–12]

- Note color, odor, consistency, amount, and frequency of stool following each bowel movement during assessment phase utilizing elimination diary or calendar. *Provides a baseline for comparison, promoting recognition of changes.*
- Auscultate abdomen for presence, location, and characteristics of bowel sounds *reflecting bowel activity.*
- Palpate abdomen for hardness, distention, and masses, *indicating possible obstruction or retention of stool.*
- Perform digital rectal examination, as indicated, *to evaluate rectal tone and detect tenderness, blood, or fecal impaction.*

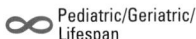

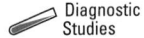

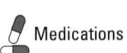

NURSING PRIORITY NO. 3 To reduce unacceptable pattern of elimination:

- Collaborate in treatment of underlying medical cause where appropriate (e.g., surgery to repair rectal prolapse, biofeedback to retrain anorectal or pelvic floor dysfunction, medications, and combinations of therapies as indicated) *to improve body and bowel function. Note: Treatment is highly individual. For example, clients with slow-transit constipation tend to benefit from fiber, osmotic laxatives, and stimulant laxatives (e.g., bisacodyl), whereas those with evacuation disorders usually do not need medication other than fiber supplementation following pelvic floor retraining.*[11,13]
- Review client's current medication regime with physician *to determine if drugs contributing to constipation can be discontinued or changed.*
- Administer medications, as indicated, such as stool softeners (e.g., docusate sodium [Colase, Surfak]) *to provide moisture to stool,* mild stimulants (e.g., bisacodyl [Dulcolax, Bisco-Lax]) *to cause rhythmic muscle contractions and improve transit time,* osmotic agents (e.g., polyethylene glycol [PEG, Miralax]) *to absorb water in intestine,* and opoid antagonist (e.g., methylanaltrexone [Relistor]) *to treat constipation in client with advanced/terminal illness necessitating long-term opioid analgesia and/or client who is unresponsive to laxatives.*
- Remove impacted stool digitally, when necessary, after applying lubricant and anesthetic ointment to anus *to soften impaction and decrease rectal pain.*
- Administer enemas (e.g., hyperosmolar agents [e.g., Fleet enema] *to draw water into colon*) or suppositories, as indicated.[4,6]
- Promote lifestyle changes:[1–12]
  - Instruct in and encourage a personalized dietary program that involves adjustment of dietary fiber and bulk in diet (e.g., fruits, vegetables, whole grains) and fiber supplements (e.g., wheat bran, psyllium) *to improve consistency of stool and increase transit time through colon if slow transit through colon is causing symptoms.*
  - Promote adequate fluid intake, including water, high-fiber fruit and vegetable juices, fruit/vegetable smoothies, and popsicles. Suggest drinking warm, stimulating fluids (e.g., decaffeinated coffee, hot water, tea) *to avoid dehydration; promote moist, soft feces; and facilitate passage of stool.*
- Instruct in/assist with other means of triggering defecation (e.g., abdominal massage, digital stimulation, placement of rectal stimulant suppositories) *to provide predictable and effective elimination and reduce evacuation problems when long-term or permanent bowel dysfunction is present.*
- Refer for physical therapy or other medical/surgical practitioners for additional interventions as indicated. *Physical therapy may be useful in improving mobility, pelvic floor retraining, and activity levels. Biofeedback treatment with muscle relaxation of anal sphincters and the puborectalis can result in a cure for constipation associated with certain evacuation disorders. Surgical interventions may be used in some instances (e.g., Malone antegrade continence enema procedure, sacral anterior root stimulation) to treat long-term, intractable constipation due to neurogenic bowel.*[5,13]

NURSING PRIORITY NO. 4 To promote wellness (Teaching/Discharge Considerations):[1–12]

- Discuss client's particular anatomy and physiology of bowel and acceptable variations in elimination.
- Provide information and resources to client/significant other about relationship of diet, exercise, fluid, and appropriate use of laxatives, as indicated,
- Provide social and emotional support *to help client manage actual or potential disabilities associated with long-term bowel management.* Discuss rationale for and encourage continuation of successful interventions.
- Encourage client to maintain elimination diary, if appropriate, *to facilitate monitoring of long-term condition and reveal most helpful interventions.*
- Collaborate with medical providers and client/caregiver in designing bowel management program to be easily replicated in home and community settings.
- Identify specific actions to be taken if problem does not resolve (e.g., return to physician for additional testing and interventions) *to promote timely intervention, thereby enhancing client's independence.*

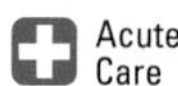

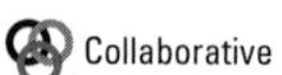

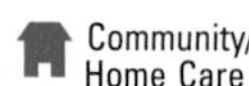

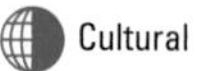

DOCUMENTATION FOCUS

Assessment/Reassessment

- Usual and current bowel pattern, duration of the problem, and interventions used.
- Characteristics of stool.
- Individual contributing factors.

Planning

- Plan of care, specific interventions or changes in lifestyle necessary to correct individual situation, and who is involved in planning.
- Teaching plan.

Implementation/Evaluation

- Responses to interventions, teaching, and actions performed.
- Change in bowel pattern, character of stool.
- Attainment or progress toward desired outcomes.
- Modifications to plan of care.

Discharge Planning

- Individual long-term needs, noting who is responsible for actions to be taken.
- Recommendations for follow-up care.
- Specific referrals made.

References

1. Longstreth, G. F., Thompson, W. G., Chey, W. D., et al. (2006). Functional bowel disorders. *Gastroenterology*, 130, 1480–1491.
2. Schmidt, F. M., Santos, V. L. (2014). Prevalence of constipation in the general adult population: An integrative review. *J Wound Ostomy Continence Nurs*, 41(1), 70–76.
3. McKay, S. L., Fravel, M., Scanlon, C. (2012). Evidence-based practice: Management of constipation. *J Gerontol Nurs*, 38(7), 9–15.
4. Camilleri, M. (1999). Functional gastrointestinal disorders: Novel insights and treatments. Retrieved August 2014 from http://www.medscape.com/viewarticle/717346_1.
5. Surrenti, E., Rath, D. M., Permberton, J. H., et al. (1995). Audit of constipation in a tertiary referral gastroenterology practice. *Am J Gastroenterol*, 90, 1471–1475.
6. Poggio, J. L., Grossman, J. G. (Updated 2014). Neurogenic bowel dysfunction. Retrieved August 2014 from http://emedicine.medscape.com/article/321172-overview.
7. Pashankar, D. S. (2005). Management of severe pediatric constipation. *Clin Colon Rectal Surg*, 18(2), 120–127.
8. Levitt, M. A., Pena, A. National Digestive Diseases Information Clearinghouse (2013). Management of severe pediatric constipation. Retrieved August 2014 from http://emedicine.medscape.com/article/937030-overview#aw2aab6b3.
9. Basson, M. D. (Updated 2014). Constipation in adults. Retrieved July 2014 from http://emedicine.medscape.com/article/184704-overview.
10. Ferry, R. J. (2013). Constipation in children. Retrieved August 2014 from http://www.emedicinehealth.com/constipation_in_children/page3_em.htm.
11. Mayo Clinic and Mayo Foundation. (1999). Functional gastrointestinal disorders: Novel insights and treatments: Functional constipation pathogenesis and management. Retrieved August 2014 from http://www.medscape.com/viewarticle/717346_5.
12. Locke, G. R., Pemberton, J. H., Phillips, S. F. (2000). American Gastroenterological Association: Medical position statement: Guidelines on constipation. *Gastroenterology*, 119(6), 1761–1778.
13. Enck, P. (1993). Biofeedback training in disordered defecation. A critical review. *Dig Dis Sci*, 38(11), 1953–1960.
14. Higgins, P. D., Johanson, J. F. (2004). Epidemiology of constipation in North America: A systematic review. *Am J Gastroenterol*, 99(4), 750–759.

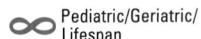

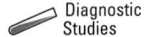

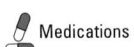

risk for chronic functional Constipation

Taxonomy II: Elimination and Exchange—Class 2 Gastrointestinal Function (000236) [**Diagnostic Division:** Elimination], Date Submitted 2013.

DEFINITION: Vulnerable to infrequent or difficult evacuation of feces, which has been present nearly 3 of the prior 12 months, which may compromise health.

RISK FACTORS

Aluminum-containing antacids; anti-epileptic drugs; antihypertensive agents; anti-Parkinsonian agents (anticholinergic or dopaminergic); calcium-channel antagonists; diuretics; iron preparations; non-steroidal anti-inflammatories (NSAIDs); opioids; tricyclic antidepressants; polypharmacy
Chronic intestinal pseudo-obstruction; slow colon transit time
Decreased food intake; diet proportionally high in protein and fat; low fiber diet, low caloric intake
Dehydration; insufficient fluid take
Impaired mobility; inactive lifestyle
Failure to thrive
Habitual ignoring of urge to defecate

PSYCHOLOGICAL

Depression
Note: A risk diagnosis is not evidenced by signs and symptoms, as the problem has not occurred; rather, nursing interventions are directed at prevention.

DESIRED OUTCOMES/EVALUATION CRITERIA

Sample NOC linkages:
Bowel Elimination: Formation and evacuation of stool
Risk Control: Personal actions to prevent, eliminate, or reduce modifiable health threats
Knowledge: Medication: Extent of understanding conveyed about the safe use of medication

Client Will (Include Specific Time Frame)

- Establish or maintain normal pattern of bowel functioning.
- Verbalize understanding of etiology and appropriate interventions or solutions for individual situation.
- Engage in behaviors or lifestyle changes to prevent constipation.

ACTIONS/INTERVENTIONS

Sample NIC linkages:
Constipation/Impaction Management: Prevention and alleviation of constipation/impaction
Bowel Management: Establishment and maintenance of a regular pattern of bowel elimination
Medication Management: Facilitation of safe and effective use of prescription and over-the-counter drugs

NURSING PRIORITY NO. 1 To identify individual risk factors:

- Review medical/surgical history *to identify conditions commonly associated with functional constipation. Note: Causes may be classified as primary and secondary. Primary causes are related to problems inherent to the intestine and are subdivided into normal-transit constipation, slow-transit constipation, and anorectal dysfunction. Secondary causes include gastrointestinal disorders, metabolic and endocrine disorders, neurologi-*

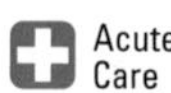
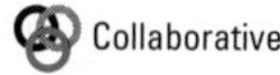
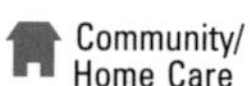
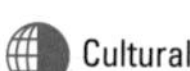

cal conditions, congestive cardiac insufficiency, psychogenic disorders, dehydration, and the use of a variety of medications.[1,2,5] *Note: Functional constipation can also be associated with symptoms arising in the mid or lower gastrointestinal tract that are not otherwise attributable to anatomic or biochemical defects. There is increasing evidence that a considerable number of individuals with constipation also have a disorder of the process of rectal evacuation.*[3,5,11]

- Note client's age, gender, and general health status. *Constipation is more likely to occur in individuals older than 65 years of age, but it may occur in client of any age with chronic or debilitating conditions. Prevalence estimates by gender support a female-to-male ratio of 2.2:1. Approximately 95% of childhood constipation is functional in nature without any obvious cause.*[3–5]
- Evaluate current medication *for agents that could slow passage of stool and cause or exacerbate constipation (e.g., opioids, anti-inflammatories, calcium channel blockers, calcium and iron supplements, anticholinergics, antidepressants, antipsychotics, antihistamines, anticonvulsants, diuretics, chemotherapy, contrast media, steroids).*[2,6]
- Review daily dietary regimen. *Imbalanced nutrition influences the amount and consistency of feces. Inadequate dietary fiber (vegetable, fruits, whole grains) and highly processed foods (e.g., fast foods, junk foods, packaged snack, or microwavable quick meals) contribute to poor intestinal function.*[1,7–9]
- Determine fluid intake *to note deficits. Most individuals do not drink enough fluids, even when healthy, reducing the speed at which stool moves through the colon. Active fluid loss through sweating, vomiting, diarrhea, or bleeding can greatly increase chances for constipation.*[2,7,9]
- Note energy and activity level and exercise pattern. *Lack of physical activity or regular exercise is often a factor in constipation.*[2,10]

NURSING PRIORITY NO. 2 To assess current pattern of elimination:

- Discuss usual elimination pattern and use of laxatives *to establish baseline and identify possible areas for intervention or instruction.*
- Note color, odor, consistency, amount, and frequency of stool following each bowel movement during assessment phase. *Provides a baseline for comparison, promoting recognition of changes.*
- Auscultate abdomen for presence, location, and characteristics of bowel sounds *reflecting bowel activity.*
- Palpate abdomen for hardness, distention, and masses, *indicating possible obstruction or retention of stool.*

NURSING PRIORITY NO. 3 To facilitate normal bowel function:

- Promote healthy lifestyle for elimination:[1–10]
  - Encourage balanced fiber and bulk (e.g., fruits, vegetables, whole grains) in diet and fiber supplements (e.g., wheat bran, psyllium) *to promote soft consistency of stool and facilitate passage through colon.*
  - Promote adequate fluid intake, including water, high-fiber fruit and vegetable juices, fruit/vegetable smoothies, and popsicles. Suggest drinking warm, stimulating fluids (e.g., decaffeinated coffee, hot water, tea) *to avoid dehydration; promote moist, soft feces; and facilitate passage of stool.*
  - Encourage daily activity and exercise within limits of individual ability to stimulate contractions of the intestines.
  - Encourage client to not ignore urge. Provide privacy and routinely scheduled time for defecation (bathroom or commode preferable to bedpan) *to promote psychological readiness and comfort.*

NURSING PRIORITY NO. 4 Promote wellness (Teaching/Discharge Considerations):[2,8,11]

- Discuss physiology and acceptable variations in elimination. *May help reduce concerns and anxiety about situation.*
- Review individual risk factors or potential problems and specific interventions for prevention of constipation.
- Promote treatment of underlying medical causes where appropriate *to improve organ function, including the bowel.*

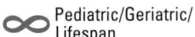

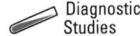

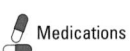

- Educate client/significant other about safe and risky practices for managing constipation. *Information can assist client to make beneficial choices when need arises.*
- Refer to NDs functional Constipation; Constipation; risk for perceived Constipation for additional interventions as appropriate.

DOCUMENTATION FOCUS

Assessment/Reassessment
- Current bowel pattern, characteristics of stool, medications.
- Individual risk factors.

Planning
- Plan of care and who is involved in planning.
- Teaching plan.

Implementation/Evaluation
- Responses to interventions, teaching, and actions performed.
- Attainment or progress toward desired outcomes.
- Modifications to plan of care.

Discharge Planning
- Individual long-term needs, noting who is responsible for actions to be taken.
- Specific referrals made.

References

1. Longstreth, G. F., Thompson, W. G., Chey, W. D., et al. (2006). Functional bowel disorders. *Gastroenterology*, 130, 1480–1491.
2. McKay, S. L., Fravel, M., Scanlon, C. (2012). Evidence-based practice: Management of constipation. *J Gerontol Nurs*, 38(7), 9–15.
3. Poggio, J. L., Grossman, J. G. (Updated 2014). Neurogenic bowel dysfunction. Retrieved August 2014 from http://emedicine.medscape.com/article/321172-overview.
4. Pashankar, D. S. (2005). Management of severe pediatric constipation. *Clin Colon Rectal Surg*, 18(2), 120–127.
5. Higgins, P. D., Johanson, J. F. (2004). Epidemiology of constipation in North America: A systematic review. *Am J Gastroenterol*, 99(4), 750–759.
6. Camilleri, M. (1999). Functional gastrointestinal disorders: Novel insights and treatments. Retrieved July 2014 from http://www.medscape.com/viewarticle/717346_1.
7. Ferry, R. J. (2013). Constipation in children. Retrieved August 2014 from http://www.emedicinehealth.com/constipation_in_children/page3_em.htm.
8. Locke, G. R., Pemberton, J. H., Phillips, S. F. (2000). American Gastroenterological Association: Medical position statement: Guidelines on constipation. *Gastroenterology*, 119(6), 1761–1778.
9. Watson, L. (2010). Childhood constipation. *Community Pract*, 83(7), 40–42.
10. Marks, J. W. (Updated 2014). Constipation. Retrieved August from http://www.medicinenet.com/constipation/article.htm.
11. Basson, M. D. (Updated 2014). Constipation in adults. Retrieved July 2014 from http://emedicine.medscape.com/article/184704-overview.

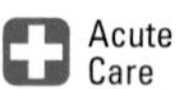

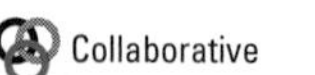

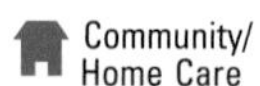

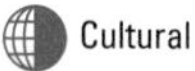

perceived Constipation

Taxonomy II: Elimination and Exchange—Class 2 Gastrointestinal Function (00012) [**Diagnostic Division:** Elimination], Submitted 1988

DEFINITION: Self-diagnosis of constipation combined with abuse of laxatives, enemas, and/or suppositories to ensure a daily bowel movement.

RELATED FACTORS

Cultural or family health beliefs
Impaired thought process

DEFINING CHARACTERISTICS

Subjective

Expects daily bowel movement
Expects daily bowel movement at same time every day
Laxative, enema, or suppository abuse

Sample Clinical Applications: Irritable bowel, confused states/dementia, hypochondriasis

DESIRED OUTCOMES/EVALUATION CRITERIA

Sample NOC linkages:

Health Beliefs: Personal convictions that influence health behaviors
Bowel Elimination: Formation and evacuation of stool
Knowledge: Health Behavior: Extent of understanding conveyed about the promotion and protection of health

Client Will (Include Specific Time Frame)

- Verbalize understanding of physiology of bowel function.
- Identify acceptable interventions to promote adequate bowel function.
- Decrease reliance on laxatives and/or enemas.
- Establish individually appropriate pattern of elimination.

ACTIONS/INTERVENTIONS

Sample NIC linkages:

Bowel Management: Establishment and maintenance of a regular pattern of bowel elimination
Counseling: Use of an interactive helping process focusing on the needs, problems, or feelings of the patient and SOs to enhance or support coping, problem solving, and interpersonal relationships
Medication Management: Facilitation of safe and effective use of prescription and over-the-counter drugs

NURSING PRIORITY NO. 1 To identify factors affecting individual beliefs:

- Determine client's understanding of a "normal" bowel pattern. Compare with client's current bowel functioning. *Helps to identify areas for discussion or intervention. For example, what is considered "normal" varies with the individual, cultural, and familial factors with differences in expectations and dietary habits.*[1] *In addition, individuals can think they are constipated when, in fact, their bowel movements are regular and soft, possibly revealing a problem with thought processes or perception. Some people believe they are constipated, or irregular, if they do not have a bowel movement every day because of ideas instilled from childhood.*[2] *The elderly client may believe that laxatives or purgatives are necessary for elimination, when in fact the problem may be long-standing habits (e.g., insufficient fluids, lack of exercise and/or fiber in the diet).*[3]

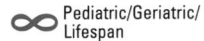

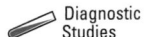

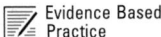

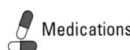

- Discuss client's use of laxatives. *Perceived constipation typically results in self-medicating with various laxatives. Although laxatives may correct the acute problem, chronic use leads to habituation, requiring ever-increasing doses that result in drug dependency and, ultimately, a hypotonic laxative colon.*[5]
- Identify interventions used by client to correct perceived problem *to establish needed changes or interventions or points for discussion and teaching.*

NURSING PRIORITY NO. 2 To promote wellness (Teaching/Discharge Considerations):

- Discuss the following with client/SO/caregiver *to clarify issues regarding actual and perceived bowel functioning and to provide support during behavior modification/bowel retraining:*[3,4]

  Review anatomy and physiology of bowel function and acceptable variations in elimination.

  Identify detrimental effects of habitual laxative or enema use and discuss alternatives.

  Provide information about relationship of diet, hydration, and exercise to improved elimination.

  Encourage client to maintain elimination calendar or diary, if appropriate.

  Provide support by active-listening and discussing client's concerns or fears.

  Provide social and emotional support *to help client manage actual or potential disabilities associated with long-term bowel management.*

  Encourage use of stress-reduction activities and refocusing of attention while client works to establish individually appropriate pattern.
- Offer educational materials and resources for client/SO to peruse at home *to assist him or her in making informed decisions regarding constipation and management options.*
- Refer to ND Constipation for additional interventions, as appropriate.

DOCUMENTATION FOCUS

Assessment/Reassessment

- Assessment findings, client's perceptions of the problem.
- Current bowel pattern, stool characteristics.

Planning

- Plan of care, specific interventions, and who is involved in the planning.
- Teaching plan.

Implementation/Evaluation

- Client's responses to interventions, teaching, and actions performed.
- Changes in bowel pattern, character of stool.
- Attainment or progress toward desired outcome(s).
- Modifications to plan of care.

Discharge Planning

- Referral for follow-up care.

References

1. Pieken, S. R. (2004). Constipation. *Gastrointestinal Health: A Self-Help Nutritional Program to Prevent, Cure, or Alleviate Irritable Bowel Syndrome, Ulcers, Heartburn, Gas, Constipation.* 3rd ed. New York: HarperCollins, 99–104.
2. National Digestive Diseases Information Clearinghouse. (Updated 2014). Constipation. Retrieved July 2014 from http://digestive.niddk.nih.gov/ddiseases/pubs/constipation/.

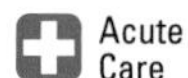

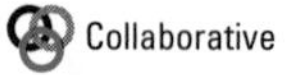

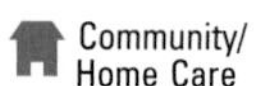

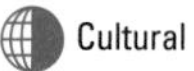

3. Stanley, M. (1999). The aging gastrointestinal system with nutritional considerations. In Stanley, M., Beare, P. G. (eds). *Gerontological Nursing: A Health Promotion/Protection Approach.* 7th ed. Philadelphia: F. A. Davis, 180–181.
4. McKay, S. L., Fravel, M., Scanlon, C. (2012). Evidence-based practice: Management of constipation. *J Gerontol Nurs*, 38(7), 9–15.
5. Basson, M. D. (Updated 2014). Constipation in adults. Retrieved July 2014 from http://emedicine.medscape.com/article/184704-overview.

risk for Constipation

Taxonomy II: Elimination and Exchange—Class 2 Gastrointestinal Function (00015) [**Diagnostic Division:** Elimination], Submitted 1998; Revised 2013

DEFINITION: Vulnerable to a decrease in normal frequency of defecation accompanied by difficult or incomplete passage of stool, which may compromise health.

RISK FACTORS

Functional
Abdominal muscle weakness
Average daily physical activity is less than recommended for gender and age
Habitually ignores urge to defecate; irregular defecation habits; inadequate toileting habits
Recent environmental change

Mechanical
Electrolyte imbalance
Hemorrhoids; pregnancy; obesity
Neurological impairment (e.g., positive EEG, head trauma, seizure disorders); Hirschsprung's disease; tumor
Prostate enlargement; postsurgical bowel obstruction
Rectal abscess, ulcer; rectal prolapse; rectal anal fissure or stricture; rectocele

Pharmacological
Pharmaceutical agent; laxative abuse

Physiological
Eating habit change (e.g., foods, eating times); insufficient dietary habits; insufficient fiber or fluid intake; dehydration
Inadequate dentition or oral hygiene
Decrease in gastrointestinal motility
NOTE: A risk diagnosis is not evidenced by signs and symptoms, as the problem has not occurred; rather, nursing interventions are directed at prevention.

DESIRED OUTCOMES/EVALUATION CRITERIA

Sample NOC linkages:
Bowel Elimination: Formation and evacuation of stool
Risk Control: Personal actions to prevent, eliminate, or reduce modifiable health threats
Knowledge: Medication: Extent of understanding conveyed about the safe use of medication

(continues on page 200)

risk for Constipation (continued)

Client Will (Include Specific Time Frame)

- Maintain effective pattern of bowel functioning.
- Verbalize understanding of risk factors and appropriate interventions or solutions related to individual situation.
- Demonstrate behaviors or lifestyle changes to prevent developing problem.

ACTIONS/INTERVENTIONS

Sample NIC linkages:

Constipation/Impaction Management: Prevention and alleviation of constipation/impaction
Bowel Management: Establishment and maintenance of a regular pattern of bowel elimination
Medication Management: Facilitation of safe and effective use of prescription and over-the-counter drugs

NURSING PRIORITY NO. 1 To identify individual risk factors/needs:

- Review medical/surgical history *to identify conditions commonly associated with constipation, including problems with colon or rectum (e.g., obstruction, scar tissue or stricture, diverticulitis, irritable bowel syndrome, tumors, anal fissure), metabolic or endocrine disorders (e.g., diabetes mellitus, hypothyroidism, uremia), limited physical activity (e.g., bedrest, poor mobility, chronic disability), chronic pain problems (especially when client is on pain medications), pregnancy and childbirth, recent abdominal or perianal surgery, and neurological disorders (e.g., stroke, traumatic brain injury, Parkinson's disease, MS, spinal cord abnormalities).*[1–3,8]
- Note client's age. *Constipation is more likely to occur in individuals older than 65 years of age, but it can occur in any age from infant to elderly. A bottle-fed infant is more prone to constipation than a breast-fed infant, especially when formula contains iron. Toddlers are at risk because of developmental factors, and children. Adolescents are at risk because of unwillingness to take break from play, poor eating and fluid intake habits, and withholding because of perceived lack of privacy. Many older adults experience constipation as a result of duller nerve sensations, immobility, dehydration, and electrolyte imbalances; incomplete emptying of the bowel; or failing to attend to signals to defecate.*[1–4]
- Discuss usual elimination pattern and use of laxatives *to establish baseline and identify possible areas for intervention or instruction.*[8]
- Ascertain client's family and cultural beliefs and practices about bowel elimination, such as "must have a bowel movement every day or I need an enema." *These factors reflect familial or cultural thinking about elimination, which affect client's lifetime patterns.*
- Review usual dietary regimen. *Imbalanced nutrition influences the amount and consistency of stool.*[2] *Inadequate dietary fiber (vegetable, fruits, whole grains) and highly processed foods contribute to poor intestinal function.*[1,3,5]
- Assess general oral and dental health. *Dental problems can impact dietary intake (e.g., loss of teeth can force individuals to eat soft foods mostly lacking in fiber).*[1,3]
- Determine fluid intake to note deficits. *Most individuals do not drink enough fluids, even when healthy, reducing the speed at which stool moves through the colon. Active fluid loss through sweating, vomiting, diarrhea, or bleeding can greatly increase chances for constipation.*[1–4,6]
- Evaluate medication or drug usage *for agents that could slow passage of stool and increase risk of constipation (e.g., narcotic pain relievers, antidepressants, anticonvulsants, aluminum-containing antacids, chemotherapy, iron supplements, contrast media, steroids).*[1–7]
- Note energy and activity level and exercise pattern. *Lack of physical activity or regular exercise is often a factor in constipation.*[1–5,7]
- Identify areas of life changes or stressors. *Factors such as pregnancy, travel, traumas, and changes in personal relationships; occupational factors; or financial concerns can cause or exacerbate constipation.*[4,7]
- Determine access to bathroom, privacy, and ability to perform self-care activities.
- Auscultate abdomen for presence, location, and characteristics of bowel sounds *reflecting bowel activity.*

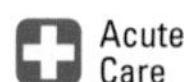

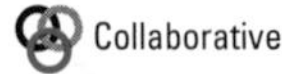

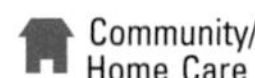

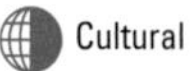

NURSING PRIORITY NO. 2 To facilitate normal bowel function:

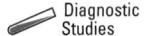

- Promote healthy lifestyle for elimination:[1–8]
  - Instruct in and encourage balanced fiber and bulk (e.g., fruits, vegetables, whole grains) in diet and fiber supplements (e.g., wheat bran, psyllium) *to improve consistency of stool and facilitate passage through colon.*
  - Limit foods with little or no fiber or diet high in fats (e.g., ice cream, cheese, meats, fast food, processed foods).
  - Promote adequate fluid intake, including water, high-fiber fruit and vegetable juices, fruit/vegetable smoothies, and popsicles. Suggest drinking warm, stimulating fluids (e.g., decaffeinated coffee, hot water, tea) *to avoid dehydration; promote moist, soft feces; and facilitate passage of stool.*
  - Encourage daily activity and exercise within limits of individual ability to stimulate contractions of the intestines.
  - Encourage client to not ignore urge. Provide privacy and routinely scheduled time for defecation (bathroom or commode preferable to bedpan) *to promote psychological readiness and comfort.*
- Recommend use of medications (stool softeners, mild stimulants, or bulk-forming agents) as needed and/or routinely when appropriate *to prevent constipation (e.g., client taking pain medications, especially opiates, or who is inactive or immobile).*[8]

NURSING PRIORITY NO. 3 Promote wellness (Teaching/Discharge Considerations):

- Discuss physiology and acceptable variations in elimination. *May help reduce concerns and anxiety about situation.*[1,5,7]
- Review individual risk factors or potential problems and specific interventions for prevention of constipation.[1,5,7]
- Encourage treatment of underlying medical causes where appropriate *to improve organ function, including the bowel.*[1,5,7]
- Educate client/significant other about safe and risky practices for managing constipation. *Information can assist client to make beneficial choices when need arises.*[1,5,7]
- Encourage client to maintain elimination diary if appropriate *to help monitor bowel pattern.*[1,5,7]
- Discuss client's current medication regime with physician *to determine if drugs that may contribute to constipation can be discontinued or changed.*[8]
- Refer to NDs Constipation; chronic functional Constipation; perceived Constipation for additional interventions as appropriate.

DOCUMENTATION FOCUS

Assessment/Reassessment

- Current bowel pattern, characteristics of stool, medications.
- Individual risk factors.

Planning

- Plan of care and who is involved in planning.
- Teaching plan.

Implementation/Evaluation

- Responses to interventions, teaching, and actions performed.
- Attainment or progress toward desired outcomes.
- Modifications to plan of care.

Discharge Planning

- Individual long-term needs, noting who is responsible for actions to be taken.
- Specific referrals made.

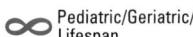

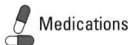

References

1. McKay, S. L., Fravel, M., Scanlon, C. (2012). Evidence-based practice: Management of constipation. *J Gerontol Nurs*, 38(7), 9–15.
2. Ferry, R. J. (Updated 2014). Constipation in children. Retrieved August 2014 from http://www.emedicinehealth.com/constipation_in_children/page3_em.htm.
3. Stanley, M. (1999). The aging gastrointestinal system, with nutritional considerations. In Beare, P. G. (ed). *Gerontological Nursing: A Health Promotion/Protection Approach*. 7th ed. Philadelphia: F. A. Davis, 180–181.
4. Watson, L. (2010). Childhood constipation. *Community Pract*, 83(7), 40–42.
5. Locke, G. R., Pemberton, J. H., Phillips, S. F. (2000). American Gastroenterological Association: Medical position statement: Guidelines on constipation. *Gastroenterology*, 119(6), 1761–1766.
6. Marks, J. W. (Updated 2014). Constipation. Retrieved August 2014 from http://www.medicinenet.com/constipation/article.htm.
7. Basson, M. D. (Updated 2014). Constipation in adults. Retrieved July 2014 from http://emedicine.medscape.com/article/184704-overview.
8. Wooten, J. M. (2006). OTC laxatives aren't all the same. *RN*, 69(9)–78.

Contamination

Taxonomy II: Safety/Protection—Class 4 Environmental Hazards (00181) [**Diagnostic Division:** Safety], Submitted 2006

DEFINITION: Exposure to environmental contaminants in doses sufficient to cause adverse health effects.

RELATED FACTORS

External

Carpeted flooring; flaking, peeling surface in presence of young children (e.g., paint, plaster); playing where environmental contaminants are used; household hygiene practices
Chemical contamination of food or water; ingestion of contaminated material (e.g., radioactive, food, water)
Economically disadvantaged
Exposure to areas with high contaminant level or atmospheric pollutants; inadequate breakdown of contaminant
Exposure to bioterrorism, or disaster (natural or man-made), or radiation; unprotected exposure to chemical (e.g., arsenic)
Inadequate municipal services (e.g., trash removal, sewage treatment facilities)
Inadequate or inappropriate use of protective clothing; personal hygiene practices
Use of environmental contaminants in the home; use of noxious material (e.g., lacquer, paint) in insufficiently ventilated area or without effective protection

Internal

Age (children < 5 years, older adults); gestational age during exposure
Female gender; pregnancy
Inadequate nutrition
Preexisting disease states; smoking
Concomitant exposure or previous exposure to contaminant

DEFINING CHARACTERISTICS

Author Note: Defining characteristics are dependent on the causative agent. Agents cause a variety of individual organ responses as well as systemic responses.

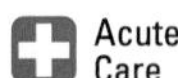

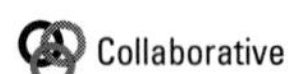

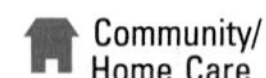

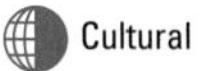

Subjective/Objective

Pesticides: [Major categories of pesticides: insecticides, herbicides, fungicides, antimicrobials, rodenticides; major pesticides: organophosphates, carbamates, organochlorines, pyrethrum, arsenic, glycophosphates, bipyridyis, chlorophenoxy compounds]

Dermatological, gastrointestinal, neurological, pulmonary, or renal effects of pesticide

Chemicals: [Major chemical agents: petroleum-based agents, anticholinesterases; type I agents act on proximal tracheobronchial portion of the respiratory tract, type II agents act on alveoli, type III agents produce systemic effects]

Dermatological, gastrointestinal, immunological, neurological, pulmonary, or renal effects of chemical exposure

Biologicals: [Toxins from living organisms—bacteria, viruses, fungi]

Dermatological, gastrointestinal, neurological, pulmonary, or renal effects of exposure to biologicals

Pollution: [Major locations: air, water, soil; major agents: asbestos, radon, tobacco (smoke), heavy metal, lead, noise, exhaust]

Neurological or pulmonary effects of pollution exposure

Waste: [Categories of waste: trash, raw sewage, industrial waste]

Dermatological, gastrointestinal, hepatic, or pulmonary effects of waste exposure

Radiation:

[External exposure through direct contact with radioactive material]

Immunological, genetic, neurological, or oncological effects of radiation exposure

Sample Clinical Applications: *Escherichia coli* infection, plague, hantavirus, asthma, botulism, cholera, lead or other heavy metal poisoning, chemical burns, asbestosis, carbon monoxide poisoning, radiation sickness

DESIRED OUTCOMES/EVALUATION CRITERIA

Sample NOC linkages:

Symptom Severity: Severity of perceived adverse changes in physical, emotional, and social functioning

Knowledge: Personal Safety: Extent of understanding conveyed about prevention of unintentional injuries

Risk Control: Personal actions to prevent, eliminate, or reduce modifiable health threats

Client Will (Include Specific Time Frame)

- Be free of injury and adverse health effects.
- Verbalize understanding of individual factors that contributed to injury and plans for correcting situation(s) where possible.
- Modify environment, as indicated, to enhance safety.

Sample NOC linkages:

Community Health Status: General state of well-being of a community or population

Community Risk Control: Lead Exposure: Community actions to reduce lead exposure and poisoning

Community Disaster Response: Community response following a natural or man-made calamitous event

Client/Community Will (Include Specific Time Frame)

- Identify hazards that led to exposure or contamination.
- Correct environmental hazards, as identified.
- Demonstrate necessary actions to promote community safety.

ACTIONS/INTERVENTIONS

In reviewing this ND, it is apparent there is overlap with other diagnoses. We have chosen to present generalized interventions. Although there are commonalities to Contamination situations, we

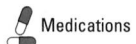

(continues on page 204)

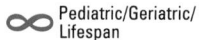

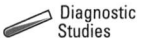

Contamination (continued)
suggest that the reader refer to other primary diagnoses, as indicated, such as ineffective Airway Clearance, ineffective Breathing Pattern, impaired Gas Exchange, impaired Home Maintenance, risk for Infection, risk for Injury, risk for Poisoning, impaired/risk for impaired Skin Integrity, risk for Suffocation, and risk for Trauma.

Sample NIC linkages:

Environmental Management: Safety: Monitoring and manipulation of the physical environment to promote safety

Community Health Development: Assisting members of a community to identify a community's health concerns, mobilize resources, and implement solutions

Environmental Risk Protection: Preventing and detecting disease and injury in populations at risk from environmental hazards

NURSING PRIORITY NO. 1 To evaluate degree/source of exposure:

- Ascertain type of contaminant(s) to which client has been exposed (e.g., chemical, biological, air pollutant), the manner of exposure (e.g., inhalation, ingestion, topical), whether exposure was accidental or intentional, and immediate or delayed reactions. *Determines course of action to be taken by all emergency and other care providers. Note: Although exposure history is often difficult to determine, national environmental agencies are working to identify types of chemicals that most humans are exposed to and the effects of those exposures. Since 1999, the Centers for Disease Control and Prevention (CDC) have measured over 300 environmental chemicals in people's blood or urine. Samples were collected from participants in CDC's National Health and Nutrition Examination Survey, which obtains and releases health-related data from a nationally representative sample in 2-year cycles.*[5] *Note: Intentional exposure to hazardous materials requires notification of law enforcement for further investigation and possible prosecution.*[1–6]
- ∞ Note age and gender. *Children (less than 5 years of age) are at greater risk for adverse effects from exposure to contaminants because (1) smaller body size causes them to receive a more concentrated "dose" than adults; (2) they spend more time outside than most adults, increasing exposure to air and soil pollutants; (3) young children spend more time on the floor, increasing exposure to toxins in carpets and low cupboards; (4) they consume more water and food per pound than adults, increasing their body-weight-to-toxin ratio; and (5) development of fetal, infant, and young children's organ systems can be disrupted. Older adults have a normal decline in function of immune, integumentary, cardiac, renal, hepatic, and pulmonary systems; an increase in adipose tissue mass; and a decline in lean body mass. Females in general have a greater proportion of body fat than men, increasing the chance of accumulating more lipid-soluble toxins.*[1–6]
- Ascertain geographical location (e.g., home, work) where exposure occurred. *Individual and/or community intervention may be needed to modify or correct problem.*
- Note socioeconomic status and availability and use of resources. *Living in poverty increases potential for multiple exposures, delayed or lack of access to healthcare, and poor general health, potentially increasing the severity of adverse effects of exposure.*[6]
- Determine factors associated with particular contaminant:

  Pesticides: Determine if client has ingested contaminated foods (e.g., fruits, vegetables, commercially raised meats) or inhaled agent (e.g., aerosol bug sprays, in vicinity of crop spraying).[2,3,9]

  Chemicals: Ascertain if client uses environmental contaminants in the home or at work (e.g., pesticides, chemicals, chlorine household cleaners) and fails to use or inappropriately uses protective clothing.[2,3,9]

  Pollution air/water: Determine if client has been exposed and is sensitive to atmospheric pollutants (e.g., radon, benzene [from gasoline], carbon monoxide, automobile emissions [numerous chemicals], chlorofluorocarbons [refrigerants, solvents], ozone or smog, particles [acids, organic chemicals, particles in smoke], commercial plants [e.g., pulp and paper mills]).[7] *Note: The Environmental Protection Agency (EPA, 2013) has identified six pollutants (carbon monoxide, lead, nitrogen oxides, ground-level ozone, particle*

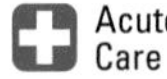

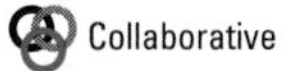

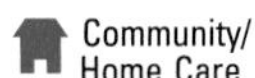

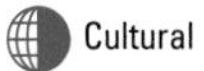

pollution [often referred to as particulate matter], sulfur oxides) as "criteria" air pollutants because it regulates them by developing human health-based and/or environmentally-based criteria for setting permissible levels.[15]

Investigate possibility of home-based exposure to air pollution. *Toxins may include carbon monoxide (e.g., poor ventilation, especially in the winter months [poor heating systems, use of charcoal grill indoors, car left running in garage], cigarette or cigar smoke indoors, ozone [spends a lot of time outdoors such as playing children, adults participating in moderate to strenuous work or recreational activities]).*[7]

Biologicals: Determine if client may have been exposed to biological agents (bacteria, viruses, fungi) or bacterial toxins (e.g., botulinum, ricin). *Exposure occurring as a result of an act of terrorism would be rare; however, individuals may be exposed to bacterial agents or toxins through contaminated or poorly prepared foods.*

Waste: Determine if client lives in area where trash and garbage accumulates or is exposed to raw sewage or industrial wastes that can contaminate soil and water.

Radiation: Ascertain if client/household member experienced accidental exposure (e.g., occupation in radiography, living near or working in nuclear industries or electrical-generating plants).

- Observe for signs and symptoms of infective agent and sepsis, such as fatigue, malaise, headache, fever, chills, diaphoresis, skin rash, and altered level of consciousness. *Initial symptoms of some diseases may mimic influenza and be misdiagnosed if healthcare providers do not maintain an index of suspicion.*
- Note presence and degree of chemical burns and initial treatment provided.
- Assist with diagnostic studies, as indicated. *Provides information about type and degree of exposure and organ involvement or damage.*
- Identify psychological response (e.g., anger, shock, acute anxiety, confusion, denial) to accidental or mass exposure incident. *Although these are normal responses, they may recycle repeatedly and result in posttrauma syndrome if not dealt with adequately.*
- Alert proper authorities to presence/exposure to contamination, as appropriate. *Depending on agent, there may be reporting requirements to local, state, and national agencies such as the local health department, the EPA, and the CDC.*

NURSING PRIORITY NO. 2 To assist in treating effects of exposure:

- Implement a coordinated decontamination plan (e.g., removal of clothing, showering with soap and water, other initial decontamination procedures) following consultation with medical toxicologist, hazardous materials team, industrial hygiene, and safety officer *to prevent further harm to client and to protect healthcare providers.*[8,9]
- Ensure availability and proper use of personal protective equipment (e.g., high-efficiency particulate air filter masks, special garments, barrier materials, including gloves and face shield) *to protect from exposure to biological, chemical, and radioactive hazards.*[8–10]
- Provide for isolation or group/cohort individuals with same diagnosis or exposure, as resources require. *Limited resources may dictate open ward-like environment; however, the need to control spread of infection still exists. Only plague, smallpox, and viral hemorrhagic fevers require more than standard infection control precautions.*
- Provide therapeutic interventions, as individually appropriate. *Specific needs of the client and the level of care available at a given time and location determine response.*
- Refer pregnant client for individually appropriate diagnostic procedures or screenings. *Helpful in determining effects of teratogenic exposure on fetus allowing for informed choices and preparations.*[14]
- Screen breast milk in lactating client following radiation exposure. *Depending on type and amount of exposure, breastfeeding may need to be briefly interrupted or occasionally terminated.*[12,13]
- Cooperate with and refer to appropriate agencies (e.g., CDC, U.S. Army Medical Research Institute of Infectious Diseases, Federal Emergency Management Agency, Department of Health and Human Services, Office of Emergency Preparedness, EPA) *to prepare for and manage mass casualty incidents.*[9,10]

NURSING PRIORITY NO. 3 To promote wellness (Teaching/Discharge Considerations):

CLIENT/CAREGIVER

- Identify individual safety needs and injury or illness prevention in home, community, and work setting.
- Install carbon monoxide monitors and other indoor air pollutant detectors in home, as appropriate.
- Review individual nutritional needs, appropriate exercise program, and need for rest. *Essentials for well-being and recovery.*
- Repair, replace, or correct unsafe household items and situations (e.g., storage of solvents in soda bottles, flaking or peeling paint or plaster, filtering unsafe tap water).
- Emphasize importance of supervising infant/child or individuals with cognitive limitations.
- Encourage removal of or proper cleaning of carpeted floors, especially for small children and persons with respiratory conditions. *Carpets hold up to 100 times as much fine particle material as a bare floor and can contain metals and pesticides.*[1]
- Identify commercial cleaning resources, if appropriate, *for safe cleaning of contaminated articles and surfaces.*
- Install dehumidifier in damp areas *to retard growth of molds.*[1]
- Encourage timely cleaning or replacement of air filters on furnace and air-conditioning unit. *Good ventilation cuts down on indoor air pollution from carpets, machines, paints, solvents, cleaning materials, and pesticides.*
- Discuss protective actions for specific "bad air" days. *Measures may include limiting or avoiding outdoor activities, especially in sensitive groups (e.g., children who are active outdoors, adults involved in moderate or strenuous outdoor activities, persons with respiratory diseases).*[6]
- Review effects of secondhand smoke and importance of refraining from smoking in home and car where others are likely to be exposed.
- Recommend periodic inspection of well water and tap water *to identify possible contaminants.*
- Encourage client/caregiver to develop a personal or family disaster plan, to gather needed supplies to provide for self/family during a community emergency, and to learn how specific public health threats might affect client and actions *to reduce the risk to health and safety.*
- Instruct client to always refer to local authorities and health experts for specific up-to-date information for community and to follow their advice.
- Refer to counselor or support groups for ongoing assistance in dealing with traumatic incident and aftereffects of exposure.
- Provide bibliotherapy including written resources and appropriate Web sites *for review and self-paced learning.*
- Refer to a smoking-cessation program, as needed.

COMMUNITY

- Promote community education programs in different modalities, languages, cultures, and educational levels geared *to increasing awareness of safety measures and resources available to individuals/community.*
- Review pertinent job-related health department and Occupational Safety and Health Administration regulations.
- Refer to local resources that provide information about air quality (e.g., pollen index, "bad air days").
- Encourage community members/groups to engage in problem-solving activities.
- Ascertain that there is a comprehensive disaster plan for the community that includes a chain of command, equipment, communication, training, decontamination area(s), and safety and security plans *to ensure an effective response to any emergency (e.g., flood, toxic spill, infectious disease outbreak, radiation release).*[11]

DOCUMENTATION FOCUS

Assessment/Reassessment

- Details of specific exposure, including location and circumstances.
- Client's/caregiver's understanding of individual risks/safety concerns.

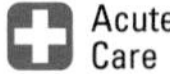
Acute Care
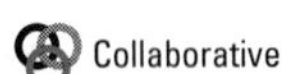
Collaborative
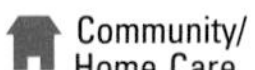
Community/ Home Care
 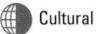
Cultural

Planning
- Plan of care and who is involved in planning.
- Teaching plan.

Implementation/Evaluation
- Individual responses to interventions, teaching, and actions performed.
- Specific actions and changes that are made.
- Attainment or progress toward desired outcome(s).
- Modifications to plan of care.

Discharge Planning
- Long-term plans for discharge needs, lifestyle and community changes, and who is responsible for actions to be taken.
- Specific referrals made.

References

1. Goldman, L. R. (1998). Linking research and policy to ensure children's environmental health. *Environ Health Perspect*, 106(13), 957–961.
2. All Family Resources. (1999). Chemical toxins safety. Retrieved March 2015 from http://www.familymanagement.com/childcare/facility/chemical.toxins.safety.html.
3. Rajen, M. (reprint 2007). Toxins everywhere. Retrieved March 2015 from http://neurotalk.psychcentral.com/thread10246.html.
4. Stabin, M. G., Breitz, H. (2000). Breast milk secretion of radiopharmaceuticals: Mechanisms, findings, and radiation dosimetry. *J Nucl Med*, 41(5), 863–873.
5. Centers for Disease Control and Prevention. (Updated 2012). Environmental chemicals. Retrieved March 2015 from http://www.cdc.gov/biomonitoring/environmental_chemicals.html.
6. Wilkinson, R., Marmot, M. (2003). *Social Determinants of Health: The Solid Facts.* 2nd ed. Copenhagen, Denmark: World Health Organization.
7. U.S. Environmental Protection Agency. (1999). Smog—Who does it hurt? What you need to know about ozone and your health. Retrieved March 2015 from http://www.epa.gov/airnow/health/smog.pdf.
8. Gum, R. M., Hoyle, J. D. (2005, updated 2013). CBRNE—Chemical warfare mass casualty management. Retrieved March 2015 from http://emedicine.medscape.com/article/831375-overview.
9. Jagminas, L. (2006, updated 2013). CBRNE—Chemical decontamination. Retrieved March 2015 from http://emedicine.medscape.com/article/831175-overview.
10. Arnold, J. L. (2006, updated 2014). Personal protective equipment. Retrieved March 2015 from http://www.emedicinehealth.com/personal_protective_equipment/article_em.htm.
11. Bauer, J., Steinhauer, R. (2002). A readied response: The emergency plan. *RN*, 65(6), 40.
12. When should a mother avoid breastfeeding? (Updated 2015). Centers for Disease Control and Prevention. Retrieved March 2015 from http://www.cdc.gov/breastfeeding/disease/.
13. UAMS College of Pharmacy: Nuclear Pharmacy. Breastfeeding guidelines following radiopharmaceutical administration. Retrieved March 2015 from http://nuclearpharmacy.uams.edu/resources/breastfeeding.asp.
14. American Academy of Family Physicians. Breastfeeding (Position paper). Retrieved March 2015 from http://www.aafp.org/about/policies/all/breastfeeding-support.html.
15. Centers for Disease Control and Prevention. EPA criteria pollutants. Retrieved March 2015 from http://www.cdc.gov/air/pollutants.htm.

risk for Contamination

Taxonomy II: Safety/Protection—Class 4 Environmental Hazards (00180) [**Diagnostic Division:** Safety], Submitted 2006; Revised 2013

DEFINITION: Vulnerable to exposure to environmental contaminants, which may compromise health.

RISK FACTORS

External

Carpeted flooring; flaking, peeling surface in presence of young children (e.g., paint, plaster); playing where environmental contaminants are used; inadequate household hygiene practices
Chemical contamination of food or water; ingestion of contaminated material (e.g., radioactive, food, water)
Economically disadvantaged
Exposure to areas with high contaminant level or atmospheric pollutants; inadequate breakdown of contaminant
Exposure to bioterrorism, or disaster (natural or man-made), or radiation; unprotected exposure to chemical (e.g., arsenic)
Inadequate municipal services (e.g., trash removal, sewage treatment facilities)
Inadequate or inappropriate use of protective clothing; inadequate personal hygiene practices
Use of environmental contaminants in the home; use of noxious material (e.g., lacquer, paint) in insufficiently ventilated area or without effective protection

Internal

Age (children < 5 years, older adults); gestational age during exposure
Female gender; pregnancy
Inadequate nutrition
Preexisting disease states; smoking
Concomitant exposure or previous exposure to contaminant
NOTE: A risk diagnosis is not evidenced by signs and symptoms, as the problem has not occurred; rather, nursing interventions are directed at prevention.
Sample Clinical Applications: *Escherichia coli* infection, plague, hantavirus, asthma, botulism, cholera, lead or other heavy metal poisoning, chemical burns, asbestosis, carbon monoxide poisoning, radiation sickness

DESIRED OUTCOMES/EVALUATION CRITERIA

Sample NOC linkages:

Knowledge: Personal Safety: Extent of understanding conveyed about prevention of unintentional injuries
Risk Control: Personal actions to prevent, eliminate, or reduce modifiable health threats

Client Will (Include Specific Time Frame)

- Verbalize understanding of individual factors that contribute to possibility of injury and take steps to correct situation(s).
- Demonstrate behaviors and lifestyle changes to reduce risk factors and protect self from injury.
- Modify environment as indicated to enhance safety.
- Be free of injury.
- Support community activities for disaster preparedness.

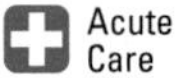

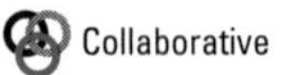

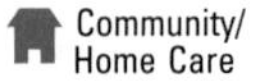

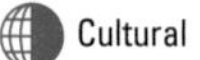

Sample NOC linkages:
Community Health Status: General state of well-being of a community or population
Community Risk Control: Lead Exposure: Community actions to reduce lead exposure and poisoning
Community Disaster Readiness: Community preparedness to respond to a natural or man-made calamitous event

Community Will (Include Specific Time Frame)
- Identify hazards that could lead to exposure or contamination.
- Correct environmental hazards as identified.
- Demonstrate necessary actions to promote community safety and disaster preparedness.

ACTIONS/INTERVENTIONS

Sample NIC linkages:
Risk Identification: Analysis of potential risk factors, determination of health risks, and prioritization of risk-reduction strategies for an individual or group
Community Health Development: Assisting members of a community to identify a community's health concerns, mobilize resources, and implement solutions
Environmental Risk Protection: Preventing and detecting disease and injury in populations at risk from environmental hazards

NURSING PRIORITY NO. 1 To evaluate degree/source of risk inherent in the home, community, and work site:

- Ascertain type of contaminant(s) and exposure routes posing a potential hazard to client or community (e.g., air, soil, or water pollutants; food source, chemical, biological, radiation) as listed in Risk Factors. *Determines course of action to be taken by client/community/care providers.*
- Note age and gender of client(s) or community base (e.g., community health clinic serving primarily economically disadvantaged children or elderly; school near large industrial plant, family living in smog-prone area). *Young children, frail elderly, and females have been found to be at higher risk for effects of exposure to many toxins.*[1,2] (Refer to ND Contamination.)
- Ascertain client's geographic location at home or work (e.g., lives where crop spraying is routine; works in nuclear plant; contract worker or soldier returning from combat area). *Individual and/or community intervention may be needed to reduce risks of accidental or intentional exposures.*
- Note socioeconomic status and availability and use of resources. *Living in poverty increases the potential for multiple exposures, delayed or lack of access to healthcare, and poor general health.*[3]
- Determine client's/significant other's (SO's) understanding of potential risk and appropriate protective measures.

NURSING PRIORITY NO. 2 To assist client to reduce or correct individual risk factors:

- Assist client to develop plan to address individual safety needs and injury or illness prevention in home, community, and work setting.
- Repair, replace, or correct unsafe household items or situations (e.g., flaking or peeling paint or plaster, filtering unsafe tap water).
- Review effects of secondhand smoke and importance of refraining from smoking in home or car *where others are likely to be exposed.*
- Encourage removal or proper cleaning of carpeted floors, especially for small children and persons with respiratory conditions. *Carpets hold up to 100 times as much fine-particle material as a bare floor and can contain metals and pesticides.*[1]

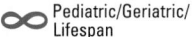

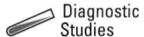

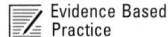

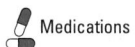

- Encourage timely cleaning or replacement of air filters on furnace and air-conditioning unit. *Good ventilation cuts down on indoor air pollution from carpets, machines, paints, solvents, cleaning materials, and pesticides.*
- Recommend periodic inspection of well water and tap water *to identify possible contaminants.*
- Encourage client to install carbon monoxide monitors and other air pollutant detectors in home as appropriate.
- Recommend placing dehumidifier in damp areas *to retard growth of molds.*
- Review proper handling of household chemicals:[4,5]

  Read chemical labels *to be aware of primary hazards (especially in commonly used household cleaning and gardening products).*

  Follow directions printed on product label (e.g., avoid use of certain chemicals on food preparation surfaces, refrain from spraying garden chemicals on windy days).

  Choose least hazardous products for the job, preferably multiuse products *to reduce number of different chemicals used and stored.* Use products labeled "nontoxic" wherever possible.

  Use form of chemical that most reduces risk of exposure (e.g., cream instead of liquid or aerosol).

  Wear protective clothing, gloves, and safety glasses when using chemicals. Avoid mixing chemicals at all times and use in well-ventilated areas.

  Store chemicals in locked cabinets. Keep chemicals in original labeled containers and do not pour into other containers.
- Place safety stickers on chemicals *to warn of harmful contents.*
- Review proper food-handling, storage, and cooking techniques.
- Stress importance of pregnant or lactating women following fish or wildlife consumption guidelines provided by state, U.S. territorial, or Native American tribes. *Ingestion of noncommercial fish or wildlife can be a significant source of pollutants.*[8]

NURSING PRIORITY NO. 3 To promote wellness (Teaching/Discharge Considerations):

HOME

- Discuss general safety concerns with client/SO/employees *to ensure that people are educated about potential risks, and ways to manage risks.*
- Stress importance of supervising infant/child or individuals with cognitive limitations *to protect those who are unable to protect themselves.*
- Post emergency and poison control numbers in a visible location.
- Encourage learning cardiopulmonary resuscitation and first aid for toxic exposures.
- Discuss protective actions for specific "bad air" days (e.g., limiting/avoiding outdoor activities).
- Review pertinent job-related safety regulations. Emphasize necessity of wearing appropriate protective equipment.
- Encourage client/caregiver to develop a personal/family disaster plan, to gather needed supplies to provide for self/family during a community emergency, and to learn how specific public health threats might affect client and actions to promote preparedness and reduce the risk to health and safety.
- Provide information and refer to appropriate resources about potential toxic hazards and protective measures. Provide bibliotherapy including written resources and appropriate Web sites *for client review and self-paced learning.*
- Refer to a smoking-cessation program as needed.

COMMUNITY

- Promote education programs geared toward increasing awareness of safety measures and resources available to individuals/community.
- Review pertinent job-related health department and Occupational Safety and Health Administration regulations *to safeguard the workplace and the community.*
- Ascertain that there is a comprehensive disaster plan in place for the community that includes a chain of command, equipment, communication, training, decontamination area(s), and safety and security plans *to ensure an effective response to any emergency (e.g., flood, toxic spill, infectious disease outbreak, radiation release).*[6]

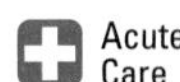

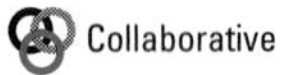

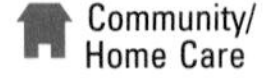

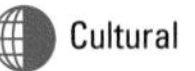

- Refer to appropriate agencies (e.g., Centers for Disease Control and Prevention, U.S. Army Medical Research Institute of Infectious Diseases, Federal Emergency Management Agency, Department of Health and Human Services, Office of Emergency Preparedness, the Evironmental Protection Agency) *to prepare for and manage mass casualty incidents.*[7]

DOCUMENTATION FOCUS

Assessment/Reassessment

- Client's/caregiver's understanding of individual risks and safety concerns.
- Community risks for exposure or contamination

Planning

- Plan of care and who is involved in planning.
- Teaching plan.

Implementation/Evaluation

- Individual responses to interventions, teaching, and actions performed.
- Specific actions and changes that are made.
- Attainment or progress toward desired outcome(s).
- Modifications to plan of care.

Discharge Planning

- Long-term plans, lifestyle and community changes, and who is responsible for actions to be taken.
- Specific referrals made.

References

1. Goldman, L. R. (1998). Linking research and policy to ensure children's environmental health. *Environ Health Perspect*, 106(13), 957–961.
2. Centers for Disease Control and Prevention. (Updated 2012). Environmental chemicals. Retrieved March 2015 from http://www.cdc.gov/biomonitoring/environmental_chemicals.html.
3. Wilkinson, R., Marmot, M. (2003). *Social Determinants of Health: The Solid Facts.* 2nd ed. Copenhagen, Denmark: World Health Organization.
4. Rajen, M. (Reprinted 2007). Toxins everywhere. Retrieved March 2015 from http://neurotalk.psychcentral.com/thread10246.html.
5. All Family Resources. (1999). Chemical toxins safety. Retrieved March 2015 from www.familymanagement.com/childcare/facility/chemical.toxins.safety.html.
6. Bauer, J., Steinhauer, R. (2002). A readied response: The emergency plan. *RN*, 65(6), 40.
7. Jagminas, L. (2006, updated 2013). CBRNE—Chemical decontamination. Retrieved March 2015 from http://emedicine.medscape.com/article/831175-overview#showall.
8. American Academy of Family Physicians. Breastfeeding (Position paper). Retrieved March 2015 from http://www.aafp.org/about/policies/all/breastfeeding-support.html.

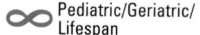

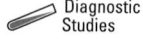

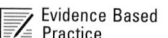

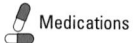

compromised family Coping

Taxonomy II: Coping/Stress Tolerance—Class 2 Coping Responses (00074) [**Diagnostic Division:** Social Interaction], Submitted 1980; Revised 1996

DEFINITION: A usually supportive primary person (family member; significant other; or close friend) provides insufficient, ineffective, or compromised support, comfort, assistance, or encouragement that may be needed by the client to manage or master adaptive tasks related to his or her health challenge.

RELATED FACTORS

Coexisting situations affecting the significant person; preoccupation by support person with concern outside of family
Developmental crisis; situational crisis faced by support person
Prolonged disease that exhausts the capacity of support person
Exhaustion of support person's capacity
Insufficient understanding/misunderstanding of information by support person
Insufficient information available to support person; misinformation obtained by support person
Insufficient reciprocal support; insufficient support given by client to support person
Family disorganization, role change

DEFINING CHARACTERISTICS

Subjective

Client complaint or concern about support person's response to health problem
Support person reports inadequate knowledge or understanding that interferes with effective supportive behaviors
Support person reports preoccupation with own reaction to client's need

Objective

Assistive behaviors by support person produce unsatisfactory results
Protective behavior by support person incongruent with client's abilities
Limitation in communication between support person and client
Support person withdraws from client
Sample Clinical Applications: Chronic conditions (e.g., chronic obstructive pulmonary disease [COPD], AIDS, Alzheimer's disease, pain, renal failure), substance abuse, cancer, depression, hypochondriasis

DESIRED OUTCOMES/EVALUATION CRITERIA

Sample NOC linkages:

Family Coping: Family actions to manage stressors that tax family resources
Family Normalization: Capacity of the family system to develop strategies for optimal functioning when a member has a chronic illness or disability
Caregiver-Patient Relationship: Positive interactions and connections between the caregiver and care recipient

Family Will (Include Specific Time Frame)

- Identify resources within themselves to deal with the situation.
- Interact appropriately with the client, providing support and assistance, as indicated.
- Provide opportunity for client to deal with situation in own way.
- Verbalize knowledge and understanding of illness, disability, or condition.

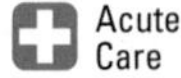

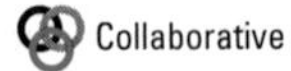

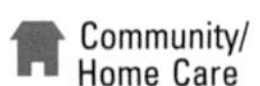

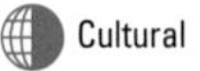

- Express feelings honestly.
- Identify need for and seek outside support.

ACTIONS/INTERVENTIONS

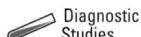

Sample NIC linkages:

Family Involvement Promotion: Facilitating family participation in the emotional and physical care of the patient

Family Support: Promotion of family values, interests, and goals

Caregiver Support: Provision of the necessary information, advocacy, and support to facilitate primary patient care by someone other than a healthcare provider

NURSING PRIORITY NO. 1 To assess causative/contributing factors:

- Identify underlying situation(s) that may contribute to the inability of family to provide needed assistance to the client. *Circumstances may have preceded the illness and now have a significant effect (e.g., client had a heart attack during sexual activity, mate is afraid of repeating).*[1]
- Note cultural factors related to family relationships that may be involved in problems of caring for member who is ill. *Family composition and structure, methods of decision making, and gender issues and expectations will affect how family deals with stress of illness/negative prognosis. Depending on role the ill client has in the family (e.g., mother or father), other members may have difficulty assuming authoritative role and managing the family.*[6]
- Note the length of illness or condition (e.g., cancer, multiple sclerosis) and/or other long-term situations that may exist. *Chronic or unresolved illness, accompanied by changes in role performance or responsibility, often exhausts supportive capacity and coping abilities of significant other (SO)/family.*[1]
- Assess information available to and understood by the family/SO(s). *Access to and understanding of information regarding the specific illness or condition, treatment, and prognosis are essential to family cooperation and care of the client.*[2,3]
- Discuss family perceptions of situation. *Expectations of client and family members may/may not be realistic and may interfere with ability to cope with situation.*[1]
- Identify role of the client in family and how illness has changed the family organization. *Illness affects how client performs usual functions in the family and affects how others in the family take over those responsibilities. These changes may result in dysfunctional behaviors, anger, hostility, and hopelessness.*[1]
- Note factors (beside the client's illness) that are affecting abilities of family members to provide needed support. *Individual members' preoccupation with own needs and concerns can interfere with providing needed care or support during stresses of long-term illness. Additionally, caregivers may incur decreased or lost income or risk losing own health insurance if they alter their work hours to care for client.*[1]

NURSING PRIORITY NO. 2 To assist family to reactivate/develop skills to deal with current situation:

- Listen to client's/SO's comments, remarks, and expression of concern(s). Note nonverbal behaviors and responses and congruency. *Provides information and promotes understanding of client's view of the illness and needs related to current situation.*[1]
- Encourage family members to verbalize feelings openly and clearly. *Promotes understanding of feelings in relationship to current events and helps them to hear what other person is saying, leading to more appropriate interactions.*[5]
- Discuss underlying reasons for client's behavior. *Helps family/SO understand and accept or deal with client behaviors that may be triggered by emotional or physical effects of illness.*[4]
- Assist the family and client to understand "who owns the problem" and who is responsible for resolution. Avoid placing blame or guilt. *When these boundaries are defined, each individual can begin to take care of own self and stop taking care of others in inappropriate ways.*[3,4]

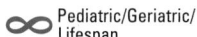

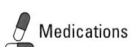

- Encourage client and family to develop problem-solving skills to deal with the situation. *Use of these skills enables each member of the family to identify what he or she sees as the problem to be dealt with and contribute ideas for solutions that are acceptable to them, promoting more effective interactions among the family members.*[4]

NURSING PRIORITY NO. 3 To promote wellness (Teaching/Discharge Considerations):

- Provide information for family/SO(s) about specific illness/condition. *Promotes better understanding of need for following therapeutic regimen to provide maximum benefit.*[8]
- Involve client and family in planning care as often as possible. *When family members are knowledgeable and understand needs, commitment to plan is enhanced.*[7,8]
- Promote assistance of family in providing client care, as appropriate. *Identifies ways of demonstrating support while maintaining client's independence (e.g., providing favorite foods, engaging in diversional activities).*[5]
- Refer to appropriate resources for assistance, as indicated (e.g., counseling, psychotherapy, financial, spiritual). *May need additional help, and getting to the appropriate resource provides accurate help for individual situation (e.g., family counseling, financial planning).*[7,8]
- Refer to NDs Anxiety, Death Anxiety, ineffective Coping, readiness for enhanced family Coping, disabled family Coping, Fear, Grieving, as appropriate.

DOCUMENTATION FOCUS

Assessment/Reassessment
- Assessment findings, including current and past coping behaviors, emotional response to situation and stressors.
- Availability and use of support systems.

Planning
- Plan of care, who is involved in planning and areas of responsibility.
- Teaching plan.

Implementation/Evaluation
- Responses of family members/client to interventions, teaching, and actions performed.
- Attainment or progress toward desired outcome(s).
- Modifications to plan of care.

Discharge Planning
- Long-term plans and who is responsible for actions.
- Specific referrals made.

References

1. Raina, P., O'Donnell, M., Rosenbaum, P., et al. (2005). The health and well-being of caregivers of children with cerebral palsy. *Pediatrics*, 115(6), 626–636.
2. Hatzmann, J., Heymans, H. S., Ferrer-i-Carbonell, A., et al. (2008). Hidden consequences of success in pediatrics: Parental health-related quality of life. *Pediatrics*, 122(5), 1030–1038.
3. Given, B., Sherwood, P., Given, C. (2008). What knowledge and skills do caregivers need? *Am J Nurs*, 108(9 (Suppl)), S28–S34.
4. Sittner, B. J., Hudson, D. B., DeFrain, J. (2007). Using the concept of family strengths to enhance nursing care. *MCN*, 32(6), 353–357.
5. Yedidia, M., Tiedemann, A. (2008). How do family caregivers describe their needs for professional help? *Am J Nurs*, 108(9 (Suppl)), S35–S37.
6. Dennis, B. P., Small, E. B. (2003). Incorporating cultural diversity in nursing care: An action plan. *ABNF*, 14(1), 17–26.
7. Feigin, R., Barnetz, Z., Davidson-Arad, B. (2008). Quality of life in family members coping with chronic illness in a relative: An exploratory study. *Families, Systems, & Health*, 26(3), 267–281.
8. Ammon, S. (2001). Managing patients with heart failure. *Am J Nurs*, 101(12), 34–40.

defensive Coping

Taxonomy II: Coping/Stress Tolerance—Class 2 Coping Responses (00071) [**Diagnostic Division:** Ego Integrity], Submitted 1988; Revised 2008

DEFINITION: Repeated projection of falsely positive self-evaluation based on a self-protective pattern that defends against underlying perceived threats to positive self-regard.

RELATED FACTORS

Conflict between self-perception and value system; uncertainty
Fear of failure, humiliation, or repercussions; insufficient self-confidence
Unrealistic self-expectations
Insufficient resilience
Insufficient confidence in others; insufficient support

DEFINING CHARACTERISTICS

Subjective

Denial of obvious problems or weaknesses
Projection of blame or responsibility
Hypersensitive to a discourtesy or criticism
Grandiosity
Rationalization of failures

Objective

Superior attitude toward others; ridicule of others; hostile laughter
Difficulty establishing or maintaining relationships
Alteration in reality testing; reality distortion
Insufficient participation in or follow-through with treatment
Sample Clinical Applications: Eating disorders, substance abuse, chronic illness; bipolar, adjustment, or dissociative disorders

DESIRED OUTCOMES/EVALUATION CRITERIA

Sample NOC linkages:
Acceptance: Health Status: Reconciliation to significant change in health circumstances
Coping: Personal actions to manage stressors that tax an individual's resources
Social Interaction Skills: An individual's use of effective interaction behaviors

Client Will (Include Specific Time Frame)

- Verbalize understanding of own problems and stressors.
- Identify areas of concern or problems.
- Demonstrate acceptance of responsibility for own actions, successes, and failures.
- Participate in treatment program or therapy.
- Maintain involvement in relationships.

ACTIONS/INTERVENTIONS

Sample NIC linkages:
Self-Awareness Enhancement: Assisting a patient to explore and understand his/her thoughts, feelings, motivations, and behaviors

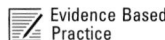

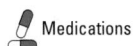

(continues on page 216)

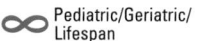

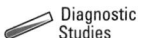

defensive Coping (continued)
Coping Enhancement: Assisting a patient to adapt to perceived stressors, changes, or threats that interfere with meeting life demands and roles
Counseling: Use of an interactive helping process focusing on the needs, problems, or feelings of the patient and significant others to enhance or support coping, problem solving, and interpersonal relationships

NURSING PRIORITY NO. 1 To determine degree of impairment:

- Assess ability to comprehend current situation, developmental level of functioning. *Crucial to planning care for this individual. Client will have difficulty functioning in these circumstances.*[1]
- Determine level of anxiety and effectiveness of current coping mechanisms. *Severe anxiety will interfere with ability to cope, and client will need to assess what is working and develop new ways to deal with current situation.*[2]
- Perform or review results of testing, such as the Taylor Manifest Anxiety Scale and Marlowe-Crowne Social Desirability Scale, as indicated. *Helps to identify coping styles, enabling more accurate therapeutic interventions.*[7]
- Determine coping mechanisms used (e.g., projection, avoidance, rationalization) and purpose of coping strategy (e.g., may mask low self-esteem). *Provides information about how these behaviors affect current situation.*[3]
- Assist client to identify and consider need to address problem differently. *Until client is willing to consider different approaches to dealing with situation, little progress can be expected.*[1]
- Describe all aspects of the problem through the use of therapeutic communication skills such as active-listening. *Provides an opportunity for the client to clarify the situation and begin to look at options for problem solving.*[2]
- Observe interactions with others. *Noting difficulties and ability to establish satisfactory relationships can provide clues to client behaviors that interfere with interactions with others.*[2]
- Note availability of family/friends support for client in current situation. *Significant others may not be supportive when person is denying problems or exhibiting unacceptable behaviors.*[6]
- Note expressions of grandiosity in the face of contrary evidence (e.g., "I'm going to buy a new car" when the individual has no job or available finances). *Evidence of distorted thinking and possibility of mental illness.*[3]
- Assess physical condition. *Defensive coping style has been connected with physical well-being and illnesses, especially chronic health concerns (e.g., congestive heart failure, diabetes, chronic fatigue syndrome).*[5]

NURSING PRIORITY NO. 2 To assist client to deal with current situation:

- Provide explanation of rules of the treatment program and discuss consequences of lack of cooperation. Encourage client participation in setting of consequences and agreement to them. *Promotes understanding and possibility of cooperation on the part of the client, especially when client has been involved in the decisions.*[2]
- Set limits on manipulative behavior; be consistent in enforcing consequences when rules are broken and limits tested. *Providing clear information and following through on identified consequences reduces the ability to manipulate staff or therapist and environment.*[3]
- Develop therapeutic relationship to enable client to test new behaviors in a safe environment. Use positive, nonjudgmental approach and "I" messages. *Promotes sense of self-esteem and enhances sense of control.*[1]
- Encourage control in all situations possible; include client in decisions and planning. *Preserves autonomy, enabling realization of sense of self-worth.*[1]
- Acknowledge individual strengths and incorporate awareness of personal assets and strengths in plan. *Promotes use of positive coping behaviors and progress toward effective solutions.*[4]
- Convey attitude of acceptance and respect (unconditional positive regard). *Avoids threatening client's self-concept, preserving existing self-esteem.*[2]
- Encourage identification and expression of feelings. *Provides opportunity for client to learn about and accept self and feelings as normal.*[2]

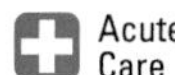

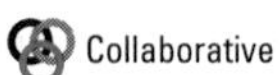

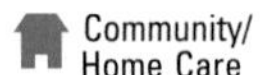

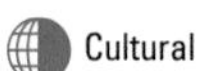

- Provide or encourage use of healthy outlets for release of hostile feelings (e.g., punching bags, pounding boards). Involve in outdoor recreation program when available. *Promotes acceptable expression of these feelings, which, when unexpressed, can lead to development of undesirable behaviors and make situation worse.*[4]
- Provide opportunities for client to interact with others in a positive manner. *Promotes self-esteem and encourages client to learn how to develop and enhance relationships.*[4]
- Assist client with problem-solving process. Identify and discuss responses to situation, maladaptive coping skills. Suggest alternative responses to situation. *Helps client select more adaptive strategies for coping.*[2]
- Use confrontation judiciously *to help client begin to identify defense mechanisms (e.g., denial, projection) that are hindering development of satisfying relationships.*[2]
- Assist with treatments for physical illnesses as appropriate. *Taking care of physical self will enable client to deal with emotional and psychological issues more effectively.*[4]

NURSING PRIORITY NO. 3 To promote wellness (Teaching/Discharge Considerations):

- Use cognitive-behavioral therapy. *Helps change negative thinking patterns when rigidly held beliefs are used by client to defend the individual against low self-esteem.*[3]
- Encourage client to learn and use relaxation techniques, guided imagery, and positive affirmation of self. *Enables client to incorporate and practice new behaviors to deal with stressors and view or respond to situation in a more realistic and positive manner.*[4]
- Promote involvement in activities or classes as appropriate. *Client can practice new skills, develop new relationships, and learn new and positive ways of interacting with others.*[1]
- Refer to additional resources (e.g., substance rehabilitation, family or marital therapy), as indicated. *Can be useful in making desired changes and developing new coping skills.*[2]
- Refer to ND ineffective Coping for additional interventions.

DOCUMENTATION FOCUS

Assessment/Reassessment

- Assessment findings, client perception of the present situation, presenting behaviors.
- Usual coping methods, degree of impairment.
- Health concerns.

Planning

- Plan of care, specific interventions, and who is involved in development of the plan.
- Teaching plan.

Implementation/Evaluation

- Response to interventions, teaching, and actions performed.
- Attainment or progress toward desired outcome(s).
- Modifications to plan of care.

Discharge Planning

- Referrals and follow-up programming.

References

1. Fowler, B. (2000). Inability to cope in Asperger's syndrome. Retrieved April 2015 from http://www.suite101.com/article.cfm/aspergers_syndrome/47938.
2. Gordon, B. N. (1981). Child temperament and adult behavior: An exploration of "goodness of fit." *Child Psychiatry Hum Dev*, 11(3), 167–178.
3. Dombeck, M., Wells-Moran, J. (Updated 2006). Coping strategies and defense mechanisms: Basic and intermediate defenses. MentalHelp.net. Retrieved April 2015 https://www.mentalhelp.net/articles/coping-strategies-and-defense-mechanisms-basic-and-intermediate-defenses/.

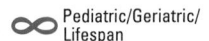

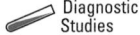

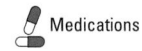

4. Vanderhyder, D. (2008). Stress management for caregivers of Alzheimer's using guided imagery. Retrieved April 2015 from http://caregiverhelp.blogspot.com/2008/06/stress-management-for-caregivers-of.html.
5. Creswell, C., Chalder, T. (2001). Defensive coping styles in chronic fatigue syndrome. *J Psychosom Res*, 51(4), 607–610.
6. Graham, M. (2011). Where to begin: Finding help during chronic illness. Retrieved April 2015 from http://invisibledisabilities.org/coping-with-invisible-disabilities/disability-benefits/finding-help/.
7. Hoyt, D. P., Magoon, T. M. (1954). A validation study of the Taylor Manifest Anxiety Scale. *J Clin Psychol*, 10(4), 357–361.

disabled family Coping

Taxonomy II: Coping/Stress Tolerance—Class 2 Coping Responses (00073) [**Diagnostic Division:** Social Interaction], Submitted 1980; Revised 1996, 2008

DEFINITION: Behavior of primary person (family member, significant other, or close friend) that disables his or her capacities and the client's capacities to effectively address tasks essential to either person's adaptation to the health challenge.

RELATED FACTORS

Chronically unexpressed feelings by support person
Differing coping styles between support person and client
Differing coping styles between support persons
Ambivalent family relationships
Inconsistent management of family's resistance to treatment

DEFINING CHARACTERISTICS

Subjective

[Expresses despair regarding family reactions or lack of involvement]

Objective

Psychosomatic symptoms
Intolerance; rejection; abandonment; desertion; agitation; aggression; hostility; depression
Performing routines without regard for client's needs; disregard for client's needs
Neglect of basic needs of client, or treatment regimen
Neglect of relationship with family member
Family behaviors detrimental to well-being
Distortion of reality about client's health problem
Impaired ability to structure a meaningful life; impaired individualization; prolonged hyperfocus on client
Adopts illness symptoms of client
Client's dependence

Sample Clinical Applications: Chronic conditions (e.g., chronic obstructive pulmonary disease [COPD], AIDS, Alzheimer's disease, chronic pain, renal failure, brain/spinal cord injury [SCI]), substance abuse, cancer, genetic conditions (e.g., Down syndrome, sickle cell disease, Huntington's disease), depression, hypochondriasis

DESIRED OUTCOMES/EVALUATION CRITERIA

Sample NOC linkages:

Family Normalization: Capacity of the family system to develop strategies for optimal functioning when a member has a chronic illness or disability
Family Coping: Family actions to manage stressors that tax family resources

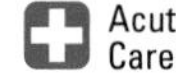

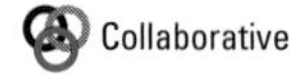

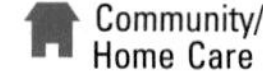

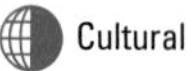

Caregiver Role Endurance: Factors that promote family care provider's capacity to sustain caregiving over extended period of time

Family Will (Include Specific Time Frame)

- Verbalize more realistic understanding and expectations of the client.
- Visit or contact client regularly.
- Participate positively in care of client, within limits of family's abilities and client's needs.
- Express feelings and expectations openly and honestly as appropriate.
- Access available resources/services to assist with required care.

ACTIONS/INTERVENTIONS

Sample NIC linkages:
Family Therapy: Assisting family members to move their family toward a more productive way of living
Family Support: Promotion of family values, interests, and goals
Family Involvement Promotion: Facilitating participation of family members in the emotional and physical care of the patient

NURSING PRIORITY NO. 1 To assess causative/contributing factors:

- Ascertain pre-illness behaviors and interactions of the family. *Provides comparative baseline for developing plan of care and determining interventions needed.*[4,8]
- Identify current behaviors of the family members (e.g., withdrawal or not visiting, brief visits, ignoring client when visiting; anger and hostility toward client and others; ways of touching between family members; expressions of guilt). *Indicators of extent of problems existing within family. Relationships among family members before and after current illness affect ability to deal with problems of caretaking and lengthy illness.*[1,8]
- Discuss family perceptions of situation. *Expectations of client and family members may not be realistic and may interfere with ability to deal with situation.*[6]
- Note cultural factors related to family relationships that may be involved in problems of caring for member who is ill. *Family composition and structure, methods of decision making, gender issues, and expectations will affect how family perceives situation and deals with stress of illness, negative prognosis.*[7]
- Note other factors that may be stressful for the family (e.g., financial difficulties or lack of community support, as when illness occurs when out of town). *Appropriate referrals can be made to provide information and assistance as needed. If not addressed, these problems can lead to caregiver burnout and compassion fatigue.*[6]
- Determine readiness of family members to be involved with care of the client. *Family members are involved in their lives, jobs, and families and may find it difficult to manage tasks necessary for helping with care of the client.*[5,6]

NURSING PRIORITY NO. 2 To provide assistance to enable family to deal with the current situation:

- Establish rapport with family members who are available. *Promotes therapeutic relationship and support for problem-solving solutions.*[1]
- Acknowledge difficulty of the situation for the family. *Communicates understanding of family's feelings and can reduce blaming and guilt feelings.*[2]
- Active-listen to concerns, note both overconcern and lack of concern. *Identifies accuracy of client's information and measure of concern, which may interfere with ability to resolve situation.*[2]
- Allow free expression of feelings, including frustration, anger, hostility, and hopelessness, while placing limits on acting out or inappropriate behaviors. *Provides opportunity to identify accuracy and validate appropriateness of feelings. Limits or minimizes risk of violent behavior.*[4]
- Give accurate information to SO(s) from the beginning. *Establishes trust and promotes opportunity for clarification and correction of misunderstandings.*[4]

- Act as liaison between family and healthcare providers. *Establishes single contact to provide explanations and clarify treatment plan, enhancing reliability of information.*[4]
- Provide brief, simple explanations about use and alarms when equipment (such as a ventilator) is required. Identify appropriate professional(s) for continued support and problem solving. *Having information and ready access to appropriate resources can reduce feelings of helplessness and promote sense of control.*[1]
- Provide time for private interaction between client and family/SO(s). *Individuals need to talk about what is happening and process new and frightening information to learn to deal with situation or diagnosis within family relationships.*[3]
- Accompany family when they visit client. *Being available for questions, concerns, and support promotes trusting relationship in which family feels free to learn all they can about situation or diagnosis.*[3]
- Assist SO(s) to initiate therapeutic communication with client. *Learning to use new methods of communication (active-listening and "I" messages) can enhance relationships and promote effective problem solving for the family.*[3]
- Include SO(s) in the plan of care. Provide instruction and demonstrate necessary skills. *Promotes family's ability to provide care and develop a sense of control over difficult situation.*[3,5]
- Refer client to protective services as necessitated by risk of physical harm or neglect. *Removing client from home is sometimes necessary to individual safety. May reduce stress on family to allow opportunity for therapeutic intervention.*[3]

NURSING PRIORITY NO. 3 To promote wellness (Teaching/Discharge Considerations):

- Assist family to identify coping skills being used and how these skills are or are not helping them deal with situation. *When family members know this information, they can begin to enhance those skills that are more effective in promoting healthy family functioning in difficult times.*[3]
- Answer family's questions patiently and honestly. Reinforce information provided by other providers. *Continues trusting relationship with family members and promotes understanding of the situation/prognosis so family members can deal more effectively with what is happening.*[1]
- Reframe negative expressions into positive whenever possible. *A positive frame contributes to supportive interactions and can lead to better outcomes.*[3]
- Respect family needs for withdrawal and intervene judiciously. *Situation may be overwhelming, and time away can be beneficial to continued participation. A brief respite can refresh family members who are serving as caregivers and permit renewed ability to manage situation.*[1]
- Encourage family to deal with the situation in small increments rather than trying to deal with the whole picture. *Reduces likelihood of individual being overwhelmed by possibilities that may face them in potentially disabling or fatal outcomes.*[1]
- Assist the family to identify familiar things that would be helpful to the client (e.g., a family picture on the wall), especially when hospitalized for a long time, such as in hospice or long-term care. *Reinforces and maintains orientation and provides a sense of home and family for client.*[1,5]
- Refer family to appropriate resources as needed (e.g., family therapy, financial counseling, spiritual advisor). *May need additional help to deal with difficult situation or illness.*[6]
- Refer to ND Grieving as appropriate.

DOCUMENTATION FOCUS

Assessment/Reassessment

- Assessment findings, current and past behaviors, family members who are directly involved and support systems available.
- Emotional response(s) to situation or stressors.
- Specific health and therapy challenges.

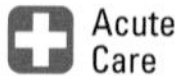

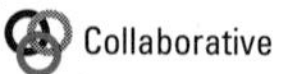

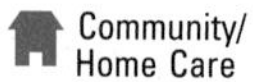

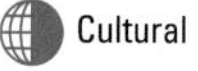

Planning

- Plan of care, specific interventions, and who is involved in planning.
- Teaching plan.

Implementation/Evaluation

- Responses of individuals to interventions, teaching, and actions performed.
- Attainment or progress toward desired outcome(s).
- Modifications to plan of care.

Discharge Planning

- Ongoing needs, available resources, other follow-up recommendations, and who is responsible for actions.
- Specific referrals made.

References

1. Schulz, R., Sherwood, P. R. (2008). Physical and mental health effects of family caregiving. *Am J Nurs*, 108(9 (Suppl)), S23–S27.
2. Feigin, R., Barnetz, Z., Davidson-Arad, B. (2008). Quality of life in family members coping with chronic illness in a relative: An exploratory study. *Families, Systems & Health*, 26(3), 267–281.
3. Murphy, E. (No date). Coping with disability. *Behavioral Health*. Retrieved April 2015 from http://www.mainlinehealth.org/Coping_with_Disability.
4. Zarit, S., Femia, E. (2008). Behavioral and psychosocial interventions for family caregivers. *Am J Nurs*, 108(9), 47–53.
5. Schumacher, K., Beck, C., Marren, J. (2006). Family caregivers: Caring for older adults, working with their families. *Am J Nurs*, 106(8), 40–49.
6. Sims, D. D. (No date). Mending the family circle: Coping with the death of a loved one. Retrieved April 2015 from http://www.touchstonesongrief.com/touchstones/articles/SURVIVING%20THE%20DEATH%20OF%20A%20LOVED%20ONE.pdf.
7. Gill, C. J. (1995). A brief history: Attitudes and treatment of persons with disabilities. Retrieved April 2015 from http://www.jik.com/ilarts.html.
8. Chawla, B. (2009). Psychosocial difficulties of parents with young children with severe disabilities. *Parenting Journals*. Retrieved April 2015 from http://www.parenting-journals.com/84/prominent-psychosocial-difficulties-that-parents-of-young-children-with-severe-disabilities-may-cope-with-during-their-child%e2%80%99s-early-years/.

ineffective Coping

Taxonomy II: Coping/Stress Tolerance—Class 2 Coping Responses (00069) [**Diagnostic Division:** Ego Integrity], Submitted 1978; Revised 1998

DEFINITION: Inability to form a valid appraisal of the stressors, inadequate choices of practiced responses, and/or inability to use available resources.

RELATED FACTORS

Situational or maturational crisis; inadequate opportunity to prepare for stressor
High degree of threat; inaccurate threat appraisal
Ineffective tension release strategies
Inadequate confidence in ability to deal with a situation; insufficient sense of control; uncertainty
Inadequate resources; insufficient social support
Ineffective tension release strategies
Inability to conserve adaptive energies

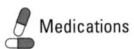

(continues on page 222)

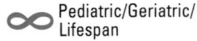

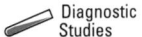

ineffective Coping (continued)
Gender differences in coping strategies
[Severe or chronic pain]

DEFINING CHARACTERISTICS

Subjective
Inability to deal with a situation, ask for help
Alteration in sleep pattern; fatigue
Substance abuse

Objective
Insufficient goal-directed behavior, problem solving, or problem resolution
Ineffective coping strategies
Inability to meet role expectation, basic needs
Insufficient access of social support
Alteration in concentration; inability to attend to information; difficulty organizing information
Change in communication pattern
Frequent illness
Risk-taking behavior
Destructive behavior toward self or others
Sample Clinical Applications: New diagnosis of major illness, chronic conditions, major depression, substance abuse, eating disorders, bipolar disorder, social anxiety disorder, pregnancy, parenting

DESIRED OUTCOMES/EVALUATION CRITERIA

Sample NOC linkages:
Coping: Personal actions to manage stressors that tax an individual's resources
Impulse Self-Control: Self-restraint of compulsive or impulsive behaviors
Decision Making: Ability to make judgments and choose between two or more alternatives

Client Will (Include Specific Time Frame)
- Assess the current situation accurately.
- Identify ineffective coping behaviors and consequences.
- Verbalize awareness of own coping abilities.
- Verbalize feelings congruent with behavior.
- Meet psychological needs as evidenced by appropriate expression of feelings, identification of options, and use of resources.

ACTIONS/INTERVENTIONS

Sample NIC linkages:
Coping Enhancement: Assisting a patient to adapt to perceived stressors, changes, or threats that interfere with meeting life demands and roles
Decision-Making Support: Providing information and support for a person who is making a decision regarding health care
Impulse Control Training: Assisting the patient to mediate impulsive behavior through application of problem-solving strategies to social and interpersonal situations

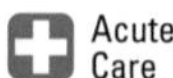
Acute Care
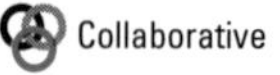
Collaborative
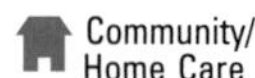
Community/ Home Care
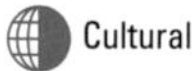
Cultural

NURSING PRIORITY NO. 1 To determine degree of impairment:

- Identify individual stressors (e.g., family, social, work environment, life changes or nursing/healthcare management). *Helps define problem(s), providing a starting point for intervention.*[1]
- Evaluate ability to understand events, provide realistic appraisal of situation. *Necessary information for developing workable plan of care.*[2]
- Identify developmental level of functioning. *People tend to regress to a lower developmental stage during illness or crisis, and recognition of client's level enables more appropriate interventions to be implemented.*[2]
- Assess current functional capacity and note how it is affecting the individual's coping ability. *Promotes identification of strategies that will be helpful in current situation.*[4]
- Determine alcohol intake, drug use, smoking habits, and sleeping and eating patterns. *Substance abuse impairs ability to deal with what is happening in current situation. Identification of impaired sleeping and eating patterns provides clues to extent of anxiety and impaired coping.*[2,3,16]
- Ascertain impact of illness on sexual needs and relationship. *Illnesses, medications, and many treatment regimens can affect sexual functioning, further stressing coping ability.*[2,3]
- Assess level of anxiety and coping on an ongoing basis. *Identifies changes in ability to cope and worsening of ability to understand at an early stage where intervention can be most effective.*[4]
- Note speech and communication patterns. Be aware of negative or catastrophizing thinking. *Identifies existing problems and assesses ability to understand situation and communicate needs.*[7,15]
- Observe and describe behavior in objective terms. Validate observations. *Promotes accuracy and assures correctness of conclusions to arrive at the best possible solutions.*[7]

NURSING PRIORITY NO. 2 To assess coping abilities and skills:

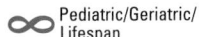

- Ascertain client's understanding of current situation and its impact on life and work. *Client may not understand situation, and being aware of these factors is necessary to planning care and identifying appropriate interventions.*[8]
- Active-listen and identify client's perceptions of what is happening and effectiveness of coping techniques. *Reflecting client's thoughts can provide a forum for understanding perceptions in relation to reality for planning care and determining accuracy of interventions needed.*[2,3]
- Discuss cultural background and whether some beliefs from family may contribute to difficulties coping with situation. *Family of origin can have a positive or negative effect on individual's ability to deal with stressful situations.*[5]
- Evaluate client's decision-making ability. *When ability to make decisions is impaired by illness or treatment regimen, it is important to take this into consideration when planning care to maximize participation and positive outcomes.*[9]
- Determine previous methods of dealing with life problems. *Identifies successful techniques that can be used in current situation. Often client is preoccupied by current concerns and does not think about previous successful skills.*[8]

NURSING PRIORITY NO. 3 To assist client to deal with current situation:

- Call client by name. Ascertain how client prefers to be addressed. *Using client's name enhances sense of self and promotes individuality and self-esteem.*[2]
- Encourage communication with staff/significant others (SOs). *Developing positive interactions between staff, SO(s), and client ensures that everyone has the same understanding.*[8]
- Use reality orientation (e.g., clocks, calendars, bulletin boards) and make frequent references to time and place as indicated. Place needed and familiar objects within sight for visual cues. *Often client can be disoriented by changes in routine, anxiety about illness and treatment regimens, and these measures help the client maintain orientation and a sense of reality.*[9]

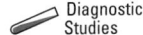

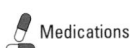

- Provide for continuity of care with same personnel taking care of the client as often as possible. *Developing relationships with same caregivers promotes trust and enables client to discuss concerns and fears freely.*[9]
- Explain disease process, procedures, or events in a simple, concise manner. Devote time for listening. *May help client to express emotions, grasp situation, and feel more in control.*[10]
- Discuss use of medications as needed. *Short-term use of anti-anxiety medication or antidepressants may be helpful for lifting mood and encouraging individual to develop new coping skills.*[6]
- Provide for a quiet environment and position equipment out of view as much as possible. *Anxiety is increased by noisy surroundings.*[8]
- Schedule activities so periods of rest alternate with nursing care. Increase activity slowly. *Client is weakened by illness and failure to cope with situation. Ensuring rest can promote ability to cope.*[8]
- Assist client in use of diversion, recreation, and relaxation techniques. *Learning new skills can be helpful for reducing stress and will be useful in the future as the client learns to cope more successfully.*[8]
- Emphasize positive body responses to medical conditions, but do not negate the seriousness of the situation (e.g., stable blood pressure during gastric bleed or improved body posture in depressed client). *Acknowledging the reality of the illness while accurately stating the facts can provide hope and encouragement.*[8]
- Encourage client to try new coping behaviors and gradually master situation. *Practicing new ways of dealing with what is happening leads to being more comfortable and can promote a positive outcome as client relaxes and handles illness and treatment regimen more successfully.*[9]
- Confront client when behavior is inappropriate, pointing out difference between words and actions. *Provides external locus of control, enhancing safety while client learns self-control.*[2]
- Assist in dealing with change in concept of body image as appropriate. (Refer to ND disturbed Body Image.) *New view of self may be negative, and client needs to incorporate change in a positive manner to enhance self-image.*[11]

NURSING PRIORITY NO. 4 To provide for meeting psychological needs:

- Treat the client with courtesy and respect. Converse at client's level, providing meaningful conversation while performing care. *Enhances therapeutic relationship.*[2]
- Take advantage of teachable moments. *Individuals learn best and are open to new information when they feel accepted and are in a comfortable environment.*[11]
- Allow client to react in own way without judgment by staff/caregivers. Provide support and diversion as indicated. *Unconditional positive regard and support promote acceptance, enabling client to deal with difficult situation in a positive way.*[8]
- Encourage verbalization of fears and anxieties and expression of feelings of denial, depression, and anger. *Free expression allows for dealing with these feelings, and when the client knows that these are normal reactions, he or she can deal with them better.*[11]
- Help client to learn how to substitute positive thoughts for negative ones (i.e., "I can do this; I am in charge of myself"). *The mind plays a significant role in one's response to stressors, and negative thoughts can actually increase the impact of the stressor.*[15]
- Provide opportunity for expression of sexual concerns. *Important aspect of person that may be difficult to express. Providing an opening for discussion by asking sensitive questions allows client to talk about concerns.*[11]
- Help client to set limits on acting-out behaviors and learn ways to express emotions in an acceptable manner. *Enables client to gain sense of self-esteem, promoting internal locus of control.*[2]

NURSING PRIORITY NO. 5 To promote wellness (Teaching/Discharge Considerations):

- Give updated or additional information needed about events, cause (if known), and potential course of illness as soon as possible. *Knowledge helps reduce anxiety or fear and allows client to deal with reality.*[8]

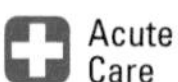

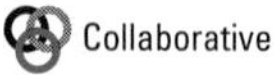

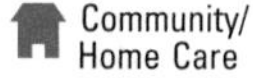

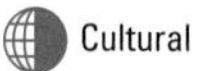

- Provide and encourage an atmosphere of realistic hope. *Promotes optimistic outlook, energizing client to address situation. Client needs to hear positive things while undergoing difficult circumstances.*[8]
- Give information about purposes and side effects of medications and treatments. *Client feels included (promoting sense of control), enabling client to cope with situation in a more positive manner.*[8]
- Emphasize importance of follow-up care. *Checkups verify that regimen is being followed accurately and that healing is progressing to promote a satisfactory outcome.*[8]
- Encourage and support client in evaluating lifestyle, occupation, and leisure activities. *Helps client to look at difficult areas that may contribute to anxiety and ability to cope, to make changes gradually without undue or debilitating anxiety.*[8,16]
- Discuss effects of stressors (e.g., family, social, work environment, or nursing/healthcare management) and ways to deal with them. *Addressing these factors will enable client to develop strategies to make changes needed to promote wellness.*[8]
- Provide for gradual implementation and continuation of necessary behavior or lifestyle changes. *Change is difficult, and beginning slowly enhances commitment to plan.*[8]
- Discuss or review anticipated procedures and client concerns, as well as postoperative expectations when surgery is recommended. *Knowledge allays fears and helps client to understand procedures and treatments and expected results. When client has prior information about what to expect during postoperative course, he or she will remain calm, anxiety will be reduced, and client will cope more effectively with situation.*[11,14]
- Refer to outside resources and professional therapy as indicated or ordered. *May be necessary to assist with long-term improvement.*[11]
- Determine desire for religious representative or spiritual counselor and facilitate arrangements for visit. *Spiritual needs are an integral part of being human, and determining and meeting individual preferences help client deal with concerns and desires for discussion or assistance in this area.*[12]
- Provide information or consultation as indicated for sexual concerns. Provide privacy when client is not in home. *Individuals are sexual beings, and concerns about role in family/relationship and ability to function are often not readily expressed. Discussion opens opportunity for clarification and understanding and helps to meet need for intimacy.*[11]
- Refer to other NDs as indicated (e.g., Anxiety, impaired verbal Communication, acute/chronic Pain, risk for self-/other-directed Violence). *Provides further assistance in area of identified need.*[13]

DOCUMENTATION FOCUS

Assessment/Reassessment

- Baseline findings, degree of impairment, and client's perceptions of situation.
- Coping abilities and previous ways of dealing with life problems.

Planning

- Plan of care, specific interventions, and who is involved in planning.
- Teaching plan.

Implementation/Evaluation

- Client's responses to interventions, teaching, and actions performed.
- Medication dose, time, and client's response.
- Attainment or progress toward desired outcome(s).
- Modifications to plan of care.

Discharge Planning

- Long-term needs and actions to be taken.
- Support systems available, specific referrals made, and who is responsible for actions to be taken.

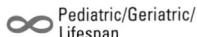

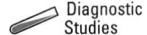

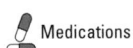

References

1. Sahel, J. A., Bandello, F., Augustin, A., et al. (2007). Health-related quality of life and utility in patients with age-related macular degeneration. *Arch Ophthalmol*, 125(7), 945–951.
2. McCoy, M. L. (2006). Care of the congestive heart failure patient: The care, cure, and core model. *J Pract Nurs*, 56(1), 5–30.
3. Murphy, E. (No date). Coping with disability. *Behavioral Health*. Retrieved April 2015 from http://www.mainlinehealth.org/Coping_with_Disability.
4. Zarit, S., Femia, E. (2008). Behavioral and psychosocial interventions for family caregivers. *Am J Nurs*, 108(9), 47–53.
5. Wilner, A. N. (2008). Patients' cultural and spiritual beliefs influence their diagnosis, treatment and management. *APA*. Retrieved March 2015 from http://www.medscape.com/viewarticle/574203_1.
6. Watkins, E. (2003). Combining cognitive therapy with medication in bipolar disorder. *Adv Psychiatr Treat*, 9, 106–110.
7. Rosland, A. M., Heisler, M., Piette, J. D. (2012). The impact of family behaviors and communication patterns on chronic illness outcomes: A systematic review. *J Behav Med*, 35(2), 221–239.
8. Cherif, M., Younis, E. I. (2000). Liver transplantation. *Clin Fam Prac*, 2(1), 117.
9. Liken, M. A. (2001). Caregivers in crisis: Moving a relative with Alzheimer's to assisted living. *Clin Nurs Res*, 10(1), 53–69.
10. Henderson, D., Henderson, K. (No date). Choosing a nutritional supplement, or multivitamin, for Meniere's Disease. Retrieved March 2015 from http://www.menieres-disease.ca/health_reports/choosing-nutritional-supplements.htm.
11. Tan, G., Waldman, K., Bostick, R. (2002). Psychosocial issues, sexuality, and cancer. *Sex Disabil*, 20(4), 297–318.
12. Geiter, H. (2002). The spiritual side of nursing. *RN*, 65(5), 43–44.
13. Maryland Department of Human Services. (2009). In-home family preservation services. Retrieved April 2015 from http://www.dhr.state.md.us/blog/?page_id=4675.
14. Headsets911. (No date). Actively coping with stress. Retrieved April 2015 from www.headsets911.com/activecoping.htm.
15. Carpenter, J. (No date). Women and leadership: The role of confidence and active coping. PP slides. Retrieved April 2015 from http://www.advance.latech.edu/pdf/Women_Leadership_Self-Confidence_and_Active_Coping.Lunch.pdf.
16. Franke, J. (1999). Stress, burnout, and addiction. *Tex Med*, 95(3), 43–52.

ineffective community Coping

Taxonomy II: Coping/Stress Tolerance—Class 2 Coping Responses (00077) [**Diagnostic Division:** Social Interaction], Submitted 1994; Revised 1998

DEFINITION: A pattern of community activities for adaptation and problem solving that is unsatisfactory for meeting the demands or needs of the community.

RELATED FACTORS

Insufficient community resources (e.g., respite, recreation, social support services)
Inadequate resources for problem solving
Nonexistent community systems
History of/exposure to disaster (e.g., natural or man-made)

DEFINING CHARACTERISTICS

Subjective

Community does not meet expectations of its members
Perceived community vulnerability, powerlessness
Excessive stress

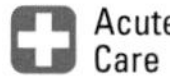
Acute Care
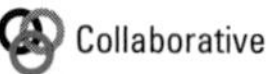
Collaborative
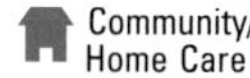
Community/ Home Care
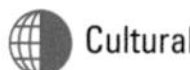
Cultural

Objective

Deficient community participation
Excessive community conflict
Elevated community illness rate
High incidence of community problems (e.g., homicides, vandalism, robbery, terrorism, abuse, unemployment, poverty, militancy, mental illness)
Sample Clinical Applications: High rate of illness, injury, or violence in community

DESIRED OUTCOMES/EVALUATION CRITERIA

Sample NOC linkages:

Community Competence: Capacity of a community to collectively problem solve to achieve community goals
Community Health Status: General state of well-being of a community or population
Community Disaster Readiness: Community preparedness to respond to a natural or man-made calamitous event

Community Will (Include Specific Time Frame)

- Recognize negative and positive factors affecting community's ability to meet its demands or needs.
- Identify alternatives to inappropriate activities for adaptation and problem solving.
- Report a measurable increase in necessary or desired activities to improve community functioning.

ACTIONS/INTERVENTIONS

Sample NIC linkages:

Community Health Development: Assisting members of a community to identify a community's health concerns, mobilize resources, and implement solutions
Environmental Management: Community: Monitoring and influencing of the physical, social, cultural, economic, and political conditions that affect the health of groups and communities
Community Disaster Preparedness: Preparing for an effective response to a large-scale disaster

NURSING PRIORITY NO. 1 To identify causative or precipitating factors:

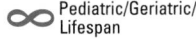

- Evaluate community activities as related to meeting collective needs within the community itself and between the community and the larger society. *Determines what activities are currently available and what needs are not being met, either by the local or county/state entities. Provides information on which to base the steps needed to begin planning for desired changes.*[1]
- Note community reports of community functioning (e.g., immunization status, transportation, water supply, financing), including areas of weakness or conflict. *Community is responsible for identifying needed changes for possible action.*[1]
- Identify effects of Related Factors on community activities. Note immediate needs (e.g., healthcare, food, shelter, funds). *Provides a baseline to determine community needs, and identifying factors that are pertinent to the community allows community to deal with current concerns.*[1,5]
- Plan for the possibility of a disaster when determined by current circumstances. *In relation to threats, terrorist activities, and natural disasters, actions need to be coordinated between the local and the larger community.*[5]
- Determine availability and use of resources. *Helpful to begin planning to correct deficiencies that have been identified. Sometimes even though resources are available, they are not being appropriately or fully used.*[2]
- Identify unmet demands or needs of the community. *Determining deficiencies is a crucial step to developing an accurate plan for correction. Sometimes elected bodies see the problems differently from the general*

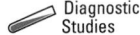

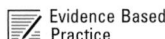

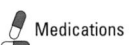

population and conflict can arise; therefore, it is important for communication to resolve the issues that are in question.[2]

NURSING PRIORITY NO. 2 To assist the community to reactivate/develop skills to deal with needs:

- Determine community strengths. *Promotes understanding of ways in which community is already meeting identified needs, and once identified, they can be built on to develop plan to improve community.*[1]
- Identify and prioritize community goals. *Goals enable the identification of actions to direct the changes that are needed to improve the community. Prioritizing enables actions to be taken in order of importance.*[1]
- Encourage community members/groups to engage in problem-solving activities. *Individuals who are involved in the problem-solving process and make a commitment to the solutions have an investment and are more apt to follow through on their commitments.*[3,5]
- Develop a plan jointly with community to deal with deficits in support. *Working together will enhance efforts and help to meet identified goals.*[3,5]

NURSING PRIORITY NO. 3 To promote wellness as related to community health:

- Create plans managing interactions within the community itself and between the community and the larger society. *These activities will meet collective needs.*[1]
- Assist the community to form partnerships within the community and between the community and the larger society. *Promotes long-term development of the community to deal with current and future problems.*[1]
- Provide channels for dissemination of information to the community as a whole (e.g., Web sites, print media; radio and TV reports, community bulletin boards; speakers' bureau; reports to committees, councils, advisory boards on file and accessible to the public). *Having information readily available for everyone provides opportunity for all members of the community to know what is being planned and have input into the planning. Keeping community informed promotes understanding of needs and plans and probability of follow-through to successful outcomes.*[1]
- Make information available in different modalities and geared to differing educational levels and cultural and ethnic populations of the community. *Ensures understanding by all members of the community and promotes cooperation with planning and follow-through.*[1]
- Seek out and evaluate underserved populations, including the homeless. *These members of the community often need to be helped to become productive citizens and be involved in the changes that are occurring.*[3]
- Work with community members to identify lifestyle changes that can be made to meet the goals identified to improve community deficits. *Changing lifestyles can promote a sense of power and encourage members to become involved in improving their community.*[4,5]

DOCUMENTATION FOCUS

Assessment/Reassessment

- Assessment findings, including perception of community members regarding problems.
- Availability of resources.

Planning

- Plan of care and who is involved in planning.
- Teaching plan.

Implementation/Evaluation

- Response of community entities to plan, interventions, and actions performed.
- Attainment or progress toward desired outcome(s).
- Modifications to plan of care.

Discharge Planning

- Long-term plans and who is responsible for actions to be taken.

References

1. Lindamer, L. A., Lebowitz, B., Hough, R. L., et al. (2009). Establishing an implementation network: Lessons learned from community-based participatory research. *Implement Science*, 4(17). Retrieved October 2015 from http://www.implementationscience.com/content/4/1/17.
2. Hunt, R. (1998). Community-based nursing. *Am J Nurs*, 98(10), 44.
3. Schraeder, C., Lamb, G., Shelton, P., et al. (1997). Community nursing organizations: A new frontier. *Am J Nurs*, 97(1), 63.
4. Lai, S. C., Cohen, M. N. (1999). Promoting lifestyle changes. *Am J Nurs*, 99(4), 63.
5. Cohn, M. (No date listed). The importance of community relations. Retrieved February 2012 from http://www.evancarmichael.com/Public-Relations/216/The-Importance-of-Community-Relations.html.

readiness for enhanced Coping

Taxonomy II: Coping/Stress Tolerance—Class 2 Coping Responses (00158) **[Diagnostic Division:** Ego Integrity], Submitted 2002; Revised 2013

DEFINITION: A pattern of cognitive and behavioral efforts to manage demands related to well-being, which can be strengthened.

DEFINING CHARACTERISTICS

Subjective

Expresses desire to enhance knowledge of stress management strategies, management of stressors
Expresses desire to enhance use of emotion-oriented/problem-oriented strategies
Expresses desire to enhance social support
Awareness of possible environmental change

Sample Clinical Applications: Chronic health conditions (e.g., asthma, diabetes mellitus, arthritis, systemic lupus, multiple sclerosis [MS], AIDS), mental health concerns (e.g., seasonal affective disorder, attention deficit disorder, Down syndrome)

DESIRED OUTCOMES/EVALUATION CRITERIA

Sample NOC linkages:

Coping: Personal actions to manage stressors that tax an individual's resources
Personal Well-Being: Extent of positive perception of one's health status
Quality of Life: Extent of positive perception of current life circumstances

Client Will (Include Specific Time Frame)

- Assess current situation accurately.
- Identify effective coping behaviors currently being used.
- Verbalize feelings congruent with behavior.
- Meet psychological needs as evidenced by appropriate expression of feelings, identification of options, and use of resources.

ACTIONS/INTERVENTIONS

Sample NIC linkages:

Coping Enhancement: Assisting a patient to adapt to perceived stressors, changes, or threats that interfere with meeting life demands and roles

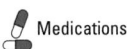

(continues on page 230)

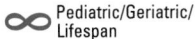

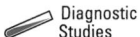

readiness for enhanced Coping (continued)

Self-Awareness Enhancement: Assisting a patient to explore and understand his or her thoughts, feelings, motivations, and behaviors

Self-Modification Assistance: Reinforcement of self-directed change initiated by the patient to achieve personally important goals

NURSING PRIORITY NO. 1 To determine needs and desire for improvement:

- Evaluate client's understanding of situation and ability to provide realistic appraisal of situation. *Provides information about client's perception, cognitive ability, and whether the client is aware of the facts of the situation, which reveals essential information for planning care.*[1]
- Determine stressors that may be affecting client. *Accurate identification of situation that client is dealing with provides information for planning interventions to enhance coping abilities.*[1]
- Ascertain motivation and expectations for change. *Motivation to improve and high expectations can encourage client to make changes that will improve his or her life. However, presence of external locus of control or unrealistic expectations may hamper efforts.*[5]
- Identify social supports available to client. *Available support systems, such as family/friends, can provide client with ability to handle current stressful events, and "talking it out" with an empathic listener will help client move forward to enhance coping skills.*[2]
- Review coping strategies client is aware of and currently using. *The desire to improve one's coping ability is based on an awareness of the status of the stressful situation.*[2]
- Determine use of alcohol or other drugs and smoking habits during times of stress. *Recognition of potential for substituting these actions or old habits to deal with anxiety increases individual's awareness of opportunity to choose new ways to cope with life stressors.*[6]
- Assess level of anxiety and coping on an ongoing basis. *Provides baseline to develop plan of care to improve coping abilities.*[2]
- Note speech and communication patterns. *Assesses ability to understand and provides information necessary to help client make progress in desire to enhance coping abilities.*[2]
- Evaluate client's decision-making ability. *Understanding client's ability provides a starting point for developing plan and determining what information client needs to develop more effective coping skills.*[1]

NURSING PRIORITY NO. 2 To assist client to develop enhanced coping skills:

- Active-listen and clarify client's perceptions of current status. *Reflecting client's statements and thoughts can provide a forum for understanding perceptions in relation to reality for planning care and determining accuracy of interventions needed.*[4]
- Review previous methods of dealing with life problems. *Enables client to identify successful techniques used in the past, promoting feelings of confidence in own ability.*[2]
- Discuss desire to improve ability to manage stressors of life. *Understanding client's decision to seek new information to enhance life will help client determine what is needed to learn new coping skills.*[2]
- Discuss understanding of concept of knowing what can and cannot be changed. *Acceptance of reality that some things cannot be changed allows client to focus energies on dealing with things that can be changed.*[6]
- Help client strengthen problem-solving skills. *Learning the process for problem solving will promote successful resolution of potentially stressful situations that arise.*[4,6]

NURSING PRIORITY NO. 3 To promote optimal well-being (Teaching/Learning Considerations):

- Discuss predisposing factors related to individual's response to stress. *Understanding that genetic influences, past experiences, and existing conditions determine whether a person's response is adaptive or maladaptive will give client a base on which to continue to learn what is needed to improve life.*[3]

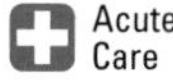

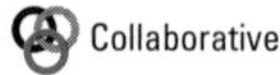

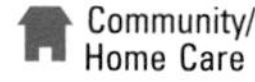

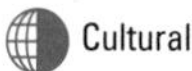

- Encourage client to develop a stress-management program. *An individualized program of relaxation, meditation, etc., enhances sense of balance in life and strengthens client's ability to manage challenging situations.*[5]
- Recommend involvement in activities of interest, such as exercise/sports, music, and art. *Individuals must decide for themselves what coping strategies are adaptive for them. Most people find enjoyment and relaxation in these kinds of activities.*[6]
- Discuss possibility of doing volunteer work in an area of the client's choosing. *Many individuals report satisfaction in giving of themselves—involvement with caring for others/pets, and client may find sense of fulfillment in service to others.*[1]
- Refer to classes and/or reading material and Web sites, as appropriate. *May be helpful to further learning and pursuing goal of enhanced coping ability.*[1]

DOCUMENTATION FOCUS

Assessment/Reassessment

- Baseline information, client's perception of need to enhance abilities.
- Coping abilities and previous ways of dealing with life problems.
- Motivation and expectation for change.

Planning

- Plan of care, specific interventions, and who is involved in planning.
- Teaching plan.

Implementation/Evaluation

- Client's responses to interventions, teaching, and actions performed.
- Attainment or progress toward desired outcome(s).
- Modifications to plan of care.

Discharge Planning

- Long-term needs and actions to be taken.
- Support systems available, specific referrals made, and who is responsible for actions to be taken.

References

1. Cancer Council NSW. (2013). Your coping toolbox. Retrieved October 2015 from http://www.cancercouncil.com.au/2448/cancer-information/general-information-cancer-information/when-you-are-first-diagnosed/emotions-and-cancer/your-coping-toolbox/.
2. Robinson, L., Smith, M. A., Segal, R. (2008). Stress management—how to reduce, prevent, and cope with stress. Retrieved October 2015 from http://www.helpguide.org/articles/stress/stress-management.htm.
3. Ryan, R. M., Deci, E. L. (2000). Self-determination theory and the facilitation of intrinsic motivation, social development, and well-being. *Am Psychol*, 55(1), 68–76.
4. Gordon, T. Getting what you need every time—Method III. Gordon Training International. Retrieved October 2015 from http://www.gordontraining.com/free-parenting-articles/get-what-you-need-every-time-method-iii/.
5. Evans, S., Tsao, J. C., Sternlieb, S., et al. (2009). Using the biopsychosocial model to understand the health benefits of yoga. *J Complement Integr Med*, 6(1), 1–22.
6. Kumarmahi, Coping—What you need to know. Retrieved October 2015 from http://www.articlesbase.com/stress-management-articles/coping-what-you-need-to-know-1346878.html.

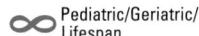

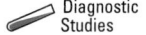

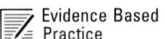

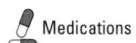

readiness for enhanced community Coping

Taxonomy II: Coping/Stress Tolerance—Class 2 Coping Responses (00076) [**Diagnostic Division:** Social Interaction], Submitted 1994; Revised 2013

DEFINITION: A pattern of community activities for adaptation and problem solving for meeting the demands or needs of the community, which can be strengthened.

DEFINING CHARACTERISTICS

Subjective

Expresses desire to enhance problem solving for identified issue, planning for predictable stressors
Expresses desire to enhance community responsibility for stress management, resources for managing stressors
Expresses desire to enhance communication among community members, between aggregates and larger community
Expresses desire to enhance availability of community recreation/relaxation programs

DESIRED OUTCOMES/EVALUATION CRITERIA

Sample NOC linkages:

Community Competence: Capacity of a community to collectively problem solve to achieve community goals
Community Health Status: General state of well-being of a community or population
Community Disaster Readiness: Community preparedness to respond to a natural or man-made calamitous event

Community Will (Include Specific Time Frame)

- Identify positive and negative factors affecting management of current and future problems/stressors.
- Have an established plan in place to deal with identified problems and stressors.
- Describe management of challenges in characteristics that indicate effective coping.
- Report a measurable increase in ability to deal with problems and stressors.

ACTIONS/INTERVENTIONS

Sample NIC linkages:

Program Development: Planning, implementing, and evaluating a coordinated set of activities designed to enhance wellness, or to prevent, reduce, or eliminate one or more health problems for a group or community
Environmental Management: Community: Monitoring and influencing of the physical, social, cultural, economic, and political conditions that affect the health of groups and communities
Health Policy Monitoring: Surveillance and influence of government and organization regulations, rules, and standards that affect nursing systems and practices to ensure quality care of patients

NURSING PRIORITY NO. 1 To determine existence of and deficits or weaknesses in management of current and future problems/stressors:

- Review community plan for dealing with problems and stressors, untoward events such as natural disaster or terrorist activity. *Provides a baseline for comparisons of preparedness with other communities and developing plan to address concerns.*[4]

Acute Care

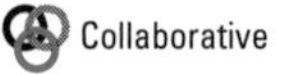
Collaborative

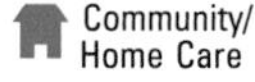
Community/ Home Care

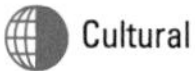
Cultural

- Assess effects of Related Factors on management of problems and stressors. *Identifying social supports available and awareness of the power of the community can enhance the plans needed to improve the community.*[1]
- Identify limitations in current pattern of community activities, such as transportation, water needs, and roads. *Recognition of the factors that can be improved through adaptation and problem solving will make it easier for the community to proceed with planning to make necessary improvements.*[3]
- Evaluate community activities as related to management of problems and stressors within the community itself and between the community and the larger society. *Disasters occurring in a community (or in the country as a whole) affect the local community and need to be recognized and addressed.*[4]

NURSING PRIORITY NO. 2 To assist the community in adaptation and problem solving for management of current and future needs/stressors:

- Define and discuss current needs and anticipated or projected concerns. *Agreement on scope and parameters of needs is essential for effective planning.*
- Determine community's strengths. *Plan can build on strengths to address areas of weakness.*
- Identify and prioritize goals to facilitate accomplishment. *Helps to bring the community together to meet a common concern or threat, maintain focus, and facilitate accomplishment.*[4]
- Identify and interact with available resources (e.g., persons, groups, financial, governmental, as well as other communities). *Promotes cooperation. Major catastrophes, such as earthquakes, floods, and terrorist activity, affect more than the local community, and communities need to work together to deal with and accomplish reconstruction and future growth.*[5]
- Make a joint plan with the community and the larger community to deal with adaptation and problem solving. *Promotes management of problems and stressors to enable most effective solution for identified concern.*[2]
- Seek out and involve underserved and at-risk groups within the community, including the homeless. *Supports communication and commitment of community as a whole.*[2]

NURSING PRIORITY NO. 3 To promote optimal well-being of community:

- Assist the community to form partnerships within the community and between the community and the larger society. *Promotes long-term developmental growth of the community.*[4]
- Support development of plans for maintaining these interactions.[5]
- Establish mechanism for self-monitoring of community needs and evaluation of efforts. *Facilitates proactive—rather than reactive—responses by the community.*[5]
- Use multiple formats to disseminate information, such as TV, radio, print media, and billboards, as well as computer bulletin boards, speakers' bureau, and reports to community leaders and groups on file and accessible to the public. *Keeps community informed regarding plans, needs, and outcomes to encourage continued understanding and participation.*[5]

DOCUMENTATION FOCUS

Assessment/Reassessment

- Assessment findings and community's perception of situation.
- Identified areas of concern, community strengths and weaknesses.

Planning

- Plan and who is involved and responsible for each action.
- Teaching plan.

Implementation/Evaluation

- Response of community entities to the actions performed.
- Attainment or progress toward desired outcomes.
- Modifications to plan.

Discharge Planning
- Short- and long-term plans to deal with current, anticipated, and potential problems and who is responsible for follow-through.
- Specific referrals made, coalitions formed.

References

1. Horowitz, C., Davis, M. H., Palermo, A. G., et al. (2000). Approaches to eliminating sociocultural disparities in health. *Health Care Financ Rev*, 21(4), 57–74.
2. Schaeder, C., Lamb, G., Shelton, P., et al. (1997). Community nursing organizations: A new frontier. *Am J Nurs*, 97(1), 63.
3. Lai, S. C., Cohen, M. N. (1999). Promoting lifestyle changes. *Am J Nurs*, 99(4), 63.
4. Gordon, T. Getting what you need every time—Method III. Gordon Training International. Retrieved October 2015 from http://www.gordontraining.com/free-parenting-articles/get-what-you-need-every-time-method-iii/.
5. Smith, K. (2002). Public heath nursing. *Encyclopedia of Public Health*. Retrieved October 2015 from http://www.encyclopedia.com/doc/1G2-3404000702.html.

readiness for enhanced family Coping

Taxonomy II: Coping/Stress Tolerance—Class 2 Coping Responses (00075) [**Diagnostic Division:** Social Interaction], Submitted 1980; Revised 2013

DEFINITION: A pattern of management of adaptive tasks by primary person (family member, significant other, or close friend) involved with the client's health change, which can be strengthened.

DEFINING CHARACTERISTICS

Subjective
Expresses desire to acknowledge growth impact of crisis
Expresses desire to enhance connection with others who have experienced a similar situation
Expresses desire to choose experiences that optimize wellness
Expresses desire to enhance health promotion, enrichment of lifestyle
Sample Clinical Applications: Genetic disorders (e.g., Down syndrome, cystic fibrosis, neural tube defects), traumatic injury (e.g., amputation, spinal cord), chronic conditions (e.g., asthma, AIDS, Alzheimer's disease)

DESIRED OUTCOMES/EVALUATION CRITERIA

Sample NOC linkages:
Family Normalization: Capacity of the family system to develop strategies for optimal functioning when a member has a chronic illness or disability
Family Coping: Family actions to manage stressors that tax family resources
Family Functioning: Capacity of the family system to meet the needs of its members during developmental transitions

Family Will (Include Specific Time Frame)
- Express willingness to look at own role in the family's growth.
- Verbalize desire to undertake tasks leading to change.
- Report feelings of self-confidence and satisfaction with progress being made.

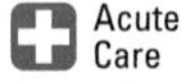

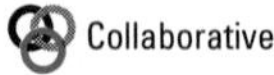

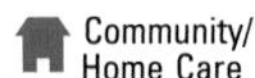

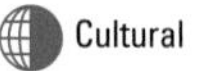

ACTIONS/INTERVENTIONS

Sample NIC linkages:
Normalization Promotion: Assisting parents and other family members of children with chronic diseases or disabilities in providing normal life experiences for their children and families
Family Support: Promotion of family values, interests, and goals
Family Involvement Promotion: Facilitating family participation in the emotional and physical care of the patient

NURSING PRIORITY NO. 1 To assess situation and adaptive skills being used by the family members:

- Determine individual situation and stage of growth family is experiencing and demonstrating. *Essential elements needed to identify family needs and develop plan of care for improving communication and interactions. Changes that are occurring may help family adapt, grow, and thrive when faced with these transitional events.*[1,6]
- Ascertain motivation and expectations for change. *Motivation to improve and high expectations can encourage individuals to make changes that will improve their lives; however, presence of external locus of control or unrealistic expectations may hamper efforts.*
- Observe communication patterns of family. Listen to family's expressions of hope, planning, and effect on relationships and life. *Provides clues to difficulties that individuals may have in expressing themselves effectively to others. Beginning to plan for the future with hope promotes changes in relationships that can enhance living for those involved.*[3]
- Note expressions such as "Life has more meaning for me since this has occurred." *Such statements identify change in values that may occur with the diagnosis or stress of a serious or potentially fatal illness.*[1]
- Identify cultural or religious health beliefs and expectations. *For example: Navajo parents may define family as nuclear, extended, or clan, and it is important to identify who are the primary child-rearing persons. Beliefs about causes of condition may affect how family interacts with client.*[5]

NURSING PRIORITY NO. 2 To assist family to develop/strengthen potential for growth:

- Provide time to talk with family to discuss their views of the situation. *Provides an opportunity to hear family's understanding and determine how realistic their ideas are for planning how they are going to deal with situation in the most positive manner.*[3]
- Establish a relationship with family/client. *Therapeutic relationships foster growth and enable family to identify skills needed for coping with difficult situation or illness.*[3]
- Provide a role model with whom the family may identify. *Setting a positive example can be a powerful influence in changing behavior, and as family members learn more effective communication skills, consideration for others, warmth, and understanding, family relationships will be enhanced.*[2]
- Discuss importance of open communication and of not having secrets. *Functional communication is clear, direct, open, and honest, with congruence between verbal and nonverbal. Dysfunctional communication is indirect, vague, and controlled, with many double-bind messages. Awareness of this information can enhance relationships among family members.*[3]
- Demonstrate techniques such as active-listening, "I" messages, and problem solving. *Learning these skills can facilitate effective communication and improve interactions within the family.*[2]
- Establish social goals of achieving and maintaining harmony with oneself, family, and community. *Enables client to interact with others in positive ways.*[3]

NURSING PRIORITY NO. 3 To promote optimum family well-being (Teaching/Discharge Considerations):

- Assist family to support the client in meeting own needs within ability or constraints of the illness or situation. *Family members may do too much for client or may not do enough, believing client "wants to be babied." With information and support, they can learn to allow client to take the lead in doing what he or she is able to do.*[3]
- Provide experiences for the family to help them learn ways of assisting and supporting client. *Learning is enhanced when individual participates in hands-on opportunities to try out new activities.*[4]
- Discuss cultural beliefs and practices that may impact family members' interaction with client and dealing with condition. *Preconceived biases may interfere with efforts toward positive growth.*[5]
- Identify other individuals/groups with similar conditions and assist client/family to make contact (groups such as Reach for Recovery, CanSurmount, Al-Anon, and so on). *Provides ongoing support for sharing common experiences, problem solving, and learning new behaviors.*
- Assist family members to learn new, more effective ways of dealing with feelings and reactions. *Growth process is essential to reach the goal of enhancing the family relationships.*[3]
- Encourage family members to pursue personal interests, hobbies, or leisure activities *to promote individual well-being and strengthen coping abilities.*[6]

DOCUMENTATION FOCUS

Assessment/Reassessment
- Adaptive skills being used, stage of growth.
- Family communication patterns.
- Motivation and expectations for change.

Planning
- Plan of care, specific interventions, and who is involved in planning.
- Teaching plan.

Implementation/Evaluation
- Client's responses to interventions, teaching, and actions performed.
- Attainment or progress toward desired outcome(s).
- Modifications to plan of care.

Discharge Planning
- Identified needs for follow-up care, support systems.
- Specific referral made.

References

1. Garbee, D. D., Gentry, J. A. (2001). Coping with the stress of surgery. *AORN J*, 73(5), 949, 949–951.
2. Gordon, T. Getting what you need every time—Method III. Gordon Training International. Retrieved October 2015 from http://www.gordontraining.com/free-parenting-articles/get-what-you-need-every-time-method-iii/.
3. Pychyl, T. A. (2009). Proactive coping: A strategy for self-regulation and enhanced well-being. *Psychology Today*. Retrieved October 2015 from http://www.psychologytoday.com/blog/dont-delay/200903/proactive-coping-strategy-self-regulation-and-enhanced-well-being.
4. Kiser, L. J., Donahue, A., Hodgkinson, S., et al. (2010). Strengthening family coping resources: The feasibility of a multifamily group intervention for families exposed to trauma. *J Trauma Stress*, 23(6), 802–806.
5. Purnell, L. D. (2011). *Guide to Culturally Competent Health Care*. 2nd ed. Philadelphia: F. A. Davis.
6. Becket, N. (1991). Clinical nurses' characterizations of patient coping problems. *Nurs Diagn*, 2(2), 72–78.

Acute Care

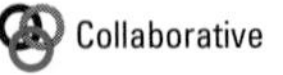

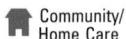

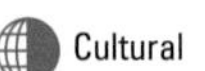

Death Anxiety

Taxonomy II: Coping/Stress Tolerance—Class 2 Coping Responses (00147) [**Diagnostic Division:** Ego Integrity], Submitted 1998; Revised 2006

DEFINITION: Vague uneasy feeling of discomfort or dread generated by perceptions of a real or imagined threat to one's existence.

RELATED FACTORS

Anticipation of: pain, suffering, adverse consequences of anesthesia, impact of death on others
Confronting the reality of terminal disease; experiencing dying process; perceived imminence of death
Discussions on the topic of death; observations related to death; near-death experience
Uncertainty of prognosis; nonacceptance of own mortality
Uncertainty about: the existence of a higher power, life after death, encountering a higher power

DEFINING CHARACTERISTICS

Subjective

Fear of: developing a terminal illness, the dying process, pain or suffering related to dying, loss of mental [or physical] abilities when dying; premature death; prolonged dying process
Negative thoughts related to death and dying
Deep sadness; powerlessness
Concern about strain on the caregiver; worried about the impact of one's death on significant other
Sample Clinical Applications: Chronic debilitating health conditions, cancer, hospital admission, impending major surgery

DESIRED OUTCOMES/EVALUATION CRITERIA

Sample NOC linkages:
Dignified Life Closure: Personal actions to maintain control during approaching end of life
Hope: Optimism that is personally satisfying and life supporting
Acceptance: Health Status: Reconciliation to significant change in health circumstances

Client Will (Include Specific Time Frame)

- Identify and express feelings (e.g., sadness, guilt, fear) freely and effectively.
- Look toward or plan for the future one day at a time.
- Formulate a plan dealing with individual concerns and eventualities of dying.

ACTIONS/INTERVENTIONS

Sample NIC linkages:
Dying Care: Promotion of physical comfort and psychological peace in the final phase of life
Spiritual Support: Assisting the patient to feel balance and connection with a greater power
Grief Work Facilitation: Assistance with the resolution of a significant loss

NURSING PRIORITY NO. 1 To assess causative/contributing factors:

- Determine how client sees self in usual lifestyle role functioning and determine perception and meaning of anticipated loss to him or her and SO(s). *Provides information that can be compared to changes that are occurring. Understanding these factors are helpful for planning.*[1]

- Ascertain current knowledge of situation. *Identifies misconceptions, lack of information, and other pertinent issues and determines accuracy of knowledge. Healthcare providers may not be anticipating death at this time or in current situation.*[1]
- Determine client's role in family constellation. Observe patterns of communication in family and response of family/SO to client's situation and concerns. *In addition to identifying areas of need or concern, this also reveals strengths useful in addressing the current concerns.*[3]
- Assess impact of client reports of subjective experiences and experience with death (or exposure to death); for example, witnessed violent death, as a child viewed body in casket, etc. *Identifies possible feelings that may be affecting current situation, thus promoting accurate planning.*[2]
- Identify cultural factors or expectations and impact on current situation and feelings. *These factors affect client attitude toward events and impending loss. Many cultures prefer to keep the client at home instead of in a long-term care facility or hospital. Growth of the hospice movement in the United States provides palliative care and comfort during the client's final days in any setting.*[4]
- Note age, physical and mental condition, and complexity of therapeutic regimen. *May affect ability to handle current situation. Younger people may handle stress of illness in more positive ways. Older people may be more accepting of possibility of death. Individuals of any age will deal with situation in own way, depending on diagnosis, condition, expectations, and situation.*[8]
- Determine ability to manage own self-care, end-of-life decisions, and other affairs, as well as awareness and use of available resources. *Information will be necessary for determining needs and planning care.*[8]
- Observe behavior indicative of the level of anxiety present (mild to panic). *The level of anxiety affects client's/SO's ability to process information and participate in activities.*[5]
- Note use of drugs (including alcohol), presence of insomnia, excessive sleeping, and avoidance of interactions with others. *Indicators of withdrawal and need for intervention to deal with symptoms or help client deal realistically with diagnosis or illness.*[6]
- Determine sense of futility, feelings of hopelessness, helplessness, and lack of motivation to help self. *Indicators of depression and need for early intervention to help client acknowledge and deal with impending death.*[7,8]
- Listen for expressions of inability to find meaning in life or suicidal ideation. *Signs of depression indicating need for referral to therapist/psychiatrist and possible pharmacological treatment to help client deal with terminal illness or situation.*[7]

NURSING PRIORITY NO. 2 To assist client to deal with situation:

- Provide open and trusting relationship. *Promotes opportunity to explore feelings about impending death.*[2]
- Make time for nonjudgmental discussion of philosophical issues or questions about spiritual impact of illness or situation. *Can help client clarify own position on these issues.*[3]
- Respect client's desire or request not to talk. Provide hope within parameters of the individual situation. *Promotes open environment that encourages client to talk freely about thoughts and feelings. Client may not be ready to talk about situation or concerns about death, or he or she may be denying the reality of what is happening.*[1,8]
- Encourage expressions of feelings (e.g., anger, fear, sadness, etc.). Acknowledge anxiety or fear. Do not deny or reassure client that everything will be all right. Be honest when answering questions and providing information. *Enhances trust and a therapeutic relationship.*[2]
- Use therapeutic communication skills of active-listening. *Technique acknowledges reality of feelings and encourages client to find own solutions.*[2]
- Provide information about normalcy of feelings and individual grief reaction. *Most individuals question their reactions and whether they are normal, and information can provide reassurance.*[3] (Refer to ND Grieving.)

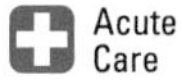

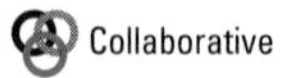

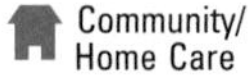

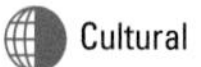

- Identify coping skills currently used and how effective they are. Be aware of defense mechanisms being used by the client. *Provides a starting point to plan care and assists client to acknowledge reality and deal more effectively with what is happening.*[3]
- Review life experiences of loss, noting client strengths and successes. *Provides opportunity to identify and use previously successful skills.*[2]
- Provide a calm, peaceful setting and privacy, as appropriate. *Promotes relaxation and enhances ability to deal with situation.*[8]
- Include family in discussions and decision making, as appropriate. *Involved family members can provide support and ideas for problem solving.*[7]
- Note client's religious or spiritual orientation, involvement in religious or church activities, and presence of conflicts regarding spiritual beliefs. *May benefit by referral to appropriate resource to help client resolve issues, if desired.*[7]
- Assist client to engage in spiritual growth activities, experience prayer or meditation, and practice forgiveness to heal past hurts. Provide information that anger with God is a normal part of the grief process. *May reduce feelings of guilt or conflict, allowing client to move forward toward resolution.*[1]
- Refer to therapists, spiritual advisors, or counselors, as appropriate. *Promotes facilitation of grief work.*
- Refer to community agencies and resources. *Assists client/SO in planning for eventualities (legal issues, hospice home care, funeral plans, etc.).*

NURSING PRIORITY NO. 3 To promote independence:

- Support client's efforts to develop realistic steps to put plans into action. *Provides sense of control over situation in which client does not have much control.*[1]
- Direct client's thoughts beyond the present state, encouraging him or her to try to enjoy each day and look to the future, as appropriate. *Being in the moment can help client enjoy this time rather than dwelling on what is ahead.*
- Provide opportunities for client to make simple decisions. *Enhances sense of control.*
- Develop individual plan using client's locus of control. *Incorporating locus of control (internal or external) enhances success of plan by enabling client/family to manage situation more effectively.*[2]
- Treat expressed decisions and desires with respect and convey to others, as appropriate. *Expresses regard for the individual and enhances sense of control in situation that is not controllable.*[8]
- Assist with completion of Advance Directives and cardiopulmonary resuscitation instructions. *Provides opportunity for client to understand options and express desires.*
- Refer to palliative, hospice, or end-of-life care resources, as appropriate. *Provides support and assistance to client and SO/family through potentially complex and difficult process. Choice of type of care is dependent on timing of care (e.g., palliative care interfaces with curative treatment, which hospice does not allow).*[1]

DOCUMENTATION FOCUS

Assessment/Reassessment

- Assessment findings, including client's fears and signs/symptoms being exhibited.
- Responses and actions of family/SOs.
- Availability and use of resources.

Planning

- Plan of care and who is involved in planning.

Implementation/Evaluation

- Client's response to interventions, teaching, and actions performed.
- Attainment or progress toward desired outcome(s).
- Modifications to plan of care.

Discharge Planning

- Identified needs and who is responsible for actions to be taken.
- Specific referrals made.

References

1. Rattan, A. (2012). The question about death and death anxiety. *HypoGenesis*. Retrieved April 2015 from http://www.hypnos.co.uk/hypnomag/rattan.htm.
2. Andrews, G., Creamer, M., Crino, R., et al. (2002). *The Treatment of Anxiety Disorders: Clinician Guides and Patient Manuals*. 2nd ed. Cambridge, UK: Cambridge University Press.
3. Feifel, H., Branscomb, B. A. (1973). Who's afraid of death? *J Abnorm Psychol*, 81(3), 282–288.
4. Lipson, J. G., Dibble, S. L., Minarik, P. A. (1996). *Culture & Nursing Care: A Pocket Guide*. San Francisco, CA: School of Nursing, UCSF Nursing Press.
5. Michelson, L., Ascher, I., eds. (1987). Death-related anxiety. *Anxiety and Stress Disorders*. New York: Guilford Press.
6. Bruera, E., Moyano, J., Seifert, L., et al. (1995). The frequency of alcoholism among patients with pain due to terminal cancer. *J Pain Symptom Manage*, 10(8), 599–603.
7. Paice, J. (2002). Managing psychological conditions in palliative care. *Am J Nurs*, 102(11), 36–43.
8. Kouch, M. (2006). Managing symptoms for a "good death." *Nursing*, 36(11), 58–63.

Decisional Conflict [specify]

Taxonomy II: Life Principles—Class 3 Value/Belief/Action Congruence (00083) [**Diagnostic Division:** Ego Integrity], Submitted 1988; Revised 2006

DEFINITION: Uncertainty about course of action to be taken when choice among competing actions involves risk, loss, or challenge to values and beliefs.

RELATED FACTORS

Unclear personal values or beliefs; perceived threat to value system
Inexperience with or interference in decision making
Insufficient information; conflicting information sources
Conflict with moral obligation
Moral principle, rule, or value supports mutually inconsistent actions
Insufficient support system
[Age, developmental stage/level of functioning]

DEFINING CHARACTERISTICS

Subjective

Uncertainty about choices; recognizes undesired consequences of actions being considered
Distress while attempting a decision
Questioning of moral principle, rule, values, or personal beliefs/values while attempting a decision

Objective

Vacillating among choices; delay in decision making
Self-focused
Physical sign of tension or distress (e.g., increase in heart rate, restlessness)

Sample Clinical Applications: Therapeutic options with undesired side effects (e.g., amputation, visible scarring) or conflicting with belief system (e.g., blood transfusion, termination of pregnancy); chronic disease states, dementia, Alzheimer's disease, terminal or end-of-life situations

DESIRED OUTCOMES/EVALUATION CRITERIA

Sample NOC linkages:

Decision-Making: Ability to make judgments; choose between two or more alternatives
Health Beliefs: Personal convictions that influence health behaviors
Psychosocial Adjustment: Life Change: Psychosocial adaptation of an individual to a life change

Client Will (Include Specific Time Frame)

- Verbalize awareness of positive and negative aspect of choices and alternative actions.
- Acknowledge and ventilate feelings of anxiety and distress associated with choice or related to making difficult decision.
- Identify personal values and beliefs concerning issues.
- Make decision(s) and express satisfaction with choices.
- Meet psychological needs as evidenced by appropriate expression of feelings, identification of options, and use of resources.
- Display relaxed manner, calm demeanor, and be free of physical signs of distress.

ACTIONS/INTERVENTIONS

Sample NIC linkages:

Decision-Making Support: Providing information and support for a person who is making a decision regarding healthcare
Values Clarification: Assisting another to clarify her/his own values in order to facilitate effective decision making
Coping Enhancement: Assisting a patient to adapt to perceived stressors, changes, or threats that interfere with meeting life demands and roles

NURSING PRIORITY NO. 1 To assess causative/contributing factors:

- ∞ Determine usual ability to manage own affairs. Clarify who has legal right to intervene on behalf of child/developmentally delayed adult (e.g., parent, other relative, or court-appointed guardian/advocate). *Family disruption or conflicts can complicate decision-making process. All adults have the right to make their own decisions unless a legal court has ruled the individual is incompetent and a guardian is appointed.*[4]
- Note expressions of indecision, dependence on others, and availability and involvement of support persons (e.g., lack of or conflicting advice). *Care providers need to be sensitive to the physical, cognitive, and emotional effects of illness on decision-making capabilities and whether the individual wants to be involved in making the decision.*[6]
- Ascertain dependency of other(s) on client and/or issues of codependency. *Influence of others may lead client to make decision that is not what is really wanted or in his or her best interest.*[1]
- Active-listen and identify reason for indecisiveness. *Helps client to clarify problem and begin looking for resolution. May talk about uncertainty—and alternative choices that can lead to risky, uncertain outcomes—and the need to make value judgments about losses versus gains.*[2,6]
- Identify cultural values and beliefs or moral obligations and principles that may be creating conflict for client and complicating decision-making process. *These issues must be addressed before client can be at peace with the decision that is made.*[5]

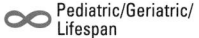

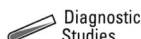

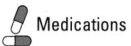

- Determine effectiveness of current problem-solving techniques. *Provides information about client's ability to make decisions that are needed or desired.*[1]
- Note presence and intensity of physical signs of anxiety (e.g., increased heart rate, muscle tension). *Client may be conflicted about the decision that is required and may need help to deal with anxiety to begin to deal with reality of situation. Different treatment decisions may have more uncertainty and generate more conflict in client.*[2,6]
- Listen for expressions of inability to find meaning in life or reason for living, feelings of futility, or alienation from God or others. (Refer to ND Spiritual Distress, as indicated.) *May need to talk about reasons for feelings of alienation to resolve concerns and may engage in questioning about own values.*[6,10]
- Review information client has to support the decision to be made. *Inaccurate or incomplete information and misinterpretations complicate the process and may result in a poor outcome.*[7,8]

NURSING PRIORITY NO. 2 To assist client to develop/effectively use problem-solving skills:

- Promote safe and hopeful environment, as needed. *Client needs to be protected and supported while he or she regains inner control.*[7]
- Encourage verbalization of conflicts and concerns. *Helps client to clarify these issues so he or she can come to a resolution of the situation.*[7,8]
- Accept verbal expressions of anger or guilt. Set limits on maladaptive behavior. *Verbalization of feelings enables client to sift through feelings and begin to deal with situation. Behavior that is inappropriate is not helpful for dealing with the situation and will lead to feelings of guilt and low self-worth.*[2]
- Clarify and prioritize individual goals, noting where the subject of the "conflict" falls on this scale. *Helps to identify importance of problems client is addressing, enabling realistic problem solving.*[2]
- Identify strengths and use of positive coping skills (e.g., use of relaxation techniques, willingness to express feelings). *Helpful for developing solutions to current situation.*[1]
- Identify positive aspects of this experience and assist client to view it as a learning opportunity. *Reframing the situation can help the client see things in a different light, enabling client to develop new and creative solutions.*[1]
- Correct misperceptions client may have and provide factual information, as needed. *Promotes understanding and enables client to make better decisions for own situation.*[1,6]
- Provide opportunities for client to make simple decisions regarding self-care and other daily activities. Accept choice not to do so. Advance complexity of choices, as tolerated. *Acceptance of what client wants to do, with gentle encouragement to progress, enhances self-esteem and ability to try more. Providing individualized decision support can help the client move to more difficult decisions.*[1,6]
- ∞ Encourage child to make developmentally appropriate decisions concerning own care. *Fosters child's sense of self-worth and enhances ability to learn and exercise coping skills.*[4]
- Discuss time considerations, setting time line for small steps and considering consequences related to not making or postponing specific decisions to facilitate resolution of conflict. *When time is a factor in making a decision, these strategies can promote movement toward solution.*[4]
- Have client list some alternatives to present situation or decisions, using a brainstorming process. Include family in this activity, as indicated (e.g., placement of parent in long-term care facility, use of intervention process with addicted member). Refer to NDs interrupted Family Processes, dysfunctional Family Processes, compromised family Coping, Moral Distress. *Involving family and looking at different options can promote successful resolution of decision to be made.*[7,8]
- Practice use of problem-solving process with current situation and decision. *Promotes identification of different possibilities that may not have been thought of otherwise.*[1]
- Discuss and clarify spiritual concerns, accepting client's values in a nonjudgmental manner. *Client will be willing to consider own situation when accepted as an individual of worth.*[5]

NURSING PRIORITY NO. 3 To promote wellness (Teaching/Discharge Considerations):

- Promote opportunities for using conflict-resolution skills, identifying steps as client does each one. *Learning this process can help to solve current dilemma and provide the person with skills he or she can use in the future.*[3]

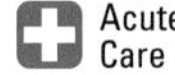

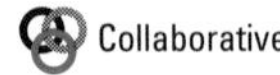

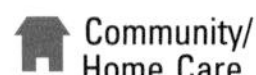

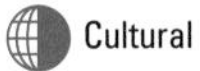

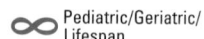

- Provide positive feedback for efforts and progress noted. *Client needs to hear he or she is doing well, and feedback promotes continuation of efforts.*[2]
- Encourage involvement of family/significant others (SOs), as desired or available. *Provides support for the client and facilitates resolution.*[9]
- Support client for decisions made, especially if consequences are unexpected or difficult to cope with. *Positive feedback promotes feelings of success even when difficult situations occur or outcome is less than desired.*[9]
- Encourage attendance at stress-reduction or assertiveness classes. *Learning these skills can help client achieve a lowered stress level that can promote ability to make decisions.*[4]
- Refer to other resources, as necessary (e.g., clergy, psychiatric clinical nurse specialist or psychiatrist, family or marital therapist, addiction support groups). *May need this additional help to deal with complicated problems and facilitate problem solving and decision making.*[2]

DOCUMENTATION FOCUS

Assessment/Reassessment

- Assessment findings, behavioral responses, degree of impairment in lifestyle functioning.
- Individuals involved in the conflict.
- Personal values and beliefs.

Planning

- Plan of care, specific interventions, and who is involved in the planning process.
- Teaching plan.

Implementation/Evaluation

- Client's and involved individuals' responses to interventions, teaching, and actions performed.
- Ability to express feelings and identify options.
- Use of resources.
- Attainment or progress toward desired outcome(s).
- Modifications to plan of care.

Discharge Planning

- Long-term needs, actions to be taken, and who is responsible for doing.
- Specific referrals made.

References

1. Tversky, A., Kahneman, D. (Updated 2012). The framing of decisions and the psychology of choice. *Science*. Retrieved April 2015 from http://rangevoting.org/TverskyK81.html.
2. Paul, M. (2009). Relationships, the art of listening. Retrieved April 2015 from http://www.innerbonding.com/show-article/2147/relationships-the-art-of-listening.html.
3. Bolstad, R., Blamlett, M. (No date). Transforming conflict. Retrieved April 2015 from http://www.nlpca.com/DCweb/winwin.html.
4. Krull, E. (2010). Family conflict power struggles. Psych Central. Retrieved April 2015 from http://blogs.psychcentral.com/family/2010/01/family-conflict-power-struggles/.
5. Purnell, L. D. (2011). *Guide to Culturally Competent Health Care*. 2nd ed. Philadelphia: F. A. Davis.
6. Osborne, H. (2004). In other words—Helping patients make difficult decisions. Retrieved April 2015 from http://www.healthliteracy.com/article.asp?PageID=3808.
7. Liken, M. A. (2001). Caregivers in crisis: Moving a relative with Alzheimer's to assisted living. *Clin Nurs Res*, 10(1), 53–69.
8. Liken, M. A. (2001). Experiences of family caregivers of a relative with Alzheimer's disease. *J Psychosoc Nurs*, 39(12), 33–37.
9. Harris, J. C., Halper, J. (2008). *Multiple Sclerosis: Best Practices in Nursing Care*. New York: Bioscience Communications.
10. Zikmund-Fisher, B. J. (2010). Deficits and variations in patients' experience with making 9 common medical decisions: The DECISIONS Survey. *Med Decis Making*, 30(5 Suppl), S85–S95.

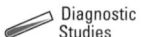

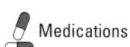

readiness for enhanced Decision-Making

Taxonomy II: Life Principles—Class 3 Value/Belief/Action Congruence (00184) [**Diagnostic Division:** Ego Integrity], Submitted 2006; Revised 2013

DEFINITION: A pattern of choosing a course of action for meeting short- and long-term health-related goals, which can be strengthened.

DEFINING CHARACTERISTICS

Subjective

Expresses desire to enhance decision making, risk-benefit analysis of decisions
Expresses desire to enhance congruency of decisions with goal/values, or sociocultural values/goal
Expresses desire to enhance understanding of choices for decision making, meaning of choices
Expresses desire to enhance use of reliable evidence for decisions

Sample Clinical Applications: Any acute or chronic condition, or healthy individual looking to improve well-being

DESIRED OUTCOMES/EVALUATION CRITERIA

Sample NOC linkages:

Decision-Making: Ability to make judgments and choose between two or more alternatives
Health Beliefs: Personal convictions that influence health beliefs
Personal Autonomy: Personal actions of a competent individual to exercise governance in life decisions
Health-Promoting Behavior: Personal actions to sustain or increase wellness

Client Will (Include Specific Time Frame)

- Identify risks and benefit of decisions.
- Express beliefs about the meaning of choices.
- Make decisions that are congruent with personal and sociocultural values and goals.
- Use reliable evidence for decisions.

ACTION/INTERVENTIONS

Sample NIC linkages:

Decision-Making Support: Providing information and support for a person who is making a decision regarding healthcare
Values Clarification: Assisting another to clarify her or his own values in order to facilitate effective decision making
Teaching: Individual: Planning, implementation, and evaluation of a teaching program to address a patient's particular needs

NURSING PRIORITY NO. 1 To assess causative/contributing factors:

- Determine usual ability to manage own affairs. *Provides baseline for understanding client's decision-making process. There may be variations in attitudes toward risk in different areas of the country that will affect this individual's decision-making preferences.*[8]
- Note expressions of decision, dependability, and availability of support persons. *Having support for decision making and having good information regarding pros and cons of choices helps client to feel comfortable with the decisions made.*[8]

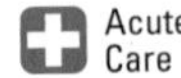

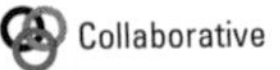

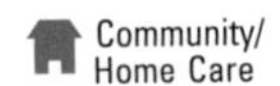

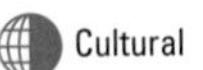

- Active-listen and identify reason(s) client would like to improve decision-making abilities and expectations for change. *As client articulates reasons for improvement, they become more clear, and direction is provided.*[2] *Motivation to improve and high expectations can encourage client to make changes that will improve his or her life. However, presence of external locus of control or unrealistic expectations may hamper efforts.*
- Note presence of physical signs of anxiety. *Client may be excited about the quest for improvement, and excitement may be interpreted as anxiety. It is important to clarify meaning of physical signs.*[2]
- Identify cultural values, beliefs, or moral obligations and principles that guide or affect the decision-making process. *Preconceived biases may color decisions and need to be recognized in order to enhance efforts toward growth.*[5]
- Discuss meaning of life, reasons for living, belief in God or higher power, and how these relate to current desire for improvement or growth. *Helps client to clarify beliefs and how they relate to decision-making process.*[6] (Refer to ND readiness for enhanced Spiritual Well-Being.)

NURSING PRIORITY NO. 2 To assist client to improve/effectively use problem-solving skills:

- Promote safe and hopeful environment and help client identify own inner control. *Will help client understand the control he or she has over decisions made.*[1]
- Encourage verbalization of ideas, concerns, and particular decisions that need to be made.[6]
- Correct misperceptions client may have and provide factual information as needed. *Promotes understanding and enables client to make better decisions for own situation.*[1,8]
- Clarify and prioritize individual's goals, noting possible conflicts or "stumbling" blocks that may be encountered. *As client weighs pros and cons of decision making, taking into account negative aspects of situation, decisions will be more realistic and acceptable to client.*[3]
- Discuss dependence on others, involvement of support persons, and possibility for conflicting advice or goals. *While it is appropriate to consider the opinions of others when making choices, one needs to be aware of the potential for conflicting views when seeking advice and make own decisions free of pressure from others.*[8]
- Identify positive aspects of this experience and assist client to view it as a learning opportunity. *As client reframes experience as an opportunity, he or she will be able to use this learning for future situations.*[3]
- Assist client in learning how to find factual information (e.g., use of the library, Internet). *Individual who takes advantage of these resources will benefit from the knowledge gained. Client will need to be cautious in evaluating information to verify accuracy.*[8]
- Discuss the process of performing a risk-benefit analysis to aid in making decisions. *The individual who learns this skill will be able to use it in many areas of life to enhance relationships, both personal and business.*[3]
- Have client list some alternatives to present decisions, using a brainstorming process. Include significant other (SO)/family in this activity if appropriate. *Looking at different options can strengthen the decision-making process.*[7]
- ∞ Encourage children to make age-appropriate decisions. *Learning problem solving at an early age will enhance sense of self-worth and ability to exercise coping skills.*
- Discuss and clarify spiritual beliefs, accepting client's values in a nonjudgmental manner. *Client may be able to decide what is really acceptable or unacceptable in the choice situation related to beliefs or values that have been expressed.*[8]

NURSING PRIORITY NO. 3 To promote optimum well-being (Teaching/Discharge Considerations):

- Identify opportunities for using conflict-resolution skills. *Emphasizing each step as it is used will help with learning these skills.*[6]
- Provide positive feedback for efforts, growth in use of skills, and learning efforts. *As individual is moving forward in learning new skills, hearing positive feedback provides reinforcement for individuals to continue efforts.*[3]

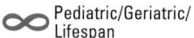

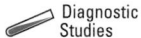

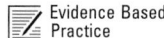

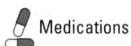

- Encourage involvement of family/SOs as desired/appropriate. *Helps all family members to improve conflict-resolution skills. When family works together, relationships are enhanced and family members can live fuller lives.*[4]
- Recommend attending stress-reduction and/or assertiveness classes as desired. *Individual can learn additional skills to enhance decision making, improving ability to make life better.*[2]
- Refer to other resources as necessary (e.g., clergy, psychiatrist, clinical psychiatric nurse specialist, family/marital therapist). *May need additional counseling to help with specific concerns.*[4]

DOCUMENTATION FOCUS

Assessment/Reassessment

- Assessment findings, behavioral responses.
- Individuals involved in improving conflict skills.
- Personal values, beliefs, and motivation for change.

Planning

- Plan of care, specific interventions, and who is involved in the planning process.
- Teaching plan.

Implementation/Evaluation

- Client's and involved individual's responses to interventions, teaching, and actions performed.
- Ability to express feelings, identify options, use resources.
- Attainment or progress toward desired outcomes(s).
- Modifications to plan of care.

Discharge Planning

- Long-term needs, actions to be taken, and who is responsible for doing.
- Specific referrals made.

References

1. Pryor, J., Jannings, W. (2004). Preparing patients to self-manage faecal continence following spinal cord injury. *Int J Ther Rehabil*, 11(2), 79–82.
2. Salem, R. (2003). Empathic listening. Beyond Intractability. Retrieved April 2015 from http://www.beyondintractability.org/essay/empathic_listening/.
3. Dunn, S. (Updated 2006). Pros and cons of researching your cancer. *CancerGuide*. Retrieved April 2015 from http://www.cancerguide.org/pros_cons.html.
4. Peterson, R., Green, S. (2009). Families first—keys to successful family functioning: Problem solving. Department of Human Development, Virginia Tech. Retrieved April 2015 from http://www.pubs.ext.vt.edu/350/350-091/350-091.html.
5. Griffin, M. (2009). Decision making: Complexities and variables. Liddy Shriver Sarcoma Initiative. Retrieved April 2015 from http://www.sarcomahelp.org/learning_center/articles/decisions.html.
6. Brandt, A. L. (2000). Transition issues for the elderly and their families. Retrieved October 2015 from http://www.ec-online.net/knowledge/articles/brandttransitions.html.
7. Liken, M. A. (2001). Caregivers in crisis: Moving a relative with Alzheimer's to assisted living. *Clin Nurs Res*, 10(1), 53–69.
8. Osborne, H. (2004). In other words. Helping patients make difficult decisions. Health Literacy Consulting. Retrieved April 2015 from http://www.healthliteracy.com/article.asp?PageID=3808.

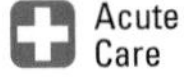

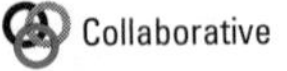

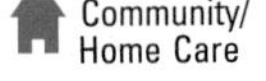

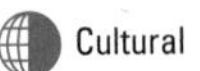

ineffective Denial

Taxonomy II: Coping/Stress Tolerance—Class 2 Coping Responses (00072) [**Diagnostic Division:** Ego Integrity], Submitted 1988; Revised 2006

DEFINITION: Conscious or unconscious attempt to disavow the knowledge or meaning of an event to reduce anxiety and/or fear, leading to the detriment of health.

RELATED FACTORS

Anxiety; perceived inadequacy in dealing with strong emotions
Insufficient sense of control; fear of losing autonomy
Excessive stress; ineffective coping strategies
Threat of unpleasant reality
Fear of separation, death
Insufficient emotional support

DEFINING CHARACTERISTICS

Subjective

Minimizes symptoms; displaces source of symptoms
Does not admit impact of disease on life
Displaces fear of impact of the condition
Denies fear of death or invalidism

Objective

Delay in seeking healthcare; refusal of healthcare
Does not perceive relevance of symptoms, danger
Use of dismissive gestures or comments when speaking of distressing event
Inappropriate affect
Use of treatment not advised by healthcare professional

Sample Clinical Applications: Chronic illnesses, eating disorders, substance abuse, Alzheimer's disease, terminal conditions, bipolar disorder, body dysmorphic disorder

DESIRED OUTCOMES/EVALUATION CRITERIA

Sample NOC linkages:

Acceptance: Health Status: Reconciliation to significant change in health circumstances
Health Beliefs: Perceived Threat: Personal conviction that a threatening health problem is serious and has potential negative consequences for lifestyle
Psychosocial Adjustment: Life Change: Adaptive psychosocial response of an individual to a significant life change

Client Will (Include Specific Time Frame)

- Acknowledge reality of situation or illness.
- Express realistic concern and feelings about symptoms or illness.
- Seek appropriate assistance for presenting problem.
- Display appropriate affect.

(continues on page 248)

ineffective Denial (continued)
ACTIONS/INTERVENTIONS

Sample NIC linkages:
Anxiety Reduction: Minimizing apprehension, dread, foreboding, or uneasiness related to an unidentified source of anticipated danger
Counseling: Use of an interactive helping process focusing on the needs, problems, or feelings of the patient and significant others to enhance or support coping, problem solving, and interpersonal relationships
Coping Enhancement: Assisting a patient to adapt to perceived stressors, changes, or threats, which interfere with meeting life demands and roles

NURSING PRIORITY NO. 1 To assess causative/contributing factors:

- Identify situational crisis or problem and client's perception of the situation. *Identification of both reality and client's perception, which may not be the same as the reality, is necessary for planning care accurately.*[1]
- Ascertain cultural values or religious beliefs affecting perception of situation and sense of personal responsibility for crisis. *Knowing that lifestyle or choices may have caused or contributed to current situation may limit client's ability to accept outcome or view event realistically. Client will make choices regarding therapeutic regimen or lifestyle changes incorporating own cultural and social factors. Conflicts may arise when provider and patient disagree on healthcare beliefs and practices.*[5,7]
- Determine stage and degree of denial. *These factors will help identify whether the client is in early stages of denial and may be more amenable to intervention than those who are well entrenched in their beliefs. Treatment needs to begin where the client is and progress from there.*[1,6]
- Compare client's description of symptoms or conditions to reality of clinical picture and impact of illness or problem on lifestyle. *Identifies extent of discrepancy between the two and where treatment needs to start to help client accept reality.*[1]

NURSING PRIORITY NO. 2 To assist client to deal appropriately with situation:

- Develop nurse-client relationship using therapeutic communication skills of active-listening and "I" messages. *Promotes trust in which client can begin to look at reality of situation and deal with it in a positive manner.*[2]
- Provide safe, nonthreatening environment. *Allows client to feel comfortable enough to talk freely without fear of judgment and to deal with issues realistically.*[2]
- Encourage expressions of feelings, accepting client's view of the situation without confrontation. Set limits on maladaptive behavior *to promote safety. Helps client to work through and understand feelings. Unacceptable behavior is counterproductive to making progress, as client will view self negatively.*[2]
- Present accurate information as appropriate, without insisting that the client accept what has been presented. *Avoids confrontation, which may further entrench client in denial. Open manner permits client to feel value of self in situation and to begin to accept reality.*[2,7]
- Discuss client's behaviors in relation to illness (e.g., diabetes mellitus, alcoholism, chronic pain conditions, terminal cancer) and point out the results of these behaviors. *Information can help client accept reality and opt to change behaviors.*[3]
- Encourage client to talk with SO(s)/friends. *May clarify concerns and reduce isolation and withdrawal. Constructive feedback from others facilitates understanding.*[4]
- Involve in group sessions. *Promotes discussion and feedback to enhance learning. Client can hear other views of reality and test own perceptions.*[4]
- Avoid agreeing with inaccurate statements or perceptions. *Prevents perpetuating false reality.*[2]

Acute Care 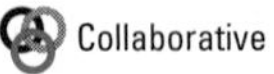 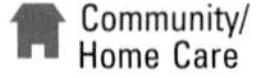 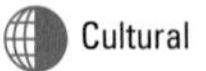

- Provide positive feedback for constructive moves toward independence. *Promotes repetition of desired behavior.*[4]

NURSING PRIORITY NO. 3 To promote wellness (Teaching/Discharge Considerations):

- Provide written information about illness or situation for client and family. *Provides client/family with reminders and resources they can refer to as they consider options.*[1]
- Involve family members/SO(s) in long-range planning. *Provides support and helps to identify and meet individual needs for the future.*[4]
- Refer to appropriate community resources (e.g., Diabetes Association, MS Society, Alcoholics Anonymous). *May be needed to help client with long-term adjustment.*
- Refer to ND ineffective Coping.

DOCUMENTATION FOCUS

Assessment/Reassessment

- Assessment findings, degree of personal vulnerability and denial.
- Impact of illness or problem on lifestyle.

Planning

- Plan of care and who is involved in the planning.
- Teaching plan.

Implementation/Evaluation

- Client's response to interventions, teaching, and actions performed.
- Use of resources.
- Attainment or progress toward desired outcome(s).
- Modifications to plan of care.

Discharge Planning

- Long-term needs and who is responsible for actions taken.
- Specific referrals made.

References

1. Mayo Clinic Staff (Updated 2014). Denial: When it helps, when it hurts. Retrieved April 2015 from http://www.mayoclinic.org/healthy-lifestyle/adult-health/in-depth/denial/art-20047926.
2. Grinstead, S. F. (2009). Overcoming resistance and denial for effective pain management. Retrieved April 2015 from http://dbhdid.ky.gov/dbh/documents/ksaods/2014/Grinstead1.pdf.
3. Burgess, E. (1994). Denial and terminal illness. *Am J Hosp Palliat Care*, 11(2), 46–48.
4. Robinson, A. W. (1999). Getting to the heart of denial. *Am J Nurs*, 99(5), 38–42.
5. Ngo-Metzger, Q., Massagli, M. P., Clarridge, B. R., et al. (2003). Linguistic and cultural barriers to care: Perspectives of Chinese and Vietnamese immigrants. *J Gen Int Med*, 18(1), 44–52.
6. Jacelon, C. S., Henneman, E. A. (2004). Profiles in dignity: Nursing perspectives on nursing and critically ill older patients. *Crit Care Nurse*, 24(4), 30–35.
7. Thomas, S. (2010). Some of mixed heritage in denial. Norfolk African American Culture Examiner. Retrieved April 2015 from http://www.examiner.com/article/some-of-mixed-heritage-denial.

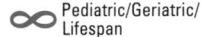

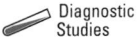

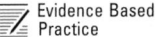

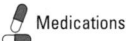

impaired Dentition

Taxonomy II: Safety/Protection—Class 2 Physical Injury (00048) [**Diagnostic Division:** Food/Fluid], Submitted 1998

DEFINITION: Disruption in tooth development/eruption patterns or structural integrity of individual teeth.

RELATED FACTORS

Insufficient dietary habits; malnutrition
Pharmaceutical agent; habitual use of staining substances (e.g., tobacco, coffee, tea, red wine); chronic vomiting
Insufficient oral hygiene; oral temperature sensitivity
Insufficient knowledge of dental health; excessive intake of fluoride or use of abrasive oral cleaning agents
Barrier to self-care; difficulty accessing dental care
Economically disadvantaged
Genetic predisposition; bruxism
[Traumatic injury to face/jaw, surgical intervention]

DEFINING CHARACTERISTICS

Subjective

Toothache

Objective

Halitosis
Enamel discoloration; erosion of enamel; excessive oral plaque/calculus
Abraded teeth; dental or root caries; tooth fracture; loose tooth; absence of teeth
Premature loss of primary teeth; incomplete tooth eruption for age
Malocclusion; tooth misalignment; facial asymmetry

Sample Clinical Applications: Facial trauma or surgery, malnutrition, eating disorders, head or neck cancer, seizure disorder

DESIRED OUTCOMES/EVALUATION CRITERIA

Sample NOC linkages:

Oral Hygiene: Condition of the mouth, teeth, gums, and tongue
Self-Care: Oral Hygiene: Ability to care for own mouth and teeth independently with or without assistive device
Knowledge: Health Behavior: Extent of understanding conveyed about the promotion and protection of health

Client/SO Will (Include Specific Time Frame)

- Display healthy gums and mucous membranes and teeth that are in good repair.
- Report adequate nutritional and fluid intake.
- Verbalize understanding of appropriate oral hygiene regimen.
- Demonstrate effective dental hygiene skills.
- Follow through on referrals for appropriate dental care.

ACTION/INTERVENTIONS

Sample NIC linkages:

Oral Health Restoration: Promotion of healing for a patient who has an oral mucosa or dental lesion

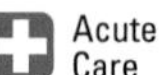

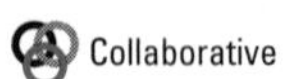

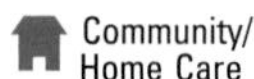

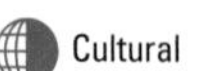

Teaching: Individual: Planning, implementation, and evaluation of a teaching program designed to address a patient's particular needs
Referral: Arrangement for services by another care provider or agency

NURSING PRIORITY NO. 1 To assess causative/contributing factors:

- Inspect oral cavity. Note presence or absence and intactness of teeth or dentures and appearance of gums. *Provides baseline for planning and interventions in terms of safety, nutritional needs, and aesthetics.*
- Evaluate current status of dental hygiene and oral health *to determine need for instruction or coaching, assistive devices, and/or referral to dental care providers.*
- Note presence of halitosis. *Bad breath may be result of numerous local or systemic conditions, including smoking, periodontal disease, dehydration, malnutrition, ketoacidosis, nasal and sinus infections, and some medications and drugs. Management can include improved mouth care or treatment of underlying conditions.*[11]
- ∞ Document age, developmental and cognitive status, and manual dexterity. Evaluate nutritional and health state, noting presence of conditions such as bulimia or chronic vomiting; musculoskeletal impairments; or problems with mouth (e.g., bleeding disorders, cancer lesions, abscesses, facial trauma). *Factors affecting client's dental health and ability to provide effective oral care.*[1,12]
- Note current situation that will affect dental health (e.g., presence of airway/endotracheal [ET] intubation, facial fractures, jaw surgery, new braces, use of anticoagulants or chemotherapy) that require special mouth care activities.[7,8]
- Document (photograph) facial injuries before treatment *to provide "pictorial baseline" for future comparison and evaluation.*

NURSING PRIORITY NO. 2 To treat/manage dental care needs:

- Ascertain client's usual method of oral care *to provide continuity of care or to build on client's existing knowledge base and current practices in developing plan of care.*
- Assist with or provide oral care, as indicated:[2,8,9,12]
  Offer tap water or saline rinses or diluted alcohol-free mouthwashes.
  Provide gentle gum massage and tongue brushing with soft toothbrush using fluoride toothpaste *to manage tartar buildup, if appropriate.*
  Use foam sticks *to swab gums and oral cavity when brushing is not possible or inadvisable.*
  Assist with brushing and flossing when client is unable to do self-care.
  Demonstrate and assist with electric or battery-powered mouth care devices (e.g., toothbrush, plaque remover) as indicated.
  Assist with or provide denture care when indicated (e.g., remove and clean after meals and at bedtime).
- ∞ Remind client to brush teeth as indicated. *Cues, modeling, or pantomime may be helpful if client is young, elderly, or cognitively or emotionally impaired.*[12]
- ✚ Reposition ET tubes and airway adjuncts routinely, carefully padding and protecting teeth and prosthetics.[7]
- Suction as needed if client is unable to manage secretions.
- Remind client of importance of maintaining good jaw and facial alignment when fractures are present.
- ∞ Encourage appropriate diet for optimal nutrition, considering client's special needs such as pregnancy, age and developmental concerns, and ability to chew (e.g., liquids or soft foods) and offering low-sugar, low-starch foods and snacks *to minimize tooth decay and improve overall health. Note: Emerging research is revealing important relationships between nutrition, tooth decay, and periodontal disease and chronic health conditions such as heart disease, diabetes, and immune-compromising conditions.*[2,9,13]
- Encourage client to avoid thermal stimuli *when teeth are sensitive* and to use specific toothpastes designed *to reduce sensitivity of teeth.*
- Administer antibiotics as needed *to treat oral or gum infections that may be present and to prevent hospital-acquired infection in the critically ill client whose teeth may be colonized by significant bacteria.*[3]

- Recommend use of analgesics and topical analgesics as needed *when dental pain is present.*
- Administer prophylactic antibiotic therapy prior to some dental procedures *in susceptible individuals* (e.g., presence of prosthetic heart valve, prior infective endocarditis, certain congenital heart defects, cardiac transplant with subsequent valvulopathy) *to reduce risk of infective endocarditis resulting from manipulation of gingival tissue or the periapical region of teeth or procedures that will perforate the oral mucosa.*[10]
- Direct client to notify dental care provider when bleeding disorder is present or anticoagulant therapy (including aspirin) is being used. *May impact choice of procedure or technique in order to prevent excess bleeding.*
- Refer to appropriate care providers (e.g., nutritionist, dental hygienists, dentists, periodontist, oral surgeon).

NURSING PRIORITY NO. 3 To promote wellness (Teaching/Discharge Considerations):

- Instruct client/caregiver to inspect oral cavity and in home-care interventions *to provide good oral care and prevent tooth decay and periodontal disease.*[4,5,9]
- Review or demonstrate proper toothbrushing techniques (e.g., spending several minutes brushing, reaching all tooth surfaces, brushing with bristles at a "45-degree angle" to teeth surfaces) after meals and daily flossing. Suggest brushing with fluoride-containing toothpaste if client is able to swallow and manage oral secretions. Avoid sharing toothbrushes. Brush child's teeth until he/she can perform alone. *This is the most effective way of reducing oral bacteria and plaque formation and preventing cavities and periodontal disease.*[8]
- Discuss dental and oral health needs, both as client perceives needs and according to professional standards. *Client's perceptions are shaped by self-image, family, and cultural expectations or conditions created by disease or trauma. Current healthcare practices and education are geared toward practices that improve client's appearance and health, including reduced consumption of refined sugars, optimal fluoridation, access to preventative and restorative dental care, prevention of oral cancers, and prevention of craniofacial injuries.*[4,5]
- Recommend that clients of all ages decrease sugary and high-carbohydrate foods in diet and snacks *to reduce buildup of plaque and risk of cavities caused by acids associated with the breakdown of sugar and starch.*[4]
- Instruct older client and caregiver(s) concerning their special needs and importance of regular dental care. *Elderly are prone to experience decay around older fillings (also have more fillings in mouth); have receding gums, exposing root surfaces, which decay easily; have reduced production of saliva and use multiple medications that can cause dry mouth with loss of tooth and gum protection; and have loosening of teeth or poorly fitting dentures associated with gum or bone loss. These factors (often compounded by disease conditions and lack of funds) affect nutrient intake, chewing, swallowing, and oral cavity health.*[5,12]
- Advise mother regarding age-appropriate concerns:[1,4–6]

  Instruct mother to refrain from allowing baby to fall asleep with bottle containing formula, milk, or sweetened beverages. Suggest use of water and pacifier during night *to prevent bottle tooth decay.*

  Determine pattern of tooth appearance and tooth loss and compare to norms for primary and secondary teeth.

  Discuss tooth discoloration and needed follow-up. *Brown or black spots on teeth usually indicate decay; gray tooth color may indicate nerve injury; and multiple cavities in adolescent could be caused from repeated vomiting or bulimia.*

  Discuss pit and fissure sealants. *Painted-on tooth surface sealants are becoming widely available to reduce number of cavities and sometimes are available through community dental programs.*

  Determine if school dental health programs are available or recommend regular professional dental examinations as child grows.

  Discuss with children/parents problems associated with oral piercing if individual is contemplating piercing or needs to know what to watch for after piercing. *Common symptoms that occur with piercing of lips, gums, and tongue include pain, swelling, infection, increased flow of saliva, and chipped or cracked teeth requiring diligent oral care or more frequent dental examination to prevent complications.*

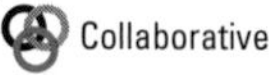

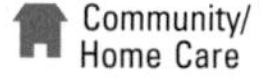

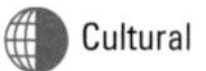

Cultural

Discuss use of or need for safety devices (e.g., helmets, face mask, mouth guards) *to prevent or limit severity of sports-related facial injuries and tooth damage or loss.*

- Discuss with pregnant women special needs and regular dental care. *Pregnant women need additional calcium and phosphorus to maintain good dental health and provide for strong teeth and bones in fetal development. Many women avoid dental care during pregnancy because of concerns for fetal health or for other reasons (including lack of financial resources). However, one research study of 400 women suggests that pregnant women who receive treatment for periodontal disease can reduce their risk of giving birth to a low-birth-weight or preterm baby.*[4]
- Review resources that are needed and available for the client to perform adequate dental hygiene care (e.g., toothbrush, paste, clean water, referral to dental care providers, access to financial assistance, personal care assistant).
- Encourage cessation of tobacco (especially smokeless) and enrolling in smoking-cessation classes *to reduce risk of oral cancers and other health problems.*
- Discuss advisability of dental checkup and care prior to instituting chemotherapy or radiation *to minimize oral, dental, or tissue damage.*

DOCUMENTATION FOCUS

Assessment/Reassessment

- Individual findings, including individual factors influencing dentition problems.
- Baseline photos and description of oral cavity or structures.

Planning

- Plan of care and who is involved in planning.
- Teaching plan.

Implementation/Evaluation

- Responses to interventions, teaching, and actions performed.
- Attainment or progress toward desired outcome(s).
- Modifications to plan of care.

Discharge Planning

- Individual long-term needs, noting who is responsible for actions to be taken.
- Specific referrals made.

References

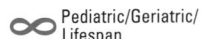

1. Gussy, M. G., Waters, E. G., Walsh, O., et al. (2006). Early childhood caries: Current evidence for aetiology and prevention. *J Paediatr Child Health*, 42, 37–43.
2. Centers for Disease Control and Prevention. Oral health: Preventing cavities, gum disease, tooth loss, and oral cancers: At a glance 2011. Retrieved October 2015 from http://198.246.124.29/chronicdisease/resources/publications/aag/pdf/2011/oral-health-aag-pdf-508.pdf.
3. Scannapieco, F. A., Stewart, E. M., Mylotte, J. M. (1992). Colonization of dental plaque by respiratory pathogens in medical intensive care patients. *Crit Care Med*, 20, 740–745.
4. Your diet and dental health; oral changes with age; sealants; oral piercing; National Academy of Sciences panel reaffirms effectiveness of fluoride. Public education pamphlets from the American Dental Association; ADA for educators. Retrieved August 2011 from http://www.ada.org/public.aspx.
5. Mount Nittany Health: A healthy smile for life. (No date). Retrieved October 2015 from http://www.mountnittany.org/articles/a-healthy-smile-for-life.
6. Engel, J. (2002). *Mosby's Pocket Guide to Pediatric Assessment*. 4th ed. St. Louis, MO: Mosby.

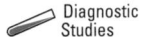

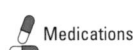

7. Truman, B., Gooch, B. F., Sulemana, I., et al. (2002). Recommendations on selected interventions to prevent dental caries, oral and pharyngeal cancers, and sports-related craniofacial injuries. *Am J Prev Med*, 23(1 Suppl), 21–54.
8. Stiefel, K. A., Damron, S., Sowers, N. J., et al. (2000). Improving oral hygiene for the seriously ill patient: Implementing research-based practice. *Medsurg Nurs*, 9(1), 40–43.
9. Healthwise Staff. (update 2015). Tooth decay: Prevention. Retrieved October 2015 from http://www.webmd.com/oral-health/tc/tooth-decay-topic-overview.
10. Stiles, S., Vega, C. P. (update 2008). AHA updates recommendations for antibiotic prophylaxis for dental procedures. Retrieved October 2015 from www.medscape.org/viewarticle/555596.
11. Porter, S. R., Scully, C. (2006). Oral malodour (halitosis). *BMJ*, 333(7569), 632–635.
12. Stein, P. S., Henry, R. G. (2009). Poor oral hygiene in long-term care. *AJN*, 109(6), 44–50.
13. Palmer, C. A., Burnett, D. J., Dean, B. (2010). It's more than just candy: Important relationships between nutrition and oral health. *Nutrition Today*, 45(4), 154–164.
14. Lopez, N. J., Smith, P. C., Guiterrez, J. (2002). Periodontal therapy may reduce the risk of preterm low birth weight in women with periodontal disease: A randomized controlled trial. *J Periodontol*, 73(8), 911–924.

risk for delayed Development

Taxonomy II: Growth/Development—Class 2 Development (00112) [**Diagnostic Division:** Teaching/Learning], Submitted 1998; Revised 2013

DEFINITION: Vulnerable to delay of 25% or more in one or more of the areas of social or self-regulatory behavior or in cognitive, language, gross, or fine motor skills, which may compromise health.

RISK FACTORS

Prenatal

Maternal age ≤15 years or ≥35 years
Unplanned or unwanted pregnancy; insufficient or late-term prenatal care
Inadequate nutrition; economically disadvantaged
Functional illiteracy
Genetic or endocrine disorder; infection; substance abuse

Individual

Prematurity; congenital or genetic disorder
Visual or hearing impairment; recurrent otitis media
Inadequate nutrition; failure to thrive
Chronic illness; treatment regimen
Brain injury (e.g., hemorrhage, shaken baby syndrome, abuse, accident); seizures
Positive drug screening; substance abuse; lead poisoning
Involvement with the foster care system; history of adoption
Behavior disorder (e.g., attention deficit, oppositional defiant)
Technology dependence (e.g., ventilator, augmentative communication)
Natural disaster

Environmental

Economically disadvantaged
Exposure to violence

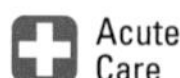 Acute Care 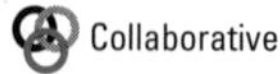 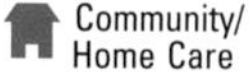 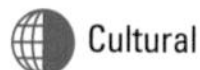

Caregiver
Learning disability
Presence of abuse (e.g., physical, psychological, sexual)
Mental health issue (e.g., depression, psychosis, personality disorder, substance abuse)
Note: A risk diagnosis is not evidenced by signs and symptoms, as the problem has not occurred; rather, nursing interventions are directed at prevention.
Sample Clinical Applications: Congenital or genetic disorders, prematurity, infection, nutritional problems (malnutrition, anorexia, failure to thrive), toxic exposures (e.g., lead), substance abuse, endocrine disorders, abuse or neglect, developmental delay

DESIRED OUTCOMES/EVALUATION CRITERIA

Sample NOC linkage:
Child Development: [specify age]: Milestones of physical, cognitive, and psychosocial progression by [specify] months or years of age

Client Will (Include Specific Time Frame)
- Perform motor, social, self-regulatory behavior, cognitive, and language skills appropriate for age or within scope of present capabilities.

Sample NOC linkages:
Knowledge: Parenting: Extent of understanding conveyed about provision of a nurturing and constructive environment for a child from 1 year through 17 years of age
Parenting Performance: Parental actions to provide a child a nurturing and constructive physical, emotional, and social environment

Parent/Caregiver Will (Include Specific Time Frame)
- Verbalize understanding of age-appropriate development and expectations.
- Identify individual risk factors for developmental delay or deviation.
- Formulate plan(s) for prevention of developmental deviation.
- Initiate interventions or lifestyle changes promoting appropriate development.

ACTIONS/INTERVENTIONS

Sample NIC linkages:
Developmental Enhancement: Child [or] Adolescent: Facilitating or teaching parents/caregivers to facilitate the optimal gross motor, fine motor, language, cognitive, social, and emotional growth of preschool and school-age children or during the transition from childhood to adulthood
Risk Identification: Analysis of potential risk factors, determination of health risks, and prioritization of risk reduction strategies for an individual or group

NURSING PRIORITY NO. 1 To assess for causative/contributing risk factors:

- Identify condition(s) that could contribute to developmental deviations. *This list is extensive and widely variable (see Risk Factors). Potential for developmental issues might be apparent at birth (e.g., neonatal brain injury, especially that occurring before or at time of birth; prematurity; extremes of maternal age; unwanted or complicated pregnancy; known prenatal substance abuse, etc.). However, risks are not confined to the child's birth events, but also encompass parent/family issues and environment (e.g., family history of developmental disorders; mother with mental illness or retardation, child with acute or chronic severe illness and lengthy hospitalizations; family poverty with inadequate living quarters, nutrition, nurturing, or supervision; family instability or violence; shaken baby syndrome and other maltreatment or child abuse; institutional home or foster system during early life or prior to adoption).*[1,11–13,16,17]

- Participate in screening child's development level by means of observation and history related by concerned parents/other significant others. *Developmental delay occurs when a child fails to achieve one or more developmental milestones within an expected time period; it may be in one or more areas (e.g., cognitive, social and emotional, speech and language, fine motor skills or gross motor skills) and may be the result of one or multiple factors.*[1,13]
- Obtain information from variety of sources. *Parents are often the first ones to think that there is a problem with their baby's development and should be encouraged to have routine well-baby checkups and screening for developmental delays. Teachers, family members, day-care or foster care providers, physicians, and others interacting with a client (older than infant) may have valuable input regarding behaviors that may indicate problems or developmental issues.*[1,2,11–13,16,17]
- Identify cultural beliefs, norms, and values, as they may impact parent/caregiver view of situation. *Culture shapes parenting practices, understanding of health and illness, perceptions related to development, and beliefs about individuals affected by developmental disorders. These cultural implications underscore the importance of having a broad array of tools for assessment and instruction, as well as a good understanding of the child's culture.*[3,12]
- Ascertain nature of required parent/caregiver activities and evaluate caregiver's abilities to perform needed activities.
- Note severity and pervasiveness of situation (e.g., potential for long-term stress leading to abuse or neglect versus situational disruption during period of crisis or transition that may eventually level out). *Situations require different interventions in terms of the intensity and length of time that assistance and support may be critical to the parent/caregiver. A crisis can produce great change within a family, some of which can be detrimental to the individual or family unit.*[4–6]
- Evaluate environment in which long-standing care will be provided. *The physical, emotional, financial, and social needs of a family are impacted and intertwined with the needs of the client. Changes may be needed in the physical structure of the home or family roles, resulting in disruption and stress, placing everyone at risk.*[4,6]
- Refer for and assist with in-depth evaluation, if indicated, using an authoritative text (e.g., Gesell, Mussen-Congor) or assessment tools (e.g., Ages and Stages Questionnaire, Parents Evaluation of Developmental Status, Temperament and Atypical Behavior Scale, Denver II Developmental Screening Test, Bender's Visual Motor Gestalt Test). *Provides guide for comparative measurement as child/individual progresses. Note: Often there is no single diagnostic test for a specific developmental delay. There are tools to evaluate child's skills in certain areas, such as motor development, speech, language, math, etc. However, a diagnosis is often determined over months or years. Also, a child who is delayed in an area at a certain age may "catch up" in later years.*[1,8–12]

NURSING PRIORITY NO. 2 To assist in preventing or limiting developmental delays:

- Note chronological age and review with parents the expectations for "normal development" in infancy and early childhood at clinic visits *to help determine developmental expectations (e.g., when child should roll over, sit up alone, speak first words, attain a certain weight or height) and how the expectations may be altered by child's condition. Ideally, children should be screened for developmental delay at the 9-, 18-, and 24- or 30-month visit, and at 15, 18, and again at 24 months for autism spectrum disorders.*[14,15] *For high-risk individuals, including children affected by biological (e.g., low birth weight) and psychosocial (e.g., foster care, homelessness) risk factors, earlier and more frequent formal developmental screening may be warranted. Note: Pediatrician may screen with a motor quotient (MQ), which is child's age calculated by milestones met divided by chronological age and multiplied by 100. An MQ between 50 and 70 requires further evaluation and intervention.*[1,7,16]

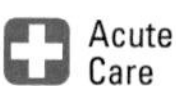

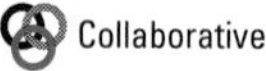

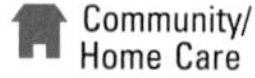

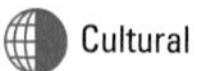

- Describe realistic, age-appropriate patterns of development to parent/caregiver and promote activities and interactions that support developmental tasks where client is at this time. *Important in planning interventions in keeping with the individual's current status and potential. Each child will have own unique strengths and challenges.*[1–3,11,17]
- Collaborate with related professional resources, as indicated (e.g., physical, occupational, rehabilitation, speech therapists; home health agencies; social services, nutritionist; special education teacher, family therapists; technological and adaptive equipment specialists; vocational counselor). *Multidisciplinary team care increases the likelihood of developing a well-rounded plan of care that meets client/family's specialized and varied needs, minimizing identified risks.*[4,10–12]

NURSING PRIORITY NO. 3 To promote wellness (Teaching/Discharge Considerations):

- Engage in and encourage prevention strategies (e.g., abstinence from drugs, alcohol, and tobacco during pregnancy, referral for treatment programs, referral for violence prevention counseling, anticipatory guidance for potential handicaps [vision, hearing, failure to thrive]). *Promoting wellness starts with preventing complications and acting early to limit severity of anticipated problems. Such strategies can often be initiated by nurses where the potential is first identified, in the community setting.*[1,4]
- Evaluate client's progress on continual basis. Identify target symptoms requiring intervention *to make referrals in a timely manner and/or to make adjustments in plan of care, as indicated.*[2]
- Emphasize importance of follow-up appointments as indicated *to promote ongoing evaluation, support, or management of situation.*[2,12]
- Discuss proactive wellness actions to take (e.g., periodic laboratory studies to monitor nutritional status, getting immunizations on schedule to prevent serious infections) *to avoid preventable complications.*[2]
- Maintain a positive, hopeful attitude. Encourage setting of short-term realistic goals for achieving developmental potential. *Small, incremental steps are often easier to deal with, and successes enhance hopefulness and well-being.*[6]
- Provide information as appropriate, including pertinent reference materials and reliable Web sites. *Bibliotherapy provides opportunity to review data at own pace, enhancing likelihood of retention.*[1,2]
- Encourage attendance at educational programs (e.g., parenting classes, infant stimulation sessions; food buying, cooking, and nutrition; home and family safety, anger management, seminars on life stresses, aging process) *to address specific learning need or desires and interact with others with similar life challenges.*[2,11]
- Refer to available community and national resources if appropriate (e.g., early intervention programs, gifted and talented programs, sheltered workshop, crippled children's services, medical equipment and supplier, caregiver support and respite services). *Can provide assistance to support family and help identify community responsibilities (e.g., services required to be provided to school-age child if developmental disabilities are diagnosed).*[1]

DOCUMENTATION FOCUS

Assessment/Reassessment

- Assessment findings, individual needs, including developmental level.
- Caregiver's understanding of situation and individual role.

Planning

- Plan of care and who is involved in the planning.
- Teaching plan.

Implementation/Evaluation

- Client's response to interventions, teaching, and actions performed.
- Caregiver response to teaching.

- Attainment or progress toward desired outcome(s).
- Modifications to plan of care.

Discharge Planning

- Identified long-term needs and who is responsible for actions to be taken.
- Specific referrals made, sources for assistive devices, educational tools.

References

1. Center for Parent Information and Resources. Developmental delay: How kids develop. Retrieved March 2015 from http://www.howkidsdevelop.com/developDevDelay.html.
2. Volkmar, F., Cook, E. H., Pomeroy, J., et al. (1999). Practice parameters for the assessment and treatment of children, adolescents, and adults with autism and other pervasive developmental disorders. *J Am Acad Child Adolesc Psychiatry*, 38(12 suppl), 32s–54s.
3. Valdivia, R. (1999). *The Implications of Culture on Developmental Delay*. Reston, VA: ERIC Clearinghouse on Disabilities and Gifted Education.
4. Doenges, M. E., Moorhouse, M. F., Murr, A. C. (2010). ND: Growth and development, delayed. *Nurse's Pocket Guide: Diagnoses, Interventions, and Rationales*. 12th ed. Philadelphia: F. A. Davis.
5. Engel, J. (2006). *Mosby's Pocket Guide to Pediatric Assessment*. 5th ed. St. Louis, MO: Mosby.
6. Newfield, S. A., Hinz, M. D., Tilley, D. S., et al. (2007). *Cox's Clinical Applications of Nursing Diagnosis: Adult, Child, Women's, Psychiatric, Gerontic, and Home Health Considerations*. 5th ed. Philadelphia: F. A. Davis.
7. North Carolina State University. (2002, updated 2011). Caring for children with special needs—Developmental delays. The National Network for Child Care. Retrieved March 2015 from www.ces.ncsu.edu/depts/fcs/pdfs/NC12.pdf.
8. Schiffman, R. F. (2004). Drug and substance use in adolescents. *MCN Am J Matern Child Nurs*, 29(1), 21–27.
9. Institute for Clinical Systems Improvement. (2005, updated 2013). Healthcare guideline: Preventive services for children and adolescents (Summary of changes). Retrieved March 2015 from https://www.icsi.org/_asset/rv9rjq/PrevSvcsKidsSoC.pdf.
10. Blann, L. E. (2005). Early intervention for children and families with special needs. *MCN Am J Matern Child Nurs*, 30(4), 263–267.
11. Mountstephen, M. (2011). *How to Detect Developmental Delay and What to Do Next: Practical Applications for Home and School*. Philadelphia: Jessica Kinsley.
12. Garzon, D. L., Thrasher, C., Tiernan, K. (2010). Providing optimal care for children with developmental disorders. *Nurse Pract*, 35(10), 30–39.
13. Narad, C., Mason, P. W. (2005, updated 2013). International adoptions: Myths and realities. Retrieved March 2015 from http://www.medscape.com/viewarticle/498588_4.
14. American Academy of Pediatrics Council on Children with Disabilities. (2006). Identifying infants and young children with developmental disorders in the medical home: An algorithm for developmental surveillance and screening. *Pediatrics*, 118(1), 405–420.
15. Drotar, D., Stancin, T., Dworkin, P. H., et al. (2008). Selecting developmental surveillance and screening tools. *Pediatr Review*, 29(10), e52–e58.
16. Aylward, G. P. (1997). Conceptual issues in developmental screening and assessment. *J Dev Behav Pediatr*, 18(5), 340–349.
17. Harden, B. J. (2004). Safety and stability for foster children: A developmental perspective. *Future Child*, 14(1), 30–47.

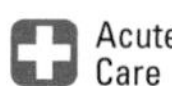

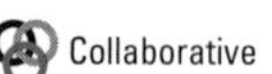

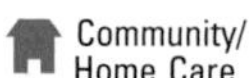

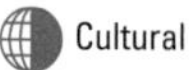

Diarrhea

Taxonomy II: Elimination and Exchange—Class 2 Gastrointestinal Function (0013) [**Diagnostic Division:** Elimination], Submitted 1975; Nursing Diagnosis Extension and Classification Revision 1998

DEFINITION: Passage of loose, unformed stools.

RELATED FACTORS

Psychological

Increase in stress level; anxiety

Situational

Laxative or substance abuse; exposure to toxin, contaminant
Treatment regimen
Enteral feedings
Travel

Physiological

Gastrointestinal inflammation, irritation
Infection; parasite
Malabsorption

DEFINING CHARACTERISTICS

Subjective

Abdominal pain
Bowel urgency; cramping

Objective

Hyperactive bowel sounds
Loose liquid stools > in 24 hours

Sample Clinical Applications: Inflammatory bowel disease, gastritis, enteral feedings, alcohol abuse, antibiotic use, food allergies or contamination, AIDS, radiation, parasites

DESIRED OUTCOMES/EVALUATION CRITERIA

Sample NOC linkages:

Bowel Elimination: Formation and evacuation of stool
Hydration: Adequate water in the intracellular and extracellular compartments of the body
Knowledge: Illness Care: Extent of understanding conveyed about illness-related information needed to achieve and maintain optimal health

Client Will (Include Specific Time Frame)

- Reestablish and maintain normal pattern of bowel functioning.
- Verbalize understanding of causative factors and rationale for treatment regimen.
- Demonstrate appropriate behavior to assist with resolution of causative factors (e.g., proper food preparation or avoidance of irritating foods).

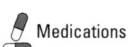

(continues on page 260)

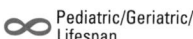

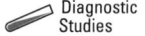

Diarrhea (continued)
ACTIONS/INTERVENTIONS

Sample NIC linkages:
Diarrhea Management: Management and alleviation of diarrhea
Fluid Monitoring: Collection and analysis of patient data to regulate fluid balance
Perineal Care: Maintenance of perineal skin integrity and relief of perineal discomfort

NURSING PRIORITY NO. 1 To assess causative factors/etiology:

- Note client's age and evaluate client's/caregiver's perception of severity of symptoms. *Acute diarrhea is usually caused by an infection, while chronic diarrhea is usually related to a functional disorder or intestinal disease. Viral diarrhea is most common among young children. Adults tend to average one bout of acute diarrhea each year. Chronic (persistent) diarrhea may be a symptom of a chronic disease and often affects adults more than children. People perceive having diarrhea in many different ways, but generally if client is having loose, watery stools occurring more than three times a day for 3 days or more, the diagnosis of diarrhea can be made. The condition can affect people of all ages, although its effect is more dangerous for infants and frail elderly (due to risk of dehydration).*[1–3]
- Obtain comprehensive history of symptoms *to help in identifying cause and treatment needs:*[1,2,4–6,13,14]
  Ascertain onset and pattern of diarrhea, noting whether it is acute or chronic. ***Acute diarrhea** is caused by (1) viral, bacterial, or parasitic infections (e.g., Norwalk virus, rotavirus; salmonella, shigella; giardia, amebiasis, respectively); (2) bacterial food-borne toxins (e.g.,* Staphylococcus aureus, Escherichia coli*); (3) medications (e.g., antibiotics, chemotherapy agents, colchicine, laxatives); and (4) enteral tube feedings. It lasts a few days up to a week.* ***Chronic diarrhea** is caused by irritable bowel syndrome, infectious diseases, inflammatory bowel disease, colon cancer and treatments, severe constipation, malabsorption disorders, laxative abuse, and certain endocrine disorders (e.g., hyperthyroidism, Addison's disease). It almost always lasts for more than 3 weeks.*
  Review history and observe stools for **characteristics** (e.g., soft to watery stools, bloody, greasy), **frequency** (e.g., more than normal number of stools/day), **time of day** (e.g., after meals), **volume**, and **duration**.
  Identify any **associated signs/symptoms** (e.g., fever/chills, abdominal cramping, emotional upset, weight loss), **aggravating factors** (e.g., stress, foods), or **mitigating factors** (e.g., changes in diet, use of prescription or over-the-counter [OTC] medications).
  Note reports of abdominal or rectal pain. *Pain is often present with inflammatory bowel disease, irritable bowel syndrome, and mesenteric ischemia.*
- Determine recent travel to developing countries or foreign environments, change in drinking water or food intake or consumption of unsafe food, swimming in untreated surface water, or similar illness of family members/others close to client *that may help identify causative environmental factors.*[2,4–6]
- Review medications, noting side effects and possible interactions. *Many drugs (e.g., antibiotics such as cephalosporins, erythromycin, penicillins, quinolones, tetracyclines, digitalis, angiotensin-converting enzyme inhibitors, NSAIDs, hypoglycemia agents, cholesterol-lowering drugs) can cause or exacerbate diarrhea, particularly in the elderly and in those who have had surgery on the intestinal tract.*[1,2,6–8]
- Evaluate diet history, noting food allergies or intolerances, and food and water safety issues, and note general nutritional, fluid, and electrolyte status *that may be causing or exacerbating diarrhea.*
- Auscultate abdomen for presence, location, and characteristics of bowel sounds. *High-pitched, rapidly occurring, and loud or tinkling bowel sounds often accompany diarrhea.*[9]
- Determine if incontinence is present. *May indicate presence of fecal impaction, particularly in the elderly, where impaction may be accompanied by diarrhea.*[3] (Refer to ND bowel Incontinence.)
- Review results of laboratory testing on stool specimens. *Can reveal presence of bacterial or viral infection, parasites, fat, blood, offending drugs, metabolic disorder, malabsorption syndrome, gastroenteritis, colitis, etc.*[1,2,4–6]

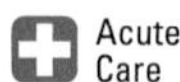

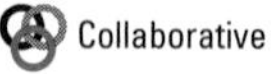

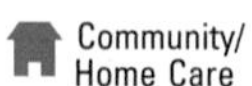

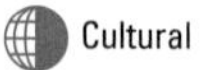

- Assist with/prepare for additional evaluation as indicated. *Chronic diarrhea may require more invasive testing, including upper and/or lower gastrointestinal radiographs, ultrasound, endoscopic evaluations, biopsy, etc.*[12]

NURSING PRIORITY NO. 2 To alleviate/limit condition:

- Assist with treatment of underlying conditions (e.g., infections, malabsorption syndrome, cancer) and complications of diarrhea. *Treatments are varied and may be as simple as allowing time for recovery from a self-limiting gastroenteritis or may require complex treatments, including antimicrobials and rehydration, or community health interventions for contaminated food or water sources.*[14]
- Encourage bedrest during an acute episode. *Rest reduces intestinal motility and metabolic rate when infection or hemorrhage is a complication.*[1–6,8,10]
- Restrict solid food intake, if indicated. *May help in short term to allow for bowel rest and reduced intestinal workload, especially if cause of diarrhea is under investigation or vomiting is present. Note: A child's preferred or usual diet may be continued to prevent or limit dehydration, with the possible limitation of fruit, fruit juices, or milk, if these factors are exacerbating the diarrhea.*[5,9]
- Limit caffeine and high-fat (e.g., butter, fried foods) or high-protein (e.g., meats) foods known to cause or aggravate diarrhea (e.g., extremely hot or cold foods, chili), milk, and fruits or fruit juices as appropriate.[1–6,8,10]
- Adjust strength and/or rate of enteral tube feedings; change formula as indicated *when diarrhea is associated with tube feedings.*[1–6,8,10]
- Consider change in infant formula. *Diarrhea may be result of or aggravated by intolerance to specific formula.*[9,10]
- Change client's routine medications as appropriate (e.g., stopping magnesium-containing antacid or antibiotic causing diarrhea).[7,8]
- Promote the use of relaxation techniques (e.g., progressive relaxation exercise, visualization techniques) *to decrease stress and anxiety.*[1–6,8,10]
- Administer medications *to treat or limit diarrhea, as indicated, depending on cause. May include use of antidiarrheals, anti-infectives, antispasmodics, etc.*[1–6,8,10,14]
- Assist client to manage situation:[12]
  Respond to call for assistance promptly.
  Place bedpan in bed with client (if desired) or commode chair near bed *to provide quick access and reduce need to wait for assistance of others.*
  Provide privacy, remove stool promptly, and use room deodorizers *to reduce noxious odors and limit embarrassment.*
  Use incontinence pads depending on the severity of the problem.
  Provide emotional and psychological support. *Diarrhea can be a source of great embarrassment and can lead to social isolation and feeling of powerlessness. Intimate relationship and sexual activity may be affected and need specific interventions to resolve.*
- Maintain skin integrity:[12]
  Assist as needed with pericare after each bowel movement *to prevent skin excoriation and breakdown.*
  Provide prompt diaper or incontinence pad change and gentle cleansing *because skin breakdown can occur quickly with diarrhea.*
  Apply lotion or skin barrier ointment as needed.
  Provide dry linen as necessary.
  Expose perineum and buttocks to air or use heat lamp with caution if needed *to keep area dry.*
  Refer to ND impaired Skin Integrity.

NURSING PRIORITY NO. 3 To restore/maintain hydration/electrolyte balance:

- Note reports of thirst, less frequent or absent urination, dry mouth and skin, weakness, light-headedness, and headache. *Signs/symptoms of dehydration and need for rehydration.*[1–3,5,6,10]

- Observe for or question parents about young child crying with no tears, fever, decreased urination or no wet diapers for 6 to 8 hours, listlessness or irritability, sunken eyes, dry mouth and tongue, and suspected or documented weight loss. *Child needs urgent or emergency treatment for dehydration if these signs are present and child is not taking fluids.*[1–3,5,6,10]
- Note presence of low blood pressure or postural hypotension, tachycardia, poor skin hydration, or turgor. *Presence of these factors indicates severe dehydration and electrolyte imbalance. The frail elderly can progress quickly to this point, especially when vomiting is present or client's normal food and fluid intake is below requirements.*[1–3,5,6,10]
- Monitor total intake and output, including stool output as possible. *Provides estimation of fluid needs.*[1,3,5,6,10]
- Weigh infant's diapers to determine output.[1–3,5,6,10]
- Offer and encourage water, plus broth or soups that contain sodium, or soft fruits or vegetables that contain potassium *to replace water and electrolytes.*[1–3,5,6,10]
- Recommend oral intake of beverages such as Gatorade, Pedialyte, Infalyte, and Smart Water. *Commercial rehydration solutions containing electrolytes may prevent or correct imbalances.*[1–3,5,6,10]
- Administer IV fluids, electrolytes, and enteral or parenteral feedings, as indicated. *IV fluids may be needed either short term to restore hydration status (e.g., acute gastroenteritis) or long term (severe osmotic diarrhea). Enteral or parenteral nutrition is reserved for clients unable to maintain adequate nutritional status because of long-term diarrhea (e.g., wasting syndrome, malnutrition states).*[1–3,5,6,10]

NURSING PRIORITY NO. 4 To promote return to normal bowel functioning:

- Encourage intake of nonirritating liquids, increasing intake as tolerated and gradually returning to normal diet.[1,2,4–6,10,11,13]
- Recommend products such as natural fiber, plain natural yogurt, and Lactinex *to restore normal bowel flora.*[1,2,4–6,10,11]
- Administer medications as ordered *to treat infectious process, decrease motility, and/or absorb water.*[1,2,4–6,10,11]

NURSING PRIORITY NO. 5 To promote wellness (Teaching/Discharge Considerations):

- Review individual's causative factors and appropriate interventions *to prevent recurrence.*
- Discuss medication regimen, including prescription and OTC drugs, *especially when client has multiple medications with potential for diarrhea as side effect or interaction.*[12]
- Encourage/refer for vaccines, as indicated. *Vaccines could include those recommended for travelers to susceptible areas of the world (e.g., cholera or typhoid vaccines) and/or could be preventative therapies for infants. For example, currently two oral live-virus vaccines are marketed in the United States for the prevention of rotavirus gastroenteritis, a major cause of severe diarrhea in infants.*[5,13]
- Instruct clients planning to travel outside the United States about traveler's diarrhea and ways to prevent or limit food- and water-borne illness *(e.g., do not drink tap water, use tap water ice cubes, or brush your teeth with tap water; avoid raw fruits and vegetables unless they can be peeled; avoid raw or rare meat or fish; discuss destination with local health department for particular recommendations, such as advisability of use of protective antibiotics).*[12,13]
- Assess home or living environment, if indicated. *Discussion with client/caregivers may be needed regarding (1) sanitation and hygiene (e.g., hand hygiene and laundry practices), (2) safe food storage and preparation (to reduce risk of foodborne infections), and (3) particular risks in select populations (e.g., persons with chronic liver disease should avoid shellfish; persons with impaired immune defenses are at increased risk for diarrhea associated with raw dairy products or unheated deli meats; pregnant women should avoid undercooked meats [infectious diarrhea]).*[12]
- Emphasize importance of hand hygiene *to prevent spread of infectious causes of diarrhea such as* Clostridium difficile, *S. aureus, etc.*[15]
- Instruct parent/caregiver in signs of dehydration and importance of fluid and electrolyte replacement, as well as simple food and fluids to provide rehydration.

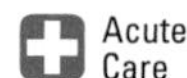

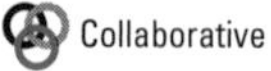

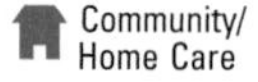

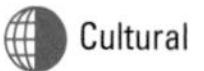

DOCUMENTATION FOCUS

Assessment/Reassessment

- Assessment findings, including characteristics and pattern of elimination.

Planning

- Plan of care and who is involved in planning.
- Teaching plan.

Implementation/Evaluation

- Client's response to treatment, teaching, and actions performed.
- Attainment or progress toward desired outcome(s).
- Modifications to plan of care.

Discharge planning

- Recommendations for follow-up care.

References

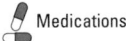

1. Hogan, C. M. (1998). The nurse's role in diarrhea management. *Oncol Nurs Forum*, 25(5), 879–885.
2. National Digestive Diseases Information Clearinghouse. (update 2013). Diarrhea. Retrieved October 2015 from http://www.niddk.nih.gov/health-information/health-topics/digestive-diseases/diarrhea/Pages/facts.aspx.
3. Carnaveli, D. L., Patrick, M. (1993). *Nursing Management for the Elderly*. 3rd ed. Philadelphia: J. B. Lippincott.
4. No author listed. (2006, update 2012). Evidence-based clinical guideline for acute gastroenteritis (AGE) in children aged 2 months through 5 years. Cincinnati Children's Hospital Medical Center. Retrieved October 2015 from http://www.guideline.gov/content.aspx?id=35123#tiptop.
5. World Gastroenterological Organization. (2012). Acute diarrhea in adults and children. Retrieved October 2015 from http://www.worldgastroenterology.org/guidelines/global-guidelines/acute-diarrhea/acute-diarrhea-english.
6. Guerrant, R. L., Van Gilder, T., Steiner, T. S., et al. (2001). Practice guidelines for the management of infectious diarrhea. *Clin Infect Dis*, 32(3), 331–351.
7. Ratnaike, R. N. (2000). Drug-induced diarrhea in older persons. *Clin Geriatr*, 8(1), 67–76.
8. Mayo Clinic Staff. (2013). Antibiotic-associated diarrhea. Retrieved October 2015 from http://www.mayoclinic.org/diseases-conditions/antibiotic-associated-diarrhea/basics/definition/con-20023556.
9. Engel, J. (2006). *Mosby's Pocket Guide to Pediatric Assessment*. 5th ed. St. Louis, MO: Mosby.
10. Larson, C. E. (2000). Evidence-based practice: Safety and efficacy of oral rehydration therapy for the treatment of diarrhea and gastroenteritis in pediatrics. *Pediatr Nurs*, 26(2), 177–179.
11. Peikin, R. (1999). *Diarrhea in Gastrointestinal Health*. New York: HarperCollins.
12. Doenges, M. E., Moorhouse, M. F., Murr, A. C. (2008). ND Diarrhea, risk for: in Gastrointestinal Disorders-Inflammatory Bowel Disease. *Nursing Care Plans: Guidelines for Individualizing Patient Care*. 8th ed. Philadelphia: F. A. Davis.
13. Guandalini, S. (2010, update 2015). Diarrhea. Retrieved October 2015 from http://emedicine.medscape.com/article/928598-overview.
14. Diskin, A. (2006, updated 2015). Emergent treatment of gastroenteritis. Retrieved October 2015 from http://emedicine.medscape.com/article/775277-overview.
15. DeNoon, D. (2006). *C. diff:* New threat from old bug: Epidemic gut infection causing rapid rise in life-threatening disease. Retrieved October 2015 from http://www.webmd.com/digestive-disorders/news/20061012/c-diff-new-threat-from-old-bug.

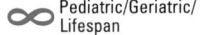

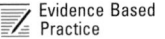

risk for Disuse Syndrome

Taxonomy II: Activity/Rest—Class 2 Activity/Exercise (00040) [**Diagnostic Division:** Activity/Rest], Submitted 1988; Revised 2013

DEFINITION: Vulnerable to deterioration of body systems as the result of prescribed or unavoidable musculoskeletal inactivity, which may compromise health.

AUTHOR NOTE: Complications from immobility can include decreased strength or endurance, activity intolerance, impaired sitting or standing or walking; pressure ulcer, impaired urinary or bowel function; respiratory complications, such as pneumonia; systemic infections; blood clots; orthostatic hypotension; and disorientation, body image disturbance, ineffective coping, and powerlessness.

RISK FACTORS

Alteration in level of consciousness
Mechanical or prescribed immobility; paralysis
Pain
Note: A risk diagnosis is not evidenced by signs and symptoms, as the problem has not occurred; rather, nursing interventions are directed at prevention.
Sample Clinical Applications: Multiple sclerosis (MS), cerebral palsy, muscular dystrophy, postpolio syndrome, brain injury or stroke, spinal cord injury (SCI), arthritis, osteoporosis, fractures, amputation, dementia

DESIRED OUTCOMES/EVALUATION CRITERIA

Sample NOC linkages:
Immobility Consequences: Physiological: Severity of compromise in physiological functioning due to impaired physical mobility
Risk Control: Personal actions to prevent, eliminate, or reduce modifiable health threats
Immobility Consequences: Psycho-Cognitive: Severity of compromise in psycho-cognitive functioning due to impaired physical mobility

Client Will (Include Specific Time Frame)
- Display intact skin and tissues or achieve timely wound healing.
- Maintain or reestablish effective elimination patterns.
- Be free of signs/symptoms of infectious processes.
- Demonstrate absence of pulmonary congestion with breath sounds clear.
- Demonstrate adequate peripheral perfusion with stable vital signs, skin warm and dry, and palpable peripheral pulses.
- Maintain usual reality orientation.
- Maintain or regain optimal level of cognitive, neurosensory, and musculoskeletal functioning.
- Express sense of control over the present situation and potential outcome.
- Recognize and incorporate change into self-concept in accurate manner without negative self-esteem.

ACTIONS/INTERVENTIONS

Sample NIC linkages:
Surveillance: Purposeful and ongoing acquisition, interpretation, and synthesis of patient data for clinical decision making
Bed Rest Care: Promotion of comfort and safety and prevention of complications for a patient unable to get out of bed

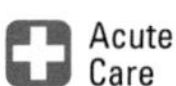

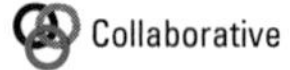

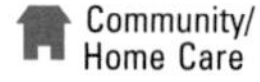

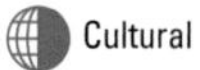

Exercise Promotion: Facilitation of regular physical exercise to maintain or advance to a higher level of fitness and health

NURSING PRIORITY NO. 1 To evaluate probability of developing complications:

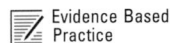

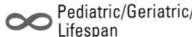

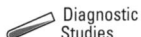

- Identify underlying conditions/pathology (e.g., cancer, trauma; fractures with casting, immobilization devices; surgery, chronic disease conditions, malnutrition; neurological conditions [e.g., stroke, brain or SCI, postpolio syndrome, MS]; chronic pain conditions; use of predisposing medications [e.g., steroids]) *that can cause or exacerbate problems associated with inactivity and immobility. Bedrest, immobility, and/or lack of physical activity (for any reason) causes a loss of protein and muscle deterioration. "Disuse syndrome" is a classic pattern of muscular deconditioning and atrophy resulting from inactivity or immobilization. Once muscle is lost, it is difficult to gain it back.*[10]
- Identify potential concerns, including cognition, mobility, and exercise status. *Disuse syndrome can be a complication of and cause for bedridden state. The syndrome can include muscle and bone atrophy, stiffening of joints, brittle bones, reduction of cardiopulmonary function, loss of red blood cells, decreased sex hormones, decreased resistance to infections, increased proportion of body fat in relation to muscle mass, and chemical changes in the brain, which adversely impact client's activities of daily living (ADLs), social life, and quality of life.*[1,2,10]
- Note client's age. *Age-related physiological changes (e.g., decrease in muscle mass and/or function, increased levels of proinflammatory cytokines, increased production of free radicals or impaired detoxification, malnutrition, low hormone output, reduced neurological drive) accompanied by chronic illness predispose older adults to functional decline related to inactivity and immobility.*[1,3,8–10]
- Determine if client's condition is acute/short term or whether it may be a long-term/permanent condition. *Relatively short-term conditions (e.g., simple fracture treated with cast) may respond quickly to rehabilitative efforts. Long-term conditions (e.g., stroke, aged person with dementia, cancers, demyelinating or degenerative diseases, SCI, psychological problems such as depression or learned helplessness) have a higher risk of complications for the client and caregiver. Note: Studies carried out with intensive-care patients supported that prolonged immobilization leads to disuse atrophy of muscles and other physiological changes that decrease patients' ability to tolerate physical activity. They also found that muscle atrophy begins within hours of immobilization, leading to a 4% to 5% loss of muscle strength for each week of bedrest.*[11,12]
- Assess and document (ongoing) client's functional status, including cognition, vision, and hearing, social support, psychological well-being, and abilities in performance of ADLs *for a comparative baseline, to evaluate response to treatment, and to identify preventative interventions or necessary services.*[8]
- Evaluate client's risk for injury. *Risk is greater in client with cognitive problems, lack of safe or stimulating environment, inadequate mobility aids, and/or sensory-perception problems.*[3]
- Ascertain attitudes of individual/significant other (SO) about condition (e.g., cultural values, stigma). Note misconceptions. *The client may be influenced (positively or negatively) by peer group, cultural, and family role expectations.*
- Evaluate client's/family's understanding and ability to manage care for prolonged period. Ascertain availability and use of support systems. *Caregivers may be influenced by their own physical or emotional limitations, degree of commitment to assisting the client toward optimal independence, or available time.*[3]
- Review psychological assessment of client's emotional status. *Potential problems that may arise from presence of condition need to be identified and dealt with to avoid further debilitation. Common associated psychological changes include depression, anxiety, and avoidance behaviors.*[2,3]

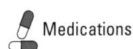

NURSING PRIORITY NO. 2 To identify/provide individually appropriate preventive or corrective interventions:

- Skin:[6,7]

  Inspect skin on a frequent basis, noting changes. Monitor skin over bony prominences.

Reposition frequently as individually indicated *to relieve pressure.*

Provide skin care daily and prn, drying well and using gentle massage and lotion *to stimulate circulation.*

Keep skin, clothing, and area clean and dry *to prevent skin irritation and breakdown.*

Initiate use of padding devices (e.g., foam, egg-crate/gel/water/air mattress or cushions) *to reduce pressure on and enhance circulation to compromised tissues.*

Review nutritional status and promote diet with adequate protein, calorie, and vitamin and mineral intake *to aid in healing and promote general good health of skin and tissues.*

Refer to NDs impaired Skin Integrity, impaired Tissue Integrity, and risk for Pressure Ulcer for additional interventions.

- Elimination:[6–8]

Observe elimination pattern, noting changes and potential problems.

Encourage a balanced diet, including fruits and vegetables high in fiber and with adequate fluids *for optimal stool consistency and to facilitate passage through colon.*

Provide or encourage adequate fluid intake, include water and cranberry juice *to reduce risk of urinary infections.*

Maximize mobility at earliest opportunity.

Evaluate need for stool softeners or bulk-forming laxatives.

Implement consistent bowel management or bladder training programs, as indicated.

Monitor urinary output and characteristics *to identify changes associated with infection.*

Refer to NDs Constipation, Diarrhea, bowel Incontinence, impaired Urinary Elimination, and Urinary Retention for additional interventions.

- Respiration:[6,7]

Monitor breath sounds and characteristics of secretions *for early detection of complications (e.g., atelectasis, pneumonia).*

Encourage ambulation and upright position. Reposition, cough, and deep breathe on a regular schedule *to facilitate clearing of secretions and improve lung function.*

Encourage use of incentive spirometry. Suction as indicated *to clear airways,*

Demonstrate techniques and assist with postural drainage when indicated for long-term airway clearance difficulties.

Assist with and instruct family and caregivers in quad coughing techniques or diaphragmatic weight training *to maximize ventilation (in presence of SCI).*

Discourage smoking. Refer for a smoking-cessation program as indicated.

Refer to NDs ineffective Airway Clearance, ineffective Breathing Pattern, impaired Gas Exchange, and impaired spontaneous Ventilation for additional interventions.

- Vascular (tissue perfusion):[6–8]

Assess cognition and mental status (ongoing). *Changes can reflect state of cardiac health or cerebral oxygenation impairment or be indicative of a mental or emotional state that could adversely affect safety and self-care.*

Determine core and skin temperature. Investigate development of cyanosis and changes in mentation *to identify changes in oxygenation status.*

Evaluate circulation and nerve function of affected body parts on a routine, ongoing basis. *Changes in temperature, color, sensation, and movement can be the effect of immobility, disease, aging, or injury.*

Encourage or provide adequate fluid *to prevent dehydration and circulatory stasis.*

Monitor blood pressure before, during, and after activity—sitting, standing, and lying if possible—*to ascertain response to and tolerance of activity.*

Assist with position changes as needed. Raise head gradually. Institute use of tilt table or sitting upright on side of bed and arising slowly where appropriate *to reduce incidence of injury that may occur as a result of orthostatic hypotension.*

Maintain proper body position; avoid use of constricting garments and restraints *to prevent vascular congestion.*

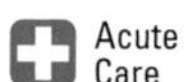

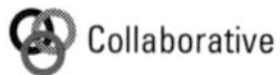

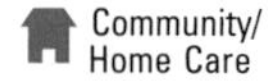

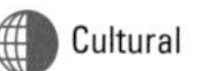

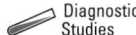

Provide range-of-motion exercise. Refer for and assist with physical therapy exercises *for strengthening, restoration of optimal range of motion, and prevention of circulatory problems related to disuse.*[4]

Mobilize quickly and as often as possible, using mobility aids and frequent rest stops to assist client in continuing activity. *Upright position and weight bearing help maintain bone strength, improve circulation, and prevent postural hypotension.*[8]

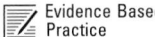

Institute peripheral vascular support measures (e.g., anti-embolism hose, Ace wraps, sequential compression devices) *to enhance venous return and reduce incidence of deep vein thrombosis. Note: With prolonged bedrest and lack of physical activity, the amount of red blood cells declines, which decreases the amount of oxygen being delivered to the tissues. Blood clots and inflammation increase.*[13]

Refer to NDs risk for Activity Intolerance, decreased Cardiac Output, risk for Peripheral Neurovascular Dysfunction, and ineffective peripheral Tissue Perfusion for additional interventions.

- Musculoskeletal (mobility, range of motion, strength, and endurance):[5–8,13]

Perform or assist with range-of-motion exercises and involve client in core strengthening and active exercises as soon as possible with physical or occupational therapy *to promote bone health, muscle strengthening, flexibility, optimal conditioning, and functional ability.*

Maximize involvement in self-care *to restore or maintain strength, functional abilities, and early independence in self-care activities.*

Intersperse activity with rest periods. Pace activities as possible *to increase strength and endurance in a gradual manner and reduce failure of planned exercise because of exhaustion or overuse of weak muscles or injured area.*

Identify need and use of supportive devices (e.g., cane, walker, functional positioning splints) as appropriate *to assist with safe mobility and functional independence.*

Evaluate role of physiological and psychological pain in mobility problem. Implement pain management program as individually indicated.

Avoid or monitor closely the use of restraints and immobilize client as little as possible *to reduce possibility of agitation and injury.*

Refer to NDs risk for Falls; impaired physical Mobility; impaired Sitting, Standing, or Walking; acute Pain; chronic Pain; and chronic Pain Syndrome for additional interventions.

- Sensory Perception:[6–8,13]

Orient client as necessary to time, place, person, and situation. Provide cues for orientation (e.g., clock, calendar). *Disturbances of sensory stimulation, interpretation, and thought processes are associated with immobility as well as aging, being ill, disease processes/treatments, and medication effects.*

Provide appropriate level of environmental stimulation (e.g., music, TV, radio, personal possessions, visitors). *Needs vary depending on the client, the nature of the current problem, and whether client is at home or in a healthcare facility. Having normal life cues can help with mental stimulation and restoration of health.*

Encourage participation in recreational or diversional activities and a regular exercise program (as tolerated) *to decrease the sensory deprivation associated with immobility and isolation.*

Promote regular sleep hours, use of sleep aids, and usual presleep rituals *to promote normal sleep and rest cycle.*

Refer to NDs chronic Confusion, deficient Diversional Activity, Insomnia, and [disturbed Sensory Perception] for additional interventions.

- Self-Esteem, Powerlessness, Hopelessness, Social Isolation:[6,7,9]

Determine factors that may contribute to impairment of client's self-esteem and social interactions. *Many factors can be involved, including the client's age, relationship status, and usual health state; presence of disabilities, including pain; financial, environmental, and physical problems; and current situation causing immobility and client's state of mind concerning the importance of the current situation in regard to the rest of client's life and desired lifestyle.*

Ascertain if changes in client's situation are likely to be short term/temporary or long term/permanent. *Can affect both the client and care provider's coping abilities and willingness to engage in activities that prevent or limit effects of immobility.*

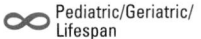

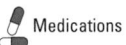

Assess living situation (e.g., lives with spouse, parents, alone) and determine factors that may positively or adversely affect client's progress, roles, and/or safety.

Explain or review all care procedures and plans. *Improves knowledge and facilitates decision making. Involves client in own care, enhances sense of control, and promotes independence.*

Encourage questions and verbalization of feelings. *Aids in reducing anxiety and promotes learning about condition and specific needs.*

Acknowledge concerns; provide presence and encouragement.

Refer for mental, psychological, or spiritual services as indicated *to provide counseling, support, and medications.*

Provide for and assist with mutual goal setting, involving SO(s). *Promotes sense of control and enhances commitment to goals.*

Ascertain that client can communicate needs adequately (e.g., call light, writing tablet, picture or letter board, interpreter).

Refer to NDs impaired verbal Communication, Powerlessness, ineffective Role Performance, Self-Esteem [specify], impaired Social Interaction, and Social Isolation for additional interventions.

- Body Image:[6,7]

Evaluate for presence or potential for physical, emotional, and behavioral conditions that may contribute to isolation and degeneration. *Disuse syndrome often affects those individuals who are already isolated for one reason or another (e.g., serious illness or injury with disfigurement, frail elderly living alone, individual with severe depression, person with unacceptable behavior or without support system).*

Orient to body changes through discussion and written information *to promote acceptance and understanding of needs.*

Promote interactions with peers and normalization of activities within individual abilities. *Physical activity and social interactions stimulate the production of chemical substances produced by the body that produce increased feelings of well-being, vitality, and alertness.*

Refer to NDs disturbed Body Image, disturbed Personal Identity, situational low Self-Esteem, and Social Isolation for additional interventions.

NURSING PRIORITY NO. 3 To promote wellness (Teaching/Discharge Considerations):

- Assist client/caregivers in development of individualized plan of care *to best meet the client's potential, enhance safety, and prevent or limit affects of disuse.*
- Provide information about individual needs and areas of concern (e.g., client's mental status, living environment, nutritional needs). *Information can help client and care providers to understand what long-term goals could be attained, what barriers may need to be overcome, and what constitutes progress or lack of progress requiring further evaluation and intervention.*[6]
- Review therapeutic regimen. *Treatment may be required for underlying condition(s), stress management, medications, therapies, and needed lifestyle changes.*
- Encourage involvement in regular exercise program, including flexibility, resistance and strengthening activities, and active or assistive range of motion *to limit consequences of disuse and maximize level of function.*[2]
- Promote self-care and SO-supported activities *to gain or maintain independence.*
- Recommend suitable balanced nutrition as well as use of supplements if needed *to provide energy for healing and maximal organ function.*
- Refer to appropriate community health providers and resources *to provide necessary assistance (e.g., help with meal preparation, financial help for groceries, dietitian or nutritionist).*[7]
- Review signs/symptoms requiring medical evaluation/follow-up *to promote timely interventions and limit adverse effects of situation.*[6]
- Identify community support services (e.g., financial, counseling, home maintenance, respite care, transportation).
- Refer to appropriate rehabilitation or home-care and support resources *to help client/care providers learn more about specific condition and acquire needed assistance, adaptive devices, and necessary equipment.*

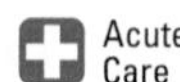

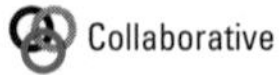

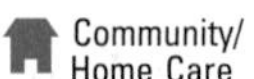

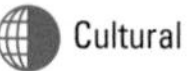

DOCUMENTATION FOCUS

Assessment/Reassessment

- Assessment findings, noting individual areas of concern, functional level, degree of independence, support systems and available resources.

Planning

- Plan of care and who is involved in planning.
- Teaching plan.

Implementation/Evaluation

- Client's response to interventions, teaching, and actions performed.
- Changes in level of functioning.
- Attainment or progress toward desired outcome(s).
- Modifications to plan of care.

Discharge Planning

- Long-term needs and who is responsible for actions to be taken.
- Specific referrals made, resources for specific equipment needs.

References

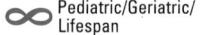

1. Eliopoulos, C. (2010). Deconditioning and sarcopenia. *Long-Term Living*. Retrieved March 2015 from http://www.ltlmagazine.com/article/deconditioning-and-sarcopenia.
2. Verbunt, J. A., Seelen, H. A., Vlaeyen, J. W., et al. (2003). Disuse and deconditioning in chronic low back pain: Concepts and hypotheses on contributing mechanisms. *Eur J Pain*, 7, 9–21.
3. Blair, K. A. (1999). Immobility and activity intolerance in older adults. In Stanley, M., Beare, P. G. (eds). *Gerontological Nursing: A Health Promotion/Protection Approach*. 2nd ed. Philadelphia: F. A. Davis.
4. Jiricka, M. K. (1994). Alterations in activity intolerance. In Port, C. M. (ed). *Pathophysiology: Concepts of Altered Health States*. Philadelphia: J. B. Lippincott.
5. Metzlar, D. J., Harr, J. (1996). Positioning your patient properly. *Am J Nurs*, 96(3), 33–37.
6. Doenges, M. E., Moorhouse, M. F., Geissler-Murr, A. C. (2004). *Nurse's Pocket Guide: Diagnoses, Interventions, and Rationales*. 9th ed. Philadelphia: F. A. Davis.
7. Newfield, S. A., Hinz, M. D., Tilley, D. S., et al. (2007). *Cox's Clinical Applications of Nursing Diagnosis: Adult, Child, Women's, Psychiatric, Gerontic, and Home Health Considerations*. 5th ed. Philadelphia: F. A. Davis.
8. Graf, C. (2006). Functional decline in hospitalized older adults. *Am J Nurs*, 106(1), 58–67.
9. Bortz, W. (2009). Disuse and aging. *J Gerontol A Bio Sci Med Sci*, 108(6), 60–72.
10. Benton, M. J., Whyte, M. D., Dyal, B. W. (2011). Sarcopenic obesity: Strategies for management. *Am J Nurs*, 111(12), 38–44.
11. Needham, M. D. (2008). Mobilizing patients in the intensive care unit: Improving neuromuscular weakness and physical function. *JAMA*, 300(14), 1685–1690.
12. Morris, P. E., Herridge, M. S. (2007). Early intensive care unit mobility: Future directions. *Crit Care Clin*, 23(1), 97–110.
13. Dysautonomia Youth Network of America, Inc. (2013). The importance of physical activity. Retrieved February 2015 from http://www.dynainc.org/living/activity.

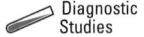

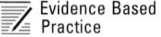

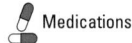

deficient Diversional Activity

Taxonomy II: Health Promotion—Class 1 Health Awareness (00097) [**Diagnostic Division:** Activity/Rest], Submitted 1980

DEFINITION: Decreased stimulation from (or interest or engagement in) recreational or leisure activities. [Note: Internal/external factors may or may not be beyond the individual's control.]

RELATED FACTORS

Insufficient diversional activity [e.g., lack of resources]
Prolonged hospitalization/institutionalization; [frequent, lengthy treatments; homebound/bedridden]
Extremes of age
[Physical limitations, fatigue, chronic pain]

DEFINING CHARACTERISTICS

Subjective

Boredom [e.g., wishes there were something to do, to read]

Objective

Current setting does not allow engagement in activities

Sample Clinical Applications: Traumatic injuries, chronic pain, prolonged recovery (e.g., postoperative, complicated fractures), cancer therapy, chronic/debilitating conditions (e.g., congestive heart failure [CHF], chronic obstructive pulmonary disease [COPD], renal failure, multiple sclerosis [MS]), awaiting organ transplantation

DESIRED OUTCOMES/EVALUATION CRITERIA

Sample NOC linkages:

Motivation: Inner urge that moves or prompts an individual to positive action
Leisure Participation: Use of relaxing, interesting, and enjoyable activities to promote well-being
Social Involvement: Social interactions with persons, groups, or organizations

Client Will (Include Specific Time Frame)

- Recognize own psychological response (e.g., hopelessness and helplessness, anger, depression) and initiate appropriate coping actions.
- Engage in satisfying activities within personal limitations.

ACTIONS/INTERVENTIONS

Sample NIC linkages:

Recreation Therapy: Purposeful use of recreation to promote relaxation and enhancement of social skills
Activity Therapy: Prescription of and assistance with specific physical, cognitive, social, and spiritual activities to increase the range, frequency, or duration of an individual's (or group's) activity
Exercise Promotion: Facilitation of regular physical exercise to maintain or advance to a higher level of fitness and health

NURSING PRIORITY NO. 1 To assess precipitating/etiological factors:

- Assess client's physical, cognitive, emotional, and environmental status. *Validates reality of diversional deprivation when it exists or identifies the potential for loss of desired diversional activity in order to plan for prevention or early intervention where possible. Note: Studies show that key problems faced by clients who are hospi-*

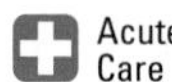

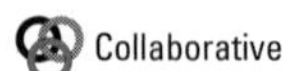

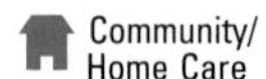

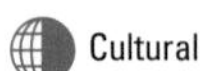

talized (or in a long-term facility, or immobilized) for extended periods of time include boredom, stress, and depression. These negative states can impede recovery and lead clients to report symptoms more frequently.[1,10]

- Observe for restlessness, flat facial expression, withdrawal, hostility, yawning, or statements of boredom as noted above, especially in individual likely to be confined either temporarily or long term. *May be indicative of need for diversional interventions.*[1]
- Note potential impact of current disability or illness on lifestyle (e.g., young child with leukemia, elderly person with fractured hip, individual with severe depression). *Provides comparative baseline for assessments and interventions.*[8]
- Be aware of age and developmental level, gender, cultural factors, and the importance of a given activity in client's life. *Cultural issues include gender roles, communication styles, privacy and personal space; expectations and views regarding time and activities; and control of the immediate environment, family traditions, and social patterns. When illness interferes with individual's ability to engage in usual activities, such as a lifelong dancer with incapacitating osteoporosis, the person may have difficulty engaging in meaningful substitute activities.*[11]
- Determine client's actual ability to participate in available activities, noting attention span, physical limitations and tolerance, level of interest or desire, and safety needs. *Presence of depression or disinterest in life; problems of immobility; protective isolation; and lack of stimulation, developmental delay, or sensory deprivation may interfere with desired activity. However, lack of involvement may not reflect client's actual abilities, but may rather be a matter of misperception about abilities.*[8]

NURSING PRIORITY NO. 2 To motivate and stimulate client involvement in solutions:

- Institute or continue appropriate actions to deal with concomitant conditions such as anxiety, depression, grief, dementia, physical injury, isolation and immobility, malnutrition, acute or chronic pain, etc. *These conditions interfere with the individual's ability to engage in meaningful activities that will stimulate his or her interest.*
- Introduce activities at client's current level of functioning, progressing to more complex activities, as tolerated. *Provides opportunity for client to experience successes, reaffirming capabilities and enhancing self-esteem.*[7]
- Establish therapeutic relationship, acknowledging reality of situation and client's feelings. *May be feeling sense of loss when unable to participate in usual activities or to interact socially as desired.*[7]
- Accept hostile expressions while limiting aggressive acting-out behavior. *Permission to express feelings of anger and hopelessness allows for beginning resolution. However, destructive behavior is counterproductive to self-esteem and problem solving.*[7]
- Involve client and parent/significant other (SO)/caregiver in determining client's needs, desires, and available resources. *Helps ensure that plan is attentive to client's interests and resources, increasing likelihood of client participation.*[2]
- Encourage parent/caregiver of young child to engage in play with confined child. *Play is essential to young child's development, can help redirect child's attention from pain of condition, and reduce child's boredom and stress.*[3,12]
- Review history of lifelong activities and hobbies client has enjoyed. Discuss reasons client is not doing these activities now and whether client can or would like to resume these activities. *Diversional activities can provide positive and productive avenues into which client can channel thoughts and time.*[4]
- Assist client/caregiver to set realistic goals for diversional activities, communicating hope and patience. *Can help client realize that this situation is not hopeless, that there are choices for improving the current situation, and that the future can hold the promise for improvement.*
- Provide instruction in relaxation techniques (e.g., meditation, sharing experiences, reminiscence, soft music, guided visualization) *to enhance coping skills.*[7]
- Participate in decisions about timing and spacing of visitors and leisure and care activities *to promote relaxation and reduce sense of boredom as well as prevent overstimulation and exhaustion.*[7]
- Encourage client to assist in scheduling required and optional activity choices. *For example, client may want to watch favorite television show at bath time; if bath can be rescheduled later, client's sense of control is enhanced.*[7]

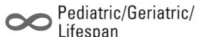

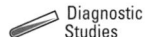

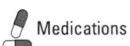

- Encourage mix of desired activities/stimuli (e.g., music, news, educational presentations, movies, computer or Internet access, books or other reading materials, visitors, games, arts and crafts, sensory enrichment [e.g., massage, aromatherapy], grooming and beauty care, cooking, social outings, gardening, discussion groups, as appropriate). *Activities need to be personally meaningful and not physically/emotionally overwhelming for client to derive the most benefit.*[4,9]
- Refrain from making changes in schedule without discussing with client. *It is important for staff to be sensitive and responsible in making and following through on commitments to client.*[7]
- Provide change of scenery (indoors and outdoors where possible). Provide for periodic changes in the personal environment when client is confined inside, eliciting the client's input for likes and desires. *Change (e.g., new pictures on the wall, seasonal colors/flowers, altering room furniture, outdoor light and air) can provide positive sensory stimulation, reduce client's boredom, and improve sense of normalcy and control.*[5]
- Suggest activities such as bird feeders/baths for bird-watching, a garden in a window box or terrarium, or a fishbowl or aquarium *to stimulate observation as well as involvement and participation in activity (e.g., bird identification, picking out feeders and seeds).*[7]
- Involve recreational, occupational, play, music, or movement therapists as appropriate *to help identify enjoyable activities for client and to procure assistive devices or modify activities for individual situation. Assists client to express needs and feelings, share experiences, escape healthcare routines, and participate in self-healing.*[1,6,9]

NURSING PRIORITY NO. 3 To promote wellness (Teaching/Discharge Considerations):

- Explore options for useful activities using the person's strengths/abilities and interests to engage the client/SO.
- Make appropriate referrals to available resources (e.g., exercise groups, senior activities, hobby clubs, volunteering, companion and service organizations) *to introduce or continue diversional activities in community/home settings.*
- Refer to NDs ineffective Coping, Hopelessness, Powerlessness, and Social Isolation for additional interventions.

DOCUMENTATION FOCUS

Assessment/Reassessment

- Specific assessment findings, including blocks to desired activities.
- Individual choices for activities.

Planning

- Plan of care, specific interventions, and who is involved in planning.

Implementation/Evaluation

- Client's responses to interventions, teaching, and actions performed.
- Attainment or progress toward desired outcome(s).
- Modifications to plan of care.

Discharge Planning

- Long-term needs and who is responsible for actions to be taken.
- Referrals made and available community resources.

References

1. Radziewicz, R. M. (1992). Using diversional activities to enhance coping. *Cancer Nurs*, 15(4), 293–298.
2. Newfield, S. A., Hinz, M. D., Tilley, D. S., et al. (2007). *Cox's Clinical Applications of Nursing Diagnosis: Adult, Child, Women's, Psychiatric, Gerontic, and Home Health Considerations*. 5th ed. Philadelphia: F. A. Davis.
3. Engel, J. (2005). *Mosby's Pocket Guide to Pediatric Assessment*. 6th ed. St. Louis, MO: Mosby.
4. Harley, K., Hunt, J., Simmons, S., et al. (2002). *Making each moment count: Developing a diversional therapies program for patients with hematologic malignancies.* (Abstract from Oncology Nursing Society Convention).

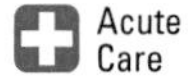

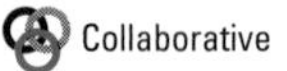

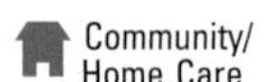

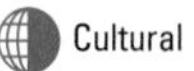

5. Dossey, B. M. (1998). Holistic modalities & healing moments. *Am J Nurs*, 98(6), 44–47.
6. Coaten, R. (2002). Movement matters: Revealing the hidden humanity within dementia through movement, dance and the imagination. *Dementia*, 1(3), 386–392.
7. Doenges, M. E., Moorhouse, M. F., Geissler-Murr, A. C. (2002). Psychosocial aspects of care. *Nursing Care Plans: Guidelines for Individualizing Patient Care*. 6th ed. Philadelphia: F. A. Davis.
8. Heriot, C. S. (1999). Developmental tasks and development in the later years of life. In Stanley, M., Bear, P. G. (eds). *Gerontological Nursing: A Health Promotion/Protection Approach*. 2nd ed. Philadelphia: F. A. Davis.
9. Wheeler, S. L., Houston, K. (2005). The role of diversional activities in the general medical hospital setting. *Holist Nurs Pract*, 19(2), 67–69.
10. Sommers, J., Vodanovich, S. J. (2000). Boredom proneness: Its relationship to psychological and physical-health symptoms. *J Clin Psych*, 56(1), 149–155.
11. Jenko, M., Moffitt, S. (2006). Transcultural nursing principles. *J Hospice & Palliative Nursing*, 8(3), 172–180.
12. Gabany, E., Shellenbarger, T. (2010). Caring for families with deployment stress. *Am J Nurs*, 110(11), 36–41.

risk for Dry Eye

Taxonomy II: Safety/Protection—Class 5 Physical Injury (00219) [**Diagnostic Division:** Safety], Submitted 2010; Revised 2013

DEFINITION: Vulnerable to eye discomfort or damage to the cornea and conjunctiva due to reduced quantity or quality of tears to moisten the eye, which may compromise health.

RISK FACTORS

Aging; female gender; hormonal change; vitamin A deficiency
Autoimmune disease (e.g., rheumatoid arthritis, diabetes mellitus); history of allergy
Contact lens wearer; ocular surface damage
Environmental factor (e.g., air conditioning, excessive wind, sunlight exposure, air pollution, low humidity)
Lifestyle choice (e.g., smoking, caffeine use, prolonged reading/[computer use])
Neurological lesion with sensory or motor reflex loss (e.g., lagophthalmos, lack of spontaneous blink reflex)
Treatment regimen; mechanical ventilation
NOTE: A risk diagnosis is not evidenced by signs and symptoms, as the problem has not occurred; rather, nursing interventions are directed at prevention.

Sample Clinical Applications: Any condition where client is unable to protect self from drying of eye tissues, including facial or general trauma or surgery; mechanical ventilation; brain injury, CVA; neurological conditions such as Parkinson's disease, Bell's palsy; diabetic retinopathy; lupus; rheumatoid arthritis

DESIRED OUTCOMES/EVALUATION CRITERIA

Sample NOC linkages:

Risk Control: Visual Impairment: Personal actions to prevent, eliminate, or reduce threats to visual function

Knowledge: Medication: Extent of understanding conveyed about the safe use of medication

Client Will (Include Specific Time Frame)

- Be free of discomfort or damage to eye related to dryness.
- Verbalize understanding of risk factors and ways to prevent dry eye.

(continues on page 274)

risk for Dry Eye (continued)
ACTIONS/INTERVENTIONS

Sample NIC linkages:
Eye Care: Prevention or minimization of threats to eye or visual integrity
Medication Administration: Eye: Preparing and instilling ophthalmic medications

NURSING PRIORITY NO. 1 To identify causative/precipitating factors related to risk:

- Obtain history of eye conditions when assessing client concerns overall. Note reports of dry sensation, burning, itching, pain, foreign body sensation, light sensitivity (photophobia), and blurred vision. *These symptoms can be associated with dry eye syndrome and, if present, require further evaluation and possible treatment.*[1]
- Note presence of conditions listed in risk factors above *to identify client with possible dry eye syndrome. Dry eye is most commonly caused by insufficient aqueous tear production. This can occur because of damage to eye surface (e.g., chemical burn) or be associated with disease conditions, neurological disorders, or environmental factors. Note: Studies have associated systemic diseases (e.g., rheumatoid arthritis and Sjögren's syndrome, allergies, thyroid disorders) with dry eye, and some studies have associated dry eye with arterial hypertension and type 2 diabetes), although not all studies are in accord regarding other risk factors noted above.*[1–4]
- Note client's gender and age. *Note: Studies show a higher incidence of dry eye syndrome in females than males, especially over the age of 50.*[1,2,4]
- Determine client's current situation (e.g., admitted to facility for procedures/surgery, recent neurological event, mechanical ventilation, facial or eye trauma; eye infections, lower eyelid malposition) *that places client at high risk for dry eye associated with low or absent blink reflex and/or decreased tear production.*[5]
- Determine client's history/presence of seasonal or environmental allergies. *which may cause or exacerbate conjunctivitis.*
- Review living and work environment *to identify factors (e.g., exposure to smoke, wind, or chemicals; poor lighting, long periods of computer use or eye-straining work) that can cause or exacerbate dry eyes.*
- Assess client's medications, noting use of certain drugs (e.g., antihistamines, beta-blockers, antidepressants, and oral contraceptives) *known to decrease tear production.*[1]
- Refer for diagnostic evaluation and interventions as indicated. *Symptom questionnaire may reveal need for further evaluation.*

NURSING PRIORITY NO. 2 To promote eye health/comfort:

- Assist in/refer for treatment of underlying cause of dry eyes. *Interventions could range from changing a medication that is causing decreased tear production to surgery to correct an anatomic abnormality of the eyelid that interferes with blinking. Referral may be needed (e.g., to rheumatologist or endocrinologist for treatment of autoimmune condition or diabetes).*[6]
- Administer artificial tears, lubricating eyedrops, or ointments as indicated *when client is unable to blink or otherwise protect eyes while in healthcare facility.*[5]

NURSING PRIORITY NO. 3 To promote wellness (Teaching/Discharge Criteria):

- Instruct high-risk client in self-management interventions *to prevent or limit symptoms of dry eye:*[6,7]
  - Avoid air blowing in eyes *such as might occur with hair dryers, car heaters, air conditioners, or fans directed toward eyes.*
  - Wear eyeglasses or safety shield glasses on windy days *to reduce effects of the wind* and goggles while swimming *to protect eyes from chemicals in the water.*
  - Take proper care of contact lenses and adhere to prescribed wearing time.
  - Add moisture to indoor air, especially in winter.
  - Take eye breaks during long reading and computer tasks or when watching TV for long periods of time.

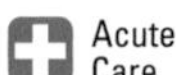
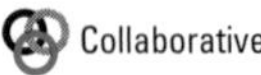
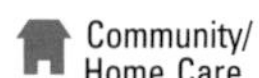
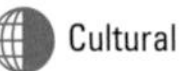

Blink repeatedly for a few seconds *to help spread tears evenly over eye.*

Position computer screen below eye level. *This may help slow the evaporation of tears between eye blinks.*

Cessation of smoking and avoidance of smoking environments. *Smoke can worsen dry eye symptoms.*

Discuss dietary changes if indicated. *Some physicians and nutritionists recommend a diet high in vitamin A, which is found in liver, carrots, and broccoli, and/or a diet high in omega-3 fatty acids, which are found in fish, walnuts, and vegetable oil, to prevent dry eye associated with vitamin A deficiency.*

DOCUMENTATION FOCUS

Assessment/Reassessment

- Individual risk factors identified.
- Client concerns or difficulty making and following through with plan.

Planning

- Plan of care and who is involved in planning.
- Teaching plan.

Implementation/Evaluation

- Response to interventions, teaching, and actions performed.
- Attainment or progress toward outcomes.

Discharge Planning

- Referrals to other resources.
- Long-term need and who is responsible for actions.

References

1. Foster, C. S., Yuksel, E., Anzaar, F., et al. (Updated 2014). Dry eye syndrome. Retrieved January 2015 from http://emedicine.medscape.com/article/1210417-overview.
2. Sendecka, M., Baryluk, A., Polz-Dacewicz, M. (2004). Prevalence and risk factors of dry eye syndrome. *Prezql Epidemiol*, 58(1), 227–233.
3. Manaviat, M. R., Rashidi, M., Afkhami-Ardekani, M., et al. (2008). Prevalence of dry eye syndrome and diabetic retinopathy in type 2 diabetic patients. *BMC Ophthalmol*, 8, 10.
4. Moss, S. E., Klein, R., Klein, B. E. (2008). Long-term-incidence of dry eye in an older population. *Optom Vis Sci*, 85(8), 668–674.
5. Schlessinger, D. A., Ulitsch, E. (2009). The eyes have it. *OR Nurse*, 3(4), 26–32.
6. Mayo Clinic Staff. (2012). Dry eye. Retrieved March 2015 from http://www.mayoclinic.org/diseases-conditions/dry-eyes/basics/definition/con-20024129.
7. Dahl, A. A. (2014). Dry eye syndrome (Dry Eyes, Keratoconjunctivitis Sicca). Retrieved January 2015 from http://www.mayoclinic.org/diseases-conditions/dry-eyes/basics/prevention/con-20024129.

risk for peripheral neurovascular Dysfunction

Taxonomy II: Safety/Protection—Class 2 Physical Injury (00086) [**Diagnostic Division:** Neurosensory], Submitted 1992; Revised 2913

DEFINITION: Vulnerable to disruption in the circulation, sensation, and motion of an extremity, which may compromise health.

RISK FACTORS

Burns; trauma; vascular obstruction
Fracture; immobilization; orthopedic surgery
Mechanical compression (e.g., tourniquet, cane, cast, brace, dressing, restraint)
Note: A risk diagnosis is not evidenced by signs and symptoms, as the problem has not occurred; rather, nursing interventions are directed at prevention.

Sample Clinical Applications:
Traumatic injuries, burns, joint replacement, laminectomy, deep vein thrombosis (DVT), peripheral vascular obstruction; compartment syndrome

DESIRED OUTCOMES/EVALUATION CRITERIA

Sample NOC linkages:
Tissue Perfusion: Peripheral: Adequacy of blood flow through the small vessels of the extremities to maintain tissue function
Neurological Status: Peripheral: Ability of the peripheral nervous system to transmit impulses to and from the central nervous system (CNS)
Risk Control: Personal actions to prevent, eliminate, or reduce modifiable health threats

Client Will (Include Specific Time Frame)

- Maintain function as evidenced by sensation and movement within normal range for individual.
- Identify individual risk factors.
- Demonstrate and participate in behaviors and activities to prevent complications.
- Relate signs/symptoms that require medical reevaluation.

ACTIONS/INTERVENTIONS

Sample NIC linkages:
Peripheral Sensation Management: Prevention or minimization of injury or discomfort in the patient with altered sensation
Circulatory Care: Arterial [or] Venous Insufficiency: Promotion of arterial [or] venous circulation

NURSING PRIORITY NO. 1 To determine significance/degree of potential for compromise:

- Assess for individual risk factors: (1) trauma to extremity that causes internal tissue damage such as crush injuries, high-velocity and penetrating trauma, and fractures (especially long-bone fractures) with hemorrhage; (2) fluid accumulation into confined space (including IV infiltration, postoperative hematoma, circumferential burns); (3) long-term pressure on tissues, such as could occur from individual being trapped under collapsed structure; (4) external pressure on tissues (e.g., tight dressings, military anti-shock trousers, splints, casts, or restraints); and (5) presence of conditions affecting peripheral circulation, such as atherosclerosis, cardiovascular or cerebrovascular disease; diabetes, sickle cell disease, DVT, and coagulation disorders or use of anticoagulants *that potentiate risk of circulation disruption, insufficiency, and occlusion.*[1–3,6,10]

Acute Care 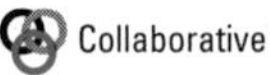 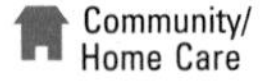 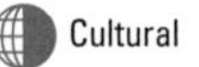

- Monitor for tissue bleeding and spread of hematoma *that can compress blood vessels and raise compartment pressures.*[1,2]
- Note position and location of casts, braces, traction apparatus, and use of restraints *to ascertain potential for pressure on tissues.*
- Review recent and current drug regimen, noting use of anticoagulants and vasoactive agents.

NURSING PRIORITY NO. 2 To assess for early signs of peripheral vascular impairment:

- Conduct a comprehensive upper or lower extremity assessment in at-risk client, including color, sensation, and functional ability. *Many individuals in this risk category are seen in the community healthcare setting for conditions not recognized as being related to peripheral vascular issues. However, early detection of circulatory issues may prevent the onset or severity of functional impairments associated with arterial or venous disorders of the extremities.*[6]
- Perform frequent neurovascular assessment in person immobilized for any reason (e.g., surgery, prolonged bedrest, diabetic neuropathy, fractures) or individuals with suspected neurovascular problems, noting differences in affected limb as compared with unaffected limb. Use the 6 Ps of assessment:[4]
  1. Pain: Using 0 to 10 (or a similar pain scale), assess for presence, location, severity, and duration of pain. *Pain may be intermittent (e.g., intermittent claudication) or more constant (e.g., compartment syndrome or arterial occlusion). Pain may range from muscle tension/tenderness and burning to severe pain. Pain may be present with exertion, with passive movement, or at rest.*[2,5,6,8]
  2. Pulses: Monitor presence (or absence) and quality of peripheral pulses (distal to injury or impairment) via palpation and/or Doppler. *Intact pulse usually indicates adequate circulation. However, occasionally a pulse may be palpated even though circulation is blocked by a soft clot; also, perfusion through larger arteries may continue after increased compartment pressure has collapsed the arteriole and venule circulation in the muscle.*[1,2,5,8]
  3. Pallor: Evaluate skin temperature, capillary refill, and color changes to assess perfusion. *Pallor with cool, shiny, taut skin and slow venous refill is indicative of circulatory impairment. Cold, pale, bluish color with purpura indicates arterial insufficiency.*[5,6]
  4. Paresthesia: Assess sensation (e.g., test peroneal nerve by pinch or pinprick in the dorsal web between first and second toe, and assess ability to dorsiflex toes in presence of leg fracture). *Changes in sensation cover a wide continuum and may include feeling of tingling, numbness, "pins and needles," burning, or diminished or absent sensation. Changes that might not be apparent to client could include loss of protective sensation in feet as determined by screening with tuning fork or percussion hammer. Sensation may be normal early in the presence of compartment syndrome because superficial circulation is not yet compromised.*[2,6,8,12]
  5. Paralysis: Evaluate for range of motion. *Movement may be limited or absent because of tissue edema and nerve compression or because of nerve impingement such as would occur with spinal nerve compression.*[2,8]
  6. Pressure: Evaluate by palpating the extremity. *Swelling or tightness may indicate obstruction, such as might occur with DVT, or compartment syndrome.*[11]

- Assist with diagnostic studies (e.g., blood studies, Doppler, ultrasound, angiography, segmental arterial pressures, intracompartmental pressures) as indicated. *Numerous diagnostic tests may be needed if diagnosis is in doubt and in view of the multitude of medical and surgical conditions associated with peripheral vascular dysfunction.*

NURSING PRIORITY NO. 3 To minimize edema formation/elevated tissue pressure:[1,3,5]

- Apply cold packs around injury/fracture site as indicated *to limit tissue swelling and hematoma formation.*
- Remove jewelry and constrictive clothing or other items from affected limb *to limit injury caused by swelling in injured tissues.*
- Elevate injured extremity(ies) unless contraindicated by confirmed presence of compartment syndrome *where elevation can actually impede arterial flow, decreasing perfusion.*[8]

- Monitor for development of infiltration of IV fluids *to prevent excessive accumulation of fluids in tissues.*[8]
- Position extremity(ies) in proper alignment *to prevent nerve impingement and elevation of tissue pressures.*[8,9]
- Monitor skin and tissues around protective and corrective devices (e.g., dressings, splint, cast, traction devices) for proper application and function *to provide support and protection without causing undue pressure on tissues.*
- Assist with or perform procedures (e.g., splitting cast, repositioning of restraints, continuous motion apparatus) *to release pressure and prevent permanent tissue damage or nerve injury.*
- Observe position and location of supporting ring of traction splints or sling and readjust as indicated *to reduce pressure on tissues and risk of nerve impingement and improve blood flow.*
- Avoid or limit use of restraints. Use padding and frequently evaluate extremity circulation, movement, and sensation when restraints are required.

NURSING PRIORITY NO. 4 To maximize circulation :[1–3,5,6]

- Position all extremities in proper alignment and keep injured extremity in neutral position *to maximize circulation.*
- Provide or assist with range-of-motion exercises. Encourage client to routinely exercise digits and joints distal to injury *to enhance circulation.*
- Administer IV fluids and blood products as needed *to maintain circulating volume and reduce potential for ischemic tissue injury associated with loss of perfusion.*
- Monitor hemoglobin/hematocrit and coagulation studies if either clotting or bleeding into tissues is known or suspected or client is receiving anticoagulant therapy.[8,9]

NURSING PRIORITY NO. 5 Prevent/limit potential for complications:[1–3,5–7]

- Assist with treatment of underlying conditions as listed in Risk Factors *to reduce risks of complications.*
- Investigate sudden changes (e.g., changes in skin temperature or color, reports of pain that are extreme for type of injury, increased pain at rest or on passive movement of extremity, development of burning or tingling sensations, tense muscles, change in pulse quality distal to injury) *that are suggestive of compartment syndrome, requiring prompt intervention.*[1,2]
- Place limb in neutral position, avoiding elevation *to enhance circulation in compartment syndrome.*
- Report symptoms to physician at once *to provide for timely evaluation and intervention.*
- Assist with and encourage early ambulation *to help prevent deep vein thrombus formation.*[9]
- Apply antiembolic hose or sequential compression devices as indicated.[9]
- Prepare for surgical intervention or other therapies (e.g., fibulectomy, fasciotomy, bypass surgery, hyperbaric oxygen therapy) as indicated *to relieve increasing pressures and restore circulation.*

NURSING PRIORITY NO. 6 To promote wellness (Teaching/Discharge Considerations) :[1–3,5,6,9]

- Encourage good nutrition with adequate calories and micronutrients *to promote healing and reduce sluggishness of circulation.*
- Review proper body alignment of limbs (e.g., elevated or neutral position) as appropriate for individual situation.
- Instruct client and family in neurovascular findings to be reported to healthcare provider when indicated (e.g., client with new fractures in cast at home, client at risk for DVT) *to limit preventable complications through early intervention.*
- Promote benefits of walking and smoking cessation *to improve circulation.*
- Discuss necessity of avoiding constrictive clothing, sharp angulation of legs, crossing ankles or legs, and thermal or mechanical trauma, *especially if client has history of peripheral vascular insufficiency or is at risk for DVT.*[8,9]
- Demonstrate proper application and removal of antiembolic hose or sequential compression devices, as indicated.

Acute Care
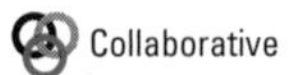
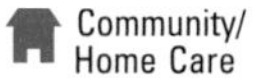
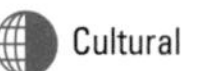

- Review safe use of heat or cold therapy, especially if client has poor sensation in extremities *to avoid thermal injury.*
- Instruct client/SO(s) to check shoes and socks for proper fit and/or wrinkles *to reduce potential for foot problems associated with neuropathies.*
- Recommend continuation of prescribed exercise program *to maintain extremity circulation and strength.*
- Review proper use and monitoring of drug regimen and safety concerns associated with anticoagulant use *to ensure maximum benefit and avoid complications and bleeding problems.*
- Recommend regular follow-up with healthcare provider *to monitor status of condition, drug efficacy, and provide for timely intervention.*

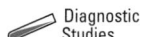

DOCUMENTATION FOCUS

Assessment/Reassessment

- Specific risk factors, nature of injury to limb.
- Assessment findings, including comparison of affected and unaffected limb, characteristics of pain in involved area.
- Doppler or compartment pressure results.

Planning

- Plan of care and who is involved in the planning.
- Teaching plan.

Implementation/Evaluation

- Response to interventions, teaching, and actions performed.
- Attainment or progress toward desired outcome(s).
- Modification of plan of care.

Discharge Planning

- Long-term needs, referrals, and who is responsible for actions to be taken.
- Specific referrals made.

References

1. Fort, C. W. (2003). How to combat 3 deadly trauma complications. *Nursing*, 33(5), 58–63.
2. Rasul, A. T. (Updated 2015). Acute compartment syndrome. Retrieved March 2015 from http://emedicine.medscape.com/article/307668-overview.
3. Bhimji, S., Hale, K. M. (Last reviewed 2014). Peripheral vascular disease. Retrieved March 2015 from http://www.emedicinehealth.com/peripheral_vascular_disease/article_em.htm.
4. ND Risk for peripheral neurovascular dysfunction. In Ackley, B. J., Ladwig, G. B. (eds). (2011). *Nursing Diagnosis Handbook: A Guide to Planning Care.* 9th ed. St. Louis, MO: Mosby.
5. Lopez-Rowe, V. (Updated 2014). Peripheral arterial occlusive disease. Retrieved March 2015 from http://emedicine.medscape.com/article/460178-overview.
6. Bonham, P. A., Flemister, B. G., Goldberg, M., et al. (2009). What's new in lower-extremity arterial disease? WOCN's 2008 Clinical Practice Guideline. *J Wound Ostomy ContinenceNurse*, 36(1), 37–44.
7. Stephens, E. (Updated 2014). Peripheral vascular disease. Retrieved March 2015 from http://emedicine.medscape.com/article/761556-overview.
8. Heron Evans, M. R. (2006). Interventions for clients with musculoskeletal trauma. In Ignatavicius, D. D., Workman, M. L. (eds). *Medical-Surgical Nursing: Critical Thinking for Collaborative Care.* 5th ed. St. Louis, MO: Elsevier-Saunders.
9. Patel, K., Chun, L. J. (Updated 2014). Deep vein thrombosis. Retrieved March 2015 from http://emedicine.medscape.com/article/1911303-overview.
10. Dougherty, A. L., Mohrie, C. R., Galarneau, M. R., et al. (2009). Battlefield extremity injuries in Operation Iraqi Freedom. *Injury*, 40(7), 772–777.
11. Bucholz, R. W., Heckman, J. P., Court-Brown, C. M. (eds). (2006). *Rockwood and Green's Fractures in Adults.* 6th ed. Philadelphia, PA: Lippincott, Williams & Wilkins.
12. Tesfaye, S., Boulton, A. J. M., Dyck, P. J. (2010). Diabetic neuropathies: Update on definitions, diagnostic criteria, estimation of severity, and treatments. *Diabetes Care*, 33(10), 2285–2293.

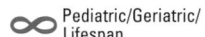

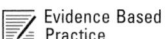

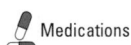

risk for Electrolyte Imbalance

Taxonomy II: Nutrition—Class 5 Hydration (00195) [**Diagnostic Division:** Food/Fluid], Submitted 2008; Revised 2013

DEFINITION: Vulnerable to changes in serum electrolyte levels, which may compromise health.

RISK FACTORS

Insufficient fluid volume; diarrhea; vomiting
Excessive fluid volume
Endocrine regulatory dysfunction (e.g., glucose intolerance, increase in IGF-1, androgen, DHEA, and cortisol); renal dysfunction
Compromised regulatory mechanism [e.g., diabetes insipidus, syndrome of inappropriate secretion of antidiuretic hormone]
Treatment regimen
Note: A risk diagnosis is not evidenced by signs and symptoms, as the problem has not occurred; rather, nursing interventions are directed at prevention.
Sample Clinical Applications: Renal failure, anorexia nervosa, diabetes mellitus, Crohn's disease; gastroenteritis, pancreatitis, traumatic brain injury, cancer, multiple trauma, burns, sickle cell disease

DESIRED OUTCOMES/EVALUATION CRITERIA

Sample NOC linkages:
Electrolyte & Acid/Base Balance: Balance of electrolytes and nonelectrolytes in the intracellular and extracellular compartments of the body
Fluid Balance: Water balance in the intracellular and extracellular compartments of the body

Client Will (Include Specific Time Frame)
- Display laboratory results within normal range for individual.
- Be free of complications resulting from electrolyte imbalance.

Sample NOC linkages:
Risk Control: Personal actions to prevent, eliminate, or reduce modifiable health threats

Client Will (Include Specific Time Frame)
- Identify and plan for individual risks.
- Engage in appropriate behaviors or lifestyle changes to prevent or reduce frequency of electrolyte imbalances.

ACTIONS/INTERVENTIONS

Sample NIC linkages:
Electrolyte Monitoring: Collection and analysis of patient data to regulate electrolyte balance
Fluid/Electrolyte Management: Regulation and prevention of complications from altered fluid and/or electrolyte levels

NURSING PRIORITY NO. 1 To assess causative/contributing factors:

- Identify client with current or newly diagnosed condition commonly associated with electrolyte imbalances, such as inability to eat or drink, febrile illness, and active bleeding or other fluid loss, including vomiting, diarrhea, gastrointestinal drainage, and burns. *The nurse taking a history on a new client, in both community health settings and acute care, should be alert to the possibility of electrolyte imbalances either being caused by an underlying condition, or actually causing the client's symptoms. Symptoms of electrolyte imbalance de-*

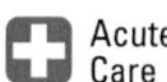
Acute Care
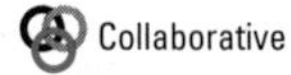
Collaborative
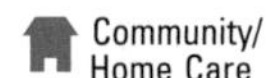
Community/ Home Care
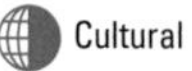
Cultural

pend upon the specific mineral affected but can include fatigue, muscle cramping, weakness, irregular heartbeat, confusion, and blood pressure changes.[10]

- Assess specific client risk, noting client age (including premature infants or sick newborn, elderly debilitated client) and chronic disease processes that may lead to electrolyte imbalance as listed in Risk Factors, including kidney disease, metabolic or endocrine disorders, chronic alcoholism, cancers or cancer treatments, conditions causing hemolysis such as massive trauma, multiple blood transfusions, and sickle cell disease.[1,18] *Electrolyte excesses are caused by factors that (1) increase electrolyte intake or absorption, (2) shift electrolytes from an electrolyte pool to the extracellular fluid, or (3) decrease electrolyte excretion.*[4] *Electrolyte deficits are caused by factors that (1) decrease electrolyte intake or absorption, (2) shift electrolytes from the extracellular fluid to an electrolyte pool, (3) increase electrolyte excretion, or (4) cause abnormal loss of electrolytes.*[4]
- Review client's medications *for those associated with electrolyte imbalance. Note: There are many such medications, including (but not limited to) diuretics, laxatives, corticosteroids, barbiturates, certain antidepressants (e.g., SSRIs), antihypertensive agents, antiepileptics, some hormones/birth control pills, and some antibiotics and antifungal agents.*

NURSING PRIORITY NO. 2 To identify potential electrolyte deficit:

- Assess mental status, noting client/caregiver report of change—altered attention span, recall of recent events, and other cognitive functions. *Altered mental status is the most common sign of sodium imbalances.*[2,18]
- Monitor heart rate and rhythm by palpation and auscultation. *Weak pulse or thready pulse can be associated with hypokalemia; tachycardia, bradycardia, and other dysrhythmias are associated with various electrolyte imbalances, including potassium, calcium, and magnesium.*[1–3,16]
- Auscultate breath sounds, assess respirations noting rate and depth and ease of respiratory effort, observe color of nailbeds and mucous membranes, and note pulse oximetry or blood gas measurement, as indicated. *Certain electrolyte imbalances, such as hypokalemia, can cause or exacerbate respiratory insufficiency.*[2]
- Review electrocardiogram (ECG). *The ECG reflects electrophysiological, anatomical, metabolic, and hemodynamic alterations and is routinely used for the diagnosis of electrolyte and metabolic disturbances, as well as myocardial ischemia, cardiac dysrhythmias, structural changes of the myocardium, and drug effects.*[1–4]
- Assess gastrointestinal symptoms, noting presence, absence, and character of bowel sounds; presence of acute or chronic diarrhea; and persistent vomiting and high nasogastric tube output. *Any disturbance of gastrointestinal (GI) functioning carries with it the potential for electrolyte imbalances.*[4,5]
- Review client's food intake. Note presence of anorexia/other eating disorders, vomiting, or recent fad or unusual diet and look for chronic malnutrition. *Can point to potential electrolyte imbalances, either deficiencies or excesses, such as high sodium content.*[5]
- Evaluate motor strength and function. *Neuromuscular function, including steadiness of gait, handgrip strength, reactivity of reflexes, and muscle weakness, can provide clues to electrolyte imbalances, including calcium, magnesium, phosphorus, sodium, and potassium.*[2,4,16]
- Assess fluid intake and output. *Many factors, such as inability to drink, large diuresis, chronic kidney failure, trauma, or surgery, affect an individual's fluid balance, thereby disrupting electrolyte transport, function, and excretion.*[1–5]
- Review laboratory results for abnormal findings. *Electrolytes include sodium, potassium, calcium, chloride, bicarbonate (carbon dioxide), and magnesium. These chemicals are absolutely essential in many bodily functions, including fluid balance, movement of fluid within and between body compartments, nerve conduction, muscle contraction—including the heart, blood clotting, and pH balance. Excitable cells, such as nerve and muscle, are particularly sensitive to electrolyte imbalances.*[4,6]
- Assess for specific imbalances:

Sodium (Na^+) *Dominant extracellular cation and cannot freely cross the cell membrane.*[6]

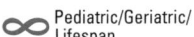

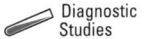

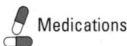

Review laboratory results—normal range in adults is 135 to 145 mEq/L. *Elevated sodium (hypernatremia) can occur if client has an overall deficit of total body water, which occurs via two mechanisms*

(inadequate fluid intake and water loss),[7,8] *and can be associated with low potassium, metabolic acidosis, and hypoglycemia.*[2]

Monitor for physical or mental disorders impacting fluid intake. *Impaired thirst sensation and inability to express thirst or obtain needed fluids may lead to hypernatremia.*[7,8]

Note presence of medical conditions that may impact sodium level. *Congestive heart failure, liver and kidney failure, pneumonia, metabolic acidosis, and intestinal conditions resulting in prolonged GI suction are associated with hyponatremia.*[4,6] *Hypernatremia can result from simple conditions such as febrile illness causing fluid loss and/or restricted fluid intake or from complicated conditions such as kidney and endocrine diseases affecting sodium intake or excretion.*[8]

Note presence of cognitive dysfunction such as confusion, restlessness, and abnormal speech *(which may be a cause or effect of sodium imbalance); orthostatic blood pressure changes, tachycardia, or low urine output; or other clinical findings such as generalized weakness, swollen tongue, weight loss, and seizures. Signs suggesting hypernatremia.*[7,8]

Assess for nausea, abdominal cramping, lethargy, and orthostatic blood pressure changes—if fluid volume is also depleted, confusion, decreased level of consciousness, or headache. *Signs and symptoms suggestive of hyponatremia, which can lead to seizures and coma if untreated.*[6]

Review drug regimen. *Drugs such as anabolic steroids, angiotensin, cisplatin, and mannitol may increase sodium level. Drugs such as diuretics, laxatives, theophylline, and triamterene can decrease sodium level.*[4]

Potassium (K^+) *Most abundant intracellular cation, obtained through diet and excreted via the kidneys.*[9]

Identify at-risk populations. *Extremes of age (premature or elderly); ingestion of unusual diet with high-potassium, low-sodium foods; clients receiving IV potassium boluses or transfusions of whole blood or packed cells; and use of potassium supplements, including over-the-counter (OTC) herbals or salt substitutes, increase possibility of hyperkalemia.*

Review laboratory results—normal range in adults is 3.5 to 5.0 mEq/L.

Obtain ECG as indicated.

Note presence of medical conditions that may impact potassium level. *Metabolic acidosis, burn or crush injuries, massive hemolysis, diabetes, kidney disease/renal failure, cancer, and sickle cell trait are associated with hyperkalemia.*[10] *Situations that may lead to hypokalemia are those that decrease potassium intake—excessive fluid resuscitation, fasting, and unbalanced diet or eating disorders/anorexia; shift potassium from the extracellular fluid into cells—alkalosis, some malignancies; or increased potassium loss through diuresis or renal disorders such as acute tubular necrosis, nasogastric suction, and diarrhea.*[1,19]

Evaluate reports of abdominal cramping, fatigue, hyperactive bowel motility, and muscle twitching and cramps followed by muscle weakness. Note presence of depressed reflexes and ascending flaccid paralysis of legs and arms. *Signs/symptoms suggesting hyperkalemia.*[2,9]

Note presence of weakness and fatigue (most common), as well as anorexia, abdominal distention, diminished bowel sounds, palpitations, postural hypotension, muscle cramps and pain (severe hypokalemia), and flaccid paralysis. *May be manifestations of hypokalemia.*[1,19]

Review drug regimen. *Use of potassium-sparing diuretics; other medications, such as NSAIDs, angiotensin-converting enzyme inhibitors, angiotensin-receptor blockers; and heparin and certain antibiotics such as pentamidine may increase potassium level.*[6,9,10] *Medications such as some COPD medications (e.g., albuterol, terbutaline), steroids, certain antimicrobials (e.g., penicillins, aminogylicides), laxatives, and some diuretics may cause hypokalemia.*[19]

Calcium (Ca^{2+}) *Most abundant cation in the body participates in almost all vital processes, working with sodium to regulate depolarization and the generation of action potentials. Disruption of these processes causes cellular irritability and dysfunction.*[2,4,10,12,15]

Laboratory results—normal range for adults is 8.5 to 10.5 mg/dL. *Elevated calcium (hypercalcemia) is associated with excessive urination (polyuria), constipation, lethargy, muscle weakness, anorexia,*

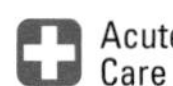

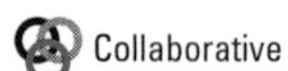

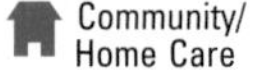

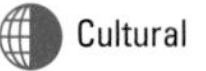

headache, and coma. Hypocalcemia can lead to cardiac dysrhythmias, hypotension, and heart failure; muscle cramps and facial spasms (positive Chvostek's sign); numbness, tingling sensations, and muscle twitching (positive Trousseau's sign); seizures; or tetany. Low serum albumin levels and vitamin D deficiency may also be associated with hypocalcemia.[4,11]

Note presence of medical conditions impacting calcium level. *Acidosis, Addison's disease, cancers (e.g., bone, lymphoma, leukemias), hyperparathyroidism, lung disease (e.g., tuberculosis, histoplasmosis), thyrotoxicosis, and polycythemia may lead to an increased calcium level. Chronic diarrhea and intestinal disorders such as Crohn's disease; pancreatitis, alcoholism, renal failure, or renal tubular disease; recent orthopedic surgery or bone healing; history of thyroid surgery or irradiation of upper middle chest and neck; and psychosis may result in hypocalcemia.*[2,4,11]

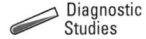

Review drug regimen. *Drugs such as anabolic steroids, some antacids, lithium, oral contraceptives, vitamins A and D, and amoxapine can increase calcium levels. Drugs such as albuterol, glucocorticoids, and insulin; laxative overuse; and phosphates, trazodone, or long-term anticonvulsant therapy can decrease calcium levels.*[4]

Magnesium (Mg^{2+}) *The second-most abundant intracellular cation after potassium, magnesium controls absorption or function of sodium, potassium, calcium, and phosphorus.*[2,4,9,10,13,14]

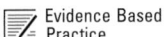

Review laboratory results—normal range in adults is 1.5 to 2.0 mEq/L. *Excess magnesium (hypermagnesemia) occurs rarely but affects the central nervous, neuromuscular, and cardiopulmonary systems.*

Note GI and renal function. *Main controlling factors of magnesium are GI absorption and renal excretion.*[12] *Low levels of potassium (most common), as well as calcium, phosphorus, and magnesium, may be manifest at the same time if GI absorption is impaired.*[14] *High levels of magnesium, calcium, phosphate, and potassium often occur together in setting of kidney disease.*[13,14]

Note presence of medical condition impacting magnesium level. *Diabetic acidosis, multiple myeloma, renal insufficiency, eclampsia, asthma, certain cardiac dysrhythmias, tumor lysis syndrome, GI hypomotility, adrenal insufficiency, neoplasms with skeletal muscle involvement, extensive soft tissue injury or necrosis, shock, sepsis, severe burns, and cardiac arrest are associated with hypermagnesemia.*[4,12,13,15] *Conditions resulting in decreased intake (e.g., starvation, alcoholism, parenteral feeding); excess gastrointestinal losses (e.g., diarrhea, vomiting, nasogastric suction, malabsorption); renal losses (e.g., inherited renal tubular defects among others); or miscellaneous other causes, including calcium abnormalities, chronic metabolic acidosis, and diabetic ketoacidosis, can lead to hypomagnesemia.*[2,4,12]

Monitor for symptoms of hypermagnesemia. *Presence of nausea, vomiting, weakness, and vasodilation suggest mild to moderate elevation of magnesium level (>3.5–5.0 mEq/L), while the presence of heart blocks, ventilatory failure, and stupor is associated with severe hypermagnesemia (>10.0 mEq/L), which can lead to coma and death.*[14]

Note muscular weakness, tremors, seizures, paresthesia, hypertension, and cardiac abnormalities. *Signs of hypomagnesemia that may lead to potentially fatal complications, including ventricular dysrhythmias, coronary artery vasospasm, and sudden death.*[9,13]

Review drug regimen. *Drugs such as aspirin and progesterone may increase magnesium level; albuterol, digoxin, diuretics, oral contraceptives, aminoglycosides, proton-pump inhibitors, immunosuppressants, cisplatin, and cyclosporines are some of the medications that may decrease magnesium levels.*[4]

NURSING PRIORITY NO. 3 To prevent imbalances:

- Collaborate in the treatment of underlying conditions *to prevent or limit effects of electrolyte imbalances caused by disease or organ dysfunction.*
- Observe and intervene with elderly hospitalized individuals upon admission and during facility stay. *Elderly are more prone to electrolyte imbalances related to fluid imbalances, the use of multiple medications including diuretics and heart and blood pressure medications, a lack of appetite or interest in eating or drinking, a lack of appropriate dietary and/or medication supervision at home, etc.*[2]

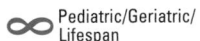

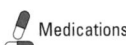

- Provide balanced nutrition to hospitalized client, using best route for feeding and monitoring intake, weight, and bowel function. *Obtaining and utilizing electrolytes and other minerals depends on client receiving them in a readily available route, preferably by oral ingestion, or by GI tube or parenteral route.*
- Measure and report all fluid losses, including emesis, diarrhea, and wound or fistula drainage. *Loss of fluids rich in electrolytes can lead to imbalances.*
- Maintain fluid balance *to prevent dehydration and shifts of electrolytes.*
- Use a pump or controller device when administering IV electrolyte solutions *to provide medication at desired rate and prevent untoward effects of excessive or too rapid delivery.*

NURSING PRIORITY NO. 4 To promote wellness (Teaching/Discharge Considerations):

- Discuss ongoing concerns for clients with chronic health problems, such as kidney disease, diabetes, and cancer; individuals taking multiple medications; and/or clients deciding to take medications or OTC drugs differently than prescribed. *By addressing these issues during each clinic visit, it may be possible to identify client at risk for electrolyte imbalances. Early intervention can help prevent serious complications.*
- Consult with dietitian or nutritionist for specific teaching needs. *Learning how to incorporate foods that increase electrolyte intake or identifying food or condiment alternatives when client is taking in too much of an electrolyte (such as client with renal failure not receiving dialysis failing to curtail high-potassium foods) increases client's self-sufficiency and likelihood of success.*
- Teach client/caregiver to take or administer drugs as prescribed—especially diuretics, antihypertensives, and cardiac drugs—*to reduce potential of complications associated with medication-induced electrolyte imbalances.*
- Instruct client/caregiver in reportable symptoms. *For example, sudden change in mentation or behavior 2 days after starting a new diuretic could indicate hyponatremia, or an elderly person taking digitalis for atrial fibrillation and a diuretic may be hypokalemic.*[2]
- Provide information regarding calcium supplements, as indicated. *It is popular wisdom to instruct people, women in particular, to take calcium for prevention of osteoporosis. However, calcium absorption cannot take place without vitamins D and K and magnesium. Client taking calcium may need additional information or resources.*[16]
- Review client's medications at each visit *for possible change in dosage or drug choice based on client's response, change in condition, or development of side effects.*
- Discuss medications with primary care provider *to determine if different pharmaceutical intervention is appropriate. For example, changing to potassium-sparing diuretic or withholding a diuretic in presence of hypokalemia may correct imbalance.*[15]

DOCUMENTATION FOCUS

Assessment/Reassessment

- Identified or potential risk factors for individual.
- Assessment findings, including vital signs, mentation, muscle strength and reflexes, presence of fatigue, respiratory distress.
- Results of laboratory tests and diagnostic studies.

Planning

- Plan of care, specific interventions, and who is involved in the planning.
- Teaching plan.

Implementation/Evaluation

- Client's responses to treatment, teaching, and actions performed.
- Attainment or progress toward desired outcome(s).
- Modifications to plan of care.

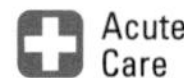

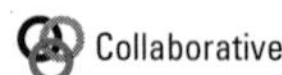

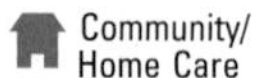

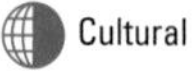

Discharge Planning

- Long-term needs, identifying who is responsible for actions to be taken.
- Specific referrals made.

References

1. Lederer, E., Alsauskas, Z. C., Mackelaite, L., et al. (Updated 2014). Hypokalemia. Retrieved March 2015 from http://emedicine.medscape.com/article/242008-overview.
2. Workman, M. L. (2006). Interventions for clients with electrolyte imbalances. In Ignatavicius, D. D., Workman, M. L. (eds). *Medical-Surgical Nursing: Critical Thinking for Collaborative Care*. 5th ed. St. Louis, MO: Elsevier Saunders.
3. Wung, S., Kozik, T. (2008). Electrocardiographic evaluation of cardiovascular status. *J Cardiovasc Nurs*, 23(2), 169–174.
4. Leeuwen, A. M., Kranpitz, T. R., Smith, L. (2006). *Davis's Comprehensive Handbook of Diagnostic Tests with Nursing Implications*. 2nd ed. Philadelphia, PA: F. A. Davis.
5. Btaiche, I. F., Khalidi, N. (2004). Metabolic complications of parenteral nutrition in adults, part 1. *Am J Health Syst Pharm*, 61(18), 1938–1949.
6. Simon, E. E., Hamrahian, S. M., Teran, F. J. (2014). Hyponatremia. Retrieved March 2015 from http://emedicine.medscape.com/article/242166-overview.
7. Elgart, H. N. (2004). Assessment of fluids and electrolytes. *AACN Clin Issues*, 15(4), 607–621.
8. Lukitsch, I., Pham, T. Q. (2014). Hypernatremia. Retrieved March 2015 from http://emedicine.medscape.com/article/241094-overview.
9. Lederer, E., Alsauskas, Z. C., Mackelaite, L., et al. (2014). Hyperkalemia. Retrieved March 2015 from http://emedicine.medscape.com/article/240903-overview.
10. Muller, A. C., Bell, A. E. (2008). Diagnostic update: Electrolyte update: Potassium, chloride and magnesium. *Crit Care Nurs*, 3(1), 5–7.
11. Felver, L., Kirkhorn, M. J. (2005). Fluid, electrolyte, and acid-base homeostatis. In Copstead, L. E. C., et al. (eds). *Pathophysiology*. 2nd ed. St. Louis, MO: Elsevier Saunders.
12. Suneja, M., Muster, H. A. (Updated 2014). Hypocalcemia. Retrieved March 2015 from http://emedicine.medscape.com/article/241893-overview.
13. Fulop, T., Agarwal, M. (Updated 2014). Hypomagnesemia. Retrieved March 2015 from http://emedicine.medscape.com/article/246366-overview.
14. Novello, N. P. (Updated 2014). Hypermagnesemia in Emergency Medicine. Retrieved March 2015 from http://emedicine.medscape.com/article/766604-overview.
15. Moe, S. M. (2008). Disorders involving calcium, phosphorus, and magnesium. *Prim Care*, 35(2), 215–237.
16. Stark, J. (2006). The renal system. In Alspach, J. G. (ed). *Core Curriculum for Critical Care Nursing*. St. Louis, MO: Saunders.
17. Fitzgerald, M. A. (2008). LAB LOGIC: Hyponatremia associated with SSRI use in a 65-year-old woman. *Nurse Pract*, 33(2), 11–12.
18. Ambalavanan, N. (2014). Fluid, electrolyte, and nutrition management of the newborn. Retrieved March 2015 from http://emedicine.medscape.com/article/976386–overview.
19. Lederer, E., Alsauskas, Z. C., Mackelaite, L., et al. (2014). Hypokalemia. Retrieved March 2015 from http://emedicine.medscape.com/article/242008-overview.

impaired urinary Elimination

Taxonomy II: Elimination and Exchange—Class 1 Urinary Function (00016) [**Diagnostic Division:** Elimination], Submitted 1973; Revised 2006

DEFINITION: Dysfunction in urine elimination.

RELATED FACTORS

Multiple causality; sensory motor impairment; anatomic obstruction; urinary tract infection; [fluid/volume states; psychogenic factors; surgical diversion]

DEFINING CHARACTERISTICS

Subjective

Frequent voiding; urinary urgency
Hesitancy
Dysuria
Nocturia; [enuresis]

Objective

Urinary incontinence
Urinary retention

Sample Clinical Applications: Urinary tract infection (UTI), benign prostatic disease (BPH), bladder cancer, interstitial cystitis, spinal cord injury (SCI), multiple sclerosis (MS), pregnancy, childbirth, pelvic trauma, abdominal surgery, dementia, Alzheimer's disease

DESIRED OUTCOMES/EVALUATION CRITERIA

Sample NOC linkages:

Urinary Elimination: Collection and drainage of urine
Urinary Continence: Control of the elimination of urine from the bladder
Self-Care: Toileting: Ability to toilet self independently with or without assistive device

Client Will (Include Specific Time Frame)

- Verbalize understanding of condition.
- Identify specific causative factors.
- Achieve normal elimination pattern or participate in measures to correct or compensate for defects.
- Demonstrate behaviors or techniques to prevent urinary infection.
- Manage care of urinary catheter or stoma and appliance following urinary diversion.

ACTIONS/INTERVENTIONS

Sample NIC linkages:

Urinary Elimination Management: Maintenance of an optimum urinary elimination pattern
Urinary Catheterization: Insertion of a catheter into the bladder for temporary or permanent drainage of urine
Perineal Care: Maintenance of perineal skin integrity and relief of perineal discomfort

NURSING PRIORITY NO. 1 To assess causative/contributing factors:

- Note presence of physical diagnoses that may be involved, such as UTI or dehydration, surgery (including urinary diversion), neurological conditions (e.g., MS, stroke, Parkinson's disease; paraplegia, tetraplegia), mental or emotional dysfunction (e.g., impaired cognition, delirium, confusion, depression, Alzheimer's disease), prostate disorders, recent or multiple pregnancies, and pelvic trauma.

- Determine pathology of bladder dysfunction relative to identified medical diagnosis. *Identifies direction for further evaluation and treatment options to discover specifics of individual situation. For example, in neurological or demyelinating diseases, such as MS, problem may be failure to store urine, empty bladder, or both.*[1,6]
- Note client's age and gender. *Incontinence and UTIs are more prevalent in women and older adults; painful bladder syndrome or interstitial cystitis (PBS/IC) is more common in women.*[3,7]
- Perform physical examination (e.g., cough test *for incontinence,* palpation *for bladder retention and masses,* prostate size, observation for urethral stricture).[8]
- Investigate reports of pain, noting location, duration, and intensity; the presence of bladder spasms; and back or flank pain, *to assist in differentiating between bladder and kidney cause of dysfunction. Note: Bladder pain located suprapubically, vaginally, in the perineum, low back, or medial aspects of the thighs that is relieved by voiding and often recurs with bladder filling suggests presence of PBS/IC.*[7]
- Have client complete standardized self-report tool, such as the Pelvic Pain and Urgency/Frequency client symptom survey, as indicated. *Helpful in evaluating the presence and severity of PBS/IC symptoms.*[7,12]
- Note reports of exacerbations (flare-ups) and spontaneous remissions of symptoms of urgency and frequency, which may/may not be accompanied by pain, pressure, or spasm. *Clients with PBS/IC void approximately 16 times per day with voided volumes usually less than normal.*[7,13]
- Determine client's usual daily fluid intake (both amount and beverage choices and use of caffeine). Note condition of skin and mucous membranes and color of urine *to determine level of hydration.*[3]
- Review medication regimen to identify drugs that can alter bladder or kidney function (e.g., some antihypertensive agents [e.g., angiotensin-converting enzyme inhibitors (ACE), beta-blockers]; anticholinergics [e.g., antihistamines, antiparkinsonian drugs]; antidepressants, antipsychotics; sedatives, hypnotics, opioids; caffeine; alcohol).[9]
- Send urine specimen (midstream clean-voided or catheterized) for culture and sensitivities in presence of signs of UTI—cloudy, foul odor, and/or bloody urine.
- Obtain specimen for antibody-coated bacteria assay. *Diagnosis of bacterial infection of the kidney or prostate is important for immediate treatment to prevent damage to these organs.*
- Review lab tests *for hyperglycemia, hyperparathyroidism, or other metabolic conditions, as well as changes in renal function, presence of infection/sexually transmitted infection, and cytology revealing cancer.*
- Rule out gonorrhea in men. *This infection needs to be considered when urethritis with a penile discharge is present and there are no bacteria in the urine.*
- Assist with or perform potassium sensitivity test (instillation of potassium solution into bladder) when appropriate. *Studies have shown that 80% of clients with PBS/IC will react positively with painful symptoms.*[14]
- Review results of other diagnostic studies (e.g., uroflowmetry; cystometogram; postvoid residual ultrasound (bladder scan), pressure flow, leak point pressure measurement; videourodynamics; electromyography; kidneys, ureters, and bladder imaging) *to identify presence and type of elimination problem.*[10]

NURSING PRIORITY NO. 2 To assess degree of interference/disability:

- Ascertain client's previous pattern of elimination and compare with current situation. Note reports of problems (e.g., frequency, urgency, painful urination; leaking or incontinence; changes in size or force of urinary stream; problems emptying bladder completely; nocturia, enuresis) *to assist in identification and treatment of particular dysfunction.*
- Ascertain client's/significant other's (SO's) perception of problem, degree of disability, and impact on self-image (e.g., client may be restricting social, employment, or travel activities; having sexual or relationship difficulties; experiencing depression).
- Note influence of culture or ethnicity, as well as gender, on client's view of problems of incontinence. *Limited evidence exists to understand and help people cope with the physical and psychosocial consequences of this chronic, socially isolating, and potentially devastating disorder.*[4]

- Have client keep a voiding diary for prescribed number of days to record fluid intake, voiding times, precise urine output, and dietary intake. *Helps determine baseline symptoms, the severity of frequency/urgency, and whether diet is a factor if symptoms worsen.*

NURSING PRIORITY NO. 3 To assist in treating/preventing urinary alteration:

- Encourage fluid intake up to 1,500 to 2,500 mL/day (within cardiac tolerance), including cranberry juice. *Maintains renal function, prevents infection and formation of urinary stones, avoids encrustation around indwelling catheter, or may be used to flush urinary diversion appliance.*[3]
- Discuss possible dietary restrictions (e.g., especially coffee, alcohol, carbonated drinks, citrus, tomatoes, and chocolate) based on individual symptoms.[7]
- Assist with developing toileting routines (e.g., timed voiding, bladder training, prompted voiding, habit retraining) as appropriate. *For adults who are cognitively intact and physically capable of self-toileting, bladder training, timed voiding, and habit retraining may be beneficial.*[3,11] *However, bladder retraining is not recommended for clients with PBS.*[7]
- Encourage client to verbalize fear or concerns (e.g., disruption in sexual activity, inability to work, concern about involvement in social activities). *Open expression allows client to talk about, deal with feelings, and begin to solve the identified problems.*[4]
- Implement and monitor interventions for specific elimination problem (e.g., pelvic floor exercises or other bladder retraining modalities; medication regimen, antimicrobials [single dose is frequently being used for UTI], sulfonamides, antispasmodics). Evaluate client's response *to modify treatment as needed.*
- Discuss possible surgical procedures and medical regimen as indicated (e.g., client with benign prostatic hypertrophy, bladder or prostatic cancer, PBS/IC). *For example, cystoscopy with bladder hydrodistention for PBS/IC or an electrical stimulator may be implanted to treat chronic urinary urge incontinence, nonobstructive urinary retention, and symptoms of urgency and frequency.*[4,7]
- Refer to specific NDs urinary Incontinence (specify) and [acute/chronic] Urinary Retention for additional interventions/treatment regimens.

NURSING PRIORITY NO. 4 To assist in management of long-term urinary dysfunction:

- Keep bladder deflated by use of an indwelling catheter connected to closed drainage. Investigate alternatives when possible. *Measures such as intermittent catheterization, surgical interventions, urinary drugs, voiding maneuvers, and condom catheter may be preferable to the indwelling catheter to provide more effective control and prevent possibility of recurrent infections.*[5]
- Use latex-free catheter and care supplies. *Reduces risk of developing sensitivity to latex, which can develop in individuals requiring frequent catheterization or who have long-term indwelling catheters.*
- Check frequently for bladder distention and observe for overflow. *Requires immediate intervention to reduce risk of infection or autonomic hyperreflexia.*
- Recommend a regular bladder or diversion appliance emptying schedule. *Avoids accidents and prevents embarrassment to the individual.*[2]
- Emphasize importance of routine diversion appliance care and assist client to recognize and deal with problems such as alkaline salt encrustation, ill-fitting appliance, malodorous urine, infection, etc. *Provides information and promotes competence in care, increasing self-confidence in dealing with appliance on a regular basis.*[2]

NURSING PRIORITY NO. 5 To promote wellness (Teaching/Discharge Considerations):

- Emphasize importance of keeping perineal area clean and dry. *Reduces risk of infection or skin breakdown.*
- Instruct female clients with UTI to drink large amounts of fluid, void immediately after intercourse, wipe from front to back, promptly treat vaginal infections, and take showers rather than tub baths as appropriate. *These measures can limit risk of or avoid reinfection.*[3]

- Recommend smoking-cessation program as appropriate. *Cigarette smoking can be a source of bladder irritation.*
- Encourage SO(s) who participate in routine care to recognize complications (including latex allergy) necessitating medical follow-up. *Client may be embarrassed to discuss symptoms, and caregivers need to be alert to changes that necessitate evaluation and treatment.*[4]
- Instruct in proper application and care of appliance for urinary diversion. Encourage liberal fluid intake, avoidance of foods and medications that produce strong odor, and use of white vinegar or deodorizer in pouch to promote odor control. *These measures help to ensure patency of device and prevent embarrassing situations for client.*[2]
- Identify sources for supplies and programs or agencies providing financial assistance. *Lack of access to necessities can be a barrier to management of incontinence and having help to obtain needed equipment can assist with daily care.*[4]
- Recommend avoidance of gas-forming foods in presence of ureterosigmoidostomy. *Flatus can cause urinary incontinence.*[1]
- Recommend use of silicone catheter. *Although these catheters are more expensive than rubber catheters, they are more comfortable and generally cause fewer problems with infection when permanent or long-term catheterization is required.*[15]
- Demonstrate proper positioning of catheter drainage tubing and bag. *Facilitates drainage and prevents reflux and complications of infection.*[2]
- Refer client/SO(s) to appropriate community resources such as ostomy specialist, support group, sex therapist, psychiatric clinical nurse specialist, etc. *May be necessary to deal with changes in body image and function.*[4]

DOCUMENTATION FOCUS

Assessment/Reassessment

- Individual findings, including previous and current pattern of voiding, nature of problem, effect on desired lifestyle.
- Cultural factors or concerns.

Planning

- Plan of care and who is involved in planning.
- Teaching plan.

Implementation/Evaluation

- Response to interventions, teaching, and actions performed.
- Attainment or progress toward desired outcome(s).
- Modifications to plan of care.

Discharge Planning

- Long-term needs and who is responsible for actions to be taken.
- Available resources and specific referrals made.
- Individual equipment needs and sources.

References

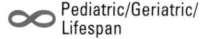

1. Newfield, S. A., Hinz, M. D., Tilley, D. S., et al. (2007). *Cox's Clinical Applications of Nursing Diagnosis: Adult, Child, Women's, Psychiatric, Gerontic, and Home Health Considerations*. 5th ed. Philadelphia: F. A. Davis.
2. Colwell, J. C. (2001). The state of the standard diversion. *J Wound Ostomy Continence Nurs*, 28(1), 6–17.
3. Wyman, J. F. (2003). Treatment of urinary incontinence in men and older women: The evidence shows the efficacy of a variety of techniques. *Am J Nurs*, 103(suppl), 26–35.
4. The state of the science on urinary incontinence. (2003). In Newman, D. K., Palmer, M. H. (eds). *Am J Nurs*, 103(3 suppl), 2–53.

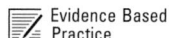

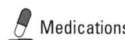

5. Beers, M. H., Berkow, R. (eds). (1999). *The Merck Manual of Diagnosis and Therapy*. 17th ed. Whitehouse Station, NJ: Merck Research Laboratories.
6. Gray, M. (2005). Overactive bladder: An overview. *J Wound Ostomy Continence Nurs*, 32(3 suppl), 1–5.
7. Panzera, A. K. (2007). Interstitial cystitis/painful bladder syndrome. *Urol Nurs*, 27(1), 13–19.
8. Bates, B. (2007). Simple questions can help uncover urinary incontinence. *Urol Nurs*, 37(4), 29–29.
9. Newman, D. K. (2005). Assessment of the patient with an overactive bladder. *J Wound Ostomy Continence Nurs*, 32(3 suppl), 5–10.
10. National Kidney and Urologic Diseases Information Clearinghouse. (Updated 2014). Urodynamic testing. Retrieved April 2015 from http://kidney.niddk.nih.gov/KUDISEASES/pubs/urodynamic/index.aspx.
11. Milne, J. L., Krissovich, M. (2004). Behavioral therapies at the primary care level: The current state of knowledge. *J Wound Ostomy Continence Nurs*, 31(6), 367–376.
12. Parsons, C. L., Dell, J., Standford, E. J. (2002). Increased prevalence of interstitial cystitis: Previously unrecognized urologic and gynecologic cases identified using a new symptom questionnaire and intravesical potassium sensitivity. *Adult Urol*, 60(4), 573–578.
13. Tchetgen, M. B., Rackley, R., Abdelmalak, J. B., et al. (2005). Interstitial cystitis. In Vasavada, S. P., Appell, R. A., Sand, P. K., et al. (eds). *Female Urology, Urogynecology, and Voiding Dysfunction*. New York: Marcel Dekker.
14. Parsons, C. L. (2002). Evidence-based strategies for recognizing and managing IC. *Contemp Urol*, 15(2), 22–35.
15. Borton, C. (Updated 2012). Catheterising bladders. Retrieved April 2015 from http://www.patient.co.uk/doctor/catheterising-bladders.

readiness for enhanced urinary Elimination

Taxonomy II: Elimination and Exchange—Class 1 Urinary Function (00166) [**Diagnostic Division:** Elimination], Submitted 2002; Revised 2013

DEFINITION: A pattern of urinary functions for meeting eliminatory needs, which can be strengthened.

DEFINING CHARACTERISTICS

Subjective

Expresses desire to enhance urinary elimination

Sample Clinical Applications: Spinal cord injury (SCI), multiple sclerosis (MS), pregnancy, childbirth, pelvic trauma, abdominal surgery, prostate disease

DESIRED OUTCOMES/EVALUATION CRITERIA

Sample NOC linkages:

Urinary Continence: Control of elimination of urine from the bladder

Knowledge: Disease Process: Extent of understanding conveyed about a specific disease process and prevention of complications

Urinary Elimination: Collection and drainage of urine

Client Will (Include Specific Time Frame)

- Verbalize understanding of condition that has potential for altering elimination.
- Maintain normal or acceptable elimination pattern, emptying bladder and voiding in appropriate amounts.
- Alter lifestyle or environment to accommodate individual needs.

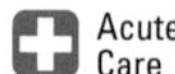

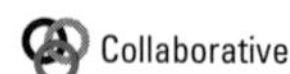

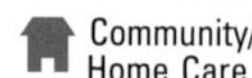

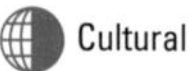

ACTIONS/INTERVENTIONS

Sample NIC linkages:
Urinary Elimination Management: Maintenance of an optimum urinary elimination pattern
Prompted Voiding: Promotion of urinary continence through the use of timed verbal toileting reminders and positive social feedback for successful toileting
Urinary Habit Training: Establishing a predictable pattern of bladder emptying to prevent incontinence for persons with limited cognitive ability who have urge, stress, or functional incontinence

NURSING PRIORITY NO. 1 To assess situation and adaptive skills being used by client:

- Note presence of physical diagnoses (e.g., surgery, childbirth, recent or multiple pregnancies, pelvic trauma, neurogenic bladder from central nervous disorders or neuropathies [stroke, SCI, diabetes], mental or emotional dysfunction, prostate disease or surgery) *that can impact client's elimination patterns.*
- Determine client's usual or previous pattern of elimination and compare with current situation *to determine client's readiness for improving elimination patterns and/or how pattern can be improved. Note: Urinary continence is a quality indicator in the Nursing Home Quality Initiative. Individual assessment and an individualized bladder management program are essential to maximizing continence.*[6]
- Observe current voiding pattern and time, color, and amount voided, as indicated (e.g., postsurgical client), *to document normalization of elimination.*
- Ascertain methods of self-management (e.g., limiting or increasing liquid intake, acting on urge in timely manner, establishing voiding schedule, regularly spaced catheterization) *to identify strengths and areas of concern in elimination management.*[1]
- Determine client's usual daily fluid intake. *Amount and timing of fluid intake, as well as beverage choices are important in managing elimination.*[1–3]
- Ascertain motivation and expectations for change. *Motivation to improve and high expectations can encourage client to make changes that will improve his or her life. However, unrealistic expectations may hamper efforts.*

NURSING PRIORITY NO. 2 To assist client to strengthen management of urinary elimination:

- Encourage fluid intake, including water and cranberry juice, *to help maintain renal function, prevent infection.*
- Regulate liquid intake at prescheduled times *to promote predictable voiding pattern.*[1,2]
- Suggest restricting fluid intake 2 to 3 hr before bedtime *to reduce voiding during the night.*[1,3,4]
- Assist with modifying current routines, as appropriate. *Client may benefit from additional information, such as responding to cues and urge to void, adjusting schedule of voiding or catheterization (shorter or longer), relaxation or distraction techniques, standing or sitting upright during voiding to ensure that bladder is completely empty, or practicing pelvic muscle-strengthening exercises.*[1,3,4]
- Provide assistance or devices as indicated. *Having means of summoning assistance; placement of bedside commode, urinal, or bedpan within client's reach; and use of elevated toilet seats or mobility devices enhance client's ability to maintain urinary function.*[4]
- Modify or recommend dietary changes if indicated. *Client may benefit from reduction of caffeine because of its bladder-irritant effect, or weight loss may help reduce overactive bladder symptoms and incontinence by decreasing pressure on the bladder.*[1,3,4]
- Modify medication regimens as appropriate. For example, administer prescribed diuretics in the morning *to lessen nighttime voiding* and reduce or eliminate use of hypnotics, if possible, *as client may be too sedated to recognize or respond to urge to void.*[4]
- Refer to appropriate resources (e.g., medical supply company, ostomy nurse, rehabilitation team) *for assistance, as desired or needed, to promote self-care.*

NURSING PRIORITY NO. 3 To promote optimum elimination:

- Encourage continuation of successful toileting program and identify possible alterations to meet individual needs (e.g., use of adult briefs for extended outing or travel with limited access to toilet). *Promotes proactive problem solving and supports self-esteem and normalization of social interactions and desired lifestyle activities.*[5]
- Instruct client/SO/caregivers in cues that client needs (e.g., voiding on routine schedule; showing client location of the bathroom; providing adequate room lighting, signs, color coding of door) *to assist client in continued continence, especially when in unfamiliar surroundings.*[2–4]
- Review expectations and prognosis of underlying condition (e.g., MS, prostate disease). *Provides information to assist client/significant other (SO) to make informed decisions and plan for possible changes.*
- Review with client/SO the signs and symptoms of urinary complications and need for medical follow-up. *Promotes timely intervention to limit or prevent adverse events.*

DOCUMENTATION FOCUS

Assessment/Reassessment

- Findings including previous and current voiding pattern, impact on lifestyle, and adaptive skills being used.
- Motivation and expectation for change.

Planning

- Plan of care and who is involved in planning.
- Teaching plan.

Implementation/Evaluation

- Responses to treatment plan, interventions, and actions performed.
- Attainment or progress toward desired outcome(s).
- Modifications to plan of care.

Discharge Planning

- Available resources, equipment needs and sources.

References

1. Sampselle, C. M. (2003). Behavioral interventions in young and middle-age women: Simple interventions to combat a complex problem. *Am J Nurs*, 103(suppl), 9–19.
2. Registered Nurses Association of Ontario. (Updated 2011). Prompting continence using prompted voiding. Nursing Best Practice Guideline Program. Retrieved April 2015 from http://rnao.ca/bpg/guidelines/promoting-continence-using-prompted-voiding.
3. Wyman, J. F., Burgio, K. L., Newman, D. K. (2009). Practical aspects of lifestyle modifications and behavioural interventions in the treatment of overactive bladder and urgency urinary incontinence. *Int J Clin Pract*, 63(8), 1171–1191.
4. Wyman, J. F. (2003). Treatment of urinary incontinence in men and older women: The evidence shows the efficacy of a variety of techniques. *Am J Nurs*, 103(suppl), 26–35.
5. Pringle-Specht, J. K. (2005). Nine myths of incontinence in older adults. *Am J Nurs*, 105(6), 58–68.
6. Palmer, M. H. (2008). Urinary incontinence quality improvement in nursing homes: Where have we been? Where are we going? *Urol Nurs*, 28(6), 444–453.

Acute Care 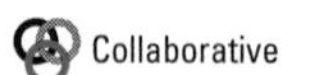 Collaborative 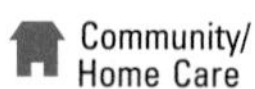 Community/Home Care 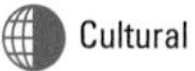 Cultural

impaired Emancipated Decision-Making

Taxonomy II: Life Principles—Class 3 Values/Belief/Action/Congruence (00242) [**Diagnostic Division:** Ego Integrity], Submitted 2013

DEFINITION: A process of choosing a healthcare decision that does not include personal knowledge and/or consideration of social norms or does not occur in a flexible environment, resulting in decisional dissatisfaction.

RELATED FACTORS

Traditional hierarchical family or healthcare systems
Limited decision-making experience
Decrease in understanding of all available healthcare options
Inability to adequately verbalize perceptions about healthcare options
Inadequate time to discuss healthcare options; insufficient privacy to openly discuss healthcare options

DEFINING CHARACTERISTICS

Subjective

Feeling constrained in describing own option
Inability to choose a healthcare option that best fits current lifestyle
Inability to describe how option will fit into current lifestyle
Excessive concern about what others think is the best decision
Excessive fear of what others think about decision

Objective

Delay in enacting chosen healthcare option
Distress when listening to other's opinion
Limited verbalization about healthcare option in other's presence
Sample Clinical Applications: Any condition/situation requiring healthcare decisions

DESIRED OUTCOMES/EVALUATION CRITERIA

Sample NOC linkages:

Decision-Making: Ability to make judgements and choose between two or more alternatives
Participation in Health Care Decisions: Personal involvement in selecting and evaluating health care options to achieve desired outcome

Client Will (Include Specific Time Frame)

- Verbalize concern about healthcare decision making.
- Express understanding of available healthcare options.
- Discuss healthcare options openly and with confidence.
- Participate in decision making freely and openly.

ACTIONS/INTERVENTIONS

Sample NIC linkages:

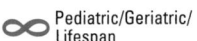

Decision-Making Support: Providing information and support for a patient who is making a decision regarding health care
Health System Guidance: Facilitating a patient's location and use of appropriate health services

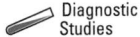

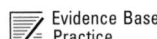

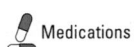

NURSING PRIORITY NO. 1 To assess causative/contributing factors (e.g., dementia or delirium):

- Determine usual ability to make decisions and factors that are currently interfering with making a personal choice. *Individual may not have sufficient knowledge or may be influenced by family pressures that may prevent making an independent decision.*[1,3]
- Note expressions of indecision, dependence on others, and availability and involvement of support persons. *Caregivers need to be sensitive to the physical, emotional, and cognitive effects of the situation on decision-making capabilities.*[2]
- Discuss issue of whether individual wants to be involved in decision making. *External influences may pressure person to give up own responsibility for the decision.*[2]
- Identify previous decisions individual has made and environment in which those and current decisions were/are made. *Provides information about client's ability and circumstances surrounding decision making.*[1]
- Active-listen and identify reasons for indecisiveness. *Helps client to clarify problem and begin to look at alternatives for situation.*[1]
- Identify cultural values, beliefs, moral obligations, or ethical concerns that may be creating conflict in current situation. *These issues need to be resolved before client will be comfortable with decision.*[5]
- Review information client has to support the decision to be made. *Provides opportunity to clarify and correct misinformation or inaccurate perceptions that can affect the outcome.*[2]

NURSING PRIORITY NO. 2 To assist client to become empowered and able to make effective decisions:

- Promote safe and hopeful environment as needed, including a therapeutic nurse-client relationship. *Client needs to feel safe and supported to be comfortable in own ability to make satisfactory decisions.*[2]
- Encourage verbalization of conflicts and concerns. *Helps to identify and clarify these issues so individual can reach a satisfying solution.*[1]
- Clarify and prioritize individual goals. *Enables client to look at the importance of the issues of the conflict and reach realistic problem solving.*[4]
- Identify strengths and use of positive coping skills, relaxation techniques, and willingness to express feelings. *Encourages individual to view themselves as a capable person who can make a desired decision.*[4]
- Discuss time constraints related to the decision to be made. *Healthcare decisions (i.e., breastfeeding) may need to be made quickly depending on the circumstances.*[1]
- Help client to learn the problem-solving process. *Provides a structure for individual to look at alternatives for making a decision in current situation and for other decisions that need to be made in the future.*[6]
- Discuss and clarify spiritual concerns, accepting client's values in a nonjudgmental manner. *Client will be willing to consider own situation when accepted as an individual of worth.*

NURSING PRIORITY NO. 3 To promote independence (Teaching/Discharge Considerations):

- Provide opportunities for practicing problem-solving skills. *Helps client to become more confident and solve current and future situations.*[4]
- Encourage family to become involved as desired/available. *Facilitates understanding of individual's needs and abilities, promoting support and acceptance of ability of family member.*[5]
- Discuss attendance at assertiveness and stress-reduction classes, if able. *Learning these skills helps client to become able to make decisions in a more decisive manner.*[1]
- Refer to other resources as indicated (e.g., public health, support group, clergy, psychiatrist, clinical specialist psychiatric nurse). *May need additional help to manage difficult decision making.*[4]

DOCUMENTATION FOCUS

Assessment/Reassessment

- Assessment findings, behavioral responses, and degree of impairment in lifestyle functioning.
- Individual involved in the conflict.
- Personal values and beliefs, moral or ethical concerns.

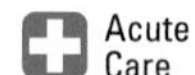

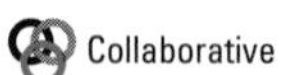

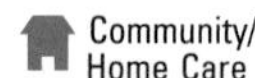

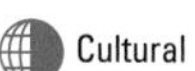

Planning
- Plan of care, specific interventions, and who is involved in the planning process.
- Teaching plan.

Implementation/Evaluation
- Client's and individuals' involved responses to interventions, teaching, and actions performed.
- Ability to express feelings and identify options.
- Use of resources.
- Attainment or progress toward desired outcome(s).
- Modifications to plan of care.

Discharge Planning
- Long-term needs, actions to be taken, and who is responsible for doing.
- Specific referrals made.

References

1. Wittman-Price, R. A. (2006). Exploring the subconcepts of the Wittman-Price Theory of Emancipated Decision-Making in woman's health care. *JNursScholarsh*, 38(4), 377–382.
2. Eggenberger, S. J., Grassley, J., Restrepo, E. (2006). Culturally competent nursing care for families. Listening to the voices of Mexican-American women. *OJIN*, 11(3). Retrieved January 2015 from http://www.nursingworld.org/MainMenuCategories/ANAMarketplace/ANAPeriodicals/OJIN/TableofContents/Volume112006/No3Sept06/ArticlePreviousTopics/CulturallyCompetentNursingCare.html.
3. Karlawish, J. (2008). Measuring decision-making capacity in cognitively impaired individuals. *Neurosignals*, 16(1), 91–98.
4. Paul, M. (2006). Relationships, the art of listening. Inner Bonding. Retrieved January 2015 from http://www.innerbonding.com/show-article/2147/relationships-the-art-of-listening.html.
5. Yuvarani, R. (2009). Family influences & decision making. Retrieved January 2015 from http://www.articlesbase.com/marketing-articles/family-influences-decision-making-family-decisionmaking-1014177.html.
6. Liken, M. (2001). Caregivers in crisis: Moving a relative with Alzheimer's to assisted living. *Clin Nurs Res*, 10(1), 53–69.

readiness for enhanced Emancipated Decision-Making

Taxonomy II: Life Principles—Class 3 Values/Belief/Action/Congruence (00243) [**Diagnostic Division:** Ego Integrity], Submitted 2013

DEFINITION: A process of choosing a healthcare decision that includes personal knowledge and/or consideration of social norms, which can be strengthened.

DEFINING CHARACTERISTICS

Subjective
Expresses desire to enhance:
Decision making; confidence in decision making
Ability to understand all available healthcare options
Privacy to discuss healthcare options; confidence to discuss healthcare options openly
Ability to verbalize own options without constraint; comfort to verbalize healthcare options in the presence of others

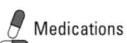

(continues on page 296)

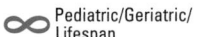

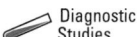

readiness for enhanced Emancipated Decision-Making (continued)
Ability to choose healthcare options that best fit current lifestyle; ability to enact chosen healthcare options
Sample Clinical Applications: Any condition/situation requiring healthcare decisions

DESIRED OUTCOMES/EVALUATION CRITERIA

Sample NOC linkages:
Decision-Making: Ability to make judgments and choose between two or more alternatives
Participation in Health Care Decisions: Personal involvement in selecting and evaluating health care options to achieve desired outcome

Client Will (Include Specific Time Frame)
- Gather information including opinions of others while making own decision.
- Express comfort with taking adequate time to make decision.
- Make decision that is congruent with lifestyle and personal and sociocultural values and goals.
- Acknowledge comfort with own decision.

ACTIONS/INTERVENTIONS

Sample NIC linkages:
Decision-Making Support: Providing information and support for a patient who is making a decision regarding healthcare
Health System Guidance: Facilitating a patient's location and use of appropriate health services

NURSING PRIORITY NO. 1 To determine current decision-making abilities and needs:

- Determine usual ability to manage own affairs and make own decisions. *Provides baseline for understanding client's usual manner of making decisions.*[1]
- Note availability of support person. *Having support can provide individual with positive feedback regarding the validity of the choice.*[3]
- Active-listen and identify reason(s) client is ready to improve decision-making ability. *Provides opportunity for individual to clarify and understand how decisions are made and how they can help to achieve desired goals.*[1]
- Identify cultural values, beliefs, moral obligations, and ethical principles that guide or affect the decision-making process. *Although individuals believe they are able to look at the issues with an unbiased eye, it has been shown that one's unconscious biases may interfere with making a decision that is desired.*[4]
- Discuss meaning of life and reasons for living and how these relate to desire for improvement. *Cutting-edge research is demonstrating that the mind within the brain affects how these issues impact the individual's decision-making process.*[5]

NURSING PRIORITY NO. 2 To assist client to improve/effectively use problem-solving skills:

- Promote safe and hopeful environment and help client identify own inner control. *The individual can take into consideration the context and pertinent facts when they feel safe and believe the decision-making is in their control and make a rational and well-thought-out decision.*[6]
- Encourage verbalization of ideas, concerns, and particular decisions that need to be made. *Identifying these issues all help client make desired choices.*[6]
- Correct misconceptions and biases client may have. *People often have unconscious biases that can interfere with decision making. Helping to clarify these ideas will make for efficient decisions.*[4]
- Identify positive aspects of this learning opportunity. *Every day individuals make decisions, often without giving thought to what is needed to make a good decision. Decision making can be developed by using rational and lateral thinking.*[6]

Acute Care
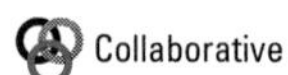
Collaborative
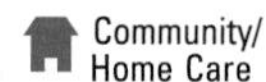
Community/Home Care
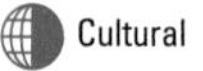
Cultural

- Discuss the process of practicing making decisions. *Decision making is a skill that we use every day at home, work, school, and in every aspect of our lives, so the more one knows about an effective process, the better one's decisions can be.*[6]
- Encourage children to make age-appropriate decisions. *The earlier they learn the problem-solving process, self-esteem and coping skills will be enhanced.*[7]
- Discuss client's spiritual beliefs and values. *Accepting these in a nonjudgmental manner can help the individual look at what they believe in relation to these issues and decision making.*[7]

NURSING PRIORITY NO. 3 To promote optimum independence (Teaching/Discharge Considerations):

- Identify opportunities for using problem-solving skills. *Emphasizing each step as it is used will facilitate the learning process.*[7]
- Involve family and significant others as desired by client. *Helps all those involved to improve their decision-making skills and enhance relationships and client can live a fuller life.*[8]
- Recommend client attend assertiveness and/or stress-reduction classes as desired. *Provides opportunity to learn new ways of dealing with problems and enhancing decision-making abilities and life in general.*[8]
- Refer to other resources as necessary (e.g., public health, healthcare providers, clergy, support group, clergy, psychiatrist/clinical specialist psychiatric nurse). *May need additional assistance for specific problems and/or support long-term needs.*[4]

DOCUMENTATION FOCUS

Assessment/Reassessment

- Assessment findings, behavioral responses.
- Motivation for change.
- Personal values, beliefs.

Planning

- Plan of care, specific interventions and actions to be performed.
- Teaching plan.

Implementation/Evaluation

- Response to interventions, teaching, and actions performed.
- Ability to express feelings and confidence in decision-making process.
- Attainment or progress toward desired outcomes.
- Modifications to plan of care.

Discharge Planning

- Long-term needs and who is responsible for actions to be taken.
- Specific referrals made.

References

1. Eisenhardt, K., Zbaracki, M. (1992). Strategic decision making. *Strategic Management Journal*, 13(52), 17–37.
2. Mazamil, J., Shubeens, A. (2008). An analysis of decision-making power among married and unmarried women. *Stud Home Comm Sci*, 2(10), 41–51. Retrieved January 2015 from http://krepublishers.com/02-Journals/S-HCS/HCS-02-0-000-08-Web/HCS-02-1-001-08-Abst-Text/HCS-02-1-043-08-036-Jan-M/HCS-02-1-043-08-036-Jan-M-Tt.pdf.
3. Stepanuk, K. M., Fisher, K. M., et al. (2013). Women's decision-making regarding medication use in pregnancy for anxiety and/or depression. *J Advanced Nursing*, 69(11), 2470–2480.
4. Banaji, M. R., Greenwald, A. G. (2013). *Blindspot: Hidden Biases of Good People*. New York: Delacorte Press.
5. Redish, A. D. (2013). *The Mind Within the Brain: How We Make Decisions and How Those Decisions Go Wrong*. New York: Oxford University Press.

6. Welthy, D. (2013). *Decide: Better Ways of Making Better Decisions.* London, UK: Kogan Page.
7. Heath, C., Heath, D. (2013). *Decisive: How to Make Better Choices in Life and Work.* New York: Crown Business. http://krepublishers.com/02-Journals/S-HCS/HCS-02-0-000-08-Web/HCS-02-1-001-08-Abst-Text/HCS-02-1-043-08-036-Jan-M/HCS-02-1-043-08-036-Jan-M-Tt.pdf.
8. Miller, W., Rollnick, S. (2008). *Motivational Interviewing in Health Care: Helping Patients Change Behavior.* New York: The Guildford Press.

risk for impaired Emancipated Decision-Making

Taxonomy II: Life Principles—Class 3 Values/Belief/Action/Congruence (00244) [**Diagnostic Division:** Ego Integrity], Submitted 2013

DEFINITION: Vulnerable to a process of choosing a healthcare decision that does not include personal knowledge and/or consideration of social norms or does not occur in a flexible environment, resulting in decisional dissatisfaction.

RISK FACTORS

Traditional hierarchical family or healthcare systems
Limited decision-making experience; insufficient self-confidence in decision making
Insufficient information regarding healthcare options
Inadequate time to discuss healthcare options
Insufficient confidence or privacy to openly discuss healthcare options
Note: A risk diagnosis is not evidenced by signs and symptoms, as the problem has not occurred; rather, nursing interventions are directed at prevention
Sample Clinical Applications: Any condition/situation requiring healthcare decisions

DESIRED OUTCOMES/EVALUATION CRITERIA

Sample NOC linkages:
Decision-Making: Ability to make judgements and choose between two or more alternatives
Participation in Health Care Decisions: Personal involvement in selecting and evaluating health care options to achieve desired outcome

Client Will (Include Specific Time Frame)
- Acknowledge awareness of difficulty in healthcare decision making.
- Seek information for making healthcare decisions.
- Discuss options openly with family/others as appropriate.
- Develop confidence as decisions are make.

ACTIONS/INTERVENTIONS

Sample NIC linkages:
Decision-Making Support: Providing information and support for a patient who is making a decision regarding health care
Health System Guidance: Facilitating a patient's location and use of appropriate health services

Refer to ND impaired Emancipated Decision Making for Interventions, Documentation, and References.

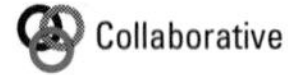

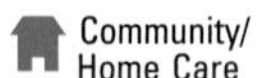

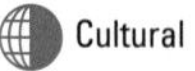

labile Emotional Control

Taxonomy II: Perceptual/Cognition—Class 4 Cognition (00251) [**Diagnostic Division:** Ego Integrity], Submitted 2013

DEFINITION: Uncontrollable outbursts of exaggerated and involuntary emotional expression.

RELATED FACTORS

Fatigue; insufficient muscle strength; musculoskeletal impairment
Functional impairment; physical disability
Stressors; social distress; alteration in self-esteem
Brain injury
Emotional disturbance; mood disorder; psychiatric disorder
Insufficient knowledge of disease or about symptom control
Pharmaceutical agent; substance abuse

DEFINING CHARACTERISTICS

Subjective

Embarrassment regarding emotional expression
Excessive laughing/crying without feeling happiness
Expression of emotion incongruent with triggering factor

Objective

Uncontrollable/involuntary crying, laughing
Tearfulness
Absence of eye contact
Difficulty in use of facial expressions
Withdrawal from social or occupational situations

Sample Clinical Applications: Traumatic brain injury, stroke, multiple sclerosis, psychiatric disorders, substance abuse

DESIRED OUTCOMES/EVALUATION CRITERIA

Sample NOC linkage:

Mood Equilibrium: Appropriate adjustment of prevailing emotional tone in response to circumstances

Client Will (Include Specific Time Frame)

- Acknowledge problem with emotional control.
- Identify feelings that occur with episodes of uncontrollable emotions.
- Follow medication regimen.
- Participate in recommended activities/rehabilitation.

ACTIONS/INTERVENTIONS

Sample NIC linkage:

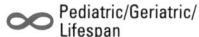

Mood Management: Providing for safety, stabilization, recovery, and maintenance of a person who is experiencing a dysfunctionally depressed or elevated mood

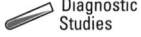

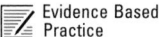

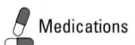

NURSING PRIORITY NO. 1 To assess causative/contributing factors:

- Determine individual factors related to client situation. *Many different physiological/psychological factors may be involved in loss of emotional control for a given person. Identifying these factors will help to develop a plan of care specific to this individual.*[1]
- Assess demographic, clinical, psychiatric, and stroke lesion characteristics. *Identifies individual areas that are affected, possibly related to injury to anterior regions of the cerebral hemispheres.*[2]
- Note when episodes of loss of control occur. *Determines frequency of incidents and factors associated with condition or with first stroke.*[2]
- Identify client's perception of incidents. *Most people are embarrassed by these outbursts, believing they could control them. Individuals with multiple sclerosis are prone to these episodes.*[1]
- Evaluate for depression. *Depression may be a factor for these individuals, but a pseudobulbar affect (PDA) needs to be recognized as different as treatments are different for these conditions.*[1]

NURSING PRIORITY NO. 2 To determine effective control of labile episodes:

- Develop a plan of care to meet the needs of the individual situation. *Provides effective care for specific problems the client is experiencing.*[1]
- Establish a therapeutic nurse/client relationship. *Promotes trust and willingness to share concerns about problems that arise.*
- Note feelings of emotional exhaustion and social isolation. *Client may not recognize that this is a medical condition and may tend to remove themselves from situations that trigger the episodes.*[4]
- Assure client that the symptoms are real and need to be treated. *Healthcare providers may not know about this condition, and the client may not recognize that these are symptoms and therefore not report them.*[4]
- Correct misperceptions and provide accurate information. *Promotes understanding and helps client to be proactive in care.*[4]

NURSING PRIORITY NO. 3 To promote wellness (Teaching/Discharge Considerations):

- Involve family in treatment plan. *Provides support for the client and promotes understanding of the uncontrollable episodes.*[4]
- Discuss use of medication. *There was no treatment until Nuedexta was recently approved to treat PDA. Its active ingredient is dextromethorphan; however, the formulation is different from any over-the-counter medications.*[4]
- Encourage involvement in social activities. *Enhances ability to participate with others.*[2]
- Refer for physical therapy and rehabilitation. *Client may exhibit emotional lability following stroke and can benefit from these activities.*[3]
- Refer to other resources as necessary such as group therapy, psychiatric therapy, and assertiveness training. *This additional help will enable client to develop a more positive lifestyle.*[1]

DOCUMENTATION FOCUS

Assessment/Reassessment

- Assessment findings, including triggering or associated factors, impact of condition on life, other pertinent information.

Planning

- Plan of care, specific interventions, and who is involved in planning process.
- Teaching plan.

Implementation/Evaluation

- Response to intervention, teaching, and actions performed.
- Ability to express feelings and control emotions.

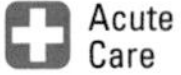

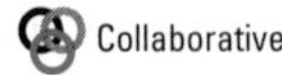

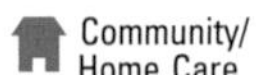

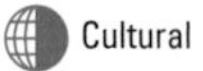

- Use of resources.
- Attainment or progress toward desired outcomes.
- Modifications to plan of care.

Discharge Planning

- Long-term needs, actions to be taken and who is responsible for doing them.
- Specific referrals made.

References

1. Arnold, C. (Spring 2000). An ocean of emotion: Mood swings, anger, and uncontrollable laughing and crying. InsideMS. Retrieved March 2015 from http://www.nationalmssociety.org/NationalMSSociety/media/MSNationalFiles/Brochures/Brochure-MS-and-the-Mind.pdf.
2. Morris, P. L., Robinson, R. G., Raphael, B. (1993). Emotional lability after stroke. *Aust, NZ J Psychiatry*, 27(4), 601–605.
3. National Stroke Association. (2014). Pseudobulbar affect (PDA). Retrieved March 2015 from http://www.strokeassociation.org/STROKEORG/LifeAfterStroke/RegainingIndependence/EmotionalBehavioralChallenges/Pseudobulbar-Affect-PBA_UCM_467457_Article.jsp.
4. DiSalva, D. (2011). Not all crying is depression: Understanding pseudobulbar affect. Psychology Today. Retrieved March 2015 from http://www.psychologytoday.com/blog/neuronarrative/201110/not-all-crying-is-depression-understanding-pseudobulbar-affect.

risk for Falls

Taxonomy II: Safety/Protection—Class 2 Physical Injury (00155) [**Diagnostic Division:** Safety], Submitted 2000; Revised 2013

DEFINITION: Vulnerable to increased susceptibility to falling, which may cause physical harm and compromise health.

RISK FACTORS

Adults

Age ≥65; living alone
History of falls
Use of assistive device (e.g., walker, cane, wheelchair)
Lower-limb prosthesis

Physiological

Acute illness; postoperative recovery period
Alteration in blood glucose level; anemia
Arthritis; condition affecting the foot; decrease in lower extremity strength; difficulty with gait
Diarrhea; incontinence; urinary urgency
Faintness when extending or turning neck; orthostatic hypotension
Hearing or visual impairment
Impaired balance or mobility; proprioceptive deficit; neuropathy
Sleeplessness

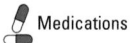

Cognitive

Alteration in cognitive functioning

(continues on page 302)

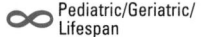

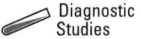

risk for Falls (continued)

Pharmaceutical Agents
Alcohol consumption
Pharmaceutical agent

Environment
Use of restraints
Exposure to unsafe weather-related condition (e.g., wet floors, ice)
Cluttered environment; use of throw rugs; insufficient antislip material in bathroom
Unfamiliar setting; insufficient lighting

Children
Age ≤2; male gender when <1 year of age [Note: Centers for Disease Control statistics suggest male gender is a factor for children age 1 to 19 but gender not significant during first year of life]
Absence of stairway gate or window guard: insufficient automobile restraints
Inadequate supervision
Note: A risk diagnosis is not evidenced by signs and symptoms, as the problem has not occurred; rather, nursing interventions are directed at prevention.
Sample Clinical Applications: Amputation, arthritis, osteoporosis, fractures, joint replacement surgery; seizure disorder, cerebrovascular disease, cataracts, dementia, paralysis, hypotension, cardiac dysrhythmias, inner ear infection, alcohol abuse or intoxication; trauma or surgery (general)

DESIRED OUTCOMES/EVALUATION CRITERIA

Sample NOC linkages:
Physical Injury Severity: Severity of injuries from accidents and trauma

Client Will (Include Specific Time Frame)
- Be free of injury.

Knowledge: Fall Prevention: Extent of understanding conveyed about prevention of falls
Fall Prevention Behavior: Personal or family caregiver actions to minimize risk factors that might precipitate falls in the personal environment

Client/Caregivers Will (Include Specific Time Frame)
- Verbalize understanding of individual risk factors that contribute to possibility of falls.
- Demonstrate behaviors and lifestyle changes to reduce risk factors and protect self from injury.
- Modify environment as indicated to enhance safety.

ACTIONS/INTERVENTIONS

Sample NIC linkages:
Fall Prevention: Instituting special precautions with patient at risk for injury from falling
Environmental Management: Safety: Monitoring and manipulation of the physical environment to promote safety
Surveillance: Safety: Purposeful and ongoing collection and analysis of information about the patient and the environment for use in promoting and maintaining patient safety

NURSING PRIORITY NO. 1 To evaluate source/degree of risk:

- Review client's general health status, *noting multiple factors that may affect safety, such as chronic/debilitating conditions, use of more than four prescriptions, recent trauma (especially a fall within the past*

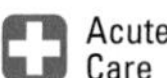
Acute Care
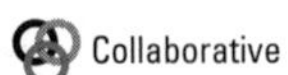
Collaborative
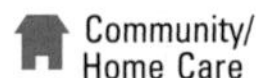
Community/ Home Care
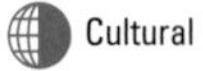
Cultural

3 to 12 months), prolonged bedrest or immobility, unstable balance on standing, and a sedentary lifestyle. Note: Many fall-risk assessment tools have been developed and compared. Best practice interventions in fall reduction have been shown to be (1) the use of a screening tool, (2) visual identification of client at high risk for falls, (3) directed multifactorial interdisciplinary risk factor interventions, and (4) client and care provider education.[1,9]

- Evaluate client's current disorders/conditions that could enhance risk potential for falls. *Acute, even short-term, situations can affect any client, such as sudden dizziness, positional blood pressure changes, new medication, change in glasses prescription, and recent use of alcohol/other drugs.*[10]
- Assess and document client's fall risk using a fall-risk scale (e.g., Morse Fall Scale [MFS], Functional Ambulation Profile, Tinetti Balance and Gait Assessment, Timed-Up-and-Go [TUG]) upon admission, change in status, transfer, and discharge. *Fall-risk scales are widely used in acute-care and long-term settings and include numbered rating scales for (1) history of falls, (2) secondary diagnosis, (3) use of ambulatory aid, (4) presence of IV, (5) gait and transfer abilities, and (6) mental status. An MFS score greater than 51 indicates the client is at high risk for falls and requires high fall-prevention interventions. A TUG scale greater than 14 seconds combined with three other risk factors (such as support needed for cognition, transportation, and attendance at multiple appointments) places a client at high risk for falls.*[1,2,7,8,10]
- Note client's age/developmental level, gender, decision-making ability, and level of competence. *Infants, young children (e.g., climbing on objects, stairs), young adults (e.g., sports activities), and elderly (e.g., significant vision, cognitive, or mobility impairments; osteoporosis; loss of muscle, fat, and subcutaneous tissue) are at greatest risk because of developmental issues or impaired/lack of ability to self-protect. Note: Tools for adult fall-risk assessment have been found to be unreliable in infants and children. Most falls in this age group occur outside the clinical setting, but assessment of facility environment and developmental issues in hospitalized children must include many factors, such as crib and play area safety, cosleeping issues, lapses of caregiver attention (such as falling asleep while feeding), medical and nursery equipment on which a toddler might climb, etc.*[2,9]
- Assess client's cognitive status (e.g., presence of brain injury, dementia, neurological disorders, visual/hearing/other sensory impairments). *Affects ability to perceive own limitations or recognize danger. If client is unable to protect self, responsibility falls upon primary care provider(s).*
- Evaluate client's general and hip muscle strength, postural stability, gait and standing balance, gross and fine motor coordination. Review history of past or current physical injuries (e.g., musculoskeletal injuries, orthopedic surgery) *that may be altering coordination, gait, and balance.*
- Review client's ongoing medication regimen, noting number and type of drugs that could impact fall potential. *Studies have confirmed that use of four or more medications (polypharmacy) increases the risk of falls. The probability of using a medication that introduces risk increased that risk from 25% when one medicine was administered to 60% when six or more medicines were being taken.*[11]
- Assess mood, coping abilities, and personality styles. *Individual's temperament, typical behavior, stressors, and level of self-esteem can affect attitude toward safety issues, resulting in carelessness or increased risk-taking without consideration of consequences.*[7–9]
- Determine client's/significant other's (SO's) level of knowledge about and attendance to safety needs. *May reveal lack of knowledge needed to provide for safety, a choice to make a different decision for some reason (e.g., "We can't hire a home assistant"; "I can't watch him every minute"; "It's not manly"), or a lack of resources to attend to safety issues in all settings.*[3,9]
- Evaluate client's use, misuse, or failure to use assistive aids when indicated. *Client may have assistive device but is at high risk for falls while adjusting to altered body state and use of unfamiliar device. Client might refuse to use devices for various reasons (e.g., waiting for help; just doesn't like it for whatever reason).*[7–9]
- Identify hazards in the care setting, home, or other environment. *Determining needs and deficits provides opportunities for environmental redesign and instruction (e.g., concerning clearing of hazards, modification of lighting, equipment placement and space management; intensifying client supervision; obtaining safety equipment; referring for vision evaluation).*[7,8,12]

- Ascertain caregiver's expectations of client (whether child, cognitively impaired, and/or elderly family member) and compare with actual abilities. *Reality of client's abilities and needs may be different from perception or desires of caregivers.*
- Note socioeconomic status and availability and use of resources in other circumstances. *Can affect current coping abilities and fall risk.*

NURSING PRIORITY NO. 2 To assist client/caregiver to reduce or correct individual risk factors:

- Collaborate in treatment of disease or condition(s) (e.g., acute illness, dementia, incontinence, neurological or musculoskeletal conditions) *to improve client's overall health and thereby reduce potential for falls.*
- Review consequences of previously determined risk factors and client/SO response (e.g., client's current fall and hip fracture caused by failure to make safety provisions for client's impairments).[3]
- Recommend or implement needed interventions and safety devices *to manage conditions that could contribute to falling and to promote safe environment for individual and others:*[1–9,12]
  Situate bed to enable client to exit toward his or her stronger side whenever possible.
  Place bed in lowest possible position, use raised-edge mattress, pad floor at side of bed, or place mattress on floor as appropriate.
  Use half siderail instead of full siderails or upright pole to assist individual in arising from bed.
  Provide chairs with firm, high seats and lifting mechanisms when indicated.
  Provide appropriate day or night lighting; evaluate vision, encourage use of prescription eyewear.
  Assist with transfers and ambulation; show client/SO ways to move safely.
  Provide and instruct in use of mobility devices and safety devices, like grab bars and call light or personal assistance systems.
  Clear environment of hazards (e.g., obstructing furniture, small items on the floor, electrical cords, throw rugs).
  Lock wheels on movable equipment (e.g., wheelchairs, beds).
  Encourage use of treaded slippers, socks, and shoes, and maintain nonskid floors and floor mats.
  Provide foot and nail care.
- Provide or encourage use of analgesics before activity if pain is interfering with desired activities. *Balance and movement can be impaired by pain associated with multiple conditions such as trauma or arthritis.*[1,2]
- Follow up with physician to review client's usual medication regimen (e.g., narcotics/opiates, psychotropics, antihypertensives, diuretics), *which can contribute to weakness, confusion, and balance and gait disturbances. May benefit from evaluating drug concentrations of certain medications (e.g., anticonvulsants, tricyclic antidepressants, antiarrhthymics) or may need an adjustment to dose, time of administration, or a change in choice of medication prescribed.*[6–11]
- Discuss benefits of supplemental estrogen, calcium, and vitamin D, as indicated. Refer for further evaluation as indicated. *Primary prevention of osteoporosis could be important in reducing falls and risk for fractures.*[12]
- Refer to physical medicine specialist, physical or occupational therapist, or recreation therapist as appropriate. *May require evaluation (e.g., balance, muscle strength) and treatment to improve client's balance, strength, or mobility; to improve or relearn ambulation; and to identify and obtain appropriate assistive devices for mobility, environmental safety, or home modification.*
- Perform home visit when appropriate. *Useful in determining client's specific needs and available resources or verifying that home safety issues are addressed, including supervision, access to emergency assistance, and client's ability to manage self-care in the home.*

NURSING PRIORITY NO. 3 To promote safety (Teaching/Discharge Considerations):[1–6]

- Educate client/SO/caregivers in fall prevention; address the need for exercise balanced with need for client/care provider safety. *While fall prevention is necessary, the need to protect the client from harm must be balanced with preserving client's independence. If the client is overly afraid of falling, the lack of activity will result in deconditioning and an even greater risk of falling.*[3]

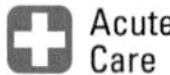
Acute Care
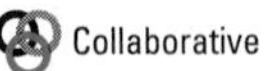
Collaborative
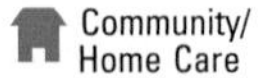
Community/ Home Care
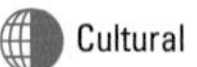
Cultural

- Discuss importance of monitoring client/intervening in conditions (e.g., client fatigue; acute illness; depression; objects that block traffic patterns in home; insufficient lighting; unfamiliar surroundings; client attempting tasks that are too difficult for present level of functioning; inability to contact someone when help is needed) *that have been shown to contribute to occurrence of falls.*[7,8]
- Address individual environmental factors associated with falling and create or instruct in a safe physical environment, such as bed height, room lighting, removal of loose carpet or throw rugs, repair of uneven flooring, and installing grab bars in bathrooms.
- Refer to community resources as indicated. Provide written material for review and reinforcement of learning. *Client/caregivers may need or desire information (now or later) about financial assistance, home modifications, referrals for counseling, home care, sources for safety equipment, or placement in an extended care facility.*
- Connect client/family with sources of assistance (e.g., neighbors, friends, support groups) *to check on client on regular basis and to assist elderly or handicapped individuals in providing such things as structural maintenance; clearing of snow, gravel, or ice from walks and steps; etc.*
- Promote community awareness about the problems of design of buildings, equipment, transportation, and workplace accidents that contribute to falls.

DOCUMENTATION FOCUS

Assessment/Reassessment

- Individual risk factors noting current physical findings (e.g., bruises, cuts, anemia; use of alcohol, drugs, and prescription medications).
- Client's/caregiver's understanding of individual risks and safety concerns.
- Caregiver's expectations of client's abilities.

Planning

- Plan of care and who is involved in planning.
- Teaching plan.

Implementation/Evaluation

- Individual responses to interventions, teaching, and actions performed.
- Specific actions and changes that are made.
- Attainment or progress toward desired outcomes.
- Modifications to plan of care.

Discharge Planning

- Long-term plans for discharge needs, lifestyle, and home setting and community changes and who is responsible for actions to be taken.
- Specific referrals made.

References

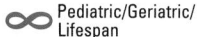

1. Institute for Clinical Systems Improvement. (Updated 2012). Guideline: Prevention of falls (acute care protocol). Retrieved March 2015 from https://www.icsi.org/_asset/dcn15z/Falls-Interactive0412.pdf.
2. VHA National Center for Patient Safety. (Updated 2014). Implementation guide for falls. Retrieved March 2014 from http://www.patientsafety.gov/CogAids/FallPrevention/index.html#page=page-1.
3. Henkel, G. (2002). Beyond the MDS. Team approach to falls assessment, prevention & management. *Caring for the Aged*, 3(4), 15–20.
4. Doenges, M. E., Moorhouse, M. F., Geissler-Murr, A. C. (2002). Nursing care plan: Extended care, falls, risk for. *Nursing Care Plans: Guidelines for Individualizing Patient Care.* (CD-ROM). 6th ed. Philadelphia: F. A. Davis.
5. Daus, C. (1999). Maintaining mobility: Assistive equipment helps the geriatric population stay active and independent. *Rehabil Manage*, 12(5), 58–61.
6. Horn, L. B. (2000). Reducing the risk of falls in the elderly. *Rehabil Manage*, 13(3), 36–38.

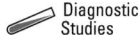

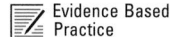

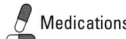

7. Bright, L. (2005). Strategies to improve the patient safety outcome indicator: Preventing or reducing falls. *Home Healthcare Nurse*, 23(1), 29–36.
8. Poe, S. S., Cvach, M. M., Gartrelu, D. G., et al. (2005). An evidence-based approach to fall risk assessment, prevention, and management: Lessons learned. *J Nurs Care Qual*, 20(2), 107–116.
9. McWilliams, J. R. (2011). An evidenced-based pediatric fall assessment tool for home health. *Home Healthcare Nurse*, 20(29), 98–105.
10. Kemle, K. (2011). Falls in older adults: Averting disaster. Retrieved March 2015 from http://www.clinicaladvisor.com/falls-in-older-adults-averting-a-disaster/article/195485/.
11. Ziere, G., Dieleman, J. P., Hofman, A., et al. (2006). Polypharmacy and falls in the middle age and elderly population. *Br J Clin Pharmacol*, 61(2), 218–223.
12. Quigley, P. A., Bulat, T., Hart-Hughes, S. (2007). Strategies to reduce risk of fall-related injuries in rehabilitation nursing. *Rehabil Nurs*, 32(3), 120–125.

dysfunctional Family Processes

Taxonomy II: Role Relationships—Class 2 Family Relationships (00063) [**Diagnostic Division:** Social Interaction], Submitted as dysfunction Family Processes: Alcoholism 1994; Revised: name change 2008, 2013

DEFINITION: Psychosocial, spiritual, and physiological functions of the family unit are chronically disorganized, which leads to conflict, denial of problems, resistance to change, ineffective problem solving, and a series of self-perpetuating crises.

RELATED FACTORS

Substance abuse
Family history of substance abuse, resistance to treatment
Ineffective coping strategies; insufficient problem-solving skills
Biochemical factors; genetic predisposition to substance abuse; addictive personality

DEFINING CHARACTERISTICS

Subjective

Feelings

Anxiety, tension, distress; low self-esteem, worthlessness; lingering resentment
Anger, frustration; shame, embarrassment; hurt; unhappiness; guilt
Emotional isolation, loneliness; powerlessness; insecurity; hopelessness; rejection
Taking responsibility for substance abuser's behavior; vulnerability; mistrust
Depression; hostility; fear; confusion; dissatisfaction; loss
Feeling different from others; feeling unloved, misunderstood
Emotionally controlled by others; loss of identity
Abandonment; confuses love and pity; moodiness; failure

Roles and Relationships

Family denial; deterioration in family relationships; disturbance in family dynamics; ineffective communication with partner; intimacy dysfunction
Change in role function; disrupted family roles or rituals; inconsistent parenting; perceived insufficient parental support; chronic family problems
Insufficient relationship skills; insufficient cohesiveness
Pattern of rejection; economically disadvantaged; neglect of obligation to family member

Objective

Feelings

Repressed emotions
Surgical procedure [?]

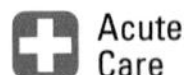

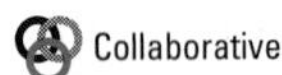

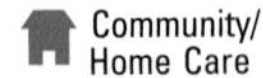

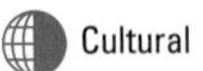

Roles and Relationships
Closed communication systems
Conflict between partners; diminished ability of family members to relate to each other for mutual growth and maturation
Insufficient family respect for individuality or autonomy of its members
Behavioral
Substance abuse; nicotine addiction
Enabling substance use pattern; insufficient knowledge about substance abuse
Special occasions centered on substance use
Rationalization; denial of problems; refusal to get help; inability to accept or receive help appropriately
Inappropriate anger expression; blaming; criticizing; verbal abuse of children/partner/parent
Lying; broken promises; unreliable behavior; manipulation; dependency
Inability to express or accept a wide range of feelings; difficulty with intimate relationship; decrease in physical contact
Harsh self-judgment; difficulty having fun; self-blaming; social isolation; complicated grieving; seeking of approval or affirmation
Ineffective communication skills; controlling, contradictory, or paradoxical communication pattern; power struggles
Insufficient problem-solving skills; conflict avoidance; orientation favors tension relief rather than goal attainment; agitation; escalating conflict; chaos
Alteration in concentration; disturbance in academic performance in children; failure to accomplish developmental tasks; difficulty with life-cycle transition
Inability to meet the emotional, security, or spiritual needs of its members
Inability to adapt to change; immaturity; stress-related physical illnesses; inability to deal constructively with traumatic experiences
Sample Clinical Applications: Alcohol abuse or withdrawal, prescription or illicit drug abuse, fetal alcohol syndrome

DESIRED OUTCOMES/EVALUATION CRITERIA

Sample NOC linkages:
Family Functioning: Capacity of the family system to meet the needs of its members during developmental transitions
Family Social Climate: Supportive milieu as characterized by family member relationships and goals
Substance Addiction Consequences: Severity of change in health status and social functioning due to substance addiction

Family Will (Include Specific Time Frame)
- Verbalize understanding of dynamics of codependence.
- Participate in individual/family treatment programs.
- Identify ineffective coping behaviors and consequences of choices or actions.
- Plan for necessary lifestyle changes.
- Take action to change self-destructive behaviors or alter behaviors that contribute to substance abuse.
- Demonstrate improvement in parenting skills.

ACTIONS/INTERVENTIONS

Sample NIC linkages:
Counseling: Use of an interactive helping process focusing on the needs, problems, or feelings of the patient and significant others to enhance or support coping, problem solving, and interpersonal relationships

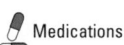

(continues on page 308)

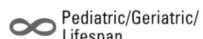

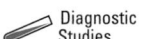

dysfunctional Family Processes (continued)

Substance Use Treatment: Supportive care of patient/family members with physical and psychosocial problems associated with the use of alcohol or drugs

Family Process Maintenance: Minimization of family process disruption effects

NURSING PRIORITY NO. 1 To assess contributing factors/underlying problem(s):

- Assess current level of functioning of family members. *Information necessary for planning care determines areas for focus and potential for change.*[2]
- Ascertain family's understanding of current situation; note results of previous involvement in treatment. *Family with a member who is addicted to alcohol has often had frequent hospitalizations in the past. Knowing what has brought about the current situation will determine a starting place for this treatment plan.*[2]
- Review family history and explore roles of family members and circumstances involving substance use. *Although one member may be identified as the client, all of the family members are participants in the problem and need to be involved in the solution.*[5]
- Determine history of accidents or violent behaviors within family and current safety issues. *Identifies family at risk and degree of concern or disregard of individual members to determine course of action to prevent further violence.*[2,4]
- Discuss current and past methods of coping. *Family members have developed coping skills to deal with behaviors of client, which may or may not be useful to changing the situation. Skills identified as useful can help to change the present situation. Those identified as not helpful (enabling behaviors) can be targeted for intervention to bring about desired changes and improve family functioning.*[1,2,5]
- Determine extent and understanding of enabling behaviors being evidenced by family members. *Family members may have developed behaviors that support the client continuing the pattern of addiction. Awareness, identification, and knowledge of these behaviors provide opportunity for individuals to begin the process of change.*[2,5]
- Identify sabotage behaviors of family members. *Issues of secondary gain (conscious or unconscious) may impede recovery. Even though family member(s) may verbalize a desire for the individual to become substance free, the reality of interactive dynamics is that they may unconsciously not want the individual to recover because this would affect the role(s) of the family member(s) in the relationship.*[2]
- Note presence and extent of behaviors of family, client, and staff that might be "too helpful," such as frequent requests for assistance, excuses for not following through on agreed-on behaviors, and feelings of anger or irritation with others. *Identification of specific behaviors (enabling) can help family members see what they do that complicates acceptance of situation by substance abuser and that need to be changed to facilitate resolution of problem.*[5]

NURSING PRIORITY NO. 2 To assist family to change destructive behaviors:

- Seek mutual agreement on behaviors and responsibilities for nurse and client/family members. *Maximizes understanding of what is expected of each person and minimizes opportunity for manipulation of each individual.*[5]
- Confront and examine denial and sabotage behaviors used by family members. *Identifies specific behaviors that individuals can be aware of and begin to change so they can move beyond blocks to recovery.*[6]
- Discuss use of anger, rationalization, or projection and ways in which these interfere with problem resolution. *Awareness of own feelings can lead to a decision to change; client then has to face the consequences of his or her own actions and may choose to get well.*[6]
- Encourage family to identify and deal with anger. Solve concerns and develop solutions. *Understanding what leads to anger and violence can lead to new behaviors and changes in the family for healthier relationships.*[3]
- Determine family strengths, areas for growth, and individual/family successes. *Family members may not realize they have strengths, and as they identify these areas, they can choose to learn and develop new strategies for a more effective family structure.*[2]

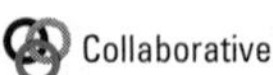

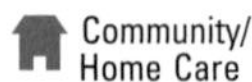

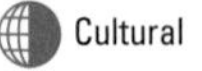

- Remain nonjudgmental in approach to family members and to member who uses alcohol or drugs. *Individual already sees self as unworthy, and judgment on the part of caregivers to family will interfere with ability to be a change agent.*[5]
- Provide information regarding effects of addiction on mood and personality of the involved person. *Family members have been dealing with client's behavior for a time, and information can help them to understand and cope with negative behaviors without being judgmental or reacting angrily.*[2]
- Distinguish between destructive aspects of enabling behavior and genuine motivation to aid the user. *Family members often want to help but need to distinguish between behavior that is helpful and that which is not to begin to solve problems of addiction.*[6]
- Identify use of manipulative behaviors and discuss ways to avoid or prevent these situations. *The client often manipulates the people around him or her to maintain the status quo. When family begins to interact in a straightforward, honest manner, manipulation is not possible and healing can begin.*[2]

NURSING PRIORITY NO. 3 To promote wellness (Teaching/Discharge Considerations):

- Provide factual information to client/family about the effects of addictive behaviors on the family and what to expect after discharge from program. *Family may have unrealistic expectations about changes that have occurred in therapy, and having information will help them deal more effectively with the difficulties of continuing the changes as they return to their new life without alcohol or substance.*[5]
- Provide information about enabling behavior and addictive disease characteristics for both the user and non-user who is codependent. *Education is a prime ingredient in treatment of addiction and can assist family members to deal realistically with these issues.*[6]
- Discuss importance of restructuring life activities, work, and leisure relationships. *Previous lifestyle and relationships supported the substance use, requiring change to prevent relapse.*[7]
- Encourage family to refocus celebrations to exclude alcohol use. *Because celebrations often include the use of alcohol, this is one area where change can be made that can reduce the risk of relapse.*[7]
- Provide support for family members; encourage participation in group work. *Support is essential to changing client and family behaviors. Participating in group provides an opportunity to practice new skills of communication and behavior.*[5]
- Encourage involvement with/refer to self-help groups, Al-Anon, AlaTeen, Narcotics Anonymous, and family therapy groups. *Regular attendance at a group can provide support; help client see how others are dealing with similar problems; and learn new skills, such as problem solving, for handling family disagreements.*[7]
- Provide bibliotherapy including reliable Web sites, as appropriate. *Reading provides helpful information for making desired changes, especially when client/family members are dedicated to making change and willing to learn new ways of interacting within the family.*[7]
- Refer to NDs compromised/disabled family Coping and interrupted Family Processes as appropriate for additional interventions.

DOCUMENTATION FOCUS

Assessment/Reassessment

- Assessment findings, including history of substance(s) that have been used and family risk factors/safety concerns.
- Family composition and involvement.
- Results of previous treatment involvement.

Planning

- Plan of care and who is involved in planning.
- Teaching plan.

Implementation/Evaluation
- Responses of family members to treatment, teaching, and actions performed.
- Attainment or progress toward desired outcome(s).
- Modifications to plan of care.

Discharge Planning
- Long-term needs and who is responsible for actions to be taken.
- Specific referrals made.

References

1. Messina, J. (2007). Eliminating manipulation: Tools for handling control issues. Retrieved October 2015 from http://coping.us/toolsforhandlingcontrol/eliminatemanipulation.html.
2. Friel, J. C., Friel, L. D. (2010). *Adult Children—The Secrets of Dysfunctional Families*. Deerfield Beach, FL: Health Communications, Inc.
3. Hollander, T. (2013). 13 Signs of anger and how to manage them in sobriety. Retrieved October 2015 from http://www.selfhelpmagazine.com/articles/alcohol-anger#sthash.AmfMkl0O.Lc1BO0gH.dpbs.
4. Moyer, V. A. (2013). Screening for intimate partner violence and abuse of elderly and vulnerable adults: U.S. Preventive Services Task Force recommendation statement. *Ann of Inter Med*, 158(6), 478–486.
5. Saaticioglu, O., Erim, R., Cakmak, D. (2006). Role of family in alcohol and substance abuse. *Psychiatry Clin Neurosci*, 60(2), 125–132.
6. Nye, C. L., Zucker, R. A., Fitzgerald, H. E. (1999). Early family-based intervention in the path to alcohol problems, rationale and relationship between treatment process characteristics and child and parenting outcomes. *J Stud Alcohol Suppl*, 13, 10–21.
7. Seilhamer, R. A., Jacob, T., Dunn, N. J. (1993). The impact of alcohol consumption on parent-child relationships in families of alcoholics. *J Stud Alcohol*, 54, 189–198.

interrupted Family Processes

Taxonomy II: Role Relationships—Class 2 Family Relationships (00060) [**Diagnostic Division:** Social Interactions], Submitted 1982; 1998

DEFINITION: Change in family relationships and/or functioning.

RELATED FACTORS

Situational transition or crisis
Developmental transition or crisis
Shift in health status of a family member
Shift in family roles; power shift among family members
Alteration in family finances
Change in family social status, or interaction with community

DEFINING CHARACTERISTICS

Subjective

Changes in relationship pattern; alteration in family satisfaction
Alteration in availability for affective responsiveness; decrease in mutual support; decrease in available emotional support; alteration in intimacy
Changes in expression of conflict with, or isolation from, community resources

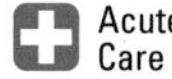

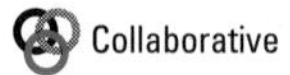

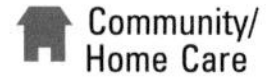

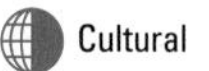

Objective

Assigned tasks change; ineffective task completion; alteration in participation for problem solving; change in participation for decision making

Change in communication pattern; alteration in family conflict resolution; power alliance changes

Change in stress-reduction behavior; change in somatization

Sample Clinical Applications: Chronic illness, cancer, surgical procedures, traumatic injury, substance abuse, Alzheimer's disease, pregnancy, adolescent rebellion, conduct disorder

DESIRED OUTCOMES/EVALUATION CRITERIA

Sample NOC linkages:

Family Functioning: Capacity of the family system to meet the needs of its members during developmental transitions

Family Normalization: Capacity of the family system to develop strategies for optimal functioning when a member has a chronic illness or disability

Family Social Climate: Supportive milieu as characterized by family member relationships and goals

Family Will (Include Specific Time Frame)

- Express feelings freely and appropriately.
- Demonstrate individual involvement in problem-solving processes directed at appropriate solutions for the situation or crisis.
- Direct energies in a purposeful manner to plan for resolution of the crisis.
- Verbalize understanding of illness/trauma, treatment regimen, and prognosis.
- Encourage and allow affected member to handle situation in own way, progressing toward independence.

ACTIONS/INTERVENTIONS

Sample NIC linkages:

Family Process Maintenance: Minimization of family process disruption effects

Family Integrity Promotion: Promotion of family cohesion and unity

Normalization Promotion: Assisting parents and other family members of children with chronic diseases or disabilities in providing normal life experiences for their children and families

NURSING PRIORITY NO. 1 To assess individual situation for causative/contributing factors:

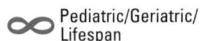

- Determine pathophysiology, illness or trauma, and developmental crisis present. *Identifies areas of need for planning care for this family.*[2]
- ∞ Identify family developmental stage (e.g., marriage, birth of a child, children leaving home, death of a spouse). *Developmental stage will affect family functioning; for instance, a couple who are newly married will be dealing with issues of learning how to live with each other, children leaving home may result in problems related to "empty-nest syndrome," or death of a spouse radically changes life for the survivor.*[2,8]
- Note components of family: parent(s), children, male/female, and extended family available. *Affects how individuals deal with current stressors. Relationships among members may be supportive or strained.*[6]
- Observe patterns of communication in this family. Are feelings expressed? Freely? Who talks to whom? Who makes decisions and for whom? Who visits? What is the interaction between family members? *Identifies not only weakness and areas of concern to be addressed, but also strengths that can be used for resolution of problem(s).*[6,9]
- Assess boundaries of family members. Do members share family identity and have little sense of individuality? Do they seem emotionally distant and not connected with one another? *These factors are critical to*

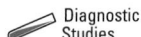

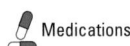

understanding family dynamics and developing strategies for change. Boundaries need to be clear so individual family members are free to be responsible for themselves.[6]

- Ascertain role expectations of family members. Who is the ill member (e.g., nurturer, provider)? How does the illness affect the roles of others? *Each person may see the situation in his or her own individual manner; clear identification and sharing of these expectations promote understanding. Family members may expect client to continue to perform usual role or may not allow client to do anything (either action can create problems for the ill member). Realistic planning can provide positive sense of self for the client.*[2,8]
- Determine "family rules" (e.g., adult concerns such as finances, illness, and so on are kept from the children). *Rules may be imposed by adults rather than through a democratic process involving all family members, leading to conflict and angry confrontations. Setting positive family rules with all family members participating can promote a functional family.*[2,3]
- Identify parenting skills and expectations. *Ineffective parenting and unrealistic expectations may contribute to abuse. Understanding normal responses and progression of developmental milestones may help parent cope with changes necessitated by current crisis.*[2,3]
- Note energy direction. Are efforts at resolution/problem solving purposeful or scattered? *Provides clues about interventions that may be appropriate to assist client and family in directing energies in a more effective manner.*[2,9]
- Listen for expressions of despair/helplessness (e.g., "I don't know what to do") to note degree of distress. *Such feelings may contribute to difficulty adjusting to situation (e.g., teenage independence, change in health status of household breadwinner, dependence of aging parent on grown child) and ability to cooperate with plan of care or treatment regimen required.*[4]
- Note cultural and/or religious beliefs and values affecting perceptions and expectations of family members. *These factors affect client/SO reactions and adjustment to situation and may limit choice of interventions and potential for successful resolution.*
- Assess support systems available outside of the family. *Having these resources can help the family begin to pull together and deal with current situation and problems they are facing.*[2]

NURSING PRIORITY NO. 2 To assist family to deal with situation/crisis:

- Deal with family members in a warm, caring, and respectful way. *Provides feelings of empathy and promotes individual's sense of worth and competence in ability to handle current situation.*[2]
- Acknowledge difficulties and realities of the situation. *Communicates message of understanding and reinforces that some degree of conflict is to be expected and can be used to promote growth.*[3]
- Encourage expressions of anger. Avoid taking them personally. *Feelings of anger are to be expected when individuals are dealing with a difficult situation. Appropriate expression enables progress toward resolution of the stages of the grieving process when indicated. Not taking their anger personally maintains boundaries between nurse and family.*[2,5]
- Stress importance of continuous, open dialogue between family members to facilitate ongoing problem solving. *Promotes understanding and assists family members to maintain clear communication and resolve problems effectively.*[6,10]
- Provide information, verbal and written, and reinforce as necessary. *Promotes understanding and opportunity to review as needed.*[2]
- Assist family to identify and encourage their use of previously successful coping behaviors. *Most people have developed effective coping skills that, when identified, can be useful in current situation.*[6,10]
- Recommend contact by family members on a regular, frequent basis. *Promotes feelings of warmth and caring and brings family closer to one another, enabling them to manage current difficult situation.*[2]

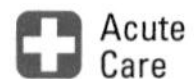

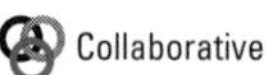

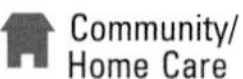

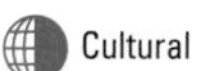

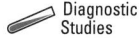

- Arrange for and encourage family participation in multidisciplinary team conference or group therapy as appropriate. *Participation in family and group therapy for an extended period increases likelihood of success as interactional issues (e.g., marital conflict, "scapegoating" of children) can be addressed and dealt with. Involvement with others can help family members to experience new ways of interacting and gain insight into their behavior, providing opportunity for change.*[2,5]
- Involve family in social support and community activities of their interest and choice. *Involvement with others outside of family constellation provides opportunity to observe how others handle problems and deal with conflict.*[2,8]

NURSING PRIORITY NO. 3 To promote wellness (Teaching/Discharge Considerations):

- Encourage use of stress-management techniques (e.g., appropriate expression of feelings, relaxation exercises). *The relaxation response helps members think more clearly, deal more effectively with conflict, and promote more effective relationships to enhance family interactions.*[4]
- Provide educational materials and information. *Learning about the problems they are facing can assist family members in resolution of current crisis.*[2]
- Refer to classes (e.g., parent effectiveness, specific disease, or disability support groups; self-help groups; clergy, psychological counseling, or family therapy as indicated). *Can assist family to effect positive change and enhance conflict-resolution skills. Presence of substance abuse problems requires all family members to seek support and assistance in dealing with situation to promote a healthy outcome.*[2,3] (Refer to ND dysfunctional Family Processes for additional interventions as appropriate.)
- Assist family to identify situations that may lead to fear or anxiety (e.g., diagnosis of chronic debilitating condition, decline in mental functioning of aging spouse/parent, sexually active teenager). (Refer to NDs Anxiety, Fear.) *Promotes opportunity to provide anticipatory guidance.*[1,5]
- Involve family in mutual goal-setting to plan for the future. *When all members of the family are involved, commitment to goals and continuation of plan are more likely to be maintained.*[3]
- Identify community agencies (e.g., Meals on Wheels, visiting nurse, trauma support group, American Cancer Society, Veterans Administration). *Provides both immediate and long-term support.*[6]

DOCUMENTATION FOCUS

Assessment/Reassessment

- Assessment findings, including family composition, developmental stage of family, and role expectations.
- Family communication patterns.
- Cultural or religious beliefs and values.

Planning

- Plan of care, specific interventions, and who is involved in planning.
- Teaching plan.

Implementation/Evaluation

- Each individual's response to interventions, teaching, and actions performed.
- Attainment or progress toward desired outcome(s).
- Modifications to plan of care.

Discharge Planning

- Long-term needs, noting who is responsible for actions to be taken.
- Specific referrals made.

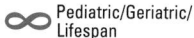

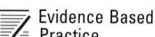

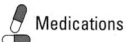

References

1. LaBier, D. (2013). Why your fears shape so much of your life. Psychology Today. Retrieved October 2015 from http://www.psychologytoday.com/blog/the-new-resilience/201303/why-your-fears-shape-so-much-your-life.
2. No author listed. (2009). Stages of family development, education, self improvement, health and medicine. Retrieved October 2015 from http://www.slideshare.net/guest74f230/stages-of-family-development.
3. Aktan, G. B., Kumpfer, K. L., Turner, C. W., et al. (1996). Effectiveness of a family skills training program for substance abuse prevention with inner city African-American families. *Subst Use Misuse*, 31(2), 157–175.
4. Reid, M. W. (1977). Counseling the disturbed family. *Aust Fam Physician*, 6(5), 474–479.
5. Rueter, M. A., Koerner, A. F. (2008). The effect of family communication patterns on adopted adolescent adjustment. *J Marriage Fam*, 70(3), 715–727.
6. Gerlach, P. (Updated 2011). Perspective on family role and rule problems. Break the Cycle. Retrieved October 2015 from http://sfhelp.org/fam/roles_rules.htm.
7. Fronk, C., Huntington, R., Chadwick, B. A. (1999). Expectations for traditional family roles: Palestinian adolescents in the West Bank and Gaza. *Sex Roles: A Journal of Research*, 41(9), 705–735.
8. Plunkett, S. (No date). Family developmental theory. Retrieved February 2012 from http://hhd.csun.edu/hillwilliams/542/Family%20Developmental%20Theory.htm.
9. Adams, L. (July 2008). How families resolve conflicts. *The Family Connection Newsletter*.
10. DaFoe Whitehead, B., Popenoe, D. (2004). The state of our unions: The social health of marriage in America 2004. *Theology Matters*, 10(2), 1–16.

readiness for enhanced Family Processes

Taxonomy II: Role Relationships—Class 2 Family Relationships (00159) [**Diagnostic Division:** Social Interactions], Submitted 2002; Revised 2013

DEFINITION: A pattern of family functioning that is sufficient to support the well-being of family members and can be strengthened.

DEFINING CHARACTERISTICS

Subjective

Expresses willingness to enhance family dynamics
Communication is adequate
Relationships are generally positive; interdependent with community; family tasks are accomplished
Energy level of family supports activities of daily living (ADLs)
Family adapts to change

Objective

Family functioning meets needs of family members
Activities support the safety or growth of family members
Family roles are appropriate or flexible for developmental stages
Respect for family members is evident; boundaries of family members are maintained
Family resilience is evident
Balance exists between autonomy and cohesiveness

Sample Clinical Applications: Chronic health conditions (e.g., asthma, diabetes mellitus, arthritis, systemic lupus, multiple sclerosis [MS], AIDS), mental health concerns (e.g., seasonal affective disorder, attention deficit disorder, Down syndrome)

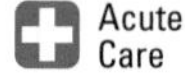

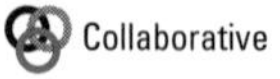

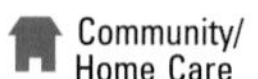

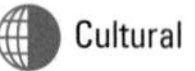

DESIRED OUTCOMES/EVALUATION CRITERIA

Sample NOC linkages:

Family Social Climate: Supportive milieu as characterized by family member relationships and goals
Family Health Status: Overall health and social competence of family unit
Family Resiliency: Positive adaptation and function of the family system following significant adversity or crisis

Client Will (Include Specific Time Frame)

- Express feelings freely and appropriately.
- Verbalize understanding of desire for enhanced family dynamics.
- Demonstrate individual involvement in problem solving to improve family communications.
- Acknowledge awareness of and respect for boundaries of family members.

ACTIONS/INTERVENTIONS

Sample NIC linkages:

Family Support: Promotion of family values, interests, and goals
Parent Education: Childrearing Family: Assisting parents to understand and promote the physical, psychological, and social growth and development of their toddler, preschool, or school-age child/children
Normalization Promotion: Assisting parents and other family members of children with chronic illnesses or disabilities in providing normal life experiences for their children and families

NURSING PRIORITY NO. 1 To determine current status of family:

- Determine family composition, such as parent(s), children, male/female, and extended family involved. *Many family forms exist in society today, such as biological, nuclear, single-parent, step-family, communal, and homosexual couple or family. A better way to determine a family may be to determine the attribute of affection, strong emotional ties, a sense of belonging, and durability of membership.*[1,6]
- Identify participating members of family, such as parent(s), children, male/female, and extended family. *Identifies members of family who need to be involved and taken into consideration in developing plan of care to improve family functioning.*[1]
- Note stage of family development. *While the North American middle-class family stages may be described as single, young adult, newly married, family with young children, family with adolescents, grown children, and later life, developmental tasks may vary greatly among cultural groups. This information provides a framework for developing a plan to enhance family processes.*[1]
- Ascertain motivation and expectations for change. *Motivation to improve and high expectations can encourage family to make changes that will improve their life. However, unrealistic expectations may hamper efforts.*[7]
- Observe patterns of communication in the family. Are feelings expressed freely? Who talks to whom? Who makes decisions? For whom? Who visits? When? What is the interaction between family members? *Identifies not only possible weakness or areas of concern to be addressed, but also strengths that can be used for planning improvement in family communication. Effective communication is that in which verbal and nonverbal messages are clear, direct, and congruent.*[1,2]
- Assess boundaries of family members. Do members share family identity and have little sense of individuality? Do they seem emotionally connected with one another? *Individuals need to respect one another, and boundaries need to be clear so family members are free to be responsible for themselves.*[1,3]
- Identify "family rules" that are accepted in the family. *Families interact in certain ways over time and develop patterns of behavior that are accepted as the way "we behave" in this family. "Functional families" rules are constructive and promote the needs of all family members.*[1]
- Note energy direction. *Efforts at problem solving, resolution of different opinions, and growth may be purposeful or may be scattered and ineffective.*[3]

- Determine cultural and/or religious factors influencing family interactions. *Expectations related to socio-economic beliefs may be different in various cultures; for instance, traditional views of marriage and family life may be strongly influenced by Roman Catholicism in Italian American and Latino American families. In some cultures, the father is considered the authority figure and the mother is the homemaker. These beliefs may be functional or dysfunctional in any given family and may change with stressors/circumstances (e.g., financial, loss or gain of a family member, personal growth).*[1,3,7]
- Note health of married individuals. *Recent reports have determined that marriage increases life expectancy by as much as 5 years.*[5]

NURSING PRIORITY NO. 2 To assist the family to improve family interactions:

- Establish nurse-family relationship. *Promotes a warm, caring atmosphere in which family members can share thoughts, ideas, and feelings openly and in a nonjudgmental manner.*[3]
- Acknowledge difficulties and realities of individual situation. *Reinforces that some degree of conflict is to be expected in family interactions that can be used to promote growth.*[1,3]
- Emphasize importance of continuous, open dialogue between family members. *Facilitates ongoing expression of open, honest feelings and opinions and effective problem solving.*[1,4]
- Assist family to identify and encourage use of previously successful coping behaviors. *Promotes recognition of previous successes and confidence in own abilities to learn and improve family interactions.*[2,4]
- Acknowledge differences among family members with open dialogue about how these differences have occurred. *Conveys an acceptance of these differences among individuals and helps to look at how they can be used to strengthen the family process.*[3]
- Identify effective parenting skills already being used and additional ways of handling difficult behaviors that may develop. *Allows the individual family members to realize that some of what has been done already was helpful and helps them to learn new skills to manage family interactions in a more effective manner.*[3]

NURSING PRIORITY NO. 3 To promote optimum well-being (Teaching/Discharge Considerations):

- Involve family members in setting goals and planning for the future. *When individuals are involved in the decision making, they are more committed to carrying through on a plan to enhance family interactions as life goes on.*[2]
- Discuss and encourage use of stress-management techniques. *Relaxation exercises, visualization, and similar skills can be useful for promoting reduction of anxiety and ability to manage stress that occurs in their lives.*[1]
- Encourage participation in learning role-reversal activities. *Helps individuals to gain insight and understanding of other person's feelings and point of view.*[3]
- Provide educational materials and information. *Enhances learning to assist in developing positive relationships among family members.*[4]
- Assist family members to identify situations that may create problems and lead to stress/anxiety. *Thinking ahead can help individuals anticipate helpful actions to handle or prevent conflict and untoward consequences.*[4]
- Refer to classes or community resources as appropriate. *Family effectiveness and self-help groups, psychotherapy, and religious affiliations can provide new information to assist family members to learn and apply to enhancing family interactions.*[4]

DOCUMENTATION FOCUS

Assessment/Reassessment

- Assessment findings, including family composition, developmental stage of family, and role expectations.
- Cultural or religious values and beliefs regarding family and family functioning.
- Family communication patterns.
- Motivation and expectations for change.

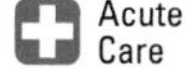

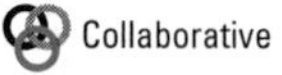

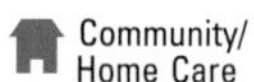

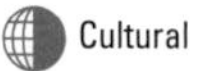

Planning
- Plan of care, specific interventions, and who is involved in planning.
- Educational plan.

Implementation/Evaluation
- Each individual's response to interventions, teaching, and actions performed.
- Attainment or progress toward desired outcome(s).
- Modifications to lifestyle and treatment plan.

Discharge Planning
- Long-term needs, noting who is responsible for actions to be taken.
- Specific referrals made.

References

1. No author listed. (2009). Stages of family development, education, self improvement, health and medicine. Retrieved October 2015 from http://www.slideshare.net/guest74f230/stages-of-family-development.
2. Gordon, T. (2011). Families need rules. Parent Programs, Gordon Training International. Retrieved October 2015 from http://www.gordontraining.com/free-parenting-articles/families-need-rules/.
3. Sophy, C. (2005). Four tips to help you set and enforce family boundaries. Retrieved October 2015 from http://ezinearticles.com/?Four-Tips-To-Help-You-Set-And-Enforce-Family-Boundaries&id=76369.
4. Sittner, B. J., Hudson, D. B., DeFrain, J. (2007). Using the concept of family strengths to enhance nursing care. *Am J Maternal/Child Nurs*, 32(6), 353–357.
5. Kaplan, R. M., Kronick, R. G. (2006). Marital status and longevity in the United States Population. *J Epidemiol Community Health*, 60(9), 760–765.
6. Hartley, R., McDonald, P. (1994). The many faces of diversity in Australian families. *Family Matters*, 37, 6–12.
7. McLeod, D. L., Wright, L. M. (2001). Conversations of spirituality: Spirituality in family systems nursing—Making the case with four clinical vignettes. *J Fam Nurs*, 7(4), 391–415.

Fatigue

Taxonomy II: Activity/Rest—Class 3 Energy Balance (00093) [**Diagnostic Division:** Activity/Rest], Submitted 1988; Nursing Diagnosis Extension and Classification Revision 1998

DEFINITION: An overwhelming sustained sense of exhaustion and decreased capacity for physical and mental work at the usual level.

RELATED FACTORS

Stressors; anxiety; depression
Nonstimulating lifestyle; negative life event; occupational demands (e.g., shift work, high level of activity, stress)
Environmental barrier (e.g., ambient noise, daylight/darkness exposure, ambient temperature/humidity, unfamiliar setting)
Increase in physical exertion; sleep deprivation
Physiological condition (e.g., pregnancy, disease, anemia); malnutrition
Physical deconditioning
[Altered body chemistry (e.g., medications, drug withdrawal, chemotherapy)]

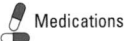

(continues on page 318)

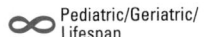

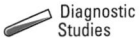

Fatigue (continued)
DEFINING CHARACTERISTICS

Subjective
Insufficient energy; impaired ability to maintain usual routines or usual physical activity
Tiredness; nonrestorative sleep pattern (i.e., due to caregiver responsibilities, parenting practices, sleep partner)
Guilt about difficulty maintaining responsibilities
Alteration in libido
Increase in physical symptoms, rest requirements

Objective
Lethargy; listlessness; drowsiness
Alteration in concentration
Disinterest in surroundings; introspection
Ineffective role performance
Sample Clinical Applications: Anemia, hypothyroidism, cancer, multiple sclerosis (MS), Lyme disease, postpolio syndrome, AIDS, chronic renal failure, chronic fatigue syndrome (CFS), depression

DESIRED OUTCOMES/EVALUATION CRITERIA

Sample NOC linkages:
Endurance: Capacity to sustain activity
Energy Conservation: Personal actions to manage energy for initiating and sustaining activity
Psychomotor Energy: Personal drive and energy to maintain activities of daily living, nutrition, and personal safety

Client Will (Include Specific Time Frame)
- Report improved sense of energy.
- Identify basis of fatigue and individual areas of control.
- Perform ADLs and participate in desired activities at level of ability.
- Participate in recommended treatment program.

ACTIONS/INTERVENTIONS

Sample NIC linkages:
Energy Management: Regulating energy use to treat or prevent fatigue and optimize function
Exercise Promotion: Facilitation of regular physical exercise to maintain or advance to a higher level of fitness and health
Nutrition Management: Assisting with or providing a balanced dietary intake of foods and fluids

NURSING PRIORITY NO. 1 To assess causative/contributing factors:

- Identify presence of physical and/or psychological conditions (e.g., pregnancy, infectious processes, blood loss, anemia, autoimmune disorders [e.g., MS, lupus, rheumatoid arthritis], trauma, chronic pain syndromes [e.g., arthritis], cardiopulmonary disorders, cancer or cancer treatments, hepatitis, AIDS, major depressive disorder, anxiety states, substance use or abuse). *Important information can be obtained from knowing if fatigue is a result of an underlying condition or disease process (acute or chronic), whether an exacerbating or remitting condition is in exacerbation, and/or whether fatigue has been present over a long time without any identifiable cause.*
- Note diagnosis or possibility of CFS, also sometimes called chronic fatigue immune dysfunction syndrome. *Defining Characteristics listed above indicate that this fatigue far exceeds feeling tired after a busy day. This condition is difficult to characterize, largely because various studies define CFS differently. Because no direct*

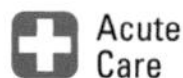

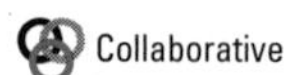

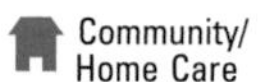

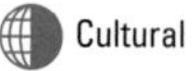

tests help in diagnosis, it is one of exclusion. CFS has been defined as a distinct disorder (affecting children and adults) characterized by chronic (often relapsing but always debilitating) fatigue, lasting for at least 6 months (often for much longer), causing impairments in overall physical and mental functioning, and without an apparent etiology.[1]

- Note client's age, gender, and developmental stage. *Some studies show a prevalence of fatigue in females more than in males, and it occurs most commonly in young to middle-aged adults.*[1,9,10]
- Assess general well-being—cardiovascular and respiratory status, musculoskeletal strength, emotional health, and nutritional and fluid status. *Underlying conditions (e.g., anemia, heart failure, depression, malnutrition) may be causing or exacerbating fatigue.*
- Note changes in life (e.g., relationship problems, family illness, injury or death; expanded responsibilities or demands of others, job-related conflicts) that can be causing or exacerbating level of fatigue. *Stress may be the result of dealing with disease or situational crises, dealing with the "unknowns," or trying to meet expectations of others.*[2] *Also, grief and depression can sap energy and cause avoidance of social and/or physical interactions that could stimulate the mind and body. Note: Persons with AIDS and the elderly are especially prone to this fatigue because they experience significant losses, often on a regular or recurring basis.*[3,4]
- Assess sleep pattern—hours and quality of sleep. *Sleep disturbance is both a contributor to and a manifestation of fatigue (e.g., a client with chronic pain or depression may be sleeping long periods but not experience refreshing sleep or may not be able to fall or stay asleep).*
- Determine ability to participate in activities and level of mobility. *While many illness conditions negatively affect client's energy and activity tolerance, if the client is not engaged in light to moderate exercise, he or she may simply adjust to more sedentary activities, which can in turn exacerbate deconditioning and debilitation. However, there are certain conditions (e.g., MS, postpolio syndrome) where the client's ability to do things diminishes as he or she does them (e.g., at the beginning of a walk the client feels okay, but fatigue sets in [out of proportion to the activity] and the client is exhausted as if running a marathon).*[5,6]
- Review medication regimen and use. *Many medications have the potential side effect of causing/exacerbating fatigue (e.g., beta-blockers, chemotherapy agents, narcotics, sedatives, muscle relaxants, antiemetics, antidepressants, antiepileptics, diuretics, cholesterol-lowering drugs, HIV treatment agents, combinations of drugs and/or substances).*
- Assess psychological and personality factors that may affect reports of fatigue level. *Client with severe or chronic fatigue may have issues affecting desire to be active (or work), resulting in over- or underactivity or concerns of secondary gain from exaggerated fatigue reports.*
- Evaluate aspect of "learned helplessness" that may be manifested by giving up. *Can perpetuate a cycle of fatigue, impaired functioning, and increased anxiety and fatigue.*

NURSING PRIORITY NO. 2 To determine degree of fatigue/impact on life:

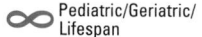

- Ask client to describe fatigue, noting particular phrases (e.g., drained, exhausted, lousy, weak, lazy, worn out, whole-body tiredness). *Helpful in clarifying client's expressions for symptoms and pattern and timing of fatigue, which varies over time and may also vary in duration, unpleasantness, and intensity from person to person.*[7]
- Have client rate fatigue (using 0 to 10 or a similar scale) and describe its effects on ability to participate in desired activities. *Fatigue may vary in intensity and is often accompanied by irritability, lack of concentration, difficulty making decisions, problems with leisure, and relationship difficulties that can add to stress level and aggravate sleep problems.*[11]
- Assess severity of fatigue using a recognized scale (e.g., Chalder Fatigue Scale, Functional Assessment of Cancer Therapy Fatigue, Multidimensional Assessment of Fatigue, Piper Fatigue Self-Report Scale, Global Fatigue Index), as appropriate. *In initial evaluations, these scales can help determine manifestation, intensity, duration, and emotional meaning of fatigue. The scales can be used in ongoing evaluations to determine current status and estimate response to treatment strategies.*[2,7–9,12]
- Measure blood pressure and heart and respiratory rate before and after activity as indicated. *Physiological response to activity (e.g., changes in blood pressure or heart or respiratory rate) may indicate need for*

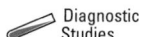

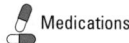

interventions to improve cardiovascular health, pulmonary status, and conditioning. (Refer to risk for Activity Intolerance for additional interventions.)

- Review availability and current use of assistance with daily activities, support systems, and resources.
- Evaluate need for individual assistance or assistive devices. *Certain conditions causing fatigue (e.g., postpolio syndrome) worsen with overuse of weakened muscles. Client may benefit from support and protection provided by braces, canes, power chairs, etc.*[6,7]

NURSING PRIORITY NO. 3 To assist client to cope with fatigue and manage with individual limitations:

- Accept reality of client's fatigue and avoid underestimating effect on quality of life the client experiences. *Fatigue is subjective and often debilitating (e.g., clients with cancer, AIDS, or MS are prone to more frequent episodes of severe fatigue following minimal energy expenditure and require longer recovery period; postpolio clients often display a cumulative effect if they fail to pace themselves and rest when early signs of fatigue are encountered).*[5,7]
- Active-listen concerns and encourage expression of feelings. *Provides support to help client deal with very frustrating and taxing situation.*
- Treat underlying conditions where possible (e.g., manage pain, depression, or anemia; treat infections; reduce numbers of interacting medications) *to reduce fatigue caused by treatable conditions.*
- Involve client/significant others (SO)/caregivers(s) in planning care *to incorporate their input, choices, and assistance.*
- Encourage client to do whatever activity possible (e.g., self-care, sit up in chair, walk for 5 minutes), pacing self and increasing activity level gradually. Schedule activities for periods when client has the most energy, *to maximize participation.*
- Structure daily routines and establish realistic activity goals with client, especially when depression is a factor in fatigue. *May enhance client's commitment to efforts and promote sense of self-esteem in accomplishing goals.*
- Instruct client/caregivers in alternate ways of doing familiar activities and methods to conserve energy, such as the following:[2,3,7–9]

  Sit instead of standing during daily care or other activities.
  Adjust the level or height of work surface for ergonomic benefit and to prevent bending over.
  Carry several small loads instead of one large load.
  Use assistive devices (e.g., wheeled walkers or chairs, power lift recliner chairs, stair-climbers).
  Plan steps of activity before beginning so that all needed materials are at hand.
  Take frequent short rest breaks and return to activity.
  Delegate tasks or duties whenever possible.
  Combine and simplify activities.
  Ask for and accept assistance.
  Say "no" or "later."
- Provide environment conducive to relief of fatigue and avoid temperature and humidity extremes. *Temperature and level of humidity are known to affect exhaustion (especially in clients with MS).*[5]
- Encourage nutritional foods; refer to a dietitian as indicated. *Nutritionally balanced diet with proteins, complex carbohydrates, vitamins, and minerals may boost energy. Frequent, small meals and simple-to-digest foods are beneficial when combating fatigue. Reduced amounts of caffeine and sugar can improve sleep and energy.*[3,7]
- Provide supplemental oxygen as needed. *If fatigue is related to oxygenation/perfusion problems, oxygen may improve energy level and ability to be active.* (Refer to ND Activity Intolerance for additional interventions.)
- Provide diversional activities (e.g., visiting with friends/family, TV/music, doing hobbies or schoolwork). *Participating in pleasurable activities can refocus energy and diminish feelings of unhappiness, sluggishness, and worthlessness, which can accompany fatigue.* (Refer to ND deficient Diversional Activity for additional interventions.)

- Avoid over/understimulation (cognitive and sensory). *Impaired concentration can limit ability to block competing stimuli and distractions.*
- Assist client/SOs to implement measures to preserve energy over longer periods of time. *Even though the client may continue to experience fatigue, his/her energy level could benefit from such things as (1) planning and organizing work tasks (e.g., delegating, combining activities, simplifying details; spending energy on important/desired tasks); (2) balancing periods of rest and work and resting before fatigue sets in; (3) pacing self and reducing sudden or prolonged strains; (4) limiting work that increases muscle tension and using good body mechanics; and (5) modifying effects of the environment such as temperature extremes and eliminating smoke and harmful fumes.*[2]
- Recommend or implement routines that promote restful sleep, such as the following:
  Regular sleep hours at night with beneficial nighttime rituals
  Short naps during day hours
  A mild, graded exercise program to include strengthening and stretching movements such as yoga or tai chi
  Quiet activities in the evening
  Meditation and/or visualization
  Warm baths
  Refer to NDs Insomnia and Sleep Deprivation for additional interventions.
- Instruct in or refer for stress-management skills of visualization, deep breathing, relaxation, and biofeedback *to deal with situation, aid in relaxation, and to reduce boredom, pain, and sense of fatigue.*
- Participate in comprehensive rehabilitation program with physical or occupational therapist and/or an exercise or rehabilitation physiologist. *Collaborative program with short-term achievable goals enhances likelihood of success and may motivate client to adopt a lifestyle for enhancement of health.*[2,7,8]
- Discuss appropriateness of other therapies (e.g., massage, acupuncture, osteopathic or chiropractic manipulations). *Complementary therapies may be helpful in reducing muscle tension and pain to promote relaxation and rest.*

NURSING PRIORITY NO. 4 To promote wellness (Teaching/Discharge Considerations):

- Discuss therapy regimen relating to individual causative factors (e.g., physical and/or psychological illnesses) and help client/SO(s) to understand relationship of fatigue to illness. Promotes acceptance of situation, allowing client to focus attention on finding ways to live with fatigue.
- Assist client/SO(s) to develop plan for activity and exercise within individual ability. *Enhances sense of control and commitment to attaining goals.*
- Emphasize necessity of allowing sufficient time to finish activities. *Client is more likely to succeed when he or she does not feel rushed and is allowed to proceed at a measured pace.*
- Instruct client in ways to monitor response to activity and significant signs/symptoms to heed. *Changes in pulse or respiratory rate or development of worsened or unrelenting fatigue is a signal to stop, rest, and then resume activity, possibly modified in some aspect, that will allow the client to proceed.*
- Promote overall health measures (e.g., good nutrition [to include reduced levels of saturated and trans fats, cholesterol, salt and added sugars], adequate fluid intake, appropriate vitamin and iron supplementation).
- Encourage client to develop assertiveness skills and prioritize goals and activities.
- Discuss burnout syndrome when appropriate and actions client can take to change individual situation.
- Assist client to identify appropriate coping behaviors. *Promotes sense of control and improves self-esteem.*
- Identify support groups and resources (e.g., condition-specific groups, reliable Web sites) *to provide information, share experiences, and enhance problem solving.*
- Refer to community resources for assistance with routine needs (e.g., Meals on Wheels, homemaker or housekeeper services, yard care, transportation options).
- Refer to counseling or psychotherapy as indicated *to deal with stressors and effects of condition.*

DOCUMENTATION FOCUS

Assessment/Reassessment

- Manifestations of fatigue and other assessment findings.
- Degree of impairment and effect on lifestyle.
- Expectations of client/SO relative to individual abilities and specific condition.

Planning

- Plan of care, specific interventions, and who is involved in the planning.
- Teaching plan.

Implementation/Evaluation

- Client's response to interventions, teaching, and actions performed.
- Attainment or progress toward desired outcome(s).
- Modifications to plan of care.

Discharge Planning

- Discharge needs and who is responsible for actions to be taken.
- Specific referrals made.

References

1. Cunha, B. A. (Updated 2015). Chronic fatigue syndrome. Retrieved October 2015 from http://emedicine.medscape.com/article/235980-overview.
2. Ratini, M. (reviewer). (Reviewed 2014). Cancer-related fatigue. WebMD. Retrieved October 2015 from http://www.webmd.com/cancer/cancer-related-fatigue.
3. Zimmerman, J. (2002). Nutrition for health and healing in HIV. ACRIA Update. Retrieved September 2011 from www.thebody.com/content/art14418.html.
4. Ackley, B. J. (2010). Fatigue. In Ackley, B. J., Ladwig, G. B. (eds). *Nursing Diagnosis Handbook: An Evidence-Based Guide to Planning Care*. 9th ed. St. Louis, MO: Mosby.
5. Lava, N. (review 2014). Multiple sclerosis fatigue: Causes and treatment. Retrieved October 2015 from http://www.webmd.com/multiple-sclerosis/guide/ms-related-fatigue.
6. National Institute of Neurological Disorders and Stroke. (2015). Post-polio syndrome fact sheet. Retrieved October 2015 from http://www.ninds.nih.gov/disorders/post_polio/detail_post_polio.htm.
7. Keeney, C. E., Head, B. A. (2011). Palliative nursing care of the patient with cancer-related fatigue. *J Hospice Palliative Nurs*, 13(5), 270–278.
8. Veterans Health Administration, Department of Defense. (2014). Clinical practice guidelines for the management of medically unexplained symptoms: Chronic pain and fatigue. Retrieved October 2015 from http://www.healthquality.va.gov/MR/mus/mus_sum.pdf.
9. Centers for Disease Control and Prevention. (Updated 2014). Chronic fatigue syndrome (CFS) in children and adolescents. Retrieved October 2015 from http://www.cdc.gov/cfs/pediatric/index.html.
10. ter Wolbeek, M., van Doornen, L. J. P., Kavelaars, A., et al. (2006). Severe fatigue in adolescents: A common phenomenon? *Pediatrics* 117(6), e1078–e1086.
11. Barton-Burke, M. (2006). Cancer-related fatigue and sleep disturbances: Further research on the prevalence of these two symptoms in long-term cancer survivors can inform education, policy, and clinical practice. *Am J Nurs*, 106(3 suppl), 72–77.
12. Trendall, J. (2005). Concept analysis: Chronic fatigue. *J Adv Nurs*, 32(5), 1126–1131.

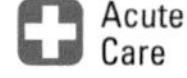

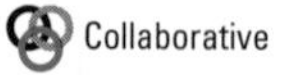

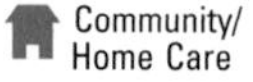

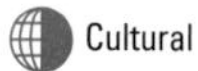

Fear [specify focus]

Taxonomy II: Coping/Stress Tolerance—Class 2 Coping Responses (00148) [**Diagnostic Division:** Ego Integrity], Submitted 1980; Revised 1996, 2000

DEFINITION: Response to perceived threat that is consciously recognized as a danger.

RELATED FACTORS

Innate response to stimuli (e.g., sudden noise, height); innate releasing mechanism to external stimuli (e.g., neurotransmitters); phobic stimulus
Learned response [e.g., conditioning, modeling from others]
Unfamiliar setting
Separation from support system
Language barrier, sensory deficit (e.g., visual, hearing)

DEFINING CHARACTERISTICS

Subjective

Apprehensiveness; excitedness; decrease in self-assurance; increase in tension; jitteriness; nausea
Cognitive: Identifies object of fear; stimulus believed to be a threat
Physiological: Anorexia; fatigue; dry mouth; dyspnea; [palpitations]

Objective

Vomiting; muscle tension; pallor; increase in blood pressure; pupil dilation
Cognitive: Decrease in productivity, learning ability, or problem-solving ability
Behaviors: Increase in alertness; avoidance [or flight] behaviors; attack behaviors; impulsiveness; focus narrowed to the source of fear
Physiological: Increased pulse; diarrhea; increase in respiratory rate; change in physiological response (e.g., blood pressure, heart rate, respiratory rate, oxygen saturation and end-tidal CO_2); increase in perspiration
Sample Clinical Applications: Phobias, hospitalization/diagnostic procedures, diagnosis of chronic or life-threatening condition

DESIRED OUTCOMES/EVALUATION CRITERIA

Sample NOC linkages:

Fear Self-Control: Personal actions to eliminate or reduce disabling feelings of apprehension, tension, or uneasiness from an identifiable source
Coping: Personal actions to manage stressors that tax an individual's resources
Fear Level: Severity of manifested apprehension, tension, or uneasiness arising from an identifiable source

Client Will (Include Specific Time Frame)

- Acknowledge and discuss fears, recognizing healthy versus unhealthy fears.
- Verbalize accurate knowledge of and sense of safety related to current situation.
- Demonstrate understanding through use of effective coping behaviors (e.g., problem solving) and resources.
- Display lessened fear as evidenced by appropriate range of feelings and relief of signs/symptoms (specific to client).

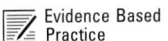

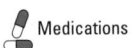

(continues on page 324)

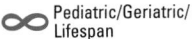

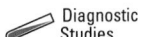

Fear (continued)
ACTIONS/INTERVENTIONS

Sample NIC linkages:
Anxiety Reduction: Minimizing apprehension, dread, foreboding, or uneasiness related to an unidentified source or anticipated danger
Security Enhancement: Intensifying a patient's sense of physical and psychological safety
Coping Enhancement: Assisting a patient to adapt to perceived stressors, changes, or threats that interfere with meeting life demands and roles

NURSING PRIORITY NO. 1 To assess degree of fear and reality of threat perceived by the client:

- Ascertain client's/significant other's (SO's) perception of what is occurring and how this affects life. *Fear is a natural reaction to frightening events, and how client views the event will determine how he or she will react. Fear differs from anxiety in that it is usually unanticipated, is dependent upon the termination of the feared object/subject, is often intense, and occurs in self-limiting episodes. Health fears may not be the "fight or flight" type, but present more like dread and anxiety.*[1,3,9]
- ∞ Determine client's age and developmental level. *Helps in understanding usual or typical fears experienced by individuals (e.g., toddler has entirely different fears than adolescent or older person with dementia being removed from home/usual living situation).*[3,11]
- Note ability to concentrate, level of attention, and degree of incapacitation (e.g., "frozen with fear," inability to engage in necessary activities). *Indicative of extent of anxiety or fear related to what is happening and need for specific interventions to reduce physiological reactions. Presence of severe reaction (panic or phobias) requires more intensive intervention.*[1,4,10]
- Compare verbal and nonverbal responses. *Noting congruencies or incongruencies can help to identify client's misperceptions of situation and what actions may be helpful. Client may be able to verbalize what he/she is afraid of, if asked, providing opportunity to address actual fears.*[1,3]
- Be alert to signs of denial or depression. *Client may deny existence of problem until overwhelmed and unable to deal with situation. Depression may be associated with fear that interferes with productive life and daily activities.*[2]
- Identify sensory deficits that may be present, such as vision or hearing impairment. *Affects reception and interpretation. Inability to correctly sense and perceive stimuli leads to misunderstanding, increasing fear.*[4]
- Measure vital signs and note physiological responses to situation. *Provides baseline information of extent of response for comparison as needed. Stabilization can indicate effectiveness of interventions by diminished response to identified fear. Note: Fear and acute anxiety can both involve sympathetic arousal (e.g., increased heart rate, respirations, and blood pressure, hyperalertness, antidiuresis, dilation of skeletal blood vessels, constriction of gut blood vessels and a surge of catecholamine release). These responses can be blunted (e.g., heart rate may not be increased if client is taking certain beta-blocking medications) and should subside as the fear state is reduced.*[6,10]
- Investigate client's reports of subjective experiences (may reflect delusions or hallucinations). *It is important to understand how the client views the situation and identify need for reality orientation and further evaluation.*[4]
- Be alert to and evaluate potential for violence. *Client who is fearful may feel need to protect himself or herself and strike out at closest person. Proactive planning can avert or manage violent behaviors.*[5]
- Assess family dynamics. *Actions and responses of family members may exacerbate or soothe fears of client; conversely, if the client is immersed in illness, whether from crisis or fear, it can take a toll on the family/involved others.*[1,11] (Refer to NDs Anxiety, readiness for enhanced family Coping, compromised/disabled family Coping, and interrupted Family Processes for additional interventions.)

NURSING PRIORITY NO. 2 To assist client/SOs in dealing with fear/situation ✚:

- Stay with the very fearful client or make arrangements to have someone else be there. *Provides nonthreatening environment in which the presence of a calm, caring person can provide reassurance that individual will be safe. Sense of abandonment can exacerbate fear.*[6]

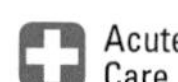
Acute Care
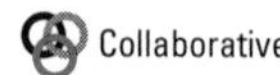
Collaborative
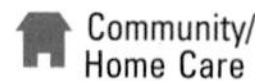
Community/Home Care
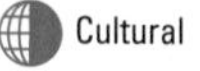
Cultural

- Active-listen client concerns. *Conveys message of belief in competence and ability of client. Promotes understanding of issues when client feels listened to so that problem solving can begin.*[2]
- Acknowledge normalcy of fear, pain, and despair and give "permission" to express feelings appropriately and freely. *Feelings are real, and it is helpful to bring them out in the open so they can be discussed and dealt with.*[6]
- Present objective information when available and allow client to use it freely. Avoid arguing about client's perceptions of the situation. *Limits conflicts when fear response may impair rational thinking.*[6]
- Speak in simple sentences and concrete terms and include written materials as appropriate. *Intense state of fear interferes with reception and interpretation of verbal information; supplementing it with written information facilitates understanding and retention of information.*[4]
- Provide opportunity for questions, answering honestly. *Enhances sense of trust and promotes positive nurse-client relationship in which individual can verbalize fears and begin to problem solve.*[1]
- ∞ Manage environmental factors, such as loud noises, harsh lighting, changing person's location without knowledge of family/SO, strangers in care area or unfamiliar people, and high traffic flow, *which can cause or exacerbate stress, especially to very young or to older individuals.*
- ∞ Be truthful with client when painful procedures are anticipated; be present and provide physical contact (e.g., hugging, refocusing attention, rocking a child) as appropriate, *to soothe fears and provide assurance.*
- Modify procedures as possible (e.g., substitute oral for intramuscular medications, combine blood draws or use finger-stick method) *to limit degree of stress and avoid overwhelming a fearful individual.*[3]
- Promote client control where possible and help client identify and accept those things over which control is not possible. *Life changes and stressful events are viewed differently by each individual. Providing the client with opportunity to make own decision when possible strengthens internal locus of control. Individual with external locus of control may attribute feelings of anxiety and fear to an external source and may perceive it as beyond his or her control.*[1]
- Provide touch, therapeutic touch, massage, and other adjunctive therapies as indicated. *Aids in meeting basic human need, decreasing sense of isolation, and assisting client to feel less anxious. Note: Therapeutic touch requires the nurse to have specific knowledge and experience to use the hands to correct energy field disturbances by redirecting human energies to help or heal.*[2,7]
- Encourage contact with a peer who has successfully dealt with a similarly fearful situation. *Provides a role model, which can enhance sense of optimism. Client is more likely to believe others who have had similar experience(s).*[1]

NURSING PRIORITY NO. 3 To assist client in learning to use own responses for problem solving:

- Acknowledge usefulness of fear for taking care of self. *Provides new idea that can be a motivator to focus on dealing appropriately with situation.*[1]
- Explain relationship between disease and symptoms if appropriate. *Providing accurate information promotes understanding of why the symptoms occur, allaying anxiety about them.*[1]
- Identify client's responsibility for the solutions while reinforcing that the nurse will be available for help if desired or needed. *Enhances sense of control, self-worth, and confidence in own ability, diminishing fear.*[8]
- Determine internal and external resources for assistance (e.g., awareness and use of effective coping skills in the past; SOs who are available for support). *Provides opportunity to recognize and build on resources client/SO may have used successfully in the past.*[1]
- Explain actions and procedures within level of client's ability to understand and handle being aware of how much information client wants *to prevent confusion or overload. Complex and/or anxiety-producing information can be given in manageable amounts over an extended period as opportunities arise and facts are given; individual will accept what he or she is ready for.*[8]
- Discuss use of anti-anxiety medications and reinforce use as prescribed. *Anti-anxiety agents may be useful for brief periods to assist client to reduce fearful feelings to manageable levels, providing opportunity for initiation of client's own coping skills.*[1]

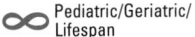

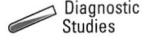

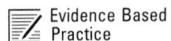

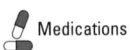

NURSING PRIORITY NO. 4 To promote wellness (Teaching/Discharge Considerations):

- Support planning for dealing with reality. *Assists in identifying areas in which control can be exercised and those in which control is not possible, enabling client to handle fearful situation or feelings.*[1]
- Assist client to learn relaxation, visualization, or guided imagery skills (e.g., imagining a pleasant place, use of music or tapes, deep breathing, meditation, mindfulness). *Promotes release of endorphins and aids in developing internal locus of control, reducing fear and anxious feelings. May enhance coping skills, allowing body to go about its work of healing. Note: Mindfulness is a method of being in the here and now, concentrating on what is happening in the moment.*[7,8]
- Encourage regular physical activity. Assist client or refer to physical therapist to develop exercise program within limits of ability. *Provides a healthy outlet for energy generated by feelings and promotes relaxation. Has been shown to raise endorphin levels to enhance sense of well-being.*[2]
- Provide for and deal with sensory deficits in appropriate manner (e.g., speak clearly and distinctly, use touch carefully as indicated by situation). *Hearing or visual impairments and other deficits can contribute to feelings of fear. Recognizing and providing for appropriate contact can enhance communication, promoting understanding.*[4]
- Refer to pastoral care, mental healthcare providers, support groups, and community agencies and organizations as indicated. *Provides information, ongoing assistance to meet individual needs, and opportunity for discussing concerns and obtaining further care when indicated.*[2]

DOCUMENTATION FOCUS

Assessment/Reassessment

- Assessment findings, noting individual factors contributing to current situation, and source of fear.
- Manifestations of fear and impact on life and ability to function.

Planning

- Plan of care and who is involved in the planning.
- Teaching plan.

Implementation/Evaluation

- Client's responses to treatment plan, interventions, and actions performed.
- Attainment or progress toward desired outcome(s).
- Modifications to plan of care.

Discharge Planning

- Long-term needs and who is responsible for actions to be taken.
- Specific referrals made.

References

1. Townsend, M. C. (2011). *Psychiatric Mental Health Nursing: Concepts of Care in Evidence-Based Practice*. 7th ed. Philadelphia: F. A. Davis.
2. Doenges, M. E., Moorhouse, M. F., Murr, A. C. (2010). *Nurse's Pocket Guide: Diagnoses, Interventions, and Rationales*. 12th ed. Philadelphia: F. A. Davis.
3. Lawrence, S. (2005). When health fears are overblown. Retrieved October 2015 from http://www.webmd.com/balance/features/when-health-fears-are-overblown.
4. Newfield, S. A., Hinz, M. D., Tilley, D. S., et al. (2007). *Cox's Clinical Applications of Nursing Diagnosis: Adult, Child, Women's, Psychiatric, Gerontic, and Home Health Considerations*. 5th ed. Philadelphia: F. A. Davis.
5. Lewis, M. I., Dehn, D. S. (1999). Violence against nurses in outpatient mental health settings. *J Psychosoc Nurs*, 37(6), 28.
6. Bay, E. J., Algase, D. L. (1999). Fear and anxiety. A simultaneous concept analysis. *Nurs Diagn*, 10, 103.

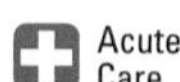
Acute Care
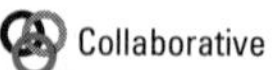
Collaborative
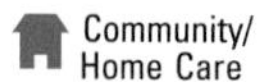
Community/ Home Care
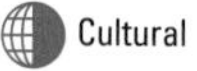
Cultural

7. Olson, M., Sneed, N. (1995). Anxiety and therapeutic touch. *Issues Ment Health Nurs*, 16(2), 97.
8. Kabat-Zinn, J. (1994). *Wherever You Go There You Are, Mindfulness Meditation in Everyday Life*. New York: Hyperion.
9. Kidd, M. (2007). What do patients fear most? Retrieved October 2015 from http://www.medscape.com/view/article/561455.
10. Craig, K. J., Brown, K. J., Baum, A. (2002). Environmental factors in the etiology of anxiety. *In Neuropsychopharmacology: The Fifth Generation of Progress*. Philadelphia: Lippincott, Williams and Wilkins.
11. Charmaz, K. (1983). Loss of self: A fundamental form of suffering in the chronically ill. *Sociol Health Illness*, 5(2), 168–195.

ineffective infant Feeding Pattern

Taxonomy II: Nutrition—Class 1 Ingestion (00107) [**Diagnostic Division:** Food/Fluid], Submitted 1992; Revised 2006

DEFINITION: Impaired ability of an infant to suck or coordinate the suck/swallow response resulting in inadequate oral nutrition for metabolic needs.

RELATED FACTORS

Prematurity
Neurological delay or impairment (e.g., positive EEG, head trauma, seizure disorder)
Oral hypersensitivity
Prolonged nil per os (NPO) status [aka nothing by mouth]
Otopharyngeal defect

DEFINING CHARACTERISTICS

Subjective

[Caregiver reports infant unable to achieve effective suck]

Objective

Inability to initiate or sustain an effective suck
Inability to coordinate sucking, swallowing, and breathing
Sample Clinical Applications: Prematurity, cleft lip/palate, thrush, hydrocephalus, cerebral palsy, fetal alcohol syndrome, respiratory distress, severe developmental delay

DESIRED OUTCOMES/EVALUATION CRITERIA

Sample NOC linkages:

Swallowing Status: Oral Phase: Preparation, containment, and posterior movement of fluids and/or solids in the mouth
Breastfeeding Establishment: Infant: Infant attachment to and sucking from the mother's breast for nourishment during the first 3 weeks of breastfeeding
Hydration: Adequate water in the intracellular and extracellular compartments of the body

Infant Will (Include Specific Time Frame)

- Display adequate output as measured by sufficient number of wet diapers daily.
- Demonstrate appropriate weight gain.
- Be free of aspiration.

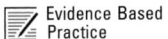

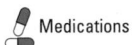

(continues on page 328)

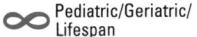

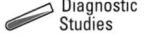

ineffective infant Feeding Pattern (continued)
ACTIONS/INTERVENTIONS

Sample NIC linkages:
Swallowing Therapy: Facilitating swallowing and preventing complications of impaired swallowing
Lactation Counseling: Use of an interactive helping process to assist in maintenance of successful breastfeeding
Bottle Feeding: Preparation and administration of fluids to an infant via a bottle

NURSING PRIORITY NO. 1 To identify contributing factors/degree of impaired function:

- Assess infant's suck, swallow, and gag reflexes. *Provides comparative baseline and useful in determining appropriate feeding method.*
- Note developmental age, structural abnormalities (e.g., cleft lip/palate), mechanical barriers (e.g., endotracheal tube, ventilator). *These factors (infant maturity and structural/mechanical barriers to infant feeding) help to determine plan of care. Note: Human milk decreases infections in preterm infants, both during hospitalization and after discharge. Human milk is the feeding of choice.*[1,2,4,6]
- Determine level of consciousness, neurological impairment, seizure activity, and presence of pain. *Provides baseline information and identifies areas of special need.*[1,2]
- Observe parent/infant interactions *to determine level of bonding and comfort that could impact stress level during feeding activity.*
- Note type and scheduling of medications. *May cause sedative effect or otherwise impair feeding activity.*[2]
- Compare birth and current weight and length measurements. *Monitors effectiveness of infant feeding technique.*[1,2,4]
- Assess signs of stress when feeding (e.g., tachypnea, cyanosis, fatigue, lethargy). *Detects areas of increased need for alternate feeding methods and/or rest periods.*[1]
- Note presence of behaviors indicating continued hunger after feeding. *Determines if infant is receiving adequate amount during feeding.*[2,4]

NURSING PRIORITY NO. 2 To promote adequate infant intake:

- Determine appropriate method for feeding (e.g., special nipple or feeding device, gavage or enteral tube feeding) and choice of breast milk or formula to meet infant needs. *Individualizes care and maintains infant health status.*[1]
- Review early infant feeding cues (e.g., rooting, lip smacking, sucking fingers or hand) versus late cue of crying with parents/caregivers. *Early recognition of infant hunger promotes timely and more rewarding feeding experience for infant and mother.*[5]
- Demonstrate techniques or procedures for feeding. Note proper positioning of infant, "latching-on" techniques, rate of delivery of feeding, and frequency of burping. (Refer to ND ineffective Breastfeeding as appropriate.) *Models appropriate feeding methods and increases parental knowledge base and confidence.*[2–4]
- Limit duration of feeding to maximum of 30 minutes based on infant's response (e.g., signs of fatigue) *to balance energy expenditure with nutrient intake.*
- Monitor caregiver's efforts. Provide feedback and assistance as indicated. *Enhances learning and encourages continuation of efforts.*[2,3]
- Refer mother to lactation specialist for assistance and support in dealing with unresolved issues (e.g., teaching infant to suck or a decrease in the mother's milk supply). *Provides resource for future needs and problem solving. Begins pattern of resource utilization.*[2–4]
- Emphasize importance of calm/relaxed environment during feeding *to reduce detrimental stimuli and enhance mother/infant's focus on feeding activity.*
- Adjust frequency and amount of feeding according to infant's response. *Prevents infant's frustration associated with under/overfeeding.*

Acute Care
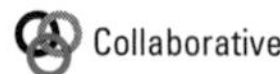
Collaborative
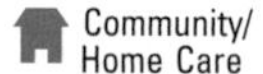
Community/ Home Care
 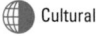
Cultural

- Advance diet, adding solids or thickening agent as appropriate for age and infant needs. *Provides for infant's nutritional and health needs.*[2,4]
- Alternate feeding techniques (e.g., nipple and gavage) according to infant's ability and level of fatigue. *Individualizes plan of care to enhance successful feeding.*[1]
- Alter medication or feeding schedules as indicated to minimize sedative effects. *Altered states of function and consciousness interfere with feeding and may lead to choking or aspirating.*[1]

NURSING PRIORITY NO. 3 To promote well-being (Teaching/Discharge Considerations):

- Encourage kangaroo care, placing infant skin-to-skin upright, tummy down, on mother's or father's chest. *Skin-to-skin care increases bonding and may promote stable heart rate, temperature, and respiration in infant.*[7]
- Instruct caregiver in techniques to prevent or alleviate aspiration. *Helps parent/caregiver feel more confident and promotes infant safety.*[1,4]
- Discuss anticipated growth and development goals for infant, as well as corresponding caloric needs. *Accommodating infant maturity and development help to individualize and update plan of care.*[1,2,5]
- Suggest recording infant's weight and nutrient intake periodically. *Monitors effectiveness of infant feeding technique by providing measurable data. Provides positive reinforcement to implementation of plan of care.*[1,2,4]
- Recommend participation in classes as indicated (e.g., first aid, infant cardiopulmonary resuscitation). *Increases knowledge base for infant safety and caregiver confidence.*[2–4]
- Refer to support groups (e.g., La Leche League, parenting support groups, stress reduction, other community resources as indicated).
- Provide bibliotherapy including appropriate Web sites for further information.

DOCUMENTATION FOCUS

Assessment/Reassessment

- Type and route of feeding, interferences to feeding and reactions.
- Infant's measurements.

Planning

- Plan of care, specific interventions, and who is involved in planning.
- Teaching plan.

Implementation/Evaluation

- Infant's response to interventions (e.g., amount of intake and output, weight gain, response to feeding) and actions performed.
- Caregiver's involvement in infant care, participation in activities, and response to teaching.
- Attainment or progress toward desired outcome(s).
- Modifications to plan of care.

Discharge Planning

- Long-term needs, referrals made, and who is responsible for follow-up actions.

References

1. Creasy, R., Resnik, R., Iams, J. D., et al. (2008). *Maternal-Fetal Medicine: Principles and Practice.* 6th ed. Philadelphia: W. B. Saunders.
2. London, M., Ladewig, P. W., Ball, J. W., et al. (2010). *Maternal & Child Nursing Care.* 3rd ed. Upper Saddle River, NJ: Prentice Hall.
3. Ladewig, P., London, M., Davidson, M., et al. (2009). *Contemporary Maternal-Newborn Nursing Care.* 7th ed. Upper Saddle River, NJ: Prentice Hall.
4. Lowdermilk, D., Cashion, M. C., Perry, S. (2011). *Maternity and Women's Health Care.* 10th ed. St. Louis, MO: Mosby.

5. American Academy of Family Physicians. Breastfeeding (Position paper). Retrieved October 2015 from www.aafp.org/online/en/home/policy/policies/b/breastfeedingpositionpaper.html.
6. Wright, N., Morton, J., Kim, J. (2008). *Best Medicine: Human Milk in the NICU*. Amarillo, TX: Hale.
7. Bergman, J. (2011). The importance of skin-to-skin contact for every newborn. *Breastfeeding Today*(6), 4–6.

readiness for enhanced Fluid Balance

Taxonomy II: Nutrition—Class 5 Hydration (00160) [**Diagnostic Division:** Food/Fluid], Submitted 2002; Revised 2013

DEFINITION: A pattern of equilibrium between fluid volume and chemical composition of body fluids, which can be strengthened.

DEFINING CHARACTERISTICS

Subjective

Expresses desire to enhance fluid balance

Sample Clinical Applications: Heart or renal failure, irritable bowel syndrome, Addison's disease, enteral or parenteral feeding

DESIRED OUTCOME/EVALUATION CRITERIA

Sample NOC linkages:

Hydration: Adequate water in the intracellular and extracellular compartments of the body

Fluid Balance: Water balance in the intracellular and extracellular compartments of the body

Risk Control: Personal actions to prevent, eliminate, or reduce modifiable health threats

Client Will (Include Specific Time Frame)

- Maintain fluid volume at a functional level as indicated by adequate urinary output, stable vital signs, moist mucous membranes, and good skin turgor.
- Demonstrate behaviors to monitor fluid balance.
- Be free of thirst.
- Be free of evidence of fluid deficit or fluid overload.

ACTIONS/INTERVENTIONS

Sample NIC linkages:

Fluid Management: Promotion of fluid balance and prevention of complications resulting from abnormal or undesired fluid levels

Fluid Monitoring: Collection and analysis of patient data to regulate fluid balance

Surveillance: Purposeful and ongoing acquisition, interpretation, and synthesis of patient data for clinical decision making

NURSING PRIORITY NO. 1 To assess potential for fluid imbalance and ways that client is managing:

- Note presence of factors with potential for fluid imbalance: (1) diagnoses or disease processes (e.g., hyperglycemia, ulcerative colitis, COPD, burns, cirrhosis of the liver, vomiting, diarrhea, hemorrhage) or situations (e.g., diuretic therapy; hot/humid climate, prolonged exercise, heat exhaustion; fever; diuretic effect of caffeine or alcohol) that may lead to deficits or (2) conditions or situations potentiating fluid excess (e.g., renal failure, cardiac failure, stroke, cerebral lesions, renal or adrenal insufficiency, psychogenic polydipsia, acute stress, anesthesia, surgical procedures, excessive or rapid infusion of IV fluids). *Body fluid balance is regulated by intake (food and fluid), output (kidney, gastrointestinal tract, skin, lungs), and regulatory hormonal mechanisms. Balance is maintained within a relatively narrow margin and can be easily disrupted by multiple factors.*[4]

- ∞ Determine potential effects of age and developmental stage. *Elderly individuals have less body water than younger adults, decreased thirst response, reduced effectiveness of compensatory mechanisms (e.g., kidneys are less efficient in conserving sodium and water), and potential for functional and environmental issues that affect their ability to manage fluid intake. Infants and children have a relatively higher percentage of total body water and metabolic rate and are often less able than adults to control their fluid intake.*[1,2,5]
- Evaluate factors that could impact client's ability to manage fluid balance. *Persons with impaired mobility, diminished vision, or who are confined to bed cannot as easily meet their own needs and may be reluctant to ask for assistance. Persons whose work environment is restrictive or outside may also have greater challenges in meeting fluid needs.*[3]
- Assess vital signs (e.g., temperature, blood pressure, heart rate), skin and mucous membrane moisture, and urine output. Weigh as indicated. *Predictors of fluid balance that should be in client's usual range in a healthy state.*[4]
- Ascertain motivation and expectations for ability to manage. *Motivation to improve and high expectations can encourage client to make changes that will improve his or her life. However, unrealistic expectations may hamper efforts.*

NURSING PRIORITY NO. 2 To prevent occurrence of imbalance:

- Monitor intake and output (I&O; e.g., frequency of voids or diaper changes) as appropriate, being aware of insensible losses (e.g., diaphoresis in hot environment, use of oxygen or permanent tracheostomy) and "hidden sources" of intake (e.g., foods high in water content), *to ensure accurate picture of fluid status.*[4]
- Weigh client regularly and compare with recent weight history. *Useful in early recognition of water retention or unexplained losses.*[1,4]
- ∞ Establish or review individual fluid needs and replacement schedule with client. Make sure client has access to fluids at all times. Teach elderly person to drink when not thirsty and to drink small amounts frequently rather than large amounts infrequently. *Enhances likelihood of meeting therapeutic goals. Note: Thirst declines with aging, but hydration needs do not.*[1,7]
- Encourage regular oral intake of fluids (e.g., between meals, additional fluids during hot weather or when exercising) interspersed with foods with a high fluid content (e.g., soup, popsicles, fruits, yogurt) of client's choice. *Adds variety to maximize intake while maintaining fluid balance.*[1]
- Provide adequate free water with enteral feedings.
- Discuss judicious use of medications as indicated (e.g., antiemetics, antidiarrheals, antipyretics, diuretics). *Medications may be indicated to prevent fluid imbalance if individual becomes ill.*[1]

NURSING PRIORITY NO. 3 To promote optimum wellness (Teaching/Discharge Considerations):

- Discuss client's individual conditions/factors that could cause occurrence of fluid imbalance as appropriate, paying special attention to environmental factors such as hot/humid climate, lack of air conditioning, and outdoor work setting *so that client/significant other (SO) can take corrective action and modify risks.*[1,3,6]
- Identify and instruct in ways to meet specific fluid needs (e.g., keep fluids near at hand, carry water bottle when leaving home, measure specific 24-hr fluid portions if restrictions apply) *to manage fluid intake over time.*[1,3]
- Instruct client/SO(s) in how to measure and record I&O, including weighing diapers or continence pads when used, *if these data are needed for home management.*
- Establish a regular schedule for weighing *to help monitor changes in fluid status.*
- Identify actions (if any) client may take to correct imbalance (e.g., limiting salt or caffeine intake, as needed use of diuretics, tight control of blood sugar).

- Review and instruct in medication regimen and administration and discuss potential for interactions or side effects that could disrupt fluid balance.[1,4,5]
- Instruct in signs and symptoms indicating need for immediate or further evaluation and follow-up to prevent complications and/or allow for timely intervention.[1,4,5]

DOCUMENTATION FOCUS

Assessment/Reassessment

- Individual findings, including factors affecting ability to manage (regulate) body fluids.
- I&O, fluid balance, changes in weight, and vital signs.
- Results of diagnostic studies and laboratory tests.
- Motivation and expectations for change.

Planning

- Plan of care and who is involved in the planning.
- Teaching plan.

Implementation/Evaluation

- Client's responses to treatment, teaching, and actions performed.
- Attainment or progress toward desired outcome(s).
- Modifications to plan of care.

Discharge Planning

- Long-term needs, noting who is responsible for actions to be taken.
- Specific referrals made.

References

1. Newfield, S. A., Hinz, M. D., Tilley, D. S., et al. (2007). *Cox's Clinical Applications of Nursing Diagnosis: Adult, Child, Women's, Psychiatric, Gerontic, and Home Health Considerations*. 5th ed. Philadelphia: F. A. Davis.
2. Miller-Huey, R. (1995–2013). Hydration in elders: More than just a glass of water. Today's Caregiver. Retrieved March 2015 from www.caregiver.com/articles/general/hydration_in_elders.htm.
3. Curtis, R. (2015). Outdoor action guide to heat and cold injuries. National Ag Safety Database. Retrieved March 2015 from http://www.princeton.edu/~oa/safety/hypocold.shtm.
4. Metheny, N. (2010). *Fluid and Electrolyte Balance: Nursing Considerations*. 5th ed. Sudbury, MA: Jones & Bartlett Learning.
5. Engle, J. (2006). *Pocket Guide to Pediatric Assessment*. 5th ed. St. Louis, MO: Mosby.
6. Bennett, J. A. (2000). Dehydration: Hazards and benefits. *Geriatr Nurs*, 21(2), 84–88.
7. Ferry, M. (2005). Strategies for ensuring good hydration in the elderly. *Nutr Rev*, 63(Suppl), s22–s29.

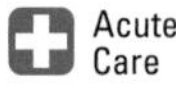

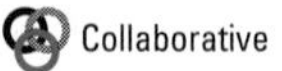

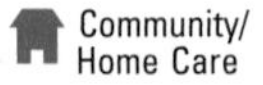

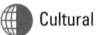

[deficient hyper/hypotonic Fluid Volume]

DEFINITION: [Decreased intravascular, interstitial, and/or intracellular fluid. This refers to dehydration with changes in sodium.]

[**NOTE:** NANDA has restricted deficient Fluid Volume to address only isotonic dehydration. For client needs related to dehydration associated with alterations in sodium, the authors have provided this second diagnostic label.]

RELATED FACTORS

[Hypertonic dehydration: uncontrolled diabetes mellitus or insipidus, hyperosmolar hyperglycemic syndrome (HHS), increased intake of hypertonic fluids or IV therapy, inability to respond to thirst reflex, inadequate free water supplementation (high-osmolarity enteral feeding formulas), renal insufficiency or failure]

[Hypotonic dehydration: chronic illness, malnutrition, excessive use of hypotonic IV solutions (e.g., D5W), renal insufficiency]

DEFINING CHARACTERISTICS

Subjective

[Reports of fatigue, nervousness, exhaustion]

[Thirst]

Objective

[Increased urine output, dilute urine (initially), or decreased output, oliguria]

[Weight loss]

[Decreased venous filling; hypotension (postural)]

[Increased pulse rate; decreased pulse volume and pressure]

[Decreased skin turgor; dry skin and mucous membranes]

[Increased body temperature]

[Change in mental status (e.g., confusion)]

[Hemoconcentration; altered serum sodium]

Sample Clinical Applications: Diabetes mellitus, diabetic ketoacidosis, renal failure, conditions requiring IV therapy or enteral feeding, heat exhaustion or stroke, presence of draining wounds or fistulas

DESIRED OUTCOMES/EVALUATION CRITERIA

Sample NOC linkages:

Fluid Balance: Water balance in the intracellular and extracellular compartments of the body

Hydration: Adequate water in the intracellular and extracellular compartments of the body

Electrolyte and Acid/Base Balance: Balance of electrolytes and nonelectrolytes in the intracellular and extracellular compartments of the body

Client Will (include Specific Time Frame)

- Maintain fluid volume at a functional level as evidenced by individually adequate urinary output, stable vital signs, moist mucous membranes, and good skin turgor.
- Verbalize understanding of causative factors and purpose of individual therapeutic interventions and medications.
- Demonstrate behaviors to monitor and correct deficit as indicated when condition is chronic.

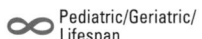

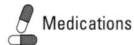

(continues on page 334)

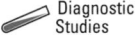

[deficient hyper/hypotonic Fluid Volume] (continued)
ACTIONS/INTERVENTIONS

Sample NIC linkages:
Fluid/Electrolyte Management: Regulation and prevention of complications from altered fluid and/or electrolyte levels
Hypovolemia Management: Expansion of intravascular fluid volume in a patient who is volume depleted
Fluid Monitoring: Collection and analysis of patient data to regulate fluid balance

NURSING PRIORITY NO. 1 To assess causative/precipitating factors:

- Note possible medical diagnoses or disease processes *that may lead to fluid deficits: (1) fluid loss (e.g., indwelling tubes, diarrhea, vomiting, fever, excessive sweating, diabetic ketoacidosis; burns, other draining wounds; gastrointestinal obstruction; use of diuretics); (2) limited intake (e.g., extremes of age, limited mobility, client dependent on others for eating and drinking; lack of knowledge related to fluid intake; heat exhaustion or stroke); (3) fluid shifts (e.g., ascites, effusions, burns, sepsis); or (4) environmental factors (e.g., isolation, restraints, very high ambient temperatures, malfunctioning air conditioning).*[5,14,15]
- Determine effects of age and gender. Obtain weight and measure subcutaneous fat and muscle mass *to ascertain total body water, which is approximately 60% of adult's weight and 75% of infant's weight. Very young and extremely elderly individuals are quickly affected by a fluid volume deficit and are least able to express need. For example, elderly people often have a decreased thirst reflex and/or may not be aware of water needs. Infants/young children and other nonverbal persons cannot describe thirst.*[1,2,15,16] *Worldwide, dehydration (secondary to diarrheal illness) is the leading cause of infant and child mortality.*[3,8]
- Evaluate nutritional status, noting current intake, weight changes, problems with oral intake, and use of supplements/tube feedings. *Factors that can negatively affect fluid intake (e.g., impaired mentation, nausea, wired jaws, immobility, insufficient time for meals, lack of finances restricting availability of food).*
- Collaborate with physician to identify or characterize the nature of fluid and electrolyte imbalance(s). *Dehydration is often categorized according to serum sodium concentration. Isonatremic (i.e., isotonic) dehydration is the most common type of dehydration. However, hypernatremic (also called "hypertonic dehydration" when relatively less sodium than water is lost) and hyponatremic (or "hypotonic dehydration" when relatively less water than sodium is lost) can both cause neurological complications and thus may be more dangerous.*[3,16] *More than one cause may exist at a given time (e.g., increased loss of salt and water caused by diuretics that leads to decreased fluid intake as a result of lethargy and confusion).*[5,9,10]
- Be aware of the difference between signs of **hypovolemia** (e.g., poor skin turgor, dizziness on standing, lethargy, delayed capillary refill, sunken eyeballs, fever, weight loss, little or no urine output) and signs of **dehydration** (e.g., lethargy, weakness, irritability, nausea, vomiting, hyperreflexia, potentially progressing to coma), *which are symptoms of the effect of elevated sodium (hypernatremia) on the central nervous system. Note: Dehydration is not always accompanied by hypovolemia, but it is almost always hypernatremic.*[8,10]
- Review client's medications, including prescription, over-the-counter drugs, herbals, and nutritional supplements, *to identify medications that can alter fluid and electrolyte balance. These may include diuretics, vasodilators, beta-blockers, aldosterone inhibitors, angiotensin-converting enzyme (ACE) inhibitors, and medications that can cause syndrome of inappropriate secretion of antidiuretic hormone (e.g., phenothiazides, vasopressin, some antineoplastic drugs).*[12]

NURSING PRIORITY NO. 2 To evaluate degree of fluid deficit:

- Obtain history of usual pattern of fluid intake and recent alterations. *Intake may be reduced because of current physical or environmental issues (e.g., swallowing problems, vomiting, severe heat wave with inadequate fluid replacement) or a behavior pattern (e.g., elderly person refuses to drink water trying to control incontinence).*

Acute Care
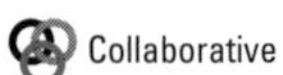
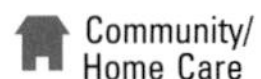
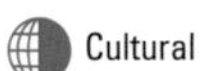

- Assess vital signs, including temperature (often elevated), pulse (elevated), respirations, and blood pressure (may be low). Measure blood pressure (lying, sitting, standing) *to evaluate orthostatic blood pressure* and monitor invasive hemodynamic parameters as indicated (e.g., central venous pressure) *to determine degree of intravascular deficit and replacement needs.*[7,8]
- Note change in usual mentation, behavior, and functional abilities (e.g., confusion, falling, loss of ability to carry out usual activities, lethargy, dizziness). *These signs indicate either sufficient hypovolemia to impair cerebral perfusion or sufficient dehydration to impair cerebral function.*[9,10]
- Observe and measure urinary output hourly or for 24 hours as indicated. Note color *(may be dark because of concentration)* and specific gravity *(high number associated with dehydration with usual range being 1.010 to 1.025).*[4]
- Estimate or measure other fluid losses (e.g., gastric, respiratory, and wound losses) *to more accurately determine fluid replacement needs.*
- Review laboratory data (e.g., hemoglobin/hematocrit; osmolality, electrolytes [sodium, potassium, chloride, bicarbonate]; blood urea nitrogen, creatinine) *to evaluate body's response to fluid loss and to determine replacement needs. Note: The dehydrated client is not always hypovolemic. An abnormal sodium level is a key marker for salt and water imbalance. For example, in* ***hypertonic*** *dehydration, blood tests may reveal osmolality greater than 300 mOsm/kg and sodium greater than 150 meq/L. The hypernatremia is the* ***result*** *of dehydration.* ***Hypotonic*** *dehydration may reveal osmolality less than 250 mOsm/kg and sodium less than 130 meq/L. Hyponatremia is the* ***result*** *of replacing water without sodium.*[4,11,17]

NURSING PRIORITY NO. 3 To correct/replace fluid losses to reverse pathophysiological mechanisms:

- Assist with treatment of underlying conditions causing or contributing to dehydration and electrolyte imbalances (e.g., change antibiotics causing diarrhea; treat fever or infection, malnutrition, or severe depression; discontinue medications contributing to dehydration).
- Administer fluids and electrolytes as indicated. *Fluid used for replacement depends on the (1) type of dehydration present and (2) degree of deficit determined by age, weight, and type of trauma or condition causing the fluid deficit. Multiple fluid resuscitation formulas (e.g., Parkland, Evans, Brooke, Slater, Monafo burn formulas) exist with variations in both the volumes per weight suggested and the type or types of crystalloid or crystalloid-colloid combinations.*[2,6,9]
- Establish 24-hr replacement schedule and routes to be used (e.g., IV, PO, tube feeding). *Entire fluid replacement may be done by IV or tube feeding if client is NPO, acutely ill, or severely dehydrated. However, if client is to be rehydrated orally, fluid replacement may be calculated to replace certain amount with meals (e.g., 75% to 80%) with the remainder offered during nonmeal times. Steady rehydration rate reduces thirst, helps to balance electrolytes, and prevents peaks and valleys in fluid level. Managing oral rehydration in this manner can replace fluids without resorting to IV therapy. These interventions should also be in place to prevent dehydration.*[2,3,5,6,8]
- Spread fluid intake throughout the day *to prevent periods of uncomfortable thirst and to promote client's ability and interest in ingesting fluids.*
- Encourage increased intake of water and other fluids based on individual needs (up to 2.5 L/day or amount determined by physician for client's age, weight, and condition).
- Provide a variety of fluids in small frequent offerings, attempting to incorporate client's preferred beverage and temperature (e.g., iced or hot) *to enhance cooperation with regimen.*
- Suggest intake of foods with a high water content (e.g., popsicles, gelatin, soup, eggnog, watermelon) and/or electrolyte replacement drinks (e.g., Gatorade, Pedialyte) as appropriate. *Variety may stimulate intake.*
- Limit intake of alcohol and caffeinated beverages that tend to exert a diuretic effect.
- Engage client, family, and all caregivers in fluid management plan. *Everyone is responsible for the prevention or treatment of dehydration and should be involved in the planning and provision of adequate fluid on a daily basis.*
- Provide nutritionally balanced diet and/or enteral feedings (avoiding use of hyperosmolar or excessively high-protein formulas) and provide adequate amount of free water with feedings.

- Maintain accurate intake and output (I&O), calculate 24-hr fluid balance, and weigh regularly (daily, in unstable client) *in order to monitor and document trends. Note: A 1 pound weight loss reflects fluid loss of about 500 mL in an adult.*[7]

NURSING PRIORITY NO. 4 To promote comfort and safety:

- Change position frequently. Bathe infrequently, using mild cleanser or soap, and provide optimal skin care with suitable emollients *to maintain skin integrity and prevent excessive dryness caused by dehydration.*
- Provide frequent oral care and eye protection *to prevent injury from dryness.*
- Provide for safety measures when client is confused. (Refer to NDs acute Confusion and chronic Confusion for additional interventions.)
- Adjust or discontinue medications (e.g., diuretics, laxatives, steroids, psychotropics, ACE inhibitors) *that may be contributing to dehydration.*[2,5]
- Observe for sudden or marked elevation of blood pressure, restlessness, moist cough, dyspnea, basilar crackles, and frothy sputum. *Too rapid a correction of fluid deficit may compromise the cardiopulmonary system, causing fluid overload and edema, especially if colloids are used in initial fluid resuscitation.*

NURSING PRIORITY NO. 5 To promote wellness (Teaching/Discharge Considerations):

- Discuss factors related to occurrence of deficit as individually appropriate. *Early identification of risk factors can decrease occurrence and severity of complications associated with hypovolemia.*[7]
- Recommend drinking more water when exercising or engaging in physical exertion or during hot weather. Suggest carrying a water bottle when away from home as appropriate.
- Identify and instruct in ways to meet specific fluid and nutritional needs.
- Offer fluids on a regular basis to infants, young children, and the elderly, *who may not sense/or be able to report thirst.*
- Instruct client/SO(s) in how to monitor color of urine *(dark urine equates with concentration and dehydration)* and/or how to measure and record I&O *(may include weighing or counting diapers in infant/toddler)* as indicated.
- Review and instruct in medication regimen and administration. Emphasize need for reporting suspected drug interactions/side effects to healthcare provider. *Facilitates timely intervention to prevent or reduce complications.*
- Instruct in signs and symptoms indicating need for emergent or further evaluation and follow-up.

DOCUMENTATION FOCUS

Assessment/Reassessment

- Individual findings, including factors affecting ability to manage (regulate) body fluids and degree of deficit.
- I&O, fluid balance, changes in weight, urine-specific gravity, and vital signs.
- Results of diagnostic studies or laboratory tests.

Planning

- Plan of care and who is involved in the planning.
- Teaching plan.

Implementation/Evaluation

- Client's responses to treatment, teaching, and actions performed.
- Attainment or progress toward desired outcome(s).
- Modifications to plan of care.

Discharge Planning

- Long-term needs, noting who is responsible for actions to be taken.
- Specific referrals made.

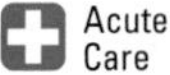

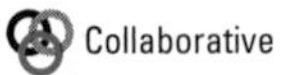

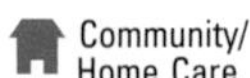

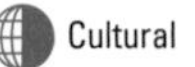

References

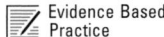

1. Newfield, S. A., Hinz, M. D., Tilley, D. S., et al. (2007). *Cox's Clinical Applications of Nursing Diagnosis: Adult, Child, Women's, Psychiatric, Gerontic, and Home Health Considerations*. 5th ed. Philadelphia: F. A. Davis.
2. Mentes, J. C. (2012). Managing oral hydration. In: Boltz, M., Capezuti, E., Fulmer, T. (Eds.). *Evidence-Based Practice Guideline Hydration Management*. 4th ed. New York: Springer.
3. Huang, L. H., Anchalla, K. P., Ellsbury, D. L., et al. (Updated 2014). Dehydration. Retrieved March 2015 from http://emedicine.medscape.com/article/906999-overview.
4. Cavanaugh, B. M. (2003). *Nurse's Manual of Laboratory and Diagnostic Tests*. 4th ed. Philadelphia: F. A. Davis.
5. American Medical Directors Association. (2009). Dehydration and fluid maintenance in the long-term care setting. Retrieved March 2015 from http://www.guideline.gov/content.aspx?id=15590.
6. Oliver, R. I. (2014). Burn resuscitation and early management. Retrieved March 2014 from http://emedicine.medscape.com/article/1277360-overview.
7. Matheny, N. (2010). *Fluid and Electrolyte Balance: Nursing Considerations*. 5th ed. Sudbury, MA: Jones & Bartlett.
8. Mayo Clinic Staff. (Updated 2014). Dehydration. Retrieved March 2015 from http://www.mayoclinic.org/diseases-conditions/dehydration/basics/definition/con-20030056.
9. Astle, S. M. (2005). Restoring electrolyte balance. *RN*, 68(5), 34–39.
10. Viele, C. S., Quin, A. M., Daly, C. F. (2006). Dehydration and electrolyte requirements in oncology care. Cancer Care Quarterly. Retrieved March 2015 from http://www.mediabistro.com/portfolios/samples_files/162412_5KaA4NawhyfT53_1903z44at_.pdf.
11. Holley, J. L. (2006). Hypovolemia and dehydration in the oncology patient—A viewpoint of salt and water imbalance. *J Support Oncol*(4), 455–456.
12. Wotton, K., Crannitch, K., Munt, R. (2008). Prevalence, risk factors and strategies to prevent dehydration in older adults. *Contemp Nurs*, 31(1), 44–56.
13. Mentes, J., Claros, E. (2006). Oral hydration in older adults. *Am J Nurs*, 106(6), 40–49.
14. Mentes, J. (2006). A typology of oral hydration problems exhibited by frail nursing home residents. *J Gerontol Nurs*, 23(1), 13–21.
15. Scholler, D. A. (1989). Changes in total body water with age. *Am J Clin Nutr*, 50(5suppl), 1176–1181.
16. Faes, M. C., Spigt, M. G., Rikkert, O. (2007). Dehydration in geriatrics. *Geriatrics and Aging*, 10(9), 590–596.
17. Modric, J. (2013). Dehydration types: Pathophysiology, lab tests and values. Retrieved March 2015 from http://www.ehealthstar.com/dehydration/types-pathophysiology.

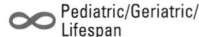

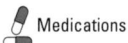

deficient [isotonic] Fluid Volume

Taxonomy II: Nutrition—Class 5 Hydration (00027) [**Diagnostic Division:** Food/Fluid], Submitted 1978; Revised 1996

DEFINITION: Decreased intravascular, interstitial, and/or intracellular fluid. This refers to dehydration, water loss alone without change in sodium.

[**NOTE:** This diagnosis has been structured to address isotonic dehydration (hypovolemia) when fluids and electrolytes are lost in even amounts and excluding states in which changes in sodium occur. For client needs related to dehydration associated with alterations in sodium, refer to deficient Fluid Volume: hyper/hypotonic.]

RELATED FACTORS

Active fluid volume loss [e.g., gastric intubation, acute or prolonged diarrhea; wounds; fistulas, ascites (third spacing), use of hyperosmotic radiopaque contrast agents]

Compromised regulatory mechanisms [e.g., fever, thermoregulatory response, renal tubule damage]

(continues on page 338)

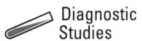

deficient [isotonic] Fluid Volume (continued)

DEFINING CHARACTERISTICS

Subjective

Thirst

Weakness

Objective

Alteration in mental status

Alteration in skin or tongue turgor; dry skin and mucous membranes

Decrease in blood pressure; decrease in pulse pressure and volume; decrease in venous filling

Decrease in urine output

Increase in body temperature and heart rate

Increase in hematocrit and urine concentration

Sudden weight loss

Sample Clinical Applications: Traumatic injury, hemorrhage, gastroenteritis (with vomiting and diarrhea), malnutrition, uncontrolled diabetes mellitus, severe burns

DESIRED OUTCOMES/EVALUATION CRITERIA

Sample NOC linkages:

Hydration: Adequate water in the intracellular and extracellular compartments of the body

Fluid Balance: Water balance in the intracellular and extracellular compartments of the body

Blood Loss Severity: Severity of internal or external bleeding/hemorrhage

Client Will (Include Specific Time Frame)

- Maintain fluid volume at a functional level as evidenced by individually adequate urinary output with normal specific gravity, stable vital signs, moist mucous membranes, good skin turgor, prompt capillary refill, and free of edema.
- Verbalize understanding of causative factors and purpose of individual therapeutic interventions and medications.
- Demonstrate behaviors to monitor and correct deficit, as indicated.

ACTIONS/INTERVENTIONS

Sample NIC linkages:

Fluid/Electrolyte Management: Regulation and prevention of complications from altered fluid and/or electrolyte levels

Hypovolemia Management: Expansion of intracellular fluid volume in a patient who is volume depleted

Shock Prevention: Detecting and treating a patient at risk for impending shock

NURSING PRIORITY NO. 1 To assess causative/precipitating factors:

- Identify relevant diagnoses *that may create a fluid volume depletion (e.g., decreased intravascular plasma volume, such as might occur with rapid blood loss or hemorrhage from trauma; vascular, pregnancy complications, gastrointestinal bleeding disorders); significant fluid (other than blood) loss such as might occur with severe gastroenteritis with vomiting and diarrhea; or extensive burns.*[1,4]
- Note presence of other factors (e.g., laryngectomy or tracheostomy tubes, drainage from wounds and fistulas or suction devices; water deprivation or fluid restrictions; decreased level of consciousness; dialysis; hot/humid climate, prolonged exercise; increased metabolic rate secondary to fever; increased caffeine or alcohol) *that may contribute to lack of fluid intake or loss of fluid by various routes.*

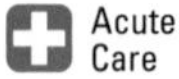
Acute Care
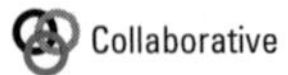
Collaborative
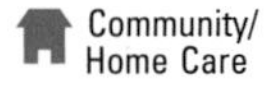
Community/ Home Care
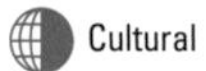
Cultural

- Prepare for and assist with diagnostic evaluations (e.g., imaging studies, x-rays) *to locate source of bleeding or cause for hypovolemia.*
- Determine effects of age, gender, weight, subcutaneous fat and muscle mass (influences total body water [TBW], which is approximately 60% of an adult's weight and 75% of an infant's weight).[11] *In general, men have higher TBW than women due to women's higher percentage of body fat and less muscle mass than men, and the elderly's TBW is less than that of a youth. Elderly individuals are often at risk for dehydration because of decreased thirst reflex, impaired renal conservation of water, increased prevalence of chronic conditions, and polypharmacy.*[2,3,8,9] *Infants/young children and other nonverbal persons cannot describe thirst. Worldwide, dehydration (secondary to diarrheal illness) is the leading cause of infant and child mortality.*[4]

NURSING PRIORITY NO. 2 To evaluate degree of fluid deficit:

- Estimate or measure traumatic or procedural fluid losses. Note possible routes of insensible fluid losses. Determine customary and current weight. *These factors are used to determine degree of volume depletion and method of fluid replacement. In burn injuries, the body surface area method states that dehydration is related to deficit of TBW and assumes that loss of weight is loss of water.*[11]
- Assess vital signs, including temperature (often elevated), pulse and respirations (elevated), and blood pressure (may be low). Measure blood pressure (lying/sitting/standing) if appropriate *to evaluate orthostatic blood pressure* and monitor invasive hemodynamic parameters as indicated (e.g., central venous pressure [CVP]) *to determine degree of intravascular deficit and replacement needs.*[1,6,7]
- Note presence of dry mucous membranes, poor skin turgor, delayed capillary refill, flat neck veins, and reports of thirst or weakness, child crying without tears, sunken eyeballs (or fontanel in infant), fever, weight loss, and little or no urine output. *Assessment signs of dehydration that client/significant other (SO) may notice. In an acute, life-threatening hemorrhage state, cold, pale, moist skin may be noted reflecting body compensatory mechanisms to profound hypovolemia.*[1,6,7]
- Note change in usual mentation, behavior, and functional abilities (e.g., confusion, falling, loss of ability to carry out usual activities, lethargy, dizziness). *These signs indicate sufficient dehydration to cause poor cerebral perfusion or can reflect the effects of electrolyte imbalance. In hypovolemic shock state, mentation changes rapidly and client may present in coma.*
- Observe/measure urinary output (hourly/24-hr totals). Note color *(may be dark greenish brown because of concentration)* and specific gravity *(high number associated with dehydration with usual range being 1.010 to 1.025).*[3,5]
- Review laboratory data (e.g., hemoglobin/hematocrit, prothrombin time, activated partial thromboplastin time; electrolytes [sodium, potassium, chloride, bicarbonate] and glucose; blood urea nitrogen, creatinine) *to evaluate body's response to bleeding/other fluid loss and to determine replacement needs.*[5] *Note: In isotonic dehydration, electrolyte levels may be lower, but concentration ratios remain near normal.*[3]

NURSING PRIORITY NO. 3 To correct/replace losses to reverse pathophysiological mechanisms:

- Control blood loss (e.g., gastric lavage with room temperature or cool saline solution, drug administration, prepare for surgical intervention).
- Stop fluid loss (e.g., administer medication to stop vomiting/diarrhea, reduce fever).[1]
- Administer fluids and electrolytes (e.g., blood, isotonic sodium chloride solution, lactated Ringer's solution, albumin, fresh frozen plasma, dextran, hetastarch). *Whether crystalloids (e.g., normal saline) or colloids (e.g., albumin) are best for fluid resuscitation continues to be a matter of discussion. A 2010 large-scale review of studies regarding effects of commonly used resuscitation fluids over the past 50 years supported the conclusion that rapid resuscitation with large-volume crystalloid is deleterious and supported slower, goal-directed resuscitation with low-volume crystalloid.*[1,7,10]
- Establish and continually reevaluate 24-hr fluid replacement needs and routes to be used *to prevent peaks and valleys in fluid level and to prevent fluid overload.*[6]

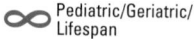

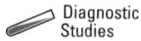

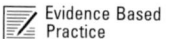

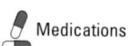

- Control humidity and ambient air temperature as appropriate, especially when major burns are present or in the presence of fever, *to reduce insensible losses.*
- Reduce bedding or clothes and provide a tepid sponge bath.
- Assist with hypothermia therapy as indicated *to decrease severe fever and elevated metabolic rate.* (Refer to ND Hyperthermia for additional interventions.)
- Maintain accurate intake and output (I&O) and weigh daily. Measure urine-specific gravity. Monitor blood pressure and invasive hemodynamic parameters as indicated (e.g., CVP) *to evaluate effectiveness of resuscitation measures.*

NURSING PRIORITY NO. 4 To promote comfort and safety:

- Change position frequently. Bathe infrequently, using mild cleanser or soap, and provide optimal skin care with emollients *to maintain skin integrity and prevent excessive dryness caused by dehydration.*
- Provide frequent oral care and eye care *to prevent injury from dryness.*
- Change dressings as needed and use adjunct appliances as indicated for draining wounds *to protect skin and to monitor losses for replacement needs.*
- Administer medications (e.g., antiemetics, antidiarrheals *to limit gastric or intestinal losses;* antipyretics *to reduce fever*). (Refer to NDs Diarrhea and Hyperthermia for additional interventions.)
- Observe for sudden or marked elevation of blood pressure, restlessness, moist cough, dyspnea, basilar crackles, and frothy sputum. *Too rapid a correction of fluid deficit may compromise the cardiopulmonary system, causing fluid overload and edema, especially if colloids are used in initial fluid resuscitation.*

NURSING PRIORITY NO. 5 To promote wellness (Teaching/Discharge Considerations):

- Discuss factors related to occurrence of fluid deficit as individually appropriate (e.g., reason for hemorrhage, potential for dehydration in children with fever or diarrhea, inadequate fluid replacement when performing strenuous work or exercise, living in hot climate, improper use of diuretics) *to reduce risk of recurrence.*
- Identify actions (if any) client may take to prevent or correct deficiencies. *Carrying a water bottle when away from home aids in maintaining fluid volume. Dressing in weather-appropriate clothing, staying in shade during heat of day, engaging in exercise during early morning or evening hours, and installation of room cooler or electric fan for hot climates helps reduce risk of heat stress or hyperthermia. In cases of mild to moderate dehydration, use of oral solutions (e.g., Gatorade, Rehydralyte), soft drinks, breast milk/formula, or Pedialyte can provide adequate rehydration.*[1]
- Instruct client/SO(s) in how to monitor color of urine (dark urine equates with concentration and dehydration) or how to measure and record I&O (may include weighing or counting diapers in infant/toddler).
- Review medications and interactions and side effects, especially medications that can cause or exacerbate fluid loss (e.g., diuretics, laxatives) and those indicated to prevent fluid loss (e.g., antidiarrheals, anticoagulants).[6]
- Discuss signs/symptoms indicating need for emergent or further evaluation and follow-up. *Promotes timely intervention.*

DOCUMENTATION FOCUS

Assessment/Reassessment

- Assessment findings, including degree of deficit and current sources of fluid intake.
- I&O, fluid balance, changes in weight or edema, urine-specific gravity, and vital signs.
- Results of diagnostic studies.

Planning

- Plan of care and who is involved in planning.
- Teaching plan.

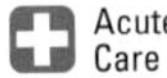

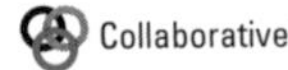

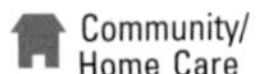

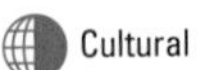

Implementation/Evaluation

- Client's responses to interventions, teaching, and actions performed.
- Attainment or progress toward desired outcome(s).
- Modifications to plan of care.

Discharge Planning

- Long-term needs, plan for correction, and who is responsible for actions to be taken.
- Specific referrals made.

References

1. Kolecki, P., Meckhoff, C. R. (Updated 2014). Hypovolemic shock. Retrieved March 2015 from http://emedicine.medscape.com/article/760145-overview.
2. Newfield, S. A., Hinz, M. D., Tilley, D. S., et al. (2007). *Cox's Clinical Applications of Nursing Diagnosis: Adult, Child, Women's, Psychiatric, Gerontic, and Home Health Considerations.* 5th ed. Philadelphia: F. A. Davis.
3. Mentes, J. C. (2012). Managing oral hydration. In: Boltz, M., Capezuti, E., Fulmer, T. (Eds.). *Evidence-Based Practice Guideline Hydration Management.* 4th ed. New York: Springer.
4. Huang, L. H., Anchalla, K. P., Ellsbury, D. L., et al. (Updated 2014). Dehydration. Retrieved March 2015 from http://emedicine.medscape.com/article/906999-overview.
5. Cavanaugh, B. M. (2003). *Nurse's Manual of Laboratory and Diagnostic Tests.* 4th ed. Philadelphia: F. A. Davis.
6. Mayo Clinic Staff. (Updated 2014). Dehydration. Retrieved March 2015 from http://www.mayoclinic.org/diseases-conditions/dehydration/basics/definition/con-20030056.
7. Diel-Oplinger, L., Kaminski, M. F. (2004). Choosing the right fluid to counter hypovolemic shock. *Nursing*, 34(3), 52–54.
8. Mentes, J., Claros, E. (2006). Oral hydration in older adults. *AJN*, 106(6), 40–49.
9. Collins, M., Claros, E. (2011). Recognizing the face of dehydration. *Nursing*, 41(8), 26–31.
10. Santry, H. P., Alam, H. B. (2014). Fluid resuscitation: Past, present, and the future. *Shock*, 33(3), 229–241.
11. Sterns, R. H. (Updated 2014). General principles of disorders of water balance (hyponatremia and hypernatremia) and sodium balance (hypovolemia and edema). Retrieved March 2015 from http://www.uptodate.com/contents/general-principles-of-disorders-of-water-balance-hyponatremia-and-hypernatremia-and-sodium-balance-hypovolemia-and-edema6.
12. Oliver, R. I. (Updated 2014). Burn resuscitation and early management. Retrieved March 2015 from http://emedicine.medscape.com/article/1277360-overview#aw2aab6b6.

excess Fluid Volume

Taxonomy II: Nutrition—Class 5 Hydration (00026) [**Diagnostic Division:** Food/Fluid], Submitted 1982; Revised 1996, 2013

DEFINITION: Increased isotonic fluid retention.

RELATED FACTORS

Compromised regulatory mechanism [e.g., syndrome of inappropriate antidiuretic hormone (SIADH), or decreased plasma proteins]
Excessive fluid intake
Excessive sodium intake

(continues on page 342)

excess Fluid Volume (continued)

DEFINING CHARACTERISTICS

Subjective

Anxiety

Orthopnea; paroxysmal nocturnal dyspnea

Objective

Edema; anasarca; weight gain over short period of time

Intake exceeds output; oliguria

Adventitious breath sounds; alteration in respiratory pattern; dyspnea

Pulmonary congestion; pleural effusion; alteration in pulmonary artery pressure (PAP)

Alteration in blood pressure

Increase in central venous pressure (CVP); jugular vein distention; positive hepatojugular reflex; hepatomegaly

Presence of S_3 heart sound

Alteration in mental status; restlessness

Decrease in hemoglobin or hematocrit; azotemia; electrolyte imbalance; alteration in urine-specific gravity

Sample Clinical Applications: Congestive heart failure, renal failure, cirrhosis of liver, cancer, toxemia of pregnancy, conditions associated with SIADH (e.g., meningitis, encephalitis, Guillain-Barré syndrome), schizophrenia (where polydipsia is a prominent feature)

DESIRED OUTCOMES/EVALUATION CRITERIA

Sample NOC linkages:

Fluid Overload Severity: Severity of excess fluids in intracellular and extracellular compartments of the body

Fluid Balance: Water balance in the intracellular and extracellular compartments of the body

Electrolyte and Acid/Base Balance: Balance of electrolytes and nonelectrolytes in the intracellular and extracellular compartments of the body

Client Will (Include Specific Time Frame)

- Stabilize fluid volume as evidenced by balanced intake and output (I&O), vital signs within client's normal limits, stable weight, and free of signs of edema.
- Verbalize understanding of individual dietary and fluid restrictions.
- Demonstrate behaviors to monitor fluid status and reduce recurrence of fluid excess.
- List signs that require further evaluation.

ACTIONS/INTERVENTIONS

Sample NIC linkages:

Hypervolemia Management: Reduction in extracellular or intracellular fluid volume and prevention of complications in a patient who is fluid overloaded

Fluid/Electrolyte Management: Regulation and prevention of complications from altered fluid and/or electrolyte levels

Peritoneal Dialysis [or] Hemodialysis Therapy: Administration and monitoring of dialysis solution into and out of the peritoneal cavity/or management of extracorporeal passage of the patient's blood through a dialyzer

NURSING PRIORITY NO. 1 To assess causative/precipitating factors:

- Note presence of medical conditions or situations (e.g., heart failure, chronic kidney disease, renal or adrenal insufficiency, excessive or rapid infusion of IV fluids, cerebral lesions, psychogenic polydipsia, acute stress,

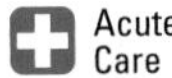

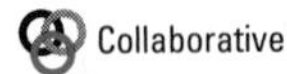

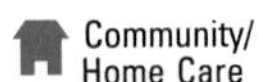

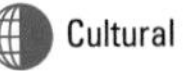

anesthesia, surgical procedures, decreased or loss of serum proteins) *that can contribute to excess fluid intake or retention.*[1,2]

- Determine or estimate amount of fluid intake from all sources: oral, intravenous, enteral or parenteral feedings, ventilator, etc. *Potential exists for fluid overload due to fluid shifts and changes in electrolyte balance. Note: Severely malnourished client can experience significant fluid shifts and electrolyte imbalances after nutritional support is initiated. This potentially lethal disorder, known as refeeding syndrome, usually is associated with parenteral nutrition, but it also can occur with enteral nutrition, oral intake, or dextrose-containing IV fluids.*[5,11]
- Review nutritional issues (e.g., intake of sodium, potassium, and protein). *Imbalances in these areas are associated with fluid imbalances.*[5]

NURSING PRIORITY NO. 2 To evaluate degree of excess:

- Compare current weight with admission or previously stated weight. Weigh daily or on a regular schedule, as indicated. *Provides a comparative baseline and evaluates the effectiveness of diuretic therapy when used (i.e., if I&O is 1 L negative, a weight loss of 2.2 lbs should be noted).*[7] *Note: Volume overload can occur over weeks to months in clients with unrecognized renal failure where lean muscle mass is lost and fluid overload occurs with relatively little change in weight.*[4]
- Measure vital signs and invasive hemodynamic parameters (e.g., CVP, PAP/pulmonary capillary wedge pressure) if available for critically ill clients. *Pressures may be high because of excess fluid volume or be low if cardiac failure is occurring.*
- Note presence of tachycardia and irregular rhythms. Auscultate heart tones for S_3, ventricular gallop. *Signs suggestive of heart failure, which results in decreased cardiac output and tissue hypoxia.*
- Auscultate breath sounds for presence of crackles or congestion. Record occurrence of exertional breathlessness, dyspnea at rest, or paroxysmal nocturnal dyspnea. *Indication of pulmonary congestion and potential of developing pulmonary edema that can interfere with oxygen–carbon dioxide exchange at the capillary level.*[3]
- Note presence and location of edema (e.g., puffy eyelids, swelling ankles and feet if ambulatory or up in chair, sacrum and posterior thighs when recumbent). Determine whether lower extremity edema is new or increasing. *Heart failure and renal failure are associated with dependent edema because of hydrostatic pressures, with dependent edema being a defining characteristic for excess fluid. Generalized edema (e.g., upper extremities and eyelids) is associated with nephrotic syndrome.*[2]
- Assess for presence of neck vein distention/hepatojugular reflux with head of bed elevated 30 to 45 deg. *Signs of increased intravascular volume.*[5]
- Measure abdominal girth *to evaluate changes that may indicate increasing fluid retention and edema.*[5]
- Evaluate mentation for restlessness, anxiety, confusion, and personality changes. *Signs of decreased cerebral oxygenation (e.g., cerebral edema) or electrolyte imbalance.*[1,8]
- Assess appetite; note presence of nausea/vomiting. Assess neuromuscular reflexes.[8]
- Observe skin and mucous membranes. *Edematous tissues are prone to ischemia and breakdown or ulceration.*
- Review laboratory data (e.g., blood urea nitrogen/creatinine, hemoglobin/hematocrit, serum albumin, proteins, electrolytes; urine-specific gravity, osmolality, sodium excretion) and chest radiograph. *These tests may be repeated not only to ascertain baseline imbalances, but also to monitor response to therapy.*

NURSING PRIORITY NO. 3 To promote mobilization/elimination of excess fluid:

- Restrict fluid intake as indicated (especially when sodium retention is less than water retention or when fluid retention is related to renal failure).[5]
- Provide for sodium restrictions if needed (as might occur in sodium retention in excess of water retention). *Restricting sodium favors renal excretion of excess fluid and may be more useful than fluid restriction.*[1]
- Set an appropriate rate of fluid intake or infusion throughout 24-hr period. Maintain steady rate of all IV infusions *to prevent exacerbation of excess fluid volume and to prevent peaks and valleys in fluid level.*[5,9]

- Administer medications (e.g., diuretics, cardiotonics, plasma or albumin volume expanders) in order to improve cardiac output and kidney function, thereby *reducing congestion and edema if heart failure is the cause of fluid overload.*
- Evaluate edematous extremities *to enhance venous return and prevent further edema formation.*
- Place in semi-Fowler's position when at bedrest as appropriate. *May promote recumbency-induced diuresis and facilitate respiratory effort when movement of the diaphragm is limited/breathing is impaired because of lung congestion.*
- Prepare for and assist with procedures as indicated (e.g., peritoneal or hemodialysis, ultrafiltration; mechanical ventilation, cardiac resynchronization therapy). *May be done to correct volume overload and electrolyte and acid-base imbalances or to improve cardiac function and support individual during shock state.*[7,10]

NURSING PRIORITY NO. 4 To maintain integrity of skin and tissues:

- Refer to NDs impaired Oral Mucous Membrane, impaired or risk for impaired Skin/Tissue Integrity, and risk for Pressure Ulcer for related interventions.

NURSING PRIORITY NO. 5 To promote wellness (Teaching/Discharge Considerations):

- Consult dietitian as needed *to develop dietary plan and identify foods to be limited or omitted:*
  Review dietary restrictions and safe substitutes for salt (e.g., lemon juice or spices such as oregano).
  Discuss fluid restrictions and "hidden sources" of fluids (e.g., foods high in water content such as fruits, ice cream, sauces, custard). Use small drinking cup or glass.
  Avoid salty or spicy foods, as they increase thirst or fluid retention. Suck ice chips, hard candy, or slices of lemon *to help allay thirst.*
- Suggest chewing gum and use of lip balm *to reduce discomforts of fluid restrictions.*
- Instruct client/family in ways to keep track of intake. For example, use a marked water bottle or container; refill as needed.[5]
- Measure output, encourage use of voiding record when it is appropriate, or weigh daily and report gain of more than 2 lb/day (or as indicated by individual situation). *If weight is rising daily, fluid is likely being retained.*[5]
- Review drug regimen and side effects of agents used to increase urine output or manage hypertension, kidney disease, or heart failure. *Many drugs have an impact on kidney function and fluid balance, especially in the elderly or those with cardiac and kidney impairments.*
- Emphasize need for mobility, frequent position changes, and early/ongoing ambulation *to prevent stasis and reduce risk of tissue injury.*
- Identify "danger" signs requiring notification of healthcare provider *to ensure timely evaluation and intervention.*[5]

DOCUMENTATION FOCUS

Assessment/Reassessment

- Assessment findings, noting existing conditions contributing to and degree of fluid retention (vital signs; amount, presence, and location of edema; weight changes).
- I&O, fluid balance.
- Results of laboratory tests and diagnostic studies.

Planning

- Plan of care and who is involved in the planning.
- Teaching plan.

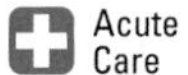
Acute Care
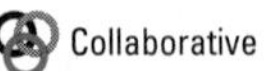
Collaborative
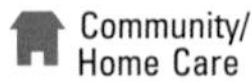
Community/ Home Care
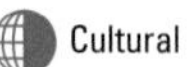
Cultural

Implementation/Evaluation

- Response to interventions, teaching, and actions performed.
- Attainment or progress toward desired outcome(s).
- Modifications to plan of care.

Discharge Planning

- Long-term needs, noting who is responsible for actions to be taken.

References

1. Harrison, T. R., Fauci, A. S. (eds). (1998). *Harrison's Principles of Internal Medicine*. 14th ed. New York: McGraw-Hill.
2. Holcomb, S. (2009). Topics in progressive care: Third-spacing: When body fluid shifts. *Nursing Crit Care*, 4(2), 9–12.
3. Matheny, N. (2010). *Fluid and Electrolyte Balance: Nursing Considerations*. 5th ed. Sudbury, MA: Jones & Bartlett Learning.
4. Veterans Health Administration, Department of Defense. (Updated 2007). VHA/DoD clinical practice guideline for the management of chronic kidney disease and pre-ESRD in the primary care setting. Retrieved March 2015 from http://f.i-md.com/medinfo/material/ce3/4eb24e6444aeb6583cc40ce3/4eb24e9544aeb6583cc40ce6.pdf.
5. South Carolina Department of Health and Environmental Control. (Updated 2006). Hydration management. Retrieved March 2015 from http://ddsn.sc.gov/providers/manualsandguidelines/Documents/HealthCareGuidelines/HydrationManagement.pdf.
6. Doenges, M. E., Moorhouse, M. F., Murr, A. C. (2010). Fluid and electrolyte imbalances. *Nursing Care Plans: Guidelines for Individualizing Client Care Across the Life Span*. 8th ed. Philadelphia: F. A. Davis.
7. Riggs, J. M. (2006). Manage heart failure. *Nurs Crit Care*, 1(4), 18–28.
8. Astle, S. M. (2005). Restoring electrolyte balance. *RN*, 68(5), 31–34.
9. Crawford, A., Harris, H. (2011). I.V. fluids: What nurses need to know. *Nursing*, 41(5), 30–38.
10. Streets, A., Vickers, S. M. (2012). Is this patient with heart failure a candidate for ultrafiltration? *Nursing*, 43(6), 30–36.
11. McCray, S., Walker, S., Parrish, C. R. (2005). Much ado about refeeding. *Pract Gastroenterol*, 30(1), 26–44.

risk for deficient Fluid Volume

Taxonomy II: Nutrition—Class 5 Hydration (00028) [**Diagnostic Division:** Food/Fluid], Submitted 1978; Revised 2010, 2013

DEFINITION: Vulnerable to experiencing decreased intravascular, interstitial, and/or intracellular fluid volumes, which may compromise health.

RISK FACTORS

Active fluid volume loss; excessive fluid loss through normal routes [e.g., diarrhea]
Barrier to accessing fluid; deviations affecting fluid intake or absorption
Extremes of age or weight
Factors influencing fluid needs [e.g., hypermetabolic state]
Fluid loss through abnormal routes [e.g., indwelling tubes]; compromised regulatory mechanism
Insufficient knowledge about fluid needs
Pharmaceutical agent [e.g., diuretics]
Note: A risk diagnosis is not evidenced by signs and symptoms, as the problem has not occurred; rather, nursing interventions are directed at prevention.

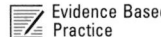

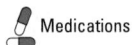

(continues on page 346)

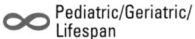

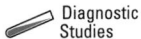

risk for deficient Fluid Volume (continued)

Sample Clinical Applications: Conditions with fever, diarrhea, nausea, vomiting; irritable bowel syndrome, draining wounds, dementia, depression, eating disorders

DESIRED OUTCOMES/EVALUATION CRITERIA

Sample NOC linkages:

Fluid Balance: Water balance in the intracellular and extracellular compartments of the body

Client Will (Include Specific Time Frame)

- Maintain fluid volume at a functional level as evidenced by individually adequate urinary output with normal specific gravity, stable vital signs, moist mucous membranes, good skin turgor, and prompt capillary refill.

Sample NOC linkages:

Risk Control: Personal actions to prevent, eliminate, or reduce modifiable health threats

Knowledge: Disease Process: Extent of understanding conveyed about a specific disease process

Client/Caregiver Will (Include Specific Time Frame)

- Identify individual risk factors and appropriate interventions.
- Demonstrate behaviors or lifestyle changes to prevent development of fluid volume deficit.

ACTIONS/INTERVENTIONS

Sample NIC linkages:

Fluid Monitoring: Collection and analysis of patient data to regulate fluid balance

Hemodynamic Regulation: Optimization of heart rate, preload, afterload, and contractility

Teaching: Disease Process: Assisting the patient to understand information related to a specific disease process

NURSING PRIORITY NO. 1 To assess causative/contributing factors:

- Note possible conditions/processes *that may lead to fluid deficits:* (1) fluid loss (e.g., indwelling tubes, diarrhea, vomiting, fever, excessive sweating, diabetic ketoacidosis; burns, other draining wounds; gastrointestinal obstruction; use of diuretics); (2) limited intake (e.g., extremes of age, limited mobility, client dependent on others for eating and drinking; lack of knowledge related to fluid intake; heat exhaustion or stroke); (3) fluid shifts (e.g., ascites, effusions, burns, sepsis); or (4) environmental factors (e.g., isolation, restraints, very high ambient temperatures, malfunctioning air conditioning).[3,6,7]
- Determine effects of age, gender, weight and subcutaneous fat/muscle mass. *These factors affect the ratio of lean body mass to body fat, influencing total body water (TBW). In general, men have higher TBW than women due to women's higher percentage of body fat and less muscle mass than men; the elderly's TBW is known to decline. Elderly individuals are often at risk for dehydration because of reduced water intake (often to less than 1 L/day), decreased thirst reflex, impaired renal conservation of water, increased prevalence of chronic conditions, and polypharmacy.*[1,10,11] *Infants, children, and developmentally delayed individuals cannot verbalize or self-manage thirst. Worldwide, dehydration (secondary to diarrheal illness) is the leading cause of infant and child mortality.*[2,6]
- Assess older client's "hydration habits" *to determine best approach if client has potential for dehydration. Note: A recent study identified four categories of nursing home residents: (1) Can drink (client is functionally capable of consuming fluids, but doesn't for any number of reasons); (2) can't drink (frailty or dysphagia makes this client incapable of consuming fluids safely); (3) won't drink (client may fear incontinence or may have never in life consumed many fluids); and (4) end of life.*[7]
- Evaluate nutritional status, noting current food intake, type of diet (e.g., client is NPO or is on a restricted or pureed diet), and *factors that can negatively affect fluid intake (e.g., impaired mentation, nausea, wired jaws, immobility, insufficient time for meals, lack of finances restricting availability of food).*

- Review client's medications, including prescription, over-the-counter (OTC) drugs, herbals, and nutritional supplements *to identify medications that can alter fluid and electrolyte balance. These may include diuretics, vasodilators, beta-blockers, aldosterone inhibitors, angiotensin-converting enzyme blockers, and medications that can cause syndrome of inappropriate secretion of antidiuretic hormone (e.g., phenothiazides, vasopressin, some antineoplastic drugs).*[8]
- Refer to NDs [deficient hyper/hypotonic Fluid Volume] or deficient [isotonic] Fluid Volume for additional interventions.

NURSING PRIORITY NO. 2 To prevent occurrence of deficit:

- Compare current fluid intake to fluid goal. Monitor intake and output balance, if indicated, being aware of changes in intake or output, as well as insensible losses, *to ensure accurate picture of fluid status.*[1,3]
- Assess skin and oral mucous membranes *for signs of dehydration, such as dry skin and mucous membranes, poor skin turgor, delayed capillary refill, and flat neck veins.*
- Monitor vital signs for changes (e.g., orthostatic hypotension, tachycardia, fever) *that may cause or be the effect of dehydration.*[3]
- Weigh client and compare with recent weight history. Perform serial weights to determine trends.
- Review laboratory data (e.g., hemoglobin/hematocrit, osmolality, electrolytes [e.g., sodium and potassium], blood urea nitrogen/creatinine) as indicated *to evaluate fluid and electrolyte status.*[2,3] *Note: Faes (2007) states that "three forms of dehydration can be distinguished on the basis of plasma tonicity: hypertonic, isotonic, and hypotonic dehydration. Hypertonic dehydration is easy to diagnose by laboratory tests (e.g., serum sodium levels >150 mmol/L or serum osmolality >300 mosmol/L), but neglects the frequently occurring isotonic and hypotonic dehydration. Isotonic dehydration results from a balanced loss of water and electrolytes (e.g., by vomiting and diarrhea) and hypotonic dehydration results when loss of electrolytes exceeds water loss (e.g., by overuse of diuretics)."*[11]
- Offer a variety of fluids and water-rich foods and make them available throughout day if client is able to take oral fluids. Assist/remind client to drink, as needed. Determine individual fluid needs and establish replacement over 24 hours *to increase client's daily fluid intake.*[9]
- Administer medications as appropriate (e.g., antiemetics, antidiarrheals, antipyretics) *to stop or limit fluid losses. Note: Some practitioners recommend avoidance of antidiarrheal agents (high incidence of side effects including lethargy, respiratory depression, and coma) or OTC antiemetics (due to side effects including drowsiness and this impaired oral rehydration).*[2,3]
- Provide nutritionally balanced diet and/or enteral feedings when indicated (avoiding use of hyperosmolar or excessively high-protein formulas) and provide adequate amount of free water with feedings.[9]
- Provide supplemental IV fluids as indicated.
- Encourage oral intake:[3–6,8]

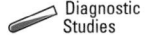

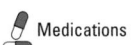

  Provide water and other fluids to a minimum amount daily (up to 2.5 L/day or amount determined by healthcare provider for client's age, weight, and condition).

  Offer fluids between meals and regularly throughout the day.

  Allow adequate time for eating and drinking at meals.

  Provide fluids in manageable cup, bottle, or with drinking straw.

  Ensure that immobile or restrained client is assisted.

  Encourage a variety of fluids in small frequent offerings, attempting to incorporate client's preferred beverage and temperature (e.g., iced or hot).

  Limit fluids that tend to exert a diuretic effect (e.g., caffeine, alcohol, high-glucose drinks).

  Promote intake of foods with a high water content (e.g., popsicles, gelatin, soup, eggnog, watermelon) or electrolyte replacement drinks (e.g., Smartwater, Gatorade, Pedialyte), as appropriate.

  Encourage client to increase fluids when engaged in exercise or physical exertion or during hot weather.
- Review diet orders to remove any nonessential fluid and salt restrictions.

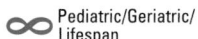

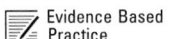

NURSING PRIORITY NO. 3 To promote wellness (Teaching/Discharge Considerations):

- Discuss individual risk factors or potential problems and specific interventions *to reduce risk of heat injury and dehydration (e.g., proper clothing and bedding for infants and elderly during hot weather, use of room cooler or fan for comfortable ambient environment).*[5]
- Review appropriate use of medications and inform client of side effects or interactions of medications *that have potential for causing or exacerbating dehydration.*
- Encourage client/caregiver to maintain diary of fluid intake, number and amount of voidings, and estimate of other fluid losses (e.g., wounds, liquid stools) as necessary *to determine replacement needs.*
- Engage client, family, and all caregivers in fluid management plan. *Enhances cooperation with regimen and achievement of goals.*

DOCUMENTATION FOCUS

Assessment/Reassessment

- Individual findings, including individual risk factors influencing fluid needs or requirements.
- Baseline weight, vital signs.
- Results of laboratory tests.
- Specific client fluid needs and preferences.

Planning

- Plan of care and who is involved in planning.
- Teaching plan.

Implementation/Evaluation

- Responses to interventions, teaching, and actions performed.
- Attainment or progress toward desired outcome(s).
- Modifications to plan of care.

Discharge Planning

- Individual long-term needs, noting who is responsible for actions to be taken.
- Specific referrals made.

References

1. Mentes, J. C. (2012). Managing oral hydration. In Boltz, M., Capezuti, E., Fulmer, T. (Eds.). *Evidence-Based Practice Guideline Hydration Management.* 4th ed. New York: Springer.
2. Huang, L. H., Anchalla, K. P., Ellsbury, D. L., et al. (Updated 2014). Dehydration. Retrieved March 2015 from http://emedicine.medscape.com/article/906999-overview.
3. American Medical Directors Association. (2009). Dehydration and fluid maintenance in the long-term care setting. Retrieved March 2015 from http://www.guideline.gov/content.aspx?id=15590.
4. Matheny, N. (2010). *Fluid and Electrolyte Balance: Nursing Considerations.* 5th ed. Sudbury, MA: Jones & Bartlett Learning.
5. Curtis, R. (1999–2010). Outdoor action guide to heat and cold injuries. National Ag Safety Database. Retrieved March 2015 from http://www.princeton.edu/~oa/safety/heatcold.shtml.
6. Mentes, J., Claros, E. (2006). Oral hydration in older adults. *Am J Nurs*, 106(6), 40–49.
7. Mentes, J. (2006). A typology of oral hydration problems exhibited by frail nursing home residents. *J Gerontol Nurs*, 23(1), 13–21.
8. Wotton, K., Crannitch, K., Munt, R. (2008). Prevalence, risk factors and strategies to prevent dehydration in older adults. *Contemp Nurs*, 31(1), 44–56.
9. Collins, M., Claros, E. (2011). Recognizing the face of dehydration. *Nursing*, 41(8), 26–31.
10. Scholler, D. A. (1989). Changes in total body water with age. *Am J Clin Nutr*, 50(5suppl), 1176–1181.
11. Faes, M. C., Spigt, M. G., Rikkert, O. (2007). Dehydration in geriatrics. *Geriatrics and Aging*, 10(9), 590–596.

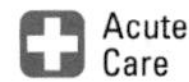

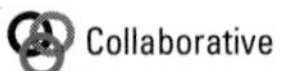

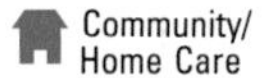

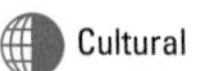

risk for imbalanced Fluid Volume

Taxonomy II: Nutrition—Class 5 Hydration (00025) [**Diagnostic Division:** Food/Fluid], Submitted 1998; Revised 2008, 2013

DEFINITION: Vulnerable to a decrease, increase, or rapid shift from one to the other of intravascular, interstitial, and/or intracellular fluid, which may compromise health. This refers to body fluid loss, gain, or both.

RISK FACTORS

Intestinal obstruction
Pancreatitis; ascites
Burns; sepsis
Trauma
Treatment regimen; apheresis
Note: A risk diagnosis is not evidenced by signs and symptoms, as the problem has not occurred; rather, nursing interventions are directed at prevention.
Sample Clinical Application: Major surgical procedures, renal dialysis, conditions requiring IV therapy or parenteral or enteral nutrition, heart failure with use of diuretic therapy

DESIRED OUTCOMES/EVALUATION CRITERIA

Sample NOC linkages:
Fluid Balance: Water balance in the intracellular and extracellular compartments of the body
Fluid Overload Severity: Severity of excess fluids in the intracellular and extracellular compartments of the body
Risk Control: Personal actions to prevent, eliminate, or reduce modifiable health threats

Client/Caregiver Will (Include Specific Time Frame)

- Demonstrate adequate fluid balance as evidenced by stable vital signs, palpable pulses of good quality, normal skin turgor, moist mucous membranes, individual appropriate urinary output, lack of excessive weight fluctuation (loss or gain), and no edema present.
- Identify individual risk factors and appropriate interventions.
- Demonstrate behaviors or lifestyle changes to prevent development of fluid imbalance.

ACTIONS/INTERVENTIONS

Sample NIC linkages:
Fluid Monitoring: Collection and analysis of patient data to regulate fluid balance
Intravenous (IV) Therapy: Administration and monitoring of IV fluids and medication
Hypervolemia Management: Reduction in extracellular and/or intracellular fluid volume and prevention of complications in a patient who is fluid overloaded

NURSING PRIORITY NO. 1 To determine risk/contributing factors:

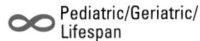

- Note presence of conditions associated with fluid imbalance (e.g., diabetes insipidus; hyperosmolar nonketotic syndrome; intestinal obstruction; heart, pancreatitis, sepsis, kidney, or liver failure).
- Note current treatment modalities, including (1) major invasive procedures (e.g., surgery, dialysis), (2) use or overuse of certain medications (e.g., heparin, diuretics), (3) use of IV fluids without a delivery device, and (4) plasmaphoresis (i.e., aphoresis) therapy. *These modalities can cause/exacerbate fluid imbalances and must be monitored for complications. Note: Therapeutic apheresis refers to extracorporeal therapies used in*

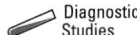

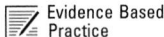

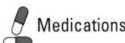

treatment of a variety of neurological, renal, hematological, and other systemic diseases caused by circulating toxic agents that cannot be cleared by other means. This may be a first-line therapy for conditions (e.g., Guillain-Barre syndrome, myasthenia gravis; therapeutic drug removal) or as a second-line therapy in conjunction with other therapies (e.g., multiple sclerosis unresponsive to steroids).[7–9]

- ∞ Note client's age, current level of hydration, and mentation. *Provides information regarding ability to tolerate fluctuations in fluid level and risk for creating or failing to respond to a problem (e.g., confused client may have inadequate intake, disconnect tubings, or readjust IV flow rate; infant or child may be unable to self-monitor or manage).*[1]

NURSING PRIORITY NO. 2 To prevent fluctuations/imbalances in fluid levels:

- Measure and record intake:
  Include all sources (e.g., oral, IV, antibiotic additives, liquids with medications).
- Measure and record output:
  Monitor urine output (hourly, or as often as needed). Report urine output less than 30 mL/hr or 0.5 mL/kg/hr *because it may indicate deficient fluid volume or cardiac or kidney failure.*
  Observe color of all excretions *to evaluate for bleeding.*
  Estimate volume or measure emesis when vomiting.
  Measure or estimate amount of liquid stool; weigh diapers or continence pads when indicated.
  ∞ Inspect dressing(s), weigh dressings, estimate blood loss in surgical sponges, and count dressings or pads saturated per hour. *Note: Small losses can be life-threatening to pediatric clients.*[2]
  Measure output from drainage devices (e.g., gastric, wound, chest).
  Estimate or calculate insensible fluid losses *to include losses in replacement calculations. Note: Losses from diffusion through skin and via respiratory tract are estimated at about 700 mL/24 hr in adults at ambient temperature,*[3] *while a diaphoretic episode requiring a full linen change may represent a fluid loss of as much as 1 L.*[5]
  Calculate 24-hr fluid balance (noting intake greater than output, or output greater than intake).
- Weigh daily or as indicated, using same scale and clothing, and evaluate changes as they relate to fluid status. *Provides for early detection and prompt intervention as needed.*
- Monitor vital signs:
  Evaluate vital signs at rest and with activities. *Blood pressure and heart and respiratory rate often increase initially when either volume deficit or fluid excess is present.*[5]
  Evaluate hemodynamic pressures when available. *Central venous pressure and pulmonary artery wedge pressure may be used in critically ill clients to determine fluid balance and fluid volume responsiveness and to guide administration of vasoactive medications. Note: Numerous studies in recent years have weighed the benefits of invasive monitoring for the purpose of evaluating fluid status (and thus cardiac output response to fluid challenge). Research is ongoing into alternate ways to perform this assessment (including the use of bioreactance, which tracks the phase of the electrical currents traversing the chest). These tests use the change in stroke volume during mechanical ventilation or after a passive leg-raising maneuver to assess fluid responsiveness. The stroke volume is measured continuously and in real time by minimally invasive or noninvasive technologies, including Doppler methods, pulse contour analysis, and bioreactance.*[2,10,11]
- Maintain IVs on volumetric infusion pumps and rapid infusion devices, as appropriate, *to deliver fluids accurately at desired rates to prevent either under/overinfusion.*[5]
- Assess for peripheral or dependent edema, adventitious breath sounds, and distended neck veins. *Clinical signs of fluid excess. Note: Intravascular volume depletion can be present at the same time as extravascular fluid excess (seen as edema) is present, so hypertension or hypotension could be found.*[4,5]
- Note increased lethargy or reports of dizziness, weakness, and muscle cramping. *Electrolyte imbalances (e.g., sodium, potassium, magnesium, calcium) may be present.*[5,6]

- Review laboratory data (e.g., electrolytes, hemoglobin/hematocrit) and chest radiograph *to determine changes indicative of electrolyte and/or fluid imbalance and fluid needs.*[5,6]
- If fluid volume deficit is possible:
  Anticipate fluid replacement needs (e.g., need for blood or plasma transfusion in client with major trauma; planned surgery where blood and fluid loss can be expected; major burn injury; person with heat stroke; vomiting, diarrhea, or inability to take fluids).[5]
  Establish and promote oral intake, incorporating beverage preferences when possible. Administer IV fluids (e.g., crystalloids, colloids, blood or blood components) *to support fluid management.*[4,5]
  Administer medications (e.g., antidiarrheals, antiemetics, agents to reduce blood loss or promote clotting) as indicated *to reduce fluid loss.*[4,5]
- Refer to NDs [deficient hypertonic/hypotonic Fluid Volume], deficient [isotonic] Fluid Volume, and risk for deficient Fluid Volume for additional interventions.
- If fluid volume excess is possible:
  Maintain fluid/sodium restrictions when needed. Offer small amounts of fluid over a 24-hr period.
  Administer medications (e.g., diuretics, cardiotonics) *to assist in management of fluid excess or edema.*[4,5]
  Assist with or prepare for procedures (e.g., dialysis, aphoresis, ultrafiltration, pacemaker, cardiac assist device) *to correct fluid overload situation*[8,9] and monitor for complications associated with fluid imbalances.
  Refer to ND excess Fluid Volume for additional interventions.

NURSING PRIORITY NO. 3 To promote wellness (Teaching/Discharge Considerations):

- Engage client, family, and all caregivers in fluid management plan. *Enhances cooperation with regimen and achievement of goals.*[5]
- Discuss individual risk factors or potential problems and specific interventions *to prevent or limit fluid imbalance and complications.*
- Instruct client/significant other in how to measure and record I/O as appropriate.
- Review and instruct in medications or nutritional regimen (e.g., enteral, parenteral) *to alert to potential complications and ways to manage.*
- Identify signs and symptoms indicating need for prompt evaluation or follow-up by primary healthcare provider *for timely intervention and correction.*[5]

DOCUMENTATION FOCUS

Assessment/Reassessment

- Individual findings, including individual factors influencing fluid needs or requirements.
- Baseline weight, vital signs.
- Specific client preferences for fluids.

Planning

- Plan of care and who is involved in planning.
- Teaching plan.

Implementation/Evaluation

- Responses to interventions, teaching, and actions performed.
- Attainment or progress toward desired outcome(s).
- Modifications to plan of care.

Discharge Planning

- Individual long-term needs, noting who is responsible for actions to be taken.
- Specific referrals made.

References

1. Newfield, S. A., Hinz, M. D., Tilley, D. S., et al. (2007). *Cox's Clinical Applications of Nursing Diagnosis: Adult, Child, Women's, Psychiatric, Gerontic, and Home Health Considerations*. 5th ed. Philadelphia: F. A. Davis.
2. Ackley, B. J., Ladwig, G. B. (2011). *Nursing Diagnosis Handbook: An Evidence-Based Guide to Planning Care*. 9th ed. St. Louis, MO: Mosby Elsevier.
3. Guyton, A. C., Hall, J. E. (2010). *Textbook of Medical Physiology*. 12th ed. Philadelphia: W. B. Saunders.
4. Matheny, N. (2010). *Fluid and Electrolyte Balance: Nursing Considerations*. 5th ed. Philadelphia: J. B. Lippincott.
5. Doenges, M. E., Moorhouse, M. F., Murr, A. C. (2014). Fluid and electrolyte imbalances. *Nursing Care Plans: Guidelines for Individualizing Client Care Across the Life Span*. 9th ed. Philadelphia: F. A. Davis.
6. Astle, S. M. (2005). Restoring electrolyte balance. *RN*, 68(5), 31–34.
7. Stieglitz, E., Huang, J. (2013). Plasmapheresis. Retrieved March 2015 from http://emedicine.medscape.com/article/1895577-overview.
8. Mokrzycki, M. H., Bolagun, R. A. (2011). Therapeutic apheresis: A review of complications and recommendations for prevention and management. *J Clin Apher*, 26(5), 243–248.
9. Mokrzycki, M. H., Bolagun, R. A. (2013). Medications and therapeutic apheresis procedures: Are we doing our best?. *J Clin Apher*, 28(1), 73–77.
10. Marik, P. E., Monnet, X., Taboul, J-L. (2011). Hemodynamic parameters to guide fluid therapy. Retrieved March 2015 from http://www.annalsofintensivecare.com/content/1/1/1.
11. Cheetah Medical. (2013). Clinical application: Tailor fluid management with CHEETAH NICOM to optimize resuscitation. Retrieved March 2015 from http://cheetah-medical.com/fluid.

Frail Elderly Syndrome

Taxonomy II: Health Promotion—Class 2: Health Management (00257) [**Diagnostic Division:** Safety], Submitted 2013

DEFINITION: Dynamic state of unstable equilibrium that affects the older individual experiencing deterioration of one or more domains of health (physical, functional, psychological, or social) and leads to increased susceptibility to adverse health effects, in particular disability.

RELATED FACTORS

Alteration in cognitive functioning; psychiatric disorder
Chronic illness; prolonged hospitalization
Malnutrition; sarcopenia; sarcopenic obesity
History of falls
Living alone
Sedentary lifestyle

DEFINING CHARACTERISTICS

Subjective

Activity intolerance
Fatigue
Hopelessness

Objective

Bathing, dressing, feeding, or toileting self-care deficit
Decreased cardiac output

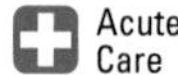

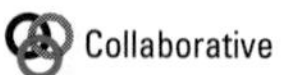

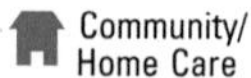

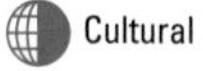

Imbalanced nutrition: less than body requirements
Impaired memory
Impaired physical mobility; impaired walking
Social isolation
Sample Clinical Applications: Chronic debilitating conditions (e.g., COPD, diabetes, AIDS, Alzheimer's disease, multiple sclerosis [MS]), cancer, terminal illnesses, major depression

DESIRED OUTCOMES/EVALUATION CRITERIA

Sample NOC linkages:
Personal Health Status: Overall physical or psychological, social, and spiritual functioning of an adult 18 years or older
Self-Management: Chronic Disease: Personal actions to manage a chronic disease progression and complications
Will to Live: Desire, determination, and effort to survive

Client/Caregiver Will (Include Specific Time Frame)

- Acknowledge presence of factors affecting well-being.
- Identify corrective/adaptive measures for individual situation.
- Demonstrate behaviors/lifestyle changes necessary to enhance functional status.

Client Will
Look to the future, expressing a sense of control.

ACTIONS/INTERVENTIONS

Sample NIC linkages:
Self-Care Assistance: Assisting another to perform activities of daily living
Resiliency Promotion: Assisting individuals, families, and communities in development, use, and strengthening of protective factors to be used in coping with environmental and societal stressors

Refer to NDs Activity Intolerance, risk-prone Health Behavior, chronic Confusion, ineffective Coping, impaired Dentition, risk for Falls, Grieving, Loneliness, imbalanced Nutrition: less than body requirements, Relocation Stress Syndrome, Self-Care Deficit (specify), chronic low Self-Esteem, risk for Spiritual Distress, and ineffective Health Management, as appropriate, for additional relevant interventions.

NURSING PRIORITY NO. 1 To identify causative/contributing factors:

- Identify presence of "frailty syndrome" (FS). *Demonstrated in elderly person by three or more symptoms together: unintentional weight loss (10 or more pounds within the past year), muscle loss and weakness, a feeling of fatigue, slow walking speed, and low levels of physical activity.*[1] *Note: The presence of FS is a predictor for hospitalization, disability, decreasing mobility, falls, and even death.*[2]
- Note individual's age and gender. *Fried's (2001) research study of more than 5,000 adults found that chances of frailty rose sharply after the age of 85. Also, women are more likely than men to be frail, possibly because women typically outlive men and "start out with less muscle mass than men and, once they lose it, they may cross the frailty threshold more rapidly than men."*[3]
- Note presence of physical complaints (e.g., fatigue/exhaustion, unintentional weight loss, muscle weakness, slow walking, inability to participate in usual physical activities, others as noted in Defining Characteristics) and presence of conditions (e.g., heart disease, undetected diabetes mellitus, dementia, stroke, renal failure, long-term period of being bedridden, terminal conditions). *Note: These factors associated with frailty may or may not be recognized by the client, but may be reported or documented by others.*

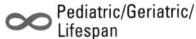

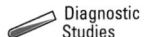

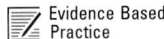

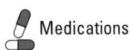

- Evaluate medication regimen. *Medications that cause electrolyte imbalances (e.g., diuretics) can exacerbate weakness. Drugs that slow reaction time (e.g., sedatives, antidepressants) can interfere with balance and coordination, as can alcohol.*[4]
- Determine nutritional status. *Malnutrition (e.g., weight loss, laboratory abnormalities, and identified micronutrient deficiencies) and factors contributing to failure to eat (e.g., chronic nausea, loss of appetite, no access to food or cooking, poorly fitting dentures, no one with whom to share meals, depression, financial problems) greatly impact health status and quality of life—especially for the elderly individual.*[2,5–7]
- Assess client's physical and cognitive status *to identify tolerance for activity and/or self-care.*
- Note client's living situation (e.g., lives alone, lives in facility). *Helps identify environmental risk factors such as risk for falls, problem with food shopping or preparation, depression, etc.*
- Evaluate client's level of adaptive behavior and client/caregiver knowledge and skills about health maintenance, environment, and safety *in order to instruct, intervene, and refer appropriately.*
- Review with client/significant other (SO) previous and current life situations, including role changes, multiple losses (e.g., death of loved ones, change in living arrangements, finances, independence), social isolation, and grieving *to identify psychological stressors that may be affecting current situation.*
- Ascertain safety of home environment and persons providing care *to identify potential for/presence of neglectful or abusive situations and/or need for referrals.*

NURSING PRIORITY NO. 2 To assess degree of impairment:

- Collaborate with multidisciplinary team to determine severity of client's limitations. *Testing may occur over period of time to identify functional and/or nutritional deficits and may include blood work, physical therapy evaluation, and nutritional studies. Note: Studies have associated certain laboratory indicators with frailty, including (but not limited to) anemia, inflammation, and clotting factors.*[6,8]
- Perform nutritional screening and/or refer for comprehensive nutritional assessment. *Studies show that person may have weight and muscle loss (sarcopenia) or weight gain/obesity with muscle function impairment and loss of strength (sarcopenic obesity).*[9] *Initial evidence indicates that when obesity and muscle impairment co-exist, they act synergistically on the risk of developing multiple health-related outcomes.*[10]

NURSING PRIORITY NO. 3 To assist client to achieve/maintain general well-being:

- Assist with treatment of underlying comorbid medical, functional, cognitive, or psychiatric conditions *that could positively influence current situation (e.g., resolution of infection, treating anemia, addressing brain injury, delirium, social isolation, depression).*[11]
- Develop plan of action with client/caregiver *to meet immediate needs for nutrition, safety, and self-care and facilitate implementation of actions.*
- Administer medications as appropriate. *Studies show that optimized management of congestive heart failure and chronic pulmonary disease or improved glycemic control of diabetes results in improved health status, fewer hospitalizations, and reductions in the physical declines associated with the frailty syndrome.*[15]
- Refer to dietitian or nutritionist to assist in planning meals to meet client's specific nutritional needs (e.g., calories, proteins, vitamins, micronutrients), taste, and abilities. *Plans could include offering client's favorite food(s), attending social events (e.g., ice cream social, happy hour), or participating in family-style meals. In addition, interventions may be geared toward treatment of depression, grief, or loss and cultural or environmental adaptation measures.*[2,7,12] (Refer to ND imbalanced Nutrition: less than body requirements for additional interventions.)
- Refer to physical and/or occupational therapist as indicated *to improve physical strength, endurance, and stamina. Note: Studies have supported that exercises (e.g., chair aerobics, stretching, resistance training, walking, tai chi) can improve balance and muscle and core strength, promoting physical function and endurance and reducing risk of falls.*[2,11]
- Discuss individual concerns about feelings of loss/loneliness and relationship between these feelings and current decline in well-being. Note desire or willingness to change situation. *Motivation or lack thereof can facilitate—or impede—achieving desired outcomes.*[12]

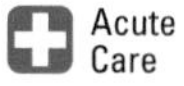

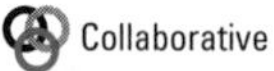

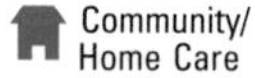

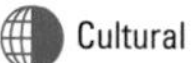

- Explore mental strengths and successful coping skills the individual has previously used and apply to current situation. Refine or develop new strategies, as appropriate. *Incorporating these into problem solving builds on past successes.*[13]
- Assist client to develop goals for dealing with life or illness situation. Involve SO in long-range planning. *Promotes commitment to goals and plan, thereby maximizing outcomes.*

NURSING PRIORITY NO. 4 To promote wellness (Teaching/Discharge Considerations):

- Assist client/SO(s) to identify and/or access useful community resources (e.g., support groups, Meals on Wheels, social worker, home care or assistive care, placement services). *Enhances coping, assists with problem solving, and may reduce risks to client and caregiver.*
- Encourage client to talk about positive aspects of life and to keep as physically active as possible *to reduce effects of dispiritedness (e.g., "feeling low," sense of being unimportant, disconnected).*[14]
- Promote socialization within individual limitations *to provide additional stimulation, reduce sense of isolation.*
- Offer opportunities to discuss life goals and support client/SO in setting/attaining new goals for this time in his or her life *to enhance hope for the future.*
- Help client explore reasons for living or begin to deal with end-of-life issues and provide support for grieving. *Enhances hope and sense of control, providing opportunity for client to take charge of own future.*[13,14]
- Assist client/SO/family to understand that frailty commonly occurs near the end of life and cannot always be reversed.[12]
- Discuss appropriateness of and refer to palliative services or hospice care, as indicated.
- Refer to pastoral care, counseling, or psychotherapy *for grief work or other issues as needed.*

DOCUMENTATION FOCUS

Assessment/Reassessment

- Individual findings, including current weight, dietary pattern, food and eating, perceptions of self, motivation for loss, support and feedback from SOs.
- Perception of losses or life changes.
- Ability to perform activities of daily living, participate in care, and meet own needs.
- Motivation for change, support and feedback from SO(s).

Planning

- Plan of care, specific interventions, and who is involved in planning.
- Teaching plan.

Implementation/Evaluation

- Responses to interventions and actions performed, general well-being, weekly weight.
- Attainment or progress toward desired outcome(s).
- Modifications to plan of care.

Discharge Planning

- Long-term needs and who is responsible for actions to be taken.
- Community resources and support groups.
- Specific referrals made.

References

1. Cimons, M. (2013). Frailty is a medical condition, not an inevitable result of aging (Op-Ed). Retrieved February 2015 from http://www.livescience.com/41602-frailty-is-medical-condition.html.
2. Cherniak, E. P., Florez, H. J., Troen, B. R., et al. (2007). Emerging therapies to treat frailty syndrome in the elderly. *Altern Med Rev*, 12(3), 246–258.

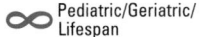

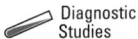

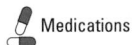

3. Fried, L. P., Tangen, C. M., Walston, J., et al. (2001). Frailty in older adults: Evidence for a phenotype. *J Gerontol A Biol Sci Med Sci*, 56(3), M146–M157.
4. Flinders, D. C. (2007). Helping elderly patients avoid frailty syndrome. Retrieved February 2015 from http://www.clinicaladvisor.com/helping-elderly-patients-avoid-frailty-syndrome/article/117361/.
5. Rehman, H. U. (2008). Involuntary weight loss in the elderly. *Clin Geriatr Med*, 13, 37–45.
6. Dawodu, S. T., Scott, D. D., Chase, M., et al. (2003, updated 2013). Nutritional management in the rehabilitation setting. Retrieved January 2015 from http://emedicine.medscape.com/article/318180-overview.
7. diMaria-Ghalili, R. A., Amelia, E. (2005). Nutrition in older adults: Interventions and assessment can help curb the growing threat of malnutrition. *Am J Nurs*, 105(3), 40–50.
8. Walston, J., McBurnie, M. A., Newman, A., et al. (2002). Frailty and activation of the inflammation and coagulation systems with and without clinical comorbidities: Results from the Cardiovascular Health Study. *Arch Intern Med*, 162(20), 2333–2341.
9. Stenholm, S., Harris, T. B., Rantanen, T., et al. (2009). Sarcopenic obesity—definition, etiology and consequences. *Curr Opin Clin Nutr Metab Care*, 11(6), 693–700.
10. Dominguez, L. J., Barbagallo, M. (2007). The cardiometabolic syndrome and sarcopenic obesity in older persons. *J Cardiometab Syndr*, 2(3), 183–189.
11. Ferrucc, L., Guralnik, J. M., Cavazzini, C., et al. (2003). The frailty syndrome: A critical issue in geriatric oncology. *Crit Rev Oncol Hematol*, 46(2), 127–137.
12. Robertson, R. G., Montagnini, M. (2004). Geriatric failure to thrive. *Am Family Med*, 70(2), 343–350.
13. Townsend, M. C. (2003). *Psychiatric Mental Health Nursing Concepts of Care*. 4th ed. Philadelphia: F. A. Davis.
14. Butcher, H. K., McGonigal-Kenney, M. (2005). Depression & dispiritedness in later life: A "gray drizzle of horror" isn't inevitable. *Am J Nurs*, 105(12), 52–61.
15. Palace, J. Z., Flood-Sukhdeo, J. (2014). The frailty syndrome. *Today's Geriatric Medicine*, 7(1), 18.

risk for Frail Elderly Syndrome

Taxonomy II: Health Promotion—Class 2 Health Management (00231) **[Diagnostic Division:** Safety], Submitted 2013

DEFINITION: Vulnerable to a dynamic state of unstable equilibrium that affects the older individual experiencing deterioration of one or more domain of health (physical, functional, psychological, or social) and leads to increased susceptibility to adverse health effects, in particular disability.

RISK FACTORS

Activity intolerance; average daily physical activity is less than recommended for gender and age; decrease in energy; exhaustion; sedentary lifestyle
Age >70 years; female gender; ethnicity other than Caucasian
Alteration in cognitive functioning
Anorexia; malnutrition; decrease in serum 25–hydroxyvitamin D concentration
Anxiety; depression; sadness
Chronic illness; prolonged hospitalization
Decrease in muscle strength; muscle weakness; walking 15 feet requires >6 seconds (4 meters >5 seconds)
Fear of falling; history of falls
Impaired balance or mobility; immobility
Sensory deficit (e.g., visual, hearing)
Sarcopenia; unintentional weight loss of 25% body weight over one year; unintentional weight loss >10 pounds (>4.5 Kg) in one year
Obesity; sarcopenic obesity
Endocrine regulatory dysfunction (e.g., glucose intolerance, increase in IGF-1, androgen, DHEA, and cortisol)
Suppressed inflammatory response (e.g., IL-6, CRP); altered clotting process (e.g., factor VII, D-dimers)

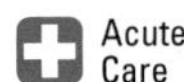

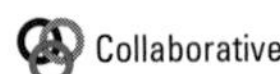

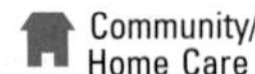

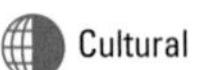

Constricted life space; economically disadvantaged; low educational level
Insufficient social support; living alone; social isolation
Social vulnerability (e.g., disempowerment, decreased life control)
Sample Clinical Applications: Chronic debilitating conditions (e.g., COPD, diabetes, AIDS, Alzheimer's disease, multiple sclerosis [MS]), cancer, terminal illnesses, major depression)
Note: A risk diagnosis is not evidenced by signs and symptoms, as the problem has not occurred; rather, nursing interventions are directed at prevention

DESIRED OUTCOMES/EVALUATION CRITERIA

Sample NOC linkages:
Personal Health Status: Overall physical, psychological, social, and spiritual functioning of an adult 18 years or older
Self-Management: Chronic Disease: Personal actions to manage a chronic disease progression and complications

Client/Caregiver Will (Include Specific Time Frame)
- Identify risk factors that can affect well-being.
- Develop plan to correct/minimize risk factors.
- Engage in behaviors/lifestyle changes necessary to maintain/enhance functional status.

Client Will
- Look to the future, expressing a sense of control.

ACTIONS/INTERVENTIONS

Sample NIC linkages:
Risk Identification: Analysis of potential risk factors, determination of health risks, and prioritization of risk-reduction strategies for an individual or group
Health Education: Developing and providing instruction and learning experiences to facilitate voluntary adaptation of behavior conducive to health in individuals, families, groups, or communities

NURSING PRIORITY NO. 1 To identify client at risk:

- Assess client upon admission to care for conditions listed in Risk Factors. *Research shows that frailty in elderly person is demonstrated by three or more symptoms together: unintentional weight loss over a year, along with muscle loss and weakness; a feeling of fatigue/exhaustion, along with slow walking speed; and low levels of physical activity.*[1]
- Note individual's age and gender. *Fried's (2001) research study of more than 5,000 adults found that chances of frailty rose sharply after the age of 85. Also, women are more likely than men to be frail, possibly because women typically outlive men and "start out with less muscle mass than men and, once they lose it, they may cross the frailty threshold more rapidly than men."*[2]
- Refer to ND Frail Elderly Syndrome for additional assessment interventions.

NURSING PRIORITY NO. 2 To promote wellness (Teaching/Discharge Considerations):

- Develop plan of action with client/caregiver *to meet immediate needs for safety and self-care.*
- Assist with treatment of underlying comorbid medical, functional, cognitive, or psychiatric conditions *that could positively influence current situation (e.g., resolution of infection, treating anemia, addressing brain injury, delirium, social isolation, depression).*[3]

- Administer medications as appropriate *Studies show that optimized management of chronic conditions results in improved health status, fewer hospitalizations, and reductions in the physical declines associated with the frailty syndrome.*[4]
- Refer to dietitian or nutritionist to assist in planning meals to meet client's specific nutritional needs (e.g., calories, proteins, vitamins, micronutrients), taste, and abilities. *Plans could include offering client's favorite food(s), attending social events (e.g., ice cream social, happy hour), or participating in family-style meals. In addition, interventions may be geared toward treatment of depression, grief, or loss and cultural or environmental adaptation measures.*[5–7]
- Refer to physical and/or occupational therapist as indicated *to improve physical strength, endurance, and stamina. Note: Studies have supported that exercises (e.g., chair aerobics, stretching, resistance training, walking, tai chi) can improve balance and muscle and core strength, promoting physical function and endurance and reducing risk of falls.*[3,5]
- Encourage client to talk about positive aspects of life and to keep as physically active as possible *to reduce effects of dispiritedness (e.g., "feeling low," sense of being unimportant, disconnected).*
- Promote socialization *to provide additional stimulation and reduce sense of isolation.*
- Assist client/significant others to identify and/or access useful community resources (e.g., support groups, Meals on Wheels, social worker, home care or assistive care, placement services). *Enhances coping, assists with problem solving, and may reduce risks to client and caregiver.*
- Refer to ND Frail Elderly Syndrome for additional interventions as indicated.

DOCUMENTATION FOCUS

Assessment/Reassessment

- Identified risk factors.
- Perception of situation and personal significance.

Planning

- Plan of care and who is involved in the planning.
- Teaching plan.

Implementation/Evaluation

- Response to interventions and teaching plan.
- Attainment or progress toward desired outcomes.

Discharge Planning

- Long-term needs and who is responsible for actions to be taken.
- Specific referral made.

References

1. Cimons, M. (2013). Frailty is a medical condition, not an inevitable result of aging (Op-Ed). Retrieved December 2014 from http://www.livescience.com/41602-frailty-is-medical-condition.html.
2. Fried, L. P., Tangen, C. M., Walston, J., et al. (2001). Frailty in older adults: Evidence for a phenotype. *J Gerontol A Biol Sci Med Sci*, 56(3), M146–M157.
3. Ferrucc, L., Guralnik, J. M., Cavazzini, C., et al. (2003). The frailty syndrome: A critical issue in geriatric oncology. *Crit Rev Oncol Hematol*, 46(2), 127–137.
4. Palace, J. Z., Flood-Sulchdeo, J. (2014). The frailty syndrome. *Today's Geriatric Medicine*, 7(1), 18.
5. Cherniak, E. P., Florez, H. J., Troen, B. R., et al. (2007). Emerging therapies to treat frailty syndrome in the elderly. *Altern Med Rev*, 12(3), 246–258.
6. DiMaria-Ghalili, R. A., Amelia, E. (2005). Nutrition in older adults: Interventions and assessment can help curb the growing threat of malnutrition. *Am J Nurs*, 105(3), 40–50.
7. Robertson, R. G., Montagnini, M. (2004). Geriatric failure to thrive. *Am Family Med*, 70(2), 343–350.

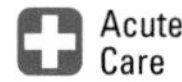

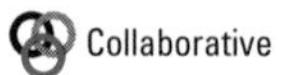

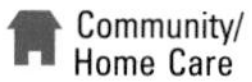

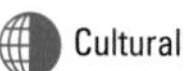

impaired Gas Exchange

Taxonomy II: Elimination and Exchange—Class 4 Respiratory Function (00030) [**Diagnostic Division:** Respiration], Submitted 1980; Revised 1996, 1998 by Nursing Diagnosis Extension and Classification

DEFINITION: Excess or deficit in oxygenation and/or carbon dioxide elimination at the alveoli-capillary membrane. [This may be an entity of its own but also may be an end result of another pathology with an interrelatedness between airway clearance and/or breathing pattern problems.]

RELATED FACTORS

Ventilation-perfusion imbalance [as in altered blood flow (e.g., pulmonary embolus, increased vascular resistance); heart failure; hypovolemic shock]
Alveolar-capillary membrane changes [e.g., acute respiratory distress syndrome; chronic conditions such as restrictive or obstructive lung disease, pneumoconiosis, asbestosis, silicosis]
[Altered oxygen supply (e.g., altitude sickness)]
[Altered oxygen-carrying capacity of blood (e.g., sickle cell or other anemia, carbon monoxide poisoning)]

DEFINING CHARACTERISTICS

Subjective

Dyspnea
Visual disturbance
Headache upon awakening
[Sense of impending doom]

Objective

Confusion
Restlessness; irritability
Somnolence
Abnormal arterial blood gases (ABGs) or arterial pH; hypoxia or hypoxemia; hypercapnia; decrease in carbon dioxide (CO_2) level
Cyanosis; abnormal skin color (e.g., pale, dusky, cyanosis)
Abnormal breathing pattern (e.g., rate, rhythm, depth); nasal flaring
Tachycardia; [dysrhythmias]
Diaphoresis
[Polycythemia]

Sample Clinical Applications: Chronic obstructive pulmonary disease (COPD), asthma, pneumonias, tuberculosis, heart failure, sickle cell anemia, acute respiratory distress syndrome (ARDS), high-altitude pulmonary edema, carbon monoxide poisoning

DESIRED OUTCOMES/EVALUATION CRITERIA

Sample NOC linkages:

Respiratory Status: Gas Exchange: Alveolar exchange of carbon dioxide and oxygen to maintain arterial blood gas concentrations
Tissue Perfusion: Pulmonary: Adequacy of blood flow through pulmonary vasculature to perfuse alveoli/capillary unit
Respiratory Status: Ventilation: Movement of air in and out of the lungs

Client Will (Include Specific Time Frame)

- Demonstrate improved ventilation and adequate oxygenation of tissues by ABGs within client's usual parameters and absence of symptoms of respiratory distress (as noted in Defining Characteristics).

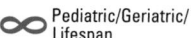

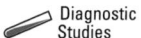

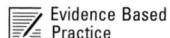

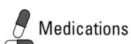

- Verbalize understanding of causative factors and appropriate interventions.
- Participate in treatment regimen (e.g., breathing exercises, effective coughing, use of oxygen) within level of ability and situation.

ACTIONS/INTERVENTIONS

Sample NIC linkages:

Respiratory Monitoring: Collection and analysis of patient data to ensure airway patency and adequate gas exchange

Oxygen Therapy: Administration of oxygen and monitoring of its effectiveness

Airway Management: Facilitation of patency of air passages

NURSING PRIORITY NO. 1 To assess causative/contributing factors:

- Note presence of factors listed in Related Factors. *Gas exchange problems can be related to multiple factors, including anemias, anesthesia, surgical procedures, high altitude, allergic response, altered level of consciousness, anxiety, fear, aspiration, decreased lung compliance, excessive or thick secretions, immobility, infection, medication and drug toxicity or overdose, neuromuscular impairment of breathing pattern, pain, and smoking.*
- Refer to NDs ineffective Airway Clearance and ineffective Breathing Pattern for additional assessment interventions as appropriate.

NURSING PRIORITY NO. 2 To evaluate degree of compromise (Acute Care):

- Evaluate respirations:

  Observe rate, rhythm, and depth. *Provides insight into the work of breathing and adequacy of alveolar ventilation. For example, increasing both rate and depth of respirations increases alveolar ventilation and occurs normally in response to exercise and stressors. Tachypnea is usually present to some degree during illness (especially with fever or upper respiratory infections), but if tachypnea is accompanied by use of accessory muscles of inspiration (e.g., external intercostals), the client may have insufficient muscle strength to sustain the work of breathing.*[1,9]

  Note client's reports/perceptions of breathing ease. *Client may report a range of symptoms (e.g., air hunger; shortness of breath with speaking, activity, or at rest).*

  Observe for dyspnea on exertion or gasping, changing positions frequently to ease breathing, and tendency to assume three-point position (bending forward while supporting self by placing one hand on each knee) *to maximize respiratory effort.*

  Note use of accessory muscles (e.g., scalene muscles, pectoralis minor, sternocleidomastoids, external intercostal muscles) *to assist diaphragm in increasing volume of thoracic cavity, which aids in inspiration.*

  (Lifespan) Observe infants/young children for nasal flaring and sternal retractions, *indicating increased work of breathing or respiratory distress.*

  Note use of abdominal muscles during expiration (normally a passive process) *to reduce thoracic dimensions and overcome airway resistance to expiration.*

- Evaluate lungs:

  Auscultate and percuss chest, describing presence or absence of breath sounds; note adventitious breath sounds. *Although air may be heard moving through the lung fields, breath sounds may be faint because of decreased airflow or areas of consolidation. In this nursing diagnosis, ventilatory effort is insufficient to deliver enough oxygen or to get rid of sufficient amounts of carbon dioxide. Abnormal breath sounds are indicative of numerous problems (e.g., hypoventilation such as might occur with atelectasis or presence of secretions, improper endotracheal [ET] tube placement, collapsed lung) and must be evaluated for further intervention.*[2,9]

- Note character and effectiveness of cough mechanism. *Affects ability to clear airways of secretions.*

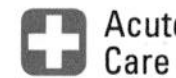 Acute Care 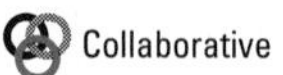 Collaborative 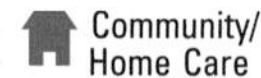 Community/ Home Care  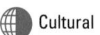 Cultural

- Evaluate skin and mucous membrane color, noting areas of pallor or cyanosis, for example, peripheral (nailbeds) versus central (around lips or earlobes) or general duskiness. *Duskiness and central cyanosis are late signs of hypoxemia.*[9]
- Evaluate behavior:
  Assess level of consciousness and mentation changes. *Decreased level of consciousness can be an indirect measurement of impaired oxygenation, but it also impairs one's ability to protect the airway, potentially further adversely affecting oxygenation.*
  Note somnolence, restlessness, and reports of headache on arising.
  Assess energy level and activity tolerance, noting reports or evidence of fatigue, weakness, and problems with sleep *that are associated with diminished oxygenation.*
- Monitor vital signs:
  Measure temperature. *A high fever greatly increases metabolic demands and oxygen consumption.*
  Monitor heart rate and rhythm. *Tachycardia and dysrhythmias may be noted as the heart reacts to cardiac ischemia and/or hypoxemia, especially during activity.*
  Monitor blood pressure (BP). *BP can be variable, depending on underlying condition and cardiopulmonary response.*
  Note increased pulmonary artery or right ventricular wedge pressures in the critically ill client with central lines. *Indicative of increased pulmonary vascular resistance.*
- Review pertinent diagnostic data (e.g., ABGs, hemoglobin, red blood cells, electrolytes) and chest radiography. Evaluate oxygen and carbon dioxide at bedside by means of pulse oximetry and end-tidal CO_2 monitoring (capnography). Note results of pulmonary function studies where available *to evaluate lung mechanics, capacities, and function. Blood studies are useful in revealing systemic reasons for problems with oxygenation and/or the results of hypoxemia and acid-base imbalances and to determine response to therapies. Point-of-care tools evaluate ventilation by providing breath-to-breath information. Recent studies have shown that capnography monitoring improves client outcomes through early recognition of hypoventilation, apnea, and airway obstruction, thus preventing hypoxic episodes. Client in respiratory failure typically shows hypoxemia and metabolic acidosis and is high risk for developing respiratory acidosis.*[4,6,9,10]

NURSING PRIORITY NO. 3 To correct/improve existing deficiencies:

- Elevate head of bed or position client appropriately. *Elevation or upright position facilitates respiratory function by gravity; however, client in severe distress will seek position of comfort. In ventilated client, prone position may be implemented in some clients to improve pulmonary perfusion and increase oxygen diffusion.*[3]
- Provide airway adjuncts and suction as indicated *to clear or maintain open airway, when client is unable to clear secretions, or to improve gas diffusion when client is showing desaturation of oxygen by oximetry or ABGs.*[3,5]
- Encourage frequent position changes, deep-breathing exercises or directed coughing, use of incentive spirometer, and chest physiotherapy as indicated. *Promotes optimal chest expansion, mobilization of secretions, and oxygen diffusion.*[3]
- Provide supplemental oxygen (via cannula, mask) using lowest concentration possible *dictated by pulse oximetry, ABGs, and client symptoms/underlying condition.*
- Ensure availability of proper emergency equipment, including ET/tracheostomy set and suction catheters appropriate for age and size of infant/child/adult. Avoid use of face mask in elderly emaciated client.
- Prepare for and assist with intubation and mechanical ventilation. *The decision to intubate and ventilate is made on a clinical diagnosis of respiratory failure, classified as hypoxemic or hypercapnic. Hypoxemic respiratory failure is the most common, associated with acute lung disorders such as pneumothorax, atelectasis, pulmonary edema, pneumonia, ARDS, and smoke inhalation. Hypercapnic respiratory failure can be seen in acute exacerbations of chronic COPD, head trauma, and spinal cord injury.*[4,11]
- Monitor and adjust ventilator settings (e.g., FIO_2, tidal volume, inspiratory and expiratory ratio, sigh, positive end–expiratory pressure) as indicated when mechanical support is being used. *The mode of ventilation*

(volume or pressure) and ventilator settings are determined by the specific needs of the client, which are determined by clinical evaluation and blood gas parameters.[11]

- Monitor for carbon dioxide narcosis (e.g., change in level of consciousness, changes in O_2 and CO_2 blood gas levels, flushing, decreased respiratory rate and headaches), *which may occur in clients receiving long-term oxygen therapy.*[6]
- Maintain adequate fluid intake *for mobilization of secretions* but avoid fluid overload *that may increase pulmonary congestion.*
- Provide psychological support, Active-listen questions and concerns. Address client's/significant other's (SO's) fears and anxiety that may be present. Maintain calm attitude while working with client/SOs. *Anxiety is contagious, and associated agitation can increase oxygen consumption and dyspnea.*
- Encourage adequate rest and limit activities to within client tolerance. Promote a calm, restful environment. *Facilitates relaxation and helps limit oxygen needs and consumption.*[3]
- Administer medications as indicated (e.g., inhaled and systemic glucocorticosteroids, antibiotics, bronchodilators, methylxanthines, antitussives/mucolytics, vasodilators). (Medications may be aerosolized or nebulized for enhanced response and limitation of side effects.) *Pharmacological agents are varied and specific to the client but are generally used to prevent and control symptoms, reduce frequency and severity of exacerbations, and improve exercise tolerance.*[11]
- Monitor therapeutic and adverse effects or interactions of drug therapy *to determine efficacy and need for change.*
- Use sedation judiciously *to avoid depressant effects on respiratory functioning.*[12]
- Minimize blood loss from procedures (e.g., blood draws—especially in neonates/infants, hemodialysis) *to limit effects of anemia and related gas diffusion impairment.*
- Assist with procedures as individually indicated (e.g., transfusion, phlebotomy, bronchoscopy) *to improve respiratory function/oxygen-carrying capacity.*
- Keep environment allergen/pollutant free *to reduce irritant effect of dust and chemicals on airways.*

NURSING PRIORITY NO. 4 To promote wellness (Teaching/Discharge Considerations):

- Review risk factors, particularly genetic, environmental, and employment-related conditions (e.g., sickle cell anemia, altitude sickness, exposure to toxins), *to help client/SO prevent complications or manage risk factors.*
- Discuss implications of smoking related to the illness or condition. Encourage client and SO(s) to stop smoking and attend cessation programs as necessary *to reduce health risks and/or prevent further decline in lung function.*[7,12]
- Review oxygen-conserving techniques (e.g., organizing tasks before beginning; sitting instead of standing to perform tasks; eating small meals; performing slower, purposeful movements) *to reduce oxygen demands.*[3]
- Reinforce need for adequate rest, while encouraging activity and exercise (e.g., upper and lower extremity endurance and strength training, and flexibility) *to decrease dyspnea and improve quality of life.*[8]
- Emphasize the importance of good general nutrition *for improving stamina and reducing the work of breathing.*[3,8]
- Refer to dietitian *for nutritional assessment and individual dietary plan as indicated.*[8,12]
- Instruct in the use of relaxation and stress-reduction techniques as appropriate.
- Review job description and work activities *to identify need for job modifications or vocational rehabilitation.*[3]
- Discuss home oxygen therapy use and instruct in safety concerns as indicated *to ensure client's safety, especially when used in the very young and fragile elderly or when cognitive or neuromuscular impairment is present.*[3]
- Identify specific supplier for supplemental oxygen and necessary respiratory devices, as well as other individually appropriate resources, such as home-care agencies, Meals on Wheels, etc., to facilitate independence.[3]

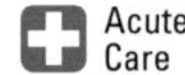

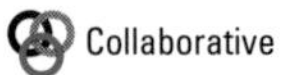

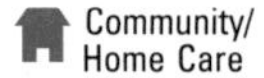

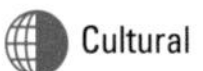

DOCUMENTATION FOCUS

Assessment/Reassessment

- Assessment findings, including respiratory rate, character of breath sounds; frequency, amount, and appearance of secretions; presence of cyanosis; laboratory findings; and mentation level.
- Conditions that may interfere with oxygen delivery or exchange.

Planning

- Plan of care, specific interventions, and who is involved in the planning.
- Liters of supplemental oxygen, ventilator settings.
- Teaching plan.

Implementation/Evaluation

- Client's responses to treatment, teaching, and actions performed.
- Attainment or progress toward desired outcome(s).
- Modifications to plan of care.

Discharge Planning

- Long-term needs, identifying who is responsible for actions to be taken.
- Community resources for equipment and supplies postdischarge.
- Specific referrals made.

References

1. Seay, S. J., Gay, S. L., Strauss, M. (2002). Tracheostomy emergencies. *Am J Nurs*, 102(3), 59.
2. Cox, H. C., Saidaromont, K., King, M., et al. (2002). *Clinical Applications of Nursing Diagnosis: Adult, Child, Women's, Psychiatric, Gerontic, and Home Health Considerations*. 4th ed. Philadelphia: F. A. Davis, 256–261.
3. Doenges, M. E., Moorhouse, M. F., Murr, A. C. (2010). *Nursing Care Plans: Guidelines for Individualizing Client Care Across the Life Span*. 8th ed. Philadelphia: F. A. Davis.
4. Carcillo, J. A., Fields, A. I. (2002). Clinical practice parameters for hemodynamic support of pediatric and neonatal patients in septic shock. *Crit Care Med*, 30(6), 1365–1378.
5. Fink, J. B., Hess, D. R. (2011). Secretion clearance techniques. In Hess, D. R., et al. (eds). *Respiratory Care: Principles and Practices*. 2nd ed. Sudbury, MA: Jones & Bartlett Learning.
6. Argyle, B. (1996). Blood gas text. Mad Scientist Software's Blood Gas Tutorial. Retrieved October 2015 from www.madsci.com/manu/gas_gen.htm.
7. Anderson, N. R. (2006). The role of the home healthcare nurse in smoking cessation: Guidelines for successful intervention. *Home Healthcare Nurse*, 24(7), 424–431.
8. McAllister, M. (2005). Promoting physiologic-physical adaptation in chronic obstructive pulmonary disease: Pharmacotherapeutic evidence-based research and guidelines. *Home Healthcare Nurse*, 23(8), 523–531.
9. Johnson, K. L., Munro, N. (2004). Diagnostic measures to evaluate oxygenation in critically ill adults: Implications and limitations. *AACN Adv Crit Care*, 15(4), 506–524.
10. Corbo, J., Bijur, P., Lahn, M., et al. (2005). Concordance between capnography and arterial blood gas measurements of carbon dioxide in acute asthma. *Ann Emerg Med*, 46(4), 323–327.
11. Byrum, D., Crabtree, C. (2009). Mechanical ventilation: Cruise control for the lungs. *Nursing Made Incredibly Easy!*, 7(5), 44–52.
12. Qaseem, A., Wilt, T. J., Weinberger, S. E., et al. (2011). Diagnosis and management of stable chronic obstructive pulmonary disease: A clinical practice guideline update. *Ann Intern Med*, 155(3), 179–191.

dysfunctional Gastrointestinal Motility

Taxonomy II: Elimination and Exchange—Class 2 Gastrointestinal Function (00196) [**Diagnostic Division:** Elimination], Submitted 2008

DEFINITION: Increased, decreased, ineffective, or lack of peristaltic activity within the gastrointestinal system.

RELATED FACTORS

Aging; prematurity
Treatment regimen
Malnutrition; enteral feedings
Food intolerance [e.g., gluten, lactose]; ingestion of contaminated material (e.g., radioactive food, water)
Sedentary lifestyle; immobility
Anxiety

DEFINING CHARACTERISTICS

Subjective

Absence of flatus
Abdominal cramping, pain
Diarrhea
Difficulty with defecation
Nausea; regurgitation

Objective

Change in bowel sounds
Abdominal distention
Acceleration of gastric emptying; diarrhea
Increase in gastric residual; bile-colored gastric residual
Hard, formed stool
Vomiting

Sample Clinical Applications: Abdominal or intestinal surgery, eating disorders, malnutrition, celiac disease, anemia, anxiety disorders, biliary cancer, cholecystectomy, Crohn's disease, irritable bowel syndrome, gastroesophageal reflux disease (GERD), gastritis, pancreatitis, quadriplegia, peritoneal dialysis, botulism, sepsis, multiple organ dysfunction syndrome, radiation therapy

DESIRED OUTCOMES/EVALUATION CRITERIA

Sample NOC linkages:

Gastrointestinal Function: Extent to which foods (ingested or tube-fed) are moved from ingestion to excretion
Knowledge: Treatment Regimen: Extent of understanding conveyed about a specific treatment regimen

Client Will (Include Specific Time Frame)

- Reestablish and maintain normal pattern of bowel functioning.
- Verbalize understanding of causative factors and rationale for treatment regimen.
- Demonstrate appropriate behaviors to assist with resolution of causative factors.

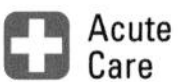

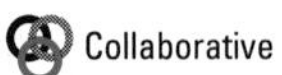

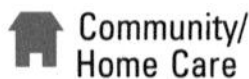

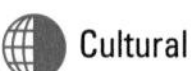

ACTIONS/INTERVENTIONS

Sample NIC linkages:
Bowel Management: Establishment and maintenance of a regular pattern of bowel elimination
Tube Care: Gastrointestinal: Management of a patient with a gastrointestinal (GI) tube
Nutrition Management: Assisting with or providing a balanced dietary intake of foods and fluids

NURSING PRIORITY NO. 1 To assess causative/contributing factors:

- Note presence of conditions (e.g., congestive heart failure, major trauma, sepsis) affecting systemic circulation and perfusion. *Blood loss or shock can result in hypoperfusion and short- or long-term GI dysfunction.*
- Determine presence of disorders causing localized or diffuse reduction in GI blood flow, such as esophageal varices, GI hemorrhage, pancreatitis, and intraperitoneal hemorrhage, *to identify client at higher risk for ineffective tissue perfusion.*
- Note presence of chronic or long-term disorders, such as GERD, hiatal hernia, inflammatory bowel (e.g., ulcerative colitis, Crohn's disease), malabsorption (e.g., dumping syndrome, celiac disease), and short-bowel syndrome, as may occur after surgical removal of portions of the small intestine. *These conditions are associated with increased, decreased, or ineffective peristaltic activity.*
- Note client's age and developmental concerns. *Children are prone to infections causing gastroenteritis, manifested by vomiting and diarrhea.*[1] *Premature or low-birth-weight neonates are at risk for developing necrotizing enterocolitis (NEC). The elderly have concerns associated with decreased motility (e.g., constipation related to slower peristalsis, lack of sufficient fiber and fluid intake, chronic use of laxatives).*[18]
- Note lifestyle issues *that can affect GI function (e.g., people who regularly engage in competitive sports such as long-distance running, cycling; persons with poor sanitary living conditions; people who travel to areas with contaminated food or water; overeating or intake of foods associated with gastric distress or intestinal distention).*[4]
- Review client's drug regimen. *Medications such as laxatives, antibiotics, anticholesterol agents, opiates, sedatives, and iron preparations may cause or exacerbate intestinal issues. In addition, the likelihood of bleeding increases from use of medications such as NSAIDs, Coumadin, and Plavix.*[2,3]
- Ascertain whether client is experiencing anxiety; acute, extreme, or chronic stress; or other psychogenic factors present in persons with emotional or psychiatric disorders (including anorexia/bulimia, etc.) *that can affect GI function.*[4,5]
- Review laboratory and other diagnostic studies. *Complete blood count may be done to evaluate for bleeding, inflammation, toxicity, and infection. Metabolic panel may reveal hepatic dysfunction, electrolyte imbalances, or low albumin levels. Computed tomography or other scans and abdominal ultrasound can help identify conditions like kidney or gallstones. X-rays may show bowel dilation or obstruction and stool and gas patterns.*[1,9,11,12] *Changes in white blood cell count with x-ray evidence of pneumoperitoneum (air in the abdominal cavity) in preterm neonate suggests NEC.*[18]

NURSING PRIORITY NO. 2 To note degree of dysfunction/organ involvement:

- Assess vital signs, noting presence of low blood pressure, elevated heart rate, and fever. *May suggest hypoperfusion or developing sepsis. Fever in presence of bright red blood in stool may indicate ischemic colitis.*
- Ascertain presence and characteristics of abdominal pain. *Pain is a common symptom of GI disorders and can vary in location, duration, and intensity.*[6] *Diffuse pain may reflect hypoperfusion of the gastrointestinal tract, which is particularly vulnerable to even small decreases in circulating volume.*[7] *Midepigastric pain immediately following meals and lasting several hours suggests abdominal angina due to atherosclerotic occlusive disease.*[19] *Tension pain caused by organ distention may develop in presence of bowel obstruction, constipation, or accumulation of pus or fluid. Inflammatory pain is deep and initially poorly localized, caused by irritation of either the visceral or the parietal peritoneum, as in acute appendicitis. Ischemic pain, the most serious type of visceral pain, has sudden onset, is intense, is progressive in severity, and is not relieved by analgesics. (Most common cause is strangulated bowel.)*[8]

- Investigate reports of pain out of proportion to degree of traumatic injury. *May reflect developing abdominal compartment syndrome.*[12]
- Inspect abdomen, noting contour. *Generalized distention may indicate presence of gas or fluid; local bulge could indicate hernia.*[7] Distention of the bowel may indicate accumulation of fluids (salivary, gastric, pancreatic, biliary, intestinal) and gases formed from bacteria, swallowed air, or any food or fluid the client has consumed.[9]
- Auscultate abdomen. *Hypoactive bowel sounds may indicate ileus. Hyperactive bowel sounds may indicate early intestinal obstruction or irritable bowel or GI bleeding. Presence of bruit may indicate blood traveling through narrowed arteries such as aorta.*[9,11]
- Palpate abdomen *to note masses, enlarged organs (e.g., spleen, liver, portions of colon), elicitation of pain with touch, and pulsation of aorta.*[9–11]
- Measure abdominal girth and compare with client's customary waist size/belt length *to monitor development or progression of distention possibly reflecting intra-abdominal bleeding, infection, or edema associated with toxins.*[10,12]
- Note frequency and characteristics of bowel movements. *Bowel movements by themselves are not necessarily diagnostic but need to be considered in total assessment because many different manifestations can occur. For example, diarrhea is the cardinal symptom of gastroenteritis, with severity depending on the causative organism. Both diarrhea and constipation can result from medications. Bloody diarrhea may indicate presence of ulcerative colitis, obstruction, or upper or lower gastrointestinal bleeding.*[1,9,14]
- Note presence of nausea, with or without vomiting, and relationship to food intake or other events, if indicated. *History of nausea and vomiting can provide important information about cause. For example, systemic conditions such as pregnancy, gastroenteritis, cancers, myocardial infarction, hepatitis, systemic infections, drug toxicity are often accompanied by nausea and vomiting. Timing of vomiting may be important, too. For example, vomiting immediately after meals could be indicative of bulimia, or vomiting large amounts several hours after eating can indicate delayed gastric emptying.*[5]
- Evaluate client's current nutritional status, noting ability to ingest and digest food. Inquire about food intolerances. Observe client's reactions to food, such as reluctance or refusal to eat, anorexia, or anxiety—wants to eat but cannot retain food. *Health depends on the intake, digestion, and absorption of nutrients, which both affects and is affected by GI function.*
- Measure intra-abdominal pressure as indicated. *Tissue edema or free fluid collecting in the abdominal cavity leads to intra-abdominal hypertension, which, if untreated, can cause abdominal compartment syndrome with end-stage organ failure.*[12]

NURSING PRIORITY NO. 3 To correct/improve existing dysfunction:

- Collaborate in treatment of underlying conditions *to correct or treat disorders associated with clients current GI dysfunction.*
- Maintain GI rest when indicated—NPO, fluids only, and gastric or intestinal decompression—*to reduce intestinal bloating and risk of vomiting.*
- Measure GI output periodically and note characteristics of drainage *to manage fluid losses and replacement needs and electrolyte balance.*
- Administer fluids and electrolytes as indicated *to replace losses and to improve GI circulation and function.*
- Encourage early ambulation. *Promotes general circulation and stimulates peristalsis and intestinal function.*
- Collaborate with dietician or nutritionist *to provide diet sufficient in nutrients by best possible route—oral, enteral, or parenteral.*
- Provide small servings of easily digested food and fluids when oral intake is tolerated.
- Encourage rest after meals *to maximize blood flow to digestive system.*
- Manage pain with medications as ordered and nonpharmacologic interventions such as positioning, back rub, and heating pad (unless contraindicated) *to enhance muscle relaxation and reduce discomfort.*[7]
- Encourage client to report changes in nature or intensity of pain *as this may indicate worsening of condition, requiring more intensive interventions.*[13]
- Collaborate with physician for medication management. *Oral medications can be absorbed erratically and can change the therapeutic effect or lead to increased side effects of a particular drug.*[15] *Dose modifica-*

 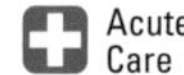 Acute Care 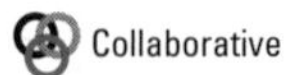 Collaborative 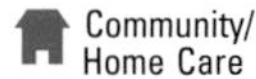 Community/Home Care 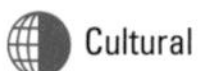 Cultural

tion, discontinuation of certain drugs (e.g., laxatives, opioids, antidepressants, iron supplements), or alternative route of administration may be required over a long period of time to improve client's GI function.[14,17]

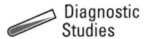

- Prepare client for procedures and surgery as indicated. *May require a variety of interventions, including endoscopic procedures, appendectomy, bowel resection with/without ostomy, percutaneous transluminal angioplasty, abdominal-aortic bypass graft, mesenteric revascularization, endarterectomy, etc., to treat problem causing or contributing to severe GI dysfunction.*

NURSING PRIORITY NO. 4 To promote wellness (Teaching/Discharge Considerations):

- Provide information regarding cause of GI dysfunction and treatment plans, utilizing best learning methods for client and including written information and bibliography of other resources for postdischarge learning. *May help client/significant other to manage symptoms in a manner more acceptable to them if this is a long-term issue.*
- Discuss normal variations in bowel patterns *to help alleviate unnecessary concern, initiate planned interventions, or seek timely medical care. This may prevent overuse of laxatives or help client understand when food, fluid, or drug modifications are needed.*[14]
- Encourage discussion of feelings regarding prognosis and long-term effects of condition. *Major or unplanned life changes can strain coping abilities, impairing functioning and jeopardizing relationships, and may even result in depression.*
- Discuss value of relaxation and distraction techniques or counseling *if anxiety or other emotional/psychiatric issue is suspected to play a role in GI dysfunction.*[5]
- Identify necessary changes in lifestyle and assist client to incorporate disease management into activities of daily living. *Promotes independence and enhances self-concept regarding ability to deal with change and manage own needs.*
- Review specific dietary changes or restrictions with client. *The client with GI disturbances may need to make various adaptations in food choices and eating habits (e.g., may need to avoid overeating in general, schedule mealtime in relation to activities and bedtime, avoid certain foods [or food element, such as wheat or gluten] and/or alcohol).*
- Suggest healthier variations in preparation of foods, as indicated—broiled instead of fried, spices added to foods instead of salt, addition of higher fiber foods, and use of lactose-free dairy products—*when these factors are affecting GI health.*[11]
- Review use of dietary fiber as a means of managing constipation and incontinence. *Studies have shown that supplementation with dietary fiber from psyllium or gum arabic is associated with a decrease in incontinence and improved stool consistency.*[16]
- Discuss fluid intake appropriate to individual situation. *Water is necessary to general health and GI function. The individual may need encouragement and instruction about how to take in enough fluids or may need fluid restrictions for certain medical conditions.*
- Recommend maintenance of normal weight, or weight loss if client is obese, *to decrease risk associated with GI disorders such as GERD or gallbladder disease.*
- Recommend smoking cessation. *Risk for acquiring or exacerbating certain GI disorders (e.g., Crohn's disease) may be increased with smoking. A recent review of relevant studies revealed various deleterious short- and long-term effects of smoking on the GI circulation and organs.*[13]
- Discuss medication regimen, including reasons for/consequences of failure to take prescribed long-term maintenance therapy (e.g., client with ulcerative colitis may require continuous treatment with 5-aminosalicylates to maintain remission). *Although many reasons are given for failing to take medications as prescribed, including denial of illness, forgetfulness, and costs of prescriptions, nonadherence negatively affects treatment efficacy and client's quality of life.*[17]
- Emphasize importance of avoiding use of NSAIDs (including aspirin), corticosteroids, some over-the-counter-drugs, vitamins containing potassium, mineral oil, or alcohol when taking anticoagulants. *These medications can be harmful to GI mucosa and increase risk of bleeding.*[9]
- Refer to NDs Constipation, bowel Incontinence, and Diarrhea for additional interventions, as needed.

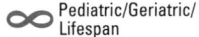

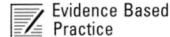

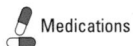

DOCUMENTATION FOCUS

Assessment/Reassessment

- Individual findings, noting nature, extent, and duration of problem; effect on independence and lifestyle.
- Dietary pattern, recent intake, food intolerances.
- Frequency and characteristics of stools.
- Characteristics of abdominal tenderness or pain, precipitators, and what relieves pain.

Planning

- Plan of care and who is involved in planning.
- Teaching plan.

Implementation/Evaluation

- Response to interventions, teaching, and actions performed.
- Attainment or progress toward desired outcome(s).
- Modifications to plan of care.

Discharge Planning

- Long-term needs and who is responsible for actions to be taken.
- Available resources, specific referrals made.

References

1. Sommers, M. S., Johnson, S. A., Beery, T. A. (2007). *Diseases and Disorders: A Nursing Therapeutics Manual*. 3rd ed. Philadelphia: F. A. Davis.
2. Neal-Boylan, L. (2007). Health assessment of the very old person at home. *Home Healthcare Nurse*, 25(6), 388–398.
3. Tabloski, P. A. (2006). *Gerontological Nursing*. Upper Saddle River, NJ: Pearson Prentice Hall.
4. Pasley, J. (2004). Introduction to gastrointestinal physiology. University of Arkansas Medical School Lecture. Retrieved March 2015 from http://www.uams.edu/m2008/notes/phys/pdf/April%2016%20Intro%20to%20GI%20Phys.pdf.
5. Muraoka, M., Mine, K., Matsumoto, K. (1990). Psychogenic vomiting: The relation between patterns of vomiting and psychiatric diagnoses. *Gut*, 31(5), 526–528.
6. Holcomb, S. S. (2008). Acute abdomen: What a pain! *Nursing*, 38(9), 34–40.
7. Sartin, J. S. (2005). Gastrointestinal disorders. In Copstead, L. E. C., Banasik, J. L. (eds). *Pathophysiology*. 3rd ed. St. Louis, MO: Elsevier Saunders.
8. Schulman, C. (2002). End points of resuscitation: Choosing the right parameters to monitor. *Dimens Crit Care Nurs*, 21(1), 2–10.
9. Miller, S. K., Alpert, P. T. (2006). Assessment and differential diagnosis of abdominal pain. *Nurs Pract*, 31(7), 39–47.
10. Held-Warmkessel, J., Schiech, L. (2008). Responding to four gastrointestinal complications in cancer patients. *Nursing*, 38(7), 32–38.
11. Hogstel, M. O., Curry, L. C. (2005). *Health Assessment Through the Life Span*. 4th ed. Philadelphia: F. A. Davis.
12. Paula, R. (Updated 2014). Abdominal compartment syndrome. Retrieved March 2015 from http://emedicine.medscape.com/article/829008-overview.
13. Massarratt, S. (2008). Smoking and the gut: Review article. *Arch Iranian Med*, 11(3), 293–305.
14. Hill, R. (2007). Don't let constipation stop you up. *Nursing Made Incredibly Easy!*, 5(5), 40–47.
15. Feigenbaum, K. (2006). Update on gastroparesis. *Gastroenterol Nurs*, 29(3), 239–244.
16. Bliss, D. Z., Jung, H. J., Savik, K., et al. (2001). Supplementation with dietary fiber improves fecal incontinence. *Nurs Res*, 50(4), 203–213.
17. Turnbough, L., Wilson, L. (2007). Take your medicine: Nonadherence issues in patients with ulcerative colitis. *Gastroenterol Nurs*, 30(3), 212–217.
18. O'Neill, J. A., Grasfeld, J., Fonkalsrud, E. (eds.) (2003). Necrotizing enterocolitis (NEC). *In Principles of Pediatric Surgery*. 2nd ed. St. Louis, MO: Mosby.
19. Aziz, F., Comerota, A. J. (2014). Abdominal angina. Retrieved March 2015 from http://emedicine.medscape.com/article/188618-overview.

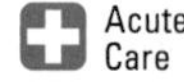

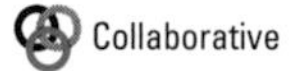

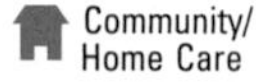

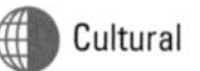

risk for dysfunctional Gastrointestinal Motility

Taxonomy II: Elimination and Exchange—Class 2 Gastrointestinal Function (00197) [**Diagnostic Division:** Elimination], Submitted 2008; Revised 2013

DEFINITION: Vulnerable to a decrease in normal frequency of defecation accompanied by difficult or incomplete passage of stool, which may compromise health.

RISK FACTORS

Aging; prematurity
Decrease in gastrointestinal (GI) circulation
Eating habit change (e.g., foods, eating times); unsanitary food preparation
Food intolerance [e.g., gluten, lactose]; change in water source
Pharmaceutical agent [e.g., antibiotics, laxatives, narcotics/opiates, proton-pump inhibitors]
Gastroesophageal reflux disease (GERD)
Diabetes mellitus
Infection
Sedentary lifestyle; immobility
Stressors; anxiety
Note: A risk diagnosis is not evidenced by signs and symptoms, as the problem has not occurred; rather, nursing interventions are directed at prevention.

Sample Clinical Applications: Abdominal or intestinal surgery, eating disorders, malnutrition, celiac disease, anemia, anxiety disorders, biliary cancer, cholecystectomy, Crohn's disease, irritable bowel syndrome, GERD, gastritis, pancreatitis, quadriplegia, peritoneal dialysis, botulism, sepsis, multiple organ dysfunction syndrome, radiation therapy

DESIRED OUTCOMES/EVALUATION CRITERIA

Sample NOC linkages:

Gastrointestinal Function: Extent to which foods (ingested or tube-fed) are moved from ingestion to excretion

Knowledge: Treatment Regimen: Extent of understanding conveyed about a specific treatment regimen

Client Will (Include Specific Time Frame)

- Maintain normal pattern of bowel functioning.
- Verbalize understanding of individual risk factors and benefits of managing condition.
- Identify preventive interventions to reduce risk and promote normal bowel pattern.

ACTIONS/INTERVENTIONS

Sample NIC linkages:

Bowel Management: Establishment and management of a regular pattern of bowel elimination

Tube Care: Gastrointestinal: Management of a patient with a GI tube

Nutrition Management: Assisting with or providing a balanced dietary intake of foods and fluids

NURSING PRIORITY NO. 1 To identify individual risk factors/needs:

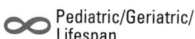

- Note presence of conditions affecting systemic circulation and perfusion such as congestive heart failure, major trauma, sepsis, etc. *Blood loss or shock can result in hypoperfusion, and short- or long-term GI dysfunction.*[1]
- Determine presence of disorders causing localized or diffuse reduction in GI blood flow (e.g., esophageal varices, intestinal cancer or obstruction; intestinal surgery; pancreatitis; prior history of bowel obstruction or

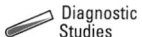

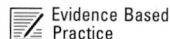

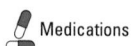

strangulated hernia; prior abdominal surgery with adhesions) *to identify client at higher risk for changes in peristaltic activity and intestinal dysfunction.*[2,13]

- Assess client's current situation with regard to prior GI history. *Client may have an isolated incident putting him or her at risk (e.g., blunt force trauma to abdomen) or at higher risk for recurrent GI dysfunction associated with history of prior GI problems.*
- Auscultate abdomen *to evaluate peristaltic activity. For example, either hypoactive or hyperactive bowel sounds may indicate developing bowel disorders.*[9,10]
- Palpate abdomen for masses, enlarged organs (e.g., spleen, liver, portions of colon), and elicitation of pain with touch *that could point to changes in organ size or function.*[9–11]
- Note frequency and characteristics of bowel movements. *Bowel movements by themselves are not necessarily diagnostic but need to be considered in total assessment because many different manifestations can occur.*[1,9,12]
- Ascertain presence and characteristics of abdominal pain. *Pain is a common symptom of GI disorders, with location and type aiding in identifying underlying problems.*[8]
- Assess vital signs for changes in blood pressure, heart rate, or body temperature. *May suggest injury or infection of the GI organs or development of a systemic infection/sepsis.*
- Evaluate client's current nutritional status, noting ability to ingest and digest food. *Health depends on the intake, digestion, and absorption of nutrients, which both affects and is affected by GI function.*
- Note client's age and developmental concerns. *Children are prone to infections causing gastroenteritis manifested by vomiting and diarrhea.*[1] *The elderly have problems associated with decreased motility (e.g., constipation is often a concern related to slower peristalsis, lack of sufficient fiber and fluid intake, chronic use of laxatives).*[3,4] *Premature or low-birth-weight neonates are at risk for developing necrotizing enterocolits.*[5]
- Note lifestyle issues *that can affect GI function (e.g., people who regularly engage in competitive sports such as long-distance running, cycling), persons with poor sanitary living conditions, people who travel to areas with contaminated food or water, overeating or intake of foods associated with gastric distress or intestinal distention, and anorexia or bulimia.*[6]
- Ascertain whether client is experiencing acute, extreme, or chronic anxiety; stress; or other psychogenic factors present in person with emotional or psychiatric disorders (including anorexia and bulimia), *which can affect GI function,*[7]
- Review client's drug regimen. *Medications such as laxatives, antibiotics, anticholesterol agents, opiates, sedatives, and iron preparations may cause or exacerbate intestinal issues. In addition, likelihood of bleeding increases from use of medications such as NSAIDs, Coumadin, and Plavix.*[3,4]
- Review laboratory and other diagnostic studies *to identify if conditions or disorders are present that may affect GI system or GI function.*

NURSING PRIORITY NO. 2 To reduce or correct individual risk factors:

- Discuss normal variations in bowel patterns *so client can initiate planned interventions or seek timely medical care. This may prevent complications, such as overuse of laxatives, or help client understand when regular exercise or food, fluid, or drug modifications are needed to improve or maintain GI health.*
- Collaborate in treatment of underlying conditions *to correct or treat disorders that could impact GI function.*
- Practice and promote hand hygiene and other infection precautions *to prevent transmission of infections that may cause/spread GI illnesses.*
- Maintain GI rest when indicated (e.g., NPO, fluids only, gastric or intestinal decompression after abdominal surgery) *to reduce intestinal bloating and reduce risk of vomiting.*
- Administer fluids and electrolytes as indicated *to replace losses and to maintain GI circulation and function.*
- Administer prescribed prophylactic medications (e.g., antiemetics, proton-pump inhibitors, antihistamines, anticholinergics, antibiotics) *to reduce potential for GI complications such as bleeding, ulceration of stomach mucosa, and viral diarrheas.*

Acute Care 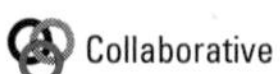 Collaborative 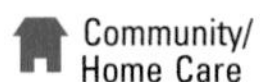 Community/ Home Care 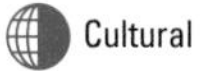 Cultural

- Collaborate with dietician or nutritionist *to provide diet sufficient in nutrients and provided by best possible route (e.g., oral, enteral, parenteral).*[2,14]
- Emphasize importance of and assist with early ambulation and ongoing exercise following surgery or other procedures. Assist client with mobility issues and refer to physical therapy as indicated *to help reduce GI complications associated with immobility and a sedentary lifestyle.*
- Encourage relaxation and distraction techniques if anxiety is suspected to play a role in GI dysfunction.[7]
- Refer to NDs Constipation, bowel Incontinence, Diarrhea, and dysfunctional Gastrointestinal Motility for additional interventions.

NURSING PRIORITY NO. 3 To promote wellness (Teaching/Discharge Considerations):

- Review measures to maintain bowel health:
  Use of dietary fiber and/or stool softeners. *Studies have shown that supplementation with dietary fiber from psyllium or gum arabic is associated with a decrease in incontinence and improved stool consistency.*[12,15]
  Fluid intake appropriate to individual. *Water is necessary to general health and GI function. The individual may need encouragement and instruction about how to take in enough fluids or may need fluid restrictions for certain medical conditions.*
  Establish or maintain regular bowel evacuation habits, incorporating privacy needs, assistance to bathroom on regular schedule, etc., as indicated.
  Emphasize benefits of regular exercise in promoting normal GI function.
- Discuss dietary recommendations with client/significant other. *The client with potential for GI disturbances may elect to make adaptations in food choices and eating habits (e.g., to avoid overeating in general, schedule mealtime in relation to activities and bedtime, avoid certain foods and/or alcohol).*
- Instruct in healthier variations in preparation of foods as indicated (e.g., broiled instead of fried, spices added to foods instead of salt, addition of higher fiber foods, lactose-free dairy products) *when these factors may affect GI health.*
- Recommend maintenance of normal weight, or weight loss if client is obese, *to decrease risk associated with GI disorders such as GERD or gallbladder disease.*
- Collaborate with physician in medication management. *Oral medications can be absorbed erratically and can change the therapeutic effect or lead to increased side effects of a particular drug.*[16] *Dose modification, discontinuation of certain drugs (e.g., laxatives, opioids, antidepressants, iron supplements), or alternative route of administration may be required over a long period of time to reduce risk of GI dysfunction.*[12,17]
- Emphasize importance of discussing with physician current and new prescribed medications and/or planned use of certain medications (e.g., NSAIDs [including aspirin], corticosteroids, some over-the-counter drugs, herbals supplements), *which can be harmful to GI mucosa.*
- Recommend smoking cessation. *Risk for acquiring or exacerbating certain GI disorders (e.g., Crohn's disease) may be increased with smoking. Note: A recent review of relevant studies reveals various deleterious short- and long-term effects of smoking on GI circulation and organs.*[19]
- Review food- and water-borne illnesses and contamination and hygiene issues, as indicated, and make needed follow-up referrals. *Many different types of viruses, bacteria, and parasites can cause GI illnesses. This can affect a household, a day-care center, a college dorm, international travelers, or a whole segment of population. Information may be given to individuals, groups, and/or public in general.*
- Refer to appropriate resources (e.g., social services, public health services) for follow-up if client is at risk for ingestion of contaminated water or food sources or would benefit from teaching concerning food preparation and storage.
- Encourage vaccinations. *The Centers for Disease Control and Prevention make recommendations for travelers and/or persons in high-risk areas or situations to receive certain vaccinations. Typhoid vaccine, for example, is indicated for travel to areas where a person might be exposed to contaminated food or water. For young children susceptible to severe gastroenteritis, the oral rotavirus vaccine can prevent 85% to 98% of rotavirus gastroenteritis.*[18,20]

DOCUMENTATION FOCUS

Assessment/Reassessment

- Individual findings, noting specific risk factors.
- Dietary pattern, recent intake, food intolerances.
- Frequency and characteristics of stools.

Planning

- Plan of care and who is involved in planning.
- Teaching plan.

Implementation/Evaluation

- Response to interventions, teaching, and actions performed.
- Attainment or progress toward desired outcome(s).
- Modifications to plan of care.

Discharge Planning

- Long-term needs and who is responsible for actions to be taken.
- Available resources and specific referrals made.

References

1. Sommers, M. S., Johnson, S. A., Beery, T. A. (2007). *Diseases and Disorders: A Nursing Therapeutics Manual.* 3rd ed. Philadelphia: F. A. Davis.
2. Goldberg, S. M. (2008). Identifying intestinal obstruction: Better safe than sorry. *Nurs Crit Care,* 3(5), 18–23.
3. Neal-Boylan, L. (2007). Health assessment of the very old person at home. *Home Healthcare Nurs,* 25(6), 388–398.
4. Tabloski, P. A. (ed.) (2006). *Gerontological Nursing.* Upper Saddle River, NJ: Pearson Prentice Hall.
5. O'Neill, J., Grasfeld, J., Fonkalsrud, E. (eds.) (2003). Necrotizing Enterocolitis (NEC). *In Principles of Pediatric Surgery.* 2nd ed. St. Louis, MO: Mosby.
6. Pasley, J. (2004). Introduction to gastrointestinal physiology. University of Arkansas Medical School Lecture. Retrieved March 2015 from http://www.uams.edu/m2008/notes/phys/pdf/April%2016%20Intro%20to%20GI%20Phys.pdf.
7. Muraoka, M., Mine, K. (1990). Psychogenic vomiting: The relation between patterns of vomiting and psychiatric diagnoses. *Gut,* 31(5), 526–528.
8. Holcomb, S. S. (2008). Acute abdomen: What a pain! *Nursing,* 38(9), 34–40.
9. Miller, S. K., Alpert, P. T. (2006). Assessment and differential diagnosis of abdominal pain. *Nurse Pract,* 31(7), 39–47.
10. Hogstel, M. O., Curry, L. C. (2005). *Health Assessment Through the Life Span.* 4th ed. Philadelphia: F. A. Davis.
11. Held-Warmkessel, J., Schiech, L. (2008). Responding to four gastrointestinal complications in cancer patients. *Nursing,* 38(7), 32–38.
12. Hill, R. (2007). Don't let constipation stop you up. *Nursing Made Incredibly Easy!,* 5(5), 40–47.
13. Paula, R. (Updated 2014). Abdominal compartment syndrome. Retrieved March 2015 from http://emedicine.medscape.com/article/829008-overview.
14. Glare, P. A., Dunwoodie, D., Clark, K., et al. (2008). Treatment of nausea and vomiting in terminally ill cancer patients. *Drugs,* 68(18), 2575–2590.
15. Bliss, D. Z., Jung, H. J., Savik, K., et al. (2001). Supplementation with dietary fiber improves fecal incontinence. *Nurs Res,* 50(4), 203–213.
16. Feigenbaum, K. (2006). Update on gastroparesis. *Gastroenterol Nurs,* 29(3), 239–244.
17. Day, M. W. (2008). Fight back against inflammatory bowel disease. *Nursing,* 38(11), 34–40.
18. Centers for Disease Control and Prevention. (Updated 2015). Vaccines and immunizations, various pages. Retrieved March 2015 from http://www.cdc.gov/vaccines/.
19. Massarratt, S. (2008). Smoking and the gut: Review article. *Arch Iranian Med,* 11(3), 34–40.
20. Cortese, M. M., Parashar, U. D. (2009). Prevention of Rotavirus Gastroenteritis Among Infants and Children. Recommendations of the Advisory Committee on Immunization Practices. *Centers for Disease Control and Prevention.* Retrieved March 2015 from http://www.cdc.gov/mmwr/preview/mmwrhtml/rr5802a1.htm.

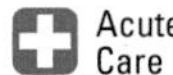

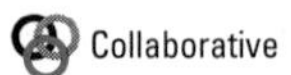

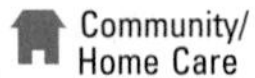

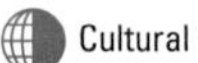

risk for ineffective Gastrointestinal Perfusion

Taxonomy II: Activity/Rest Class 4: Cardiovascular/Pulmonary Responses (00202) [**Diagnostic Division:** Circulation], Submitted 2008; revised 2013

DEFINITION: Vulnerable to decrease in gastrointestinal circulation, which may compromise health.

RISK FACTORS

Abdominal aortic aneurysm; abdominal compartment syndrome
Abnormal prothrombin time (PT); abnormal partial thromboplastin time (PTT); coagulopathy (e.g., sickle cell anemia); anemia; disseminated intravascular coagulopathy; hemodynamic instability
Age >60 years; female gender
Cerebral vascular accident; vascular disease; diabetes mellitus
Gastrointestinal (GI) condition (e.g., ulcer, ischemic colitis or pancreatitis); acute gastrointestinal hemorrhage; gastroesophageal varices
Impaired liver function (e.g., cirrhosis, hepatitis)
Myocardial infarction; decrease in left ventricular performance
Renal disease (e.g., polycystic kidney, renal artery stenosis, failure)
Smoking
Trauma; treatment regimen
Note: A risk diagnosis is not evidenced by signs and symptoms, as the problem has not occurred; rather, nursing interventions are directed at prevention.
Sample Clinical Applications: Gastrointestinal (GI) bleed, atherosclerosis, sickle cell anemia, diabetes, pancreatitis, congestive heart failure (CHF), cirrhosis, hemorrhage shock

DESIRED OUTCOMES/EVALUATION CRITERIA

Sample NOC linkages:
Tissue Perfusion: Abdominal Organs: Adequacy of blood flow through the small vessels of the abdominal viscera to maintain organ function
Gastrointestinal Function: Extent to which foods (ingested or tube-fed) are moved from ingestion to evacuation

Client Will (Include Specific Time Frame)
- Demonstrate adequate tissue perfusion as evidenced by active bowel sounds and absence of abdominal pain, nausea, and vomiting.
- Verbalize understanding of condition, therapy regimen, side effects of medication, and when to contact healthcare provider.
- Engage in behaviors or lifestyle changes to improve circulation (e.g., smoking cessation, diabetic glucose control, medication management).

ACTIONS/INTERVENTIONS

Sample NIC linkages:
Surveillance: Purposeful and ongoing acquisition, interpretation, and synthesis of patient data for clinical decision making
Circulatory Care: Arterial Insufficiency: Promotion of arterial circulation
Gastrointestinal Intubation: Insertion of a tube into the GI tract

NURSING PRIORITY NO. 1 To assess causative/contributing factors:

- Note presence of conditions affecting systemic circulation/perfusion such as heart failure with left ventricular dysfunction, major trauma with hypotension, surgery with major blood loss, septic shock, and so forth. *Blood loss and hypovolemic or hypotensive shock can result in GI hypoperfusion and bowel ischemia.*[1]
- Determine presence of disorders such as esophageal varices, pancreatitis, abdominal or chest trauma, increase of intra-abdominal pressure or abdominal hypertension, prior history of bowel obstruction or strangulated hernia, or prior abdominal surgery with adhesions *that could cause local or regional reduction in GI blood flow.*[2–5,22]
- Identify client with history of bleeding or coagulation disorders, such as prior GI bleed, sickle cell anemia, or other coagulopathies and cancer, *to identify risk for potential bleeding problems complicating current situation (e.g., client having elective surgical procedure) or exacerbation of comorbidities.*
- Note client's age and gender. *Studies suggest that risk increases with age in both sexes and that risk is higher in men than women when assessing risk for GI bleed and abdominal aortic aneurysm.*[1,6] *Premature or low-birth-weight neonates are at risk for developing necrotizing enterocolitis.*[21]
- Investigate reports of abdominal pain, noting location, intensity, duration, and relationship to activities (e.g., eating, lifting heavy objects), trauma, surgery, or acute or chronic conditions causing displacement of abdominal organs accompanied by abdominal distention (e.g., peritonitis, cirrhosis, ascites), etc. *Many disorders can result in abdominal pain, some of which can include conditions affecting GI perfusion, such as postprandial abdominal angina due to occlusive mesenteric vascular disease, abdominal compartment syndrome, or other potential perforating disorders such as a duodenal or gastric ulcer or ischemic pancreatitis.*[4,7,8]
- Review routine medication regimen (e.g., NSAIDs, Coumadin, low-dose aspirin such as used for prophylaxis in certain cardiovascular conditions, corticosteroids). *Likelihood of bleeding increases from use of such medications.*[9–11]
- Note history of smoking, *which can potentiate vasoconstriction, or* excessive alcohol use or abuse, *which can cause general inflammation of the stomach mucosa and potentiate risk of GI bleeding or liver involvement and esophageal varices.*
- Auscultate abdomen to evaluate peristaltic activity. *Hypoactive or absent bowel sounds may indicate intraperitoneal injury and bowel perforation and bleeding. Abdominal bruit can indicate abdominal aortic injury or aneurysm.*[5]
- Palpate abdomen for distension, masses, enlarged organs (e.g., spleen, liver, or portions of colon), elicitation of pain with touch, and pulsation of aorta, *which could identify problem in GI organs or circulation system.*[12–14]
- Percuss abdomen for fixed or shifting dullness over regions that normally contain air. *Can indicate accumulated blood or fluid.*[15]
- Measure and monitor progression of abdominal girth as indicated. *Abdominal distention can reflect bowel problems such as ileus or other bowel obstruction. It may also be indicative of organ failure (e.g., heart, liver, kidney) or organ injury or enlargement/displacement with intra-abdominal fluid and gas accumulation. These conditions can cause or exacerbate GI perfusion problems.*[8]
- Note reports of nausea or vomiting along with problems with elimination. *May reflect hypoperfusion of the GI tract, which is particularly vulnerable to even small decreases in circulating volume.*[16]
- Assess client with severe or prolonged vomiting, forceful coughing, lifting and straining activities, or childbirth, *which can result in a tear in the esophageal or stomach wall resulting in hemorrhage.*
- Evaluate stools for color and consistency. Test for occult blood, as indicated. *If bleeding is present, stools may be black or "tarry," currant-colored, or bright red. Consistency can range from normal with occult blood to thick liquid stools.*[1]
- Assess vital signs noting sustained hypotension, *which can result in hypoperfusion of abdominal organs.*
- Test gastric suction contents for blood when tube is used to decompress stomach and/or manage vomiting. *Can help in early identification of bleeding complications.*
- Review laboratory tests and other diagnostic studies (e.g., complete blood count, bilirubin, liver enzymes, electrolytes, stool guaiac; endoscopy, abdominal ultrasound or computed tomography, aortic angiogra-

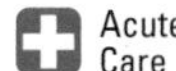

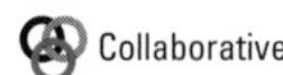

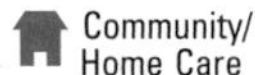

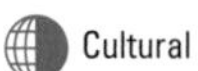

phy, paracentesis) *to identify if conditions or disorders are present that may affect GI perfusion and function.*[8,13]
- Measure intra-abdominal pressure as indicated. *Tissue edema or free fluid collecting in the abdominal cavity leads to intra-abdominal hypertension, which, if untreated, can cause abdominal compartment syndrome with end-stage organ failure.*[23]

NURSING PRIORITY NO. 2 To reduce or correct individual risk factors:

- Collaborate in treatment of underlying conditions *to correct or treat disorders that could affect GI perfusion.*
- Administer fluids and electrolytes as indicated *to replace losses and to maintain GI circulation and function.*
- Administer prescribed prophylactic medications in at-risk clients during illness and hospitalization (e.g., antiemetics, proton-pump inhibitors, antihistamines, anticholinergics, antibiotics) *to reduce potential for stress-related GI complications such as bleeding and ulceration of stomach mucosa.*[17,18]
- Maintain gastric or intestinal decompression; when indicated, measure output periodically and note characteristics of drainage.
- Provide small and easily digested food and fluids when oral intake is tolerated.
- Encourage rest after meals *to maximize blood flow to digestive system.*
- Prepare client for surgery as indicated. *May be a surgical emergency (e.g., gastric resection, bypass graft, mesenteric endarterectomy).*
- Refer to NDs dysfunctional Gastrointestinal Motility, risk for Bleeding, Nausea, and imbalanced Nutrition: less than body requirements for additional interventions.

NURSING PRIORITY NO. 3 To promote wellness (Teaching/Discharge Considerations):

- Discuss individual risk factors (e.g., family history, obesity, age, smoking, hypertension, diabetes, clotting disorders) and potential outcomes of atherosclerosis (e.g., systemic and peripheral vascular disease conditions). *Information necessary for client to make informed choices about remedial risk factors and commit to lifestyle changes as appropriate to prevent onset of complications or manage symptoms when condition is present.*
- Identify necessary changes in lifestyle and assist client to incorporate disease management into activities of daily living. *Promotes independence and enhances self-concept regarding ability to deal with change and manage own needs.*
- Encourage client to quit smoking and join Smoke-out or another smoking-cessation program.
- Establish regular exercise program *to enhance circulation and promote general well-being.*[19]
- Emphasize importance of routine follow-up and laboratory monitoring as indicated. *Important for effective disease management and possible changes in therapeutic regimen.*
- Emphasize importance of discussing with primary care provider current and new prescribed medications and/or planned use of certain medications (e.g., anticoagulants, NSAIDs including aspirin; corticosteroids, some over-the-counter drugs, herbal supplements), *which can be harmful to GI mucosa or cause bleeding.*[20]

DOCUMENTATION FOCUS

Assessment/Reassessment

- Individual findings, noting specific risk factors.
- Vital signs, adequacy of circulation.
- Abdominal assessment, characteristics of emesis/gastric drainage and stools.

Planning

- Plan of care and who is involved in planning.
- Teaching plan.

Implementation/Evaluation

- Response to interventions, teaching, and actions performed.
- Attainment or progress toward desired outcome(s).
- Modifications to plan of care.

Discharge Planning

- Long-term needs and who is responsible for actions to be taken.
- Available resources, specific referrals made.

References

1. Sommers, M. S., Johnson, S. A., Beery, T. A. (2007). *Diseases and Disorders: A Nursing Therapeutics Manual.* 3rd ed. Philadelphia: F. A. Davis.
2. Goldberg, S. M. (2008). Identifying intestinal obstruction: Better safe than sorry. *Nurs Crit Care*, 3(5), 18–25.
3. Feigenbaum, K. (2006). Update on gastroparesis. *Gastroenterol Nurs*, 29(3), 239–244.
4. Kelso, L. A. (2008). Cirrhosis: Caring for patients with end-stage liver failure. *Nurse Pract*, 33(7), 24–30.
5. Blank-Reid, C. (2007). Abdominal trauma: Dealing with the damage. *Nursing*, 37(4Suppl: ED), 4–11.
6. Tan, W. A., Powell, S., Nanjundappa, A. (Updated 2014). Abdominal aortic aneurysm, rupture imaging. Retrieved March 2015 from http://emedicine.medscape.com/article/416397-overview.
7. Aziz, F., Comerota, A. J. (Updated 2014). Abdominal angina. Retrieved March 2015 from http://emedicine.medscape.com/article/188618-overview.
8. Paula, R. (Updated 2014). Compartment syndrome, abdominal. Retrieved March 2015 from http://emedicine.medscape.com/article/829008-overview.
9. Neal-Boylan, L. (2007). Health assessment of the very old person at home. *Home Healthcare Nurse*, 25(6), 388–398.
10. Tabloski, P. A. (ed.) (2006). *Gerontological Nursing*. Upper Saddle River, NJ: Pearson Prentice Hall.
11. Estes, K., Thomure, J. (2008). Aspirin for the primary prevention of adverse cardiovascular events. *Crit Care Nurs Q*, 31(4), 324–338.
12. Miller, S. K., Alpert, P. T. (2006). Assessment and differential diagnosis of abdominal pain. *Nurse Pract*, 31(7), 39–47.
13. Hogstel, M. O., Curry, L. C. (2005). *Health Assessment Through the Life Span*. 4th ed. Philadelphia: F. A. Davis.
14. Held-Warmkessel, J., Schiech, L. (2008). Responding to 4 gastrointestinal complications in cancer patients. *Nursing*, 38(7), 32–38.
15. Dietzen, K. K. (2006). Assessment of the gastrointestinal system. In Ignatavicius, D. D., Workman, M. L. (eds). *Medical-Surgical Nursing: Critical Thinking for Collaborative Care*. 5th ed. St. Louis, MO: Elsevier Saunders.
16. Schulman, J., Schiech, C. (2002). End points of resuscitation: Choosing the right parameters to monitor. *Dimens Crit Care Nurs*, 21(1), 2–10.
17. Singh, H., Houy, T. L., Singh, N., et al. (2008). Gastrointestinal prophylaxis in critically ill patients. *Crit Care Nurs Q*, 31(4), 291–301.
18. Chey, W. D., Wong, B. C. Y. (2007). American College of Gastroenterology guideline on the management of *Helicobacter pylori* infection. *Am J Gastroenterology*, 102, 1808–1825.
19. Frost, K. L., Topp, R. (2006). A physical activity Rx for the hypertensive patient. *Nurse Pract*, 31(4), 29–37.
20. Turnbough, L., Wilson, L. (2007). Take your medicine: Nonadherence issues in patients with ulcerative colitis. *Gastroenterol Nurs*, 30(3), 212–217.
21. Bin-Nun, A., Bromiker, R., Wilschanski, M. (2005). Oral probiotics prevent necrotizing enterocolitis in very low birth weight neonates. *J Pediatr*, 147(2), 192–196.
22. Cheatham, M. L. (2009). Abdominal compartment syndrome: Pathophysiology and definitions. *Scand J Trauma, Resusc Emer Med*, 17(10).
23. Hunter, J. D., Damani, Z. (2004). Intra-abdominal hypertension and the abdominal compartment syndrome. *Anaesthesia*, 59(9), 899–907.

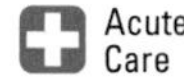

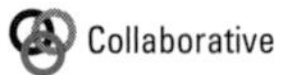

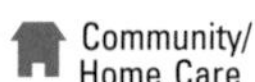

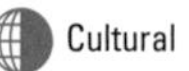

Grieving

Taxonomy II: Coping/Stress Tolerance—Class 2 Coping Responses (00136) [**Diagnostic Division:** Ego Integrity], Submitted as anticipatory Grieving 1980; Revised 1996, 2006

DEFINITION: A normal complex process that includes emotional, physical, spiritual, social, and intellectual responses and behaviors by which individuals, families, and communities incorporate an actual, anticipated, or perceived loss into their daily lives.

RELATED FACTORS

Anticipatory loss/loss of significant object (e.g., possession, job, status, home, body part)
Anticipatory loss or death of a significant other

DEFINING CHARACTERISTICS

Subjective

Anger; pain; suffering; despair; blaming
Alteration in activity level, sleep pattern, dream pattern
Finding meaning in a loss; personal growth
Guilt about feeling relief

Objective

Detachment; disorganization; psychological distress; panic behavior
Maintaining a connection to the deceased
Alterations in immune or neuroendocrine functioning

Sample Clinical Applications: Cancer, traumatic injuries (e.g., brain or spinal cord), amputation, chronic or debilitating conditions (e.g., renal failure, chronic obstructive pulmonary disease [COPD], multiple sclerosis [MS], amyotrophic lateral sclerosis [ALS]), genetic or birth defects, community disaster

DESIRED OUTCOMES/EVALUATION CRITERIA

Sample NOC linkages:

Grief Resolution: Adjustment to actual or impending loss

Psychosocial Adjustment: Life Change: Adaptive psychosocial response of an individual to a significant life change

Caregiver Emotional Health: Emotional well-being of a family care provider while caring for a family member

Client Will (Include Specific Time Frame)

- Identify and express feelings (e.g., sadness, guilt, fear) freely and effectively.
- Acknowledge impact or effect of the grieving process (e.g., physical problems of eating, sleeping) and seek appropriate help.
- Look toward and plan for future 1 day at a time.

Sample NOC linkages:

Community Competence: Capacity of a community to collectively problem solve to achieve community goals

Community Will (Include Specific Time Frame)

- Recognize needs of citizens, including underserved population.
- Activate or develop plan to address identified needs.

(continues on page 378)

Grieving (continued)
ACTIONS/INTERVENTIONS

Sample NIC linkages:
Grief Work Facilitation: Assistance with the resolution of a significant loss
Grief Work Facilitation: Perinatal Death: Assistance with the resolution of a perinatal loss
Dying Care: Promotion of physical comfort and psychological peace in the final phase of life

NURSING PRIORITY NO. 1 To assess causative/contributing factors:

- Determine circumstances of current situation (e.g., sudden death, prolonged fatal illness, loved one kept alive by extreme medical interventions). *Grief can be anticipatory (mourning the loss of loved one's former self before actual death) or actual. Both types of grief can provoke a wide range of intense and often conflicting feelings. Grief also follows losses other than death (e.g., traumatic loss of a limb, or loss of home by a tornado, loss of known self due to brain injury).*[11]
- Determine significance of loss to community (e.g., school bus accident with loss of life, major storm with damage to community infrastructure, financial failure of major employer).
- Determine client's perception of anticipated or actual loss and meaning to him or her. "What are your concerns?" "What are your fears? Your greatest fear?" "How do you see this affecting you and your lifestyle?" *Identifying the needs to be addressed and acknowledging the client's responses are integral to planning care.*[9] *Some individuals may use anticipatory grieving as a defense against the inevitable loss. While some people may find this helpful when the loss occurs, many people find that intense feelings occur regardless of the period of anticipation.*[2]
- Ascertain response of family/significant others (SOs) to client's situation/concerns. *Family concerns affect client and need to be listened to and appropriate interventions taken. Problems may arise if family completes grieving prematurely and disengages from the dying member, who then feels abandoned at a time when the support is needed.*[2]

NURSING PRIORITY NO. 2 To determine current response:

- Note emotional responses, such as withdrawal, angry behavior, and crying. Provide information about normal stages of grieving. *Awareness allows for appropriate choice of interventions because individuals handle grief in different ways. Knowledge promotes understanding of emotional responses.*[4]
- Observe client's body language and check out meaning with the client. Note congruency of body language with verbalizations. *Body language is open to interpretation and needs to be validated so that misinterpretation does not occur. Client may be saying one thing, but often body language is saying something else; identifying incongruencies can provide opportunity for individual to understand self in relation to grieving process.*[2]
- Note cultural and religious factors and expectations that may impact client's responses to situation. *Beliefs vary with the individual/community and will affect responses to the situation.*[5,8]
- Determine impact on general well-being (e.g., increased frequency of minor illnesses, exacerbation of chronic condition, problems with eating, activity level, sexual desire, role performance [e.g., work, parenting]). *Indicators of severity of feelings client is experiencing and need for specific interventions to resolve these issues.*[5]
- Note family communication and interaction patterns. *Dysfunctional patterns of communication such as avoidance, preaching, and giving advice, can block effective communication and isolate family members.*[3]
- Discuss with client and family/SOs, and others as appropriate plans that need to be made as well as anticipated adjustments and role changes related to the situation. Encourage and answer questions as needed. *This type of discussion will bring concerns out in the open and help with adaptation to the loss.*[5,11]
- Determine availability and use of community resources and support groups. *Appropriate use of support can help the individual feel less isolated and can promote feelings of inclusion and comfort.*[2]

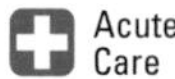

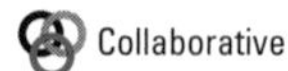

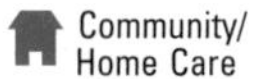

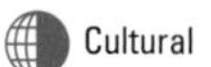

- Note community plans in place to deal with major loss (e.g., team of crisis counselors stationed at a school to address the loss of classmates, vocational counselors or retraining programs, outreach of services from neighboring communities).

NURSING PRIORITY NO. 3 To assist client/community to deal with situation:

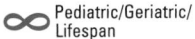

- Provide open environment and trusting relationship. *Promotes a free discussion of feelings and concerns in a safe environment where client can reveal innermost fears and beliefs about anticipated loss.*[2]
- Use therapeutic communication skills of active-listening, silence, and acknowledgment. Respect client desire or request not to talk. *These skills convey belief in ability of client to deal with situation and develop a sense of competence. Client may not be ready to discuss feelings and situation, and respecting client's own time line conveys confidence.*[2]
- Inform children about the anticipated or actual death or loss in age-appropriate language. *Providing accurate information about loss or change in life situation will help the child begin the mourning process.*[10]
- Give permission to child to express feelings about situation and ask questions, being careful to provide honest answers within child's understanding. *Adults may be uncomfortable or upset talking about death or loss, and children may be excluded from adult conversation about what is happening.*[10]
- Provide puppets or play therapy for toddlers/young children. *Young children do not have the ability to express their feelings verbally; use of play may help them express grief and help deal with loss in ways that are appropriate to the age.*[2]
- Permit appropriate expressions of anger, fear. Note hostility toward spiritual power or feelings of abandonment. *Anger is a normal part of the grieving process, and talking about these feelings allows individual to think about them and move on, coming to some resolution regarding the anticipated loss.*[2] (Refer to ND Spiritual Distress for additional interventions.)
- Provide information about normalcy of individual grief reaction. *Many people are not familiar with grief and are concerned that what they are experiencing is not normal. Letting them know that grief takes many forms and what they are feeling is all right helps them deal with what is happening.*[6,9]
- Be honest when answering questions, providing information. *Enhances nurse-client relationship, promoting trust and confidence.*[2]
- Provide assurance to child that cause for situation is not his or her own doing, bearing in mind age and developmental level. *May lessen sense of guilt and affirm there is no need to assign blame to self or any family member.*[2]
- Provide hope within parameters of individual situation. *Assisting client to find the positives will help with management of current situation.* Do not give false reassurance. *Comments such as "Everything will be all right" or "Don't worry" are not helpful and convey lack of understanding to the client.*[2]
- Review past life experiences and previous loss(es), role changes, and coping skills used, noting strengths and successes. *Useful in dealing with current situation and problem solving existing needs.*[4]
- Discuss control issues, such as what is in the power of the individual to change and what is beyond control. *Recognition of these factors helps client focus energy for maximal benefit and outcome on what can be done.*[4]
- Incorporate family/SO(s) in problem solving. *Encourages family to support and assist client to deal with situation while meeting needs of family members.*[2]
- Determine client's status and role in family (e.g., parent, sibling, child) and address loss of family member role. *Client's illness affects usual activities in the role he or she has in the family and inevitably affects all the other family members as responsibilities are taken over by them.*[2]
- Instruct in use of visualization and relaxation techniques. *These skills can be helpful to reduce anxiety and stress and help client and family members manage grief more effectively.*[7]
- Use sedatives or tranquilizers with caution. *While the use of these medications may be helpful in the short term, too much dependence on them may retard passage through the grief process.*[2,6]
- Mobilize resources when client is the community. *When anticipated loss affects community as a whole, such as closing of manufacturing plant, impending disaster (e.g., wildfire, terrorist concerns), multiple*

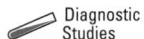

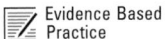

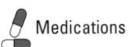

supports will be required to deal with size and complexity of situation. Indeed, when more people are directly or indirectly involved in the anticipated or actual loss, emotions and anxiety tend to be amplified and transmitted, thus complicating the situation.[1]

- Encourage community members/groups to engage in talking about event or loss and verbalizing feelings. Seek out underserved populations to include in process. *Increases likelihood that the needs of the entire community are identified and addressed.*
- Encourage individuals to participate in activities to deal with loss and rebuild community. *Exercising control in a productive manner empowers individuals and promotes rebuilding of life and community.*

NURSING PRIORITY NO. 4 To promote wellness (Teaching/Discharge Considerations):

- Provide information that feelings are okay and are to be expressed appropriately. Set limits regarding destructive behavior. *Talking about feelings can facilitate the grieving process, but destructive behavior can be damaging to self-esteem.*[2]
- Discuss recurring nature of grief reactions. *On birthdays, major holidays, at times of significant personal events, or anniversary of loss, intense grief reactions may occur for a long time after the loss. If these reactions start to disrupt day-to-day functioning, client may need to seek help.*[1] (Refer to NDs such as ineffective community Coping, complicated Grieving.)
- Encourage continuation of usual activities and schedule and involvement in appropriate exercise program, as appropriate and able. *Promotes sense of control and self-worth, enabling client to feel more positive about ability to handle situation.*[2]
- Identify and promote involvement of family and social support systems. *A supportive environment enhances the effectiveness of interventions and promotes a successful grieving process.*[4]
- Discuss and assist with planning for future or funeral, as appropriate. *Involving family members in this discussion ensures that everyone knows what is desired and what is planned, thus avoiding unexpected disagreements.*[4]
- Refer to additional resources, such as pastoral care, counseling or psychotherapy, organized community support groups, as indicated, for both client and family/SO. *Useful for ongoing needs and facilitation of grieving process.*[2,8]
- Identify resources and develop community plan to address anticipated large-scale losses. *Preparation for complex challenges facilitates prompt response as needs occur.*
- Support community efforts to strengthen support and develop plan to foster recovery and growth.

DOCUMENTATION FOCUS

Assessment/reassessment

- Assessment findings, including client's perception of anticipated loss and signs/symptoms that are being exhibited.
- Responses of family/SO(s) or community members, as indicated.
- Availability and use of resources.

Planning

- Plan of care and who is involved in planning.
- Teaching plan.

Implementation/Evaluation

- Client's response to interventions, teaching, and actions performed.
- Attainment or progress toward desired outcome(s).
- Modifications to plan of care.

Discharge planning

- Long-term needs and who is responsible for actions to be taken.
- Specific referrals made.

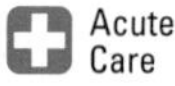

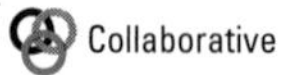

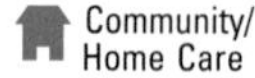

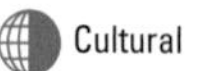

References

1. Sharma, V. P. (1996). Normal mourning and "complicated grief." Retrieved October 2015 from www.Mindpub.com/art045.htm.
2. Townsend, M. C. (2010). *Essentials of Psychiatric Mental Health Nursing: Concepts of Care in Evidence Based Practice*. 5th ed. Philadelphia: F. A. Davis.
3. Kissane, D. W., Bloch, S. (2002). *Family Focused Grief Therapy*. Berkshire, UK: Open University Press.
4. Cox, H. C., Sridaromont, K., King, M., et al. (2002). *Clinical Applications of Nursing Diagnosis: Adult, Child, Women's, Psychiatric, Gerontic, and Home Health Considerations*. 5th ed. Philadelphia: F. A. Davis.
5. Purnell, L. D., Paulanka, B. J. (2008). *Transcultural Health Care: A Culturally Competent Approach*. 3rd ed. Philadelphia: F. A. Davis.
6. No author listed. (Revised 2013). Grief, bereavement, and coping with loss: Treatment. National Cancer Institute. Retrieved October 2015 from http://www.cancer.gov/about-cancer/advanced-cancer/caregivers/planning/bereavement-pdq.
7. Pearce, J. C. (2004). *The Biology of Transcendence: A Blueprint of the Human Spirit*. Rochester, VT: Park Street Press.
8. Matzo, M., Sherman, D. W., Mazanec, P., et al. (2002). Teaching cultural consideration at the end of life. End of Life Nursing Education Consortium program recommendations. *J Contin Educ Nurs*, 33(6), 270–278.
9. Neeld, E. H. (2003). *Seven Choices*. 4th ed. Austin, TX: Centerpoint Press.
10. Riely, M. (2003). Facilitating children's grief. *J School Nurs*, 19(4), 212–218.
11. Family Caregiver Alliance: National Center on Caregiving. Grief and loss. Retrieved October 2015 from http://caregiver.org/grief-and-loss.

complicated Grieving

Taxonomy II: Coping/Stress Tolerance—Class 2 Coping Responses (00135) [**Diagnostic Division:** Ego Integrity], Submitted 1980; Revised 1986, 2004, 2006

DEFINITION: A disorder that occurs after the death of a significant other, in which the experience of distress accompanying bereavement fails to follow normative expectations and manifests in functional impairment.

RELATED FACTORS

Death of significant other
Emotional disturbance
Insufficient social support
[Loss of significant object (e.g., possessions, job, status, home, parts and processes of body)]

DEFINING CHARACTERISTICS

Subjective

Anxiety, anger, disbelief: feeling of emptiness or detached from others
Feeling dazed or stunned; feeling of shock
Distress about the diseased person; longing or yearning for deceased person
Insufficient sense of well-being; fatigue; low levels of intimacy; depression
Nonacceptance of a death; persistent painful memories, distress about the deceased person

Objective

Avoidance of grieving
Decrease in functioning in life roles
Excessive stress; separation or traumatic distress

(continues on page 382)

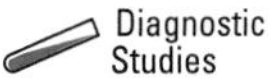
Diagnostic Studies
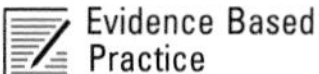
Evidence Based Practice
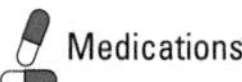
Medications
 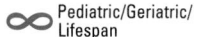
Pediatric/Geriatric/Lifespan

complicated Grieving (continued)
Experiencing symptoms the deceased experienced
Preoccupation with thoughts about a deceased person; rumination; searching for the deceased; self-blame
Sample Clinical Applications: Death of significant other, traumatic loss, depression, attempted suicide

DESIRED OUTCOMES/EVALUATION CRITERIA

Sample NOC linkages:
Depression Level: Severity of melancholic mood and loss of interest in life events
Grief Resolution: Adjustment to actual or impending loss
Psychosocial Adjustment: Life Change: Adaptive psychosocial responses of an individual to a significant life change

Client Will (Include Specific Time Frame)

- Acknowledge presence and impact of dysfunctional situation.
- Demonstrate progress in dealing with stages of grief at own pace.
- Participate in work and self-care and activities, as able.
- Verbalize a sense of progress toward resolution of the grief and hope for the future.

ACTIONS/INTERVENTIONS

Sample NIC linkages:
Grief Work Facilitation: Assistance with the resolution of a significant loss
Grief Work Facilitation: Perinatal Death: Assistance with the resolution of a perinatal loss
Coping Enhancement: Assisting a patient to adapt to perceived stressors, changes, or threats that interfere with meeting life demands and roles

NURSING PRIORITY NO. 1 To determine causative/contributing factors:

- Identify loss that is present. Note circumstances of death such as sudden or traumatic (e.g., fatal accident, homicide), related to socially sensitive issue (e.g., AIDS, suicide), or associated with unfinished business (e.g., spouse died during time of crisis in marriage, son has not spoken to parent for years). *These situations can sometimes cause individual to become stuck in grief and unable to move forward with life.*[11–13]
- Determine significance of the loss to client (e.g., presence of chronic condition leading to divorce or disruption of family unit and change in lifestyle or financial security). *The more complicated or devastating the loss is to the individual, the more likely she or he will have difficulty reaching resolution.*[15]
- Identify cultural or religious beliefs and expectations *that may impact or dictate client's response to loss.*[15]
- Ascertain response of family/significant others (SOs) to situation (e.g., sympathetic or urging client to "just get over it"). Assess needs of SO(s). *Response of family members will affect how client is dealing with situation—functional families are supportive or conflict resolving in nature while dysfunctional families tend to be sullen, hostile, or immediate functioning. This information is important for planning care and choosing resources to enable all members to effectively cope with events.*[6,9]

NURSING PRIORITY NO. 2 To determine degree of impairment/dysfunction:

- Observe for cues of sadness (e.g., sighing, faraway look, unkempt appearance, inattention to conversation, somatic complaints such as exhaustion, headaches). *Indicators of the extent of grief and how individual is dealing with situation.*[12,14]
- Identify stage of grief being expressed: denial, isolation, anger, bargaining, depression, and acceptance. *Helps to establish how client is dealing with grieving and degree of difficulty client is having adjusting to the death or loss.*[10]

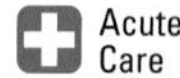
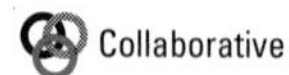
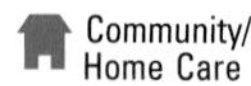
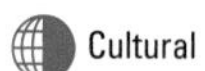

- Listen to words and communications indicative of renewed or intense grief (e.g., constantly bringing up death or loss even in casual conversation long after event; outbursts of anger at relatively minor events; expressing desire to die) *indicating person is possibly unable to adjust/move on from feelings of intense grief.*[12] *Note: Complicated grief therapy utilizes the concept of revisiting the loss through storytelling of the death especially for individuals prone to avoid thinking about the trauma of the loss.*[6]
- Determine level of functioning, ability to care for self, and use of support systems and community resources. *Individual may be incapacitated by depth of loss and be unable to manage day-to-day activities adequately, necessitating intervention and assistance.*[14]
- Be aware of avoidance behaviors (e.g., anger; withdrawal; long periods of sleeping or refusing to interact with family; sudden or radical changes in lifestyle; inability to handle everyday responsibilities at home, work, or school; conflict). *Additional indicators of depth of grieving being experienced and need for more intensive support and monitoring to help client deal effectively with death or loss.*[10–12]
- Determine if client is engaging in reckless or self-destructive behaviors (e.g., substance abuse, heavy drinking, promiscuity, aggression) *to identify safety issues.*[1]
- Identify cultural factors and ways individual(s) has dealt with previous loss(es). *Way of expressing self may reflect cultural background and religious beliefs. Understanding cultural expectations will help put current behavior and responses in context and determine the nature and degree of dysfunction.*[8]
- Perform or refer for psychological testing, as indicated (e.g., Beck's Depression Scale). *Determines degree of depression and possible need for medication.*[2]

NURSING PRIORITY NO. 3 To assist client/others to deal appropriately with loss:

- Encourage verbalization without confrontation about realities. *It is helpful to listen without correcting misperceptions in the beginning, allowing free flow of expression. Provides opportunity for reflection aiding resolution and acceptance.*[2]
- Encourage client to choose topics of conversation and refrain from forcing client to "face the facts." *Talking freely about concerns can help client identify what is important to deal with and how to cope with situation.*[9]
- Active-listen feelings and be available for support or assistance. Speak in a soft, caring voice. *Communicates acceptance and caring, enabling client to seek own answers to current situation.*[2]
- Encourage expression of anger, fear, and anxiety. (Refer to appropriate NDs.) *These feelings are part of the grieving process, and to accomplish the work of grieving, they need to be expressed and accepted.*[9]
- Permit verbalization of anger with acknowledgment of feelings and setting of limits regarding destructive behavior. *Enhances client safety, promotes resolution of grief process by encouraging expression of feelings that are not usually accepted, and supports self-esteem.*[2]
- Acknowledge reality of feelings of guilt or blame, including hostility toward spiritual power. Do not minimize loss; avoid clichés and easy answers. (Refer to ND Spiritual Distress.) *Reinforces that feelings are acceptable and allows client to become aware of own thoughts and begin to deal with feelings.*[1,7]
- Respect the client's needs and wishes for quiet, privacy, talking, or silence. *Individual may not be ready to talk about or share grief and needs to be allowed to make own time line.*[2]
- Give "permission" to be at this point when the client is depressed. *Assures client that feelings are normal and can be a starting point to deal in a positive manner with loss/death that has occurred.*[9]
- Provide comfort and availability as well as caring for physical needs. *Client needs to know he or she will be supported and helped when not able to care for self.*[2]
- Reinforce use of previously effective coping skills. Instruct in and encourage use of visualization and relaxation techniques. *Identifying and discussing how client has dealt with loss in the past can provide opportunities in the current situation. Use of these techniques helps client to learn to relax and consider options for dealing with loss.*[2]
- Assist SOs to cope with client's response. Include age-specific interventions. *Family/SO(s) may not understand/be intolerant of client's distress and inadvertently hamper client's progress. Family members, including children, may express their feelings in anger, resulting in punishment for behavior that is deemed unacceptable rather than recognized as the basis in grief.*[10]

- Include family/SO(s) in setting realistic goals for meeting needs of client and family members. *Involving all members enhances the probability that each member will express their needs and hear what the needs of others are, ensuring a more effective outcome.*[2]
- Encourage family members to participate in support group or family-focused therapy as indicated. *Technique of family-focused grief therapy focuses on emotional expression of grief and family functioning to strengthen the family's adaptive capacity and promote cohesiveness.*[3]
- Use sedatives or tranquilizers with caution. *While the use of these medications may be of limited benefit in the short term, too much dependence on them may retard passage through the grief process.*[2,4]
- Refer to mental health provider for counseling. *Standard individual psychotherapy identifies and addresses symptoms, relationship problems, and their connections to grief. Research suggests the complicated grief therapy technique may be more effective by supporting the idea of dual processing (i.e., alternating attention between the loss and a focus on restoration and the future).*[6–13]
- Refer to ND Grieving for additional interventions as appropriate.

NURSING PRIORITY NO. 4 To promote wellness (Teaching/Discharge Considerations):

- Discuss with client/SO healthy ways of dealing with difficult situations. *Identifying ways individual(s) has dealt with losses in the past will help identify strengths and successes and what might be useful in the current situation.*[2]
- Have individual(s) identify familial, religious, and cultural factors that have meaning. *One's family of origin has a major impact on what the individuals learn about these issues and how to deal with losses. Identifying and discussing how they affect the current situation may help bring loss into perspective and facilitate grief resolution.*[5,8]
- Encourage involvement in usual activities, exercise, and socialization within limits of physical ability and psychological state. *Keeping life to a somewhat normal routine can provide individual(s) with some sense of control over events that are not controllable.*
- Suggest client keep a journal of experiences and feelings. *As client writes about what is happening, new insights may occur. Reading over what has been written can help individual see progress that has been made and begin to have hope for the future.*[9]
- Advocate planning for the future as appropriate to individual situation (e.g., staying in own home after death of spouse, returning to sporting activities following traumatic amputation, choice to have another child or to adopt, rebuilding home following a disaster). *Provides a sense of control and purpose and ensures that individual's wishes will be heard and respected.*[10]
- Identify volunteer opportunities (e.g., working with children at risk, raising funds for favorite charity, investigating new employment or relocation opportunities, participating in community reorganization or clean up). *Exercising control in a productive manner empowers individuals and promotes rebuilding of life and community.*
- Refer to other resources (e.g., pastoral care, family counseling, psychotherapy, organized support groups—widow's group) as indicated. *Provides additional support to resolve situation and continue grief work.*[4]

DOCUMENTATION FOCUS

Assessment/Reassessment

- Assessment findings, including meaning of loss to the client, current stage of the grieving process, and responses of family/SOs.
- Cultural or religious beliefs and expectations.
- Availability and use of resources.

Planning

- Plan of care and who is involved in the planning.
- Teaching plan.

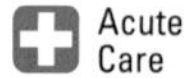

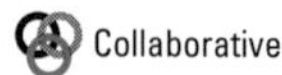

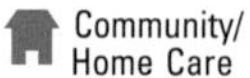

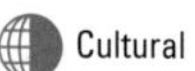

Implementation/Evaluation
- Client's response to interventions, teaching, and actions performed.
- Attainment or progress toward desired outcome(s).
- Modifications to plan of care.

Discharge Planning
- Long-term needs and who is responsible for actions to be taken.
- Specific referrals made.

References

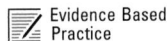

1. Lubit, R. H. (Updated 2008). Acute treatment of disaster survivors. Retrieved March 2015 from http://babyhealthcaretips.blogspot.com/2010/01/acute-treatment-of-disaster-survivors.html.
2. Townsend, M. C. (2010). *Essentials of Psychiatric Mental Health Nursing Concepts of Care in Evidence Based Practice*. 5th ed. Philadelphia: F. A. Davis, 585–601.
3. Kissane, D. W., Bloch, S. (2002). *Family Focused Grief Therapy*. Berkshire, UK: Open University Press.
4. Newfield, S. A., Hinz, M. D., Tilley, D. S., et al. (2007). *Cox's Clinical Applications of Nursing Diagnosis: Adult, Child, Women's, Psychiatric, Gerontic, and Home Health Considerations*. 5th ed. Philadelphia: F. A. Davis.
5. Purnell, L. D., Paulanka, B. J. (2008). *Transcultural Health Care: A Culturally Competent Approach*. 3rd ed. Philadelphia: F. A. Davis.
6. National Cancer Institute. (Updated 2014). Grief, bereavement, and coping with loss: Treatment. Retrieved March 2015 from http://www.cancer.gov/cancertopics/pdq/supportivecare/bereavement/HealthProfessional/page5.
7. Pearce, J. C. (2004). *The Biology of Transcendence: A Blueprint of the Human Spirit*. Rochester, VT: Park Street Press.
8. Matzo, M., Sherman, D. W., Mazanec, P., et al. (2002). Teaching cultural consideration at the end of life. End of Life Nursing Education Consortium program recommendations. *J Contin Educ Nurs*, 33(6), 270–278.
9. Neeld, E. H. (2003). *Seven Choices*. 4th ed. Austin, TX: Centerpoint Press.
10. Riely, M. (2003). Facilitating children's grief. *J School Nurs*, 19(4), 212–218.
11. Sharma, V. P. (1996). Normal mourning and "complicated grief." Retrieved March 2015 from www.Mindpub.com/art045.htm.
12. No author listed. (2006). Grief becomes complicated, unresolved or stuck. Retrieved March 2015 from https://crumblingwalls.wordpress.com/2006/09/16/grief-becomes-complicated-unresolved-or-stuck/.
13. Kersting, K. (2004). A new approach to complicated grief. *Monitor on Psychology*, 35(10), 51.
14. National Cancer Institute. (Updated 2014). Types of grief reactions. Retrieved March 2015 from http://www.cancer.gov/cancertopics/pdq/supportivecare/bereavement/HealthProfessional/page3.
15. National Cancer Institute. (Updated 2013). Factors that affect complicated grief. Retrieved March 2015 from http://www.cancer.gov/cancertopics/pdq/supportivecare/bereavement/Patient/page4.

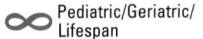

risk for complicated Grieving

Taxonomy II: Coping/Stress Tolerance—Class 2 Coping Responses (00172) [**Diagnostic Division:** Ego Integrity], Submitted 2004; Revised 2006, 2013

DEFINITION: Vulnerable to a disorder that occurs after the death of a significant other, in which the experience of distress accompanying bereavement fails to follow normative expectations and manifests in functional impairment, which may compromise health.

RISK FACTORS
Death of significant other
Emotional disturbance

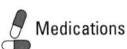

(continues on page 386)

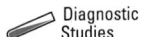

risk for complicated Grieving (continued)
Insufficient social support
[Loss of significant object (e.g., possessions, job, status, home, parts and processes of body)]
Note: A risk diagnosis is not evidenced by signs and symptoms, as the problem has not occurred; rather, nursing interventions are directed at prevention.
Sample Clinical Applications: Death of significant other, depression

DESIRED OUTCOMES/EVALUATION CRITERIA

Sample NOC linkages:
Personal Resiliency: Positive adaptation and function of an individual following significant adversity or crisis
Grief Resolution: Adjustment to actual or impending loss
Psychosocial Adjustment: Life Change: Psychosocial adaptation of an individual to a life change

Client Will (Include Specific Time Frame)
- Acknowledge awareness of individual factors affecting client in this situation (see Risk Factors).
- Identify emotional responses and behaviors occurring after the death or loss.
- Participate in therapy to learn new ways of dealing with anxiety and feelings of inadequacy.
- Discuss meaning of loss to individual or family.
- Verbalize a sense of beginning to deal with grief process.

ACTIONS/INTERVENTIONS

Sample NIC linkages:
Grief Work Facilitation: Assistance with the resolution of a significant loss
Grief Work Facilitation: Perinatal Death: Assistance with the resolution of a perinatal loss
Coping Enhancement: Assisting a patient to adapt to perceived stressors, changes, or threats that interfere with meeting life demands and roles

NURSING PRIORITY NO. 1 To identify risk/contributing factors:
- Determine loss that has occurred and meaning to client. Note if death was sudden or traumatic (e.g., fatal accident, homicide), related to socially sensitive issue (e.g., AIDS, suicide), or associated with unfinished business (e.g., spouse died during time of crisis in marriage, son has not spoken to parent for years). *These situations can sometimes cause individual to become stuck in grief and unable to move forward with life.*[1,2]
- ∞ Ascertain circumstances surrounding loss of fetus, infant, or child (e.g., gestational age of fetus, multiple miscarriages, death due to violence or fatal illness). *Repeated losses and/or violent death can increase client's/significant other's (SO's) sense of futility and compromise resolution of grieving process.*[2,7]
- ∞ Meet with both parents following loss of child *to determine how they are dealing with the loss together and individually. Death of a child is often more difficult for parents/family, based on individual values and sense of life unlived.*[2]
- Note stage of grief client is experiencing (e.g., denial, anger, bargaining, depression). *Stages of grief may progress in a predictable manner or stages may be random or revisited.*[3]
- Assess client's ability to manage activities of daily living and period of time since loss has occurred. *Periods of crying, feelings of overwhelming sadness, loss of appetite, and insomnia can occur with grieving; however, when they persist and interfere with normal activities, client may need additional assistance.*[3]
- Note availability and use of support systems and community resources.
- Listen to words and communications indicative of renewed or intense grief (e.g., constantly bringing up death or loss even in casual conversation long after event, outbursts of anger at relatively minor events, expressing desire to die), *indicating person is possibly unable to adjust or move on from feelings of intense grief.*[4]

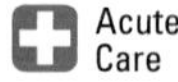

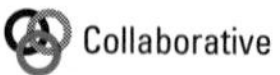

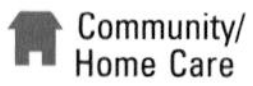

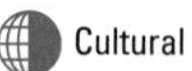

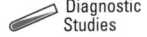

- Identify cultural or religious beliefs and expectations that may impact or dictate client's response to loss. *These factors affect current situation and may help bring loss into perspective and promote grief resolution.*[2,5]
- Assess status of relationships or marital difficulties and adjustments to loss. *Responses of family/SOs affect how client deals with situation.*[6]

NURSING PRIORITY NO. 2 To assist client to deal appropriately with loss:

- Discuss meaning of loss to client, Active-listen to responses without judgment. *The more complicated or devastating the loss is to the individual, the more likely she or he will have difficulty reaching resolution.*
- Respect client's desire for quiet, privacy, talking, or silence. *Individual may not be ready to talk about or share grief and needs to be allowed to make own time line.*[3]
- Encourage expression of feelings, including anger, fear, and anxiety. Let client know that all feelings are okay, while setting limits on destructive behavior. *These feelings are part of the grieving process, and to accomplish the work of grieving, they need to be expressed and accepted.*[3,6]
- Acknowledge client's sense of relief when death follows a long and debilitating course. *Sadness and loss are still there, but the death may be a release, or client may feel guilty about having a sense of relief.*
- Assist SOs/family to understand and be tolerant of client's feelings and behavior. *Family/SO(s) may not understand or be intolerant of client's distress and inadvertently hamper client's progress. Family members, including children, may express their feelings in anger, resulting in punishment for behavior that is deemed unacceptable, rather than recognizing the basis in grief.*[8]

NURSING PRIORITY NO. 3 To promote wellness (Teaching/Discharge Considerations):

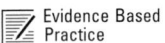

- Assist client/SOs to identify successful coping skills they have used in the past. *These can be used in current situation to facilitate dealing with grief.*[3]
- Support client and family in setting goals for meeting needs of members for moving on beyond the grieving process.
- Encourage resuming involvement in usual activities, exercise, and socialization within physical and psychological abilities. *Keeping life to a somewhat normal routine can provide individual with some sense of control over events that are not controllable.*[5]
- Advocate planning for the future as appropriate to individual situation (e.g., staying in own home after death of spouse, returning to sporting activities following traumatic amputation, choice to have another child or to adopt, rebuilding home following a disaster). *Provides a sense of control and purpose and ensures that individual's wishes will be heard and respected.*[8]
- Refer to other resources, as needed, such as psychotherapy, family counseling, religious references or pastor, or a grief support group. *Depending upon meaning of the loss, individual may require ongoing support to work through grief.*[5]

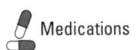

DOCUMENTATION FOCUS

Assessment/Reassessment

- Assessment findings, including meaning of loss to the client, current stage of the grieving process, psychological status, and responses of family/SOs.
- Cultural or religious beliefs, expectations, and rituals.
- Availability and use of resources.

Planning

- Plan of care and who is involved in the planning.
- Teaching plan.

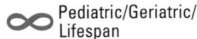

Implementation/Evaluation

- Client's response to interventions, teaching, and actions performed.
- Attainment or progress toward desired outcome(s).
- Modifications to plan of care.

Discharge Planning

- Long-term needs and who is responsible for actions to be taken.
- Specific referrals made.

References

1. Sharma, V. P. (1996). Normal mourning and "complicated grief." Retrieved March 2015 from www.Mindpub.com/art045.htm.
2. National Cancer Institute. (Updated 2014). Risk factors for complicated grief and other negative bereavement outcomes. Retrieved March 2015 from http://www.cancer.gov/cancertopics/pdq/supportivecare/bereavement/HealthProfessional/page4.
3. Townsend, M. C. (2010). *Essentials of Psychiatric Mental Health Nursing Concepts of Care in Evidence Based Practice*. 5th ed. Philadelphia: F. A. Davis, 585–601.
4. No author listed. (2006). Grief becomes complicated, unresolved or stuck. Retrieved March 2015 from https://crumblingwalls.wordpress.com/2006/09/16/grief-becomes-complicated-unresolved-or-stuck/.
5. Matzo, M., Sherman, D. W., Mazenec, P., et al. (2002). Teaching cultural considerations at the end of life. End of Life Nursing Education Consortium program recommendations. *J Contin Educ Nurs*, 33(6), 212–218.
6. Neeld, E. H. (2003). *Seven Choices*. 4th ed. Austin, TX: Centerpoint Press.
7. Kersting, K. (2004). A new approach to complicated grief. *Monitor on Psychology*, 35(10), 51.
8. Riely, M. (2003). Facilitating children's grief. *J School Nurs*, 19(4), 212–218.

risk for disproportionate Growth

Taxonomy II: Growth/Development—Class 1 Growth (00113) [**Diagnostic Division:** Teaching/Learning], Submitted 2013

DEFINITION: Vulnerable to growth above the 97th percentile or below the 3rd percentile for age, crossing two percentile channels, which may compromise health.

RISK FACTORS

Prenatal

Inadequate maternal nutrition; maternal infection; multiple gestation
Substance abuse; exposure to teratogen
Congenital or genetic disorder

Individual

Prematurity
Malnutrition; maladaptive feeding behavior by caregiver, or self-feeding; insatiable appetite; anorexia
Infection; chronic illness
Substance abuse [including anabolic steroids]

Environmental

Deprivation, economically disadvantaged
Exposure to violence, natural disasters
Exposure to teratogen; lead poisoning

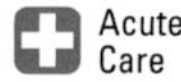

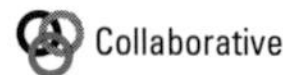

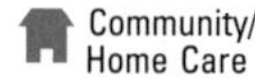

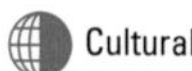

Caregiver

Presence of abuse (e.g., physical, psychological, sexual)

Mental health issue (e.g., depression, psychosis, personality disorder, substance abuse)

Learning disability; alteration in cognitive functioning

Note: A risk diagnosis is not evidenced by signs and symptoms, as the problem has not occurred; rather, nursing interventions are directed at prevention.

Sample Clinical Applications: Congenital or genetic disorders, prematurity, infection, nutritional problems (malnutrition, anorexia, failure to thrive, excessive intake or obesity), toxic exposures (e.g., lead), abuse or neglect, endocrine disorders, pituitary tumor

DESIRED OUTCOMES/EVALUATION CRITERIA

Sample NOC linkages:

Growth: Normal increase in bone size and body weight during growth years

Weight: Body Mass: Extent to which body weight, muscle, and fat are congruent to height, frame, gender, and age

Client Will (Include Specific Time Frame)

- Receive appropriate nutrition as dictated by individual needs.
- Demonstrate weight and growth stabilizing or progressing toward age-appropriate size.
- Participate in plan of care as appropriate for age and ability.

Sample NOC linkages:

Child Development: [specify age group]: Milestones of physical, cognitive, and psychosocial progression by [specify] months/years of age

Client/Caregiver Will (Include Specific Time Frame)

- Verbalize understanding of potential for growth delay or deviation and plan for prevention.

ACTIONS/INTERVENTIONS

Sample NIC linkages:

Nutritional Monitoring: Collection and analysis of patient data to prevent or minimize malnourishment

Teaching: Infant [or] Toddler Nutrition [specify age]: Instruction on nutrition and feeding practices during the first, second, and third years of life

Weight Management: Facilitating maintenance of optimal body weight and percent body fat

NURSING PRIORITY NO. 1 To assess causative/contributing factors:

- Determine factors or condition(s) existing that could contribute to growth deviation as listed in Risk Factors, including familial history (e.g., pituitary tumors, Marfan's syndrome, genetic anomalies), prematurity with complications, use of certain drugs or substances during pregnancy, maternal diabetes or other chronic illness, poverty or inability to attend to nutritional issues, eating disorders, etc. *Information essential to developing plan of care.*
- Identify nature and effectiveness of parenting and caregiving activities. *Inadequate, inconsistent caregiving; unrealistic or insufficient expectations; lack of stimulation; inadequate limit setting; and lack of responsiveness indicates problems in parent-child relationship.*[4]
- Note severity and pervasiveness of situation (e.g., individual/significant other showing effects of long-term physical or emotional abuse or neglect vs. individual experiencing recent-onset situational disruption or inadequate resources during period of crisis or transition).

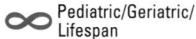

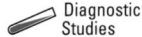

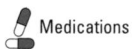

- Evaluate nutritional status. *Overfeeding or malnutrition (protein and other basic nutrients) on a constant basis prevents individual from reaching healthy growth potential, even if no disorder or disease exists. Malnutrition is the most common cause of growth failure worldwide. In industrialized nations, children continue to have nutritional deficiencies that can impair growth or development.*[12]
- Review results of studies such as skull and hand x-rays; bone scans, such as computed tomography or magnetic resonance imaging; and chest or abdominal imaging *to determine bone age and extent of bone and soft tissue overgrowth and the presence of pituitary or other growth hormone–secreting tumor.* Note laboratory studies (e.g., growth hormone levels, glucose tolerance, thyroid and other endocrine studies, serum transferrin and prealbumin) *to identify pathology.*[8,11,12]
- Determine cultural, familial, and societal values *that may impact situation or parental expectations (e.g., some cultures equate a "plump" baby with a healthy baby; childhood obesity is now a risk for American children and parents are concerned about child's food intake; expectations for "normal growth").*[13]
- Assess cognition, awareness, orientation, and behavior of the client/caregiver. *Actions such as withdrawal or aggression and reactions to environment and stimuli provide information for identifying needs and planning care.*[1]
- Active-listen concerns about body size and ability to perform competitively (e.g., sports, body building) *to ascertain the potential for inappropriate use of anabolic steroids or other drugs.*

NURSING PRIORITY NO. 2 To prevent/limit deviation from growth norms:

- Determine chronological age and note reported losses or alterations in functional level. *Provides comparative baseline.*
- Note familial factors (e.g., parent's body build and stature) *to help determine individual growth expectations (e.g., when child should attain a certain weight and height) and how the expectations may be altered by child's condition.*[12]
- Review expectations for current height and weight percentiles and degree of deviation. Plan for periodic evaluations. *Growth rates are measured in terms of how much a child grows within a specified time. These rates vary dramatically as a child grows (normal growth is a discontinuous process) and must be evaluated periodically over time to ascertain that child has definite growth disturbance. Accelerated or slowed growth rates are rarely normal and warrant further evaluation.*[1]
- Investigate deviations in height, weight, and head size. *Deviations may include weight only (increased or decreased) or height (increased or decreased) and head size (disproportionate to rest of body). These deviations may be seen alone or in combination, all requiring additional testing over time to determine cause and effect on child's growth and development. Some are more urgent than others (e.g., small head size is evaluated further/treated as soon as identified, whereas short stature may require a longer evaluation period to determine if developmental problem exists).*[1]
- Determine if child's growth is above 97th percentile (very tall and large) for age. *Child should be further evaluated for endocrine disorders or pituitary tumor (could result in gigantism). Other disorders may be characterized by excessive weight for height (e.g., hypothyroidism, Cushing's syndrome) and abnormal sexual maturation or abnormal body/limb proportions.*[2,8]
- Determine if child's growth is below third percentile (very short and small) for age. *Child should have further evaluations for failure to thrive related to intrauterine growth retardation, prematurity or very low birth weight, small parents, poor nutrition, stress or trauma, endocrine disorders (e.g., growth hormone or thyroid deficiency), or medical condition (e.g., intestinal disorders with malabsorption, diseases of heart, kidneys, diabetes mellitus). Treatment of underlying condition may alter or improve child's growth pattern.*[3,9,10]
- Assist with therapies to treat or correct underlying conditions (e.g., Crohn's disease, cardiac problems, or renal disease), endocrine problems (e.g., hyperpituitarism, hypothyroidism, type 1 diabetes mellitus, growth hormone abnormalities), genetic or intrauterine growth retardation, and infant feeding problems and nutritional deficits.

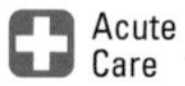

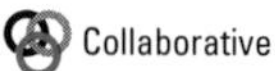

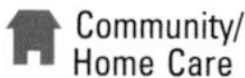

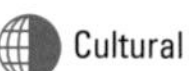

- Include nutritionist and other specialists as indicated (e.g., physical or occupational therapist) in developing plan of care. *Helpful in determining specific dietary needs for growth and weight issues as well as child's issues with foods (e.g., child who is sensory overresponsive may be bothered by food textures, child with posture problems may need to stand to eat, etc.); child may require assistive devices and appropriate exercise and rehabilitation programs.*[6]
- Note reports of changes in facial features, joint pain, lethargy, sexual dysfunction, or progressive increase in hat, glove, ring, or shoe size in adults, especially after age 40. *Individual should be referred for further evaluation for hyperpituitarism or growth hormone imbalance and acromegaly.*[8]

NURSING PRIORITY NO. 3 To promote wellness (Teaching/Discharge Considerations):

- Provide information regarding growth issues, as appropriate, including pertinent reference materials such as books, audiovisual materials, credible Web sites, etc. *Provides opportunity to review data at own pace, enhancing likelihood of retention, and opportunity to make informed decisions.*
- Discuss with pregnant women and adolescents consequences of substance use or abuse. *Prevention of growth disturbances depends on many factors but includes the cessation of smoking, alcohol, and many drugs that have the potential for causing central nervous system or orthopedic disorders in the fetus.*[5,7]
- Refer for genetic screening as appropriate. *There are many reasons for referral, including (and not limited to) positive family history of a genetic disorder (e.g., fragile X syndrome, muscular dystrophy), pregnant female with exposure to toxins or potential teratogenic agents, women older than 35 years at delivery, previous child born with congenital anomalies, history of intrauterine growth retardation, etc.*
- Address parent/caregiver issues (e.g., parental abuse, learning deficiencies, environment of poverty) *where they could impact client's ability to thrive.*
- Promote client lifestyle that prevents or limits complications (e.g., management of obesity, hypertension, sensory or perceptual impairments), regular medical follow-up, nutritionally balanced meals, socialization for age and development, etc., *to enhance functional independence and quality of life.*
- Recommend involvement in regular monitored exercise and/or sports programs *to enhance muscle tone and strength, and appropriate body building.*
- Review medications being considered (e.g., appetite stimulant, growth hormone, thyroid replacement, antidepressant), noting potential side effects/adverse reactions *to promote adherence to regimen and reduce risk of untoward responses.*
- Identify available community resources as appropriate (e.g., public health programs such as the Women, Infants, and Children program; medical equipment suppliers; nutritionist; substance abuse programs; specialists in endocrine problems/genetics).
- Emphasize importance of periodic reassessment of growth and development (e.g., periodic lab studies to monitor hormone levels, bone maturation, and nutritional status). *Aids in evaluating effectiveness of interventions over time, promotes early identification of need for additional actions, and helps to avoid preventable complications.*

DOCUMENTATION FOCUS

Assessment/Reassessment

- Assessment findings, individual needs, current growth status and trends.
- Caregiver's understanding of situation and individual role.
- Cultural or familial values and expectations.

Planning

- Plan of care and who is involved in the planning.
- Teaching plan.

Implementation/Evaluation

- Client's responses to interventions, teaching, and actions performed.
- Caregiver response to teaching.
- Attainment or progress toward desired outcome(s).
- Modifications to plan of care.

Discharge Planning

- Identified long-term needs and who is responsible for actions to be taken.
- Specific referrals made, sources for assistive devices, educational tools.

References

1. Legler, J. D., Rose, L. C. (1999). Assessment of abnormal growth curves. *Am Fam Physician*, 58(1), 1–9.
2. National Institutes of Health Genetic and Rare Diseases Information Center. (Updated 2010). Gigantism. Retrieved March 2015 from http://rarediseases.info.nih.gov/gard/6506/gigantism/case/28765/case-questions.
3. Child Growth Foundation. (No date). Endocrine gland disorders. Retrieved March 2015 from http://www.childgrowthfoundation.org/Default.aspx?page=ConditionsGHD.
4. Gordon, T. (2000). *Parent Effectiveness Training*. Updated ed. 30th anniversary New York: Three Rivers Press.
5. Maloni, J. A., Albrecht, S. A., Thomas, K. K., et al. (2003). Implementing evidence-based practice: Reducing risk for low birth weight through pregnancy smoking cessation. *J Obstet Gynecol Neonat Nurs*, 32(5), 676–682.
6. American Dietetic Association. (1997). Nutrition in comprehensive program planning for persons with developmental disabilities. *J Am Diet Assoc*, 97(2), 189–193.
7. Schiffman, R. F. (2004). Drug and substance use in adolescents. *MCN Am J Matern Child Nurs*, 29(1), 21–27.
8. Diaz-Thompson, A., Shim, M., Schwartz, R. A. (Updated 2015). Gigantism and acromegaly. Retrieved March 2015 from http://emedicine.medscape.com/article/925446-overview.
9. Kemp, S., Gungor, N. (Updated 2014). Growth failure. Retrieved March 2015 from http://emedicine.medscape.com/article/920446-overview.
10. Mannheim, J. K. (Updated 2013). Delayed growth. Various pages. Retrieved March 2015 from http://www.nlm.nih.gov/medlineplus/ency/article/003021.htm.
11. Sinha, S. (2014). Short stature. Retrieved March 2015 from http://emedicine.medscape.com/article/924411-overview.
12. Falkenstern, S. K., Bauer, L. A. (2009). Helping kids grow. *The Nurse Pract*, 34(3), 30–41.
13. Kumanyika, S. K. (2008). Environmental influences on childhood obesity: Ethnic and cultural influences context. *Physiol Behav*, 94(1), 61–70.

deficient community Health

Taxonomy II: Health Promotion—Class 2 Health Management (00215) [**Diagnostic Division:** Teaching/Learning], Submitted 2010

DEFINITION: Presence of one or more health problems or factors that deter wellness or increase the risk of health problems experienced by an aggregate

RELATED FACTORS

Insufficient access to healthcare providers; insufficient resources (e.g., financial, social, knowledge)
Insufficient community experts
Inadequate program budget, outcome data, or evaluation plan
Inadequate social support or consumer satisfaction with program

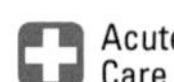

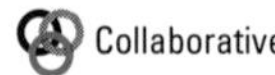

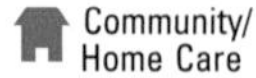

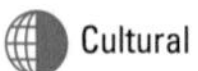

DEFINING CHARACTERISTICS

Subjective

[Community members or agencies verbalize overburdening of resources or inability to meet therapeutic needs of all members]

Objective

Risk of hospitalization experienced by aggregates or populations
Risk of physiological or psychological states experienced by aggregates or populations
Health problem experienced by aggregates or populations
Program unavailable to enhance wellness of an aggregate or population
Program unavailable to prevent, reduce, or eliminate health problem(s) of an aggregate or population
Sample Clinical Applications: HIV/AIDS, substance abuse, sexually transmitted infections, teen pregnancy, prematurity, acute lead poisoning, influenza, severe acute respiratory syndrome (SARS)

DESIRED OUTCOMES/EVALUATION CRITERIA

Sample NOC linkages:
Community Competence: Capacity of a community to collectively problem solve to achieve community goals
Community Health Status: General state of well-being of a community or population
Community Risk Control: Communicable Disease: Community actions to eliminate or reduce the spread of infectious agents that threaten public health

Community Will (Include Specific Time Frame)

- Identify both strengths and limitations affecting community programs for meeting health-related goals.
- Participate in problem solving of factors interfering with regulating and integrating community programs.
- Develop plans to address identified community health needs.

ACTIONS/INTERVENTIONS

Sample NIC linkages:
Community Health Development: Assisting members of a community to identify a community's health concerns, mobilize resources, and implement solutions
Program Development: Planning, implementing, and evaluating a coordinated set of activities designed to enhance wellness, or to prevent, reduce, or eliminate one or more health problems for a group or community
Health Policy Monitoring: Surveillance and influence of government and organization regulations, rules, and standards that affect nursing systems and practices to ensure quality care of patients

NURSING PRIORITY NO. 1 To identify causative/precipitating factors:

- Determine healthcare providers' understanding, terminology, and practice policies relating to community (populations and aggregate). *Population-based practice considers the broad determinants of health, such as income/social status, housing, employment/working conditions, social support networks, education, neighborhood safety/violence issues, physical environment, personal health practices and coping skills, cultural customs/values, and community capacity to support family and economic growth.*[6]
- Investigate health problems, unexpected outbreaks or acceleration of illness, and health hazards in the community. *Identifying specific problems allows for population-based interventions emphasizing primary prevention, promoting health, and preventing problems before they occur.*[2,6,7]
- Evaluate strengths and limitations of community healthcare resources for wellness, illness, or sequelae of illness. *Knowledge of currently available resources and ease of access provide a starting point to determine needs of the community and plan for future needs.*

- Note reports from members of the community regarding ineffective or inadequate community functioning. *Provides feedback from people who live in the community and avail themselves of resources, thus presenting a realistic picture of problem areas.*
- Determine areas of conflict among members of community. *Cultural or religious beliefs, values, social mores, and lack of a shared vision may limit dialogue or creative problem solving if not addressed.*[5,7]
- Ascertain effect of related factors on community. *Issues of safety, poor air quality, lack of education or information, and lack of sufficient healthcare facilities affect citizens and how they view their community—whether it is a healthy, positive environment in which to live or lacks adequate healthcare or safety resources.*[1]
- Determine knowledge and understanding of treatment regimen. *Citizens need to know and understand what is being proposed to correct the identified deficiencies before they are willing to be involved and actively support goals of the treatment regimen.*
- Note use of resources available to community for developing and funding programs. *May require creative program planning to utilize/maximize resources to meet multiple needs.*

NURSING PRIORITY NO. 2 To assist community to develop strategies to improve community functioning and management:

- Foster cooperative spirit of community without negating individuality of members/groups. *As individuals feel valued and respected, they are more willing to work together with others to develop a plan for identifying and improving healthcare for the community.*[2]
- Involve community in determining healthcare goals and prioritizing them to facilitate planning process. *The goal is healthy people in a healthy community, and as community members become involved and see that by prioritizing the identified goals, progress can be seen as individuals become healthier and needed services become readily available.*[2]
- Link people to needed services and assure the provision of healthcare to extent possible. Plan together with community health and social agencies to problem-solve solutions identified and anticipated problems and needs. *Interventions may be directed at an entire population within a community, the systems that affect the health of those populations, and/or the individuals and families within at-risk populations. Working together promotes a sense of involvement and control, helping people implement more effective problem solving.*[2,3]
- Identify specific populations at risk or underserved (e.g., chronically ill or disabled persons; elder adults; mentally ill persons; substance abusers; veterans; economically disadvantaged families; rural, migrant, immigrant, and homeless persons; racial and ethnic minorities) to actively involve them in the planning and evaluation processes. *These groups are often marginalized and may lack knowledge of available services, or lack resources to access services. Being part of the solution enhances sense of being heard, empowering these groups and promoting continued participation in the process.*[3,4,7,8]
- Network with others involved in educating healthcare providers and healthcare consumers regarding community needs. Create a teaching plan and form a speakers' bureau. Provide accurate information and demonstrate desired action. Present information in a culturally appropriate manner. *Disseminating information to community members regarding value of treatment or preventive programs helps people know and understand the importance of these actions and be willing to support the programs.*[1,3,7]

NURSING PRIORITY NO. 3 To promote wellness (Teaching/Discharge Considerations):

- Assist community to develop a plan for continued assessment of community needs and functioning (e.g., access to adequate healthcare; education regarding disease prevention, public health threats, and immunization; local warning system and evacuation plan in event of disaster; emergency contact numbers; planning for community members with special needs [elderly, handicapped, low-income persons]; violence prevention, personal or property protection; water, sanitation, toxic substance management; mobilization of local, state, and national resources). *Promotes proactive approach in planning for the future and continuation of efforts to improve healthy behaviors and necessary services. Note: Networks may be internal to the agency (e.g., with*

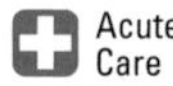

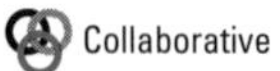

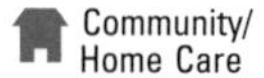

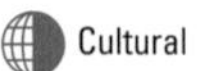

epidemiologists; public health nurses and educators; in-house laboratories; plumbing, electrical, and building inspectors) community-wide (e.g., with nongovernmental organizations, industry, academia, labs), or within the government's public health/environmental protection system (Environmental Protection Agency, the Centers for Disease Control and Protection, other federal agencies; state offices such as State Engineer and Attorney General; local agencies).[1,4,7]

- Encourage community to form partnerships within the community and between the community and the larger society. *Aids in long-term planning for anticipated and projected needs and concerns to ensure the quality and accessibility of health services.*[1]

DOCUMENTATION FOCUS

Assessment/Reassessment

- Assessment findings, including members' perceptions of community problems, healthcare resources.
- Community use of available resources.

Planning

- Plan and who is involved in planning process.
- Teaching plan.

Implementation/Evaluation

- Community's response to plan, interventions, and actions performed.
- Attainment or progress toward desired outcome(s).
- Modifications to plan.

Discharge Planning

- Long-term goals and who is responsible for actions to be taken.
- Specific referrals made.

References

1. American Public Health Association. (2012). Environmental health competency project: Draft recommendations for non-technical competencies at the local level. Retrieved May 2012 from http://www.apha.org/programs/standards/healthcompproject/corenontechnicalcompetencies.htmtx.
2. American Public Health Association. (2008). Public health in America. Retrieved May 2012 from http://www.health.gov/phfunctions/public.htm.
3. *Healthy People 2010 Toolkit: A Field Guide to Health Planning*. (2002). Washington, DC: Public Health Foundation.
4. Centers for Disease Control and Prevention. (2010). CDC vision for the 21st century: "Health protection....health equality." Retrieved May 2012 from http://www.cdc.gov/about/organization/mission.htm.
5. Bokinskie, J. C., Evanson, T. A. (2009). The stranger among us: Ministering health to migrants. *J Christian Nurs*, 26(4), 202–209.
6. Keller, L. O., Schaffer, M. A., Lia-Hoagberg, M. A. (2002). Assessment, program planning, and evaluation in population-based public health practice. *J Public Health Manage & Pract*, 8(5), 30–43.
7. de Chesnay, M., Anderson, B. A. (2012). Chapter 1: Vulnerable populations: Vulnerable people. *Caring for the Vulnerable: Perspectives in Nursing Theory, Practice, and Research*. 3rd ed. Burlington, MA: Jones & Bartlett Learning.
8. Phillips, C. D., McLeroy, K. R. (2004). Health in rural America: Remembering the importance of place. *Am J Public Health*, 94(10), 1661–1663.

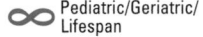

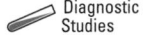

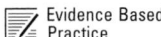

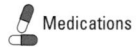

risk-prone Health Behavior

Taxonomy II: Health Promotion—Class 2 Health Management (00188) [**Diagnostic Division:** Teaching/Learning], Submitted as impaired Adjustment 1986; Revised 1998; Revised/Renamed 2006, 2008

DEFINITION: Impaired ability to modify lifestyle/behavior in a manner that improves health status.

RELATED FACTORS

Inadequate comprehension; low self-efficacy
Stressors
Smoking; substance abuse
Insufficient social support; economically disadvantaged
Negative attitude toward healthcare

DEFINING CHARACTERISTICS

Subjective

Minimizes health status change
Failure to achieve optimal sense of control

Objective

Failure to take action that prevents health problem
Nonacceptance of health status change

Sample Clinical Applications: New diagnosis/life changes for client, Alzheimer's disease, brain injury, personality or psychotic disorders, postpartum depression/psychosis, substance use/abuse

DESIRED OUTCOMES/EVALUATION CRITERIA

Sample NOC linkages:

Acceptance: Health Status: Reconciliation to significant change in health circumstances

Psychosocial Adjustment: Life Change: Adaptive psychosocial response of an individual to a significant life change

Treatment Behavior: Illness or Injury: Personal actions to palliate or eliminate pathology

Client Will (Include Specific Time Frame)

- Demonstrate increasing interest or participation in self-care.
- Develop ability to assume responsibility for personal needs when possible.
- Identify stress situations leading to difficulties in adapting to change in health status and specific actions for dealing with them.
- Initiate lifestyle changes that will permit adaptation to present life situations.
- Identify and use appropriate support systems.

ACTIONS/INTERVENTIONS

Sample NIC linkages:

Coping Enhancement: Assisting a patient to adapt to perceived stressors, changes, or threats that interfere with meeting life demands and roles

Counseling: Use of an interactive helping process focusing on the needs, problems, or feelings of the patient and significant others to enhance or support coping, problem solving, and interpersonal relationships

Teaching: Disease Process: Assisting the patient to understand information related to a specific disease process

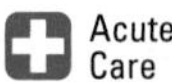

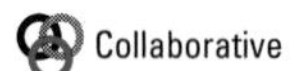

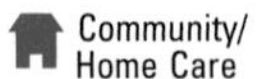

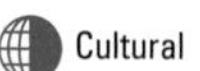

NURSING PRIORITY NO. 1 To assess degree of impaired function:

- Perform a physical and/or psychosocial assessment. *Determines the extent of the limitation(s) of the present condition.*[1]
- Listen to the client's perception of inability or reluctance to adapt to situations that are occurring at present. *Perceptions are reality to the client and need to be identified so they may be addressed and dealt with.*[3]
- Survey (with the client) past and present significant support systems (family, church, groups, organizations). *Identifies helpful resources that may be needed in current situation or change in health status.*[2]
- Explore the expressions of emotions signifying impaired adjustment by client/significant others (SOs). *Overwhelming anxiety, fear, anger, worry, passive or active denial can be experienced by the client who is having difficulty adjusting to a change in health or a feared diagnosis.*[4]
- Note child's interaction with parent/caregiver. *Interactions can be indicative of problems when family is dealing with major health issues and change in family functioning. Development of coping behaviors is limited at this age, and primary caregivers provide support for the child and serve as role models.*[5]
- Determine whether child displays problems with school performance, withdraws from family/peers, or demonstrates aggressive behavior toward others/self. *Indicators of poor coping and need for specific interventions to help child deal with own health issues or what is happening in the family.*[6]

NURSING PRIORITY NO. 2 To identify the causative/contributing factors relating to the impaired adjustment:

- Listen to client's perception of factors leading to the present dilemma, noting onset, duration, presence or absence of physical complaints, and social withdrawal. *Change often creates a feeling of disequilibrium, and the individual may respond with irrational or unfounded fears. Client may benefit from feedback that corrects misperceptions about how life will be with the change in health status.*[7]
- Note substance use or abuse (e.g., smoking, alcohol, prescription medications, street drugs) *that may be used as a coping mechanism, exacerbate health problem, or impair client's comprehension of situation.*
- Identify possible cultural beliefs or values influencing client's response to change. *Different cultures deal with change of health issues, such as cancer, chronic obstructive pulmonary disease, and diabetes mellitus, in different ways.*[12]
- Assess affective climate within family system and how it determines family members' response to adjustment to major health challenge. *Families who are high-strung and nervous may interfere with client's dealing with illness in a rational manner, while those who are more sedate and phlegmatic may be more helpful to the client in accepting the current circumstances.*[2]
- Determine lack of or inability to use available resources. *The high degree of anxiety that usually accompanies a major lifestyle change often interferes with ability to deal with problems created by the change or loss. Helping client learn to use these resources enables him or her to take control of own illness.*[8]
- Discuss normalcy of anger as life is being changed and encourage channeling anger to healthy activities. *The increased energy of anger can be used to accomplish other tasks and enhance feelings of self-esteem.*[2]
- Review available documentation and resources to determine actual life experiences (e.g., medical records, statements of SOs, consultants' notes). *In situations of great stress (physical or emotional), the client may not accurately assess occurrences leading to the present situation.*[9]

NURSING PRIORITY NO. 3 To assist client in coping/dealing with impairment:

- Organize a team conference (including client and ancillary services). *Individuals who are involved and knowledgeable can focus on contributing factors that are affecting client's adjustment to the current situation and can plan for management as indicated.*[10]

- Explain disease process or causative factors and prognosis as appropriate, promote questioning, and provide written and other resource materials. *Enhances understanding, clarifies information, and provides opportunity to review information at individual's leisure.*
- Share information with adolescent's peers with client's permission and involvement when illness or injury affects body image or function. *Peers are primary support for this age group, and sharing information promotes understanding and compassion.*[5]
- Provide an open environment encouraging communication. *Supports expression of feelings concerning impaired function so they can be dealt with realistically.*[2]
- Use therapeutic communication skills (e.g., Active-listening, acknowledgment, silence, "I" statements). *Promotes open relationship in which client can explore possibilities and solutions for changing lifestyle situation.*[13]
- Acknowledge client's efforts to adjust: "You have done your best." *May reduce feelings of blame or guilt and defensive responses.*[11]
- Discuss and evaluate resources that have been useful to the client in adapting to changes in other life situations. *Vocational rehabilitation, employment experiences, and psychosocial support services may be useful in current situation.*[11]
- Develop a plan of action with client to meet immediate needs (e.g., physical safety and hygiene, emotional support of professionals and SOs) and assist in implementation of the plan. *Provides a starting point to deal with current situation for moving ahead with plan for adjusting to change in life circumstances and for evaluation of progress toward goals.*
- Reinforce structure in daily life. Include exercise as part of routine. *Routines help the client focus. Exercise improves sense of wellness and enhances immune response.*
- Review with client coping skills used in previous life situations and role changes. *Identifies the strengths that may be used to facilitate adaptation to change or loss that has occurred.*[8]
- Refine or develop new coping strategies as appropriate. *Strengthens skills for dealing with change in health or lifestyle.*
- Identify and problem solve with the client frustrations in daily care. *Focusing on the smaller factors of concern gives the individual the ability to perceive the impaired function from a less threatening perspective (one-step-at-a-time concept). Also promotes sense of control over situation.*
- Involve SO(s) in long-range planning for emotional, psychological, physical, and social needs. *Change that is occurring when illness is long term or permanent indicates that lifestyle changes will need to be dealt with on an ongoing basis, which may be difficult for client and family to adjust to.*[12]
- Refer for individual/family counseling as indicated. *May need additional assistance to cope with current situation.*

NURSING PRIORITY NO. 4 To promote wellness (Teaching/Discharge Considerations):

- Identify strengths the client perceives in present life situation. Keep focus on the present. *Unknowns of the future may be too overwhelming when diagnosis or injury means permanent changes in lifestyle and long-term management.*
- Assist SOs to learn methods of managing present needs. (Refer to NDs specific to client's deficits.) *Promotes internal locus of control and helps develop plan for long-term needs reflecting changes required by illness or changes in health status.*[2]
- Pace and time learning sessions to meet client's needs, providing for feedback during and after learning experiences (e.g., self-catheterization, range-of-motion exercises, wound care, therapeutic communication). Promotes skill and enhances retention, thereby improving confidence.[1]
- Refer to other resources in the long-range plan of care. *Long-term assistance may include such elements as home care, transportation alternatives, occupational therapy, or vocational rehabilitation that may be useful for making indicated changes in life and assisting with adjustment to new situation as needed.*[2]

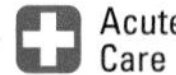

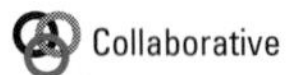

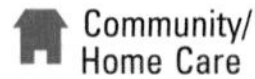

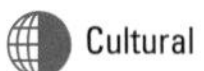

- Assist client/SO(s) to see appropriate alternatives and potential changes in locus of control. *Often major change in health status results in loss of sense of control, and client needs to begin to look at possibilities for managing illness and what abilities can make life go on in a positive manner.*

DOCUMENTATION FOCUS

Assessment/Reassessment

- Reasons for and degree of impairment.
- Client's/SO's perception of the situation.
- Effect of behavior on health status or condition.

Planning

- Plan for adjustments and interventions for achieving the plan and who is involved.
- Teaching plan.

Implementation/Evaluation

- Client responses to the interventions, teaching, and actions performed.
- Attainment or progress toward desired outcome(s).
- Modifications to plan of care.

Discharge Planning

- Resources that are available for the client and SO(s) and referrals that are made.

References

1. Klopf, J., Kofler-Westergren, B., Mitterauer, B. (2007). Towards an action-oriented criteria in risk assessment. *Int J Forensic Ment Health*, 6(1), 47–56.
2. Tucker, J. S., Orlando, M., Elliott, M. N., et al. (2006). Affective and behavioral responses to health-related social control. *Health Psychol*, 25(6), 715–722.
3. Locher, J. L., Burgio, K. L., Goode, P. S., et al. (2002). Effects of age and causal attribution to aging on health-related behaviors associated with urinary incontinence in older women. *Gerontologist*, 42(4), 515–521.
4. Koton, S., Tanne, D., Bornstein, M. N., et al. (2004). Triggering risk factors for ischemic stroke: A case-crossover study. *Neurology*, 63(11), 2006–2010.
5. Pinhas-Hamiel, O., Dolan, L. M., Daniels, S. R., et al. (1996). Increased incidence of non-insulin-dependent diabetes mellitus among adolescents. *J Pediatr*, 128(8), 608–615.
6. Deckelbaum, R. J., Williams, C. L. (2001). Childhood obesity: The health issue. *Obesity Res*, 9(5), S239–S243.
7. Badger, J. M. (2001). Burns: The psychological aspect. *Am J Nurs*, 101(11), 38–41.
8. Bartol, T. (2002). Putting a patient with diabetes in the driver's seat. *Nursing*, 32(2), 53–55.
9. Konigova, R. (1992). The psychological problems of burned patients. The Rudy Hermans Lecture 1991. *Burns*, 18(3), 189–199.
10. Grady, K. L. (2006). Management of heart failure in older adults. *J Cardiovasc Nurs*, 21(5 Suppl), S10–S14.
11. Burke, V., Mansour, J., Mori, T. A., et al. (2008). Changes in cognitive measures associated with a lifestyle program for treated hypertensives: A randomized controlled trial (ADAPT). *Health Educ Res*, 23(2), 202–217.
12. Chang, M., Kelly, A. E. (2007). Patient education: Addressing cultural diversity and health literacy issues. *Urol Nurs*, 27(5).
13. Pilgrim, G. (2010). Therapeutic communication techniques. Retrieved March 2015 from http://www.buzzle.com/articles/therapeutic-communication-techniques.html.

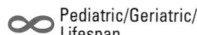

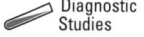

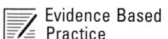

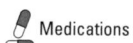

ineffective Health Maintenance

Taxonomy II: Health Promotion—Class 2 Health Management (00099) [**Diagnostic Division:** Safety], Submitted 1982

DEFINITION: Inability to identify, manage, and/or seek out help to maintain health
[Author note: This diagnosis contains components of other NDs. We recommend subsuming health maintenance interventions under the "basic" nursing diagnosis when a single causative factor is identified (e.g., deficient Knowledge [specify], ineffective Health Management, chronic Confusion, impaired verbal Communication, ineffective Coping, compromised family Coping, risk for delayed Development).]

RELATED FACTORS

Ineffective communication skills
Unachieved developmental tasks
Alteration in cognitive functioning; impaired decision making
Perceptual impairment
Decrease in gross or fine motor skills
Ineffective coping strategies; complicated grieving; spiritual distress
Insufficient resources (e.g., financial, social, knowledge)

DEFINING CHARACTERISTICS

Objective

Insufficient knowledge about basic health practices
Absence of interest in improving health behaviors; pattern of lack of health-seeking behavior
Absence of adaptive behaviors to environmental changes
Insufficient social support

Sample Clinical Applications: Chronic conditions (e.g., multiple sclerosis [MS], rheumatoid arthritis, chronic pain), brain injury or stroke, spinal cord injury or paralysis, laryngectomy, dementia, Alzheimer's disease, developmental delay

DESIRED OUTCOMES/EVALUATION CRITERIA

Sample NOC linkages:

Health-Promoting Behavior: Personal actions to sustain or increase wellness

Knowledge: Health Behavior: Extent of understanding conveyed about the promotion and protection of health

Participation in Health Care Decisions: Personal involvement in selecting and evaluating healthcare options to achieve desired outcome

Client Will (Include Specific Time Frame)

- Identify necessary health maintenance activities.
- Verbalize understanding of factors contributing to current situation.
- Assume responsibility for own healthcare needs within level of ability.
- Adopt lifestyle changes supporting individual healthcare goals.

Sample NOC linkages:

Risk Detection: Personal actions to identify personal health threats

Social Support: Reliable assistance from others

SO/Caregiver Will (Include Specific Time Frame)

- Verbalize ability to cope adequately with existing situation and provide support and monitoring as indicated.

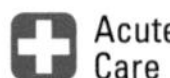

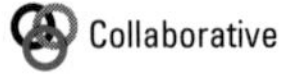

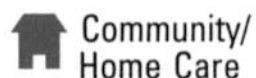

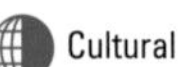

ACTIONS/INTERVENTIONS

Sample NIC linkages:
Health System Guidance: Facilitating a patient's location and use of appropriate health services
Support System Enhancement: Facilitation of support to patient by family, friends, and community
Health Education: Developing and providing instruction and learning experiences to facilitate voluntary adaptation of behavior conducive to health in individuals, families, groups, or communities

NURSING PRIORITY NO. 1 To assess causative/contributing factors:

- Recognize differing perceptions regarding health issues between healthcare providers and clients. Explore ways to partner. *Awareness that healthcare provider's goals may not be the same as a client's goals can provide opportunities to explore and communicate. Left undone, the door is open for frustration on both sides, affecting client care experience and/or perceived outcome of care. Note: For example, one study found that healthcare staff rated client's self-responsibility as the most important variable (out of 17) while the patients rated it 11th.*[13,14]
- Identify health practices and beliefs in client's personal and family history, including health values, religious or cultural beliefs, and expectations regarding healthcare. *Clients and healthcare providers do not always view a health risk in the same way. The client may not view current situation as a problem or may be unaware of routine health maintenance practices and needs. Note: In one study researchers found that information designed to meet unique characteristics of the individual through culturally relevant tailoring increased the adherent rate of interventions significantly.*[11,12]
- Note client's age (e.g., very young or elderly age); cognitive, emotional, physical, and developmental status; and level of dependence and independence. *Client's status may range from complete dependence (dysfunctional) to partial or relative independence and determines type of interventions/support needed.*
- Note whether impairment is related to an acute or sudden onset situation or a progressive illness or long-term health problem. *Determines type and intensity and length of time support may be required.*[4]
- Ascertain client's ability and desire to learn. Determine barriers to learning (e.g., can't read, speaks or understands different language, is overcome with stress or grief). *The client may not be physically, emotionally, or mentally capable at present because of current situation or may need information in small, manageable increments.*[1]
- Assess communication skills and ability or need for interpreter. Identify support person requiring or willing to accept information. *Ability to understand is essential to identification of needs and planning care. May need to provide the information to another individual if client is unable to comprehend.*[9]
- Evaluate medication regimen and also for substance use/abuse (e.g., alcohol/other drugs) as indicated. *Can affect client's understanding of information or desire and ability to accept responsibility for self.*[6]
- Note client's desire and level of ability to meet health maintenance needs as well as self-care activities of daily living. *Care may begin with helping client make a decision to improve situation, as well as identifying factors that are currently interfering with meeting needs.*[3]
- Note setting where client lives (e.g., long-term/other residential care facility, rural vs. urban setting; homebound, or homeless). *Socioeconomic status and geographic location contribute to an individual's ability to achieve or maintain good health.*[10]
- Ascertain recent changes in lifestyle. *For instance, a man whose spouse dies and who has no skills for taking care of his own/family's health needs may need assistance to learn how to manage new situation, or a newly unemployed individual without healthcare benefits may require referral to public assistance agencies.*[8]
- Determine level of adaptive behavior, knowledge, and skills about health maintenance, environment, and safety. *Will determine beginning point for planning and intervening to help client learn necessary skills to maintain health in a positive manner.*[7]

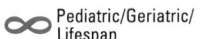

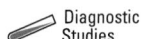

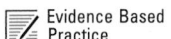

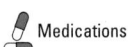

- Evaluate home environment, as indicated, *to note individual adaptation needs (e.g., supplemental humidity, air purifier, change in heating system).*[1]
- Note client's use of professional services and resources (i.e., appropriate or inappropriate, nonexistent).[9]

NURSING PRIORITY NO. 2 To assist client/caregiver(s) to maintain and manage desired health practices:

- Discuss with client/significant others (SOs) beliefs about health and reasons for not following prescribed plan of care. *Determines client's view about current situation and potential for change. Provides opportunity for discussion about alternate plan of care that client may find more suitable or may help identify a compromise that could improve client's participation in a particular course of treatment.*
- Identify realistic health goals and develop plan with client/SO(s) for self-care. *Allows for incorporating existing disabilities with client's/SO's desires, adapting and organizing care as necessary.*[1]
- Involve comprehensive specialty health teams when available or indicated (e.g., pulmonary, psychiatric, enterostomal, IV therapy, nutritional support, substance abuse counselors).
- Provide time to active-listen concerns of client/SO(s). *Provides opportunity to clarify expectations and misconceptions.*
- Provide anticipatory guidance *to maintain and manage effective health practices during periods of wellness and to identify ways client can adapt when progressive illness or long-term health problems occur.*[9,11]
- Encourage socialization, "buddy system," and personal involvement *to enhance support system, provide pleasant stimuli, and limit permanent regression.*[2]
- Provide for communication and coordination between healthcare facility teams and community healthcare providers *to promote continuation of care and maximize outcomes.*[2]
- Monitor adherence to prescribed medical regimen *to problem solve difficulties in adherence and alter the plan of care as needed.*[1]

NURSING PRIORITY NO. 3 To promote wellness (Teaching/Discharge Considerations):

- Provide information about individual healthcare needs, using client's preferred learning style (e.g., pictures, words, video, Internet). *Can help client to understand own situation and enhance cooperation with the plan of care.*[8]
- Limit amount of information presented at one time, especially when dealing with elderly or cognitively impaired client. Present new material through self-paced instruction when possible. *Allows client time to process and store new information.*[8]
- Help client/SO(s) prioritize healthcare goals. Provide a written copy to those involved in planning process *for future reference/revision as appropriate. Promotes planning to enable the client to maintain a healthy and productive lifestyle.*[10]
- Assist client/SO(s) to develop stress-management skills. *Knowing ways to manage stress helps individual to develop and maintain a healthy lifestyle.*[3]
- Identify ways to make adaptations in exercise program *to meet client's changing needs and abilities and environmental concerns.*[5]
- Identify signs and symptoms requiring further screening, evaluation, and follow-up. Essential to identify developing problems that could interfere with maintaining well-being.[10,11]
- Make referral as needed for community support services (e.g., homemaker or home attendant, Meals on Wheels, skilled nursing care, community or free clinic, Well-Baby Clinic, senior citizen healthcare activities). *Client may need additional assistance to maintain self-sufficiency.*[9]
- Refer to social services as indicated. *May need assistance with financial, housing, or legal concerns (e.g., conservatorship).*[2]
- Refer to support groups as appropriate (e.g., senior citizen groups, Alcoholics or Narcotics Anonymous, Red Cross, Salvation Army). *Provides information and help for specific needs or at times of crisis.*[9]
- Arrange for hospice service for client with terminal illness. *Will help client and family deal with end-of-life issues in a positive manner.*[3,4]

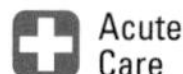

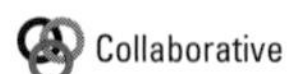

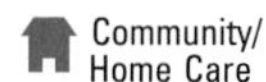

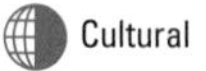

DOCUMENTATION FOCUS

Assessment/Reassessment

- Assessment findings, including individual abilities, family involvement, and support factors.
- Cultural or religious beliefs, healthcare values, and expectations.
- Availability and use of resources.

Planning

- Plan of care and who is involved in planning.
- Teaching plan.

Implementation/Evaluation

- Responses of client/SO(s) to plan, interventions, teaching, and actions performed.
- Attainment or progress toward desired outcome(s).
- Modifications to plan of care.

Discharge Planning

- Long-term needs and who is responsible for actions to be taken.
- Specific referrals made.

References

1. Bohny, B. (1997). A time for self-care: Role of the home healthcare nurse. *Home Healthcare Nurs*, 15(4), 281–286.
2. Callaghan, P., Morrissey, G. (1993). Social support and health: A review. *J Adv Nurs*, 18(2), 203–210.
3. Dossey, B. M., Dossey, L. (1998). Body-mind-spirit: Attending to holistic care. *Am J Nurs*, 98(8), 35–38.
4. Gregory, C. M. (1997). Caring for caregivers: Proactive planning eases burden on caregivers. *AWHONN Lifelines*, 1(2), 51–53.
5. Lai, S. C., Cohen, M. N. (1999). Promoting lifestyle changes. *Am J Nurs*, 99(4), 63–67.
6. Larsen, L. S. (1998). Effectiveness of counseling intervention to assist family caregivers of chronically ill relatives. *J Psychosoc Nurs*, 36(8), 26–32.
7. MacNeill, D., Weis, T. (1998). Case study: Coordinating care. *Continuing Care*, 17(4), 78.
8. McCrory Pocinki, K. (1991). Writing for an older audience: Ways to maximize understanding and acceptance. *J Nutr Elder*, 11(1–2), 69–77.
9. Stuifbergen, A. (1997). Health promotion: An essential component of rehabilitation for persons with chronic disabling conditions. *Adv Nurs Sci*, 19(4), 138–147.
10. U.S. Department of Health and Human Services: Public Health Foundation *About Healthy People*. Retrieved October 2015 from http://www.healthypeople.gov/2020/About-Healthy-People.
11. Health maintenance evaluation: Replacing the "annual physical" (No date listed). Fact sheet for Palo Alto Medical Foundation. Retrieved October 2015 from http://www.pamf.org/preventive/healtheval.html.
12. Kreuter, M. W., Sugg-Skinner, C., Holt, C. L., et al. (2005). Cultural tailoring for mammography and fruit and vegetable intake among low-income African-American women in urban public health centers. *Prev Med*, 4(1), 53–61.
13. Quill, T., Norton, S., Shah, M., et al. (2006). What is most important for you to achieve? An analysis of patient responses when receiving palliative care consultation. *J Palliat Med*, 9(2), 382–388.
14. Antoniazzi, M., Celinski, M., Alcock, J. (2002). Self-responsibility and coping with pain: Disparate attitudes toward psychosocial issues in recovery from work place injury. *Disabil Rehabil*, 24(18), 948–953.

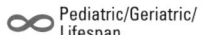

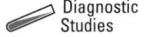

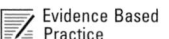

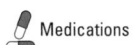

ineffective Health Management

Taxonomy II: Health Promotion—Class 2 Health Management (00078) [**Diagnostic Division:** Teaching/Learning], Submitted 1994; Revised 2008

DEFINITION: Pattern of regulating and integrating into daily living a therapeutic regimen for the treatment of illness and its sequelae that is unsatisfactory for meeting specific health goals.

RELATED FACTORS

Complexity of healthcare system or therapeutic regimen
Decisional conflicts
Economically disadvantaged
Excessive demands; family conflict
Family pattern of healthcare
Inadequate number of cues to action
Insufficient knowledge of therapeutic regimen
Perceived seriousness of condition, susceptibility, benefit, or barrier
Powerlessness
Insufficient social support

DEFINING CHARACTERISTICS

Subjective

Difficulty with prescribed regimen

Objective

Failure to include treatment regimen in daily living, or take action to reduce risk factors
Ineffective choices in daily living for meeting health goal
[Unexpected acceleration of illness symptoms; development of avoidable complications]

Sample Clinical Applications: Chronic conditions (e.g., cancer, chronic obstructive pulmonary disease [COPD], multiple sclerosis [MS], arthritis, chronic pain, end-stage heart, liver, or renal failure) or new diagnoses necessitating lifestyle changes

DESIRED OUTCOMES/EVALUATION CRITERIA

Sample NOC linkages:

Treatment Behavior: Illness or Injury: Personal actions to palliate or eliminate pathology
Health Beliefs: Personal convictions that influence health behaviors
Adherence Behavior: Self-initiated actions to promote wellness, recovery, and rehabilitation

Client Will (Include Specific Time Frame)

- Verbalize acceptance of need or desire to change actions to achieve agreed-on health goals.
- Verbalize understanding of factors and blocks involved in individual situation.
- Participate in problem solving of factors interfering with integration of therapeutic regimen.
- Demonstrate behaviors or changes in lifestyle necessary to maintain therapeutic regimen.
- Identify and use available resources.

ACTIONS/INTERVENTIONS

Sample NIC linkages:

Self-Modification Assistance: Reinforcement of self-directed change initiated by the patient to achieve personally important goals

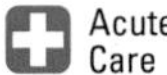
Acute Care
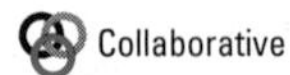
Collaborative
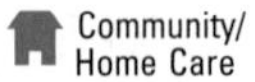
Community/ Home Care
 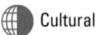
Cultural

Health System Guidance: Facilitating a patient's location and use of appropriate health services
Patient Contracting: Negotiating an agreement with an individual that reinforces a specific behavior change

NURSING PRIORITY NO. 1 To identify causative/contributing factors:

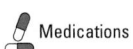

- Determine whether client has acute or chronic illness; if chronic, note whether more than one condition is present at the same time and assess the complexity of care needs. *These factors affect how client views and manages self-care. Client may be overwhelmed, in denial, depressed, or have complications exacerbating care needs. Note: For example, diabetes is considered a biopsychosocial illness, meaning there are not only biological factors, including cause of illness and the toll it takes on the body, but also psychological, social, and economic components for the client dealing with a chronic progressive disease over a long time, usually with comorbidities.*[10]
- Ascertain client's knowledge/understanding of condition and treatment needs. *Provides a baseline so planning care can begin where the client is in relation to condition or illness and current regimen.*[1]
- Determine client's/family's health goals and patterns of healthcare. *Provides information about current behaviors and misperceptions that may be potential areas of conflict, values, or financial considerations.*[1]
- Identify health practices and beliefs in client's personal and family history, including health values, religious or cultural beliefs, and expectations regarding healthcare. *The client may not view current situation as a problem or be unaware of health management needs. Expectations of others may dictate client's adaptation to situation and willingness to modify life. Note: In one study, researchers found that information designed to meet unique characteristics of the individual through culturally relevant tailoring significantly increased adherence rate with interventions.*[1,8,9]
- Identify client locus of control. *Those with an internal locus of control (e.g., expressions of responsibility for self and ability to control outcomes, such as "I didn't quit smoking") are more likely to take charge of situation, whereas individuals with an external locus of control (e.g., expressions of lack of control over self and environment, such as "Nothing ever works out" or "What bad luck to get lung cancer") may perceive difficulties as beyond his or her control and will look to others or external source to solve his or her problems and take care of them.*[7]
- Identify individual perceptions and expectations of treatment regimen. *May reveal misinformation, unrealistic expectations, or other factors that may be interfering with client's willingness to follow therapeutic regimen.*[1,10]
- Determine issues of secondary gain for the client/significant others (SOs). *Marital/family concern or attention, school or work issues, or financial considerations may cause client to subconsciously desire to remain ill or disabled. This can interfere with complying with prescribed treatment plans, prolong recovery time, and create frustrating medical-legal issues.*[11]
- Review complexity of treatment regimen (e.g., number of expected tasks, such as taking medication several times/day, visiting multiple healthcare providers with treatment or follow-up appointments; abundant, often conflicting information sources). Evaluate how difficult tasks might be for client (e.g., must stop smoking or must follow strict dialysis diet even when feeling well, must manage limitations while remaining active in life roles). *These factors are often involved in lack of participation in treatment plan.*[12]
- Note availability and use of resources for assistance and caregiving or respite care services. *Client may not have, be aware of, or know how to access resources that may be available.*[6]

NURSING PRIORITY NO. 2 To assist client/SO(s) to develop strategies to improve management of therapeutic regimen:

- Use therapeutic communication skills to assist client to problem-solve solution(s). *Active listening promotes accurate identification of the problem, ensuring that problem solving is directed to the correct solution.*[7]
- Explore client involvement in or lack of mutual goal setting. *Understanding client's willingness to be involved or not provides insight into the reasons for these actions and appropriate interventions.*[7]

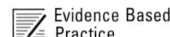

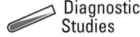

- Have client identify consequences of current behaviors/ineffective management of condition. *May help client visualize the "cost" of lack of commitment to therapeutic regimen.*
- Use client's locus of control to develop individual plan to adapt regimen. *For client with internal control, encourage client to take control of own care, and for those with external control, begin with small tasks and add as tolerated.*[7]
- Identify steps necessary to reach desired goal(s). *Specifying steps to take requires discussion and the use of critical-thinking skills to determine how to best reach the agreed-on goals.*[4]
- Contract with the client for participation in care, as appropriate. *By making a contract, client commits self to therapeutic regimen and is more likely to follow through because of commitment.*[6]
- Accept client's evaluation of own strengths and limitations while working together to improve abilities. State belief in client's ability to cope and/or adapt to situation. *Individuals may minimize own strengths and exaggerate limitations when faced with the difficulties of a chronic illness. By helping in concrete ways, client can begin to accept reality of strengths. Stating your belief in positive terms lets client hear someone else's evaluation and begin to accept that he or she can manage the situation.*[3]
- Acknowledge individual efforts and capabilities. *Positive reinforcement encourages continuation of desired behaviors and facilitates movement toward attainment of desired outcomes.*[5,7]
- Provide information and help client to know where and how to find it on own. Reinforce previous instructions and rationale, using a variety of learning modalities, including role-playing, demonstration, written materials, etc. *Incorporating multiple modalities promotes retention of information. Developing client's skill at finding own information encourages self-sufficiency and sense of self-worth.*[2]

NURSING PRIORITY NO. 3 To promote optimal health (Teaching/Discharge Considerations):

- Emphasize importance of client knowledge and understanding of the need for treatment or medication as well as consequences of actions and choices. *Reinforces client's role in success of therapeutic regimen, encouraging continuation of competent behaviors.*[1]
- Promote client/caregiver/SO(s) participation in planning and evaluating process. *Enhances commitment to plan and promotes competent self-management, optimizing outcomes.*[1]
- Assist client to develop strategies for monitoring symptoms and response to therapeutic regimen. *Promotes early recognition of changes, allowing proactive response.*[5]
- Mobilize support systems, including family/SO(s), social services, financial assistance, etc. *Success of therapeutic regimen is enhanced by using support systems effectively, avoiding or reducing stress and worry of dealing with unresolved problems.*[2]
- Refer to counseling or therapy (group and individual) as indicated. *Client may need additional help to deal with stress and anxiety of chronic condition or illness.*[1]
- Identify home- and community-based nursing services. *These agencies can provide services for assessment, follow-up care, and education in client's home to promote more effective management of therapeutic regimen.*[1]

DOCUMENTATION FOCUS

Assessment/Reassessment

- Assessment findings, including underlying dynamics of individual situation, client's perception of problem or needs, locus of control.
- Cultural values or religious beliefs.
- Family involvement and needs.
- Individual strengths and limitations.
- Availability and use of resources.

Planning

- Plan of care and who is involved in planning.
- Teaching plan.

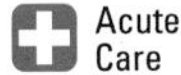
Acute Care
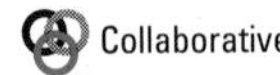
Collaborative
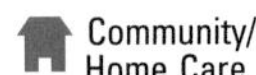
Community/ Home Care
 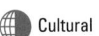
Cultural

Implementation/Evaluation

- Response to interventions, teaching, and actions performed.
- Attainment or progress toward desired outcome(s).
- Modifications to plan of care.

Discharge Planning

- Long-term needs and who is responsible for actions to be taken.
- Available resources, specific referrals made.

References

1. Newfield, S. A., Hinz, M. D., Scott-Tilley, D. S., et al. (2007). *Cox's Clinical Applications of Nursing Diagnosis: Adult, Child, Women's, Psychiatric, Gerontic, and Home Health Considerations*. 5th ed. Philadelphia: F. A. Davis.
2. U.S. Department of Health and Human Services: Public Health Foundation. About healthy people (various pages). Retrieved October 2015 from http://healthypeople.gov/2020/About-Healthy-People.
3. Stuifbergen, A. (1997). Health promotion: An essential component of rehabilitation for persons with chronic disabling conditions. *Adv Nurs Sci*, 19(4), 147–148.
4. Larsen, L. S. (1998). Effectiveness of counseling intervention to assist family caregivers of chronically ill relatives. *J Psychosoc Nurs*, 36(8), 26–32.
5. Lai, S. C., Cohen, M. N. (1999). Promoting lifestyle changes. *Am J Nurs*, 99(4), 63–67.
6. Miller, J. F. (1999). *Coping with Chronic Illness: Overcoming Powerlessness*. 3rd ed. Philadelphia: F. A. Davis.
7. Townsend, M. C. (2011). *Psychiatric Mental Health Nursing Concepts of Care in Evidence-Based Practice*. 7th ed. Philadelphia: F. A. Davis.
8. Purnell, L. D. (2009). *Guide to Culturally Competent Health Care*. 2nd ed. Philadelphia: F. A. Davis.
9. Krueter, M. W., Sugg-Skinner, C., Holt, C. L., et al. (2005). Cultural tailoring for mammography and fruit and vegetable intake among low-income African-American women in urban public health centers, 4(1), 53–61.
10. Zinzer, K. A., Mulhern, J. L., Kareem, A. A. (2011). The implementation of the Chronic Care Model with respect to dealing with the biopsychosocial aspects of the chronic disease of diabetes. *Adv Skin Wound Care*, 24(10), 475–484.
11. Dersh, J., Polatin, P. B., Leeman, G., et al. (2004). The management of secondary gain and loss in medicolegal settings: Strengths and weaknesses. *J Occup Rehabil*, 14(4), 267–279.
12. Corser, W., Dontje, K. (2011). Self-management perspectives of heavily comorbid primary care adults. *Prof Case Manag*, 16(1), 6–15.

ineffective family Health Management

Taxonomy II: Health Promotion—Class 2 Health Management (00080) [**Diagnostic Division:** Teaching/Learning], Submitted 1992

DEFINITION: A pattern of regulating and integrating into family processes a program for the treatment of illness and its sequelae that is unsatisfactory for meeting specific health goals.

RELATED FACTORS

Complexity of therapeutic regimen, or healthcare system
Decisional conflict
Economically disadvantaged
Family conflicts

(continues on page 408)

ineffective family Health Management (continued)

DEFINING CHARACTERISTICS

Subjective

Difficulty with prescribed regimen

Objective

Inappropriate family activities for meeting health goal

Acceleration of illness symptoms of a family member

Failure to take action to reduce risk factors; decrease in attention to illness

Sample Clinical Applications: Chronic conditions (e.g., chronic obstructive pulmonary disease [COPD], multiple sclerosis [MS], arthritis, chronic pain, substance abuse, end-stage liver or renal failure) or new diagnoses necessitating lifestyle changes

DESIRED OUTCOMES/EVALUATION CRITERIA

Sample NOC linkages:

Family Health Status: Overall health and social competence of family unit

Family Normalization: Capacity of the family system to develop strategies for optimal functioning when a member has a chronic illness or disability

Family Participation in Professional Care: Family involvement in decision making, delivery, and evaluation of care provided by health-care personnel

Family Will (Include Specific Time Frame)

- Identify individual factors affecting regulation/integration of treatment program.
- Participate in problem solving of identified factors.
- Engage in mutual goal setting for care/treatment plan.
- Verbalize acceptance of need or desire to change actions to achieve agreed-on outcomes or health goals.
- Demonstrate behaviors/changes in lifestyle necessary to maintain therapeutic regimen.

ACTIONS/INTERVENTIONS

Sample NIC linkages:

Family Involvement Promotion: Facilitating participation of family members in the emotional and physical care of the patient

Family Mobilization: Utilization of family strengths to influence patient's health in a positive direction

Health System Guidance: Facilitating a patient's location and use of appropriate health services

NURSING PRIORITY NO. 1 To identify causative/precipitating factors:

- Ascertain family's perception of efforts to date. *Perceptions are more important than facts, and by getting family's point of view, realistic goals can be set and family can look to the future.*[2]
- Evaluate family functioning and activities, including frequency and effectiveness of family communication, promotion of autonomy, adaptations to meet changing needs, health of home environment and lifestyle, problem-solving abilities, and ties to the community. *Understanding the family and the context in which it lives allows for more personalized support of the family and choosing coping strategies in partnership with the family to meet individualized goals.*[7]
- Note family health goals and agreement of individual members. *Presence of conflict interferes with problem solving and needs to be addressed before family can move forward to meet goals.*[2]

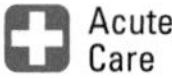

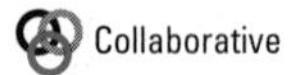

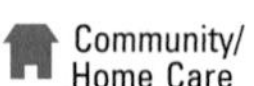

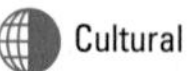

- Determine understanding and value of the treatment regimen to the family. *Individual members may misunderstand either the cause of the illness or the prescribed regimen and may disagree with what is happening, thereby promoting dissension within the family group and causing distress for the identified client.*[1]
- Identify cultural values and religious beliefs affecting view of situation and willingness to make necessary changes. *May influence choice of interventions.*
- Identify availability and use of resources. *Knowing who is available to help and support the family will help in planning care to maximize positive outcomes.*[2]

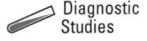

NURSING PRIORITY NO. 2 To assist family to develop strategies to improve management of therapeutic regimen:

- Provide family-centered education addressing management of condition/chronic illness, treatment plan, and self-care needs. *Accurate information helps family make informed decisions, see the connection between illness and treatment, facilitate treatment adherence, and improve client outcomes.*[3,8]
- Encourage incorporation of care strategies into family's lifestyle. *Assisting family to manage needs on a daily basis can instill confidence, decrease anxiety, and provide a degree of predictability to daily life.*[8]
- Assist family members to recognize inappropriate family activities. Help the members identify both togetherness and individual needs and behavior. *Effective interactions can be enhanced and perpetuated when these factors are identified and used to improve family behaviors.*[2]
- Make a plan jointly with family members to deal with complexity of healthcare regimen or system and other related factors. *Enhances commitment to plan, optimizing outcomes when family and caregivers work together to plan therapeutic regimen.*[2,5] *Engaging all family members as able empowers family to build new competencies and shared confidence in own abilities enabling more effective coping.*[6]
- Identify community resources as needed using the three strategies of education, problem solving, and resource linking to address specific deficits. *Providing information and helping family members learn effective problem-solving techniques and how to access needed resources can help them deal successfully with the chronically ill family member.*[4]

NURSING PRIORITY NO. 3 To promote wellness as related to future health and well-being of family members (Teaching/Discharge Considerations):

- Help family identify criteria to promote ongoing self-evaluation of situation and effectiveness and family progress. *Involvement promotes sense of control and provides the opportunity to be proactive in meeting needs.*[2]
- Assist family to plan for potential problems or complications. *Helping families anticipate likely challenges allows them to plan more effective coping strategies.*[6]
- Make referrals to and/or jointly plan with other health, social, and community resources. *Problems often are multifaceted, requiring involvement of numerous providers or agencies to plan appropriate regimen to meet family/individual needs.*[3]
- Encourage involvement in disease/condition support groups. *Family resiliency is gained/supported through contact with other families dealing with similar challenges and from learning from one another.*[6]
- Provide contact person or case manager for one-on-one assistance as needed. *Having a single contact to coordinate care, provide support, and assist with problem solving maintains continuity and prevents misunderstandings and errors in managing the family's regimen.*[1]
- Refer to NDs caregiver Role Strain and ineffective Health Management, as indicated.

DOCUMENTATION FOCUS

Assessment/Reassessment

- Individual findings, including nature of problem and degree of impairment, family values, health goals, and level of participation and commitment of family members.

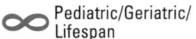

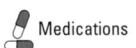

- Cultural values, religious beliefs.
- Availability and use of resources.

Planning

- Plan of care and who is involved in planning.
- Teaching plan.

Implementation/Evaluation

- Response to interventions, teaching, and actions performed.
- Attainment or progress toward desired outcome(s).
- Modifications of plan of care.

Discharge Planning

- Long-term needs, plan for meeting and who is responsible for actions.
- Specific referrals made.

References

1. Cox, H. C., Hinz, M. D., Lubno, M. A., et al. (2002). *Clinical Applications of Nursing Diagnosis: Adult, Child, Women's, Psychiatric, Gerontic, and Home Health Considerations*. 4th ed. Philadelphia: F. A. Davis.
2. Healthy People 2010 Toolkit: A Field Guide to Health Planning. (2002). Washington, DC: Public Health Foundation.
3. Stuifbergen, A. (1997). Health promotion: An essential component of rehabilitation for persons with chronic disabling conditions. *Adv Nurs Sci*, 19(4), 147–148.
4. Larsen, L. S. (1998). Effectiveness of counseling intervention to assist family caregivers of chronically ill relatives. *J Psychosoc Nurs*, 36(8), 26–32.
5. Gance-Cleveland, B. (2005). Motivational interviewing as a strategy to increase families' adherence to treatment regimens. *J Spec Pediatr Nurs*, 10(3), 151–155.
6. Walsh, F. (1996). The concept of family resilience: Crisis and challenge. *Family Process*, 35(3), 261–281.
7. Jokinen, P. (2004). The family life-path theory: A tool for nurses working in partnership with families. *J Child Health Care*, 8(2), 124–133.
8. Kumar, C., Edelman, M., Ficorelli, C. (2005). Children with asthma. *MCN*, 30(5), 305–311.

readiness for enhanced Health Management

Taxonomy II: Health Promotion—Class 2 Health Management (00162) [**Diagnostic Division:** Teaching/Learning], Submitted 2002; Revised 2010, 2013

DEFINITION: A pattern of regulating and integrating into daily living a therapeutic regimen for treatment of illness and its sequelae, which can be strengthened.

DEFINING CHARACTERISTICS

Subjective

Expresses desire to enhance management of illness, symptoms, or risk factors
Expresses desire to enhance management of prescribed regimens
Expresses desire to enhance immunization/vaccination status
Expresses desire to enhance choices of daily living for meeting goals

Sample Clinical Applications: Diabetes mellitus, congestive heart failure (CHF), chronic obstructive pulmonary disease (COPD), asthma, multiple sclerosis (MS), systemic lupus, HIV positive, AIDS, premature newborn

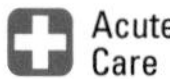

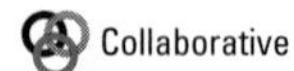

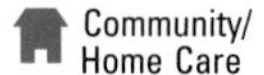

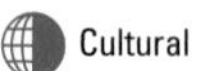

DESIRED OUTCOMES/EVALUATION CRITERIA

Sample NOC linkages:

Adherence Behavior: Self-initiated actions to promote optimal wellness, recovery, and rehabilitation
Knowledge: Treatment Regimen: Extent of understanding conveyed about a specific treatment regimen
Participation in Health-Care Decisions: Personal involvement in selecting and evaluating health-care options to achieve desired outcomes

Client Will (Include Specific Time Frame)

- Assume responsibility for managing treatment regimen.
- Demonstrate proactive management by anticipating and planning for eventualities of condition or potential complications.
- Identify and use additional resources, as appropriate.
- Remain free of preventable complications and progression of illness and sequelae.

ACTIONS/INTERVENTIONS

Sample NIC linkages:

Health System Guidance: Facilitating a patient's location and use of appropriate health services
Health Education: Developing and providing instruction and learning experiences to facilitate voluntary adaptation of behavior conducive to health in individuals, families, groups, or communities
Anticipatory Guidance: Preparation of patient for an anticipated developmental or situational crisis

NURSING PRIORITY NO. 1 To determine motivation for continued growth:

- Ascertain client's beliefs about health and his/her ability to maintain health. *Belief in ability to accomplish desired action is predictive of performance.*
- Verify client's level of knowledge and understanding of therapeutic regimen. Note specific health goals and what measures client has been using to achieve his/her goals. *Provides opportunity to ensure accuracy and completeness of information for future learning.*[1]
- Determine source(s) individuals use when seeking health information and what is done with this information (e.g., incorporated into self-management, used as basis for seeking healthcare). *The manner in which people access and use healthcare information varies widely, with variables including age, race/culture, location, literacy, and computer use. Although the Internet is utilized by many individuals to learn about their health and healthcare needs, studies show that the most common and trusted sources of information are still healthcare professionals. Many people supplement information received from healthcare professionals with information from TV, radio, newspapers, magazines, and family/friends/coworkers.*[9,10]
- Determine individual's perceptions of adaptation to treatment, anticipated changes, or possible threats to well-being. *How client sees the situation is important to discussing what is happening in regard to the treatment regimen and planning for the future.*[1]
- Identify individual's expectations of long-term treatment needs and anticipated changes. *Knowing expectations identifies understanding and acceptance of what is realistic for own situation.*[3]
- Determine influence of cultural beliefs on client/caregiver(s) participation in regimen. *These factors influence the way people view health issues and management.*

NURSING PRIORITY NO. 2 To assist client/SO(s) to develop plan to meet individual needs:

- Active-listen concerns to identify underlying issues (e.g., physical or emotional stressors, external factors such as environmental pollutants or other hazards) *that could impact client's ability to control own health.*

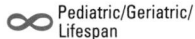

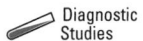

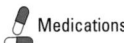

- Identify steps necessary to reach desired health goal(s). *Understanding the process enhances commitment and the likelihood of achieving the goals.*[4]
- Discuss resources presently used by client *to note whether changes can be arranged (e.g., increased hours of home-care assistance, access to case manager to support complex or long-term program). Helps with planning for improved therapeutic regimen.*[3]
- Accept client's evaluation of own strengths/limitations while working together to improve abilities. *Promotes sense of self-esteem and confidence to continue efforts to manage therapeutic regimen, such as diabetes and MS, more effectively.*[6]
- Incorporate client's cultural values or religious beliefs that support attainment of health goals. Problem solve conflicts *to facilitate growth.*
- Provide information and bibliotherapy. Help client/significant others (SOs) identify and evaluate resources they can access on their own. *Promotes sense of confidence in own ability to learn about illness or condition. When referencing the Internet and nontraditional or unproven resources, the individual must exercise some restraint and determine the reliability of the source and information provided before acting on it.*[5]
- Acknowledge individual's efforts, capabilities, and skills to acquire or maintain interpersonal, self-care, and coping skills. *Provides positive reinforcement, encouraging continued progress toward desired goals to enhance therapeutic regimen.*[3,5,8]

NURSING PRIORITY NO. 3 To promote optimum health management (Teaching/Discharge Considerations) :

- Promote client/caregiver choices and involvement in planning for and implementing added tasks or responsibilities. *Being involved in planning and knowing that he or she can make own choices promotes commitment to program and enhances probability that client will follow through with change.*[1,8]
- Assist in implementing strategies for monitoring progress and responses to therapeutic regimen. *Promotes proactive problem solving, enabling client/caregiver to identify problems as they arise and deal appropriately with them so regimen is maintained.*[1,8]
- Identify additional community resources and support groups. *Provides additional opportunities for role modeling, skill training, anticipatory problem solving, etc.*[2,6]

DOCUMENTATION FOCUS

Assessment/Reassessment

- Findings, including dynamics of individual situation.
- Individual strengths and additional needs.
- Cultural values or religious beliefs.

Planning

- Plan of care and who is involved in planning.
- Teaching plan.

Implementation/Evaluation

- Response to interventions, teaching, and actions performed.
- Attainment or progress toward desired outcome(s).
- Modifications to plan of care.

Discharge Planning

- Short- and long-term needs and who is responsible for actions.
- Available resources, specific referrals made.

References

1. Newfield, S. A., Hinz, M. D., Scott-Tilley, D. S., et al. (2007). *Cox's Clinical Applications of Nursing Diagnosis: Adult, Child, Women's, Psychiatric, Gerontic, and Home Health Considerations*. 5th ed. Philadelphia: F. A. Davis.
2. U.S. Department of Health and Human Services: Public Health Foundation. About healthy people (various pages). Retrieved October 2015 from http://www.healthypeople.gov/2020/About-Healthy-People.
3. Stuifbergen, A. (1997). Health promotion: An essential component of rehabilitation for persons with chronic disabling conditions. *Adv Nurs Sci*, 19(4), 147–148.
4. Larsen, L. S. (1998). Effectiveness of counseling intervention to assist family caregivers of chronically ill relatives. *J Psychosoc Nurs*, 36(8), 26–32.
5. Lai, S. C., Cohen, M. N. (1999). Promoting lifestyle changes. *Am J Nurs*, 99(4), 63–67.
6. Miller, J. F. (1999). *Coping with Chronic Illness: Overcoming Powerlessness*. 3rd ed. Philadelphia: F. A. Davis.
7. Purnell, L. D. (2009). *Guide to Culturally Competent Health Care*. 2nd ed. Philadelphia: F. A. Davis.
8. Agency for Healthcare Research and Quality. Strategies to support self-management in chronic conditions. Retrieved October 2015 from http://www.guideline.gov/content.aspx?id=34758.
9. Dart, J., Gallois, C., Yellowlees, P. (2008). Community health information sources: A survey in three disparate communities. *Aust Health Rev*, 32(1), 186–196.
10. Cutilli, C. C. (2010). Patient Education Center: Seeking health information: What sources do your patients use? *Orthop Nurs*, 29(3), 214–219.

impaired Home Maintenance

Taxonomy II: Activity/Rest—Class 5 Self-Care (00098) [**Diagnostic Division:** Safety], Submitted 1980

DEFINITION: Inability to independently maintain a safe growth-promoting immediate environment.

RELATED FACTORS

Condition impacting ability to maintain home (e.g., disease; illness; injury)
Illness/injury impacting ability to maintain home
Alteration in cognitive functioning
Insufficient role model, support system
Insufficient knowledge of home maintenance, neighborhood resources

DEFINING CHARACTERISTICS

Subjective

Difficulty maintaining a comfortable [safe] environment
Request for assistance with home maintenance
Excessive family responsibilities
Financial crisis (e.g., debt, insufficient finances)

Objective

Unsanitary environment
Pattern of disease or infection caused by unhygienic conditions
Insufficient equipment for maintaining home; insufficient cooking equipment, clothing, or linen

Sample Clinical Applications: Chronic conditions (e.g., AIDS, multiple sclerosis [MS], rheumatoid arthritis), depression, dementia, developmental delay

(continues on page 414)

impaired Home Maintenance (continued)

DESIRED OUTCOMES/EVALUATION CRITERIA

Sample NOC linkages:

Self-Care: Instrumental Activities of Daily Living [IADLs]: Ability to perform activities needed to function in the home or community independently with or without assistive device

Family Functioning: Capacity of the family system to meet the needs of its members during developmental transitions

Safe Home Environment: Physical arrangements to minimize environmental factors that might cause physical harm or injury in the home

Client/Caregiver Will (Include Specific Time Frame)

- Identify individual factors related to difficulty in maintaining a safe environment.
- Verbalize plan to eliminate health and safety hazards.
- Adopt behaviors reflecting lifestyle changes to create and sustain a healthy and growth-promoting environment.
- Demonstrate appropriate, effective use of resources.

ACTIONS/INTERVENTIONS

Sample NIC linkages:

Home Maintenance Assistance: Helping the patient/family to maintain the home as a clean and pleasant place to live

Environmental Management: Safety: Monitoring and manipulation of the physical environment to promote safety

Support System Enhancement: Facilitation of support to patient by family, friends, and community

NURSING PRIORITY NO. 1 To assess causative/contributing factors:

- Identify presence of or potential for conditions such as diabetes, fractures, spinal cord injury, amputation, MS, arthritis, stroke, Parkinson's disease, dementia, and mental illness, *which can compromise client's/significant other's (SO's) functional abilities in taking care of home.*[3]
- Note personal or environmental factors (e.g., family member with multiple care tasks, addition of family member(s) [e.g., new baby, ill parent moving in]; substance abuse; poverty/inadequate financial resources; absence of family/support systems; lifestyle of self-neglect; client comfortable with home environment or has no desire for change) *that can contribute to neglect of home cleanliness or repair.*[2,5]
- Determine problems in the household and degree of discomfort or unsafe conditions noted by client/SO. *Some safety problems may be immediately obvious (e.g., lack of heat, water; need for laundry, garbage disposal, etc.), while other problems may be more subtle and difficult to manage (e.g., lack of sufficient finances for home repairs, lack of knowledge about food storage, indoor air and fire safety, rodent control). Client/SO may need assistance or teaching regarding safety of his or her environment, especially if it is negatively impacting the client's health.*[2,6]
- Assess client's/SO's level of cognitive, emotional, and physical functioning *to ascertain client's needs and caregiver's capabilities when developing plan of care for preventive, supportive, and therapeutic care.*[1,2]
- Identify lack of interest or knowledge or misinformation *to determine need for health education/home safety program or other intervention.*
- Identify support systems available to client/SO(s) *to determine needs and initiate referrals (e.g., companionship, daily care, respite care, homemaking, running errands, meal preparation or meal-service program, financial assistance).*[1]
- Determine financial resources to meet needs of individual situation. *May need referral to social services for funds, necessary equipment, home repairs, transportation, etc.*[2]

NURSING PRIORITY NO. 2 To help client/SO(s) to create/maintain a safe, growth-promoting environment:

- Coordinate planning with multidisciplinary team and client/SO as appropriate. *Coordination and cooperation of team improves motivation and maximizes outcomes.*
- Assist client/SO(s) to develop plan for restoring/maintaining a clean, healthful environment. *Activities such as sharing of household tasks or repairs between family members, contract services, exterminators, and trash removal can promote ongoing maintenance.*
- Educate and assist client/family to address lifestyle adjustments that may be required, such as personal/home hygiene practices, elimination of substance abuse or unsafe smoking habits, proper food storage, stress management, etc. *Individuals may not be aware of impact of these factors on their health or welfare; they may be overwhelmed and in need of specific assistance for varying periods of time.*
- Discuss home environment or perform home visit as indicated *to determine client's ability to care for self, to identify potential health and safety hazards, and to determine adaptations that may be needed (e.g., wheelchair-accessible doors and hallways, safety bars in bathroom, safe place for child play, clean water available, working cook stove or microwave, screens on windows).*[2]
- Assist client/SO(s) to identify and acquire necessary equipment and services (e.g., chair or stair lifts; commode chair; safety grab bar; structural adaptations; service animals; aids for hearing, seeing, mobility; trash removal; cleaning supplies) *to meet individual needs.*[3]
- Identify resources available for appropriate assistance (e.g., visiting nurse, budget counseling, homemaker, Meals on Wheels, physical or occupational therapy, social services).[2]
- Discuss options for financial assistance with housing needs. *Client may be able to stay in home with minimal assistance or may need significant assistance over a wide range of possibilities, including removal from the home.*[2]

NURSING PRIORITY NO. 3 To promote wellness (Teaching/Discharge Considerations):

- Evaluate client at each community contact or before facility discharge *to determine if home maintenance needs are ongoing in order to initiate appropriate referrals.*[3]
- Discuss environmental hazards *that may negatively affect health or ability to perform desired activities.*
- Discuss long-term plan *for taking care of environmental needs (e.g., assistive personnel, specialized controls for electrical equipment, trash removal and pest control services).*[4]
- Provide information necessary for the individual situation. *Helps client/family decide what can be done to improve situation.*[3]
- Identify ways to access/use community resources and support systems (e.g., extended family, neighbors, church group, seniors program).
- Refer to NDs caregiver Role Strain, compromised family Coping, ineffective Coping, risk for Injury, deficient Knowledge [specify], and Self-Care Deficit [specify] for additional interventions as appropriate.

DOCUMENTATION FOCUS

Assessment/Reassessment

- Assessment findings include individual (cognitive, emotional, and physical functioning) and environmental factors, specific safety concerns.
- Availability and use of support systems.

Planning

- Plan of care and who is involved in planning; support systems and community resources identified.
- Teaching plan.

Implementation/Evaluation

- Client's/SO's responses to interventions, teaching, and actions performed.
- Attainment or progress toward desired outcome(s).
- Modifications to plan of care.

Discharge Planning

- Long-term needs and who is responsible for actions to be taken.
- Specific referrals made, equipment needs/resources.

References

1. Townsend, M. C. (2011). *Psychiatric Mental Health Nursing Concepts of Care in Evidence-Based Practice*. 7th ed. Philadelphia: F. A. Davis.
2. Newfield, S. A., Hinz, M. D., Tilley, D. S., et al. (2007). *Cox's Clinical Applications of Nursing Diagnosis: Adult, Child, Women's, Mental Health, Gerontic, and Home Health Considerations*. 5th ed. Philadelphia: F. A. Davis.
3. Fenn, M. (1998). Health promotion: Theoretical perspectives and clinical application. *Holis Nurs Pract*, 19(2), 1–7.
4. Schmelling, S. (2005). Home, adapted home. *Rehabil Manage*, 18(6), 12–19.
5. Gibbons, S., Lauder, W., Ludwick, R. (2006). Self-neglect: A proposed new NANDA diagnosis. *Int J Nurs Terminol Classif*, 17(1), 10–18.
6. Centers for Disease Control and Prevention. (2009). Healthy homes; Health issues related to community design (fact sheets). Retrieved October 2015 from http://www.cdc.gov/healthyplaces/factsheets/health_issues_related_to_community_design_factsheet_final.pdf.

readiness for enhanced Hope

Taxonomy II: Self–Perception Class 1 Self—Concept (00185) [**Diagnostic Division:** Ego Integrity], Submitted 2006; Revised 2013

DEFINITION: A pattern of expectations and desires for mobilizing energy on one's own behalf, which can be strengthened.

DEFINING CHARACTERISTICS

Subjective

Expresses desire to enhance: hope; belief in possibilities; congruency of expectation with goal; ability to set achievable goals; problem solving to meet goals

Expresses desire to enhance: sense of meaning in life; connectedness with others; spirituality

Sample Clinical Applications: Any acute or chronic condition, or healthy individual looking to improve well-being

DESIRED OUTCOMES/EVALUATION CRITERIA

Sample NOC linkages:

Hope: Optimism that is personally satisfying and life supporting

Quality of Life: Extent of positive perception of current life circumstances

Personal Well-Being: Extent of positive perception of one's health status

Client Will (Include Specific Time Frame)

- Identify and verbalize feelings related to expectations and desires.
- Verbalize belief in possibilities for the future.
- Discuss current situation and desire to enhance hope.
- Set short-term goals that will lead to behavioral changes to meet desire for enhanced hope.

ACTIONS/INTERVENTIONS

Sample NIC linkages:
Hope Inspiration: Enhancing the belief in one's capacity to initiate and sustain actions
Self-Awareness Enhancement: Assisting a patient to explore and understand his or her thoughts, feelings, motivations, and behaviors
Spiritual Growth Facilitation: Facilitation of growth in patient's capacity to identify, connect with, and call upon the source of meaning, purpose, comfort, strength, and hope in their lives

NURSING PRIORITY NO. 1 To determine needs and desire for improvement:

- Review familial and social history to identify past situations (e.g., illness, emotional conflicts, alcoholism) that have led to decision to improve life. *When trials of life have been resolved, individuals may look toward making life better.*[1]
- Determine current physical condition of client/significant other (SO). *Treatment regimen and indicators of healing can influence ability to promote positive feelings of hope.*[2]
- Ascertain client's perception of current state and expectations or goals for the future (e.g., general well-being, prosperity, independence). *Perception is more important than reality in individual's mind and can help to pursue realistic goals for self.*[3]
- Identify spiritual beliefs/cultural values that guide or influence client's spirituality and view of self. *Influences sense of hope and connectedness.*[4]
- Determine meaning of life or reasons for living, belief in God or higher power. *Helps client to clarify beliefs and how they relate to desire for improvement in life.*
- Ascertain motivation and expectations for change. Note congruency of expectations with desires for change. *Motivation to improve and high expectations can encourage client to make changes that will improve his or her life. However, presence of unrealistic expectations may hamper efforts.*[3,4]
- Note degree of involvement in activities and relationships with others. *Interactions with others can promote a sense of connectedness and enjoyment of relationships.*[3]

NURSING PRIORITY NO. 2 To assist client to achieve goals and strengthen sense of hope:

- Establish a therapeutic relationship, showing positive regard and hopefulness for the client. *Enhances feelings of worth and comfort, inspiring client to continue pursuit of goals.*[3]
- Help client recognize areas that are in his or her control versus those that are not. *To be most effective, client needs to expend energy in those areas where he or she has control and let the others go.*[2]
- Assist client to develop manageable short-term goals. *Success at short-term goals that are manageable will lead to attainment of long-term goals too.*[2]
- Identify activities to achieve goals and facilitate contingency planning. *Promotes dealing with situation in manageable steps, enhancing chances for success and sense of control.*[5]
- Explore interrelatedness of relationship between unresolved emotions, anxieties, fears, and guilt. *Provides opportunity to address issues that may be limiting individual's ability to improve life situation.*[5]
- Assist client to acknowledge current coping behaviors and defense mechanisms that may hamper moving toward goals. *Allows client to focus on coping mechanisms that are more successful in problem solving.*[3]
- Encourage client to concentrate on progress not perfection. *If client can accept that perfection is difficult or not always the desirable outcome, he or she may be able to view own accomplishments with pride.*[3]
- Involve client in care and explain all procedures thoroughly, answering questions truthfully. *Enhances trust and relationship, promoting hope for a positive outcome.*[2]
- Express hope to client and encourage SO(s) and other health team members to do so. *Enhances client's sense of hope and belief in possibilities of a positive outcome.*[1]
- Identify ways to strengthen sense of interconnectedness or harmony with others *to support sense of belonging and connection that promotes feelings of wholeness and hopefulness.*[1]

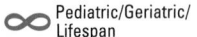

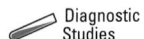

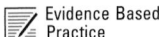

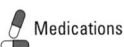

NURSING PRIORITY NO. 3 To promote optimum wellness:

- Demonstrate and encourage use of relaxation techniques, guided imagery, and meditation activities. *Learning to relax can help client decrease tension resulting in refreshment of body and mind, enabling individual to perform and think more successfully.*[3]
- Provide positive feedback for efforts taken to improve situation, growth in use of skills, and learning efforts. *Acknowledges client's efforts as individual is moving forward in learning new skills and reinforces gains.*[3]
- Explore ways that beliefs give meaning and value to daily living. *As client's understanding of these issues improves, hope for the future is strengthened.*[1]
- Encourage life-review by client. *Acknowledges own successes, identifies opportunity for change, and clarifies meaning in life.*[5]
- Identify ways for spiritual expression, strengthening spirituality. *There are many options for enhancing spirituality through connectedness with self and others (e.g., volunteering, mentoring, involvement in religious activities).*[5] (Refer to ND readiness for enhanced Spiritual Well-Being.)
- Encourage client to join groups with similar or new interests. *Expanding knowledge and making friendships with new people will widen horizons for the individual.*
- Refer to community resources and support groups, and spiritual advisor as indicated.

DOCUMENTATION FOCUS

Assessment/Reassessment

- Assessment findings, including client's perceptions of current situation, relationships, sense of desire for enhancing life.
- Cultural or spiritual values and beliefs.
- Motivation and expectations for improvement.

Planning

- Plan of care and who is involved in planning.
- Teaching plan.

Implementation/Evaluation

- Responses to interventions, teaching, and actions performed.
- Attainment or progress toward desired outcome(s).
- Modifications to plan of care.

Discharge Planning

- Identified long-term needs, individual goals for change, and who is responsible for actions to be taken.
- Specific referrals made.

References

1. Laudet, A. B., Morgen, K., White, W. L. (2006). The role of social supports, spirituality, religiousness, life meaning and affiliation with 12-step fellowships in quality of life satisfaction among individuals in recovery from alcohol and drug problems. *Alcohol Treat Q*, 24(1–2), 33–73.
2. Davison, S. N., Simpson, C. (2006). Hope and advance care planning in patients with end stage renal disease: Qualitative interview study. *BMJ*, 333, 886–889.
3. Saltz, L. B. (2008). Progress in cancer care—The hype, hope and the gap between perception and reality. *J Clin Oncol*, 26(31), 520–521.
4. Blagen, M., Yang, J. (2008). Courage and hope as factors for client change: Important cultural implications and spiritual considerations. Retrieved October 2015 from https://www.counseling.org/docs/default-source/vistas/vistas_2008_blagen.pdf?sfvrsn=11.
5. Rousseau, P. (2000). Hope in the terminally ill. *West J Med*, 173(2), 117–118.

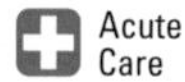

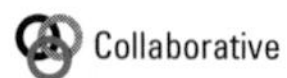

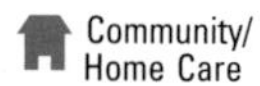

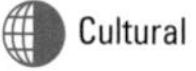

Hopelessness

Taxonomy II: Self-Perception—Class 1 Self-Concept (00124) [**Diagnostic Division:** Ego Integrity], Submitted 1986

DEFINITION: Subjective state in which an individual sees limited or no alternatives or personal choices available and is unable to mobilize energy on own behalf.

RELATED FACTORS

Prolonged activity restriction; social isolation
Deteriorating physiological condition
Chronic stress; history of abandonment
Loss of belief in spiritual power or transcendent values

DEFINING CHARACTERISTICS

Subjective

Despondent verbal cues (e.g., "I can't," sighing); [believes things will not change]

Objective

Passivity; decrease in verbalization
Decrease in affect, appetite, or response to stimuli
Decrease in initiative; inadequate involvement in care
Alteration in sleep pattern
Turning away from speaker; shrugging in response to speaker; poor eye contact
Sample Clinical Applications: Chronic conditions, terminal diagnoses, infertility

DESIRED OUTCOMES/EVALUATION CRITERIA

Sample NOC linkages:

Depression Self-Control: Personal actions to minimize melancholy and maintain interest in life events
Hope: Optimism that is personally satisfying and life supporting
Quality of Life: Extent of positive perception of current life circumstances

Client Will (Include Specific Time Frame)

- Recognize and verbalize feelings.
- Identify and use coping mechanisms to counteract feelings of hopelessness.
- Involve self in and control (within limits of the individual situation) own self-care and activities of daily living.
- Set progressive short-term goals that develop, foster, and sustain behavioral changes and positive outlook.
- Participate in diversional activities of own choice.

ACTIONS/INTERVENTIONS

Sample NIC linkages:

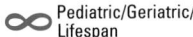

Hope Inspiration: Enhancing the belief in one's capacity to initiate and sustain actions
Emotional Support: Provision of reassurance, acceptance, and encouragement during times of stress
Mood Management: Providing for safety, stabilization, recovery, and maintenance of a patient who is experiencing dysfunctionally depressed or elevated mood

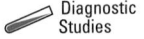

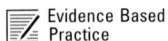

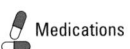

NURSING PRIORITY NO. 1 To identify causative/contributing factors:

- Review familial/social history and physiological history contributing to current problems. *History of poor coping abilities, disorder of familial relating patterns, emotional problems, language or cultural barriers (leading to feelings of isolation), recent or long-term illness of client or family member, and multiple social and/or physiological traumas to individual or family members can all affect client's feelings of hopelessness.*[2,5]
- Identify current familial, social, and physical factors contributing to sense of hopelessness. *Issues such as a newly diagnosed chronic/terminal disease, lack of support system, recent job loss, loss of spiritual or religious faith, and recent multiple traumas can result in an individual giving up. Identification of the issues involved in each person's situation is necessary to appropriately plan for care.*[2]
- Determine client's locus of control (internal or external) and associated cultural factors influencing self-view. Note expressions of responsibility for self versus expressions of lack of control over self and environment. *Individuals view life change and stressful events differently. Those with internal locus of control tend to be more optimistic about their ability to deal with adversity even in the face of current difficulties. Individual with external locus of control may attribute feelings of hopelessness to an external source, perceiving it as beyond his or her control, and will look to others to solve problems and take care of them.*[2,5]
- Identify coping behaviors and defense mechanisms displayed previously and in current situation as well as client's perception of effectiveness then and now. *It is important to identify client's strengths and encourage their use as client begins to deal with what is currently happening.*[2]
- Have client describe events that lead to feeling inadequate or having no control. *Identifies sources of frustration and defines problem areas so action can be taken to learn how to deal with them in more positive ways.*[6]
- Determine presence of suicidal ideation, availability of plan, and means to follow through with plan. (Refer to ND risk for Suicide.) *Hopelessness is identified as a central underlying factor in the predisposition to suicide, and the client sees no other way out of a hopeless situation.*[7]
- Perform physical examination and review results of lab tests and diagnostic studies. *Current situation may be the result of a decline in physical well-being or progression of a chronic condition, or physical symptoms may be associated with effects of depression (e.g., loss of appetite, lack of sleep).*[7]

NURSING PRIORITY NO. 2 To assess level of hopelessness:

- Note behaviors indicative of hopelessness as listed in Defining Characteristics. *Identifies problem areas to be addressed in developing an effective plan of care and suggests possible resources needed.*[6]
- Evaluate and discuss use of defense mechanisms (useful or not). *Identifying behaviors such as increased sleeping, dependence on medications, illness behaviors, eating disorders, denial, forgetfulness, daydreaming, ineffectual organizational efforts, exploiting own goal-setting, and regression can provide accurate information for client to begin changing behavior or inaccurate beliefs.*[6]
- Discuss problem and duration of alcohol or drug abuse as indicated. *Behavior may be an effort to provide psychological numbing in an attempt to lessen pain of situation or may have preceded and contributed to sense of hopelessness. Client may feel hopeless about stopping behavior and believe that it is impossible.*[2]
- Evaluate degree of hopelessness using psychological testing such as Beck's Depression Scale. Note client's feelings about life not being worth living and other signs of hopelessness and worthlessness. *Identifying the degree of hopelessness and possible suicidal thoughts is crucial to instituting appropriate treatment to protect client.*[10]

NURSING PRIORITY NO. 3 To assist client to identify feelings and to begin to cope with problems as perceived by the client:

- Establish a therapeutic and facilitative relationship showing positive regard for the client. Answer questions truthfully. *Enhances trust so that client may feel safe to disclose feelings, talk openly about concerns, and feel understood and listened to.*[2,3,10]
- Encourage client to verbalize and explore feelings and perceptions of what is happening. *Talking about feelings of anger, helplessness, powerlessness, confusion, despondency, isolation, and grief (which can lead to a*

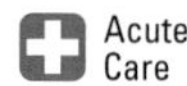

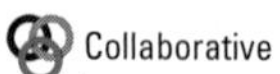

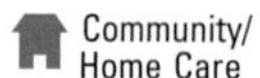

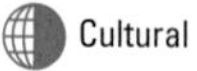

sense of hopelessness and the belief that nothing can be done) provides opportunity for reflection and enables client to begin to understand self and that there are actions that can be helpful.[3]

- ∞ Provide opportunity for children to "play out" feelings (e.g., puppets or art for preschooler, peer discussions for adolescents). *Provides insight into perceptions and can give direction for developing coping strategies.*[2]
- ∞ Engage teens and parents in discussions and arrange to do activities with them. *Parents can make a difference in their children's lives by being with them, discussing sensitive topics, and going different places with them.*[3,4]
- Express hope to client and encourage significant others and other health-team members to do so as well. Avoid expressions of false hope. *Client may not identify positives in own situation and may find it difficult to accept them from others, but will hear them. False reassurances will undermine sense of security.*[2]
- Help client recognize areas in which he or she has control versus those that are not within his or her control. *Often the individual who is feeling hopeless is focusing on issues that cannot be changed. When the client begins to focus energy in those areas where he or she has control, a sense of hope can be nurtured.*[6]
- Use client's locus of control to develop individual plan of care. *Tailoring care to the individual's ability will maximize effectiveness. For instance, client with internal control can take control of own destiny, and those with external control may need to begin with small tasks and add as tolerated, moving toward learning to take more control of personal choices.*[13]
- Encourage client to identify short-term goals. Promote activities to achieve goals and facilitate contingency planning. *Dealing with situation in manageable steps enhances chances for success, promotes sense of control, and encourages belief that there is hope for resolution of situation/moving forward.*[6]
- Discuss current options with client and list actions that can be taken. Correct misconceptions expressed by the client. *Encourages use of own actions, validates reality, and promotes sense of control of the situation.*[2]
- Endeavor to prevent situations that might lead to feelings of isolation or lack of control in client's perception. *Client will interpret these occurrences as further proof that there is no hope.*[6]
- Promote client control in establishing time, place, and frequency of treatment/therapy sessions. Involve family members in the appointments as appropriate. *Allows individual to assume control over own situation, engendering positive feelings of ability to manage what is happening. Involvement of family members provides source of support and encouragement for client.*[2]
- Encourage risk-taking in situations in which the client can succeed. *Succeeding in new ventures can improve self-esteem and hope for more successful actions.*[2]
- Help client begin to develop new coping mechanisms. *New skills need to be learned and used effectively to counteract hopelessness.*[3]
- Encourage structured and controlled increase in physical activity as tolerated. *Promotes the release of endorphins, enhancing sense of well-being.*[2]
- Demonstrate and encourage use of relaxation exercises, guided imagery. *Anxious feelings create tension, and learning to relax can help client begin to look at possibilities of feeling more hopeful.*[9]
- Discuss safe use of prescribed antidepressants. *May require short-term use to elevate mood while client pursues other therapeutic measures to regain sense of hope.*[2]

NURSING PRIORITY NO. 4 To promote wellness (Teaching/Discharge Considerations):

- Provide positive feedback for actions taken to deal with and overcome feelings of hopelessness. *Encourages changes in thinking patterns and continuation of desired behaviors.*[10,12]
- Assist client/family to become aware of factors or situations leading to feelings of hopelessness. *Helps individuals to identify precipitating events and provides opportunities to avoid or modify situation, promoting sense of control over life.*[8]
- Discuss initial signs of hopelessness. *Helps client to identify behaviors such as procrastination, increased need for sleep, decreased physical activity, or withdrawal from social or familial activities and how they have affected thinking and ability to deal with current situation. Awareness provides the opportunity to begin to change.*[9]

- Facilitate client's incorporation of personal loss. *Often prior losses in individual's life result in feelings of hopelessness and lack of control in current events. Hopelessness means a loss of hope rather than just an absence of hope. Enhancing grief work and promoting resolution of feelings help client to begin to feel hope again and look forward to life.*[9]
- Encourage client/family to develop support systems in the immediate community. *Having support nearby provides individuals with assistance and advocacy for moving forward, enabling them to look toward future with hope.*[4,6]
- Help client to become aware of, nurture, and expand spiritual self. (Refer to ND Spiritual Distress.) *Spiritual needs are an integral part of being human. Acknowledging and learning about spiritual aspect of self can help client look toward the future with hope for improved sense of well-being.*[11]
- Encourage and facilitate interaction with religious representative or spiritual counselor as indicated. *Client's sense of hopelessness may include the loss of spiritual connectedness or client may view spiritual being as responsible for current situation.*[1]
- Introduce the client into a support group before the individual therapy is terminated for continuation of therapeutic process. *Provides for a smooth transition so client feels accepted and comfortable in the presence of others.*[6]
- Stress need for continued monitoring of medication regimen by healthcare provider. *Necessary to evaluate effectiveness and prevent or minimize possible side effects. Antidepressant agents are not to be discontinued abruptly without consulting healthcare provider.*[2]
- Refer to other resources for assistance as indicated (e.g., clinical nurse specialist, psychiatrist, social services, Alcoholics or Narcotics Anonymous, Al-Anon or Alateen). *May need additional help to develop hope for the future, sustain efforts for change.*[2]

DOCUMENTATION FOCUS

Assessment/Reassessment

- Assessment findings, including what has been lost in hopelessness, degree of impairment, locus of control, use of coping skills.
- Cultural or religious beliefs and expectations.
- Spiritual concerns.
- Availability and use of resources or support systems.

Planning

- Plan of care and who is involved in planning.
- Teaching plan.

Implementation/Evaluation

- Responses to interventions, teaching, and actions performed.
- Attainment or progress toward desired outcome(s).
- Modifications to plan of care.

Discharge Planning

- Identified long-term needs, client's goals for change, and who is responsible for actions to be taken.
- Specific referrals made.

References

1. Geiter, H. (2002). The spiritual side of nursing. *RN*, 65(5), 43–44.
2. Reznikoff, P. T. M. (1982). Perceived peer and family relationships, hopelessness and locus of control as factors in adolescent suicide attempts. *Suicide Life Threat Behav*, 12(3), 141–150.
3. Gordon, T. Families need rules. Gordon Training International. Retrieved October 2015 from http://www.gordontraining.com/free-parenting-articles/families-need-rules/.
4. Clark, C. M. Relations between social support and physical health. Rochester Institute of Technology. Re-

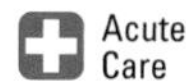

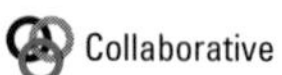

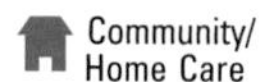

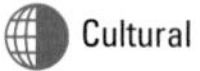

trieved October 2015 from http://www.personalityresearch.org/papers/clark.html.

5. McLeod, D., Wright, L. M. (2001). Conversations of spirituality: Spirituality in family systems nursing—Making the case with four clinical vignettes. *J Fam Nurs*, 7(4), 391–415.
6. Kwon, P. (2002). Hope, defense mechanisms, and adjustment: Implications for false hope and defensive hopelessness. *J Pers*, 70(2), 207–231.
7. Ghosh, T. B., Victor, B. S. (1994). Suicide. In Hales, R. R., et al. (eds). *The American Psychiatric Press Textbook of Psychiatry*. 2nd ed. Washington, DC: American Psychiatric Press.
8. Drew, B. (1990). Differentiation of hopelessness, helplessness, and powerlessness using Erik Erikson's "Roots of Virtue." *Arch Psychiatr Nurs*, 4, 332–337.
9. Patterson, B. (2009). A Buddhist approach to grief counseling. Navigating Life's Changes. Retrieved February 2012 from http://bethspatterson.wordpress.com/2009/09/06/a-buddhist-approach-to-grief-counseling/.
10. Beck, A. T., Brown, G., Berchick, R. J. (1990). Relationship between hopelessness and ultimate suicide: A replication with psychiatric out-patients. *Am J Psychiatry*, 147, 190–195.
11. Sharma, Y. R. S. Scientific research studies on spiritual science and philosophy. SelfGrowth.com. Retrieved October 2015 from http://www.articlesfactory.com/articles/metaphysical/scientific-research-studies-on-spiritual-science-and-philosophy.html.
12. Seligman, M. Positive health. Authentic Happiness, University of Pennsylvania. Retrieved October 2015 from https://www.authentichappiness.sas.upenn.edu/learn/positivehealth.
13. Kunert, P. K. (2002). Stress and adaptation. In Porth, C. M. (ed). *Pathophysiology: Concepts of Altered Health States*. Philadelphia: J. B. Lippincott.

risk for compromised Human Dignity

Taxonomy II: Self-Perception—Class 1 Self-Concept (00174) [**Diagnostic Division:** Ego Integrity], Submitted 2006; Revised 2013

DEFINITION: Vulnerable for perceived loss of respect and honor, which may compromise health.

RISK FACTORS

Loss of control over body function; exposure of the body
Humiliation; invasion of privacy
Disclosure of confidential information; stigmatization
Dehumanizing treatment; intrusion by clinician
Insufficient comprehension of health information
Little decision-making experience
Cultural incongruence
Note: A risk diagnosis is not evidenced by signs and symptoms, as the problem has not occurred; rather, nursing interventions are directed at prevention.
Sample Clinical Applications: Chronic conditions (e.g., multiple sclerosis [MS], stroke, quadriplegia, amyotrophic lateral sclerosis [ALS])

DESIRED OUTCOMES/EVALUATION CRITERIA

Sample NOC linkages:
Client Satisfaction: Protection of Rights: Extent of positive perception of protection of a patient's legal and moral rights provided by nursing staff
Client Satisfaction: Cultural Needs Fulfillment: Extent of positive perception of integration of cultural beliefs, values, and social structures into nursing care

Client Will (Include Specific Time Frame)
- Verbalize awareness of specific problem.
- Identify positive ways to deal with situation.

(continues on page 424)

risk for compromised Human Dignity (continued)

- Demonstrate problem-solving skills.
- Express desire to increase participation in decision-making process.
- Express sense of dignity in situation.

ACTIONS/INTERVENTIONS

Sample NIC linkages:

Cultural Brokerage: The deliberate use of culturally competent strategies to bridge or mediate between the patient's culture and the biomedical healthcare system

Patient Rights Protection: Protection of healthcare rights of a patient, especially a minor, incapacitated, or incompetent patient unable to make decisions

Emotional Support: Provision of reassurance, acceptance, and encouragement during times of stress

NURSING PRIORITY NO. 1 To determine individual situation as perceived by client:

- Determine client's perception and specific factors that could lead to sense of loss of dignity. *Human dignity is a totality of the individual's uniqueness—mind, body, and spirit—and all components must be considered.*[4]
- Note names, labels, or items used by staff, friends/family that stigmatize the client. *Human dignity is threatened by insensitive as well as inadequate healthcare and lack of client participation in care decisions.*[4]
- Identify cultural beliefs or values and degree of importance to client. *Individuals cling to their basic beliefs and values, especially during times of stress, which may result in conflict with current circumstances.*[7]
- Identify client's/significant other's (SO's) healthcare goals and expectations. *Clarifies client's (or SO's/family's) vision, provides framework for planning care, and identifies possible conflicts.*[2]
- Note availability of support systems. *Client will feel loved and valued and will be able to manage difficult circumstances better when the support of family and friends surrounds individual.*[2]
- Ascertain response of family/SOs to client's situation. *It is important that family supports and values client to enable him or her to manage situation. If they are not supportive or conflicts arise, client may need to separate self from family members who are negative.*[3]

NURSING PRIORITY NO. 2 To assist client to deal with situation in positive ways:

- Ask client by what name he or she would like to be addressed. *Name is important to a person's identity and recognizes his or her individuality. Many older people prefer to be addressed in a formal manner (e.g., Mr. or Mrs.).*[2,7]
- Active-listen feelings, encouraging client to verbalize concerns. Be available for support and assistance. *Can help client to discover underlying reasons for feelings and seek solutions to problems.*[5]
- Respect the client's needs and wishes for quiet, privacy, talking, or silence. *Conveys respect and concern for client's dignity.*[3]
- Provide for privacy when discussing sensitive or personal issues. *Demonstrates respect for client and promotes sense of safe environment for free exchange of thoughts and feelings.*[3]
- Use understandable terms when talking to client/family about the medical condition, procedures, and treatments (component of informed consent). *Most lay people do not understand medical terms and may be hesitant to ask what is meant.*[6]
- Encourage family/SO(s) to treat client with respect and understanding, especially when the client is older and may be irritable and difficult to deal with. *Everyone needs to be treated with respect and dignity, regardless of individual abilities or frailty.*[4]
- Include client and family in decision making, especially regarding end-of-life issues. *Helps the individual feel respected or valued and involved in the care process.*[2]
- Involve facility or local ethics committee as appropriate *to facilitate mediation or resolution of conflicts between client/family and staff or client and family members.*[5]

- Protect client's privacy when providing personal care and during procedures. *Prevents embarrassment over unnecessary exposure and conveys a message of caring and preserves client dignity.*

NURSING PRIORITY NO. 3 To promote wellness (Teaching/Discharge Considerations):

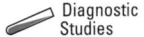

- Discuss client's rights as an individual. *While hospitals and other care settings have a Client's Bill of Rights, a broader view of human dignity is stated in the U.S. Constitution.*[1,6]
- Assist with planning for the future, taking into account client's desires and rights. *As the client plans for the future, the needs of the self as a human who has dignity are considered and incorporated to preserve that dignity.*[4]
- Incorporate familial, religious, and cultural factors that have meaning for client in planning process. *When these issues are addressed and incorporated in plan of care, they add to the feelings of inclusion for the client.*[4,7]
- Refer to other resources (e.g., pastoral care, counseling, organized support groups, classes), as appropriate. *May need additional assistance to deal with illness/situation.*

DOCUMENTATION FOCUS

Assessment/Reassessment

- Assessment findings, including individual risk factors, client's perceptions, and concerns about involvement in care.
- Individual cultural or religious beliefs and values, healthcare goals.
- Responses and involvement of family/SOs.

Planning

- Plan of care and who is involved in planning.
- Teaching plan.

Implementation/Evaluation

- Client's response to interventions, teaching, and actions performed.
- Attainment or progress toward desired outcome(s).
- Modifications to plan of care.

Discharge Planning

- Long-term needs and who is responsible for actions to be taken.
- Specific referrals made.

References

1. Bush, G. W. (2002). Champion aspirations for human dignity. Retrieved March 2015 from http://2001-2009.state.gov/r/pa/ei/wh/15422.htm.
2. Schulman, A. (2009). Bioethics and the question of human dignity. University of Notre Dame Press. Retrieved March 2015 from http://www3.nd.edu/~undpress/excerpts/P01307-ex.pdf.
3. Cheshire, W. P. (2007). Grey matters when eloquence is inarticulate. *Ethics & Medicine: An International Journal of Bioethics*. Retrieved March 2015 from https://cbhd.org/content/grey-matters-when-eloquence-inarticulate.
4. Moran, G. Dignity, uniqueness and rights. Retrieved March 2015 from http://www.nyu.edu/classes/gmoran/EXC-RIGH.pdf.
5. Pilgrim, G. (2011). Therapeutic communication techniques. Retrieved March 2015 from http://www.buzzle.com/articles/therapeutic-communication-techniques.html.
6. No author listed Patient's Bill of Rights. Retrieved March 2015 http://www.healthsourceglobal.com/docs/patient%20bill%20of%20rights_merged.pdf.
7. Chang, M., Kelley, A. (2007). Patient education: Addressing cultural diversity and health literacy issues. *Urol Nurs*, 27(5), 411–417.

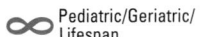

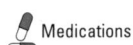

Hyperthermia

Taxonomy II: Safety/Protection—Class 6 Thermoregulation (00007) [**Diagnostic Division:** Safety], Submitted 1986; Revised 2013

DEFINITION: Core body temperature elevated above the normal diurnal range due to failure of thermoregulation.

RELATED FACTORS

Decreased sweat response; dehydration vigorous activity
High environmental temperature; inappropriate clothing
Illness; increase in metabolic rate; ischemia; sepsis
Pharmaceutical agent
Trauma

DEFINING CHARACTERISTICS

Objective

Abnormal posturing; convulsion, seizure
Flushed skin; skin warm to touch; vasodilation
Hypotension; tachycardia; tachypnea; apnea
Irritability; lethargy; stupor; coma
Infant does not maintain suck
Sample Clinical Applications: Infectious diseases, head trauma, hyperthyroidism, heat exhaustion or heatstroke, surgical procedure, anesthesia

DESIRED OUTCOMES/EVALUATION CRITERIA

Sample NOC linkages:

Thermoregulation: Balance among heat production, heat gain, and heat loss
Thermoregulation: Newborn: Balance among heat production, heat gain, and heat loss during the first 28 days of life
Personal Safety Behavior: Personal actions that prevent physical injury to self

Client Will (Include Specific Time Frame)

- Maintain core temperature within normal range.
- Be free of complications such as irreversible brain or neurological damage and acute renal failure.
- Identify underlying cause or contributing factors and importance of treatment as well as signs/symptoms requiring further evaluation or intervention.
- Demonstrate behaviors to monitor and promote normothermia.
- Be free of seizure activity.

ACTIONS/INTERVENTIONS

Sample NIC linkages:

Temperature Regulation: Attaining and/or maintaining body temperature within a normal range
Fever Treatment: Management of a patient with hyperpyrexia caused by nonenvironmental factors
Malignant Hyperthermia Precautions: Prevention or reduction of hypermetabolic response to pharmacological agents used during surgery

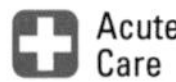

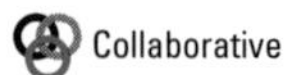

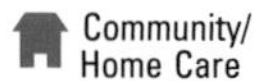

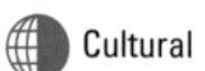

NURSING PRIORITY NO. 1 To assess causative/contributing factors:

- Identify underlying cause. *These factors can include* ***excessive heat production*** *such as occurs with strenuous exercise, fever, shivering, tremors, convulsions, hyperthyroid state, and infection or sepsis and malignant hyperpyrexia, heatstroke, and sympathomimetic drugs;* ***impaired heat dissipation*** *such as occurs with heatstroke, dermatological diseases, burns, and inability to perspire such as occurs with spinal cord injury and certain medications (e.g., diuretics, sedatives, certain heart and blood pressure medications); and* ***loss of thermoregulation*** *such as may occur in infections, brain lesions, and drug overdose.*[1,8,9]
- Note chronological and developmental age of client. *Infants, young children, and elderly persons are most susceptible to damaging hyperthermia. Environmental factors and relatively minor infections can produce a much higher temperature in infants and young children than in older children and adults. Infants, children, or impaired individuals are not able to protect themselves and cannot recognize and/or act on symptoms of hyperthermia. Elderly persons have age-related risk factors (e.g., poor circulation, inefficient sweat glands, skin changes caused by normal aging, chronic diseases).*[1–4,9]

NURSING PRIORITY NO. 2 To evaluate effects/degree of hyperthermia:

- Monitor core temperature by appropriate route (e.g., tympanic, rectal). Note presence of temperature elevation (>98.6°F [37°C]) or fever (100.4°F [38°C]). *Rectal and tympanic temperatures most closely approximate core temperature; however, shell temperatures (oral, axillary, touch) are often measured at home and are predictive of fever. Rectal temperature measurement may be the most accurate but is not always expedient (e.g., client declines, is agitated, has rectal lesions or surgery). Abdominal temperature monitoring may be done in the premature neonate.*[1–4]
- Assess whether body temperature reflects heatstroke. *Defined as body temperature higher than 105°F (40.5°C) that is associated with neurological dysfunction and is potentially life threatening.*[9,11]
- Assess neurological response, noting level of consciousness and orientation, reaction to stimuli, reaction of pupils, and presence of posturing or seizures. *High fever accompanied by changes in mentation (from confusion to delirium) may indicate septic state or heatstroke.*[1–3,5]
- Monitor blood pressure and invasive hemodynamic parameters if available (e.g., cardiac output, arterial pressures). *Hyperdynamic state (high central venous pressure, low systemic vascular resistance, tachycardia, elevated blood pressure, which may later fall) can occur, especially in person with preexisting cardiovascular disease if heat-related illness (e.g., heatstroke or malignant hyperthermia reaction to anesthesia) has rendered the client critically ill.*[1–3,5]
- Monitor heart rate and rhythm. *Tachycardia, dysrhythmias, and electrocardiogram changes are common due to electrolyte and acid-base imbalance, dehydration, specific action of catecholamines, and direct effects of hyperthermia on blood and cardiac tissue.*[1–3,5]
- *Monitor respirations. Hyperventilation may initially be present, but ventilatory effort may eventually be impaired by seizures and hypermetabolic state (shock and acidosis).*
- Auscultate breath sounds *to note presence and progression of adventitious sounds such as crackles (rales), especially when heart failure or pneumonia is present.*[1–3,5]
- Monitor and record all sources of fluid loss such as urine *(oliguria or renal failure may occur due to hypotension, dehydration, shock, and tissue necrosis),* vomiting and diarrhea, wounds or fistulas, and insensible losses *(potentiates fluid and electrolyte losses).*[1–3,5]
- Note presence or absence of sweating. *The body attempts to increase heat loss by evaporation, conduction, and diffusion. Evaporation is decreased by environmental factors of high humidity and high ambient temperature as well as body factors producing loss of ability to sweat or sweat gland dysfunction (e.g., spinal cord transection, cystic fibrosis, dehydration, vasoconstriction).*[8,9]
- Monitor laboratory studies such as arterial blood gases, electrolytes and cardiac and liver enzymes *(may reveal tissue degeneration)*; glucose *(hypoglycemia)*; blood urea nitrogen/creatinine *(acute renal failure)*; and urinalysis *(myoglobinuria, proteinuria, and hemoglobinuria can occur as products of tissue necrosis).*[1,11]

NURSING PRIORITY NO. 3 To assist with measures to reduce body temperature/restore normal body/organ function:[1–3,5,8,9,11]

- Administer antipyretics, orally or rectally (e.g., acetaminophen, ibuprofen), as ordered. Avoid use of aspirin products in children *(may cause Reye's syndrome or liver failure)*[13] or in individuals with a clotting disorder or receiving anticoagulant therapy.
- Promote cooling by means of:
  Limit clothing and dress in lightweight, loose-fitting clothes. *Encourages heat loss by radiation and conduction.*
  Cool the environment with air-conditioning or fans. *Promotes heat loss by convection.*
  Provide cool or tepid sponge baths, spray bottle, or immersion if temperature is greater than 104°F (40°C) *(heat loss by evaporation and conduction)* or local ice packs, especially in groin and axillae *(areas of high blood flow). Note: Immersion in very cold/ice water is good for exertional heatstroke (such as with athletes or military recruits in training) but use with caution in treatment of classic heatstroke (such as in elderly client or client with alcoholism), which has been associated with a high mortality rate.*[12] *In pediatric clients, alcohol sponge baths are contraindicated because they increase peripheral vascular constriction and central nervous system depression; cold water sponges or immersion can increase shivering, producing heat.*[13]
  Keep clothing and linens dry *to reduce shivering.*
  Monitor use of hypothermia blanket and wrap extremities with bath towels *to minimize shivering.* Turn off hypothermia blanket when core temperature is within 1 to 3 degrees of desired temperature *to allow for downward drift.*
  Administer medications (e.g., dantrolene, chlorpromazine, diazepam) as ordered, *to manage hyperthermia and control shivering and seizures.*
  Assist with internal cooling methods in presence of malignant hyperthermia *to promote rapid core cooling.*
- Provide hydration:
  Offer or force plenty of fluids by appropriate route even if client is not thirsty *to replace fluids lost through perspiration and respiration.*
  Avoid alcohol and caffeinated beverages *(increases fluid loss by diuresis).*
  Administer replacement IV fluids and electrolytes *to support circulating volume and tissue perfusion and treat acid-base imbalance.*
- Promote client safety (e.g., maintain patent airway, padded siderails, quiet environment, mouth care for dry mucous membranes, skin protection from cold when hypothermia blanket is used, observation of equipment safety measures).
- Maintain bedrest *to reduce metabolic demands and oxygen consumption.*
- Provide supplemental oxygen *to offset increased oxygen demands and consumption.*
- Administer medications as indicated to treat underlying cause, such as antibiotics *(for infection)*, dantrolene *(for malignant hyperthermia)*, and beta blockers *(for thyroid storm).*
- Provide high-calorie diet and enteral or parenteral nutrition *to meet increased metabolic demands.*

NURSING PRIORITY NO. 4 To promote wellness (Teaching/Discharge Considerations):

- Instruct parents in how to measure child's temperature, at what body temperature to give antipyretic medications, and what symptoms to report to physician. *Low-grade fever enhances immune system functioning in presence of infection and is not harmful as long as individual is not dehydrated or susceptible to febrile seizures.*[3] *Fever may be treated at home to relieve the general discomfort and lethargy associated with fever. Fever is reportable, however, especially in infants or very young children with or without other symptoms and in older children or adults if it is unresponsive to antipyretics and fluids because it often accompanies a treatable infection (viral or bacterial).*[13]
- Review with client/significant other specific cause of hyperthermia. *Helps to identify those factors that client can control (if any), such as correction of underlying disease process (e.g., thyroid suppression medication), ways to protect oneself from excessive exposure to environmental heat (e.g., proper clothing, restriction of*

Acute Care 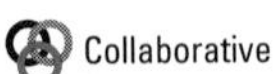 Collaborative 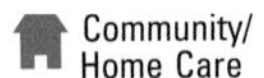 Community/Home Care 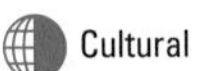 Cultural

activity, scheduling outings during cooler part of day), and understanding of family traits (e.g., malignant hyperthermia reaction to anesthesia is often familial).[7,9]

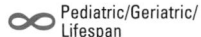

- Discuss importance of adequate fluid intake at all times and ways to improve hydration status when ill or when under stress (e.g., exercise, hot environment).
- ∞ Instruct families/caregivers (of young children, persons who are outdoors in very hot climate, elderly living alone) in dangers of heat exhaustion and heatstroke and ways to manage hot environments. Caution parents to avoid leaving young children in unattended car, emphasizing the extreme hazard to the child in a very short period of time depending on outdoor temperature and humidity, whether the car is parked in direct sunlight, and air and surface temperatures in the car. *Heat injuries can be immediately life threatening. Being aware of environmental hazards and hydration levels can save one's life.*[6,10]
- Recommend avoidance of hot tubs/saunas as appropriate (e.g., client with cardiac conditions compromised by decreased cardiac output associated with peripheral vasodilation, pregnancy that may affect fetal development or increase maternal cardiac workload).
- Review signs/symptoms of hyperthermia (e.g., flushed skin, increased body temperature, increased respiratory and heart rate; fainting, loss of consciousness, seizures). *Indicates need for prompt intervention.*
- ∞ Identify community resources, especially for elderly clients, to address specific needs *(e.g., provision of fans for individual use, location of cooling rooms—usually in a community center—during heat waves, daily telephone contact to assess wellness).*

DOCUMENTATION FOCUS

Assessment/Reassessment

- Temperature and other assessment findings, including vital signs and state of mentation.

Planning

- Plan of care, specific interventions, and who is involved in the planning.
- Teaching plan.

Implementation/Evaluation

- Responses to interventions, teaching, and actions performed.
- Attainment or progress toward desired outcome(s).
- Modifications to plan of care.

Discharge Planning

- Specific referrals made and those responsible for actions to be taken.

References

1. Stoppler, M. C. (2002, updated 2015). Heatstroke. Retrieved October 2015 from http://www.medicinenet.com/heat_stroke/article.htm.
2. Sur, D. K., Bukont, E. L. (2007). Evaluating fever of unidentifiable source in young children. *Am Fam Physician*, 75(12), 1805–1811.
3. Engel, J. (2006). *Mosby's Pocket Guide to Pediatric Assessment.* 5th ed. St. Louis, MO: Mosby.
4. Kare, J., Shneiderman, A. (2001). Hyperthermia and hypothermia in the older population, 23(3), 39–52.
5. Doenges, M. E., Moorhouse, M. F., Murr, A. C. (2010). Sepsis/Septicemia. *Nursing Care Plans: Guidelines for Individualizing Patient Care Across the Life Span.* 8th ed. Philadelphia: F. A. Davis.
6. Occupational Safety and Health Administration (OSHA). (2014). Portecting workers from heat stress. Retrieved October 2015 from https://www.osha.gov/Publications/osha3154.pdf.
7. Malignant Hyperthermia Association of the United States. (Updated 2013). Guideline statement for malignant hyperthermia in the perioperative environment. Retrieved October 2015 from http://www.ast.org/uploadedFiles/Main_Site/Content/About_Us/Guideline_Malignant_Hyperthermia.pdf.
8. Cunha, J. P. (2015). Heat cramps. Retrieved October 2015 from http://www.emedicinehealth.com/heat_cramps/article_em.htm.

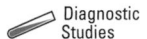

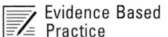

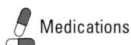

9. Hyperthermia: Too hot for your health. (2010, updated 2015). National Institute on Aging. Retrieved October 2015 from https://www.nia.nih.gov/health/publication/hyperthermia.
10. Grundstein, A., Dowd, J., Meentemeyer, V. (2001). Quantifying the heat related hazard for children in motor vehicles. *American Meteorological Society*, 91(9), 1183.
11. Schraga, E. D., Kates, L. W. (2011). Cooling techniques for hyperthermia. Retrieved October 2015 from http://emedicine.medscape.com/article/149546-overview.
12. Casa, D. J., McDermott, B. P., Lee, E. C., et al. (2007). Cold water immersion: The gold standard for exertional heatstroke treatment. *Exerc Sport Sci Rev*, 35(3), 141–149.
13. Ferry, R. (2010, reviewed 2015). Fever in children. Retrieved October 2015 from http://www.emedicinehealth.com/fever_in_children/article_em.htm.

Hypothermia

Taxonomy II: Safety/Protection—Class 6 Thermoregulation (00006) [**Diagnostic Division:** Safety], Submitted 1986; Revised 1988, 2013

DEFINITION: Core body temperature below the normal diurnal range due to failure of thermoregulation.

RELATED FACTORS

Alcohol consumption
Economically disadvantaged
Extremes of age or weight
Insufficient clothing
Heat transfer (e.g., conduction, convection, evaporation, radiation)
Insufficient knowledge of hypothermia prevention
Malnutrition; decrease in metabolic rate; insufficient supply of subcutaneous fat; inactivity
Pharmaceutical agent, [drug overdose]
Trauma; damage to hypothalamus; radiation

Neonates

High risk or unplanned out-of-hospital birth; early bathing of newborn; delay in breastfeeding
Immature stratum corneum
Increased body surface area to weight ratio
Increase in oxygen demand; increase in pulmonary vascular resistance (PVR); ineffective vascular control
Insufficient nonshivering thermogenesis

DEFINING CHARACTERISTICS

Objective

Acrocyanosis, cyanotic nail beds; peripheral vasoconstriction; hypoxia
Bradycardia; tachycardia
Decrease in blood glucose level; hypoglycemia
Increase in metabolic rate; increase in oxygen consumption
Shivering; piloerection
Skin cool to touch; slow capillary refill

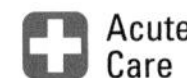

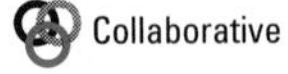

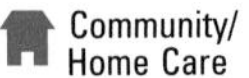

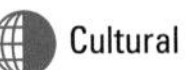

Accidental Low Body Temperature in Children and Adults
Mild hypothermia, core temperature 32°–35°C (89.6°–95°F)
Moderate hypothermia, core temperature 30°–32°C (86°–89.6°F)
Severe hypothermia, core temperature <30°C (86°F)
Injured Adults and Children
Hypothermia, core temperature <35°C (95°F)
Severe hypothermia, core temperature <32°C (89.6°F)
Neonates
Grade 1 hypothermia, core temperature 36°–36.5° C (96.8°–97.7°F)
Grade 2 hypothermia, core temperature 35°–35.9°C (95°–96.6°F)
Grade 3 hypothermia, core temperature 34°–34.9° C (93.2°–94.8°F)
Grade 4 hypothermia, core temperature <34°C (93.2°F)
Infant with insufficient energy to maintain sucking; or with insufficient weight gain (<30 g/d)
Irritability
Jaundice, pallor
Respiratory distress; metabolic acidosis
Sample Clinical Applications: Dementia, malnutrition, anorexia nervosa, brain trauma, stroke, endocrine disorders, some surgical procedures (e.g., craniotomy), alcohol intoxication, abuse or neglect, prematurity, near drowning

DESIRED OUTCOMES/EVALUATION CRITERIA

Sample NOC linkages:
Thermoregulation: Balance among heat production, heat gain, and heat loss
Thermoregulation: Newborn: Balance among heat production, heat gain, and heat loss during the first 28 days of life

Client Will (Include Specific Time Frame)
- Display core temperature within normal range.
- Be free of complications such as cardiac failure, respiratory infection or failure, and thromboembolic phenomena.

Sample NOC linkages:
Personal Safety Behavior: Personal actions that prevent physical injury to self

Client/Caregiver Will (Include Specific Time Frame)
- Maintain safe environment.
- Identify underlying cause or contributing factors that are within caregiver control.
- Verbalize understanding of specific interventions to prevent hypothermia.
- Demonstrate behaviors to monitor and promote normothermia.

ACTIONS/INTERVENTIONS

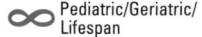

Sample NIC linkages:
Hypothermia Treatment: Rewarming and surveillance of a patient whose core body temperature is below 35°C [95°F]
Temperature Regulation: Attaining and/or maintaining body temperature within a normal range

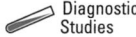

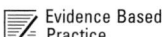

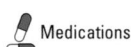

NURSING PRIORITY NO. 1 To assess causative/contributing factors:

- Note underlying cause, for example, (1) ***decreased heat production*** *such as occurs with hypopituitary, hypoadrenal and hypothyroid conditions, and hypoglycemia and neuromuscular inefficiencies seen in extremes of age;* (2) ***increased heat loss*** *(e.g., exposure to cold weather, winter outdoor activities; cold water drenching or immersion; improper clothing, shelter, or food for conditions; vasodilation from medications, drugs, or poisons; skin-surface problems such as burns or psoriasis; fluid losses, dehydration; surgery, open wounds, exposed skin or viscera; multiple rapid infusions of cold solutions or transfusions of banked blood; overtreatment of hyperthermia);* and (3) ***impaired thermoregulation.*** *The hypothalamus is sensitive to blood temperature changes of as little as 0.5°C and also reacts to nerve impulses received from nerve endings in the skin. Hypothalamus failure might occur with central nervous system [CNS] trauma or tumor; intracranial bleeding or stroke; toxicological and metabolic disorders; and Parkinson's disease and multiple sclerosis.*[1,2]
- ∞ Note contributing factors: **age of client** (e.g., premature neonate, child, elderly person), **concurrent or co-existing medical problems** (e.g., brainstem injury, CNS trauma; near drowning, sepsis, hypothyroidism), **other factors** (e.g., alcohol or other drug use or abuse, homelessness), **nutrition status** (e.g., thin, tall person loses heat easier than short stature, overweight person), and **living condition and relationship status** (e.g., aged or cognitive impaired client living alone).[1,2,6]

NURSING PRIORITY NO. 2 To prevent further decrease in body temperature:

MILD-TO-MODERATE HYPOTHERMIA:[1–6]

- Remove wet clothing and bedding.
- Add layers of clothing and wrap in warm blankets.
- Increase physical activity if possible.
- Provide warm liquids after shivering stops if client is alert and can swallow.
- Provide warm nutrient-dense food (carbohydrates, proteins, fats) and fluids (hot, sweet liquids are easily digestible and absorbable).
- Avoid alcohol, caffeine, and tobacco *to prevent vasodilation, diuresis, or vasoconstriction, respectively.*
- Place in warm ambient temperature environment and protect from drafts; provide external heat sources.
- ∞ Provide barriers to heat loss, as well as active rewarming for newborns, especially preterm and/or low-birth-weight infants, monitoring temperature closely. *Measures might include use of protective hats, open radiant warmer or Isolette, and/or heating blanket. Note: In Cochrane Neonatal Reviews, McCall et al. (2010) found that plastic wraps or bags were effective in reducing heat losses in infants less than 28 weeks' gestation but not in infants between 28 to 31 week's gestation. Plastic caps were effective in reducing heat losses in infants less than 29 weeks. Stockinet caps were not effective in reducing heat losses. Skin-to-skin care was shown to be effective in reducing the risk of hypothermia when compared to conventional incubator care for infants. The transwarmer mattress reduced the incidence of hypothermia on admission to NICU in very low-birth-weight infants.*[7]

SEVERE HYPOTHERMIA:[1–6]

- Remove client from causative or contributing factors.
- Dry the skin, cover with blankets, and provide shelter with warm ambient temperature; use radiant lights.
- Provide heat to trunk, not to extremities, initially. Avoid use of heat lamps or hot water bottles. *Surface rewarming can result in rewarming shock due to surface vasodilation.*
- Keep individual lying down. Avoid jarring *(can trigger an abnormal heart rhythm).*

NURSING PRIORITY NO. 3 To evaluate effects of hypothermia ✚:

- Measure core temperature with low register thermometer (measuring below 34.4°C [94°F]).
- Assess respiratory effort *(rate and tidal volume are reduced when metabolic rate decreases and respiratory acidosis occurs).*
- Auscultate lungs, noting adventitious sounds. *Pulmonary edema, respiratory infection, and pulmonary embolus are potential complications of hypothermia.*

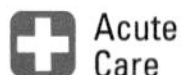

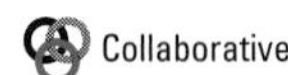

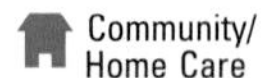

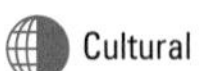

- Monitor heart rate and rhythm. *Cold stress reduces pacemaker function, and bradycardia (unresponsive to atropine), atrial fibrillation, atrioventricular blocks, and ventricular tachycardia can occur. Ventricular fibrillation occurs most frequently when core temperature is 27.7°C (82°F) or below.*[1,2,4]
- Monitor blood pressure, noting hypotension. *Can occur due to vasoconstriction, and shunting of fluids as a result of cold injury effect on capillary permeability.*
- Measure urine output. *Oliguria or renal failure can occur due to a low flow state and/or following hypothermic osmotic diuresis.*
- Note CNS effects (e.g., mood changes, sluggish thinking, amnesia, complete obtundation) and peripheral CNS effects (e.g., paralysis—30.9°C [87.7°F]; dilated pupils—below 30°C [86°F]; flat electroencephalogram—20°C [68°F]).[1,2,4]
- Monitor laboratory studies such as arterial blood gases *(respiratory and metabolic acidosis)*, electrolytes *(hyperkalemia initially, followed by hypokalemia after hypothermia-induced diuresis)*, complete blood count *(increased hematocrit, decreased white blood cell count)*, cardiac enzymes *(myocardial infarct may occur owing to electrolyte imbalance, cold stress catecholamine release, hypoxia, or acidosis)*, coagulation profile *(late hypothermia associated with increased prothrombin time and partial prothrombin time)*, and glucose *(hyperglycemia occurs initially, followed by hypoglycemia)*, as well as pharmacological profile *(for toxicology [alcohol/other drugs]; possible cumulative drug effects).*[2]

NURSING PRIORITY NO. 4 To restore normal body temperature/organ function:

- Assist with surface warming. Cover head, neck, and thorax, leaving extremities uncovered as appropriate *to maintain peripheral vasoconstriction.* Note: Do not institute surface rewarming prior to core rewarming in severe hypothermia *(causes afterdrop of temperature by shunting cold blood back to heart in addition to rewarming shock as a result of surface vasodilation).*[1–4]
- Assist with core rewarming measures, such as warmed IV solutions and warm-solution lavage of body cavities (gastric, peritoneal, bladder) or cardiopulmonary bypass if indicated to normalize core temperature. Rewarm no faster than 1°F to 2°F per hour *to avoid sudden vasodilation, increased metabolic demands on heart, and hypotension (rewarming shock).*[2]
- Protect skin and tissues by repositioning, applying lotion or lubricants, and avoiding direct contact with heating appliance or blanket. *Impaired circulation can result in severe tissue damage.*
- Keep client quiet; handle gently *to reduce potential for fibrillation in cold heart.*[2]
- Provide cardiopulmonary resuscitation as necessary, with compressions initially at one-half the normal heart rate. *Severe hypothermia causes slowed conduction, and cold heart may be unresponsive to medications, pacing, and defibrillation.*[2,4,5]
- Maintain patent airway. Assist with intubation if indicated. Provide heated, humidified oxygen when used.
- Turn off warming blanket when temperature is within 1°F to 3°F of desired temperature *to accommodate drift and avoid hyperthermia situation.*
- Administer IV fluids with caution *to prevent overload as the vascular bed expands.*[2] *Cold heart is slow to compensate for increased volume.*
- Avoid vigorous pharmacological therapy. *As rewarming occurs, organ function returns, correcting endocrine abnormalities, and tissues become more receptive to the effects of drugs previously administered, creating risk for overdose.*
- Perform range-of-motion exercises, provide support hose or sequential compression device, reposition, encourage coughing and deep-breathing exercises, and avoid restrictive clothing or restraints *to reduce effects of circulatory stasis.*
- Provide well-balanced, high-calorie diet or feedings *to replenish glycogen stores and nutritional balance.*

NURSING PRIORITY NO. 5 To promote wellness (Teaching/Discharge Considerations):

- Review specific risk factors or causes of hypothermia. Note that hypothermia can be accidental or intentional *(e.g., when induced-hypothermia therapy is used after cardiac arrest or brain injury)*, requiring interventions to protect client from adverse affects.[5]

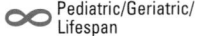

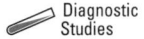

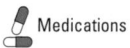

- Identify factors that client can control (if any), such as protection from environment and adequate heat in home, layering of clothing and blankets, minimizing heat loss from head with hat or scarf, appropriate cold weather clothing, avoidance of alcohol or other drugs if anticipating exposure to cold, potential risks for future hypersensitivity to cold, etc.
- Discuss signs/symptoms of early hypothermia (e.g., changes in mentation, somnolence, impaired coordination, slurred speech) *to facilitate recognition of problem and timely intervention. Information may be especially important if client works or plays outdoors (e.g., camping, skiing, hiking).*[1,2]
- Identify assistive community resources, as indicated (e.g., social services, emergency shelters, clothing suppliers, food bank, public service company, financial resources). *Individual/significant other may be in need of numerous resources if hypothermia was associated with inadequate housing, homelessness, or malnutrition.*

DOCUMENTATION FOCUS

Assessment/Reassessment

- Findings, noting degree of system involvement.
- Graph temperature.

Planning

- Plan of care and who is involved in planning.
- Teaching plan.

Implementation/Evaluation

- Responses to interventions, teaching, and actions performed.
- Attainment or progress toward desired outcome(s).
- Modifications to plan of care.

Discharge Planning

- Long-term needs, identifying who is responsible for each action.
- Specific referrals made.

References

1. Curtis, R. (2002, updated 2015). Outdoor Action guide to hypothermia and cold weather injuries. Princeton University Outdoor Action. Retrieved January 2015 from http://www.princeton.edu/~oa/safety/hypocold.shtml.
2. Li, J., Silverberg, M. A., Decker, W., et al. (2001, updated 2014). Hypothermia. Retrieved January 2015 from http://emedicine.medscape.com/article/770542-overview.
3. Doenges, M. E., Moorhouse, M. F., Murr, A. C. (2010). Surgical intervention: Risk for imbalanced body temperature. *Nursing Care Plans: Guidelines for Individualizing Client Care Across the Life Span.* 8th ed. Philadelphia: F. A. Davis, 792.
4. State of Alaska cold injuries and cold water near drowning guidelines. (2003, updated 2005). Retrieved January 2015 from http://www.hypothermia.org/protocol.htm.
5. Calver, P., Braungardt, T., Kupchik, N., et al. (2005). The big chill: Improving the odds after cardiac arrest. CE Home Study Program for RNweb. Retrieved January 2015 from http://www.modernmedicine.com/modern-medicine/content/big-chill-improving-odds-after-cardiac-arrest?page=full.
6. Soreide, E., Smith, C. E. (2004). Hypothermia in trauma victims—Friend or foe? *Indian J Crit Care Med (IJCCM)*, 8(2), 116–119.
7. McCall, E. M., Alderdice, F., Halliday, H. L., et al. (2010). Interventions to prevent hypothermia at birth in preterm and/or low birthweight infants. Cochrane Database of Systematic Reviews 2010. Retrieved January 2015 from https://www.nichd.nih.gov/cochrane_data/mccalle_01/mccalle_01.html.

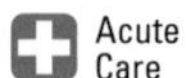

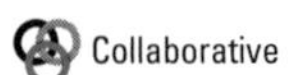

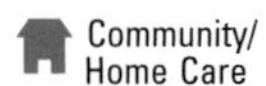

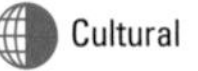

risk for Hypothermia

Taxonomy II: Safety/Protection—Class 6 Thermoregulation (00253) [**Diagnostic Division:** Safety], Submitted 2013

DEFINITION: Vulnerable to a failure of thermoregulation that may result in a core body temperature below the normal diurnal range, which may compromise health.

RISK FACTORS

Alcohol consumption
Damage to hypothalamus; radiation
Economically disadvantaged; insufficient clothing
Extremes of age or weight; insufficient supply of subcutaneous fat; malnutrition
Heat transfer (e.g., conduction, convection, evaporation, radiation)
Inactivity
Insufficient caregiver knowledge of hypothermia prevention
Low environmental temperature
Trauma; radiation, pharmaceutical agent

Children and Adults: Accidental

Mild hypothermia, core temperature approaching 35°C (95°F)
Moderate hypothermia, core temperature approaching 32°C (89.6°F)
Severe hypothermia, core temperature approaching 30°C (86°F)

Children and Adults: Injured Patients

Hypothermia, core temperature approaching 35°C (95°F)
Severe hypothermia, core temperature approaching 32°C (89.6°F)

Neonates

High risk or unplanned out-of-hospital birth
Delay in breastfeeding
Early bathing of newborn
Immature stratum corneum
Increased body surface area to weight ratio
Increase in oxygen demand; increase in pulmonary vascular resistance (PVR); ineffective vascular control
Insufficient nonshivering thermogenesis
Grade 1 hypothermia, core temperature approaching 36.5°C (97°F)
Grade 2 hypothermia, core temperature approaching 36°C (96.8°F)
Grade 3 hypothermia, core temperature approaching 35°C (95°F)
Grade 4 hypothermia, core temperature approaching 34°C (93.2°F)

NOTE: A risk diagnosis is not evidenced by signs and symptoms as the problem has not occurred; rather, nursing interventions are directed at prevention.

Sample Clinical Applications: Dementia, malnutrition, anorexia nervosa, brain trauma, stroke, endocrine disorders, some surgical procedures (e.g., craniotomy), alcohol intoxication, abuse or neglect, prematurity, near-drowning

(continues on page 436)

risk for Hypothermia (continued)

DESIRED OUTCOMES/EVALUATION CRITERIA

Sample NOC linkages:

Thermoregulation: Balance among heat production, heat gain, and heat loss

Client Will (Include Specific Time Frame)

- Display core temperature within normal range.

Sample NOC linkages:

Risk Control: Hypothermia: Personal actions to understand, prevent, eliminate, or reduce the threat of low body temperature

Client/Caregiver Will (Include Specific Time Frame)

- Maintain safe environment.
- Identify underlying cause or contributing factors that can be controlled.
- Verbalize understanding of specific interventions to prevent hypothermia.
- Demonstrate behaviors to monitor and promote normothermia.

ACTIONS/INTERVENTIONS

Sample NIC linkages:

Temperature Regulation: Attaining or maintaining body temperature within a normal range

Risk Identification: Analysis of potential risk factors, determination of health risks, and prioritization of risk reduction strategies for an individual or group

NURSING PRIORITY NO. 1 To assess risk factors:

- Note presence of risk factors as related to current situation, for example (1) ***decreased heat production*** *such as occurs with hypopituitary, hypoadrenal and hypothyroid conditions, and hypoglycemia and neuromuscular inefficiencies seen in extremes of age;* (2) ***increased heat loss*** *(e.g., exposure to cold weather, winter outdoor activities; cold water drenching or immersion; improper clothing, shelter, or food for weather conditions; problems such as could occur with burns; fluid losses, dehydration; surgery, open wounds, exposed skin or viscera);* and (3) ***impaired thermoregulation*** *as might occur with central nervous system trauma or tumor, intracranial bleeding or stroke, toxicological and metabolic disorders, and Parkinson's disease and multiple sclerosis.*[1,2]
- ∞ Note age of client (e.g., premature neonate, child, elderly person) and other associated conditions, such as nutrition status (e.g., thin, tall person loses heat easier than short stature, overweight person) and living condition and relationship status (e.g., aged or cognitive impaired client living alone or homeless alcoholic).[1–3]
- Measure core temperature with low register thermometer (measuring below 94°F [34.4°C]) *to identify client approaching hypothermia range as listed in Risk Factors.*
- Monitor for change in vital signs and mental status.

NURSING PRIORITY NO. 2 To prevent hypothermia (Teaching/Discharge Considerations):

- Review specific risk factors or causes of hypothermia *to assist client/caregivers in identifying safety concerns.*
- Identify factors that client can control (if any), such as protection from environment and adequate heat in home, layering clothing and blankets, minimizing heat loss from head with hat or scarf, appropriate cold

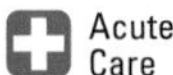

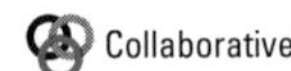

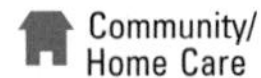

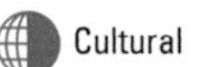

weather clothing, avoidance of alcohol or other drugs if anticipating exposure to cold, potential risks for future hypersensitivity to cold, etc.

- Discuss signs/symptoms of early hypothermia (e.g., changes in mentation, somnolence, impaired coordination, slurred speech) *to facilitate recognition of problem and timely intervention. Information may be especially important if client works or plays outdoors (e.g., camping, skiing, hiking).*[1,2]
- Identify assistive community resources, as indicated (e.g., social services, emergency shelters, clothing suppliers, food bank, public service company, financial resources). *Individual/significant other may be in need of numerous resources if risk for hypothermia is associated with inadequate housing, homelessness, or malnutrition.*

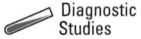

DOCUMENTATION FOCUS

Assessment/Reassessment

- Individual risks identified.
- Available Resources.

Planning

- Plan of care and who is involved in planning.
- Teaching plan.

Implementation/Evaluation

- Responses to interventions, teaching, and actions performed.
- Attainment or progress toward desired outcome(s).
- Modifications to plan of care.

Discharge Planning

- Long-term needs, identifying who is responsible for each action.
- Specific referrals made.

References

1. Curtis, R. (2002, updated 2015). Outdoor Action guide to hypothermia and cold weather injuries. Princeton University Outdoor Action. Retrieved January 2015 from http://www.princeton.edu/~oa/safety/hypocold.shtml.
2. Li, J., Silverberg, M. A., Decker, W., et al. (2001, updated 2014). Hypothermia. Retrieved January 2015 from http://emedicine.medscape.com/article/770542-overview.
3. Soreide, E., Smith, C. E. (2004). Hypothermia in trauma victims - Friend or foe? *Indian J Crit Care Med*, 8, 116–119.

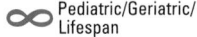

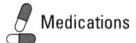

risk for perioperative Hypothermia

Taxonomy II: Safety/Protection—Class 6 Thermoregulation (00254) [**Diagnostic Division:** Safety], Submitted 2013

DEFINITION: Vulnerable to an inadvertent drop in core body temperature below 36°C (96.8°F) occurring 1 hour before to 24 hours after surgery, which may compromise health.

RISK FACTORS

American Society of Anesthesiologists (ASA) Physical Status classification score >1
Cardiovascular complications
Combined regional and general anesthesia
Diabetic neuropathy
Heat transfer (e.g., high volume of unwarmed infusion, unwarmed irrigation >20 liters)
Low body weight
Low environmental temperature
Low preoperative temperature (<36°C [96.8°F])
Surgical procedure

NOTE: A risk diagnosis is not evidenced by signs and symptoms as the problem has not occurred; rather, nursing interventions are directed at prevention.

Sample Clinical Applications: Surgical procedures where therapeutic hypothermia is not planned

DESIRED OUTCOMES/EVALUATION CRITERIA

Sample NOC linkages:

Thermoregulation: Balance among heat production, heat gain, and heat loss

Client Will (Include Specific Time Frame)

- Display core temperature within normal range.
- Be free of complications such as cardiac failure, respiratory infection or failure, thromboembolic phenomena, and delayed healing.

Sample NOC linkages:

Risk Control: Hypothermia: Personal actions to understand, prevent, eliminate, or reduce the threat of low body temperature

Care Provider Will (Include Specific Time Frame)

- Identify client condition/situations that may lead to problems with temperature regulation.
- Engage in protective actions to control body temperature.

ACTIONS/INTERVENTIONS

Sample NIC linkages:

Temperature Regulation: Intraoperative: Attaining and/or maintaining desired intraoperative body temperature

NURSING PRIORITY NO. 1 To identify risk factors affecting current situation:

- Ascertain type of surgical procedure client is having. *Helps in identifying elements of risk. For example, some procedures carry higher risk of hypothermia (e.g., laparoscopic abdominal procedure with carbon dioxide insufflation; large volume liposuction; extensive surgical procedure of any sort with prolonged exposure of body surfaces and long period of anesthesia).*[1–3]

- Assess client conditions/comorbidities (e.g., diabetes, impaired skin and tissue integrity, respiratory, cardiac, vascular, neurologic disorders) *that may place client at higher risk for perioperative complications, including hypothermia.*[4]
- Note client's body type and age. *Very thin, malnourished or dehydrated individuals, as well as those who are very young or elderly, are more susceptible to perioperative hypothermia. The body's ability to regulate temperature may lessen with age.*[5,6]
- Note client's medication regimen. *Medications including some vasodilators, antipsychotics, and sedatives can impair the body's ability to regulate its temperature.*[6]

NURSING PRIORITY NO. 2 To maintain appropriate body temperature/prevent hypothermia complications:

- Measure client's temperature preoperatively and confirm that continuous monitoring of temperature is occurring during procedure. Report preoperative temperature below ideal range to surgical team/anesthesiologist.
- Implement preventive warming techniques in the operating room. *Evidence supports commencement of active warming preoperatively and monitoring it throughout the intraoperative period. Single strategies such as forced-air warming are more effective than passive warming (e.g., blankets from a warmer); however, combined strategies, including preoperative commencement, use of warmed fluids plus forced-air warming, and other active strategies, were more effective in vulnerable groups.*[13]
  - Consider administering warmed IV fluids. *The Association of Perioperative Registered Nurses states "warming IV fluids to near 37°C (98.6°F) prevents heat loss from the administration of cold IV fluids and should be considered as an adjunct to skin surface warming. When less than two liters of volume is given, fluid warming is of limited value because fluid-induced cooling is minimal."*[7]
  - Use heated blankets from warming cabinet. *Note: while easy to use and effective, blankets on top of client can limit access to surgical site. Also, adding too many layers of warmed cotton blankets is ineffective in raising the patient's body temperature. The first blanket can reduce heat loss by 33%, but adding another blanket only adds another 18% reduction in heat loss. Adding three or more blankets adds no further warming.*[8]
  - Use conductive warming devices. *One type of warming pad is an electrical resistive/conductive device that warms underneath the client's body. The anesthesiologist can select one of five preset temperatures. Because the client is warming from underneath, blankets need not be placed on top, allowing for greater surgical access.*[9]
  - Provide forced-air warming blanket. *Warm air is pumped through a hose into a disposable blanket that covers the client. Heat transfer results from the movement of warm air across the surface of the patient's skin, which allows forced-air blankets to transfer more heat at a lower temperature.*[7,13,14]
  - Use warm water garment or mattress. *Research has shown that circulating water garments and energy transfer pads warm about 50% better than forced air because they warm both over and under the body. Note: Care must be exercised when the mattress is used, as the heat of the fluid mattress combined with body weight and static position increases the risk of pressure ulcers or necrosis.*[10,11]
  - Increase operating room temperature, as indicated. *It is currently thought that optimal operating room temperatures for the client should be no less than 20°C (68°F) to reduce risk of hypothermia complications while still providing comfortable environment for scrubbed personnel under surgical lights. Recovery room temperatures of 20°C to 24°C (68°F to 75°F) may be ideal for rewarming client.*[12]

DOCUMENTATION FOCUS

Assessment/Reassessment

- Findings, noting degree of system involvement.
- Graph temperature.

Planning

- Plan of care.

Implementation/Evaluation

- Responses to interventions and actions performed.
- Attainment of desired outcome(s).
- Modifications to plan of care.

References

1. Shermak, M. A., Mahaffey, G. (2010). Preventing liposuction complications. *OR Nurse 2105*, 4(1), 14–19.
2. Conner, R. (Ed.) (2008). Recommended practices for endoscopic minimally invasive surgery. *Perioperative Standards and Recommended Practices.* Denver: AORN, Inc.
3. Paulikas, C. A. (2008). Prevention of unplanned perioperative hypothermia. *AORN J*, 88(3), 358–364.
4. Fletcher, H. C. (2014). Preventing skin injury in the OR. *OR Nurse 2015*, 8(3), 28–34.
5. Lynch, S., Dixon, J., Leary, D. (2010). Reducing the risk of unplanned perioperative hypothermia. *AORN J*, 92(5), 553–562.
6. Surgical Care Improvement Project Steering Committee. (2011). Turn up the heat: Avoiding surgical complications with adequate patient warming. The OR Connection. Retrieved January 2015 from http://www.medlineuniversity.com/DesktopModules/Documents/ViewDocument.aspx.
7. Association of periOperative Registered Nurses (AORN). (2010). Recommended practices for prevention of unplanned perioperative hypothermia. In (ed). *2010 Perioperative Standards and Recommended Practices*. Denver: AORN, Inc.
8. Weirich, T. L. (2008). Hypothermia warming protocols: Why are they not widely used in the OR? *AORN J*, 87(2), 333–344.
9. Mathias, J. M. (2006). Taking steps to keep OR patients warm. *OR Manager*, 22(12), 14–16.
10. Sessler, D., Todd, M. (2000). Perioperative heat balance. *Anesthesiology*, 92(2), 578–596.
11. Zangrillo, A., Pappalardo, F., Talo, G., et al. (2006). Temperature management during off-pump coronary artery bypass graft surgery: A randomized clinical trial on the efficacy of a circulating water system versus a forced-air system. *J Cardiothorac Vasc Anesth*, 20(6), 788–792.
12. Good, K. K., Verble, J. A., Secrest, J., et al. (2006). Postoperative hypothermia—the chilling consequences. *AORN J*, 83(5), 1054–1066.
13. Moola, S., Lockwood, C. (2011). Effectiveness of strategies for the management and/or prevention of hypothermia within the adult perioperative environment. *Int J Evid Based Healthc*, 9(4), 337–345.
14. Stevens, M. H. (2011). Forced-air warming: An effective tool in fighting SSI. Infection Control Today. Retrieved January 2015 from http://www.infectioncontroltoday.com/articles/2011/03/forced-air-warming-an-effective-tool-in-fighting-ssi.aspx.

ineffective Impulse Control

Taxonomy II: Perception/Cognition—Class 4 Cognition (00222) [**Diagnostic Division:** Ego Integrity], Submitted 2010

DEFINITION: A pattern of performing rapid, unplanned reactions to internal or external stimuli without regard for the negative consequences of these reactions to the impulsive individual or to others.

RELATED FACTORS

Anger; denial; delusion
Insomnia; fatigue
Chronic low self-esteem; disturbed body image; hopelessness
Stress vulnerability; environment that might cause irritation, frustration
Ineffective coping; co-dependency
Smoker; substance abuse
Economically disadvantaged
Social isolation; suicidal feeling

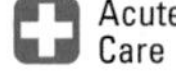

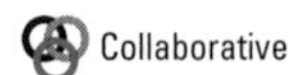

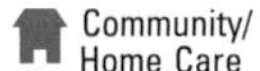

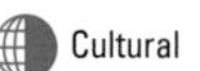

Compunction [i.e., feeling of uneasiness about rightness of action]; unpleasant physical symptoms
Organic brain disorders; disorder of: cognition, development, mood, personality

DEFINING CHARACTERISTICS

Subjective

Inability to save money or regulate finances
Asking personal questions of others despite their discomfort

Objective

Acting without thinking
Sensation seeking; sexual promiscuity
Sharing personal details inappropriately; too familiar with strangers
Irritability; temper outbursts
Pathological gambling
Violence

Sample Clinical Applications: Eating disorders, addictions—substance/sexual, bipolar disorders, dementia, attention deficit hyperactivity disorder (ADHD), oppositional defiant disorder, traumatic brain injury, Down syndrome, Asperger's syndrome

DESIRED OUTCOMES/EVALUATION CRITERIA

Sample NOC linkages:

Impulse Self-Control: Self-restraint of compulsive behaviors
Mood Equilibrium: Appropriate adjustment of prevailing emotional tone in response to circumstances

Client Will (Include Specific Time Frame)

- Acknowledge problem with impulse control.
- Identify feelings that precede desire to engage in impulsive actions.
- Verbalize desire to learn new ways of controlling impulsive behavior.
- Participate in anger management therapy.

ACTIONS/INTERVENTIONS

Sample NIC linkages:

Impulse Control Training: Assisting the patient to mediate impulsive behavior through application of problem-solving strategies to social and interpersonal situations
Anger Control Assistance: Facilitation of the expression of anger in an adaptive, nonviolent manner

NURSING PRIORITY NO. 1 To assess causative/contributing factors:

- Investigate causes/individual factors that may be involved in client's situation. *Impulse disorders are a group of mental health disorders generally believed to be the result of biological, social, and psychological factors. It is theorized that unbalanced neurotransmitters in the brain may be a cause, as well as the hormone imbalances implicated in violent and aggressive behavior.*[1–4,7,9]
- Evaluate for underlying neurological conditions. *Presence of traumatic brain injury, strokes, brain tumors, etc., may result in poor impulse control, affecting therapeutic choices.*[11]
- Explore individual's inability to control actions. *Healthy people are aware of an impulse and are able to make a decision about whether to follow the urge. The key differentiation between healthy impulsiveness and an impulse disorder is the negative consequences that follow.*[1,7,9]

- Note negative consequences incurred by client's impulsive actions, such as repeat detentions or suspensions from school, loss of employment, financial ruin, arrests/convictions, and civil litigation. *Regardless of the form of the impulsive disorder—predisposition to rapid unplanned reactions (e.g., ADHD, bipolar, substance use, explosive behavior) or impaired ability to resist impulses (e.g., compulsive buying, kleptomania, pathological gambling, pyromania)—individuals with poor control engage in the activity even if they know that there will be negative consequences.*[1–3,7,9,10]
- Ascertain degree of anxiety client experiences when having an impulse to act on the desire. *Not acting on the impulse creates intense anxiety or arousal in the individual. Engaging in the behavior produces release of the anxiety and possibly pleasure or gratification. This may be followed by remorse; regret; or, conversely, satisfaction.*[1–3,7]
- Identify behaviors indicative of attention-deficit disorder for further evaluation. *This diagnosis needs to be made by a physician based on reports of behaviors of inattention, hyperactivity, and impulsivity by multiple sources (e.g., parent, teachers, employer) in more than one setting and lasting at least 6 months.*[4]
- Evaluate for co-occurring psychiatric conditions. *The presence of comorbidities has treatment implications and, if left untreated, will complicate and/or limit successful outcomes for impulse control therapy.*[4,7,9]

NURSING PRIORITY NO. 2 To assist client to develop strategies to manage impulsive behaviors:

- Collaborate with treatment of condition, as indicated. *Individuals with impulsive control disorders do not necessarily present for treatment. Those with kleptomania, fire starters, and compulsive gamblers usually come to the attention of court authorities and may be referred for mental health services.*[1–5,7,9]
- Encourage client to make the decision to change and set personally achievable goals. *Making this decision can enable the client to enter therapy and be willing to stay with the program.*[2,4,7]
- Encourage client to identify negative consequences of behavior by expressing own feelings and anxieties regarding the adverse impact on his/her life. *Helps individual begin to understand problems of impulsive behavior.*[7]
- Help client take responsibility and control in situation. *Recognizing own control over impulsive behavior can help client begin to manage problems.*[3,4,7]
- Develop a treatment plan for child with ADHD in conjunction with the parents, teachers, and physician. *Medications and behavioral therapy can be helpful, along with monitoring the child and setting goals that are realistic and achievable.*[4]
- Organize a routine schedule for the child with Asperger's syndrome. *Deficits in cognitive functioning make it difficult for the child to see the big picture, process information, see the consequences of an action, and understand the concept of time.*[5,6]
- Plan for problem with "melt downs," tantrums, or rage in children with Asperger's syndrome. *These children do not recognize feelings, and parents and caregivers need to maintain a calm manner, remove child in a nonpunitive fashion, move closer, redirect, etc. These actions are calming; however, the child may begin acting out and need to go to a safe room where he or she can regain control.*[5,6]
- Discuss issue of hypersexuality. *It can be difficult to determine whether this term applies to an individual because people have differing definitions for what is too much sexual behavior.*[8]
- Determine use of medications. *No specific medications have been approved by the FDA for use with impulse control disorders, but some medications such as selective serotonin reuptake inhibitor antidepressants are being used successfully.*[1,4,7]

NURSING PRIORITY NO. 3 To promote wellness (Teaching/Discharge Considerations):

- Involve in cognitive/behavioral therapy. *Having client identify behavioral patterns that result in negative consequences or harmful effects for self or others allows the individual to recognize and avoid these situations and use techniques that facilitate self-restraint.*[3–5,7]
- Discuss the use of exposure therapy. *This helps the client build up a tolerance for the trigger situation while using self-control.*[3,7]

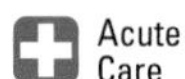

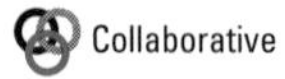

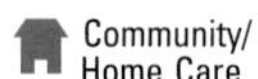

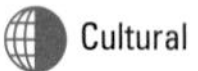

• Encourage client to become involved in group or community activities. *Provides opportunity to learn new social skills and feel better about self.*[7]

DOCUMENTATION FOCUS

Assessment/Reassessment

• Individual findings, including type of situation involved in client's loss of control.
• Negative consequences incurred due to behavior.
• Client awareness of consequences of actions.

Planning

• Plan of care, specific interventions, and who is involved in planning.
• Individual teaching plan.

Implementation/Evaluation

• Responses to interventions, teaching, and actions performed.
• Attainment or progress toward desired outcome(s).
• Any modifications to plan of care.

Discharge Planning

• Long-term needs and who is responsible for actions to be taken.
• Specific referrals made.

References

1. Bose, D. (2009). Impulse control disorders. Retrieved October 2015 from http://www.buzzle.com/articles/impulse-control-disorder.html.
2. Pal, S. (2009). Unable to control impulses. Culturally Sensitive Rehabilitation in Mental Health. Retrieved October 2015 from http://www.csrmh.com/index.php?news=309.
3. Aboujaoude, E., Koran, L. M. (eds.) (2010). *Impulse Control Disorders*. New York, NY: Cambridge University Press.
4. National Institute of Mental Health (NIMH). (No date). Attention deficit hyperactivity disorder (ADHD). Retrieved October 2015 from http://www.nimh.nih.gov/health/topics/attention-deficit-hyperactivity-disorder-adhd/index.shtml.
5. No author. (2015). Asperger syndrome fact sheet. National Institute of Neurological Disorders and Stroke. NIH Publication No. 13-5624. Retrieved October 2015 from http://www.ninds.nih.gov/disorders/asperger/detail_asperger.htm.
6. Hutten, M. (2012). Aspergers children who worry excessively: Tips for parents. Retrieved October 2015 from http://www.myaspergerschild.com/2012/06/aspergers-children-who-worry.html.
7. No author. (No date). Impulse control disorders. PsychSolve. Retrieved October 2015 from https://www.newharbinger.com/psychsolve/impulse-control-disorders.
8. Kaplan, M., Krueger, R. (2010). Diagnosis, assessment, and treatment of hypersexuality. *J Sex Res*, 47(2), 181–198.
9. Grant, J. E., Levine, L., Kim, D. (2005). Impulse control disorders in adult psychiatric inpatients. *Am J Psychiatry*, 162(11), 2184–2188.
10. Grant, J. E., Potenza, M. N., Weinstein, A., et al. (2010). Introduction to behavioral addictions. *Am J Drug Alcohol Abuse*, 36(5), 233–241.
11. Yudofsky, S. C., Silver, J. M. (1985). Psychiatric aspects of brain injury: Trauma, stroke and tumor. In Hales, R. E., Frances, A. J. (eds). *Psychiatric Update—American Psychiatric Association Annual Review*, Vol. IV. Washington, DC: American Psychiatric Press.

bowel Incontinence

Taxonomy II: Elimination and Exchange—Class 2 Gastrointestinal Function (00014) [**Diagnostic Division:** Elimination], Submitted 1975; Revised 1998

DEFINITION: Change in normal bowel habits characterized by involuntary passage of stool.

RELATED FACTORS

Abnormal increase in abdominal or intestinal pressure
Alteration in cognitive functioning; stressors
Chronic diarrhea; impaction; incomplete emptying of the bowel
Colorectal lesion; dysfunctional or abnormal rectal sphincter; impaired reservoir capacity; upper or lower motor nerve damage
Deficient dietary habits
Difficulty in toileting self-care
Environmental factor (e.g., inaccessible bathroom)
Generalized decline in muscle tone; immobility
Pharmaceutical agent; laxative abuse

DEFINING CHARACTERISTICS

Subjective

Inability to expel formed stool despite recognition of rectal fullness
Bowel urgency; inability to delay defecation
Inability to recognize rectal fullness

Objective

Constant passage of soft stool
Fecal staining of clothing, bedding
Fecal odor
Reddened perianal skin
Does not recognize or inattentive to urge to defecate

Sample Clinical Applications: Hemorrhoids, rectal prolapse, anal/gynecological surgery, childbirth injuries/uterine prolapse, spinal cord injury (SCI), stroke, multiple sclerosis (MS), ulcerative colitis, dementia

DESIRED OUTCOMES/EVALUATION CRITERIA

Sample NOC linkages:

Bowel Continence: Control of passage of stool from the bowel
Bowel Elimination: Formation and evacuation of stool
Neurological Status: Ability of the peripheral and central nervous system (CNS) to receive, process, and respond to internal and external stimuli

Client Will (Include Specific Time Frame)

- Verbalize understanding of causative or controlling factors.
- Identify individually appropriate interventions.
- Participate in therapeutic regimen to control incontinence.
- Establish and maintain as regular a pattern of bowel functioning as possible.

ACTIONS/INTERVENTIONS

Sample NIC linkages:
Bowel Incontinence Care: Promotion of bowel continence and maintenance of perineal skin integrity
Bowel Incontinence Care: Encopresis: Promotion of bowel continence in children
Bowel Training: Assisting the patient to train the bowel to evacuate at specific intervals

NURSING PRIORITY NO. 1 To assess causative/contributing factors:

- Determine type of bowel incontinence present, as possible: *(1) loss of anal sphincter control (such as might occur with sphincter trauma), (2) stool seepage (as may occur with fistula and prolapse), or (3) poor bowel control (as might occur with inflammatory bowel disease, following intestinal surgery; chronic constipation with weakening musculature; laxative abuse, parasitic infection, toxins).*[8]
- Determine historical aspects of incontinence with preceding/precipitating events. *Common factors are (1) structural changes in the sphincter muscle (e.g., hemorrhoids, rectal prolapse; prostate, anal, or gynecological surgery; vaginal delivery with inadequate repair of obstetric sphincter disruption); (2) injuries to sensory nerves (e.g., spinal cord injury, multiple sclerosis); major trauma; stroke, tumor, or radiation therapy; (3) strong-urge or severe prolonged diarrhea (e.g., ulcerative colitis, Crohn's disease, infectious diarrhea); (4) dementia (e.g., acute or chronic cognitive impairment, not necessarily related to sphincter control); (5) result of toxins (e.g., salmonella); (6) aging, particularly in menopausal women; and (7) effects of improper diet or type and rate of enteral feedings.*[1–8]
- Note client's age and gender. *Bowel incontinence is more common in children, women of childbirth age, and elderly adults (difficulty responding to urge in a timely manner, problems walking or undoing zippers, decrease of maximum squeeze pressure); it is more common in boys than girls, but more common in elderly women than elderly men.*[1,2,7]
- Review medication regimen, including over-the-counter drugs. *Laxative abuse and drugs with a side effect of diarrhea (e.g., antibiotics) or constipation (e.g., sedatives, hypnotics, opioids, muscle relaxants) may impact bowel control.*
- Review diagnostic studies. *Pelvic and/or anal ultrasound may be used to identify structural abnormalities; endoscopy may be used to visualize lower gastrointestinal tract; manometry may be used to measure pressure and strength of anal muscles; and nerve studies may be used to check for nerve damage. Blood tests and stool cultures may be done to identify presence of bacteria and toxins.*[1–3,5,6]

NURSING PRIORITY NO. 2 To determine current pattern of elimination:

- Ascertain timing and characteristic aspects of incontinent occurrence, noting preceding or precipitating events. *Helps to identify patterns or worsening trends. Interventions are different for a sudden acute accident than for chronic long-term incontinence problems. Note: Client may have passive incontinence and be unaware that stool is being passed (related to poorly functioning sphincter muscle) or urge incontinence in which the individual is aware but unable to prevent passage of stool (sphincter muscle normal). Problem may have been present for a long time, either because of client/caregiver sense of embarrassment or failure to realize that effective treatment may be available.*[2,5]
- Determine stool characteristics, including **consistency** (may be liquid, hard formed, or hard at first and then soft), **amount** (may be a small amount of liquid or entire solid bowel movement), and **frequency**. *Provides information that can help differentiate type of incontinence present and provides comparative baseline for response to interventions.*
- Note where bowel accidents occur and what client is experiencing at the time. *Changes in usual routines or surrounding environment, general health condition, and the addition of emotional stressors (such as a new baby in the home or increased confusion in a dementia client) can cause or exacerbate incontinence behaviors.*[5]

NURSING PRIORITY NO. 3 To promote control/management of incontinence:

- Assist in treatment of underlying factors (e.g., as listed in Related Factors and Defining Characteristics). *While incontinence is a symptom and not a disease, appropriate treatment can often correct the problem or at least improve the client's quality of life.*[2]
- Administer medications, as indicated, such as stool softeners or bulk formers and laxatives *(may be used when the cause is constipation)* or antidiarrheals, including cholinergics *(may be used to decrease intestinal secretions and bowel motility if diarrhea is cause for incontinence).*[1,2]
- Establish a toileting program as early as possible *to maximize success of program and preserve comfort and self-esteem.*[1–5,7]

  Take client to the bathroom or place on commode or bedpan at specified intervals, taking into consideration individual needs and incontinence patterns.

  Use the same type of facility for toileting as much as possible.

  Make sure bathroom is safe for impaired person (good lighting, support rails, good height for getting onto and up from stool).

  Provide time and privacy for elimination.

  Demonstrate techniques and assist client/caregiver to practice contracting abdominal muscles, leaning forward on commode *to increase intra-abdominal pressure during defecation,* and left to right abdominal massage *to stimulate peristalsis.*
- Encourage and instruct client/caregiver in providing diet high in natural bulk and fiber, with fruits, vegetables, grains, and reduced fatty foods. Identify and eliminate problem foods *to avoid diarrhea, constipation, or gas formation.*[2]
- Adjust enteral feedings and/or change formula, as indicated, *to reduce diarrhea effect.*[7]
- Encourage adequate fluid intake (at least 2,000 mL/d) within client's need and tolerance, including fruit juices *to help manage constipation.* Encourage warm fluids after meals *to promote intestinal motility.* Avoid caffeine and alcohol *to reduce diarrhea.*[7]
- Recommend walking and a regular exercise program, pelvic floor exercises, and biofeedback, as individually indicated, *to improve abdominal and pelvic muscles and strengthen rectal sphincter tone.*[2,7]
- Encourage or provide perineal care with frequent gentle cleansing and use of emollients after incontinent stools *to reduce excoriation of skin.*[6]
- Provide incontinence aids or pads until control is obtained. Change pads frequently *to reduce incidence of skin rashes or breakdown.*[6]
- Refer to ND Diarrhea *if incontinence is due to uncontrolled diarrhea* and ND Constipation *if incontinence is due to impaction.*

NURSING PRIORITY NO. 4 To promote wellness (Teaching/Discharge Considerations):

- Review and encourage continuation of successful interventions as individually identified.
- Instruct in use of suppositories or laxatives or stool softeners, when indicated, *to stimulate timed defecation.*
- Identify foods (e.g., daily bran muffins or prunes) *that promote soft stool consistency and bowel regularity.* Recommend avoidance of problem foods dependent on individual reactions.
- Refer client/caregivers to outside resources when condition is long term or chronic *to obtain care assistance and emotional support and respite.*
- Encourage scheduling of social activities within time frame of bowel program, as indicated (e.g., avoid a 4-hr excursion with no access to appropriate facilities if bowel program requires toileting every 3 hr), *to maximize social functioning and success of bowel program.*

DOCUMENTATION FOCUS

Assessment/Reassessment

- Current and previous pattern of elimination, physical findings, character of stool, actions tried.

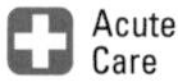

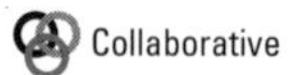

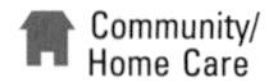

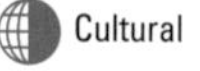

Planning
- Plan of care and who is involved in planning.
- Teaching plan.

Implementation/Evaluation
- Client's/caregiver's responses to interventions, teaching, and actions performed.
- Changes in pattern of elimination, characteristics of stool.
- Attainment or progress toward desired outcome(s).
- Modifications to plan of care.

Discharge Planning
- Identified long-term needs, noting who is responsible for each action.
- Specific bowel program at time of discharge.

References

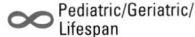

1. Ranganath, S., Ferzandi, T. R. (2015). Fecal incontinence. Retrieved March 2015 from http://emedicine.medscape.com/article/268674-overview#a0102.
2. Cleveland Clinic Health System. (2012). Bowel incontinence. Retrieved March 2015 from http://my.clevelandclinic.org/health/diseases_conditions/hic_Bowel_Incontinence.
3. Bowel incontinence. (1996, updated 2008). *Patient & Public Information.* Arlington Heights, IL: American Society of Colon and Rectal Surgeons.
4. Doenges, M. E., Moorhouse, M. F., Murr, A. C. (2010). Spinal cord injury (acute rehabilitative phase). *Nursing Care Plans: Guidelines for Individualizing Client Care Across the Life Span.* 8th ed. Philadelphia: F. A. Davis.
5. Monicken, D. (1989). *Special Care Problems: Bowel Incontinence*, 5th ed. Department of Veterans Affairs, Veterans Health Services and Research Administration, Office of Geriatrics and Extended Care.
6. Langemo, D., Hanson, D., Hunter, S., et al. (2011). Incontinence and incontinence-associated dermatitis. *Adv Skin Wound Care*, 24(3), 126–140.
7. Dugdale, D. D. (reviewer) (2010). Bowel incontinence. Retrieved March 2015 from http://www.nlm.nih.gov/medlineplus/ency/article/003135.htm.
8. Bharucha, A. E., Dunivan, G., Goode, P. S., et al. (2015). Epidemiology, pathophysiology, and classification of fecal incontinence: State of the science summary for the National Institute of Diabetes and Digestive and Kidney Diseases (NIDDK) workshop. *Am J Gastroenterology*, 110(1), 27–36.

functional urinary Incontinence

Taxonomy II: Elimination and Exchange—Class 1 Urinary Function (00020) [**Diagnostic Division:** Elimination], Submitted 1986; Revised 1998

DEFINITION: Inability of usually continent person to reach the toilet in time to avoid unintentional loss of urine.

RELATED FACTORS

Alteration in environmental factor
Neuromuscular impairment
Weakened supporting pelvic structure
Impaired vision
Psychological disorder; alteration in cognitive functioning; [reluctance to request assistance or use bedpan]

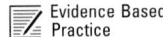

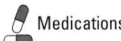

(continues on page 448)

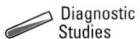

functional urinary Incontinence (continued)
DEFINING CHARACTERISTICS

Subjective

Sensation of need to void

Objective

Voiding prior to reaching toilet; time between sensation of urge and ability to reach toilet is too short
Completely empties bladder
Early morning urinary incontinence

Sample Clinical Applications: Diabetes mellitus, congestive heart failure (CHF) (diuretic use), arthritis, bladder prolapse or cystocele, stroke

DESIRED OUTCOMES/EVALUATION CRITERIA

Sample NOC linkages:

Urinary Elimination: Collection and discharge of urine
Urinary Continence: Control of the elimination of urine from the bladder
Self-Care: Toileting: Ability to toilet self independently with or without assistive device

Client/Caregiver Will (Include Specific Time Frame)

- Verbalize understanding of condition and identify interventions to prevent incontinence.
- Alter environment to accommodate individual needs.
- Report voiding in individually appropriate amounts.
- Void at acceptable times and places.

ACTIONS/INTERVENTIONS

Sample NIC linkages:

Prompted Voiding: Promotion of urinary continence through the use of timed verbal toileting reminders and positive social feedback for successful toileting
Urinary Habit Training: Establishing a predictable pattern of bladder emptying to prevent incontinence for persons with limited cognitive ability who have urge, stress, or functional incontinence
Self-Care Assistance: Toileting: Assisting another with elimination

NURSING PRIORITY NO. 1 To assess causative/contributing factors:

- ∞ Identify or differentiate client with functional incontinence (e.g., bladder and urethra are functioning normally, but client either cannot get to toilet or fails to recognize need to urinate in time to get to the toilet) from other types of incontinence. *Many causes are transient and reversible but can often occur in elderly hospitalized client. Note: A mnemonic to help remember the functional contributors to incontinence is as follows: DIAPPERS: D–delirium; I–infection (urinary); A–atrophic urethritis or vaginitis; P–pharmacologic agents; P–psychiatric illness; E–excess urine output (due to excess fluid intake, alcoholic or caffeinated beverages, diuretics, peripheral edema, congestive heart failure, metabolic disorders such as hyperglycemia or hypercalcemia); R–reduced mobility; S–stool impaction.*[5]
- Determine if client is voluntarily postponing urination. *Often the demands of the work setting (such as restrictions on bathroom breaks, working alone [e.g., pharmacist, nurse, teacher], or demands of the job [heavy workload and unable to find time for a bathroom break]) make it difficult for individuals to go to the bathroom when the need arises, resulting in frequent urinary tract infections and incontinence.*[1,5]
- Evaluate cognition. *Delirium or acute confusion or psychosis can affect mental status—orientation to place, recognition of urge to void, or its significance.*[1,5]

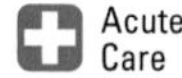

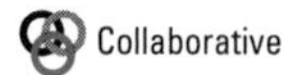

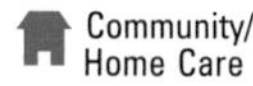

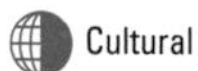

- Note presence and type of functional impairments (e.g., poor eyesight, mobility difficulties, dexterity problems, self-care deficits) *that can hinder ability to get to bathroom.*[4]
- Identify environmental conditions that interfere with timely access to bathroom or successful toileting process. *Unfamiliar surroundings, poor lighting, improperly fitted chair walker, low toilet seat, absence of safety bars, and travel distance to toilet may affect self-care ability.*
- Review medical history for conditions known to increase urine output or alter bladder tone. *For example, diabetes mellitus, prolapsed bladder, and multiple sclerosis can affect frequency of urination and ability to hold urine until individual can reach the bathroom.*[1]
- Note use of medications or agents that can increase urine formation. *Diuretics, alcohol, and caffeine are several substances that can increase amount and frequency of voiding.*
- Test urine for presence of glucose. *Hyperglycemia can cause polyuria and overdistention of the bladder, resulting in problem with continence.*

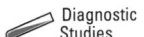

NURSING PRIORITY NO. 2 To assess degree of interference/disability:

- Determine the frequency and timing of continent and incontinent voids. Note time of day or night when incontinence occurs, as well as timing issues (e.g., difference between the time it takes to get to bathroom and remove clothing and involuntary loss of urine). *Information will be used to plan program to manage incontinence.*[2]
- Initiate voiding diary. Note time of day or night when incontinence occurs as well as timing issues (e.g., difference between the time it takes to get to bathroom and remove clothing and involuntary loss of urine).
- Measure or estimate amount of urine voided or lost with incontinent episodes *to help determine options for managing problem.*
- Ascertain effect on lifestyle (including socialization and sexuality) and self-esteem. *There is a general belief that incontinence is an inevitable result of aging and that nothing can be done about it. However, individuals with incontinence problems are often embarrassed, withdraw from social activities and relationships, and hesitate to discuss the problem—even with their healthcare provider.*[1]

NURSING PRIORITY NO. 3 To assist in treating/preventing incontinence:

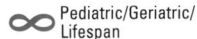

- Remind client to void when needed and schedule voiding times (e.g., cognitive decline, client who ambulates slowly because of physical limitations) *to reduce incontinence episodes and promote comfort.*[4,6]
- Administer prescribed diuretics in the morning. *The effect of these medications diminishes by bedtime, thus resulting in fewer nighttime voidings.*
- Reduce or eliminate use of hypnotics, if possible. *Client may be too sedated to recognize or respond to urge to void.*[3,5]
- Provide means of summoning assistance and respond immediately to summons. *Ready placement of a call light when hospitalized or a bell in the home setting enables client to obtain toileting help, as needed. Quick response to summons can promote continence.*[3]
- Use night lights to mark bathroom location. *Elderly person may become confused upon arising and be unable to locate bathroom in the dark. Lighting will facilitate access, reducing the possibility of accidents.*[3]
- Provide cues such as adequate room lighting, signs, and color coding of door. *Assists disoriented client to find the bathroom.*[3]
- Remove throw rugs and excess furniture in travel path to bathroom. *Reduces risk of falls and facilitates access to bathroom.*[3]
- Adapt clothes for quick removal. *Velcro fasteners, full skirts, crotchless panties or no panties, and suspenders or elastic waists instead of belts on pants facilitate toileting once urge to void is noted.*[3]
- Provide raised toilet seat or easily accessible bedside commode, urinal, or bedpan as indicated. *Facilitates toileting when individual has difficulty with movement.*[1]
- Schedule voiding on regular time schedule (e.g., every 2–3 hr). Encourage client to resist ignoring urge to urinate or have a bowel movement. *Emptying bladder on a regular schedule or when feeling urge reduces risk*

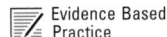

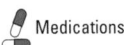

for incontinence. Since urge to void may be difficult to differentiate from urge to defecate, advise client to respond to urge.[1,6]

- Assist client to assume normal anatomic position *for ease of complete bladder emptying.*[3]
- Restrict fluid intake 2 to 3 hr before bedtime. *May reduce need to waken to void during the night.*[1,6]
- Include physical or occupational therapist in determining ways to alter environment, appropriate assistive devices. *Useful in meeting individual needs of client.*[1]
- Refer to urologist or continence specialist as indicated for interventions such as pelvic floor strengthening exercises, biofeedback techniques, vaginal weight training. *May be useful/needed to meet individual needs of client.*

NURSING PRIORITY NO. 4 To promote wellness (Teaching/Discharge Considerations):

- Discuss with client/significant other need for prompted and scheduled voidings *to manage continence when client is unable to respond immediately to urge to void.*[1]
- Suggest limiting intake of coffee, tea, and alcohol. *Diuretic effect of these substances impacts voiding pattern and can contribute to incontinence.*[1]
- Maintain positive regard when incontinence occurs. *Reduces embarrassment associated with incontinence, need for assistance, and use of bedpan.*[1]
- Promote participation in developing long-term plan of care. *Encourages involvement in follow-through of plan, thus increasing possibility of success and confidence in own ability to manage program.*[1]
- Refer to NDs reflex/stress/urge urinary Incontinence for additional interventions, as appropriate.

DOCUMENTATION FOCUS

Assessment/Reassessment

- Current elimination pattern, assessment findings, and effect on lifestyle and self-esteem.

Planning

- Plan of care and who is involved in planning.
- Teaching plan.

Implementation/Evaluation

- Response to interventions, teaching, and actions performed.
- Attainment or progress toward desired outcome(s).
- Modifications to plan of care.

Discharge Planning

- Long-term needs and who is responsible for actions to be taken.
- Specific referrals made.

References

1. The state of the science on urinary incontinence. (2003). In Newman, D. K., Palmer, M. H. (eds). *Am J Nurs*, 3(suppl), 2–53.
2. Wyman, J. F. (2003). Treatment of urinary incontinence in men and older women: The evidence shows the efficacy of a variety of techniques. *Am J Nurs*, 103(suppl), 26–35.
3. Newfield, S. A., Hinz, M. D., Tilley, D. S., et al. (2007). *Cox's Clinical Applications of Nursing Diagnosis: Adult, Child, Women's, Psychiatric, Gerontic, and Home Health Considerations*. 5th ed. Philadelphia, PA: F. A. Davis.
4. Pringle-Specht, J. K. (2005). Nine myths of incontinence in older adults. *Am J Nurs*, 105(6), 58–68.
5. Vasavada, S. P., Carmel, M. E., Rackley, R. (Updated 2014). Urinary incontinence. Retrieved March 2015 from http://emedicine.medscape.com/article/452289-overview.
6. Lazarou, G. (Updated 2014). Bladder control problems. Retrieved March 2015 from http://www.emedicinehealth.com/bladder_control_problems/article_em.htm.

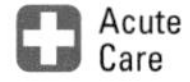

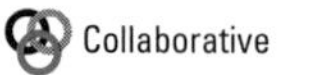

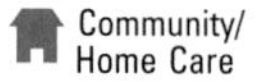

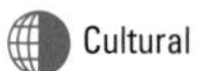

overflow urinary Incontinence

Taxonomy II: Elimination and Exchange—Class 1 Urinary Function (00176) [**Diagnostic Division:** Elimination], Submitted 2006

DEFINITION: Involuntary loss of urine associated with overdistention of the bladder.

RELATED FACTORS

Bladder outlet obstruction; fecal impaction
Urethral obstruction; severe pelvic prolapse
Detrusor external sphincter dyssynergia; detrusor hypocontractility
Treatment regimen [e.g., side effects of medications]

DEFINING CHARACTERISTICS

Subjective

Involuntary leakage of small volume of urine
Nocturia

Objective

Bladder distention
High post-void residual volume
Sample Clinical Applications: Uterine prolapse, benign prostatic hypertrophy, diabetes mellitus, multiple sclerosis (MS), spinal cord injury (SCI), pelvic fractures, urinary stones

DESIRED OUTCOMES/EVALUATION CRITERIA

Sample NOC linkages:
Urinary Continence: Control of elimination of urine from the bladder
Urinary Elimination: Collection and discharge of urine
Knowledge: Disease Process: Extent of understanding conveyed about a specific disease process and prevention of complications

Client Will (Include Specific Time Frame)

- Verbalize understanding of causative factors and appropriate interventions for individual situation.
- Demonstrate techniques or behaviors to alleviate or prevent overflow incontinence.
- Void in sufficient amounts with no palpable bladder distention, experience no postvoid residuals greater than 50 mL, and have no dribbling or overflow.

ACTIONS/INTERVENTIONS

Sample NIC linkages:
Urinary Incontinence Care: Assistance in promoting continence and maintaining perineal skin integrity
Urinary Catheterization: Intermittent: Regular periodic use of a catheter to empty the bladder

NURSING PRIORITY NO. 1 To assess causative/contributing factors:

- Review client's history for (1) bladder outlet obstruction (e.g., prostatic hypertrophy, urethral stricture, urinary stones or tumors), (2) nonfunctioning detrusor muscle (i.e., sensory or motor paralytic bladder due to underlying neurological disease), or (3) atonic bladder that has lost its muscular tone (i.e., chronic overdistention) *to identify potential for or presence of conditions associated with overflow incontinence.*[5,6]

- Note client's age and gender. *Urinary incontinence due to overflow bladder is more common in older men because of the prevalence of obstructive prostate gland enlargement. However, age and sex are not factors in other conditions affecting overflow bladder incontinence, such as nerve damage from diseases such as diabetes, alcoholism, Parkinson's disease, multiple sclerosis, or spina bifida.*[1,5,6]
- Review medication regimen *for drugs that can cause or exacerbate retention and overflow incontinence (e.g., anticholinergics, calcium channel blockers, psychotropics, anesthesia, opiates, sedatives, alpha- and beta-blockers, antihistamines, neuroleptics).*[2,4,5]

NURSING PRIORITY NO. 2 To determine degree of interference/disability:

- Note client reports of symptoms common to overflow incontinence:[3,5,6]
  Feeling no need to urinate, while simultaneously losing urine; frequent leaking or dribbling.
  Feeling the urge to urinate but not being able to.
  Feeling as though the bladder is never completely empty.
  Passing a dribbling stream of urine, even after spending a long time at the toilet.
  Frequently getting up at night to urinate.
- Prepare for or assist with urodynamic testing (e.g., uroflowmetry *to assess urine speed and volume*; cystometrogram *to measure bladder pressure and volume*; bladder scan *to measure retention or postvoid residual, leak point pressure*).[1,5]

NURSING PRIORITY NO. 3 To assist in treating/preventing overflow incontinence:

- Collaborate in treatment of underlying conditions (e.g., medications or surgery for prostatic hypertrophy or severe pelvic prolapse; use of medication, such as terazosin, to relax urinary sphincter; altering dose or discontinuing medications contributing to retention). *If the underlying cause of the overflow problem can be treated or eliminated, client may be able to return to normal voiding pattern.*
- Collaborate with physician regarding client's medications (e.g., anticholinergics, antidepressants, antipsychotics, sedatives, narcotics, alpha-adrenergic blockers) *that could be discontinued or altered to reduce/limit their effects on cognition and/or innervation and function of the bladder.*[9]
- Administer medications, as indicated. *For some men with an enlarged prostate, treatment with an alpha-adrenergic blocker (e.g., doxazosin [Cardura], tamulosin [Flomax]) can help relax the muscle at the base of the urethra and allow urine to pass from the bladder.*[5]
- Administer stool softeners, laxatives, enema/other treatments as indicated. *Chronic constipation is a factor in weakening muscles that control urination. Fecal impaction can be a cause of urinary retention and overflow incontinence, especially in elderly clients.*[6]
- Demonstrate and encourage use of gentle massage over bladder (Credé's maneuver). *May facilitate bladder emptying when cause is detrusor weakness.*
- Implement intermittent or continuous catheterization. *Short-term use may be required while acute conditions are treated (e.g., infection, surgery for enlarged prostate); long-term use is required for permanent conditions (e.g., SCI or other neuromuscular conditions resulting in permanent bladder dysfunction). Note: Sterile intermittent catheterization is preferred when possible in overflow incontinence to promote the return to normal bladder emptying and to reduce risk of infection and other complications associated with long-term indwelling catheter.*[5,7,8]
- Refer to NDs urge urinary Incontinence, stress urinary Incontinence, and [acute/chronic] Urinary Retention for additional interventions.

NURSING PRIORITY NO. 4 To promote wellness (Teaching/Discharge Considerations):

- Identify and continue client's successful self-management of incontinence, where possible. *Continuation of successful strategies (e.g., allowing plenty of time for voiding, double voiding, self-catherization) can reduce risk of recurrence/failure of continence.*

 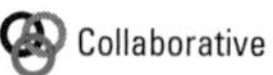 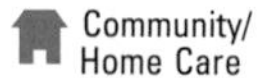  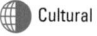

- Establish regular schedule for bladder emptying whether voiding or using catheter.
- Emphasize need for adequate fluid intake, including use of acidifying fruit juices or ingestion of vitamin C *to discourage bacterial growth and stone formation.*
- Instruct client/significant others in clean intermittent self-catheterization techniques *to prevent reflux or increased renal pressures and to enhance independence.*
- Review signs/symptoms of complications requiring prompt medical evaluation *to promote timely intervention and prevent complications.*

DOCUMENTATION FOCUS

Assessment/Reassessment

- Current elimination pattern, assessment findings, and effect on lifestyle and sleep.

Planning

- Plan of care and who is involved in planning.
- Teaching plan.

Implementation/Evaluation

- Response to interventions, teaching, and actions performed.
- Attainment or progress toward desired outcome(s).
- Modifications to plan of care.

Discharge Planning

- Long-term needs and who is responsible for actions to be taken.
- Specific referrals made.

References

1. Merkelj, I. (2001). Urinary incontinence in the elderly. *South Med J*, 94(10), 952–957.
2. National Association for Continence (NAFC). (No date). Continence management (Various pages). Retrieved October 2015 from http://www.nafc.org/management.
3. Gray, M. (2005). Overactive bladder: An overview. *J Wound Ostomy Continence Nurs*, 32(3 suppl), 1–5.
4. Goode, P. S., Burgio, K. L. (2001). Managing incontinence in the geriatric patient. In Kursh, E. D., et al. (eds). *Office Urology: The Clinician's Guide*. Totawa, NJ: Humana Press.
5. Ratini, M. (Updated 2014). Overflow incontinence. Retrieved March 2015 from http://www.webmd.com/urinary-incontinence-oab/overflow-incontinence.
6. Lazarou, G. (Updated 2014). Bladder control problems. Retrieved March 2015 from http://www.emedicinehealth.com/bladder_control_problems/article_em.htm.
7. Terpenning, M. S., Allada, R., Kauffman, C. A. (1989). Intermittent urethral catheterization in the elderly: (Evidence Level IV: Nonexperimental study). *J Am Geriatr Soc*, 37(5), 411–416.
8. Dowling-Castronovo, A., Bradway, C. (2012). Urinary incontinence (UI) in older adults admitted to acute care. In Capezuti, E., et al. (eds). *Evidence-Based Geriatric Nursing Protocols for Best Practice*. 4th ed. New York, NY: Springer.
9. Simon, H., Zieve, D. (reviewers) (update 2012). Urinary incontinence (section on overflow incontinence). Retrieved October 2015 from https://umm.edu/health/medical/reports/articles/urinary-incontinence.

reflex urinary Incontinence

Taxonomy II: Elimination and Exchange—Class 1 Urinary Function (00018) [**Diagnostic Division:** Elimination], Submitted 1986; Revised 1998

DEFINITION: Involuntary loss of urine at somewhat predictable intervals when a specific bladder volume is reached.

RELATED FACTORS

Tissue damage [e.g., due to radiation cystitis, radical pelvic surgery]
Neurological impairment above level of sacral or pontine micturition center

DEFINING CHARACTERISTICS

Subjective

Absence of sensation of bladder fullness, urge to void, or of voiding sensation
Sensation of urgency to void without voluntary inhibition of bladder contraction
Sensation of bladder fullness

Objective

Predictable pattern of voiding
Inability to voluntarily inhibit or initiate voiding
Incomplete emptying of bladder with [brain] lesion above pontine micturition center
Sample Clinical Applications: Spinal cord injury (SCI), multiple sclerosis (MS), bladder or pelvic cancer, Parkinson's disease, dementia

DESIRED OUTCOMES/EVALUATION CRITERIA

Sample NOC linkages:

Urinary Continence: Control of the elimination of urine from the bladder
Neurological Status: Autonomic: Ability of the autonomic nervous system to coordinate visceral and hemostatic function
Urinary Elimination: Collection and discharge of urine

Client Will (Include Specific Time Frame)

- Verbalize understanding of condition or contributing factors.
- Establish bladder regimen appropriate for individual situation.
- Demonstrate behaviors or techniques to manage condition and prevent complications.
- Void at acceptable times and places.

ACTIONS/INTERVENTIONS

Sample NIC linkages:

Urinary Incontinence Care: Assistance in promoting continence and maintaining perineal skin integrity
Urinary Catheterization: Intermittent: Regular periodic use of a catheter to empty the bladder

NURSING PRIORITY NO. 1 To assess degree of interference/disability:

- Identify pathology of problem (e.g., pelvic cancer, central nervous system disorder, SCI, stroke, Parkinson's disease, diabetes with bladder neuropathy, brain tumor) *that results in either hypotonic or spastic neuro-*

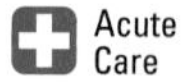

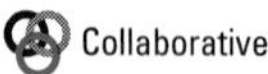

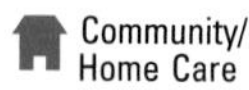

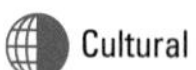

genic bladder, thereby affecting bladder storage, emptying, and control. Note: The causes of reflex incontinence are often mixed (e.g., most people with reflex incontinence experience symptoms of urinary frequency, urgency, and nocturia). In this situation, the bladder empties urine as it fills.[3–5,7,8]

- Ascertain whether client experiences any sense of bladder fullness or awareness of incontinence. *Individuals with reflex incontinence have little, if any, awareness of need to void. Loss of sensation of bladder filling can result in overfilling, inadequate emptying (retention), and/or constant dribbling.*[5,8] (Refer to NDs [acute/chronic] Urinary Retention and overflow urinary Incontinence for additional interventions.)
- Review voiding diary, if available, or record frequency and time of urination. Compare timing of voidings, particularly in relation to certain factors (e.g., liquid intake and medications). *Aids in targeting interventions to meet individual situation.*[1]
- Measure amount of each voiding during assessment phase. *Incontinence often occurs once a specific bladder volume is reached and may indicate need for insertion of a permanent or intermittent catheter.*[2,8]
- Determine postvoid residual volume (via bladder scan) in client with incomplete emptying or on scheduled catheterization *to evaluate for urinary retention when attempting toilet training, to establish schedule for intermittent catheterization, and to avoid unnecessary catheterization.*[6] *Note: Often the bladder is not completely emptied because there is no voluntary control of the bladder.*[8]
- Refer to urologist or appropriate specialist for testing. *Urinalysis, ultrasound, radiographs, and urine flowmetry are standard to measure urine flow. A urodynamic evaluation measuring bladder capacity, pressure, and rate of urinary flow may also be indicated.*

NURSING PRIORITY NO. 2 To assist in managing incontinence:

- Evaluate client's ability to manipulate or use urinary collection device or catheter. *Type and degree of neurological impairment (i.e., SCI, MS, dementia) may interfere with client's ability to be self-sufficient.*[7]
- Collaborate in treatment of underlying cause or management of incontinence. *Of all the types of urinary incontinence, reflex incontinence is probably the most difficult to treat; however, this condition may be treated with medications, neuromodulation (electrical stimulation of specific nerves to influence the nerve circuit that controls urination), botulinum-A toxin (BTA) injection, bladder surgery, or indwelling bladder catheters. Note: A European study has shown promising results of BTA injections into the detrusor muscle to treat neurogenic incontinence due to detrusor overactivity.*[8,9] *Pentosan polysulfate sodium (Elmiron) has been approved by the FDA for moderate or better improvement in overall symptoms in interstitial cystitis (IC), and low-dose amitriptyline (Elavil) may increase bladder capacity through beta-adrenergic receptors on the bladder.*[10]
- Involve client/significant other/caregiver in creating plan of care *to develop mutually agreed-upon goals and ensure individual needs are met, enhancing commitment to plan.*[1–8]
- Encourage minimum of 1,500 to 2,000 mL of fluid intake daily. *Reduces risk of bladder and kidney infection/stone formation and may reduce symptoms of IC when caused by concentrated urine.*[10]
- Remind or assist client to go to toilet before the expected time of incontinence *in an attempt to stimulate the reflexes for voiding.*[1]
- Engage in bladder retraining program as appropriate. *Suppression of urgency and progressive small increases in intervals between voiding may help reduce urinary frequency in clients with IC.*[10]
- Set alarm to awaken during night, if necessary, to maintain catheterization schedule or use external catheter or collection device, as appropriate. *Developing a regular time to empty the bladder may prevent urinary retention or overflow incontinence during the night.*
- Implement continuous or intermittent catheterization schedule, if condition indicates, *to prevent bladder overdistention and detrusor muscle damage. Note: Experience has shown that intermittent catheterization is preferable to indwelling catheters in young persons (both male and female) with SCI. It is also a valuable alternative for individuals with chronic urinary retention due to an obstructed, weak, or nonfunctioning bladder.*[1,4,7]

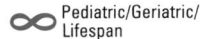

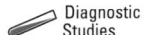

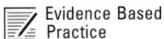

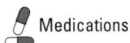

NURSING PRIORITY NO. 3 To promote wellness (Teaching/Discharge Considerations):

- Encourage continuation of regularly timed bladder program. *May be able to establish a schedule that takes advantage of whatever ability remains, even though the neurological impairment is affecting bladder sensation.*
- Suggest use of incontinence pads/pants during day and with social contact, if appropriate. *Depending on client's activity level, amount of urine loss, manual dexterity, and cognitive ability, these devices provide security and comfort and protect the skin and clothing from urine leakage, reduce odor, and are generally unnoticeable under clothing.*[7,8]
- Emphasize importance of perineal care following voiding and frequent changing of incontinence pads, if used. *Maintains cleanliness and prevents skin irritation or breakdown and odor.*[7,8]
- Encourage limited intake of coffee, tea, and alcohol, as well as avoidance of citrus foods, artificial sweeteners, tomatoes, and spicy foods. *Diuretic effect of these beverages may affect predictability of voiding pattern and the substances may cause flare-ups/exacerbate symptoms of IC.*[10]
- Instruct in proper care of catheter and cleaning techniques when used. *Reduces risk of infection.*[7,8]
- Review signs/symptoms of urinary complications and need for medical follow-up. *Provides immediate attention preventing exacerbation of problem or extension of infection into kidneys.*

DOCUMENTATION FOCUS

Assessment/Reassessment
- Findings including degree of disability and effect on lifestyle.
- Availability of resources or support person.

Planning
- Plan of care and who is involved in planning.
- Teaching plan.

Implementation/Evaluation
- Responses to treatment plan, interventions, and actions performed.
- Attainment or progress toward desired outcome(s).
- Modifications to plan of care.

Discharge Planning
- Long-term needs and who is responsible for actions to be taken.
- Available resources, equipment needs and sources.

References

1. The state of the science on urinary incontinence. (2003). In Newman, D. K., Palmer, M. H. (eds). *Am J Nurs*, 103(suppl), 20.
2. Newfield, S. A., Hinz, M. D., Tilley, D. S., et al. (2007). *Cox's Clinical Applications of Nursing Diagnosis: Adult, Child, Women's, Psychiatric, Gerontic, and Home Health Considerations.* 5th ed. Philadelphia: F. A. Davis.
3. Beers, M. H., Berkow, R. (eds). (1999). *The Merck Manual of Diagnosis and Therapy.* 17th ed. Whitehouse Station, NJ: Merck Research Laboratories.
4. Gray, M. (2005). Assessment and management of urinary incontinence. *Nurse Pract*, 30(7), 32–43.
5. Vasavada, S. P., Carmel, M. E., Rackley, R. (Updated 2014). Urinary incontinence. Retrieved March 2015 from http://emedicine.medscape.com/article/452289-overview.
6. Newman, D. K. (2009). Using the BladderScan™ for bladder volume assessment. Retrieved March 2015 from http://www.seekwellness.com/incontinence/using_the_bladderscan.htm.
7. No author listed. (Updated 2014). Living with spinal cord injury-bladder care. Retrieved March 2015 from http://www.webmd.com/brain/tc/living-with-a-spinal-cord-injury-bladder-care.

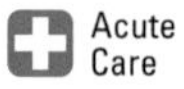

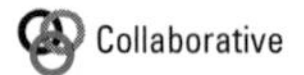

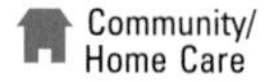

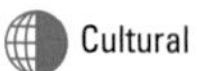

8. Stoppler, M. C. (Updated 2014). Urinary incontinence. Retrieved March 2015 from http://www.emedicinehealth.com/incontinence/article_em.htm.
9. Reitz, A., Stöhrer, M., Kramer, G., et al. (2004). European experience of 200 cases treated with botulinum-A toxin injections into the detrusor muscle for urinary incontinence due to neurogenic detrusor overactivity. *European Urol*, 45(4), 510–515.
10. Butrick, C. W., Howard, F. M., Sand, P. K. (2010). Diagnosis and management of interstitial cystitis/painful bladder syndrome. *J Womens Health*, 19(6), 1185–1193.

stress urinary Incontinence

Taxonomy II: Elimination and Exchange—Class 1 Urinary Function (00017) [**Diagnostic Division:** Elimination], Submitted 1986; Revised 2006

DEFINITION: Sudden leakage of urine with activities that increase intra-abdominal pressure.

RELATED FACTORS

Degenerative changes in pelvic muscles; weak pelvic muscles
Increase in intra-abdominal pressure [e.g., obesity, gravid uterus]
Intrinsic urethral sphincter deficiency

DEFINING CHARACTERISTICS

Subjective

Involuntary leakage of small volume of urine (e.g., with sneezing, laughing, coughing, on exertion)

Objective

Involuntary leakage of small volume of urine in the absence of detrusor contraction or an overdistended bladder

DESIRED OUTCOMES/EVALUATION CRITERIA

Sample NOC linkages:

Urinary Continence: Control of elimination of urine from the bladder
Symptom Control: Personal actions to minimize perceived adverse changes in physical and emotional functioning

Client Will (Include Specific Time Frame)

- Verbalize understanding of condition and interventions for bladder conditioning.
- Demonstrate behaviors or techniques to strengthen pelvic floor musculature.
- Remain continent even with increased intra-abdominal pressure.

ACTIONS/INTERVENTIONS

Sample NIC linkages:

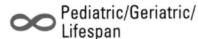

Pelvic Muscle Exercise: Strengthening and training the levator ani and urogenital muscles through voluntary, repetitive contraction to decrease stress, urge, or mixed types of urinary incontinence
Urinary Incontinence Care: Assistance in promoting continence and maintaining perineal skin integrity
Urinary Habit Training: Establishing a predictable pattern of bladder emptying to prevent incontinence for persons with limited cognitive ability who have urge, stress, or functional incontinence

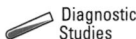

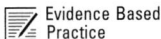

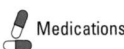

NURSING PRIORITY NO. 1 To assess causative/contributing factors:

- Identify physiological causes of increased intra-abdominal pressure (e.g., obesity, gravid uterus; repeated heavy lifting [occupational risk]), contributing history (e.g., multiple births, bladder or pelvic trauma/fractures), surgery (e.g., radical prostatectomy, bladder or other pelvic surgeries that may damage sphincter muscles), and participation in high-impact athletic or military field activities (particularly women). *Identification of specifics of individual situation provides for developing an accurate plan of care.*[2,6,7]
- Assess for urine loss (usually in small amounts) with coughing, sneezing, or sports activities; relaxed pelvic musculature and support, noting inability to start and stop stream while voiding; and bulging of perineum when bearing down. *Severity of symptoms may indicate need for more specialized evaluation.*
- Note client's sex and age. *Note: The majority of clients with stress urinary incontinence are women, although men who undergo surgical prostatectomy may also experience it. Although pregnancy and childbirth are known to cause stress incontinence in younger women, it is also common in older women, possibly related to loss of estrogen and weakened muscles in the pelvic organs.*[11]
- Review client's medications (e.g., alpha-blockers, angiotensin-converting enzyme inhibitors, loop diuretics) *for those that may cause or exacerbate stress incontinence. Note: The urge incontinence effect with these agents is usually transient.*[1,7]
- Assess for mixed incontinence (consisting of two or more kinds of incontinence), noting whether bladder irritability, reduced bladder capacity, or voluntary overdistention is present. *The most common combinations are urge with stress incontinence and urge or stress with functional incontinence. These impact treatment choices.*[1,11] (Refer to NDs urge and reflex urinary Incontinence; [acute/chronic] Urinary Retention.)

NURSING PRIORITY NO. 2 To assess degree of interference/disability:

- Observe voiding patterns, time and amount voided, and note the stimulus provoking incontinence. Review voiding diary if available. *Provides information that can help determine type of incontinence and type of treatment indicated.*
- Prepare for and assist with testing or refer to urology specialist as indicated. *Diagnosing urinary incontinence often requires comprehensive evaluation (e.g., measuring bladder filling and capacity, leak-point pressure, rate of urinary flow, pelvic ultrasound, cystogram/other scans) to differentiate stress incontinence from other types.*[1–12]
- Determine effect on lifestyle (including daily activities, participation in sports or exercise and recreation, socialization, sexuality) and self-esteem. *Untreated incontinence can have emotional and physical consequences. Client may limit or abstain from sports or recreational activities. Urinary tract infections, skin rashes, and sores can occur. Self-esteem is affected, and the client may suffer from depression and withdraw from social functions.*[6]
- Ascertain methods of self-management. *Client may already be limiting liquid intake, voiding before any activity, or using undergarment protection.*
- Perform bladder scan to determine postvoid residuals as indicated. *Presence of volumes greater than 200 mL (or 150 mL in elder clients) suggests incomplete emptying of bladder, requiring further evaluation.*[8]

NURSING PRIORITY NO. 3 To assist in treating/preventing incontinence:

- Implement nonsurgical treatment techniques:
  Keep a voiding diary, as indicated. *The use of a frequency/volume chart is helpful in bladder training. A review of urine output in relation to fluid intake record can reveal need to modify fluid intake in client who is resistant to fluid management efforts. The contribution of dietary items that may precipitate incontinence may become obvious after reviewing the voiding log.*[12]
  Practice timed voidings (e.g., 3-hr intervals during the day) *to keep bladder relatively empty.*
  Extend time between voidings to 3- to 4-hr intervals. *May improve bladder capacity and retention time.*[12]
  Limit use of coffee, tea, and alcohol. *Diuretic effect of these substances may lead to bladder distention, increasing likelihood of incontinence.*[4]

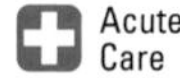
Acute Care
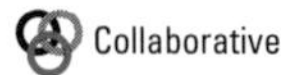
Collaborative
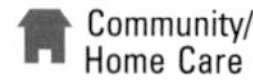
Community/ Home Care
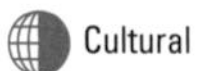
Cultural

Encourage weight loss as indicated *to reduce pressure on intra-abdominal and pelvic organs.*[1]
Void before physical exertion such as exercise or sports activities *to reduce potential for incontinence.*[9]
Encourage regular pelvic floor strengthening exercises (Kegel exercises). *These exercises involve tightening the muscles of the pelvic floor and need to be done numerous times throughout the day.*[2]
Avoid or limit heavy lifting and high-impact aerobics or sports *to decrease incontinence associated with elevated intra-abdominal pressures.*[4]
Incorporate "bent-knee sit-ups" into exercise program. *Increasing abdominal muscle tone can help relieve stress incontinence.*[3]

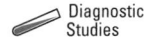

- Assist with medical treatment of underlying urological condition, as indicated. *Stress incontinence may be treated with surgical intervention (e.g., bladder neck suspension, pubovaginal sling to reposition bladder and strengthen pelvic musculature; prostate surgery) and nonsurgical therapies (e.g., behavioral modification, pelvic muscle exercises, medications, use of pessary, vaginal cones; electrical stimulation; biofeedback).*[7,9,11]
- Administer medications, as indicated, such as midodrine (ProAmatine), oxybutynin (Ditropan), tolterodine (Detrol), or solifenacin (Vesicare). *May improve bladder tone and capacity and increase effectiveness of bladder sphincter and proximal urethra contractions.*[1,5,11]

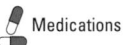

NURSING PRIORITY NO. 4 To promote wellness (Teaching/Discharge Considerations):

- Suggest use of incontinence pads or pants as needed. *Considering client's activity level, amount of urine loss, physical size, manual dexterity, and cognitive ability to determine specific product choices best suited to individual situation and needs may be necessary when leakage continues to occur in spite of other measures.*
- Emphasize importance of perineal care following voiding and frequent changing of incontinence pads. Recommend application of oil-based emollient. *Prevents infection and protects skin from irritation.*
- Discuss participation in incontinence management for activities such as heavy lifting and strenuous sports activities that increase intra-abdominal pressure. *Substituting swimming or other low-impact exercises may help reduce frequency of incontinence and maintain active life.*
- Recommend or refer for behavioral training, as indicated. *Research indicates that combining pelvic floor muscle exercises with biofeedback is more effective than simple verbal or written instructions.*[10]

DOCUMENTATION FOCUS

Assessment/Reassessment
- Findings including pattern of incontinence and physical factors present.
- Effect on lifestyle and self-esteem.
- Client understanding of condition.

Planning
- Plan of care and who is involved in the planning.
- Teaching plan.

Implementation/Evaluation
- Responses to interventions, teaching, actions performed, and changes that are identified.
- Attainment or progress toward desired outcome(s).
- Modifications to plan of care.

Discharge Planning
- Long-term needs, referrals, and who is responsible for specific actions.
- Specific referrals made.

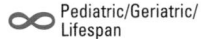

References

1. Shenot, P. J. (Updated 2014). Urinary incontinence in adults. *The Merck Manual for Health Care Professionals*. Retrieved March 2015 from http://www.merckmanuals.com/professional/genitourinary_disorders/voiding_disorders/urinary_incontinence.html.
2. Wyman, J. F. (2003). Treatment of urinary incontinence in men and older women: The evidence shows the efficacy of a variety of techniques. *Am J Nurs*, 103(suppl), 26–35.
3. Newfield, S. A., Hinz, M. D., Tilley, D. S., et al. (2007). ND: Urinary Incontinence, stress. *Cox's Clinical Applications of Nursing Diagnosis: Adult, Child, Women's, Psychiatric, Gerontic, and Home Health Considerations*. 5th ed. Philadelphia: F. A. Davis.
4. The state of the science on urinary incontinence. (2003). In Newman, D. K., Palmer, M. H. (eds). *Am J Nurs*, 3(suppl), 2–53.
5. Booth, C. (2002). Introduction to urinary incontinence. *Hosp Pharmacist*, 9(3), 65–68.
6. Carls, C. (2007). The prevalence of stress urinary incontinence in high school and college-age female athletes in the Midwest: Implications for education and prevention. *Urol Nurs*, 27(1), 21–24.
7. Vasavada, S. P., Carmel, M. E., Rackley, R. (Updated 2014). Urinary incontinence. Retrieved March 2015 from http://emedicine.medscape.com/article/452289-overview.
8. Newman, D. K. (2009). Using the BladderScan™ for bladder volume assessment. Retrieved March 2015 from http://www.seekwellness.com/incontinence/using_the_bladderscan.htm.
9. Bray, B., Van Sell, S. L., Miller-Anderson, M. (2007). Stress incontinence: It's no laughing matter. *RN*, 70(4), 25–29.
10. Bump, R. C., Hurt, W. G., Fantl, J. A. (1991). Assessment of Kegel pelvic muscle exercise performance after brief verbal instruction. *Am J Obstet Gynecol*, 165(2), 322–327.
11. National Association for Continence. (2010). Continence management (various pages). Retrieved March 2015 from http://www.nafc.org/urinary-incontinence.
12. Rovner, E. S., Wein, A. J. (2004). Treatment options for stress urinary incontinence. *Rev Urol*, 6(Suppl 3), S29–S47.

urge urinary Incontinence

Taxonomy II: Elimination and Exchange—Class 1 Urinary Function (00019) [**Diagnostic Division:** Elimination], Submitted 1986; Revised 2006

DEFINITION: Involuntary passage of urine occurring soon after a strong sense of urgency to void.

RELATED FACTORS

Decrease in bladder capacity
Bladder infection; atrophic urethritis or vaginitis
Alcohol consumption; caffeine intake; [increased fluid intake]
Treatment regimen [e.g., diuretic use]
Fecal impaction
Detrusor hyperactivity with impaired bladder contractility

DEFINING CHARACTERISTICS

Subjective

Urinary urgency; involuntary loss of urine with bladder contractions or spasms
Inability to reach toilet in time to avoid urine loss

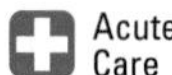
Acute Care
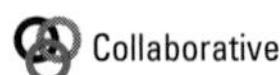
Collaborative
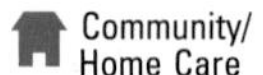
Community/ Home Care
 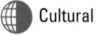
Cultural

Sample Clinical Applications: Abdominal trauma/surgery, pelvic inflammatory disease (PID), recurrent urinary tract infections (UTIs), brain injury, stroke, multiple sclerosis (MS), Parkinson's disease, diabetes mellitus, dementia

DESIRED OUTCOMES/EVALUATION CRITERIA

Sample NOC linkages:
Urinary Continence: Control of elimination of urine from the bladder
Cognition: Ability to execute complex mental processes
Self-Care: Toileting: Ability to toilet self independently with or without assistive device

Client Will (Include Specific Time Frame)

- Verbalize understanding of condition.
- Demonstrate behaviors or techniques to control or correct situation.
- Report increase in interval between urge and involuntary loss of urine.
- Void every 3 to 4 hrs in individually appropriate amounts.

ACTIONS/INTERVENTIONS

Sample NIC linkages:
Urinary Bladder Training: Improving bladder function for those with urge incontinence by increasing the bladder's ability to hold urine and the patient's ability to suppress urination
Urinary Habit Training: Establishing a predictable pattern of bladder emptying to prevent incontinence for persons with limited cognitive ability who have urge, stress, or functional incontinence
Urinary Incontinence Care: Assistance in promoting continence and maintaining perineal skin integrity

NURSING PRIORITY NO. 1 To assess causative/contributing factors:

- Note presence of conditions often associated with urgent voiding (e.g., UTI; pregnancy; pelvic or gynecological surgery; prostatitis, or prostate surgery; obesity; bladder tumors or stones; nerve damage from conditions such as diabetes, stroke, Parkinson's, MS; certain cancers, including the bladder and prostate; recent or lengthy use of indwelling urinary catheter) *affecting bladder capacity, pelvic musculature tone, or innervation.*[7,8,13]
- Ask client about urgency (more than just normal desire to void). *Urgency (also called overactive bladder) is a sudden, compelling need to void that is difficult to defer, can occur frequently (e.g., eight or more times in 24 hr), and may be accompanied by leaking or urge incontinence.*[6–8,13]
- Note factors that may affect ability to respond to urge to void in timely manner. *Impaired mobility, use of sedation, or cognitive impairments may result in client failing to recognize need to void or moving too slowly to make it to the bathroom, with subsequent loss of urine.*
- Determine use or presence of bladder irritants. *A significant intake of alcohol, caffeine, acidic or spicy food and fluids can result in increased output or urge symptoms and can contribute to the possibility of incontinence.*[5]
- Review client's medications for affect on bladder function, such as beta-blockers and cholinergic drugs *(can increase detrusor tone)*; neuroleptics, antidepressants, sedatives, and opiates *(can cause detrusor relaxation)*; muscle relaxants and psychoactive drugs *(can cause sphincter relaxation)*; and diuretics *(can increase urine production).*[15]
- Assess for cloudy, odorous urine associated with acute, painful urgency symptoms. *Incontinence often reflects presence of infection.*[1]
- Test urine for glucose. *Presence of glucose in urine causes polyuria, resulting in overdistention of the bladder and inability to hold urine until reaching the bathroom.*[2]

- Assist with appropriate diagnostic testing (e.g., pre/postvoid bladder scanning; pelvic examination *for strictures, impaired perineal sensation or musculature*; urinalysis, uroflowmetry voiding pressures; cystoscopy, cystometrogram) *to determine anatomic and functional status of bladder and urethra.*[2,3,8]
- Assess for concomitant stress or functional incontinence. *Older women often have a mix of stress and urge incontinence, whereas individuals with dementia or disabling neurological disorders tend to have urge and functional incontinence.* (Refer to NDs stress/functional urinary Incontinence for additional interventions.)

NURSING PRIORITY NO. 2 To assess degree of interference/disability:

- Measure amount of urine voided, especially noting amounts less than 100 mL or greater than 550 mL. *Bladder capacity may be impaired, or bladder contractions facilitating emptying may be ineffective.* (Refer to ND [acute/chronic] Urinary Retention.)
- Record frequency of voiding during a typical day and typical night. *Maintaining a voiding diary identifies degree of difficulty being experienced by client.*[2,4]
- Note length of warning time between initial urge and loss of urine. *Overactivity or irritability shortens the length of time between urge and urine loss and helps clarify the type of incontinence.*
- Ascertain if client experiences triggers (e.g., sound of running water, putting hands in water, seeing a restroom sign, "key-in-the lock" syndrome).[8]
- Ascertain effect on lifestyle including daily activities, sleep, socialization, sexuality, and self-esteem. *There is a considerable impact on the quality of life of individuals with an incontinence problem, affecting socialization and view of themselves as sexual beings and sense of self-esteem.*[2]

NURSING PRIORITY NO. 3 To assist in treating/preventing incontinence:

- Implement continence management interventions:
  - Establish voiding schedule (habit and bladder training) based on client's usual voiding pattern. *Bladder retraining program is often successful in the control of urge incontinence. Note: One review of multiple studies revealed a strongly positive effect on continence using a combination of behavioral interventions (including pelvic muscle exercises) and medications in older women. However, it appears that clients have difficulty sustaining the effort of behavioral modification, and thus the positive effect is lost.*[1,4,9,14]
  - Recommend consciously delaying voiding by using distraction (e.g., slow, deep breathing), self-statements (e.g., "I can wait"), and contracting pelvic muscles when exposed to triggers. *Behavioral techniques for urge suppression.*[2,9]
  - Combine pelvic floor strengthening exercise with biofeedback, as appropriate. *Enhances effectiveness of training and success at controlling incontinence.*[4,9]
  - Instruct client to tighten pelvic floor muscles before arising from bed. *Helps prevent loss of urine as abdominal pressure changes.*[4,13]
  - Set alarm to awaken during night, if indicated. *May be useful in maintaining continence during training schedule.*[4]
  - Manage fluid intake (e.g., increase fluid intake to 1,500 to 2,000 mL/d or as indicated) *to prevent dehydration and promote good urine flow*[4] *(e.g., reduce fluid intake if indicated). Note: Too much water can also increase bladder irritation, so amount of intake needs to be determined by individual response.*[12]
  - Regulate liquid intake at prescheduled times, and limit fluids 2 to 3 hr prior to bedtime. *Promotes a predictable voiding pattern and can help limit nocturia.*
  - Modify diet, as indicated (e.g., reduce acidic/citrus juices, chocolate and caffeine-containing drinks, carbonated beverages, spicy foods, artificial sweeteners), *to reduce bladder irritants.*[12]
  - Suggest limiting intake of coffee, tea, and alcohol *to reduce diuretic effect, urge symptoms, and nighttime incontinence.*[12]
  - Manage bowel elimination *to prevent continence problems associated with constipation or fecal impaction.*
- Offer assistance to cognitively impaired client (e.g., prompt client or take to bathroom on regularly timed schedule) *to reduce frequency of incontinence episodes and promote comfort.*

Acute Care 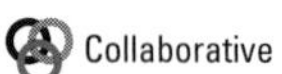

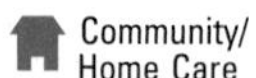

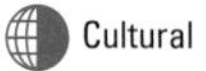

- Provide assistance or devices, as indicated, for clients who are mobility impaired. *Providing means of summoning assistance, and placing bedside commode, urinal, or bedpan within reach helps to avoid unintended loss of urine and promotes sense of control over situation.*[4]
- Collaborate in treating underlying cause. *Urgency symptoms may resolve with treatment of medical problem (e.g., infection; recovery from surgery, childbirth, or pelvic trauma) or may be resistant to resolution (e.g., incontinence associated with neurogenic bladder).*
- Refer to specialist or treatment program, as indicated, for additional or specialized interventions (e.g., biofeedback, use of vaginal cones, electronic stimulation therapy). *Significant reduction in incontinence episodes is reported with use of combined therapies (e.g., electronic stimulation therapy plus pelvic muscle exercises).*[12–14]
- Administer medications (e.g., antibiotics, antimuscarinics [oxybutynin (Ditropan), tolterodine (Detrol), solifenacin (VESIcare)]) *to reduce incidence of UTIs and reduce voiding frequency and urgency by blocking overactive detrusor contractions.*[6,10,13]
- Discuss possible surgical interventions. *Urinary incontinence surgery includes a variety of procedures, from minimally invasive injections of bulking agents to major surgical interventions to change position of or enlarge the bladder, add support to weakened pelvic muscles, replace the urinary sphincter, or implant a sacral nerve stimulator that acts as a bladder pacemaker.*[2,11,13]

NURSING PRIORITY NO. 4 To promote wellness (Teaching/Discharge Considerations):

- Encourage comfort measures (e.g., use of incontinence pads or adult briefs, wearing loose-fitting or especially adapted clothing) *to prepare for or manage urge incontinence symptoms over the long term as well as to enhance sense of security and confidence in abilities to be socially active.*[5]
- Emphasize importance of perineal care after each voiding. *Prevents skin irritation and reduces potential for bladder infection and incontinence-related dermatitis.*[5]
- Identify signs/symptoms indicating urinary complications and need for medical follow-up care. *Helps client be aware of and seek intervention in a timely manner to prevent more serious problems from developing.*[4]

DOCUMENTATION FOCUS

Assessment/Reassessment

- Individual findings, including pattern of incontinence, effect on lifestyle and self-esteem.

Planning

- Plan of care, specific interventions, and who is involved in planning.
- Teaching plan.

Implementation/Evaluation

- Response to interventions, teaching, and actions performed.
- Attainment or progress toward desired outcome(s).
- Modifications to plan of care.

Discharge Planning

- Discharge needs and who is responsible for actions to be taken.
- Specific referrals made.

References

1. Wyman, J. F. (2003). Treatment of urinary incontinence in men and older women: The evidence shows the efficacy of a variety of techniques. *Am J Nurs*, 103(suppl), 26–35.
2. Booth, C. (2002). Introduction to urinary incontinence. *Hosp Pharmacist*, 9(3), 65–68.
3. Beers, M. H., Berkow, R. (eds). (1999). *The Merck Manual of Diagnosis and Therapy*. 17th ed. Whitehouse Station, NJ: Merck Research Laboratories.
4. The state of the science on urinary incontinence. (2003). In Newman, D. K., Palmer, M. H. (eds). *Am J Nurs*, 103(3 Suppl), 2–53.
5. Newfield, S. A., Hinz, M. D., Tilley, D. S., et al. (2007). ND: Urinary incontinence. *Cox's Clinical Applications of Nursing Diagnosis: Adult, Child, Women's, Psychiatric, Gerontic, and Home Health Considerations*. 5th ed. Philadelphia: F. A. Davis.
6. Gray, M. (2005). Assessment and management of urinary incontinence. *Nurse Pract*, 30(7), 32–43.
7. Gray, M. (2005). Overactive bladder: An overview. *J Wound Ostomy Continence Nurs*, 32(3 suppl), 1–5.
8. Newman, D. K. (2005). Assessment of the patient with an overactive bladder. *J Wound Ostomy Continence Nurs*, 32(3 suppl), 5–10.
9. Wyman, J. F. (2005). Behavioral interventions for the patient with overactive bladder. *J Wound Ostomy Continence Nurs*, 32(3 suppl), 11–15.
10. Mauk, K. L. (2005). Pharmacology update: Medications for bladder management. *ARN Network*, 21(3), 3–10.
11. Foundation for Medical Education and Research. (2011). Urinary incontinence surgery: When other treatments aren't enough. Retrieved March 2015 from http://www.riversideonline.com/health_reference/Womens-Health/WO00126.cfm.
12. Stoppler, M. C. (Updated 2014). Urinary incontinence. Retrieved March 2015 from http://www.emedicinehealth.com/incontinence/article_em.htm.
13. Karriem-Norwood, V. (reviewer) (Updated 2014). Urge Incontinence. Retrieved March 2015 from http://www.webmd.com/urinary-incontinence-oab/america-asks-11/urge?page=1.
14. Burgio, K. L., Locher, J. L., Goode, P. S. (2000). Combined behavioral and drug therapy for urge incontinence in older women. *Obstetrical & Gynecological Survey*, 55(8), 485–486.
15. Porter Health Care System: Health Education. (2014). Urinary incontinence. Retrieved March 2015 from http://www.porterhealth.com/health-education/85,P01528.

risk for urge urinary Incontinence

Taxonomy II: Elimination and Exchange—Class 1 Urinary Function (00022) [**Diagnostic Division:** Elimination], Submitted 1998; Revised 2008, 2013

DEFINITION: Vulnerable to involuntary passage of urine occurring soon after a strong sensation of urgency to void, which may compromise health.

RISK FACTORS

Alcohol consumption
Atrophic urethritis or vaginitis
Detrusor hyperactivity with impaired bladder contractility
Impaired bladder contractility; involuntary sphincter relaxation
Ineffective toileting habits
Small bladder capacity; fecal impaction
Treatment regimen

Note: A risk diagnosis is not evidenced by signs and symptoms, as the problem has not occurred; rather, nursing interventions are directed at prevention.

Sample Clinical Applications: Multiple sclerosis (MS), benign prostatic hypertrophy (BPH), recurrent urinary tract infections (UTIs), renal calculi, pelvic surgery or radiation, Guillain-Barré syndrome, dementia, major depression

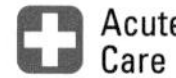

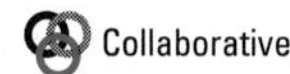

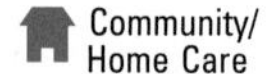

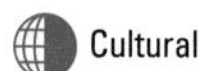

DESIRED OUTCOMES/EVALUATION CRITERIA

Sample NOC linkages:

Urinary Continence: Control of elimination of urine from the bladder

Risk Control: Personal actions to prevent, eliminate, or reduce modifiable health threats

Client Will (Include Specific Time Frame)

- Identify individual risk factors and appropriate interventions.
- Demonstrate behaviors or lifestyle changes to prevent development of problem.

ACTIONS/INTERVENTIONS

Sample NIC linkages:

Urinary Bladder Training: Improving bladder function for those with urge incontinence by increasing the bladder's ability to hold urine and the patient's ability to suppress urination

Urinary Habit Training: Establishing a predictable pattern of bladder emptying to prevent incontinence for persons with limited cognitive ability who have urge, stress, or functional incontinence

Self-Care Assistance: Toileting: Assisting another with elimination

NURSING PRIORITY NO. 1 To assess potential for developing incontinence:

- Note presence of diagnoses often associated with urgent voiding (e.g., UTI; pregnancy; pelvic or gynecological surgery; prostatitis, or prostate surgery; obesity; bladder tumors or stones; nerve damage from conditions such as diabetes, stroke, Parkinson's, MS; certain cancers, including the bladder and prostate; recent or lengthy use of indwelling urinary catheter). *Such conditions can affect bladder capacity; pelvic, bladder, or urethral musculature tone; and/or innervation.*[1–3,10]
- Ask client about urgency (more than just normal desire to void). *Urgency (also called overactive bladder [OAB]) is a sudden, compelling need to void that is difficult to defer, can occur frequently (e.g., eight or more times in 24 hr), and may be accompanied by leaking or urge incontinence.*[11–14]
- Note factors that may affect ability to respond to urge to void in a timely manner. *Impaired mobility, use of sedation, or cognitive impairments may result in client failing to recognize need to void or moving too slowly to make it to the bathroom, with subsequent loss of urine.*[2,10]
- Determine use or presence of bladder irritants. *A significant intake of alcohol, caffeine, acidic or spicy food and fluids can result in increased output or urge symptoms and contribute to the possibility of incontinence.*[5]
- Review client's medications for affect on bladder function, such as beta-blockers and cholinergic drugs *(can increase detrusor tone)*; neuroleptics, antidepressants, sedatives, and opiates *(can cause detrusor relaxation)*; muscle relaxants and psychoactive drugs *(can cause sphincter relaxation)*; and diuretics *(can increase urine production)*.[7,8]
- Measure amount of urine voided, especially noting amounts less than 100 mL or greater than 550 mL, *to determine bladder capacity and effectiveness of bladder contractions to facilitate emptying.*[6]
- Prepare for and assist with appropriate testing (e.g., urinalysis, noninvasive bladder scanning, urine culture, urine and serum glucose, voiding cystometrogram). *Accurate assessment and diagnosis can determine voiding pattern and identify pathology that may lead to the development of incontinence.*[2,4,8]

NURSING PRIORITY NO. 2 To prevent occurrence of problem:

- Assist in treatment of underlying conditions that may contribute to urge incontinence. *Urgency symptoms may resolve with treatment of medical problem (e.g., UTI; recovery from pelvic surgery, childbirth, or pelvic trauma; use of estrogen-based oral or topical products for atrophic vaginitis; etc.).*
- Record intake along with frequency and degree of urgency of voiding. *May reveal developing incontinence problem when need to void is more frequent and urgent relative to normal fluid intake.*

- Ascertain client's awareness and concerns about developing problem and whether lifestyle is affected (e.g., daily activities, socialization, sexual patterns). *Provides information regarding the degree of concern client is experiencing and need for preventive measures to be instituted.*
- Regulate liquid intake at prescheduled times (with and between meals). *Promotes a predictable voiding pattern to establish a bladder-training program to prevent incontinence.*[4]
- Establish schedule for voiding (habit training) based on client's usual voiding pattern. *Can successfully reduce risk for incontinence.*
- Manage bowel elimination *to prevent continence problems associated with constipation or fecal impaction.*
- Provide assistance or devices, as indicated, for clients who are mobility impaired. *Providing means of summoning assistance and placing bedside commode, urinal, or bedpan within client's reach can promote sense of control in self-managing voiding.*[5]
- Encourage regular pelvic floor strengthening exercises (Kegel exercises or use of vaginal cones). *Can improve pelvic musculature tone and strength, preventing or halting incontinence. Note: Studies reveal a positive effect on urge incontinence using a combination of behavioral interventions (including pelvic muscle exercises) and medications in older women.*[4,6,9]

NURSING PRIORITY NO. 3 To promote wellness (Teaching/Discharge Considerations):

- Provide information to client/significant other about potential for urge incontinence (also called OAB) and lifestyle measures to prevent development of incontinence, as individually indicated.
- Recommend limiting intake of coffee, tea, and alcohol. *These substances have an irritating effect on the bladder and may contribute to incontinence.*[10]
- Suggest wearing loose-fitting or especially adapted clothing. *Facilitates response to voiding urge, especially in elderly or infirm individuals, enabling them to reach the toilet without loss of urine.*[6]
- Emphasize importance of perineal care after each voiding. *Reduces risk of ascending infection and incontinence-related dermatitis.*[5]
- Identify signs/symptoms indicating urinary complications and need for medical follow-up care. *Helps client be aware and seek intervention in a timely manner to prevent more serious problems from developing.*

DOCUMENTATION FOCUS

Assessment/Reassessment

- Individual findings, including specific risk factors and pattern of voiding.

Planning

- Plan of care, specific interventions, and who is involved in planning.
- Teaching plan.

Implementation/Evaluation

- Response to interventions, teaching, and actions performed.
- Attainment or progress toward desired outcome(s).
- Modifications to plan of care.

Discharge Planning

- Discharge needs and who is responsible for actions to be taken.
- Specific referrals made.

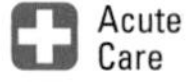

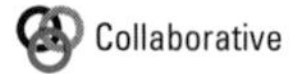

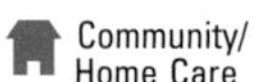

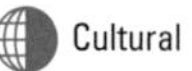

References

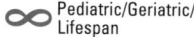

1. Vasavada, S. P., Carmel, M. E., Rackley, R. (Updated 2014). Urinary incontinence. Retrieved March 2015 from http://emedicine.medscape.com/article/452289-overview.
2. Booth, C. (2002). Introduction to urinary incontinence. *Hosp Pharmacist*, 9(3), 65–68.
3. Continence for women: Evaluation of AWHONN's third research utilization project. (2000). In Sampsell, C. M., Wyman, J. F., Thomas, K. K., et al. (eds). *JOGNN*, 29, 9–17.
4. The state of the science on urinary incontinence. (2003). In Newman, D. K., Palmer, M. H. (eds). *Am J Nurs*, 3(Suppl), 2–53.
5. Newfield, S. A., Hinz, M. D., Tilley, D. S., et al. (2007). ND: Urinary Incontinence. *Cox's Clinical Applications of Nursing Diagnosis: Adult, Child, Women's, Psychiatric, Gerontic, and Home Health Considerations*. 5th ed. Philadelphia: F. A. Davis.
6. Wyman, J. F. (2003). Treatment of urinary incontinence in men and older women: The evidence shows the efficacy of a variety of techniques. *Am J Nurs*, 103(suppl), 26–35.
7. Porter Health Care System: Health Education. (2014). Urinary incontinence. Retrieved March 2015 from http://www.porterhealth.com/health-education/85,P01528.
8. Newman, D. K. (2009). Using the BladderScan™ for bladder volume assessment. Retrieved March 2015 from http://www.seekwellness.com/incontinence/using_the_bladderscan.htm.
9. Burgio, K. L., Locher, J. L., Goode, P. S. (2000). Combined behavioral and drug therapy for urge incontinence in older women. *Obstet Gynecol Surv*, 55(8), 485–486.
10. Stoppler, M. C. (Updated 2014). Urinary incontinence. Retrieved March 2015 from http://www.emedicinehealth.com/incontinence/article_em.htm.
11. Gray, M. (2005). Assessment and management of urinary incontinence. *Nurse Pract*, 30(7), 32–43.
12. Gray, M. (2005). Overactive bladder: An overview. *J Wound Ostomy Continence Nurs*, 32(3 suppl), 1–5.
13. Newman, D. K. (2005). Assessment of the patient with an overactive bladder. *J Wound Ostomy Continence Nurs*, 32(3 suppl), 5–10.
14. Karriem-Norwood, V. (reviewer) (Updated 2014). Urge Incontinence. Retrieved March 2015 from http://www.webmd.com/urinary-incontinence-oab/america-asks-11/urge?page=1.

risk for Infection

Taxonomy II: Safety/Protection—Class 1 Infection (00004) [**Diagnostic Division:** Safety], Submitted 1986; Revised 1986, 2013

DEFINITION: Vulnerable to invasion and multiplication of pathogenic organisms, which may compromise health.

RISK FACTORS

Chronic illness (e.g., diabetes mellitus)
Inadequate vaccination
Insufficient knowledge to avoid exposure to pathogens

Inadequate Primary Defenses:

Alteration in peristalsis
Alteration in pH of secretions; status of body fluids
Alteration in skin integrity
Decrease in ciliary action
Premature or prolonged rupture of amniotic membrane
Smoking

Inadequate Secondary Defenses:

Decrease in hemoglobin; leukopenia, suppressed inflammatory response (e.g., IL-6, CRP); immunosuppression

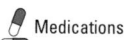

(continues on page 468)

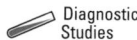

risk for Infection (continued)
Inadequate vaccination
Increased Environmental Exposure to Pathogens:
Exposure to disease outbreak
[Exposure to multiple healthcare workers, multiple care settings]
Note: A risk diagnosis is not evidenced by signs and symptoms, as the problem has not occurred; rather, nursing interventions are directed at prevention.
Sample Clinical Applications: Immune suppressed conditions (e.g., HIV positive, AIDS, cancer), chronic obstructive pulmonary disease (COPD), long-term use of steroids (e.g., asthma, rheumatoid arthritis, systemic lupus erythematosus [SLE]), diabetes mellitus, malnutrition, surgical or invasive procedures, substance abuse, burns, pregnancy/preterm labor

DESIRED OUTCOMES/EVALUATION CRITERIA

Sample NOC linkages:
Knowledge: Infection Management: Extent of understanding conveyed about infection, its treatment, and the prevention of complications
Risk Control: Personal actions to prevent, eliminate, or reduce modifiable health threats
Infection Severity: Severity of infection and associated symptoms

Client Will (Include Specific Time Frame)
- Verbalize understanding of individual causative or risk factor(s).
- Identify interventions to prevent or reduce risk of infection.
- Demonstrate techniques and lifestyle changes to promote safe environment.
- Achieve timely wound healing, be free of purulent drainage or erythema, and be afebrile.

ACTIONS/INTERVENTIONS

Sample NIC linkages:
Infection Protection: Prevention and early detection of infection in a patient at risk
Infection Control: Minimizing the acquisition and transmission of infectious agents
Surveillance: Purposeful and ongoing acquisition, interpretation, and synthesis of patient data for clinical decision making

NURSING PRIORITY NO. 1 To determine risk/contributing factors:

- Assess for presence of host-specific factors that affect immunity:[1,7–9]
  - **Extremes of age:** *Newborns and the elderly are more susceptible to disease and infection than the general population. Studies reported by the Centers for Disease Control and Prevention (CDC) in 2015 showed that between 1 and 3 million infections occur annually in nursing homes and assisted living facilities.*[1,18] *Infections that are regularly found (endemic) in this population include urinary tract infections (UTIs), lower respiratory tract infections, and outbreaks of respiratory and gastrointestinal (GI) infections.*[22]
  - **Presence of underlying disease:** *Client may have disease that directly impacts immune system (e.g., cancer, AIDS, autoimmune disorder) or may be weakened by prolonged disease conditions (e.g., diabetes, kidney disease, heart failure) or treatments.*
  - **Certain treatment settings/modalities:** *Client in acute/critical-care setting and/or on mechanical ventilation may have a prolonged exposure to risk factors for infection, including problems with breathing and circulation, GI motility disorders, and use of analgesics and sedatives, causing a higher rate of acquired infections. Note: The National and State Healthcare-Associated Infections Progress Report (2013) to the CDC reported progress in several areas, including preventing "central line-associated bloodstream infec-*

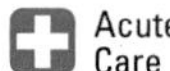
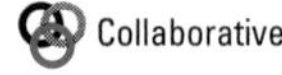
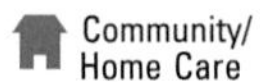
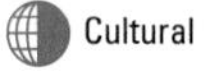

tions (CLABSI), select surgical site infections (SSI), hospital-onset Clostridium difficile infections (C. difficile), and hospital-onset methicillin-resistant Staphylococcus aureus (MRSA) bacteremia (bloodstream infections)." There was, however, a 6% increase in catheter-associated urinary tract infections (CAUTIs) between 2009 and 2013.[17,20] *However, recent data also reported that infections from gram-negative bacteria (e.g., 13% of* E. coli *and* Klebsiella, *17% of* P. aeruginosa *and 74% of* A. baumannii*) in intensive-care units were multidrug resistant (CDC, 2011).*[21]

Lifestyle: *Personal habits or living situations, such as persons sharing close quarters and/or equipment (e.g., college dorm, group home, long-term care facility, day care, correctional facility); persons/groups with inadequate vaccination protection; and IV drug use, shared needles, and unprotected sex can increase susceptibility to infections.*

Nutritional status: *Malnutrition weakens the immune system; elevated serum glucose levels (e.g., administration of total parenteral nutrition or poorly controlled diabetes mellitus) provide growth media for pathogens.*

Trauma: *Loss of skin or mucous membrane integrity or invasive surgical or diagnostic procedures; premature rupture of amniotic membranes; urinary catheterizations; and parenteral injection, sharps, and needle sticks are common paths of pathogen entry.*

Certain medications: *Steroids and chemotherapeutic agents directly affect the immune system. Long-term or improper antibiotic treatment can disrupt body's normal flora and result in increased susceptibility to antibiotic-resistant organisms.*

Presence or absence of immunity: *Natural immunity may be acquired as a result of development of antibodies to a specific agent following infection, preventing recurrence of specific disease (e.g., chicken pox). Active immunization (via vaccination; e.g., measles, polio) and passive immunization (e.g., antitoxin or immunoglobulin administration) can prevent certain communicable diseases.*

Environmental exposure: *May be accidental or intentional. Exposure can occur in different ways, such as use of specific microorganisms (in laboratories, biotechnological industries, acts of bioterrorism). Accidental exposure can result from exposure to contaminants arising from commonplace processes (e.g., waste water recycling) or through animal contact (e.g., agriculture, animal food processing) and through contact with humans (e.g., healthcare, education, mass transit, close contact living, etc.).*[23]

- Observe skin/tissues surrounding injuries (e.g., knife cuts, toe injuries, insect or animal bites); also inspect insertion sites of invasive lines, sutures, surgical incisions, and wounds. *Redness, warmth, swelling, pain, and red streaks are signs of developing localized infection that may have systemic implications if treatment is delayed.*[4,5,9,12]
- Assess and document skin conditions around insertions of orthopedic pins, wires, and tongs. *Direct connection to bone increases the risk of infections in bone sites that can lead to osteomyelitis, bone loss, and long-term delays of healing.*[4,5,9,12]
- Review laboratory values (e.g., white blood cell count and differential, blood, urine, sputum, or wound cultures) *to identify presence of pathogens and treatment options.*
- Refer to NDs risk for Aspiration, risk for Contamination, risk for urinary tract Injury, risk for impaired oral Mucous Membranes, and risk for impaired Skin or Tissue Integrity for related assessments and interventions.

NURSING PRIORITY NO. 2 To reduce/correct existing risk factors:

HEALTHCARE ENVIRONMENT

- Practice and emphasize constant and proper hand-washing techniques (using antibacterial soap and running water) before and after all care contacts and after contact with items likely to be contaminated. Wear gloves where appropriate to minimize contamination of hands and discard after each client. Wash hands after glove removal. Instruct client/significant others (SOs)/visitors to wash hands, as indicated. *This is a first-line defense against healthcare-associated infections (HAIs).*[1,10]
- Provide a clean, well-ventilated environment (may require turning off central air-conditioning and opening window for good ventilation, room with negative air pressure, etc.).

- Post visual alerts in healthcare settings instructing clients/SOs to inform healthcare providers if they have symptoms of respiratory infections or influenza-like symptoms. *Can limit or prevent transmission to and from client and may reveal additional cases.*[1,3,6,7,10]
- Monitor client's visitors/caregivers for respiratory illnesses. Offer masks and tissues to client/visitors who are coughing or sneezing *to limit exposures and reduce cross-contamination.*[1]
- Encourage parents of sick children to keep them away from child-care settings and school until afebrile for 24 hr.
- Provide for isolation as indicated (e.g., contact, droplet, and airborne precautions). Educate staff in infection-control procedures. *Reduces risk of cross-contamination.*[1,13]
- Emphasize proper use of personal protective equipment by staff/visitors as dictated by agency policy *for particular exposure risk (e.g., airborne, droplet, splash risk), including mask or respiratory filter of appropriate particulate regulator, gowns, aprons, head covers, face shields, and protective eyewear.*[1,3,8]
- Include information in preoperative teaching about ways *to reduce potential for postoperative infection (e.g., respiratory measures to prevent pneumonia, wound or dressing care, avoidance of others with infection).*[4,14]
- Encourage early ambulation, deep breathing, coughing, position changes, and early removal of endotracheal and/or nasal or oral feeding tubes *for mobilization of respiratory secretions and prevention of aspiration and respiratory infections.*[10,11]
- Monitor and assist with use of adjuncts (e.g., respiratory aids such as incentive spirometry) *to prevent pneumonia.*[10,11]
- Maintain adequate hydration and electrolyte balance *to prevent imbalances that would predispose to infection.*
- Provide or encourage balanced diet, emphasizing proteins to feed the immune system. *Immune function is affected by protein intake; the balance between omega-6 and omega-3 fatty acid intake; and adequate amounts of vitamins A, C, and E and the minerals zinc and iron. A deficiency of these nutrients puts the client at an increased risk of infection.*
- Handle and properly package tissue and fluid specimens.[1,2]
- Administer prophylactic antibiotics and immunizations as indicated.
- Assist with medical procedures (e.g., wound or joint aspiration, incision and drainage of abscess, bronchoscopy) as indicated.
- Administer and monitor medication regimen (e.g., antimicrobials, drip infusion into osteomyelitis, subeschar clysis, topical antibiotics) and note client's response *to determine effectiveness of therapy and presence of side effects.*

MEDICAL DEVICES

- Maintain sterile technique for invasive procedures (e.g., IV, urinary catheter, tracheostomy care, pulmonary suctioning).[1,2]
- Use disposable equipment whenever possible. Disinfect or sterilize reusable equipment and surfaces according to manufacturer recommendations.[1–3]
- Dispose of needles and sharps in approved containers *to reduce risk of needlestick or sharps injury.*[1,3]
- Choose proper vascular access device based on anticipated treatment duration and solution or medication to be infused and best available aseptic insertion techniques; cleanse incisions and insertion sites daily/per facility protocol with appropriate solution *to reduce potential for catheter-related bloodstream infections.*[12]
- Maintain appropriate hang times for parenteral solutions (IVs, additives, nutritional solutions) *to reduce opportunity for contamination and bacterial growth.*
- Assist with monitoring client on ventilator for signs of bacterial infections and wean from mechanical ventilator as soon as possible *to reduce risk of ventilator-associated pneumonia.*[13]
- Fill bubbling humidifiers or nebulizers with sterile water—not distilled or tap water. Use heat and moisture exchangers instead of a heated humidifier with mechanical ventilator.[11,13]

SKIN/TISSUES

- Change surgical or other wound dressings as needed or indicated, using proper technique for changing and disposing of contaminated materials.[1,3,4,14,19]

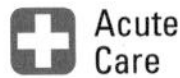
Acute Care
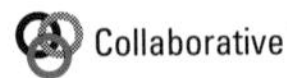
Collaborative
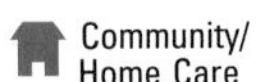
Community/ Home Care
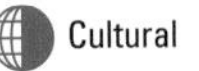
Cultural

- Cleanse incisions and insertion sites as indicated with appropriate antimicrobial topical or solution *to prevent growth of bacteria.*[4,19]
- Separate touching surfaces of excoriated skin (e.g., in herpes zoster, burns, weeping dermatitis) and apply appropriate skin barriers. Use gloves when caring for open lesions *to minimize autoinoculation or transmission of viral diseases.*[4]
- Perform or instruct in daily mouth care. Include use of antiseptic mouthwash for individuals in acute or long-term care settings *at high risk for HAIs.*[13]
- Provide regular urinary catheter and perineal care when client requires assistance with these actions. *Reduces risk of ascending urinary tract infection.*
- Cover perineal and pelvic region dressings or casts with plastic when using bedpan *to prevent contamination when wound is in perineal or pelvic region.*
- Discuss routine or preoperative antiseptic body shower or scrubs when indicated (e.g., orthopedic, plastic surgery) *to reduce bacterial colonization.*[10,19]

COMMUNITY

- Recommend individuals/staff isolate self at home when ill *to prevent spread of infection to others, including coworkers.*[1,6]
- Alert infection control officer/proper authorities to presence of specific infectious agents and number of cases as required. *Provides for case finding and helps curtail outbreak.*[6,16]
- Group/cohort individuals with same diagnosis or exposure as resources require. *Limited resources (as may occur with an outbreak or epidemic) may dictate a ward-like environment, but need for regular precautions to control spread of infection still exists.*[6]
- Encourage contacting healthcare provider for prophylactic therapy as indicated following exposure to individuals with infectious disease (e.g., tuberculosis, hepatitis, influenza).

NURSING PRIORITY NO. 3 To promote wellness (Teaching/Discharge Considerations):

- Review individual nutritional needs, appropriate exercise program, and need for rest *to enhance immune system function and healing.*[5,6]
- Instruct client/SO(s) in techniques to protect the integrity of skin, care for lesions, temperature measurement, and prevention of spread of infection in the home setting. *Provides basic knowledge for self-help and self-protection.*[2,5]
- Emphasize necessity of taking medications such as antivirals or antibiotics as directed (e.g., dosage and length of therapy). *Premature discontinuation of treatment when client begins to feel well may result in return of infection and potentiate drug-resistant strains.*[15]
- Discuss importance of not taking antibiotics prescribed for another person or using "leftover" drugs unless specifically instructed by healthcare provider. *Inappropriate use can lead to development of drug-resistant strains or secondary infections.*[5]
- Discuss the role of smoking and secondhand smoke in respiratory infections and in postoperative healing. Refer to smoking cessation programs as indicated.[19]
- Promote safer-sex practices and reporting sexual contacts of infected individuals *to prevent the spread of HIV or other sexually transmitted infections.*[1,5,15]
- Encourage high-risk persons, including healthcare workers, to have influenza and pneumonia vaccinations *to reduce individual risk as well as help prevent spread of flu and viral pneumonias to others.*[1,6,16]
- Promote childhood immunization program. Encourage adults to update immunizations as appropriate.[7]
- Discuss precautions with client engaged in international travel and refer for immunizations *to reduce incidence and transmission of global infections.*[8]
- Review use of prophylactic antibiotics if appropriate *(e.g., before dental work for clients with history of rheumatic fever, heart valve replacements).*[5]
- Identify resources available to the individual (e.g., substance abuse or rehabilitation, needle-exchange program as appropriate; available or free condoms).

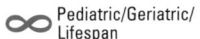

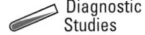

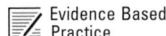

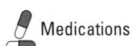

- Provide information and involve in appropriate community and national education programs *to increase awareness of and prevention of communicable diseases*.[1,5,6]
- Refer to NDs ineffective Health Maintenance and impaired Home Maintenance for additional interventions as appropriate.

DOCUMENTATION FOCUS

Assessment/Reassessment

- Individual risk factors that are present, including recent and current antibiotic therapy.
- Wound and/or insertion sites, character of drainage or body secretions.
- Signs/symptoms of infectious process.

Planning

- Plan of care, specific interventions, and who is involved in planning.
- Teaching plan.

Implementation/Evaluation

- Responses to interventions, teaching, and actions performed.
- Attainment or progress toward desired outcome(s).
- Modifications to plan of care.

Discharge Planning

- Discharge needs and who is responsible for actions to be taken.
- Specific referrals made.

References

1. McDonald, M., Robinson, A. A. (2012). Infection control. Retrieved March 2015 from http://www.nursingceu.com/courses/375/index_nceu.html.
2. Friedman, M. M. (2002). Improving infection control in home care: From ritual to science-based practice. *Home Healthcare Nurse*, 18(2), 99–106.
3. World Health Organization. Hospital hygiene and infection control. Retrieved March 2015 from http://www.who.int/water_sanitation_health/medicalwaste/148to158.pdfhttp://www.who.int/water_sanitation_health/medicalwaste/148to158.pdf.
4. Thompson, J. (2000). A practical guide to wound care. *RN*, 63(1), 48–52.
5. Androwich, I., Burkhart, L., Gettrust, K. V. (1996). *Community and Home Health Nursing*. Albany, NY: Delmar.
6. Doenges, M. E., Moorhouse, M. F., Murr, A. C. (2010). Care plan: Disaster considerations; and ND infection, risk for, in numerous care plans. *Nursing Care Plans: Guidelines for Individualizing Client Care Across the Life Span*. 8th ed. Philadelphia: F. A. Davis.
7. Goldrick, B. A., Goetz, A. M. (2006). 'Tis the season for influenza. *Nurse Pract*, 31(12), 24–33.
8. Hunter, A., Denman-Vitale, S., Garzon, L. (2007). Global infections: Recognition, management, and prevention. *Nurse Pract*, 32(2), 34–41.
9. Romero, D. V., Treston, J., O'Sullivan, A. L. (2006). Hand-to-hand combat: Preventing MRSA infection. *Adv Wound Care*, 19(6), 328–333.
10. Houghton, D. (2006). HAI prevention: The power is in your hands. *Nurs Manage*, 37(5 suppl), 1–7.
11. Lorente, L., Lecuona, M., Jimenez, A., et al. (2006). Ventilator-associated pneumonia using a heated humidifier or a heat and moisture exchanger: A randomized controlled trial. *Crit Care*, 10(4), R116.
12. Rosenthal, K. (2006). Guarding against vascular site infection. *Nurs Manage*, 37(4), 54–66.
13. Ventilator-associated pneumonia (VAP) event. (Updated 2015). *CDC and Healthcare Infection Control Practices Manual*. Retrieved March 2015 from http://www.cdc.gov/nhsn/PDFs/pscManual/6pscVAPcurrent.pdf.
14. Odom-Forren, J. (2006). Preventing surgical site infections. *Nursing*, 36(6), 59–63.
15. Kirton, C. (2005). The HIV/AIDS epidemic: A case of good news/bad news. *Nursing Made Incredibly Easy!*, 3(2), 28–40.
16. Lashley, F. R. (2006). Emerging infectious diseases at the beginning of the 21st century. *Online J Issues Nurs*, 11(1). Retrieved March 2015 from http://www.medscape.com/viewarticle/528306.
17. Nseir, S., Makris, C., Mathieu, D., et al. (2010). Intensive care unit–acquired infection as a side effect of sedation. *Crit Care*, 14(2), R30.

18. Centers for Disease Control and Prevention: National Healthcare Safety Network. (Updated 2015). Tracking infections in long-term care facilities. Retrieved March 2015 from http://www.cdc.gov/nhsn/LTC/.
19. Alexander, J. W., Solomkin, J. S., Edwards, M. J. (2011). Updated recommendations for control of surgical site infections. *Ann Surg*, 253(6), 1082–1093.
20. Centers for Disease Control and Prevention. (2013). Healthcare-associated Infections (HAIs). *The National and State Healthcare-Associated Infections Progress Report (2013)*. Retrieved March 2015 from http://www.cdc.gov/HAI/surveillance/index.html.
21. Centers for Disease Control and Prevention. (2011). Gram-negative bacteria infections in healthcare settings. Retrieved March 2015 from http://www.cdc.gov/hai/organisms/gram-negative-bacteria.html.
22. Strausbaugh, L. J., Sukumar, S. R., Joseph, C. L. (2003). Infectious disease outbreaks in nursing homes: An unappreciated hazard for frail elderly persons. *Clin Infect Dis*, 36(7), 870–876.
23. Haagmus, J. A., Tariq, D. J., Heederik, D. J. (2012). Infectious disease risks associated with occupational exposure: A systematic review of the literature. *Occup Environ Med*, 69(2), 140–146.

risk for Injury

Taxonomy II: Safety/Protection—Class 2 Physical Injury (00035) [**Diagnostic Division:** Safety], Submitted 1978, Revised 2013

DEFINITION: Vulnerable to physical damage due to environmental conditions interacting with the individual's adaptive and defensive resources, which may compromise health.

RISK FACTORS

Internal

Abnormal blood profile [e.g., leukocytosis/leukopenia, altered clotting factors, thrombocytopenia, sickle cell, thalassemia, decreased hemoglobin]; immune/autoimmune dysfunction; biochemical dysfunction
Alteration in affective orientation; effector dysfunction
Alteration in sensation (resulting from spinal cord injury, diabetes mellitus, etc.)
Extremes of age
Impaired primary defense mechanisms (e.g., broken skin); tissue hypoxia; malnutrition

External

Alteration in cognitive or psychomotor functioning
Compromised nutritional source (e.g., vitamins, food types)
Exposure to pathogen or toxic chemical [pollutants, poisons, drugs, pharmaceutical agents, alcohol, nicotine, preservatives, cosmetics, dyes]
Immunization level within community; nosocomial agent
Physical barrier (e.g., design, structure, and arrangement of community, building, equipment); unsafe mode of transport

NOTE: A risk diagnosis is not evidenced by signs and symptoms, as the problem has not occurred; rather, nursing interventions are directed at prevention.

Sample Clinical Applications: Burns, seizure disorder, dementia, AIDS, cataracts, glaucoma, Parkinson's disease, substance abuse, malnutrition, developmental delay, para/quadraplegia, neuropathy.

[Note: In reviewing this ND, it is apparent there is much overlap with other diagnoses. We have chosen to present generalized interventions. Although there are commonalities to injury situations, we suggest that the reader refer to other primary diagnoses as indicated, such as risk for Bleeding; risk for acute Confusion; chronic Confusion; risk for Contamination; risk for Falls; ineffective Health Maintenance; impaired Home

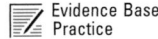

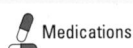

(continues on page 474)

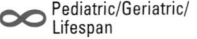

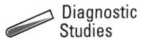

risk for Injury (continued)

Maintenance; risk for Infection; impaired physical Mobility; impaired/risk for impaired Parenting; ineffective Protection; risk for Poisoning; impaired/risk for impaired Skin/Tissue Integrity; Rape-Trauma Syndrome; risk for Pressure Ulcer; ineffective Tissue Perfusion; risk for Trauma; risk for self and other-directed Violence; Wandering for additional interventions.]

DESIRED OUTCOMES/EVALUATION CRITERIA

Sample NOC linkage:

Physical Injury Severity: Severity of injuries from accidents and trauma

Client Will (Include Specific Time Frame)

- Be free of injury.

Sample NOC linkages:

Personal Safety Behavior: Personal actions that prevent physical injury to self

Risk Control [specify]: Personal actions to prevent, eliminate, or reduce modifiable health threats [e.g., alcohol/drug use, altered visual function, sun exposure]

Client/Caregivers Will (Include Specific Time Frame)

- Verbalize understanding of individual factors that contribute to possibility of injury.
- Demonstrate behaviors, lifestyle changes to reduce risk factors and protect self from injury.
- Modify environment as indicated to enhance safety.

ACTIONS/INTERVENTIONS

Sample NIC linkages:

Surveillance: Safety: Purposeful and ongoing collection and analysis of information about the patient and the environment for use in promoting and maintaining client safety

Risk Identification: Analysis of potential risk factors, determination of health risks, and prioritization of risk reduction strategies for an individual or group

Environmental Management: Safety: Monitoring and manipulation of the physical environment to promote safety

NURSING PRIORITY NO. 1 To evaluate degree/source of risk inherent in the individual situation:

- Identify client at risk (e.g., acute illness, surgery, trauma; chronic illness conditions with weakness, immunosuppression, abnormal blood profiles, or prolonged immobility; acute or chronic confusion, dementia, head injury; use of multiple medications; use of alcohol or other drugs; mental illness, emotional liability; cultural, familial, and socioeconomic factors adversely affecting lifestyle and home; exposure to environmental chemicals or other hazards).
- Perform thorough assessments regarding safety issues when planning for client care and discharge. *Failure to accurately assess and intervene or refer regarding these issues can place the client at needless risk and creates negligence issues for the healthcare practitioner. Note: Research has identified 30 safe practices that evidence shows can work to reduce or prevent adverse events and medical errors regarding client safety, including (and not limited to) adequate numbers of nursing personnel; ensuring that written documentation of the client's preference for life-sustaining treatments is prominently displayed in chart; evaluating each person upon admission, and regularly thereafter, for the risk of developing pressure ulcers; employing clinically appropriate strategies to prevent malnutrition; vaccinating healthcare workers against influenza to protect both them and clients; and standardizing methods for labeling, packaging, and storing medications.*[14]

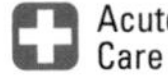
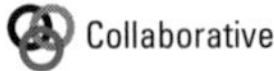
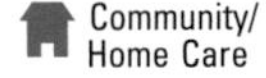
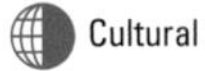

- Note age, developmental stage, and gender. *Children, young adults, elderly persons, and men are at greater risk for injury, which may reflect client's ability or desire to protect self and influences choice of interventions or teaching.*[15,16]
- Evaluate developmental level, decision-making ability, level of cognition, competence, and independence. *Determines client's/significant other's (SO's) ability to attend to safety issues.*
- Assess mood, coping abilities, and personality styles (i.e., temperament, aggression, impulsive behavior, level of self-esteem). *May result in carelessness or increased risk-taking without consideration of consequences.*[1,2]
- Evaluate individual's emotional and behavioral response to violence in surroundings (e.g., neighborhood, television, peer group). *May affect client's view of and regard for own or others' safety.*[1,2,15]
- Assess muscle strength and gross and fine motor coordination *to identify risk for falls. Note: The frequency of falls increases with age and frailty level. Risk factors for falls lie in four categories: (1) biological, (2) behavioral, (3) environmental, and (4) socioeconomic. In each of these areas, some risk factors can be modified to decrease fall risk. Protective factors for falls in older age are related to behavioral change and environmental modification.*[17]
- Observe client for signs of injury and ascertain age of injury (e.g., old or new bruises, history of fractures, frequent absences from school or work). Determine potential for abusive behavior by intimate partner/family members/peers. *Client or care providers may require further evaluation or investigation for abuse; prevention strategies may be indicated.*[5,7]
- Ascertain knowledge of safety needs and injury prevention and motivation to prevent injury in home, community, and work settings. *Information may reveal areas of misinformation, lack of knowledge, and need for teaching.*[6]
- Note socioeconomic status and availability and use of resources.

NURSING PRIORITY NO. 2 To assist client/caregiver to reduce or correct individual risk factors:

- Provide healthcare within a culture of safety (e.g., adherence to nursing standards of care and facility safe-care policies) *to prevent errors resulting in client injury, to promote client safety, and to model safety behaviors for client/SO. Note: A culture of safety encompasses the following elements (adapted from Kizer, 2001): shared beliefs and values about the healthcare delivery system; recruitment and training with patient safety in mind; organizational commitment to detecting and analyzing patient injuries and near misses; open communication regarding patient injury results, both within and outside the organization; and the establishment of a just culture.*[14]

  Practice hand hygiene at all times and device safety when client has IV lines and catheters *to prevent nosocomial infections and potential for blood-borne pathogens.*

  Administer medications and infusions using the "6 rights" system (right client, right medication, right route, right dose, right time, right documentation).[8]

  Inform and educate client/SO regarding all treatments and medications.

  Adhere to measures to prevent blood clots, especially in client with abnormal blood profile, surgical procedures, or immobility.

  Monitor environment for potentially unsafe conditions or hazards, modify as needed.

  Prevent falls:[6,9]

  - Orient or reorient client to environment, as needed.
  - Place confused elderly client or young child near nurses' station *to provide for frequent observation.*
  - Instruct client/SO to request assistance, as needed; make sure call light is within reach and client knows how to operate.
  - Utilize bed/chair alarms *that alert when client is trying to get up alone.*
  - Maintain bed or chair in lowest position with wheels locked. Provide covered cribs for enclosed bed or wall bed on floor, where indicated.
  - Provide seat raisers for chairs and use stand-assist, repositioning, or lifting devices as indicated *to prevent injury to both client and care providers.*

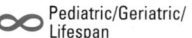

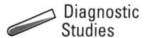

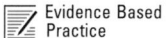

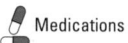

Ensure that all floors are clear of tripping hazards and that pathway to bathroom is unobstructed and properly lighted.
Place assistive devices (e.g., walker, cane, glasses, hearing aid) within reach and ascertain that client is using them appropriately.
Safety-lock exit and stairwell doors *when client can wander away.*

- Avoid use of restraints as much as possible when client is confused. *Restraints can increase client's agitation and risk of entrapment and death.*
- Provide client/SO information regarding client's specific disease or condition and consequences of continuing unhealthy behaviors (e.g., increase in oral cancer among teenagers using smokeless tobacco; fetal alcohol syndrome or neonatal addiction in prenatal women using tobacco, alcohol, or other drugs) *to enhance decision making and clarify expectations and individual needs.*
- Review consequences of previously determined risk factors that client is reluctant to modify. *Many consequences could occur, such as oral cancer in teenager using smokeless tobacco; occurrence of spontaneous abortion, fetal alcohol syndrome, or neonatal addiction in prenatal woman using drugs; fall related to failure to use assistive equipment; toddler getting into medicine cabinet; binge drinking while skiing; health and legal implications of illicit drug use; and working too many hours for safe operation of machinery or vehicles.*
- Determine if risk-prone behavior is occurring or likely to occur *to initiate appropriate wellness counseling and referrals.*
- Review client's history of immunization and understanding of the importance of immunization to self/family. Refer to ND readiness for enhanced Health Management *to determine changes or adaptations that may be desired/required.*
- Review client's level of physical activity in his or her lifestyle *to determine changes or adaptations that may be required by current situation.*
- Refer to physical or occupational therapist as appropriate *to identify high-risk tasks; conduct site visits; select, create, and modify equipment or assistive devices; and provide education about body mechanics and musculoskeletal injuries in addition to providing therapies as indicated.*[6]
- Perform home assessment and recommend actions (or take steps) to correct unsafe conditions, such as:[1–13]

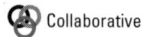

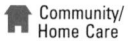

  locking up medications and poisonous substances;
  using window grates or locks and safety gates at top and bottom of stairs *to prevent young children from falling*;
  installing handrails on stairs/steps, ramps, and bathtub safety products (e.g., grab bars/handles, non-skid mats or stickers);
  using electrical outlet covers or lockouts;
  locking exterior doors *to prevent confused individual from wandering off while SO is engaged in other household activities;*
  removing matches, smoking materials, and knobs from the stove *so young children or confused individuals do not turn on burner and leave it unattended;*
  properly placing lights, alarms (e.g., fire, carbon monoxide, and intruder), and fire extinguishers;
  discussing safe use of oxygen; and
  obtaining medical alert device or home monitoring service.
- Review specific employment concerns or worksite issues and needs (e.g., ergonomic chairs and workstations, properly fitting safety equipment and footwear, regular use of safety glasses or goggles and ear protectors, safe storage of hazardous substances, number of hours worked per shift/week).
- Demonstrate and encourage use of techniques to reduce or manage stress and vent emotions such as anger and hostility. *Identifying and dealing with emotions appropriately enables individual to maintain control of behavior and avoid possibility of violent outbursts.*[2,5,7]
- Discuss importance of self-monitoring of factors that can contribute to occurrence of injury (e.g., fatigue, anger, irritability). *Client/SO may be able to modify risk through monitoring of actions or postponement of certain actions, especially during times when client is likely to be highly stressed.*
- Encourage participation in self-help programs, such as assertiveness training, anger management, and positive self-image *to enhance self-esteem.*

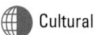

- Review expectations caregivers have of children, cognitively impaired, and/or elderly family members. Discuss concerns about discipline practices.[13]
- Discuss need for and sources of supervision (e.g., before- and after-school programs, elderly day care).

NURSING PRIORITY NO. 3 To promote wellness (Teaching/Discharge Considerations):

- Identify individual needs and resources for safety education (e.g., home hazard information, fall prevention, water safety [including burns or drowning hazards], firearm safety, cardiopulmonary resuscitation/first aid).[3,10,11]
- Emphasize importance of correct use of baby gates, cabinet door locks, child safety seats, car seat belts, bicycle or other helmets, regular use of sports safety equipment, etc.
- Provide instruction or refer to classes for back safety and proper use of injury-prevention devices. Recommend use of ergonomic bed and chair as appropriate.
- Provide telephone numbers and other contact numbers as individually indicated (e.g., doctor, 911, poison control, police, elder advocate).
- Provide bibliotherapy including written resource lists and reliable Web sites *for later review and self-paced learning.*
- Refer to professional resources as indicated (e.g., counseling or psychotherapy, budget counseling, substance recovery, anger management, parenting classes).
- Refer to or assist with community education programs *to increase awareness of safety measures and resources available to the individual. Note: Many evidence-based programs are being implemented nationally to promote safe environments for children, adolescents, and adults. These may include (and are not limited to) education about bullying and Internet safety issues, suicide prevention, use of helmets when riding bicycles or skateboarding, drowning prevention, gun safety, substance abuse, and intimate partner violence and anger management.*[2–5,7,9,11,12]
- Promote community awareness about the problems of the design of buildings, equipment, transportation, and workplace practices that contribute to accidents.[4]
- Identify community resources, neighbors, or friends to assist elderly or handicapped individuals in providing such things as structural maintenance, removal of snow and ice from walks and steps, etc.
- Identify emergency escape plans and routes for home and community *to be prepared in the event of natural or man-made disaster (e.g., fire, hurricane, earthquake, toxic chemical release).*[4]

DOCUMENTATION FOCUS

Assessment/Reassessment

- Individual risk factors, noting current physical findings (e.g., bruises, cuts).
- Client's/caregiver's understanding of individual risks and safety concerns.
- Availability and use of resources.

Planning

- Plan of care and who is involved in planning.
- Teaching plan.

Implementation/Evaluation

- Individual responses to interventions, teaching, and actions performed.
- Specific actions and changes that are made.
- Attainment or progress toward desired outcome(s).
- Modifications to plan of care.

Discharge Planning

- Long-term plans for discharge needs, lifestyle and community changes, and who is responsible for actions to be taken.
- Specific referrals made.

References

1. Gorman-Smith, D., Henry, D. B., Tolan, P. H. (2004). Exposure to community violence and violence perpetration: The protective effects of family functioning. *J Clin Child Psychol*, 33(3), 439–449.
2. Centers for Disease Control and Prevention. (2012). Understanding youth violence. Injury Center: Violence Prevention. Retrieved February 2015 from http://www.cdc.gov/ViolencePrevention/pdf/YV-FactSheet-a.pdf.
3. Emergency Nurses Association. (2012). Firearm safety and injury prevention: Position statement. Retrieved February 2015 from http://www.ena.org/SiteCollectionDocuments/Position%20Statements/FirearmInjuryPrevention.pdf.
4. Doenges, M. E., Moorhouse, M. F., Murr, A. C. (2010). Care plan: Disaster considerations; and ND infection, risk for, in numerous care plans. *Nursing Care Plans: Guidelines for Individualizing Client Care Across the Life Span*. 8th ed. Philadelphia: F. A. Davis.
5. Centers for Disease Control and Prevention. (2010). Intimate partner violence. National Center for Injury Prevention and Control. Retrieved February 2015 from http://www.cdc.gov/violenceprevention/pdf/nisvs_report2010-a.pdf.
6. Nelson, A., Owen, B., Lloyd, J. D., et al. (2003). Safe patient handling & movement. *Am J Nurs*, 103(3), 32–43.
7. Centers for Disease Control and Prevention. Sexual violence. National Center for Injury Prevention and Control. Retrieved February 2015 from http://www.cdc.gov/violenceprevention/pdf/SV_factsheet-a.pdf.
8. Gozdan, M. J. (2009). Using technology to reduce medication errors. *Nursing*, 39(6), 57–58.
9. Mayo Clinic Staff. Intracranial hematoma prevention. Retrieved February 2015 from http://www.mayoclinic.org/diseases-conditions/intracranial-hematoma/basics/prevention/con-20019654.
10. Lassman, J. (2002). Water safety. *J Emerg Nurs*, 28(3), 241–243.
11. Centers for Disease Control and Prevention. Drowning risks in natural water settings. Retrieved February 2015 from http://www.cdc.gov/Features/dsDrowningRisks/.
12. Centers for Disease Control and Prevention. Preventing suicide. Retrieved February 2015 from http://www.cdc.gov/features/preventingsuicide/.
13. Safety for older consumers' home safety checklist. Consumer Product Safety Commission (CPSC) document no. 701. Retrieved February 2015 from http://www.cpsc.gov/PageFiles/122038/701.pdf.
14. The National Quality Forum and Agency for Healthcare Research and Quality. (2005). 30 Safe Practices for Better Health Care. Retrieved February 2015 from http://archive.ahrq.gov/research/findings/factsheets/errors-safety/30safe/30-safe-practices.pdf.
15. Schwebel, D. C., Barton, B. K. (2005). Contributions of multiple risk factors to child injury. *J Pediatr Psychol*, 30(7), 553–561.
16. Ristolainen, L., Heinonen, A., Waller, B., et al. (2009). Gender differences in sport injury risk and types of injuries: A retrospective twelve-month study on cross-country skiers, long distance runners and soccer players. *J Sports Sci Med*, 8, 443–451.
17. World Health Organization. (2007). WHO global report on falls prevention in older age. Section 2.5. Retrieved February 2015 from http://www.who.int/ageing/publications/Falls_prevention7March.pdf.

risk for corneal Injury

Taxonomy II: Safety/Protection—Class 5 Physical Injury (00245) [**Diagnostic Division:** Safety], Submitted: 2013

DEFINITION: Vulnerable to infection or inflammatory lesion in the corneal tissue that can affect superficial or deep layers, which may compromise health.

RISK FACTORS

Blinking <5 times per minute
Exposure of the eyeball; periorbital edema
Glasgow Coma Scale score <7
Pharmaceutical agent
Prolonged hospitalization

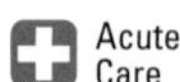

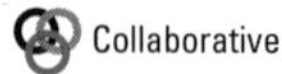

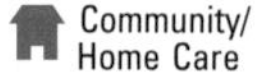

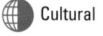

Use of supplemental oxygen; intubation; mechanical ventilation; tracheostomy
Note: A risk diagnosis is not evidenced by signs and symptoms, as the problem has not occurred; rather, nursing interventions are directed at prevention.
Sample Clinical Applications: Any condition where client is unable to protect self from drying of eye tissues, including facial or general trauma or surgery; mechanical ventilation; brain injury, CVA; neurological conditions such as Parkinson's disease, Bell's palsy; diabetic retinopathy; lupus; rheumatoid arthritis

DESIRED OUTCOMES/EVALUATION CRITERIA

Sample NOC linkage:
Risk Control: Personal actions to understand, prevent, eliminate, or reduce modifiable health threats

Client/Caregiver Will (Include Specific Time Frame)
- Identify/monitor personal risk factors.
- Engage in risk control strategies.

Sample NOC linkage:
Dry Eye Severity: Severity of signs and symptoms of insufficient tears

Client Will (Include Specific Time Frame)
Be free of discomfort or damage to corneal tissues.

ACTIONS/INTERVENTIONS

Sample NIC linkages:
Risk Identification: Analysis of potential risk factors, determination of health risks, and prioritization of risk reduction strategies for an individual or group
Eye Care: Prevention or minimization of threats to eye or visual integrity

NURSING PRIORITY NO. 1 To identify causative/precipitating factors related to risk:

- Obtain history of eye conditions when assessing client concerns overall. Listen for reports of eye pain, foreign body sensation, light sensitivity (photophobia), and blurred vision. *These symptoms can be associated with corneal injury and, if present, require further evaluation and possible treatment.*[1]
- Note presence of conditions (e.g., recent neurological event, facial trauma or burns; use of contact lenses, failure to use safety glasses in high-risk employment situation) or treatment environments (e.g., intubated client on mechanical ventilation; use of therapeutic hypothermia; sedated, anesthetized, or obtunded client with absent blink reflex) *to identify client at high risk for corneal injury. Note: Mercieca, et al. found that 75% of sedated/paralyzed patients on mechanical ventilation in intensive care units have incomplete closure of the eyelids (lagophthalmos), predisposing them to corneal dryness and inflammation.*[2,3]
- Obtain history of events from client/others when trauma (e.g., facial blunt force trauma, car crash with airbag deployment, accidental or intentional gun shot wounds; accidents with fireworks or hot metal) has occurred. *Eye injury (including corneal abrasions and lacerations) may not be immediately discovered but should be suspected.*[4]
- Evaluate current drug regimen, noting pharmaceutical agents (e.g., topical drugs, preservatives in eye drops; beta blockers, antihistamines, phenothiazides; diruetics, steroids, sedatives, neuromuscular blocking agents) *that can contribute to dry eye, thereby increasing risk of corneal inflammation or injury in high-risk clients.*[5]

NURSING PRIORITY NO. 2 To promote eye health/comfort:

- Refer for diagnostic evaluation and interventions as indicated. *A standard eye exam and visual acuity testing may be performed, and other diagnostic studies (e.g., radiography, computed tomography, magnetic resonance imaging) may be indicated to locate foreign bodies or associated orbital, cranial, or facial trauma.*[4]

- Assist in/refer for treatment of underlying conditions that might be affecting corneal health.
- Perform routine assessment of eyes and preventive interventions in critically ill client:[2,6,8,9]
  Evaluate client's ability to maintain eyelid closure on daily basis and as needed.
  Perform actions to maintain eyelid closure in client that cannot do it for self (e.g., taping).
  Perform eye care (e.g., cleaning with saline soaked gauze, administration of eye-specific lubricant, where indicated).
  Observe for developing complications.
  Ascertain that client undergoing anesthesia has proper eye protection (e.g., lubricant, eyelids taped, goggles), especially when placed in prone position. *The cornea is easily abraded because of reduced lacrimation during anesthesia, if face masks are improperly applied, or if surgical drapes are manipulated while the eyes remain. In some positions, such as prone, a significant amount of pressure can be applied to the eyes.*

NURSING PRIORITY NO. 3 To promote wellness (Teaching/Discharge Criteria):

- Instruct high-risk client/caregivers in self-management interventions *to prevent corneal inflammation symptoms:*[1,5,7,10]
  Avoid rubbing eyes with fingers or harsh cloths.
  Protect eyes from blowing air or oxygen; discuss benefit of redirecting air flow.
  Wear protective eyewear in situations or sports where objects may fly into eyes or face.
  Wear protective eyewear that gives 180-degree protection while using a grinding wheel or hammering on metal.
  Wear sunglasses that block ultraviolet radiation when in bright sunlight or under sunlamps.
  Follow prescribed wear time for contact lenses.
  Add moisture to indoor air, especially in winter, to *reduce corneal irritation associated with dryness.*
  Blink repeatedly for a few seconds when using computer for any length of time *to prevent dryness and help spread tears evenly over eye.*
- Instruct in use of eye drops or ointments as indicated *to prevent inflammation/infection or to protect corneal surface.*
- Refer to appropriate healthcare provider concerning glasses, contact lenses, or other safety eyewear and offer information about suppliers.

DOCUMENTATION FOCUS

Assessment/Reassessment

- Individual risk factors identified.
- Client concerns or difficulty making and following through with plan.

Planning

- Plan of care and who is involved in planning.
- Teaching plan.

Implementation/Evaluation

- Response to interventions, teaching, and actions performed.
- Attainment or progress toward outcomes.

Discharge Planning

- Referrals to other resources.
- Long-term need and who is responsible for actions.

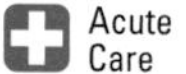
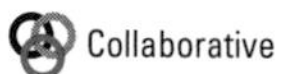
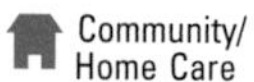
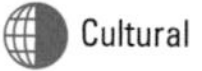

References

1. Verma, A., Khan, F. H. (2014). Corneal abrasion. Retrieved January 2015 from http://emedicine.medscape.com/article/1195402-overview.
2. Rosenberg, J. B., Eisen, L. A. (2008). Eye care in the intensive care unit: Narrative review and meta-analysis. *Crit Care Med*, 36(2), 3151–3155.
3. Schlessinger, D. A., Ulitsch, E. (2009). The eyes have it. *OR Nurse*, 3(4), 26–32.
4. Aronson, A. A., Yang, N. M. (2013). Corneal laceration. Retrieved January 2015 from http://emedicine.medscape.com/article/798005-overview.
5. Foster, C. S., Yuksel, E., Anzaar, F., et al. (2013). Dry eye syndrome. Retrieved January 2015 from http://emedicine.medscape.com/article/1210417-overview#showall.
6. Intensive Care Coordination & Monitoring Unit. (2007, updated 2010). Provision of eye care for the critically ill adult: NSWHealth Guidelines for Intensive Care. Retrieved January 2015 from http://intensivecare.hsnet.nsw.gove.au/five/doc/intensive%20care%20collaborative%20guidelines/Eye%20Care%20CPG%20Final%20version.pdf.
7. Mayo Clinic Staff. (2014). Dry eye (prevention). Retrieved January 2015 from http://www.mayoclinic.org/diseases-conditions/dry-eyes/basics/prevention/con-20024129.
8. Cucchiara, R. F., Faust, J. P. (1994). Patient positioning. In Miller, R. D. (eds.). *Anesthesia*. New York: Churchill Livingstone, 1057–1073.
9. Roth, S., Thisted, R. A., Erickson, J. P., et al. (1996). Eye injuries after nonocular surgery. A study of 60,965 anesthetics from 1988 to 1992. *Anesthesiology*, 85(5), 1020–1027.
10. Dahl, A. A. (2014). Corneal abrasion. Retrieved January 2015 from http://www.emedicinehealth.com/corneal_abrasion/article_em.htm.

risk for urinary tract Injury

Taxonomy II: Safety/Protection—Class 2 Physical Injury (00250) [**Diagnostic Division:** Safety], Submitted 2013

DEFINITION: Vulnerable to damage of the urinary tract structures from use of catheters, which may compromise health.

RISK FACTORS

Condition preventing ability to secure catheter (e.g., burn, trauma, amputation)
Long-term use of urinary catheters; multiple catheterizations
Retention balloon inflated to ≥30 ml
Use of large caliber urinary catheter
Note: A risk diagnosis is not evidenced by signs and symptoms, as the problem has not occurred; rather, nursing interventions are directed at prevention.

DESIRED OUTCOMES/EVALUATION CRITERIA

Sample NOC linkages:
Physical Injury Severity: Severity of signs and symptoms of bodily injuries

Client Will (Include Specific Time Frame)
• Be free of injury.
Sample NOC linkages:
Personal Safety Behavior: Personal actions that prevent physical injury to self
Risk Control [specify]: Personal actions to prevent, eliminate, or reduce modifiable health threats

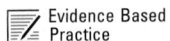

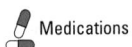

(continues on page 482)

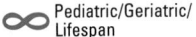

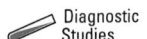

risk for urinary tract Injury (continued)

Client/Caregivers Will (Include Specific Time Frame)
- Verbalize understanding of individual factors that contribute to possibility of injury.
- Demonstrate behaviors and lifestyle changes to reduce risk factors and protect from injury.

ACTIONS/INTERVENTIONS

Sample NIC linkages:
Urinary Catheterization: Insertion of a catheter into the bladder for temporary or permanent drainage of urine
Urinary Catheterization: Intermittent: Regular periodic use of a catheter to empty the bladder

NURSING PRIORITY NO. 1 To assess causative/contributing factors:

- Identify conditions potentially affecting client need for/response to catheterization (e.g., acute illness, presence of infection, surgery, trauma including skin and tissue problems; chronic illness, including neurological conditions with paralysis or weakness; prolonged immobility; acute or chronic confusion, dementia, sedation, or use of multiple medications affecting mental acuity). *These conditions could require indwelling catheter for varying lengths of time with attendant potential for complications. Risk factors include longer duration of catheterization, bacterial colonization of the drainage bag, errors in catheter care, catheterization late in the hospital course, and immunocompromised or debilitated states. Note: About 80% of hospital-acquired urinary tract infections (UTIs) are related to urethral catheterization.*[1]
- Determine type of catheterization client is likely to require. *Client might require one-time or intermittent, long-term single catheterization for any number of reasons (e.g., relief of acute urinary retention, management of voiding issues associated with multiple sclerosis or spinal cord injury). These procedures may be done by either the client or a caregiver. Indwelling urinary catheters are generally used when longer-term urinary management issues are expected. Use of indwelling catheter should be limited to (1) urinary retention, (2) close monitoring of urine output in critically ill patients, (3) fluid challenge in patients with acute renal insufficiency, (4) open wound in sacral or perineal area in client with urinary incontinence, and (5) comfort care in terminally ill client.*[2,3]
- Note client's age, developmental level, decision-making ability, level of cognition, competence, and independence. *Determines client's/significant other's (SO's) ability to attend to safety issues and influences choice of interventions or teaching about catheterization.*
- Check for allergies to latex and select appropriate catheter (e.g., coated). *Latex allergic reactions are implicated in the development of urethritis and urethral stricture or anaphylaxis. Materials that are commonly used for the long term (such as silver alloy or hydrogel coated) may be used to overcome irritation and microscopic lacerations or stricture development associated with latex.*[4,5]

NURSING PRIORITY NO. 2 To reduce potential for complications:

- Avoid catheterization when possible. Refer to NDs pertaining to impaired urinary Elimination and Incontinence for related interventions. *Studies have shown that urinary catheters often are placed unnecessarily, remain in use without physician awareness, and are not removed promptly when no longer needed.*[2,6,7]
- Perform catheterization using best practices:

Use strict aseptic technique when inserting indwelling catheter (clean technique may be implemented for long-term intermittent catheterization). *Note: The Centers for Disease Control and Prevention's 2009 recommendations stated, "In the acute care hospital setting, insert urinary catheters using aseptic technique and sterile equipment," but "In the non-acute care setting, clean (i.e., non-sterile) technique for intermittent catheterization is an acceptable and more practical alternative to sterile technique for patients requiring chronic intermittent catheterization."*[8]

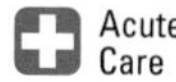

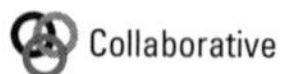

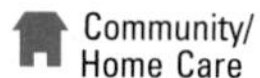

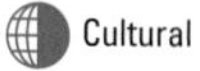

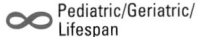

Select the smallest bore catheter possible that will allow for adequate drainage, using size guidelines. *Appropriate selection of catheter size will help reduce the likelihood of bladder spasm. Adult sizes are typically 14 Fr or 16 Fr. Guidelines are available for each pediatric age group from neonate (5–6 Fr.) to adolescent (10, 12, 14 Fr). Note: Large-size catheters (18 Fr or larger) can increase erosion of the bladder neck and urethral mucosa, cause the formation of strictures, and impede adequate drainage of periurethral gland secretions.*[3,9–11]

Ascertain good urine is established before inflating balloon. *Ensures that catheter has been correctly inserted into the bladder. Note: If the balloon is opened before catheter is completely inserted into the bladder, bleeding, damage and even rupture of the urethra can occur.*[13]

Inflate balloon, using correct amount of sterile liquid (usually 10 cc but check actual balloon size). *Balloon size is relevant to levels of bladder irritation. Although balloons are thin walled to reduce irritation to the bladder, it is still important to use the smallest size possible, usually with a 5- to 10-mL capacity. The use of 30-mL balloons is not recommended.*[12,13] *Note: Large balloons (20 to 30 cc) are useful in chronically catheterized client with lax pelvic muscles, but in most people, they can cause bladder irritation and leaking.*[14]

Secure catheter to thigh or abdomen, as indicated. Inspect the skin underneath the securement device with each reapplication to monitor for irritation or dermatitis. *Catheter/tubing can be held in place with adhesive tapes, safety pins, sutures, or non-adhesive devices. Latex-free non-adhesive products secure with a soft hook-and-loop closure strap. There are many reasons for this intervention, including (1) reducing bladder irritability/spasms, (2) preventing metal erosion or inflammation, (3) managing discomfort related to catheter movement and traction, (4) preventing inadvertent migration of balloon from bladder into urethra or accidental removal of catheter, (5) avoiding obstruction of urine flow secondary to catheter kinking, and (6) preventing retention of urine and risk for catheter-associated UTIs. [Note: Unsecured and displaced catheters can also cause pressure ulcers on the perineum and buttocks.]*[15–20]

Position the collection bag level *to facilitate gravity drainage of the bladder and to prevent reflux of urine into the bladder. Note: A Belly Bag™ abdominal drainage bag may be chosen over affixing tubing to leg in some instances (e.g., extremity trauma such as burns or amputation). The bag fastens around the waist by means of a woven belt with a quick release buckle. An anti-reflux valve behind the catheter port prevents reflux urine flow.*[13,19]

Perform ongoing evaluation of catheter function and monitor color and characteristics of urine *to assess for developing complications. A properly maintained closed drainage system and unobstructed urine flow are essential for prevention of urinary tract infection.*[5]

- Ascertain if client is experiencing discomfort or pain (e.g., bladder spasms). *Bladder spasms are caused by the irritation of the bladder, bladder neck, or urethral mucosa. Spasms are a distressing complication, but are usually self-limiting when procedure is followed (e.g., proper size and insertion of catheter, appropriate size and inflation of balloon). Note: Contractions may intensify when large indwelling urinary catheters with large-capacity balloons are inserted.*[10,20,21]

NURSING PRIORITY NO. 3 To promote wellness (Teaching/Discharge Instructions):

- Review individual needs regarding catheter self-management with client/SO[22] *to reduce risk of complications:*

Always wash hands before and after handling catheter.

Make sure that urine is flowing out of the catheter into collection bag.

Keep urine collection bag below level of bladder.

Make sure that catheter tubing does not get twisted or kinked.

Check for inflammation or signs of infection (e.g., pus or irritated, swollen, red, or tender skin) in the area around the catheter.

Clean the area around the catheter twice a day using soap and water. Dry with clean towel afterward.

Do not apply powder or lotion to the skin around the catheter.

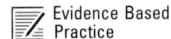

Do not tug or pull on the catheter.

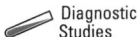

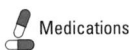

Follow physician instructions regarding catheter cleaning and/or replacement (if long-term indwelling), frequency of catheterization (if intermittent).

- Instruct client/caregiver in techniques to protect the integrity of skin. Refer to NDs risk for impaired Skin/Tissue Integrity and risk for Pressure Ulcer for related interventions.
- Instruct client/caregiver in reportable problems, such as leaking, sediment in urine, absence of urine, presence of pain, etc. *In one large-scale study regarding catheter problems, 43% experienced leakage, 31% had a UTI, 24% had blockage of the catheter, 23% had catheter-associated pain, and 12% had accidental dislodgement of the catheter.*[23]
- Identify resources available to the individual (e.g., substance abuse or rehabilitation, needle-exchange program as appropriate; available or free condoms).

DOCUMENTATION FOCUS

Assessment/Reassessment

- Individual risk factors, noting current physical findings.
- Client's/caregiver's understanding of individual risks and safety concerns.

Planning

- Plan of care and who is involved in planning.
- Teaching plan.

Implementation/Evaluation

- Individual responses to interventions, teaching, and actions performed.
- Specific actions and changes that are made.
- Attainment or progress toward desired outcome(s).
- Modifications to plan of care.

Discharge Planning

- Long-term plans for discharge needs, lifestyle and community changes, and who is responsible for actions to be taken.
- Specific referrals made.

References

1. Brusch, J. L. (2013). Catheter-related urinary tract infection. Medscape. Retrieved February 2015 from http://emedicine.medscape.com/article/2040035-overview#showall.
2. Jain, P., Parada, A., Smith, L. G. (1995). Overuse of the indwelling urinary tract catheter in hospitalized medical patients. *Arch Intern Med*, 155(13), 1425–1429.
3. Hart, S. (2008). Urinary catheterization. *Nursing Standard*, 22(27), 44–48.
4. Crippa, M., Belleri, L., Mistrello, G., et al. (2006). Prevention of latex allergy among health care workers and in the general population: Latex protein content in devices commonly used in hospitals and general practice. *Int Arch Occup Environ Health*, 79(7), 550–557.
5. Schumm, K., Lam, T. B. (2008). Types of urethral catheters for management of short-term voiding problems in hospitalised adults. *Cochrane Database Syst Rev*, April 16(2), CD004013.
6. Saint, S., Wiese, J., Amory, J. K., et al. (2000). Are physicians aware of which of their patients have indwelling urinary catheters? *Am J Med*, 109(6), 476–480.
7. Fakih, M. G., Dueweke, C., Miesner, S., et al. (2008). Effect of nurse-led multidisciplinary rounds on reducing the unnecessary use of urinary catheterization in hospitalized patients. *Infect Control Hosp*, 29(9), 815–819.
8. Centers for Disease Control and Prevention. (2009). Guideline for prevention of catheter-associated urinary tract infections, 2009. Retrieved February 2015 from http://www.cdc.gov/hicpac/cauti/02_cauti2009_abbrev.html.
9. Carlson, D., Mowery, B. D. (1997). Standards to prevent complications of urinary catheterization in children: Should and should-knots. *J Soc Pediatr Nurs*, 2(1), 37–41.

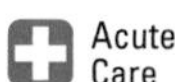
Acute Care
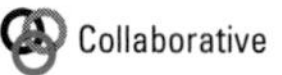
Collaborative
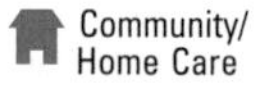
Community/Home Care
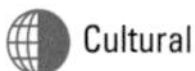
Cultural

10. Winson, L. (1997). Catheterization: A need for improved patient management. *Br J Nurs*, 6(21), 1229–1252.
11. Chen, A. K. (No date). Catheterization without tears: Expert offers a guide to bladder catheterization in children. Advance Healthcare Network for Nurses. Retrieved February 2015 from http://nursing.advanceweb.com/article/catheterization-without-tears.aspx.
12. Westbrook, I. P. (2000). Catheter design and selection. In *Introduction to Urological Nursing*. Downey, P. (ed.). Hoboken, NJ: John Wiley & Sons.
13. No author listed. (No date). Foley catheter placement. Retrieved February 2015 from professionals.sw.org/resources/docs/authorized/ome/foleycatheterplacement2.pdf.
14. Hospice Education Institute. (No date). Urinary catheters. Retrieved February 2015 from https://www.hospiceworld.org/book/urinary-catheters.htm.
15. Macaulay, M. (1994). Urinary drainage systems. In *Urol Nursing*. Laker, C. (ed.). London, UK: Scutari Press.
16. Wound, Ostomy and Continence Nurses Society. (2012). Indwelling urinary catheter securement: Best practice for clinicians. Retrieved February 2015 from http://www.faet.org/docs/indwellingurinarycathetersecurement.pdf.
17. Gray, M. L. (2008). Securing the indwelling catheter. *Am J Nurs*, 108(12), 44–50.
18. Siegel, T. J. (2008). The ins and outs of urinary catheters. Evidence-based management. *Advance Nurs Pract*, 16(8), 57–60.
19. Care Pathways. (No date). Belly Bag urinary drainage bag. Retrieved February 2015 from http://www.carepathways.com/estore-cat-Incon.cfm?Title=Belly+Bag+Urinary+Drainage+Bag.
20. Kelly, T. W., Griffiths, G. L. (1983). Balloon problems with foley catheters. *Lancet*, 2(8362), 1310.
21. Sulzbach, L. M. (2002). Ask the Experts (questions regarding catheter management). *Crit Care Nurse*, 22(84), 87.
22. WebMD Staff. (2013). Care for an indwelling urinary catheter: Fact sheet for public education. Retrieved February 2015 from http://www.webmd.com/a-to-z-guides/care-for-an-indwelling-urinary-catheter-topic-overview.
23. Wilde, M., McDonald, M. V., Brasch, J., et al. (2013). Long term users self-care practices and problems. *J Clin Nurs*, 22(356), 367.

Insomnia

Taxonomy II: Activity/Rest—Class 1 Sleep/Rest (00095) [**Diagnostic Division:** Activity/Rest], Submitted 2006

DEFINITION: A disruption in amount and quality of sleep that impairs functioning.

RELATED FACTORS

Alcohol consumption; pharmaceutical agent; hormonal change
Stressors; depression; fear; anxiety; grieving
Inadequate sleep hygiene; frequent naps
Average daily physical activity is less than recommended for gender and age
Physical discomfort
Environmental barrier (e.g., ambient noise, daylight/darkness exposure, ambient temperature/humidity, unfamiliar setting)

DEFINING CHARACTERISTICS

Subjective

Difficulty initiating or maintaining sleep; early awaking; alteration in sleep pattern
Dissatisfaction with sleep; nonrestorative sleep pattern (e.g., due to caregiver responsibilities, parenting practices, sleep partner)
Sleep disturbance producing next-day consequences; insufficient energy

(continues on page 486)

Insomnia (continued)
Decrease in quality of life; compromised health status
Increase in accidents

Objective
Alteration in concentration
Alteration in mood/affect
Increase in absenteeism
Sample Clinical Applications: Chronic pain, substance use or abuse, hyperthyroidism, pulmonary diseases (e.g., COPD, asthma), sleep apnea, restless leg syndrome, depression, Alzheimer's disease, senile dementia, anxiety disorders, bipolar disorders, pregnancy—prenatal or postnatal period

DESIRED OUTCOMES/EVALUATION CRITERIA

Sample NOC linkages:
Fatigue Level: Severity of observed or reported prolonged generalized fatigue
Sleep: Natural periodic suspension of consciousness during which the body is restored
Rest: Quality and pattern of diminished activity for mental and physical rejuvenation

Client Will (Include Specific Time Frame)
- Verbalize understanding of sleep impairment.
- Identify individually appropriate interventions to promote sleep.
- Adjust lifestyle to accommodate chronobiological rhythms.
- Report improvement in sleep or rest pattern.
- Report increased sense of well-being and feeling rested.

ACTIONS/INTERVENTIONS

Sample NIC linkages:
Sleep Enhancement: Facilitation of regular sleep/wake cycles
Relaxation Therapy: Use of techniques to encourage and elicit relaxation for the purpose of decreasing undesirable signs and symptoms such as pain, muscle tension, or anxiety
Environmental Management: Manipulation of the patient's surroundings for therapeutic benefit, sensory appeal, and psychological well-being; promotion of optimal comfort

NURSING PRIORITY NO. 1 To identify causative/contributing factors:

- Identify presence of Related Factors that can contribute to insomnia (e.g., chronic pain, arthritis, dyspnea; movement disorders; dementia; obesity; pregnancy, menopause; psychiatric disorders); metabolic diseases (e.g., hyperthyroidism and diabetes); prescribed and over-the-counter (OTC) drugs; alcohol, stimulant, or other recreational drug use; circadian rhythm disorders (e.g., shift work, jet lag); environmental factors (e.g., noise, no control over thermostat, uncomfortable bed); major life stressors (e.g., grief, loss, finances).[1–5,9,10]
- Note client age. *Increased sleep latency (time required to fall asleep), decreased sleep efficiency, and increased awakenings are common in the elderly. Two primary sleep disorders that increase with age are sleep apnea and periodic limb movements in sleep.*[2,9]
- Observe parent-infant interactions and provision of emotional support. Note mother's sleep-wake pattern. *Lack of knowledge of infant cues or problem relationships may create tension interfering with sleep. Structured sleep routines based on adult schedules may not meet child's needs.*[6]
- Ascertain presence and frequency of enuresis, incontinence, or need for frequent nighttime voidings, thus interrupting sleep.[2,9]

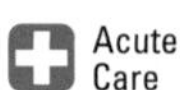

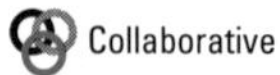

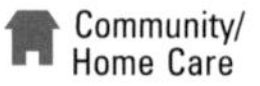

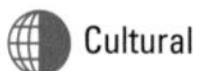

- Assist with or review psychological assessment, noting individual and personality characteristics *if anxiety disorders or depression could be affecting sleep.*[2,8,9,13]
- Determine recent traumatic events in client's life (e.g., a death in family, loss of job). *Physical and emotional trauma often affects client's sleep patterns and quality for a short period of time. This disruption can become long term and require more intensive assessment and intervention.*[2,3]
- Review client's medication regimen, including prescription (e.g., beta-blockers [e.g., metoprolol, propranolol], sedative antidepressants [e.g., amitriptyline], sedative neuroleptics [e.g., chlorpramazine, clozapine]; other antidepressants [e.g., floxetine]; steroids, antihypertensives, bronchodilators, weight-loss drugs, thyroid preparations, sedatives), OTC products (e.g., decongestants), and herbal remedies. *Use or timing may be interfering with falling asleep or staying asleep requiring adjustments such as change in dose or time medication is taken or choice of drug prescribed.*[7,9,10]
- Note caffeine and alcohol intake. *May interfere with falling asleep or duration and quality of sleep.*
- Assist with diagnostic testing (e.g., polysomnography, daytime multiple sleep latency testing, actigraphy, full-night sleep studies) *to determine cause and type of sleep disturbance. Note: Insomnia is a clinical diagnosis. Diagnostic studies are indicated principally for clarification of comorbid disorders.*[14]

NURSING PRIORITY NO. 2 To determine sleep pattern and dysfunction(s):

- Review sleep diary (where available); observe or obtain feedback from client/significant others (SOs) regarding client's sleep problems, usual bedtime, rituals or routines, number of hours of sleep, time of arising, and environmental needs *to determine usual sleep pattern and provide comparative baseline.*
- Listen to subjective reports of sleep quality (e.g., client never feels rested or feels excessively sleepy during day). *Provides opportunity to address misconceptions or unrealistic expectations and plan for interventions.*
- Determine type of insomnia (e.g., transient, short term, chronic). *Transient episodes are occasional restless nights caused by such factors as jet lag, first night in a new bed, and so forth. Short-term insomnia lasts a few weeks and arises from temporary stressful experience, such as pressures at work, loss of job, and death in family, and usually resolves over time as client adapts to stressor. Chronic insomnia lasts for more than 6 months and can be caused by many physical and psychological factors as well as use/misuse of medications and drugs.*[9,13]
- Investigate whether client snores and in what position(s) this occurs. Also determine if obese individual experiences loud periodic snoring, along with unusual nighttime activities (e.g., sitting upright, sleepwalking), and morning headaches, sleepiness, and/or depression. *Sleep studies may need to be done to rule out obstructive sleep disorder.*[2,4,14]
- Note alteration of habitual sleep time, such as change of work pattern or rotating shifts or change in normal bedtime (hospitalization). *Helps identify circumstances that are known to interrupt sleep patterns resulting in mental and physical fatigue, affecting concentration, interest, energy, and appetite.*[5]
- Observe physical signs of fatigue (e.g., restlessness, hand tremors, thick speech, drowsiness).
- Assist with diagnostic testing (e.g., electroencephalogram, electrooculogram, electromyogram; psychological assessment/testing, chronological chart). *Polysomnography tests (the three electrical tests noted above) are performed in a sleep laboratory to measure several parameters of sleep, including brain wave activity, eye movement, and leg muscle tone. These tests may be performed after initial clinical evaluation or symptom management fails to discover or resolve a particular sleep disturbance or point to appropriate interventions and treatments.*[1,2,4]

NURSING PRIORITY NO. 3 To assist client to establish optimal sleep/rest patterns:

- Collaborate in treatment of underlying medical and psychiatric problem (e.g., obstructive sleep apnea, pain, gastroesophageal reflux disease, lower urinary tract infection/prostatic hypertropy; depression, bipolar disorder; complicated grief).
- Assist client with implementing measures to manage sleep problems when in facility care:[9,11,14]
Arrange care to provide for uninterrupted periods of rest. *Allows for longer periods of sleep, especially during night.*

Provide quiet environment and comfort measures (e.g., back rub, washing hands and face, cleaning and straightening sheets). *Promotes relaxation and readiness for sleep.*

Administer pain medications (if required) 1 hr before sleep *to relieve discomfort and take maximum advantage of analgesic and sedative effect.*

Discuss and implement effective age-appropriate bedtime rituals (e.g., going to bed at same time each night, drinking warm milk, rocking, story reading, cuddling, favorite blanket or toy) *to enhance client's relaxation, reinforce that bed is a place to sleep, and promote sense of security for child or confused elder.*[6,9]

- Limit fluid intake in evening if nocturia is a problem *to reduce need for nighttime elimination.* Suggest avowing chocolate and caffeinated or alcoholic beverages, especially prior to bedtime. *Substances known to impair falling asleep or staying asleep. Alcohol may help individual fall asleep, but ensuing sleep is fragmented.*[6]
- Explore other sleep aids (e.g., warm bath or milk, light protein snack before bedtime, soothing music, favorite TV show). *Nonpharmaceutical aids may enhance falling asleep free of concern of medication side effects such as morning hangover or drug dependence.*
- Develop behavioral program for insomnia, such as:[1–5,9,10,14,15]
  establishing regular sleeping and waking-up time, and maintaining a routine at bedtime and arising;
  thinking relaxing thoughts when in bed;
  avoiding napping in the daytime;
  exercising daily, but not immediately before bedtime;
  avoiding heavy meals at bedtime;
  using bed only for sleeping or sex;
  wearing comfortable, loose-fitting clothing to bed;
  refraining from reading or watching TV in bed;
  getting out of bed if not asleep in 15 to 30 min and participating in relaxing activity until sleepy;
  getting up at the same time each day—even on weekends and days off;
  getting adequate exposure to bright light during day; and
  individually tailoring a stress-reduction program, music therapy, and/or relaxation routine.
- Recommend and assist with implementing program to "reset" sleep clock (chronotherapy when client has delayed sleep-onset insomnia). *These sleep-wake problems are common among shift workers and airplane travelers. Shift workers can benefit by adhering to a set routine and ensuring that noises and interruptions are kept to a minimum. Those who travel across time zones can benefit by adjusting their sleep time to match the time zone of their arrival and avoiding caffeine and alcohol.*[5]
- Use barbiturates or other sleeping medications sparingly. *Research indicates long-term use of these medications, especially in the absence of cognitive behavioral therapy (CBT), fails to show long-term benefit and can actually induce sleep disturbances.*[16]
- Encourage routine use of continuous positive airway pressure therapy when indicated *to obtain optimal benefit of treatment for sleep apnea.*
- Monitor effects of therapeutic use of amphetamines or stimulants (such as may be used for attention deficit disorder or narcolepsy). *Use of these medications can induce or potentiate sleep disturbances.*[7]
- Administer and monitor effects of prescribed medications to promote sleep (e.g., *benzodiazapines* such as zolpidem [Ambien], zaleplon [Sonata], eszopiclone [Lunesta]), *antidepressants* (e.g., trazodone [Desyrel], nefazodone [Serzone]), and *melatonin agonists* (e.g., ramelteon [Rozrem]). *Many medications may be tried to manage insomnia. While most are effective in the short term, many lose effectiveness over time. The client may have adverse side effects or develop tolerance and misuse the drug. Many drug regimens are most effective when combined with CBT, in which the client can be weaned off medications at some point.*[9,14]
- Refer to sleep specialist as indicated or desired. *Follow-up evaluation and intervention may be needed when insomnia is having a serious impact on client's quality of life, productivity, and safety (e.g., on the job, at home, on the road). Note: Studies show that the most effective treatment for primary insomnia is CBT. Techniques are used to ameliorate factors that perpetuate or exacerbate chronic insomnia, such as poor sleep habits, hyperarousal, irregular sleep schedules, inadequate sleep hygiene, and misconceptions about sleep and the consequences of insomnia.*[2,12,16]

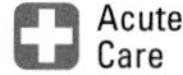

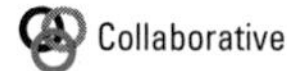

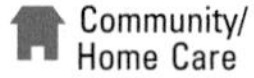

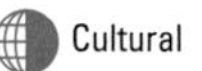

NURSING PRIORITY NO. 4 To promote wellness (Teaching/Discharge Considerations):

- Assure client that occasional sleeplessness should not threaten health. *Knowledge that occasional insomnia is universal and usually not harmful may promote relaxation and relief from worry, which can perpetuate the problem.*[4]
- Assist client to develop individual program of relaxation. Demonstrate techniques (e.g., biofeedback, self-hypnosis, visualization, progressive muscle relaxation). *Methods that reduce sympathetic response and decrease stress can help induce sleep, particularly in persons suffering from chronic and long-term sleep disturbances.*[3]
- Encourage participation in regular exercise program during day *to aid in stress control and release of energy. Note: Exercise at bedtime may stimulate rather than relax client and actually interfere with sleep.*[2]
- Investigate use of aids (e.g., sleep mask, darkening shades or curtains, earplugs, monotonous sounds [white noise]) *to block out ambient light and noise.*
- Assist individuals with insomnia associated with shift work to develop individual schedule *to take advantage of peak performance times as identified in chronobiological chart.*
- Recommend midmorning nap if one is required. *Napping, especially in the afternoon, can disrupt normal sleep patterns.*
- Assist client to deal with grieving process if grief is causing or exacerbating insomnia. (Refer to ND Grieving.)

DOCUMENTATION FOCUS

Assessment/Reassessment

- Assessment findings, including specifics of sleep pattern (current and past) and effects on lifestyle and level of functioning.
- Medications, interventions, and previous therapies tried.
- Results of testing.

Planning

- Plan of care and who is involved in planning.
- Teaching plan.

Implementation/Evaluation

- Client's response to interventions, teaching, and actions performed.
- Attainment or progress toward desired outcome(s).
- Modifications to plan of care.

Discharge Planning

- Long-term needs and who is responsible for actions to be taken.
- Specific referrals made.

References

1. National Sleep Foundation. What to do when you can't sleep. Retrieved October 2015 from https://sleepfoundation.org/insomnia/content/what-do-when-you-cant-sleep.
2. Krishnan, P., Hawranik, P. (2008). Diagnosis and management of geriatric insomnia: A guide for nurse practitioners. *Nurse Pract*, 20(12), 590–599.
3. Newfield, S. A., Hinz, M. D., Tilley, D. S., et al. (2007). *Cox's Clinical Applications of Nursing Diagnosis: Adult, Child, Women's, Psychiatric, Gerontic, and Home Health Considerations.* 5th ed. Philadelphia: F. A. Davis.
4. Brain basics: Understanding sleep. (Update 2014). National Institute of Neurological Disorders and Stroke. Retrieved October 2015 from www.ninds.nih.gov/disorders/brain_basics/understanding_sleep.htm.
5. Kam, K. (2011). Sleep and the night shift: Could you have work sleep disorder? Retrieved October 2015 from http://www.webmd.com/sleep-disorders/excessive-sleepiness-10/night-shift-sleep.
6. London, M., Ladewig, P. W., Ball, J. W., et al. (2010). *Maternal and Child Nursing Care.* 3rd ed. Upper Saddle River, NJ: Prentice Hall.

7. Deglin, J. H., Vallerand, A. H., Sanoski, C. A. (2011). *Davis's Drug Guide for Nurses.* 12th ed. Philadelphia: F. A. Davis.
8. Townsend, M. C. (2011). *Psychiatric Mental Health Nursing: Concepts of Care in Evidence-Based Practice.* 7th ed. Philadelphia: F. A. Davis.
9. Gentili, A., Brannon, G. E., Vij, S. (Updated 2014). Geriatric sleep disorder. Retrieved October 2015 from http://emedicine.medscape.com/article/292498-overview.
10. Hertz, G., Cataletto, M. E. (Updated 2014). Sleep dysfunction in women. Retrieved October 2015 from http://emedicine.medscape.com/article/1189087-overview.
11. Turkowski, B. B. (2006). Managing insomnia. *Orthop Nurs*, 25(5), 339–345.
12. Nadolski, M. (2005). Getting a good night's sleep: Diagnosing and treating insomnia. *Plast Surg Nurs*, 25(4), 167–173.
13. Spielman, A. J., Caruso, L. S., Glovinsky, P. B. (1987). A behavioral perspective on insomnia treatment. *Psychiatr Clin North Am*, 10(4), 541–543.
14. Chawla, J., Passaro, E. A., Park, Y., et al. (2015). Insomnia. Retrieved October 2015 from http://emedicine.medscape.com/article/1187829-overview.
15. Schutte-Rodin, S., Broch, L., Buysse, D., et al. (2008). Clinical guideline for the evaluation and management of chronic insomnia in adults. *J Clin Sleep Med*, 15(4), 487–504.
16. Morin, C. M., Vallieres, A., Guay, B., et al. (2009). Cognitive behavioral therapy, singly and combined with medication, for persistent insomnia. *JAMA*, 301(19), 2005–2015.

neonatal Jaundice

Taxonomy II: Nutrition—Class 4 Metabolism (00194) [**Diagnostic Division:** Safety], Submitted 2008; Revised 2010

DEFINITION: The yellow-orange tint of the neonate's skin and mucous membranes that occurs after 24 hours of life as a result of unconjugated bilirubin in the circulation.

RELATED FACTORS

Age <7 days
Deficient feeding pattern
Unintentional weight loss [>7%–8% in breastfeeding newborn; 15% in term infant]
Delay in meconium passage
Infant experiences difficulty making the transition to extrauterine life

DEFINING CHARACTERISTICS

Objective

Yellow-orange skin color; yellow sclera, mucous membranes
Bruised skin
Abnormal blood profile [e.g., hemolysis; total serum bilirubin >2 mg/dL; total serum bilirubin in high-risk range on age in hour-specific nomogram]
Sample Clinical Applications: Newborn, premature infant

DESIRED OUTCOMES/EVALUATION CRITERIA

Sample NOC linkages:

Newborn Adaptation: Adaptive response to the extrauterine environment by a physiologically mature newborn during the first 28 days

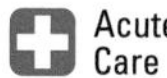
Acute Care
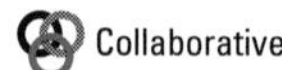
Collaborative
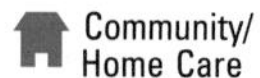
Community/ Home Care
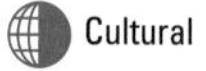
Cultural

Infant Will (Include Specific Time Frame):

- Display decreasing bilirubin levels with resolution of jaundice.
- Be free of central nervous system (CNS) involvement or complications associated with therapeutic regimen.

Sample NOC linkages:

Knowledge: Treatment Procedure: Extent of understanding conveyed about a procedure required as part of a treatment regimen

Parent/Caregiver Will (Include Specific Time Frame):

- Verbalize understanding of cause, treatment, and possible outcomes of hyperbilirubinemia.
- Demonstrate appropriate care of infant.

ACTIONS/INTERVENTIONS

Sample NIC linkages:

Newborn Monitoring: Measurement and interpretation of physiology status of the neonate for the first 24 hours after delivery

Phototherapy: Neonate: Use of light therapy to reduce bilirubin levels in newborn infants

Breastfeeding Assistance: Preparing a new mother to breastfeed her infant

NURSING PRIORITY NO. 1 To assess causative/contributing factors:

- Determine infant and maternal blood group and blood type. *ABO incompatibilities affect 20% of all pregnancies and most commonly occur in mothers with type O blood, whose anti-A and anti-B antibodies pass into fetal circulation, causing red blood cell (RBC) agglutination and hemolysis.*[1]
- Note gender, race, and place of birth. *Risk of developing jaundice is higher in males, infants of East Asian or American Indian descent, and those living at high altitudes. Incidence is lower for African American infants.*[2]
- Review intrapartal record for specific risk factors, such as low birth weight (LBW) or intrauterine growth retardation, prematurity, abnormal metabolic processes, vascular injuries, abnormal circulation, sepsis, or polycythemia. *The risk of significant neonatal jaundice is increased in LBW or premature infants, presence of congenital infection, or maternal diabetes.*[2] *Studies suggest neonates at 36 to 37 weeks' gestation are four to five times more likely to develop hyperbilirubinemia than those born at 40 weeks.*[3] *Also, certain clinical conditions may cause a reversal of the blood-brain barrier, allowing bound bilirubin to separate either at the level of the cell membrane or within the cell itself, increasing the risk of CNS involvement.*
- Note use of instruments or vacuum extractor for delivery. Assess infant for presence of birth trauma, cephalohematoma, and excessive ecchymosis or petechiae. *Resorption of blood trapped in fetal scalp tissue and excessive hemolysis may increase the amount of bilirubin being released and cause jaundice.*[7]
- Review infant's condition at birth, noting need for resuscitation or evidence of excessive ecchymosis or petechiae, cold stress, asphyxia, or acidosis. *Asphyxia and acidosis reduce affinity of bilirubin to albumin increasing the amount of unbound circulating (indirect) bilirubin, which may cross the blood-brain barrier, causing CNS toxicity.*[2]
- Evaluate maternal and prenatal nutritional levels; note possible neonatal hypoproteinemia, especially in the preterm infant. *One gram of albumin carries 16 mg of unconjugated bilirubin; therefore, lack of sufficient albumin (hypoproteinemia) in the newborn increases risk of jaundice.*
- Assess infant for signs of hypoglycemia such as jitteriness, irritability, and lethargy. Obtain heelstick glucose levels as indicated. *Hypoglycemia necessitates use of fat stores for energy-releasing fatty acids, which compete with bilirubin for binding sites on albumin.*
- Determine successful initiation and adequacy of breastfeeding. *Poor caloric intake and dehydration associated with ineffective breastfeeding increase risk of developing hyperbilirubinemia.*[1]

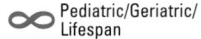

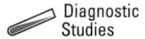

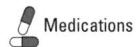

- Evaluate infant for pallor, edema, or hepatosplenomegaly. *These signs may be associated with hydrops fetalis, Rh incompatibility, and in utero hemolysis of fetal RBCs.*
- Evaluate for jaundice in natural light, noting sclera and oral mucosa, yellowing of skin immediately after blanching, and specific body parts involved. Assess oral mucosa, posterior portion of hard palate, and conjunctival sacs in dark-skinned newborns. *Detects evidence/degree of jaundice generally first noted on face and progressing to trunk and then extremities.*[1,6] *Clinical appearance of jaundice is evident at bilirubin levels greater than 5 mg/dL in the full-term infant. Estimated degree of jaundice is as follows: face, 4 to 8 mg/dL; trunk, 10 to 12 mg/dL; groin, 8 to 16 mg/dL; arms/legs, 11 to 18 mg/dL; and hands/feet, 15 to 20 mg/dL. Note: Yellow underlying pigment may be normal in dark-skinned infants.*[1,6,7]
- Note infant's age at onset of jaundice. *Aids in differentiating type of jaundice (i.e., physiological, breast milk induced, or pathological). Physiological jaundice usually appears between the second and third days of life, as excess RBCs needed to maintain adequate oxygenation for the fetus are no longer required in the newborn and are hemolyzed, thereby releasing bilirubin.*[2,6] *Breast milk jaundice usually appears between the fourth and the seventh days of life, affecting approximately 14% of breastfed infants.*[6] *Pathological jaundice occurs within the first 24 hours of life or when the total serum bilirubin level rises by more than 5 mg/dL per day.*[2,7]

NURSING PRIORITY NO. 2 To evaluate degree of compromise:

- Review laboratory studies, including total serum bilirubin and albumin levels, hemoglobin/hematocrit, and reticulocyte count, *to monitor severity of problem and need for, or effectiveness, of therapy.*[2] *Note: Excessive unconjugated bilirubin has an affinity for extravascular tissue, including the basal ganglia of brain tissue.*[7]
- Calculate plasma bilirubin-albumin–binding capacity. *Aids in determining risk of kernicterus and treatment needs.*[1] *When total bilirubin value divided by total serum protein level is less than 3.7, the danger of kernicterus is very low. However, the risk of injury is dependent on factors such as degree of prematurity, presence of hypoxia or acidosis, and drug regimen (e.g., sulfonamides, chloramphenicol).*[7]
- Assess infant for progression of signs and behavioral changes associated with bilirubin toxicity. *Early-stage toxicity involves neurodepression (lethargy, poor feeding, high-pitched cry, diminished or absent reflexes), late-stage hypotonia, and neuro-hyperreflexia (twitching, convulsions, opisthotonos, fever). Behavior changes associated with kernicterus usually occur between the 3rd and 10th days of life and rarely occur prior to 36 hours of life.*
- Evaluate appearance of skin and urine, noting brownish-black color. *An uncommon side effect of phototherapy, particularly in presence of cholestatic jaundice, involves exaggerated pigment changes (bronze baby syndrome), which may occur if conjugated bilirubin levels rise. The changes in skin color may last for 2 to 4 months but are not associated with harmful sequelae.*

NURSING PRIORITY NO. 3 To correct hyperbilirubinemia and prevent associated complications:

- Keep infant warm and dry; monitor skin and core temperature frequently. *Prevents cold stress and the release of fatty acids that compete for binding sites on albumin, thus increasing the level of freely circulating bilirubin.*
- Initiate early oral feedings within 4 to 6 hours following birth, especially if infant is to be breastfed. *Establishes proper intestinal flora necessary for reduction of bilirubin to urobilinogen and decreases reabsorption of bilirubin from bowel by promoting passage of meconium stool.*[7]
- Encourage frequent breastfeeding—8 to 12 times per day. Assist mother with pumping of breasts as needed to maintain milk production. *Interruption of breastfeeding is rarely necessary unless serum levels reach 20 mg/dL; however, breastfeeding support may increase frequency and efficacy of intake.*[2,5–7]
- Administer small amounts of breast milk substitute (L-aspartic acid or enzymatically hydrolyzed casein) for 24 to 48 hours if indicated. *Use of feeding additives is under investigation with mixed results for inhibition of beta-glucuronidase leading to increased fecal excretion of bilirubin.*[4,5]
- Apply transcutaneous jaundice meter, as indicated. *Provides noninvasive screening of jaundice, quantifying skin color in relation to total serum bilirubin.*

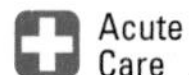

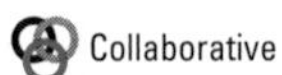

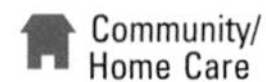

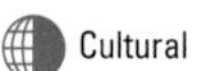

- Initiate phototherapy per protocol, using fluorescent bulbs placed above the infant or a fiberoptic pad or blanket (except for newborn with Rh disease). *Primary therapy for neonates with unconjugated hyperbilirubinemia. Three separate processes work to convert bilirubin isomers to water-soluble isomers and the formation of lumirubin. The photoisomers are then excreted in urine, stool, and bile.*[2]
- Apply eye patches ensuring correct fit during periods of phototherapy *to prevent retinal injury*. Remove eye covering during feedings or other care activities as appropriate *to provide visual stimulation and interaction with caregivers/parents.*[8]
- Avoid application of lotion or oils to skin of infant receiving phototherapy *to prevent dermal irritation or injury.*[8]
- Reposition infant every 2 hours *to ensure all areas of skin are exposed to bili light when fiberoptic pad or blanket is not used.*[8]
- Cover male groin with small pad *to protect from heat-related injury to testes.*[8]
- Monitor infant's weight loss, urine output and specific gravity, and fecal water loss from loose stools associated with phototherapy *to determine adequacy of fluid intake.*[2] *Note: Infant may sleep for longer periods in conjunction with phototherapy, increasing risk of dehydration if frequent feeding schedule is not maintained.*
- Administer intravenous immunoglobulin (IVIG) to neonates with Rh or ABO isoimmunization. *Rate of hemolysis in Rh disease or other cases of immune hemolytic jaundice usually exceeds the rate of bilirubin reduction related to phototherapy. IVIG inhibits antibodies that cause red cell destruction helping to limit the rise in bilirubin levels.*[2–5]
- Administer enzyme induction agent (phenobarbital) as appropriate. *May be used on occasion to stimulate hepatic enzymes to enhance clearance of bilirubin.*[2]
- Assist with preparation and administration of exchange transfusion. *Exchange transfusions are occasionally required in cases of severe hemolytic anemia unresponsive to other treatment options or in the presence of acute bilirubin encephalopathy, as evidenced by hypertonia, arching, retrocollis, opisthotonos, fever, and high-pitched cry.*[1,2] *Procedure removes serum bilirubin and provides bilirubin-free albumin, increasing binding sites for bilirubin, and it treats anemia by providing RBCs that are not susceptible to maternal antibodies.*
- Document events during transfusion, carefully recording amount of blood withdrawn and injected (usually 7–20 mL at a time). *Helps prevent errors in fluid replacement. Amount of blood exchanged is approximately 170 mL/kg of body weight. A double-volume exchange ensures that between 75% and 90% of circulating RBCs are replaced.*

NURSING PRIORITY NO. 4 To promote wellness (Teaching/Discharge Considerations):

- Provide information about types of jaundice and pathophysiological factors and future implications of hyperbilirubinemia. *Promotes understanding, corrects misconceptions, and may reduce fear and feelings of guilt.*
- Review means of assessing infant status (feedings, intake/output, stools, temperature, serial weights if scale available) and for monitoring increasing bilirubin levels (e.g., observing blanching of skin over bony prominence or behavior changes), especially if infant is to be discharged early. *Enables parents to monitor infant's progress and to recognize signs of increasing bilirubin levels. Note: Persistence of jaundice beyond 2 weeks in formula-fed infant or 3 weeks in breastfed infant requires further evaluation.*[7]
- Provide parents with 24-hour emergency telephone number and name of contact person, stressing importance of reporting increased jaundice or changes in behavior. *Promotes independence and provides for timely evaluation and intervention.* Refer to lactation specialist *to enhance or reestablish breastfeeding process.*[6]
- Arrange appropriate referral for home phototherapy program if necessary. *Lack of available support systems may necessitate use of visiting nurse to monitor home phototherapy program.*
- Provide written explanation of home phototherapy, safety precautions, and potential problems. *Home phototherapy is recommended only for full-term infants after the first 48 hours of life whose serum bilirubin levels are between 14 and 18 mg/dL, with no increase in direct-reacting bilirubin concentration.*
- Make appropriate arrangements for follow-up testing of serum bilirubin at same laboratory facility. *Treatment is discontinued once serum bilirubin concentrations fall below 14 mg/dL. Untreated or chronic*

hyperbilirubinemia can lead to permanent damage, such as high-pitch hearing loss, cerebral palsy, or mental retardation. [7]

- Discuss possible long-term effects of hyperbilirubinemia and the need for continued assessment and early intervention. *Neurologic damage associated with kernicterus includes cerebral palsy, mental retardation, sensory difficulties, delayed speech, learning difficulties, and death.*

DOCUMENTATION FOCUS

Assessment/Reassessment

- Assessment findings, risk or related factors.
- Adequacy of intake—hydration level, character and number of stools.
- Laboratory results—bilirubin trends.

Planning

- Plan of care, specific interventions, and who is involved in the planning.
- Teaching plan and resources provided.

Implementation/Evaluation

- Client's responses to treatment and actions performed.
- Parents' understanding of teaching.
- Attainment or progress toward desired outcome(s).
- Modifications to plan of care.

Discharge Planning

- Long-term needs, identifying who is responsible for actions to be taken.
- Community resources for equipment and supplies postdischarge.
- Specific referrals made.

References

1. American Academy of Pediatrics. (2004). Treatment of hyperbilirubinema in the newborn infant 35 or more weeks of gestation. *Pediatrics*, 114(1), 297–316.
2. Hansen, T. W. R. (Updated 2014). Neonatal jaundice. Retrieved March 2015 from http://emedicine.medscape.com/article/974786-overview.
3. Sarici, S. U., Serdar, M. A., Korkmaz, A., et al. (2004). Incidence, course, and prediction of hyperbilirubinemia in near-term and term newborns. *Pediatrics*, 113(4), 775–780.
4. Gourley, G. R., Li, Z., Kreamer, B. L., et al. (2005). A controlled, randomized, double-blind trial of prophylaxis against jaundice among breastfed newborns. *Pediatrics*, 116(2), 385–391.
5. Canadian Paediatric Society Position Statement. (2007). Guidelines for detection, management and prevention of hyperbilirubinemia in term and late preterm newborn infants (35 or more weeks' gestation). *Paediatr Child Health*, 12(suppl B), 1B–12B.
6. Deshpande, P. G. (Updated 2014). Breast milk jaundice. Retrieved March 2015 from http://emedicine.medscape.com/article/973629-overview.
7. Porter, M. L., Dennis, B. L. (2002). Hyperbilirubinemia in the term newborn. *Am Fam Physician*, 65(4), 599–606.
8. Springhouse (eds.). (2008). Phototherapy. *Lippincott's Nursing Procedures*. 5th ed. Philadelphia: Lippincott Williams & Wilkins.

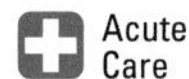

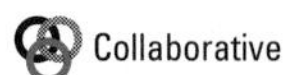

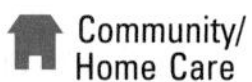

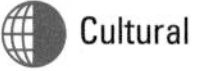

risk for neonatal Jaundice

Taxonomy II: Nutrition—Class 4 Metabolism (00230) [**Diagnostic Division:** Safety], Submitted 2010; Revised 2013

DEFINITION: Vulnerable to the yellow-orange tint of the neonate's skin and mucous membranes that occur after 24 hours of life as a result of unconjugated bilirubin in the circulation, which may compromise health.

RISK FACTORS

Age < 7 days; prematurity
Feeding pattern not well established
Abnormal weight loss (>7%–8% in breastfeeding newborn; 15% in nonbreastfeeding newborn)
Delay in meconium passage
Infant experiences difficulty making the transition to extrauterine life
Note: A risk diagnosis is not evidenced by signs and symptoms, as the problem has not occurred; rather, nursing interventions are directed at prevention.
Sample Clinical Applications: Newborn, premature infant

DESIRED OUTCOMES/EVALUATION CRITERIA

Sample NOC linkages:
Newborn Adaptation: Adaptive response to the extrauterine environment by a physiologically mature newborn during the first 28 days

Infant Will (Include Specific Time Frame)
- Be free of signs of hyperbilirubinemia with normal bilirubin level
- Establish effective feeding pattern

Sample NOC linkages:
Risk Control: Personal actions to prevent, eliminate, or reduce modifiable health threats

Parent/Caregiver Will (Include Specific Time Frame)
- Verbalize understanding of cause, treatment, and possible outcomes of hyperbilirubinemia.
- Demonstrate appropriate care of infant.

ACTIONS/INTERVENTIONS

Sample NIC linkages:
Newborn Monitoring: Measurement and interpretation of physiologic status of the neonate the first 24 hours after delivery
Breastfeeding Assistance: Preparing a new mother to breastfeed her infant
Bottle Feeding: Preparation and administration of fluids to an infant via a bottle

NURSING PRIORITY NO. 1 To determine individual risk factors:

- Determine infant and maternal blood group and blood type. *ABO incompatibilities affect 20% of all pregnancies and most commonly occur in mothers with type O blood, whose anti-A and anti-B antibodies pass into fetal circulation, causing red blood cell (RBC) agglutination and hemolysis.*[1]
- Note gender, race, and place of birth. *Risk of developing jaundice is higher in males, infants of East Asian or American Indian descent, and those living at high altitudes. Incidence is lower for African American infants.*[2]

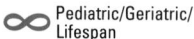

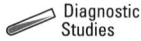

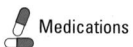

- Review intrapartal record for specific risk factors, such as low birth weight (LBW) or intrauterine growth retardation, prematurity, abnormal metabolic processes, vascular injuries, abnormal circulation, sepsis, or polycythemia. *The risk of significant neonatal jaundice is increased in LBW or premature infants, presence of congenital infection, or maternal diabetes.*[2] *Studies suggest neonates at 36 to 37 weeks' gestation are four to five times more likely to develop hyperbilirubinemia than those born at 40 weeks.*[3] *Also, certain clinical conditions may cause a reversal of the blood-brain barrier, allowing bound bilirubin to separate either at the level of the cell membrane or within the cell itself, increasing the risk of central nervous system (CNS) involvement.*
- Note use of instruments or vacuum extractor for delivery. Assess infant for presence of birth trauma, cephalohematoma, and excessive ecchymosis or petechiae. *Resorption of blood trapped in fetal scalp tissue and excessive hemolysis may increase the amount of bilirubin being released and cause jaundice.*[4]
- Review infant's condition at birth, noting need for resuscitation or evidence of excessive ecchymosis or petechiae, cold stress, asphyxia, or acidosis. *Asphyxia and acidosis reduce affinity of bilirubin to albumin increasing the amount of unbound circulating (indirect) bilirubin, which may cross the blood-brain barrier, causing CNS toxicity.*[2]
- Evaluate maternal and prenatal nutritional levels; note possible neonatal hypoproteinemia, especially in preterm infant. *One gram of albumin carries 16 mg of unconjugated bilirubin; therefore, lack of sufficient albumin (hypoproteinemia) in the newborn increases risk of jaundice.*
- Assess infant for signs of hypoglycemia such as jitteriness, irritability, and lethargy. Obtain heelstick glucose levels as indicated. *Hypoglycemia necessitates use of fat stores for energy-releasing fatty acids, which compete with bilirubin for binding sites on albumin.*
- Determine successful initiation and adequacy of breastfeeding. *Poor caloric intake and dehydration associated with ineffective breastfeeding increase risk of developing hyperbilirubinemia.*[1]
- Examine infant for pallor, edema, or hepatosplenomegaly. *These signs may be associated with hydrops fetalis, Rh incompatibility, and in-utero hemolysis of fetal RBCs.*
- Evaluate for jaundice in natural light, noting sclera and oral mucosa, yellowing of skin immediately after blanching, and specific body parts involved. Assess oral mucosa, posterior portion of hard palate, and conjunctival sacs in dark-skinned newborns. *Detects evidence/degree of jaundice generally first noted on face and progressing to trunk and then extremities.*[1,6] *Clinical appearance of jaundice is evident at bilirubin levels greater than 5 mg/dL in full-term infant. Estimated degree of jaundice is as follows: face, 4 to 8 mg/dL; trunk, 10 to 12 mg/dL; groin, 8 to 16 mg/dL; arms/legs, 11 to 18 mg/dL; and hands/feet, 15 to 20 mg/dL. Note: Yellow underlying pigment may be normal in dark-skinned infants.*[1,4,6]

NURSING PRIORITY NO. 2 To prevent onset of hyperbilirubinemia:

- Review laboratory studies, including total serum bilirubin and albumin levels, hemoglobin/hematocrit, and reticulocyte count, as indicated.
- Keep infant warm and dry; monitor skin and core temperature frequently. *Prevents cold stress and the release of fatty acids that compete for binding sites on albumin, thus increasing the level of freely circulating bilirubin.*
- Initiate early oral feedings within 4 to 6 hours following birth, especially if infant is to be breastfed. *Establishes proper intestinal flora necessary for reduction of bilirubin to urobilinogen and decreases reabsorption of bilirubin from bowel by promoting passage of meconium stool.*[4]
- Encourage frequent breastfeeding—8 to 12 times per day. Assist mother with pumping of breasts as needed to maintain milk production for hospitalized preterm infant. *Breastfeeding support may increase frequency and efficacy of intake.*[2,4,5]
- Administer intravenous immunoglobulin (IVIG) to neonates with Rh or ABO isoimmunization. *Rate of hemolysis in Rh disease or other cases of immune hemolytic jaundice usually exceeds the rate of bilirubin reduction related to phototherapy. IVIG inhibits antibodies that cause red cell destruction helping to limit the rise in bilirubin levels.*[2,5]

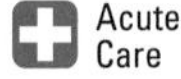

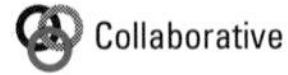

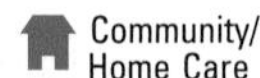

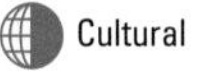

NURSING PRIORITY NO. 3 To promote wellness (Teaching/Discharge Considerations):

- Review means of assessing infant status (feedings, intake/output, stools, temperature, serial weights if scale available) and for monitoring increasing bilirubin levels (e.g., observing blanching of skin over bony prominence or behavior changes), especially if infant is to be discharged early. *Enables parents to monitor infant for early signs of increasing bilirubin levels.*[4]
- Provide parents with 24-hour emergency telephone number and name of contact person, stressing importance of reporting signs of jaundice or changes in infant's behavior. *Promotes independence and provides for timely evaluation and intervention.*
- Refer to lactation specialist as indicated *to assist with establishing/enhancing breastfeeding process.*
- Review proper formula preparation/storage and demonstrate feeding techniques *to meet nutritional and fluid needs.*
- Make arrangements for follow-up testing of serum bilirubin at same laboratory facility.

DOCUMENTATION FOCUS

Assessment/Reassessment

- Assessment findings, risk or related factors.
- Adequacy of intake—hydration level, character and number of stools.
- Laboratory results—bilirubin level.

Planning

- Plan of care, specific interventions, and who is involved in the planning.
- Teaching plan and resources provided.

Implementation/Evaluation

- Parents understanding of teaching.
- Attainment or progress toward desired outcome(s).
- Modifications to plan of care.

Discharge Planning

- Home care needs and who is responsible for actions to be taken.
- Any referrals made.

References

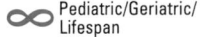

1. American Academy of Pediatrics. (2004). Treatment of hyperbilirubinema in the newborn infant 35 or more weeks of gestation. *Pediatrics*, 114(1), 297–316.
2. Hansen, T. W. R. (Updated 2014). Neonatal jaundice. Retrieved March 2015 from http://emedicine.medscape.com/article/974786-overview.
3. Sarici, S. U., Serdar, M. A., Korkmaz, A., et al. (2004). Incidence, course, and prediction of hyperbilirubinemia in near-term and term newborns. *Pediatrics*, 113(4), 775–780.
4. Porter, M. L., Dennis, B. L. (2002). Hyperbilirubinemia in the term newborn. *Am Fam Physician*, 65(4), 599–606.
5. Canadian Paediatric Society. (2007). Position Statement: Guidelines for detection, management and prevention of hyperbilirubinemia in term and late preterm newborn infants (35 or more weeks' gestation). *Paediatr Child Health*, 12(suppl B), 1B–12B.
6. Deshpande, P. G. (Updated 2014). Breast milk jaundice. Retrieved March 2015 from http://emedicine.medscape.com/article/973629-overview.

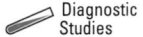

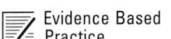

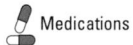

deficient Knowledge [Learning Need] [specify]

Taxonomy II: Perception/Cognition—Class 4 Cognition (00126) [**Diagnostic Division:** Teaching/Learning], Submitted 1980

DEFINITION: Absence or deficiency of cognitive information related to specific topic.

RELATED FACTORS

Insufficient information; insufficient knowledge of resources
Insufficient interest in learning
Misinformation presented by others
Alteration in cognitive functioning or memory
Insufficient interest in learning

DEFINING CHARACTERISTICS

Subjective

Insufficient knowledge

Objective

Inaccurate follow-through of instruction or performance on a test
Inappropriate behavior (e.g., hysterical, hostile, agitated, apathetic)
[Development of preventable complication)
Sample Clinical Applications: Any newly diagnosed disease or traumatic injury, progression of or deterioration in a chronic condition

DESIRED OUTCOMES/EVALUATION CRITERIA

Sample NOC linkages:
Knowledge: [specify—42 choices]: Extent of understanding conveyed about a specific disease process, the promotion and protection of health, maintaining optimal health, etc.
Information Processing: Ability to acquire, organize, and use information
Client Satisfaction: Teaching: Extent of positive perception of instruction provided by nursing staff to improve knowledge, understanding, and participation in care

Client Will (Include Specific Time Frame)

- Participate in learning process.
- Identify interferences to learning and specific action(s) to deal with them.
- Exhibit increased interest and assume responsibility for own learning by beginning to look for information and ask questions.
- Verbalize understanding of condition or disease process and treatment.
- Identify relationship of signs/symptoms to the disease process and correlate symptoms with causative factors.
- Perform necessary procedures correctly and explain reasons for the actions.
- Initiate necessary lifestyle changes and participate in treatment regimen.

ACTIONS/INTERVENTIONS

Sample NIC linkages:
Teaching: Individual [or 29 other choices]: Planning, implementation, and evaluation of a teaching program designed to address a patient's particular needs
Learning Facilitation: Promoting the ability to process and comprehend information
Learning Readiness Enhancement: Improving the ability and willingness to receive information

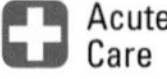

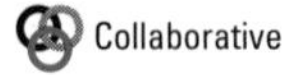

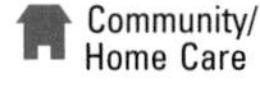

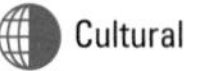

NURSING PRIORITY NO. 1 To assess readiness to learn and individual learning needs:

- Ascertain level of knowledge, including anticipatory needs. *Learning needs can include many things (e.g., disease cause and process, factors contributing to symptoms, procedures for symptom control, needed alterations in lifestyle, ways to prevent complications). Client may or may not ask for information or may express inaccurate perceptions of health status and needed behaviors to manage self-care.*[1]
- Engage in active listening. *Conveys expectation of confidence in client's ability to determine learning needs and best ways of meeting them.*[5]
- Determine client's ability and readiness and barriers to learning. *Client may not be physically, emotionally, or mentally capable at this time and may need time to work through and express emotions before learning.*[1]
- Be alert to signs of avoidance. *May need to allow client to suffer the consequences of lack of knowledge before client is ready to accept information.*[1]
- Identify significant others (SOs)/family members requiring information. Providing appropriate information to others can provide reinforcement for learning, as everyone will understand what is to be expected.[4]

NURSING PRIORITY NO. 2 To determine other factors pertinent to the learning process:

- Note personal factors (e.g., age, developmental level, gender, social and cultural influences, religion, life experiences, level of education, emotional stability) *that affect ability and desire to learn and assimilate new information, take control of situation, and accept responsibility for change.*[2,11]
- Determine blocks to learning, including (1) language barriers (e.g., can't read or write, speaks or understands a different language than that spoken by teacher); (2) physical factors (e.g., cognitive impairment, sensory deficits [e.g., aphasia, dyslexia, hearing or vision impairment]); (3) physical constraints (e.g., acute illness, activity intolerance, impaired thought processes); (4) complexity of material to be learned (e.g., caring for colostomy, giving own insulin injections); (5) forced change in lifestyle (e.g., smoking cessation); or (6) have stated no need or desire to learn. *Many factors affect the client's ability and desire to learn, and his or her expectations of the learning process must be addressed if learning is to be successful.*[1,11]
- Assess the level of the client's capabilities and the possibilities of the situation. *May need to assist SO(s) or caregivers to learn by introducing one new idea, by building on previous information, by finding pictures to demonstrate an idea, etc., to adapt teaching to client's specific needs.*[6]

NURSING PRIORITY NO. 3 To assess the client's/SO's motivation:

- Identify motivating factors for the individual (e.g., client needs to stop smoking because of advanced lung cancer, client wants to lose weight because family member died of complications of obesity). *Motivation may be negative (e.g., smoking causes lung cancer) or positive (e.g., client wants to promote health/prevent disease). Provides information that can guide content specific to client's situation and motivations.*[3,12]
- Provide information relevant only to the situation. *Reducing the amount of information at any one given time helps to keep the client focused and prevents client from feeling overwhelmed.*[4]
- Provide positive reinforcement rather than negative reinforcers (e.g., criticism and threats). *Enhances cooperation and encourages continuation of efforts.*[5]

NURSING PRIORITY NO. 4 To establish priorities in conjunction with client:

- Determine client's most urgent need from both client's and nurse's viewpoints. *Identifies whether client and nurse are together in their thinking and provides a starting point for teaching and outcome planning for optimal success.*[6]
- Discuss client's perception of need. *Takes into account the client's personal desires/needs and values/beliefs, providing a basis for planning appropriate care.*[6]
- Differentiate "critical" content from "desirable" content. *Identifies information that must be learned now as well as content that could be addressed at a later time. Client's emotional state may preclude hearing much of what is presented, and by only providing what is essential, client may hear it.*[3]

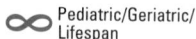

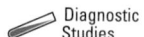

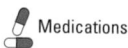

NURSING PRIORITY NO. 5 To determine the content to be included:

- Identify information that needs to be remembered (cognitive) at client's level of development and education. *Enhances possibility that information will be heard and understood.*[6]
- Identify information having to do with emotions, attitudes, and values (affective). *The affective learning domain addresses a learner's emotions toward learning experiences, and attitudes, interest, attention, awareness, and values are demonstrated by affective behaviors. Knowing the client's affective state enhances learning possibilities.*[7,12]
- Identify psychomotor skills that are necessary for learning. *Psychomotor learning involves both cognitive learning and muscular movement. The phases for learning these skills are cognitive (what), associative (how), and autonomous (practice to automaticity). Learners need to know what, why, and how they will learn. For example, if papers need to be typed, the psychomotor skill will be touch typing. The individual will learn touch typing finger placement and how to type smoothly and rhythmically.*[8]

NURSING PRIORITY NO. 6 To develop learner's objectives:

- State objectives clearly in learner's terms to meet learner's (not instructor's) needs. *Understanding why the material is important to the learner provides motivation to learn.*[8]
- Identify outcomes (results) to be achieved. *Understanding what the outcomes will be helps the client realize the importance of learning the material, providing the motivation necessary to learning.*[8]
- Recognize level of achievement, time factors, and short-term and long-term goals. *Learning progresses in stages. Stage 1: unconsciously unskilled where we don't know that we don't know. Stage 2: consciously unskilled, we know that we don't know and start to learn. Stage 3: consciously skilled, we know how to do it but need to think and work hard to do it. Stage 4: we become unconsciously skilled, where the new skills are easier and even seem natural.*[9]
- Include the affective goals (e.g., reduction of stress). *The learner's emotional behaviors affect the learning experience and need to be actively addressed for maximum effectiveness.*[7]

NURSING PRIORITY NO. 7 To identify teaching methods to be used:

- Determine client's/SO's method of accessing information and preferred learning mode (e.g., auditory, visual, kinesthetic; group classes, one-to-one instruction, online) and include in teaching plan. *Using multiple modes of instruction facilitates learning and enhances retention, especially when faced with a stressful situation, illness, or new treatment regimen.*[3,10]
- Involve the client/SO(s) by using age-appropriate materials tailored to client's interest and literacy skills (e.g., interactive programmed books, questions, dialogue, audio/visual materials). *Accesses familiar mental images at client's developmental level to help individual learn more effectively.*[3,12,13]
- Involve with others who have same problems, needs, or concerns. *Group presentations and support groups provide role models and opportunity for sharing of information to enhance learning.*
- Use team and group teaching as appropriate.

NURSING PRIORITY NO. 8 To facilitate learning:

- Provide mutual goal-setting and learning contracts. Clarifies expectations of teacher and learner.
- Provide written information/guidelines and self-learning modules for client to refer to as necessary. *Reinforces learning process.*
- Pace and time learning sessions and learning activities to individual's needs. Involve and evaluate effectiveness of learning activities with client. *Client statements, questions, comments provide feedback about ability to grasp information being presented.*
- Provide an environment that is conducive to learning *to limit distractions and allow client to focus on the material presented.*

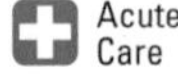

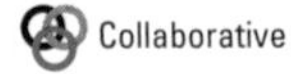

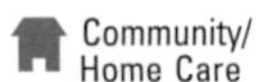

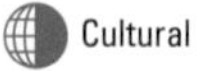

- Be aware of factors related to teacher in the situation (e.g., vocabulary, dress, style, knowledge of the subject, and ability to impart information effectively) *that may affect client's reaction to teacher or ability to learn from this individual.*
- Begin with information the client already knows and move to what the client does not know, progressing from simple to complex. *Can arouse interest and limit sense of being overwhelmed.*[12]
- Deal with the client's anxiety or other strong emotions. Present information out of sequence, if necessary, dealing first with material that is most anxiety producing *when the anxiety is interfering with the client's learning process.*
- Provide active role for client in learning process, including questions and discussion. *Promotes sense of control over situation.*
- Have client paraphrase content in own words, perform return demonstration, and explain how learning can be applied in own situation *to enhance internalization of material and to evaluate learning.*[3]
- Provide for feedback (positive reinforcement) and evaluation of learning and acquisition of skills. *Validates current level of understanding and identifies areas requiring follow-up.*[5]
- Be aware of informal teaching and role modeling that takes place on an ongoing basis. *Answering specific questions and reinforcing previous teaching during routine contacts or care enhances learning on a regular basis.*[1]
- Assist client to use information in all applicable areas (e.g., situational, environmental, personal). *Enhances learning to promote better understanding of situation or illness.*[1]

NURSING PRIORITY NO. 9 To promote wellness (Teaching/Discharge Considerations):

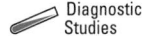

- Provide access information for contact person *to answer questions and validate information after discharge.*[1]
- Identify available community resources and support groups *to assist with problem solving, provide role models, and support personal growth/change.*[4]
- Provide additional learning resources (e.g., bibliography, reliable Web sites, audio/visual media), as appropriate. *May assist with further learning and promote learning at own pace.*[7]

DOCUMENTATION FOCUS

Assessment/Reassessment

- Individual findings, learning style, and identified needs; presence of learning blocks (e.g., hostility, inappropriate behavior).

Planning

- Plan for learning, methods to be used, and who is involved in the planning.
- Teaching plan.

Implementation/Evaluation

- Responses of the client/SO(s) to the learning plan and actions performed.
- How the learning is demonstrated.
- Attainment or progress toward desired outcome(s).
- Modifications to plan of care.

Discharge Planning

- Additional learning and referral needs.

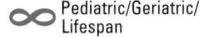

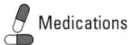

References

1. Bohny, B. A. (1997). A time for self-care: Role of the home healthcare nurse. *Home Healthcare Nurse*, 15(4), 281–286.
2. Purnell, L. D. (2011). *Guide to Culturally Competent Health Care*. 2nd ed. Philadelphia: F. A. Davis.
3. Duffy, B. (1997). Using a creative teaching process with adult patients. *Home Healthcare Nurse*, 15(2), 102–108.
4. Bartholomew, L. K. (2000). Watch, discover, think, and act: A model for patient education program development. *Patient Educ Couns*, 39(2–3), 269–280.
5. Lieb, S. (2010). Principles of adult learning. Retrieved October 2015 from http://www.life-slc.org/learningprinciples/Principles_of_Adult_Learning.pdf.
6. Townsend, M. C. (2011). *Psychiatric Mental Health Nursing: Concepts of Care in Evidence-Based Practice*. 7th ed. Philadelphia: F. A. Davis.
7. No author listed. Bloom's taxonomy of learning domains. The three types of learning. Retrieved October 2015 from http://www.learningandteaching.info/learning/bloomtax.htm.
8. Selwyn, N. *Education in a Digital World: Global Perspective*. New York: Routledge.
9. Adams, L. Learning a new skill is easier said than done. Gordon Training International. Retrieved October 2015 from http://www.gordontraining.com/free-workplace-articles/learning-a-new-skill-is-easier-said-than-done/.
10. No author. (2000, updated 2011). Kolb's learning styles and experiential learning model. Retrieved October 2015 from http://www.nwlink.com/~donclark/hrd/styles/kolb.html.
11. Understanding transcultural nursing. (2005). *Nursing*, 35(1), 14–23. Suppl: Career Directory.
12. Anderson, N. R. (2006). The role of the home healthcare nurse in smoking cessation: Guidelines for successful intervention. *Home Health Nurse*, 24(7), 424–431.
13. Pieper, B., Sieggreen, M., Freeland, B. (2006). Discharge information needs of clients after surgery. *J Wound, Ostomy Continence Nurs*, 33(3), 281–290.

readiness for enhanced Knowledge [specify]

Taxonomy II: Perception/Cognition—Class 4 Cognition (00161) [**Diagnostic Division:** Teaching/Learning], Submitted 2002; Revised 2013

DEFINITION: A pattern of cognitive information related to a specific topic, or its acquisition, which can be strengthened.

DEFINING CHARACTERISTICS

Subjective

Expresses desire to enhance learning

Behaviors congruent with expressed knowledge

Sample Clinical Applications: As a health-seeking behavior, the patient may be healthy or this diagnosis can occur in any clinical condition

DESIRED OUTCOMES/EVALUATION CRITERIA

Sample NOC linkages:

Knowledge: [specify—42 choices]: Extent of understanding conveyed about a specific disease process, the promotion and protection of health, maintaining optimal health, etc.

Information Processing: Ability to acquire, organize, and use information

Client Satisfaction: Teaching: Extent of positive perception of instruction provided by nursing staff to improve knowledge, understanding, and participation in care

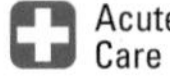
Acute Care
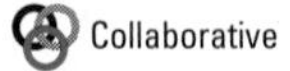
Collaborative
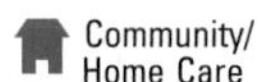
Community/ Home Care
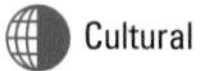
Cultural

Client Will (Include Specific Time Frame)

- Exhibit responsibility for own learning by seeking answers to questions.
- Verify accuracy of informational resources.
- Verbalize understanding of information gained.
- Use information to develop individual plan to meet healthcare needs/goals.

ACTIONS/INTERVENTIONS

Sample NIC linkages:

Teaching: Individual [or 29 other choices]: Planning, implementation, and evaluation of a teaching program designed to address a patient's particular needs
Learning Facilitation: Promoting the ability to process and comprehend information
Learning Readiness Enhancement: Improving the ability and willingness to receive information

NURSING PRIORITY NO. 1 To develop plan for learning:

- Verify client's level of knowledge about specific topic. *Provides opportunity to ensure accuracy and completeness of knowledge base for future learning.*[4]
- Determine motivation and expectation for learning. *Provides insight useful in developing goals and identifying information needs.*[4]
- Assist client to identify learning goals and measurable outcomes. *Helps to frame or focus content to be learned. Provides motivation for learning and a measure to evaluate learning process.*[5,8]
- Ascertain preferred methods of learning (e.g., auditory, visual, interactive, or "hands-on"). *Identifies best approaches for the individual to facilitate learning process.*[5]
- Note personal factors (e.g., age and developmental level, gender, social and cultural influences, religion, life experiences, level of education) *that may impact learning style, choice of informational resources, willingness to take control of situation, accept responsibility for change.*[2]
- Determine challenges to learning, such as language barriers (e.g., client cannot read, speaks or understands language other than that of care provider, dyslexia), physical factors (e.g., sensory deficits such as vision or hearing impairments, aphasia), physical stability (e.g., acute illness, activity intolerance), or difficulty of material to be learned. *Identifies special needs to be addressed if learning is to be successful.*[6]

NURSING PRIORITY NO. 2 To facilitate learning:

- Provide information in varied formats appropriate to client's learning style (e.g., audiotapes, print materials, videos, classes or seminars, online). *Use of multiple formats increases learning and retention of material.*[3]
- Provide information about additional or outside learning resources (e.g., bibliotherapy, pertinent Web sites). *Promotes ongoing learning at own pace.*[7]
- Discuss ways to verify accuracy of informational resources. *Encourages independent search for learning opportunities while reducing likelihood of acting on erroneous or unproven data that could be detrimental to client's well-being.*[4]
- Identify available community resources and support groups. *Provides additional opportunities for role modeling, skill training, anticipatory problem solving, etc.*[1]
- Be aware of and discuss informal teaching and role modeling that takes place on an ongoing basis. *Incongruencies in community or peer role models and support group feedback and print advertisements, popular music, and videos may exist, creating questions and potentially undermining learning process.*[4]
- Assist client to identify ways to integrate and use information in all applicable areas (e.g., situational, environmental, personal). *Ability to apply or use information increases desire to learn and retention of information.*[5]
- Encourage client to journal, keep a log, or graph as appropriate. *Provides opportunity for self-evaluation of effects of learning, such as better management of chronic condition, reduction of risk factors, and acquisition of new skills.*[6,9]

DOCUMENTATION FOCUS

Assessment/Reassessment

- Individual findings, learning style and identified needs, presence of challenges to learning.
- Motivation and expectations for learning.

Planning

- Plan for learning, methods to be used, and who is involved in the planning.
- Educational plan.

Implementation/Evaluation

- Responses of the client/significant other(s) to the educational plan and actions performed.
- How the learning is demonstrated.
- Attainment or progress toward desired outcome(s).
- Modifications to lifestyle or treatment plan.

Discharge Planning

- Additional learning and referral needs.

References

1. Bohny, B. A. (1997). A time for self-care: Role of the home healthcare nurse. *Home Health Nurse*, 15(4), 281–286.
2. Purnell, L. D. (2011). *Guide to Culturally Competent Health Care*. 2nd ed. Philadelphia: F. A. Davis.
3. Duffy, B. (1997). Using a creative teaching process with adult patients. *Home Health Nurse*, 15(2), 102–108.
4. Bartholomew, L. K. (2000). Watch, discover, think, and act: A model for patient education program development. *Patient Educ Couns*, 39(2–3), 269–280.
5. Clark, D. (2000, updated 2014). Learning styles and preferences. Retrieved October 2015 from http://www.nwlink.com/~donclark/hrd/styles.html.
6. Townsend, M. C. (2011). *Psychiatric Mental Health Nursing: Concepts of Care in Evidence-Based Practice*. 7th ed. Philadelphia: F. A. Davis, 377–533.
7. No author listed. Bloom's taxonomy of learning domains. The three types of learning. Retrieved October 2015 from http://www.learningandteaching.info/learning/bloomtax.htm.
8. Selwyn, N. *Education in a Digital World: Global Perspective*. New York: Routledge.
9. Adams, L. Learning a new skill is easier said than done. Gordon Training International. Retrieved October 2015 from http://www.gordontraining.com/free-workplace-articles/learning-a-new-skill-is-easier-said-than-done/.

Latex Allergy Response

Taxonomy II: Safety/Protection—Class 5 Defensive Processes (00041) [**Diagnostic Division:** Safety], Submitted 1998; Revised 2006

DEFINITION: A hypersensitive reaction to natural latex rubber products.

RELATED FACTORS

Hypersensitivity to natural latex rubber protein

DEFINING CHARACTERISTICS

Subjective

Life-Threatening Reactions Within 1 Hour of Exposure:
Chest tightness
Type IV Reactions Occurring ≥1 hour After Exposure:
Discomfort reaction to additives (e.g., thiurams and carbamates)
Gastrointestinal Characteristics: Abdominal pain; nausea
Orofacial Characteristics: Itching (e.g., eyes; facial, nasal, oral); nasal congestion
Generalized Characteristics: Generalized discomfort; total body warmth

Objective

Life-Threatening Reactions Within 1 Hour of Exposure:
Contact urticaria progressing to generalized symptoms
Edema (e.g., lips, throat, tongue, uvula)
Dyspnea; wheezing; bronchospasm; respiratory arrest
Hypotension; syncope; myocardial infarction
Type IV Reactions Occurring ≥1 Hour After Exposure:
Eczema; skin irritation and/or redness
Orofacial Characteristics: Erythema (e.g., eyes, facial, nasal); periorbital edema; rhinorrhea, tearing of the eyes
Generalized Characteristics: Skin flushing; generalized edema; restlessness

Sample Clinical Applications: Multiple allergies, neural tube defects (e.g., spina bifida, myelomeningoceles), multiple surgeries at early age, chronic urological conditions (e.g., neurogenic bladder, exstrophy of bladder), spinal cord trauma

DESIRED OUTCOMES/EVALUATION CRITERIA

Sample NOC linkages:

Allergic Response: Localized: Severity of localized hypersensitive immune response to a specific environmental (exogenous) antigen
Allergic Response: Systemic: Severity of systemic hypersensitive immune response to a specific environmental (exogenous) antigen
Knowledge: Treatment Regimen: Extent of understanding conveyed about a specific treatment regimen

Client Will (Include Specific Time Frame)

- Be free of signs of hypersensitive response.
- Verbalize understanding of individual risks and responsibilities in avoiding exposure.
- Identify signs/symptoms requiring prompt intervention.

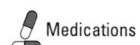

(continues on page 506)

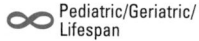

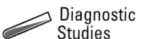

Latex Allergy Response (continued)
ACTIONS/INTERVENTIONS

Sample NIC linkages:
Latex Precautions: Reducing the risk of a systemic reaction to latex
Allergy Management: Identification, treatment, and prevention of allergic responses to food, medications, insect bites, contrast material, blood, or other substances
Environmental Management: Manipulation of the patient's surroundings for therapeutic benefit, sensory appeal, and psychological well-being

NURSING PRIORITY NO. 1 To assess contributing factors:

- Identify persons in high-risk categories such as (1) those with history of certain food allergies (e.g., banana, avocado, chestnut, kiwi, papaya, peach, nectarine); (2) prior allergies, asthma, and skin conditions (e.g., eczema and other dermatitis); (3) those occupationally exposed to latex products (e.g., healthcare workers, police, firefighters, emergency medical technicians [EMTs], food handlers, hairdressers, cleaning staff, factory workers in plants that manufacture latex-containing products); and (4) those with neural tube defects (e.g., spina bifida) or congenital urological conditions requiring frequent surgeries and/or catheterizations (e.g., exstrophy of the bladder). *Studies have shown that latex allergy is present in 1% to 5% of the general population, found in 8% to 12% of healthcare workers, and in at least 10% of rubber industry workers. Symptoms of latex allergy have been described in 14% of a group of EMTs and in 54% of a pediatric emergency department staff.*[7,15,16]
- Question client regarding latex allergy upon admission to healthcare facility, especially when procedures are anticipated (e.g., laboratory, emergency department, operating room, wound care management, 1-day surgery, dentist). *Basic safety information to help healthcare providers prevent/prepare for safe environment for client and themselves while providing care.*[2,4,7]
- Discuss history of exposure; e.g., client works in environment where latex is manufactured or latex gloves are used frequently, child was blowing up balloons (may be an acute reaction to the powder), use of condoms (may affect either partner), or individual requires frequent catheterizations. *Finding cause of reaction may be simple or complex but often requires diligent investigation and history-taking from multiple sources.*
- Administer or note presence of positive skin-prick test, when performed. *Sensitive, specific, and rapid test but should be used with caution in persons with suspected sensitivity, as it carries risk of anaphylaxis.*[10]
- Perform challenge or patch test, if appropriate, *to identify specific allergens in client with known type IV hypersensitivity. Note: Emergency department diagnosis and management depend on the history and physical examination as the following tests are not available in a useful time frame.*[10]
- Note response to radioallergosorbent test or enzyme-linked latex-specific IgE. *Performed to measure the quantity of IgE antibodies in serum after exposure to specific antigens and has generally replaced skin tests and provocation tests, which are inconvenient, often painful, and/or hazardous to the client. Note: These tests are useful in nonemergent evaluations.*[1,10,11]

NURSING PRIORITY NO. 2 To take measures to reduce/limit allergic response/avoid exposure to allergens:

- Ascertain client's current symptoms, noting rash, hives, and itching; red, teary eyes; and edema, diarrhea, nausea, and feeling of faintness. *Baseline for determining where the client is along a continuum of symptoms so that appropriate treatments can be initiated. Note: The most severe reactions tend to occur with latex proteins contacting internal tissues during invasive procedures and when they touch mucous membranes of the mouth, vagina, urethra, or rectum.*[7,9,12]
- Determine time since exposure (e.g., immediate or delayed onset such as 24–48 hrs).
- Assess skin (usually hands but may be anywhere) for dry, crusty, hard bumps and horizontal cracks caused by irritation from chemicals used in/on the latex item (e.g., latex or powder used in latex gloves, condoms). *Dry,*

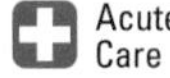
Acute Care
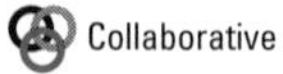
Collaborative
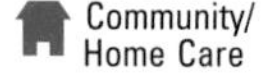
Community/ Home Care
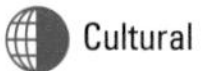
Cultural

itchy rash (contact irritation) is the most common response and is not a true allergic reaction but can progress to a delayed type of allergic contact dermatitis with oozing blisters and spread in a way similar to poison ivy.[2,12]

- Assist with treatment of contact dermatitis/type IV reaction:
  Wash affected skin with mild soap and water.
  Avoid latex gloves where possible; wear cotton glove liners where latex gloves must be used.
  Wash hands between glove changes and after each glove removal.
  Avoid powder, oil-based salves or lotions when using latex gloves. *Note: Powdered latex gloves are associated with higher amounts of aerosolized latex particles in the air. Those concerned with managing risks should minimize concentration of latex protein in the air in order to reduce respiratory and eye symptoms.*[5]
  Consider application of topical ointments such as corticosteroid, and antihistimine.
  Inform client that the most common cause is latex gloves but that many other products contain latex and could aggravate condition.
  Monitor closely for signs of systemic reactions (e.g., difficulty breathing or swallowing; wheezing; hoarseness; stridor; hypotension; tremors; chest pain; tachycardia; dysrhythmias; edema of face, eyelids, lips, tongue, and mucous membranes). *Type IV response can progress to type I anaphylaxis. A systematic review of studies found that a type I allergic reaction may be immediate in sensitized individuals and that acute treatment must be carried out in a latex-free environment.*[14]
  Note behavior such as agitation, restlessness, and expressions of fearfulness in the presence of above listed symptoms. *Indicative of severe allergic response that can result in anaphylactic reaction and lead to respiratory or cardiac arrest.*[6]
  Administer treatment, as appropriate, if severe or life-threatening reaction occurs:
    Stop treatment or procedure, if needed.
    Support airway and administer 100% oxygen or mechanical ventilation, if needed.
    Administer emergency medications and treatments per protocol (e.g., antihistamines, epinephrine, corticosteroids, IV fluids).
- Educate care providers in ways to prevent inadvertent exposure (e.g., post latex precaution signs in client's room, document allergy to latex in chart, routinely monitor client's environment for latex-containing products and remove them promptly) and in emergency treatment measures should they be needed.
- Ascertain that latex-safe environment (e.g., surgical suite, hospital room) and products are available according to recommended facility guidelines and standards, including equipment and supplies (e.g., powder-free, low-protein latex products) and latex-free items (e.g., gloves, syringes, catheters, tubings, tape, thermometers, electrodes, oxygen cannulas, underpads, storage bags, diapers, feeding nipples), as appropriate.[2,9,10,13]
- Notify physicians, colleagues, and medical products suppliers of client's condition (e.g., pharmacy *so that medications can be prepared in latex-free environment,* home-care oxygen company *to provide latex-free cannulas*). *Users of latex gloves and purchasers should be aware that the risk of developing latex allergy is highest with the use of* ***powdered*** *latex gloves and that examination gloves may contain more latex allergen than surgical gloves.*[5]
- Encourage client to wear medical ID bracelet *to alert providers to condition if client is unresponsive.*[3,4,7]

NURSING PRIORITY NO. 3 To promote wellness (Teaching/Learning):

- Instruct in signs of reaction and emergency treatment needs. *Reactions range from skin irritation to anaphylaxis. Reaction may be gradual but progressive, affecting multiple body systems, or may be sudden, requiring lifesaving treatment. Allergy can result in chronic illness, disability, career loss, hardship, and death. There is no cure except complete avoidance of latex.*
- Emphasize the critical importance of taking immediate action for type I reaction *to limit life-threatening symptoms.*
- Demonstrate equipment and injection procedure and recommend client carry auto-injectable epinephrine *to provide timely emergency treatment, as needed.*

- Emphasize necessity of informing all new care providers of hypersensitivity *to reduce preventable exposures.*
- Instruct client/family/significant other (SO) that latex exposure occurs through contact with skin or mucous membrane, by inhalation, parenteral injection, or wound inoculation.
- Instruct client/SO to survey and routinely monitor environment for latex-containing products and replace as needed.
- Provide printed lists or Web sites for identifying common household products that may contain latex (e.g., carpet backing, hoses, rubber grip utensils, diapers, undergarments, shoes, toys, pacifiers, computer mouse pads, erasers, rubber bands, etc.) and where to obtain latex-free products and supplies.[4,7]
- Provide resource and assistance numbers for emergencies. *When allergy is suspected or the potential for allergy exists, protection must begin with identification and removal of possible sources of latex.*
- Provide worksite review, where indicated, and recommendations to prevent exposure. *Latex allergy can be a disabling occupational disorder. Education about the problem promotes prevention of allergic reaction, facilitates timely intervention, and helps nurse to protect clients, latex-sensitive colleagues, and themselves.*[3,4]
- Recommend full medical work-up for client presenting with hand dermatitis, especially if job tasks include use of latex.[8]
- Contact suppliers to verify that latex-free equipment, products, and supplies are available, including (but not limited to) low-allergen or powder-free synthetic gloves, airways, masks, stethoscope tubings, IV tubing, tape, thermometers, urinary catheters, stomach and intestinal tubes, electrodes, oxygen cannulas, pencil erasers, wrist name bands, and rubber bands.[7]
- Ascertain that procedures are in place to identify and resolve problems with medical devices relevant to allergic reactions or glove performance.[4]
- Advise client to be aware of potential for related food allergies (e.g., bananas, kiwis, melons, tomatoes, avocados, nuts). *These foods can trigger a latex-like allergic reaction because the proteins in them mimic latex proteins as they break down in the body.*
- Refer to resources, including, but not limited to, ALERT (Allergy to Latex Education & Resource Team, Inc.), Latex Allergy News, Spina Bifida Association, National Institute for Occupational Safety and Health, Kendall's Healthcare Products (Web site), and Hudson RCI (Web site), *for further information about common latex products in the home, latex-free products, and assistance.*

DOCUMENTATION FOCUS

Assessment/Reassessment

- Assessment findings including type and extent of symptoms.
- Pertinent history of contact with latex products and frequency of exposure.

Planning

- Plan of care and interventions and who is involved in planning.
- Teaching plan.

Implementation/Evaluation

- Response to interventions, teaching, and actions performed.
- Attainment or progress toward desired outcome(s).
- Modifications to plan of care.

Discharge Planning

- Discharge needs, specific referrals made, and additional resources available.

Acute Care 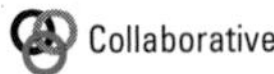 Collaborative 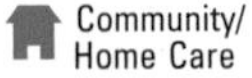 Community/Home Care 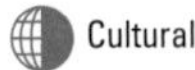 Cultural

References

1. Cavanaugh, B. M. (2003). *Nurse's Manual of Diagnostic Tests*. 4th ed. Philadelphia, PA: F. A. Davis.
2. Author unknown. (1996). Latex allergy: Protect yourself, protect your patients. *Oreg Nurse*, 61(3), 14.
3. National Institutes for Occupational Safety and Health, DHHS. (Updated 2014). Latex allergy: A prevention guide. Retrieved March 2015 http://www.cdc.gov/niosh/docs/98-113/.
4. American Nurses' Association: Nursing World. (No date listed). Workplace issues: Latex allergy. Retrieved March 2015 http://www.nursingworld.org/MainMenuCategories/Policy-Advocacy/ExpiredContent-GOVA/OSHA/SHLATEX11704.html.
5. Agency for Healthcare Research and Quality/National Guideline Clearinghouse. (Updated 2010). Occupational contact dermatitis and urticaria. Retrieved March 2015 from http://www.guideline.gov/content.aspx?id=36827.
6. Urticaria and angioedema. In Sommers, M. S., Johnson, S. A. (eds). (1997). *Davis's Manual of Nursing Therapeutics for Diseases and Disorders*. Philadelphia, PA: F. A. Davis.
7. Occupational Safety and Health Administration. (2008). Potential for sensitization and possible allergic reaction to natural rubber latex gloves and other natural rubber products. Retrieved March 2015 from http://www.https://www.osha.gov/dts/shib/shib012808.html.
8. Worthington, K., Wilburn, S. (2001). Latex allergy: What's the facility's responsibility and what's yours? *Am J Nurs*, 101(7), 88.
9. Klotter, J. (2006). *Latex allergy prevention*. Townsend Letter for Doctors and Patients, May 1, 2006.
10. Behrman, A. J. (Updated 2013). Latex allergy. Retrieved March 2015 from http://emedicine.medscape.com/article/756632-overview.
11. Allergy testing. (Updated 2014). Article for Lab Tests Online (various pages). Retrieved March 2015 from http://labtestsonline.org/understanding/analytes/allergy/tab/test.
12. Gavin, M., Patti, P. J. (2009). Issues in latex allergy in children and adults receiving home healthcare. *Home Healthc Nurse*, 27(4), 231–239.
13. AORN Latex Guideline: 2004 standards, recommended practices, and guidelines. *AORN J*, 79(3), 653–672.
14. Hepner, D. L., Castells, M. C. (2003). Latex allergy: An update. *Anesth Analg*, 96(5(Suppl)), 1219–1229.
15. Dorevitch, S., Forst, M. C. (2000). The occupational hazards of emergency physicians. *Am J Emerg Med*, 18(3), 300–311.
16. Galindo, M. J., Quirce, S., Garcia, O. L., et al. (2011). Latex allergy in primary care providers. *J Investig Allergol Clin Immunol*, 21(6), 459–465.

risk for Latex Allergy Response

Taxonomy II: Safety/Protection—Class 5 Defensive Processes (00042) [**Diagnostic Division:** Safety], Submitted 1998; Revised 2006, 2013

DEFINITION: Vulnerable to a hypersensitivity to natural latex rubber products, which may compromise health.

RISK FACTORS

History of allergy or latex reaction
Frequent exposure to latex product
Food allergy (e.g., avocado, banana, chestnut, kiwi, peanut, shellfish, mushroom, tropical fruit)
Allergy to poinsettia plant
Asthma
Multiple surgical procedures; history of surgery during infancy
Note: A risk diagnosis is not evidenced by signs and symptoms, as the problem has not occurred; rather, nursing interventions are directed at prevention.

Sample Clinical Applications: Multiple allergies, neural tube defects (e.g., spina bifida, myelomeningoceles), multiple surgeries at early age, chronic urological conditions (e.g., neurogenic bladder, exstrophy of bladder), spinal cord trauma

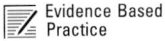

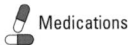

(continues on page 510)

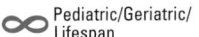

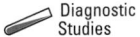

risk for Latex Allergy Response (continued)

DESIRED OUTCOMES/EVALUATION CRITERIA

Sample NOC linkages:

Allergic Response: Localized: Severity of localized hypersensitive immune response to a specific environmental (exogenous) antigen

Risk Control: Personal actions to prevent, eliminate, or reduce modifiable health threats

Knowledge: Health Behavior: Extent of understanding conveyed about the promotion and protection of health

Client Will (Include Specific Time Frame)

- Identify and correct potential risk factors in the environment.
- Demonstrate appropriate lifestyle changes to reduce risk of exposure.
- Identify resources to assist in promoting a safe environment.
- Recognize need for and seek assistance to limit response or complications.

ACTIONS/INTERVENTIONS

Sample NIC linkages:

Latex Precautions: Reducing the risk of a systemic reaction to latex

Allergy Management: Identification, treatment, and prevention of allergic responses to food, medications, insect bites, contrast material, blood, or other substances

Risk Identification: Analysis of potential risk factors, determination of health risks, and prioritization of risk-reduction strategies for an individual or group

NURSING PRIORITY NO. 1 To assess causative/contributing factors:

- Identify persons in high-risk categories such as (1) those with history of certain food allergies (e.g., banana, avocado, chestnut, kiwi, papaya, peach, nectarine), (2) those with asthma or skin conditions (e.g., eczema), (3) those occupationally exposed to latex products (e.g., healthcare workers, police/firefighters, emergency medical technicians [EMTs], food handlers, hairdressers, cleaning staff, factory workers in plants that manufacture latex-containing products), and (4) those with neural tube defects (e.g., spina bifida) or congenital urological conditions requiring frequent surgeries and/or catheterizations (e.g., exstrophy of the bladder). *Most latex allergies are diagnosed by a detailed client history plus physical examination. Studies have shown that latex allergy is present in 1% to 5% of the general population, found in 8% to 12% of healthcare workers, and in at least 10% of rubber industry workers. Symptoms of latex allergy have been described in 14% of a group of EMTs and in 54% of a pediatric emergency department staff.*[2,10–12] *Note: The most severe reactions tend to occur with latex proteins contacting internal tissues during invasive procedures and when they touch mucous membranes of the mouth, vagina, urethra, or rectum.*[2,5–7]
- Question client regarding latex allergy upon admission to each healthcare facility, especially when procedures are anticipated (e.g., new physician/healthcare provider, laboratory, emergency department, operating room, wound care management, 1-day surgery, dentist). *Current information indicates that natural latex is found in thousands of medical supplies; however, most manufacturers are now using synthetic latex for products, and new synthetic latex is under development. These products are associated with fewer allergic reactions among individuals who are sensitive to natural latex.*[1,2]

NURSING PRIORITY NO. 2 To assist in correcting factors that could lead to latex allergy:

- Ascertain that facilities have established policies and procedures. *Promotes awareness in the workplace to address safety and reduce risk to workers and clients.*[3]

- Create latex-safe environments in care setting (e.g., substitute nonlatex products, such as natural rubber gloves, PVC IV tubing, latex-free tape, thermometers, electrodes, oxygen cannulas). *Reduces risk of exposure.*[8,9]
- Promote good skin care when latex gloves may be preferred/required for barrier protection (e.g., in specific disease conditions such as HIV or during surgery). Use powder-free gloves, change gloves frequently, and wash hands immediately after glove removal; refrain from use of oil-based hand cream. *Reduces dermal and respiratory exposure to latex proteins that bind to the powder in gloves.*[2,4]
- Discuss necessity of avoiding latex exposure. Recommend or assist high-risk client/family to survey environment and remove any medical or household products containing latex. *Avoidance of latex is the only way to prevent the allergic reaction.*[2]
- Provide worksite review, where indicated, and recommendations to prevent exposure. *Latex allergy can be a disabling occupational disorder. Education about the problem promotes prevention of allergic reaction, facilitates timely intervention, and helps nurse to protect clients, latex-sensitive colleagues, and themselves.*[1,4]

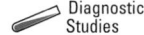

NURSING PRIORITY NO. 3 To promote wellness (Teaching/Discharge Considerations):

- Instruct client/caregivers about types of potential reactions. *Reaction may be gradual and progressive (e.g., irritant contact rash with gloves); can be progressive, affecting multiple body systems; or may be sudden and anaphylactic, requiring lifesaving treatment.*[1,3]
- Identify measures to take if reactions occur and ways to avoid exposure to latex products *to reduce risk of injury and provide for prompt intervention.* (Refer to ND Latex Allergy Response.)
- Refer to allergist for testing as appropriate. *Testing may include the challenge test with latex gloves, a skin patch test, or a blood test for IgE.*
- Encourage client to wear medical ID bracelet/necklace and emphasize the importance of informing all new care providers of hypersensitivity *to reduce preventable exposures.*[1,4]
- Refer to resources (e.g., Latex Allergy News, National Institute for Occupational Safety and Health, Kendall's Healthcare Products [Web site], Hudson RCI [Web site]) *for further information about common latex products in the home, latex-free products, and assistance.*

DOCUMENTATION FOCUS

Assessment/Reassessment

- Assessment findings, pertinent history of contact with latex products, and frequency of exposure.

Planning

- Plan of care and who is involved in planning.
- Teaching plan.

Implementation/Evaluation

- Response to interventions, teaching, and actions performed.
- Attainment or progress toward desired outcome(s).
- Modifications to plan of care.

Discharge Planning

- Long-term needs and who is responsible for actions to be taken.
- Specific referrals made.

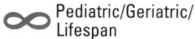

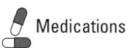

References

1. American Nurses' Association: Nursing World. (No date). Workplace issues: Latex allergy. Retrieved March 2015 from http://www.nursingworld.org/MainMenuCategories/Policy-Advocacy/ExpiredContent-GOVA/OSHA/SHLATEX11704.html.
2. Lenehan, G. P. (2002). Latex allergy: Separating fact from fiction. *Nursing*, 32(3), 58–64.
3. No author listed. (1996). Latex allergy: Protect yourself, protect your patients. *Oreg Nurse*, 61(3), 14.
4. National Institutes for Occupational Safety and Health, DHHS. (Updated 2014). Latex allergy: A prevention guide. Retrieved March 2015 http://www.cdc.gov/niosh/docs/98-113/.
5. Klotter, J. (May 1, 2006). Latex allergy prevention. *Townsend Letter for Doctors and Patients.*
6. Behrman, A. J. (Updated 2013). Latex allergy. Retrieved March 2015 from http://emedicine.medscape.com/article/756632-overview.
7. Karriem-Norwood, V. (reviewer) (updated 2014). Latex allergies. Retrieved March 2015 from www.webmd.com/allergies/guide/latex-allergies.
8. Association of Operating Room Nurses. (2006). Standards, recommended practices and guidelines. *AORN J*, 79(3), 199–214.
9. Molnlycke Health Care, US, LLC. (2006). Latex-safe is best gloving practice against latex allergy. PR Newswire. Retrieved March 2015 from http://www.prnewswire.com/news-releases/latex-safe-is-best-gloving-practice-against-latex-allergy-molnlycke-says-56008667.html.
10. Occupational Safety and Health Administration. (2008). Potential for sensitization and possible allergic reaction to natural rubber latex gloves and other natural rubber products. Retrieved March 2015 from http://www.https://www.osha.gov/dts/shib/shib012808.html.
11. Dorevitch, S., Forst, M. C. (2000). The occupational hazards of emergency physicians. *Am J Emerg Med*, 18(3), 300–311.
12. Galindo, M. J., Quirce, S., Garcia, O. L. (2011). Latex allergy in primary care providers. *J Investig Allergol Clin Immunol*, 21(6), 459–465.

sedentary Lifestyle

Taxonomy II: Health Promotion—Class 1 Health Awareness (00168) [**Diagnostic Division:** Activity/Rest], Submitted 2004

DEFINITION: Reports a habit of life that is characterized by a low physical activity level.

RELATED FACTORS

Insufficient interest in, motivation, or resources [e.g., time, money, companionship, facilities] for physical activity

Insufficient training for physical exercise

Insufficient knowledge of health benefits associated with physical exercise

DEFINING CHARACTERISTICS

Subjective

Preference for activity low in physical activity

Objective

Average daily physical activity is less than recommended for gender and age

Physical deconditioning

Sample Clinical Applications: Chronic or debilitating conditions (e.g., arthritis, multiple sclerosis [MS], chronic obstructive pulmonary disease [COPD], heart failure, paralysis), chronic pain, obesity, depression

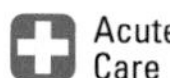

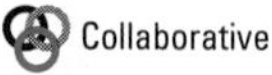

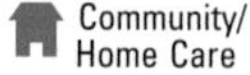

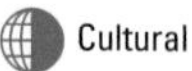

DESIRED OUTCOMES/EVALUATION CRITERIA

Sample NOC linkages:

Knowledge: Prescribed Activity: Extent of understanding conveyed about prescribed activity and exercise
Physical Fitness: Performance of physical activities with vigor
Motivation: Inner urge that moves or promotes an individual to positive action

Client Will (Include Specific Time Frame)

- Verbalize understanding of importance of regular exercise to general well-being.
- Identify necessary precautions, safety concerns, and self-monitoring techniques.
- Formulate and implement realistic exercise program with gradual increase in activity.

ACTIONS/INTERVENTIONS

Sample NIC linkages:

Exercise Promotion: Facilitation of regular physical activity to maintain or advance to a higher level of fitness and health
Teaching: Prescribed Activity/Exercise: Preparing a patient to achieve and/or maintain a prescribed level of activity
Self-Modification Assistance: Reinforcement of self-directed change initiated by the patient to achieve personally important goals

NURSING PRIORITY NO. 1 To assess precipitating/etiological factors:

- Identify client's specific condition(s) (e.g., obesity, depression, MS, arthritis, Parkinson's disease, surgery, hemiplegia or paraplegia, chronic pain, brain injury) *that may contribute to immobility or the onset and continuation of inactivity or sedentary lifestyle.*
- ∞ Assess client's age, developmental level, motor skills, ease and capability of movement, and posture and gait. *Determines type and intensity of needed interventions related to activity.*[1]
- Determine client's current weight and body mass index (BMI); note dietary habits. *If client is overweight and BMI is not in healthy range, a weight-loss program should be suggested along with exercise. Note: In general, BMI is considered a reliable measure of body fat for men and women. However, changes in body composition and stature that occur with aging can influence the reliability of BMI as a marker of body fat.*[8,12]
- Assess physical capabilities to participate in exercise/activities, noting attention span, physical limitations and tolerance, level of interest or desire, and safety needs. *Identifies barriers that need to be addressed.*[1,6]
- Review usual activities and work requirements/environment. Absence of regular exercise and the presence of a stressful job with little physical exercise increases likelihood of deconditioning and affects choice of interventions and need for involvement of the primary healthcare provider in determining a safe program.[8]
- Note emotional and behavioral responses to problems associated with a self- or condition-imposed sedentary lifestyle. *Feelings of disinterest, frustration, and powerlessness may impede attainment of goals.*[2]
- Determine family dynamics and support provided by family/friends. *Major lifestyle change may require support of others to achieve and maintain goals or client may be at increased risk of slipping back into "old" ways.*[8]
- Ascertain availability of resources (e.g., finances for gym membership, transportation, exercise facility or gym at work site, proximity of walking trail or bike path, safety of neighborhood for outdoor activity).

NURSING PRIORITY NO. 2 To motivate and stimulate client involvement:

- Establish therapeutic relationship, acknowledging reality of situation and client's feelings. *Changing a lifelong habit can be difficult, and client may feel discouraged with body and hopeless to turn situation into a positive experience.*[2]

- Ascertain client's perception of current activity and exercise patterns, impact on life, and cultural expectations of client/others. *Helps to determine whether or not client perceives need for change and potential limitations in choices for activities.*[8]
- Discuss client's stated motivation for change. *Concerns of client/significant others (SOs) regarding threats to personal health/longevity or acceptance by teen peers may be sufficient to cause client to initiate change; however, client must want to change for himself or herself in order to sustain change.*[4,8]
- Review necessity for and benefits of regular exercise. *Research confirms that exercise has benefits for the whole body (e.g., can boost energy, enhance coordination, reduce muscle deterioration, improve circulation, lower blood pressure, produce healthier skin and a toned body, prolong youthful appearance). Regular exercise has also been found to boost cardiac fitness in both conditioned and out-of-shape individuals.*[4,13]
- Counsel client regarding individual health risks. *Focuses attention on own situation and helps prioritize needs, making change more manageable.*[8]
- Involve client, SO/parent, or caregiver in developing exercise plan and goals *to meet individual needs, desires, and available resources. Also increases commitment to program and successful attainment of goals.*
- Introduce activities at client's current level of functioning, progressing to more complex activities, as tolerated. *Reduces likelihood of overwhelming client at the beginning and maintains interest over time.*
- Recommend mix of age- and gender-appropriate activities or stimuli (e.g., movement classes, walking, hiking, jazzercise, swimming, biking, skating, bowling, golf, weight training). *Activities need to be personally meaningful for client to derive the most enjoyment and to sustain motivation to continue with program.*[2,6]
- Encourage change of scenery (indoors and outdoors where possible) and periodic changes in the personal environment when client is confined inside.

NURSING PRIORITY NO. 3 To promote optimal level of function and prevent exercise failure:

- Assist with treatment of underlying condition impacting participation in activities *to maximize function within limitations of situation.* Refer to dietitian for weight-loss program, as indicated.
- Collaborate with physical medicine specialist or occupational or physical therapist in providing active or passive range-of-motion exercises and isotonic muscle contractions. *Techniques such as gait training, strength training, and exercise to improve balance and coordination can be helpful in rehabilitating client.*[1]
- Schedule ample time to perform exercise activities balanced with adequate rest periods.[1]
- Provide for safety measures as indicated by individual situation, including environmental management and fall prevention. (Refer to ND risk for Falls.)
- Reevaluate ability/commitment periodically. *Changes in strength or endurance signal readiness for progression of activities or possibly to decrease exercise if overly fatigued. Wavering commitment may require change in types of activities and/or the addition of a workout buddy to reenergize involvement.*[2,5]
- Discuss discrepancies in planned and performed activities with client aware and unaware of observation. Suggest methods for dealing with identified problems. *May be necessary when client is using avoidance or controlling behavior or is not aware of own abilities due to anxiety or fear.*[2,5]

NURSING PRIORITY NO. 4 To promote wellness (Teaching/Discharge Considerations):

- Educate client/SO about benefits of physical activity as it relates to client's particular situation. *Many studies have shown the health benefits of physical activity in the setting of chronic illness (e.g., it increases function in arthritis, improves glycemic control in type 2 diabetes, and can enhance quality of life).*[10,11]
- Review components of physical fitness: (1) muscle strength and endurance, (2) flexibility, (3) body composition (muscle mass, percentage of body fat), and (4) cardiovascular health. *Fitness routines need to include all elements to attain maximized benefits and prevent deconditioning.*[4,5,7]
- Instruct in safety measures, as individually indicated (e.g., warm-up and cool-down activities; taking pulse before, during, and after activity; adequate intake of fluids, especially during hot weather or strenuous activity; wearing reflective clothing when jogging or reflectors on bicycle; locking wheelchair before transfers; judicious use of medications; supervision, as indicated).[1]

- Recommend keeping an activity or exercise log, including physical and psychological responses and changes in weight, endurance, and body mass. *Provides visual evidence of progress or goal attainment and encouragement to continue with program.*[2,6]
- Encourage client to involve self in exercise *as part of wellness management for the whole person.*[3,6]
- Encourage parents to set a positive example for children *by participating in exercise and engaging in an active lifestyle.*[3,6]
- Identify community resources, charity activities, and support groups. *Community walking/hiking trails, sports leagues, etc., provide free/low-cost options. Activities such as 5k walks for charity, participation in Special Olympics, or age-related competitive games provide goals to work toward. Note: Some individuals may prefer solitary activities; however, most individuals enjoy supportive companionship when exercising.*[3,4]
- Discuss alternatives for exercise program in changing circumstances (e.g., walking the mall during inclement weather, using exercise facilities at hotel when traveling, water aerobics at local swimming pool, joining a gym).
- Promote individual participation in community awareness of problem and discussion of solutions. *Physical inactivity (and associated diseases) is a major public health problem that affects large numbers of people in all regions of the world. Recognizing the problem and future consequences may empower the global community to develop effective measures to promote physical activity and improve public health.*[7]
- Promote community goals for increasing physical activity, such as school-based physical education; the Sports, Play, and Active Recreation for Kids program; a "buddy" system or contracting for specific physical activities; and the Physician-Based Assessment and Counseling for Exercise, *to address national concerns about obesity and major barriers to physical activity, such as time constraints, lack of training in physical activity, behavioral change methods, and lack of standard protocols.*[3,6,7,9]

DOCUMENTATION FOCUS

Assessment/Reassessment

- Individual findings, including level of function and ability to participate in specific or desired activities, motivation for change.

Planning

- Plan of care and who is involved in the planning.
- Teaching plan.

Implementation/Evaluation

- Responses to interventions, teaching, and actions performed.
- Attainment or progress toward desired outcome(s).
- Modifications to plan of care.

Discharge Planning

- Discharge and long-term needs, noting who is responsible for each action to be taken.
- Specific referrals made.
- Sources of and maintenance for assistive devices.

References

1. Boesch, C., Meyers, J., Habersaat, A. (2005). Maintenance of exercise capacity and physical activity patterns after cardiac rehabilitation. *Cardiopulm Rehabil*, 25(1), 14–21.
2. Sallis, J. F. (1996). The role of behavioral science in improving health through physical activity. *Summary of presentation. Science Writers Briefing, December 1996*. Sponsored by OBSSR and the American Psychological Association.
3. Wehling-Weepie, A. K., McCarthy, A. (2002). A healthy lifestyle program: Promoting child health in schools. *J School Nurs*, 18(6), 322–328.
4. McCormack, B. N., Yorkey, M. (2005). *Ten Great Things Exercise Can Do for You*. New York, NY: Wiley, American Media.
5. Lai, S. C., Cohen, M. N. (1999). Promoting lifestyle changes. *Am J Nurs*, 99(4), 63.

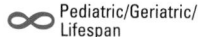

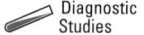

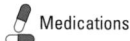

6. Fries, W. C. (2005). Family fitness across the generations. Retrieved November 2015 from http://www.medicinenet.com/script/main/art.asp?articlekey=56090.
7. World Health Organization. (2007). Sedentary lifestyle: A global public health problem. "Move for health" information sheet. Retrieved January 2012 from http://www.who.int/hpr/gs.fs.pa.shtml#.
8. Morantz, C., Torrey, B. (2004). Obesity and sedentary lifestyle guidelines. *Am Fam Physician*, 69(10), 2479–2480.
9. Task Force on Community Preventive Services—Independent Expert Panel. (2002). Recommendations to increase physical activities in communities. *Am J Prev Med*, 22(2 suppl), 67–72.
10. Conn, V. S., Hafdahl, A. R., Minor, M. A., et al. (2008). Physical activity interventions among adults with arthritis: Meta-analysis of outcomes. *Semin Arthritis Rheum*, 37(5), 307–316.
11. Conn, V. S., Hafdahl, A. R., Mehr, D. R., et al. (2007). Metabolic effects of interventions to increase physical exercise in adults with type 2 diabetes. *Diabetologia*, 50(5), 913–921.
12. Zamboni, M., Zoico, E., Scartezzini, T., et al. (2003). Body composition changes in stable-weight elderly subjects: The effect of sex. *Aging Clin Exp Res*, 15(4), 321–327.
13. Warburtin, D. E. R., Nicol, C. W., Bredin, S. S. D. (2006). Narrative review: Health benefits of physical activity: The evidence. *CMAJ*, 174(6), 801–809.

risk for impaired Liver Function

Taxonomy II: Nutrition—Class 4 Metabolism (0000178) [**Diagnostic Division:** Food/Fluid], Submitted 2006; Revised 2008, 2013

DEFINITION: Vulnerable to a decrease in liver function, which may compromise health.

RISK FACTORS

Viral infection [e.g., hepatitis A/B/C, Epstein-Barr); HIV co-infection
Pharmaceutical agent [e.g., acetaminophen, statins]
Substance abuse

Note: A risk diagnosis is not evidenced by signs and symptoms, as the problem has not occurred; rather, nursing interventions are directed at prevention.

Sample Clinical Applications: Hepatitis, HIV, substance abuse, drug overdose (acetaminophen), Epstein-Barr infection

DESIRED OUTCOMES/EVALUATION CRITERIA

Sample NOC linkages:

Knowledge: Disease Process: Extent of understanding conveyed about a specific disease process
Risk Control: Personal actions to prevent, eliminate, or reduce modifiable health threats
Infection Severity: Severity of infection and associated symptoms

Client Will (Include Specific Time Frame)

- Verbalize understanding of individual risk factors that contribute to possibility of liver damage/failure.
- Demonstrate behaviors, lifestyle changes to reduce risk factors and protect self from injury.
- Be free of signs of liver failure as evidenced by liver function studies within normal range, and absence of jaundice, hepatic enlargement, or altered mental status.

ACTIONS/INTERVENTIONS

Sample NIC linkages:

Risk Identification: Analysis of potential risk factors, determination of health risk, and prioritization of risk-reduction strategies for an individual or group

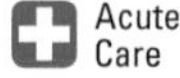

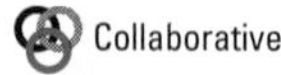

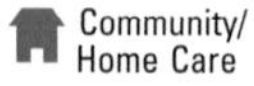

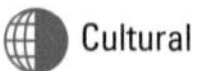

Infection Protection: Prevention and early detection of infection in a patient at risk
Substance Use Treatment: Supportive care of patient/family members with physical and psychosocial problems with the use of alcohol or drugs

NURSING PRIORITY NO. 1 To identify individual risk factors/needs:

- Determine presence of condition(s) as listed in Risk Factors, noting whether problem is acute (e.g., viral hepatitis, acetaminophen overdose) or chronic (e.g., alcoholic cirrhosis). *Influences choice of interventions.*
- Note client history of known/possible exposure to virus, bacteria, or toxins *that can damage liver:*[1–5,12,13]
  Works in high-risk occupation (e.g., performs tasks that involve contact with blood, blood-contaminated body fluids, other body fluids, or sharps). *Carries high risk for exposure to hepatitis B and C.*
  Injects drugs, especially if client shared a needle; received tattoo or piercing with an unsterile needle.
  Received blood or blood products prior to 1989.
  Ingested contaminated food or water or experienced poor sanitation practices by food service workers. *Poses risk for exposure to enteric viruses (hepatitis A and E).*
  Close contact (e.g., lives with or has sex with infected person or carrier; infant born to infected mother).
  Regular exposure to toxic chemicals (e.g., carbon tetrachloride cleaning agents, bug spray, paint fumes, tobacco smoke).
  Uses prescription drugs (e.g., sulfonamides, phenothiazines, isoniazid).
  Ingests certain herbal remedies or mega doses of vitamins.
  Uses alcohol with medications (including over-the-counter [OTC] medications).
  Consumes alcohol heavily and/or over long period of time.
  Ingested acetaminophen (accidentally, as may occur when client takes too large a dose or has several medications containing acetaminophen over time, or intentionally, as may occur with suicide attempt).
  Travels internationally to or emigrates from countries such as Africa, Southeast Asia, Korea, China, Vietnam, Eastern Europe, Mediterranean countries, or the Caribbean *(where hepatitis is endemic).*
- Review results of laboratory tests (e.g., liver function studies, such as hepatic function panel including alanine aminotransferase, alkaline phosphatase, aspartate aminotransferase; bilirubin, gamma-glutamyl transferase, lactic acid dehydrogenase, albumin, total protein and prothrombin time; drug levels, hepatitis screening tests and titers) and other diagnostic studies (e.g., ultrasonography, CT scanning, MRI imaging) *that indicate presence of hepatotoxic condition and need for medical treatment.*[6,15]

NURSING PRIORITY NO. 2 To assist client to reduce or correct individual risk factors:

- Assist with medical treatment of underlying condition (e.g., hepatitis, alcoholism, drug overdose) *to support organ function and minimize liver damage.*
- Educate client/significant other on way(s) to prevent exposure to or incidence of hepatitis infections and limit damage to liver:[4,9,17]
  Practice safer sex (e.g., avoid multiple-partner sex, wear condoms, avoid sex with partners known to be infected).
  Wash hands well after using the bathroom or changing soiled diapers.
  Avoid injecting drugs or sharing needles.
  Avoid sharing razors, toothbrushes, or nail clippers.
  Make sure needles and inks are sterile for tattooing and body piercing.
  Use proper precautions and appropriate protective equipment when working in high-risk occupations (e.g., healthcare, police and fire departments, emergency services, day-care services, chemical manufacturing) *where most at risk for inhalation of toxins or needlesticks or body fluid exposures.*
  Avoid tap water and practice good hygiene and sanitation when traveling internationally.
  Use harsh cleansers and aerosol products in well-ventilated room; wear mask and gloves, cover skin, and wash well afterward. *Insecticides and other chemicals can reach the liver through skin and destroy liver cells.*

Obtain vaccinations when appropriate. *Some hepatitis strains (e.g., A and B) are preventable, thus minimizing risk of liver damage.*

- Discuss safe use and concerns about client's medication regimen (e.g., acetaminophen, NSAIDs, herbal or vitamin supplements, phenobarbital, cholesterol-lowering drugs such as statins, certain antibiotics [e.g., sulfonamides, isonicotinyl hydrazine], certain cardiovascular drugs [e.g., amiodarone, hydralazine], certain antidepressants [e.g., tricyclics]) *known to cause hepatotoxicity, either alone or in combination or in overdose situation. Note: Many OTC and prescription medicines, even "natural" or herbal remedies, contain chemicals that can harm the liver over time. Very high doses of certain pain relievers (e.g., acetaminophen) can cause liver failure.*[6–9]
- Encourage client to read labels, especially when taking acetaminophen for pain, to determine strength of medication, note safe number of doses over 24 hr, and become familiar with "hidden" sources of acetaminophen (e.g., Nyquil, Vicodin). Limit alcohol intake *to avoid or reduce risk of liver damage. Note: Studies have demonstrated that alcoholic clients may develop severe, even fatal, toxic liver injury after ingestion of standard therapeutic doses of acetaminophen.*[5,13,14]
- Emphasize importance of responsible drinking (e.g., men should limit alcohol to no more than two drinks/day, and women, one drink/day) or avoid alcohol altogether when indicated (if client has any kind of liver disease) *to reduce incidence of cirrhosis and severity of liver damage or failure.*[4,11]
- Encourage smoking cessation. *The additives in cigarettes pose a challenge to the liver by reducing it's ability to eliminate toxins.*[15]
- Encourage client with liver dysfunction to avoid fatty foods. *Fat interferes with normal function of liver cells and can cause additional damage and permanent scarring to liver cells when they can no longer regenerate.*[8]
- Refer to nutritionist, as indicated, for dietary needs, including calories, proteins, vitamins, and trace minerals *to promote healing and limit effects of deficiencies. Note: A balanced diet for liver health includes proteins, fruits, and vegetables and is low in cholesterol, fats, carbohydrates, and simple sugars.*[16,17]
- Discuss signs/symptoms (e.g., increased abdominal girth; rapid weight loss or gain; increased peripheral edema; dyspnea, fever; blood in stool or urine; excess bleeding of any kind; jaundice) *that warrant prompt notification of healthcare provider for evaluation and treatment of severe liver dysfunction and possible organ failure.*[9]
- Refer to specialist or liver treatment center, as indicated. *May be beneficial for client with chronic liver disease when decompensating, for client with hepatitis and other co-existing disease condition (e.g., HIV), or for client with intolerance to treatment due to side effects.*

NURSING PRIORITY NO. 3 To promote wellness (Teaching/Discharge Considerations):

- Emphasize importance of hand hygiene, use of bottled water, and avoidance of fresh produce and raw meat/seafood *if client is traveling to area where hepatitis A is endemic or food/waterborne illness is a risk.*[10]
- Instruct in measures including protection from blood or other body fluids and sharps safety, safer-sex practices, avoiding needle sharing, and body tattoos and piercings *to prevent occupational and nonoccupational exposures to hepatitis.*
- Discuss need for vaccination, as indicated (e.g., healthcare and public safety worker, children under 18, international traveler, recreational drug user, men who have sex with other men, client with clotting disorders or liver disease, anyone sharing household with an infected person) *to prevent exposure and transmission of blood or body fluid hepatitis and limit risk of liver injury.*[10]
- Discuss appropriateness of prophylaxis immunizations. *Although the best way to protect against hepatitis B and C infections is to prevent exposure to viruses, postexposure prophylaxis should be initiated promptly to prevent or limit severity of infection, especially in persons with close contact with infected individual or in client with compromised immune system.*[11]
- Provide information regarding availability of gamma globulin, immune serum globulin, hepatitis B immune globulin, and HB vaccine (Recombivax HB, Engerix-B) through the health department or family physician.

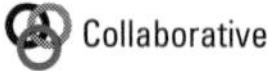

Collaborative
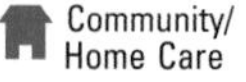

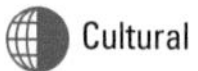

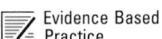

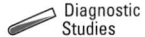

- Emphasize necessity of follow-up care (in client with chronic liver disease) *to monitor liver function and effectiveness of interventions* and importance of adherence to therapeutic regimen *to prevent or minimize permanent liver damage.*
- Refer to community resources for immunizations/drug/alcohol treatment program, as indicated.

DOCUMENTATION FOCUS

Assessment/Reassessment
- Assessment findings, including individual risk factors.
- Results of laboratory tests and diagnostic studies.

Planning
- Plan of care and who is involved in planning.
- Teaching plan.

Implementation/Evaluation
- Response to interventions, teaching, and actions performed.
- Attainment or progress toward desired outcome(s).
- Modifications to plan of care.

Discharge Planning
- Long-term needs, plan for follow-up, and who is responsible for actions to be taken.
- Specific referrals made.

References

1. Bockhold, K. M. (2000). Who's afraid of hepatitis C? *Am J Nurs*, 100(5), 26–32.
2. Shovein, J. T., Camozo, R. J., Hyams, I. (2000). Hepatitis A: How benign is it? *Am J Nurs*, 100(3), 43–47.
3. National Digestive Diseases Information Clearinghouse. (Updated 2012). Viral hepatitis: A through E and beyond. NIH Publication No. 03-4762. Retrieved March 2015 from digestive.niddk.nih.gov/ddiseases/pubs/viralhepatitis/.
4. American Liver Foundation. (2015). The progression of liver disease. Retrieved March 2015 from http://www.liverfoundation.org/abouttheliver/info/progression/.
5. Hawthorne, S. (reviewer) (Updated 2014). Acetaminophen (Tylenol) liver damage. MedicineNet. Retrieved March 2015 from http://www.medicinenet.com/tylenol_liver_damage/article.htm.
6. American Association for Clinical Chemistry. (Updated 2014). Liver panel. Lab Tests Online. Retrieved March 2015 from http://labtestsonline.org/understanding/analytes/liver-panel/tab/glance/.
7. Nabili, S. T. (Updated 2014). Liver blood test. MedicineNet. Retrieved March 2015 from http://www.emedicinehealth.com/liver_blood_tests/article_em.htm.
8. Cormier, M. (2005). The role of hepatitis C support groups. *Gastroenterol Nurs*, 28(3 suppl), S4–S9.
9. Whiteman, K., McCormick, C. (2005). When your patient is in liver failure. *Nursing*, 35(4), 58–63.
10. Durston, S. (2005). What you need to know about viral hepatitis. *Nursing*, 35(8), 36–41.
11. Kania, D. S., Scott, C. M. (2007). Postexposure prophylaxis considerations for occupational and nonoccupational exposures. *Adv Emerg Nurs J*, 29(1), 20–32.
12. Bates, B. (2009). Hepatitis C will be "the big virus" over next 20 years. Reprint and comment for jfponline by J. Evans. Retrieved March 2015 from http://www.jfponline.com/fileadmin/content_pdf/imn/archive_pdf/vol42iss18/70742_main.pdf.
13. Heuman, D. M., Mihaus, A. A., Hung, P. D. (Updated 2014). Alcoholic hepatitis. Retrieved March 2015 from http://emedicine.medscape.com/article/170539-overview.
14. Zimmerman, H. J., Maddrey, W. J. (1995). Acetaminophen (paracetamol) hepatotoxicity with regular intake of alcohol: Analyses of instances of therapeutic misadventure. *Hepatology*, 22(3), 767–773.
15. El-Zayadi, A. R. (2006). Heavy smoking and liver. *World J Gastroenterol*, 12(38), 6089–6101.
16. O'Shea, R. S., Dasarathy, S., McCullough, R. S. (2010). Alcoholic liver disease. *Am J Gastroenterol*, 105(1), 14–32.
17. Holcomb, S. S. (2008). Caring for the patient with chronic hepatitis C. *Nursing*, 38(12), 32–37.

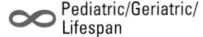

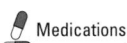

risk for Loneliness

Taxonomy II: Comfort—Class 3 Social Comfort (00054) [**Diagnostic Division:** Social Interaction], Submitted 1994; Revised 2006, 2013

DEFINITION: Vulnerable to experiencing discomfort associated with a desire or need for more contact with others, which may compromise health.

RISK FACTORS

Affectional deprivation
Physical or social isolation
Emotional deprivation
Note: A risk diagnosis is not evidenced by signs and symptoms, as the problem has not occurred; rather, nursing interventions are directed at prevention.
Sample Clinical Applications: Debilitating conditions (e.g., multiple sclerosis [MS], chronic obstructive pulmonary disease [COPD], renal failure), cancer, AIDS; major depression

DESIRED OUTCOMES/EVALUATION CRITERIA

Sample NOC linkages:
Loneliness Severity: Severity of emotional, social, or existential isolation response
Social Involvement: Social interactions with persons, groups, or organizations

Client Will (Include Specific Time Frame)
- Identify individual difficulties and ways to address them.
- Engage in desired social activities.
- Report involvement in interactions or relationships that client views as meaningful.

Sample NOC linkages:
Knowledge: Parenting: Extent of understanding conveyed about provision of a nurturing and constructive environment for a child from 1 year through 17 years of age

Parent Will (Include Specific Time Frame)
- Provide infant/child with consistent and loving caregiving.
- Participate in programs for adolescents and families.

ACTIONS/INTERVENTIONS

Sample NIC linkages:
Socialization Enhancement: Facilitation of another person's ability to interact with others
Hope Inspiration: Enhancing the belief in one's capacity to initiate and sustain actions
Family Integrity Promotion: Promotion of family cohesion and unity

NURSING PRIORITY NO. 1 To identify causative/precipitating factors:
- Differentiate between ordinary loneliness and a state of constant sense of dysphoria. *Being alone is a different state than loneliness.*[3]
- ∞ Note client's age and duration of problem—that is, situational (e.g., leaving home for college) or chronic. *Adolescents may experience lonely feelings related to the changes that are happening as they become adults. Elderly individuals incur multiple losses associated with aging, loss of spouse, decline in physical health, and changes in roles, thus intensifying feelings of loneliness.*[3,12]

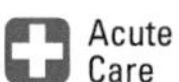

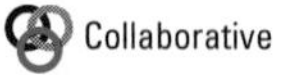

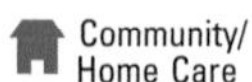

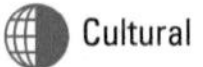

- Determine degree of distress, tension, anxiety, and restlessness present. Note history of frequent illnesses, accidents, and crises. *Identifies somatic complaints that can result from loneliness. Individuals under stress tend to have more illnesses and accidents related to inattention and anxiety.*[6]
- Note presence and proximity of family/significant others (SOs). *Loneliness may not be related to being alone, but knowing that family is available can help with planning care. Client may be estranged from other family members or they may not be willing to be involved with client.*[1,6]
- Discuss with client whether there is a person(s) in his or her life who is trustworthy and who will listen with empathy to the feelings that are expressed. *Identifying someone in the individual's life who can fill this role can help client talk about and understand feelings.*[1]
- Determine how individual perceives and deals with solitude. *Client may see being alone as positive, allowing time to pursue own interests, or may view solitude as sad and long for lost people, lifestyle pattern, or events.*[6,13]
- Review issues of separation from parents as a child or loss of SO(s)/spouse. *Early separation from parents often affects the individual as other losses occur throughout life, leading to feelings of inadequacy and inability to deal with current situation.*[6,13]
- Assess sleep and appetite disturbances and ability to concentrate. *Feelings of loneliness often accompany depression, and identifying whether client is adequately taking care of self is important to planning care.*[7]
- Note expressions of "yearning" for an emotional partnership. *Widows and widowers are particularly prone to feelings of loneliness. Going from being a "couple" to being alone is a difficult transition, and these feelings are indicative of a desire to return to the "couple" state.*[7]
- Assess feelings of loneliness in client who is receiving palliative/hospice care. *These individuals often feel alienated and lonely as they face the end of their life and may need additional socialization to help them feel valued.*[5]

NURSING PRIORITY NO. 2 To assist client to identify feelings and situations in which he or she experiences loneliness:

- Establish therapeutic nurse-client relationship. *Provides a sense of connection with someone, thereby enabling client to feel free to talk about feelings of loneliness and current situation that is related to these feelings.*[1,10]
- Discuss individual concerns about feelings of loneliness and relationship between loneliness and lack of SOs. Note desire and willingness to change situation. *Motivation or lack thereof can facilitate or impede achieving desired outcomes. Often feelings of loneliness arise from underlying depression related to loss, thus affecting individual's coping abilities.*[7]
- Support expression of negative perceptions of others and whether client believes they are true. *Provides opportunity for client to clarify reality of situation and recognize own denial. Individual's view of the world is colored by feelings of loneliness and depression.*[1]
- Accept client's expressions of loneliness as a primary condition and not necessarily as a symptom of some underlying condition. *Provides a beginning point, which will allow the client to look at what loneliness means in life without having to search for deeper meaning.*[1,2]

NURSING PRIORITY NO. 3 To assist client to become involved:

- Discuss reality versus perception of situation. Have client identify people with whom he or she interacts on a regular basis. *Provides opportunity for reality check and beginning to understand own feelings of loneliness related to what is happening in own life.*[2,13]
- Discuss importance of emotional bonding (attachment) between infants/young children, parents/caregivers, as appropriate. *Understanding the importance of attachment provides parents with information that will help them take measures to ensure that this bonding occurs.*[2]
- Involve in classes such as assertiveness, language and communication, and social skills. *Addressing individual needs will enhance socialization and provide client with the skills to become involved in social activities, thus promoting self-confidence and alleviating feelings of loneliness.*[3,8,11]

- Role-play situations that are new or are anxiety provoking for client. *Practicing new situations helps develop self-confidence and provides client with information about what to expect and how to deal with the unexpected in a positive manner.*[2]
- Discuss positive health habits, including personal hygiene, and exercise activity of client's choosing. *Improves feelings of self-esteem, thus enabling client to feel more confident in social situations.*[7]
- Identify individual strengths and areas of interest that client identifies and is willing to pursue. *Provides opportunities for involvement with others to develop new social skills.*[7,11]
- Encourage attendance at support groups (e.g., therapy, separation or grief, religious). *Participating in these activities can meet individual needs and help client begin to deal with feelings of loneliness.*[7]
- Help client establish plan for progressive involvement, beginning with a simple activity, such as calling an old friend or speaking to a neighbor, and then leading to more complicated interactions and activities. *Taking small steps promotes success, and confidence is gained as each step is taken, thus helping the client to be more involved and to resolve feelings of loneliness.*[7]
- Provide opportunities for interactions in a supportive environment (e.g., have client accompanied as in a "buddy system") during initial attempts to socialize. *Helps reduce stress, provides positive reinforcement, and facilitates successful outcome.*[7]

NURSING PRIORITY NO. 4 To promote wellness (Teaching/Discharge Considerations):

- Let client know that loneliness can be overcome. *It is up to the individual to build self-esteem and learn to feel good about self.*[4,13]
- Encourage involvement in special interest groups (e.g., computers, bird watchers) or charitable services (e.g., serving in a soup kitchen, youth groups, animal shelter). *Becoming involved with others takes focus off of self and own concerns, promotes feelings of self-worth, and encourages client to again be an active part of society.*[7]
- Suggest volunteering for church committee or choir, attending community events with friends and family, becoming involved in political issues or campaigns, or enrolling in classes at local college or continuing education programs, as able. *When client is willing to become involved in these kinds of activities, perception of loneliness fades into the background, and even though individual may still be lonely, the sense of loneliness is not so pervasive.*[7]
- Refer to appropriate counselors for help with relationships, social skills, or other identified needs. *May provide additional assistance to help client deal with feelings of loneliness and isolation.*[9,10]
- Refer to NDs Anxiety, Hopelessness, and Social Isolation for additional interventions, as appropriate.

DOCUMENTATION FOCUS

Assessment/Reassessment

- Assessment findings, including client's perception of problem, availability of resources or support systems.
- Client's desire and commitment to change.

Planning

- Plan of care and who is involved in planning.
- Teaching plan.

Implementation/Evaluation

- Response to interventions, teaching, and actions performed.
- Attainment or progress toward desired outcome(s).
- Modifications to plan of care.

Discharge Planning

- Long-term needs, plan for follow-up, and who is responsible for actions to be taken.
- Specific referrals made.

References

1. JMag Editor. (2011). The new face and facts of loneliness. *JMag*. Retrieved March 2015 from http://www.jdate.com/jmag/2009/08/the-new-face-and-facts-of-loneliness/.
2. No author listed. (2006). One is the loneliest number. *The Oprah Magazine*. Retrieved March 2015 from http://www.oprah.com/relationships/Loneliness-Research-How-Loneliness-Affects-Health-How-to-Help.
3. Herbert, W. (2007). The aging of loneliness. We're Only Human. Retrieved March 2015 from http://www.psychologicalscience.org/onlyhuman/2007/08/aging-of-loneliness.cfm.
4. Burnett, P. (2009). Loneliness and low self-esteem. Retrieved March 2015 from http://ezinearticles.com/?Loneliness-and-Low-Self-Esteem&id=2499357.
5. Paice, J. (2002). Managing psychological conditions in palliative care. *Am J Nurs*, 102(11), 36–43.
6. Hauge, S., Kirkevold, M. (2010). Older Norwegians' understanding of loneliness. *Int J Qual Stud Health Well-Being*. Retrieved March 2015 from http://www.ncbi.nlm.nih.gov/pmc/articles/PMC2879870/.
7. McAuley, E., Blissmer, B., Marquez, D. X., et al. (2000). Social relations, physical activity, and well-being in older adults. *Prev Med*, 31(5), 608–617.
8. Acorn, S., Bampton, E. (1992). Patient's loneliness: A challenge for rehabilitation nurses. *Rehabil Nurs*, 17(1), 22–25.
9. Davidson, L., Stayner, D. (1997). Loss, loneliness, and the desire for love: Perspectives on the social lives of people with schizophrenia. *Psychiatr Rehabil J*, 20(3), 3–12.
10. Robinson, K. (1994). Loneliness. University of New York at Buffalo. Retrieved March 2015 from http://ub-counseling.buffalo.edu/loneliness.shtml.
11. Finch, A. (2007). Fed up with feeling alone? Retrieved March 2015 from http://www.selfgrowth.com/articles/Finch3.html.
12. Nagar, A. (2008). Elderly perception of loneliness and ways of resolving it. Retrieved March 2015 from http://www.articlesbase.com/psychology-articles/elderly-perception-of-loneliness-and-ways-of-resolving-it-403625.html.
13. Seepersad, S., Choi, M., Shin, N. (2008). How does culture influence the degree of romantic loneliness and closeness. *J Psychol*, 142(2), 209–221.

risk for disturbed Maternal-Fetal Dyad

Taxonomy II: Sexuality—Class 3 Reproduction (00209) [**Diagnostic Division:** Safety], Submitted 2008; Revised 2013

DEFINITION: Vulnerable to disruption of the symbiotic maternal-fetal dyad as a result of comorbid or pregnancy-related conditions, which may compromise health.

RISK FACTORS

Pregnancy complication (e.g., premature rupture of membranes [PROM], placenta previa or abruption, multiple gestation)
Compromised fetal oxygen transport (due to anemia, [sickle cell anemia], cardiac disease, asthma, hypertension, seizures, premature labor, hemorrhage, etc.)
Alteration in glucose metabolism (e.g., diabetes, steroid use)
Presence of abuse (e.g., physical, psychological, sexual)
Substance abuse
Treatment regimen [e.g., pharmaceutical agents, surgery]
Note: A risk diagnosis is not evidenced by signs and symptoms, as the problem has not occurred; rather, nursing interventions are directed at prevention.
Sample Clinical Applications: High-risk pregnancy, prenatal substance abuse, gestational hypertension, maternal diabetes mellitus, prenatal hemorrhage, prenatal infection, premature dilatation of cervix, abdominal trauma, domestic violence

(continues on page 524)

risk for disturbed Maternal-Fetal Dyad (continued)

DESIRED OUTCOMES/EVALUATION CRITERIA

Sample NOC linkages:

Maternal Status Antepartum: Extent to which maternal well-being is within normal limits from conception to the onset of labor

Fetal Status Antepartum: Extent to which fetal signs are within normal limits from conception to the onset of labor

Prenatal Health Behavior: Personal action to promote a healthy pregnancy and a healthy newborn

Client Will (Include Specific Time Frame)

- Verbalize understanding of individual risk factors or condition(s) that may impact pregnancy.
- Engage in necessary alterations in lifestyle and daily activities to manage risks.
- Participate in screening procedures as indicated.
- Identify signs/symptoms requiring medical evaluation or intervention.
- Display fetal growth within normal limits and carry pregnancy to term.

ACTIONS/INTERVENTIONS

Sample NIC linkages:

High-Risk Pregnancy Care: Identification and management of a high-risk pregnancy to promote healthy outcomes for mother and baby

Surveillance: Late Pregnancy: Purposeful and ongoing acquisition, interpretation, and synthesis of maternal/fetal data for treatment, observation, or admission

NURSING PRIORITY NO. 1 To identify individual risk/contributing factors:

- Review history of previous pregnancies for presence of complications, such as PROM, placenta previa, miscarriage or pregnancy losses due to premature dilation of the cervix, preterm labor and deliveries, previous birth defects, hyperemesis gravidarum, or repeated urinary tract or vaginal infections.[22,23]
- Obtain history about prenatal screening and amount and timing of care. *Prenatal screening can detect inherited and congenital abnormalities long before birth, providing opportunities for informed parental decisions, such as repair of abnormality in utero or helping mother understand a procedure. Lack of prenatal care or late prenatal care may be result of ignorance of or fear about pregnancy or the result of inadequate finances or other support and can place both mother and fetus at risk.*[9,23]
- Note conditions potentiating vascular changes and reduced placental circulation (e.g., diabetes, gestational hypertension, cardiac problems, smoking) or those that alter oxygen-carrying capacity (e.g., asthma, anemia, Rh incompatibility, hemorrhage). *Extent of maternal vascular involvement and reduction of oxygen-carrying capacity have a direct influence on uteroplacental circulation and gas exchange.*[8,10]
- Note maternal age. *Maternal age above 35 years is associated with increased risk of placental separation or abruptio placentae, spontaneous abortions, preterm delivery or stillbirths, fetal chromosomal abnormalities and malformations, and intrauterine growth retardation (IUGR). The most common maternal complications in this age group are gestational hypertension and gestational diabetes. In pregnant adolescents (younger than 15) the most common high-risk conditions include gestational hypertension, anemia, labor dysfunction, cephalopelvic disproportion and low birth weight, and preterm delivery.*[2,5,8,11,14,23]
- Ascertain current and past dietary patterns and practices. *Client may be malnourished, underweight or obese (weight less than 100 lb or greater than 200 lb), or may reveal preconception eating disorders that can have a negative impact on fetal organ development—especially brain tissue in the early weeks of pregnancy.*[1,3,15,23]
- Assess for severe, unremitting nausea and vomiting, especially when it persists after the first trimester. *Hyperemesis gravidarum places mother at risk for substantial weight loss and fluid and electrolyte imbalances and*

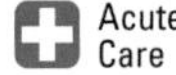

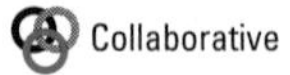

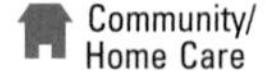

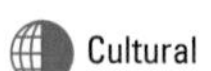

exposes the developing fetus to acidotic state and malnutrition. Development of hyperemesis gravidarum may require hospitalization.[14,19,23]

- Note history of exposure to teratogenic agents and infectious diseases (e.g., tuberculosis, influenza, measles); high-risk occupations; exposure to toxic substances such as lead, organic solvents, and carbon monoxide; use of certain over-the-counter or prescription medications; and substance use or abuse (including illicit drugs and alcohol).[4,6,7,14,18]
- Identify family or cultural influences in pregnancy. *Family history may include multiple births, congenital diseases, generational abuse, or lack of support or finances. Cultural background may identify health risks associated with nationality (e.g., sickle cell anemia in people of African descent or Tay-Sachs disease in people of Eastern European Jewish ancestry) or religious practices (e.g., exclusion of dairy products, no maternal immunizations for rubella), which can impact health of mother or fetal development.*[11,14]
- Review laboratory studies. *Low hemoglobin suggests anemia, which is associated with hypoxia. Blood type and Rh group may reveal incompatibility risks, elevated serum glucose seen in gestational diabetes mellitus (GDM) and elevated liver function studies suggest hypertensive liver involvement, and drop in platelet count may be associated with gestational hypertension and HELLP (hemolysis, elevated liver enzymes, and low platelet) syndrome. Nutritional studies may reveal decreased levels of serum proteins, electrolytes, minerals, and vitamins essential to maternal health and fetal development.*[8,9,15,23]
- Review vaginal, cervical, or rectal cultures and serology results. *May reveal presence of sexually transmitted infections, a virus of the TORCH group (e.g., toxoplasmosis, other, rubella, cytomegalovirus, herpes simplex), or Listeria; identify active/carrier state of hepatitis, HIV, and AIDS.*[12,13,22]
- Assist in screening for and identifying genetic or chromosomal disorders. *Disorders such as phenylketonuria or sickle cell anemia necessitate special treatment to prevent negative effects on fetal growth.*[11]
- Investigate current home situation. *May have history of unstable relationship or inadequate/lack of housing, which affects safety as well as general well-being.*[20]

NURSING PRIORITY NO. 2 To monitor maternal/fetal status:

- Weigh client and compare current weight with pregravid weight. Have client record weight between visits. *Underweight clients are at risk for anemia, inadequate protein/calorie intake, vitamin or mineral deficiencies, and gestational hypertension. Overweight women are at risk for possible changes in the cardiovascular system that create risks for development of gestational hypertension, GDM, and hyperinsulinemia of the fetus, resulting in macrosomia. Research indicates increased risk of fetal distress and cesarean delivery. A sudden weight gain of 2 or more pounds in a week may indicate gestational hypertension.*[3,8,15,23]
- Assess fetal heart rate (FHR), noting rate and regularity. Have client monitor fetal movement daily as indicated. *Tachycardia in a term infant may indicate a compensatory mechanism to reduced oxygen levels and/or presence of sepsis. A reduction in fetal activity occurs before bradycardia.*[23]
- Test urine for presence of ketones. *Indicates inadequate glucose utilization and breakdown of fats for metabolic processes.*[10,23]
- Provide information and assist with procedures as indicated, for example:[9,14,23]

  Amniocentesis: *May be performed for genetic purposes or to assess fetal lung maturity. Spectrophotometric analysis of the fluid may be done to detect bilirubin after 26 weeks' gestation.*

  Ultrasonography: *Assesses gestational age of fetus and detects presence of multiples or fetal abnormalities. Locates placenta (and amniotic fluid pockets before amniocentesis, if performed), and monitors clients at risk for reduced/inadequate placental perfusion (such as adolescents; clients older than 35 years; clients with diabetes, gestational hypertension, cardiac/kidney disease, anemia, or respiratory disorders).*

  Biophysical profile: *Assesses fetal well-being through ultrasound evaluation to measure amniotic fluid index, FHR and nonstress test reactivity, fetal breathing movement, body movement (large limbs), and muscle tone (flexion and extension).*

  Contraction stress test (CST): *A positive CST with late decelerations indicates a high-risk client/fetus with possible reduced uteroplacental reserves.*

- Screen for abuse during pregnancy. *Prenatal abuse is correlated with a low maternal weight gain, infections, anemia, delay in seeking prenatal care until the third trimester, and preterm delivery.*[20]
- Screen for preterm uterine contractions, which may or may not be accompanied by cervical dilatation. *Occurs in 6% to 7% of all pregnancies and may result in delivery of a preterm infant if tocolytic management is not successful in reducing uterine contractility and irritability.*[21]

NURSING PRIORITY NO. 3 To maintain or improve maternal and fetal well-being:

- Instruct client in reportable symptoms and monitor for unusual symptoms at each prenatal visit (e.g., vaginal bleeding, headache along with blurred vision and ankle swelling, faintness, persistent vomiting). *Provides opportunity for early intervention in event of developing complications.*[15,23]
- Assist in treatment of underlying medical condition(s) that have potential for causing maternal or fetal harm.[10]
- Assess perceived impact of complication on client and family members. Encourage verbalization of concerns. *Family stress often occurs in an uncomplicated pregnancy, and it is amplified in a high-risk pregnancy, where concerns focus on the health of both the client and the fetus. Family is strengthened if all members have a chance to express fears openly and work cooperatively.*[23]
- Facilitate positive adaptation to situation through active listening, acceptance, and problem solving. *Helps in successful accomplishment of the psychological tasks of pregnancy, although the high-risk couple may remain ambivalent as a self-protective mechanism against possible loss of the pregnancy or fetal death.*[23]
- Develop dietary plan with client that provides necessary nutrients (calories, protein, vitamins, and minerals) *to create new tissue and to meet increased maternal metabolic needs.*[16,18]
- Promote fluid intake of at least 2 qt of noncaffeinated fluid per day. *Prevents dehydration, which may compromise optimal uterine and placental functioning and increase uterine irritability, which could potentiate premature labor.*
- Encourage client to participate in individually appropriate adaptations and self-care techniques, such as scheduling rest periods two to three times a day, avoiding overexertion or heavy lifting, or maintaining contact with family and daily life if bedrest is required. *Medical problems necessitating special therapy or restrictions at home or hospitalization significantly disrupt normal routines and cause stress. Preventive problem solving promotes participation in own care and enhances self-confidence, sense of control, and client/couple satisfaction.*[23,25]
- Review medication regimen. *Prepregnancy treatment for chronic conditions may require alteration for maternal/fetal safety.*
- Review availability and use of resources. *Presence or absence of supportive resources can make the difference for the client and family in being able to manage the situation.*
- Administer Rh immune globulin (RhIgG) to client at 28 weeks' gestation in Rh-negative clients with Rh-positive partners or following amniocentesis, if indicated. *RhIgG helps reduce incidence of maternal isoimmunization in nonsensitized mothers and helps prevent erythroblastosis fetalis and fetal red blood cell (RBC) hemolysis.*[23,24]
- Encourage modified or complete bedrest as indicated. *Activity level may need modification, depending on symptoms of uterine activity, cervical changes, or bleeding. Side-lying position increases renal and placental perfusion, which is effective in preventing supine hypotensive syndrome.*[23] *Note: Bedrest may result in generalized weakness, raising safety concerns when client is out of bed.*
- Provide supplemental oxygen as appropriate. *Increases the oxygen available for fetal uptake, especially in presence of severe anemia or sickle cell crisis or when maternal/fetal circulation is compromised.*
- Prepare for and assist with intrauterine fetal exchange transfusion as indicated by titers (Kleihauer-Betke test). *If excess fetal RBC hemolysis occurs, transfusion into fetal peritoneal cavity with RhO-negative blood replaces hemolyzed RBCs when fetus is determined at risk of dying before 32 weeks' gestation.*[24]

Acute Care 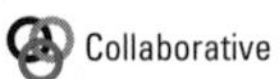 Collaborative 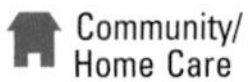 Community/ Home Care 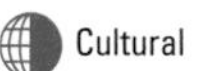 Cultural

NURSING PRIORITY NO. 4 To promote wellness (Teaching/Discharge Considerations):

- Emphasize the normalcy of pregnancy, focus on pregnancy milestones, and "count down" to birth. *Avoids or limits perception of "sick role" and promotes sense of hope that modifications or restrictions serve a worthwhile purpose.*[23]
- Discuss implications of preexisting condition and possible impact on pregnancy. *Pregnancy may have no effect or may reduce or exacerbate severity of symptoms of chronic conditions. Repeat sickle cell crises predispose client and fetus to increased mortality and morbidity rates. Client with multiple sclerosis or spinal cord injury may have decreased ability to sense uterine contractions or presence of labor, necessitating closer monitoring.*[10]
- Provide information about risks of weight reduction during pregnancy and about nourishment needs of client and fetus. *Prenatal calorie restriction and resultant weight loss may result in nutrient deficiency or ketonemia, with negative effects on fetal central nervous system and possible IUGR.*[18]
- Encourage smoking cessation, refer to community program or support group as indicated. *Severe adverse effects of smoking on the fetus may be reduced if mother quits smoking early in pregnancy, and pregnancy outcomes can still be improved if mother stops smoking as late as 32 weeks' gestation.*[17]
- Help client/couple plan restructuring of roles or activities necessitated by complication of pregnancy. *Education, support, and assistance in maintenance of family integrity help foster growth of its individual members and reduce stress that the client may feel from her dependent role.*[23]
- Have client demonstrate new behaviors or therapeutic techniques. *During pregnancy, control of condition may require specific modified or new behaviors. Demonstration allows accurate assessment of learning.*
- Recommend client assess uterine tone and presence of contractions for 1 hr once or twice a day as indicated *to monitor uterine irritability or early indication of premature labor.*[21]
- Encourage close monitoring of blood glucose levels, as appropriate. *Clients with type I or insulin-dependent-diabetes mellitus generally need to check blood glucose levels 4 to 12 times/day because insulin needs may increase two to three times above pregravid baseline.*[10]
- Demonstrate technique and specific equipment used when FHR monitoring is done in the home setting. *Provides opportunity for more detailed information regarding fetal well-being in a less stressful environment. Enhances sense of active involvement.*
- Identify danger signals requiring immediate notification of healthcare provider (e.g., PROM, preterm labor, vaginal drainage or bleeding). *Recognizing risk situations encourages prompt evaluation and intervention, which may prevent or limit untoward outcomes.*[21,22]
- Review availability and use of resources. *Presence or absence of supportive resources can make the difference for the client and family in being able to manage the situation.*[22]
- Refer to community service agencies (e.g., visiting nurse, social service) or resources, such as Sidelines. *Community supports may be needed for ongoing assessment of medical problem, family status, coping behaviors, and financial stressors. Note: Sidelines is a national telephone support group for pregnant women on bedrest.*
- Refer for counseling if family does not sustain positive coping and growth. *May be necessary to promote growth and to prevent family disintegration.*

DOCUMENTATION FOCUS

Assessment/Reassessment

- Assessment findings, weight, signs of pregnancy, and safety concerns.
- Specific risk factors, comorbidities, and treatment regimen.
- Results of screening laboratory tests and diagnostic studies.
- Participation in prenatal care.
- Cultural beliefs and practices.

Planning

- Plan of care, specific interventions, and who is involved in the planning.
- Community resources for equipment or supplies.
- Specific referrals made.
- Teaching plan.

Implementation/Evaluation

- Client/fetal response to treatment and actions performed.
- Client's response to teaching provided.
- Attainment or progress toward desired outcome(s).
- Modifications to plan of care.

References

1. National Institute of Child Health and Human Development. (Updated 2013). What are the factors that put a pregnancy at risk? Retrieved March 2015 from https://www.nichd.nih.gov/health/topics/high-risk/conditioninfo/Pages/factors.aspx.
2. Cleary-Goldman, J., Malone, F. D., Vidaver, J., et al. (2005). Impact of maternal age on obstetric outcome. *Obstet Gynecol*, 105(5), 983–990.
3. Ehrenberg, H. M., Iams, J. D., Goldenberg, R. L., et al. (2009). Maternal obesity, uterine activity, and the risk of spontaneous preterm birth. *Obstet Gynecol*, 113(1), 48–52.
4. No author listed. (Updated 2015). Surgeon General's advisory on alcohol use in pregnancy. Retrieved March 2015 from http://come-over.to/FAS/SurGenAdvisory.htm.
5. Miller, D. A. (2005). Is advanced maternal age an independent risk factor for uteroplacental insufficiency? *Am J Obstet Gynecol*, 192(6), 1974–1982.
6. March of Dimes. (2008). Street drugs and during pregnancy. Retrieved March 2015 from http://www.marchofdimes.org/pregnancy/print/illicit-drug-use-during-pregnancy.html.
7. Acharya, K. S., Grotegut, C. A. (Updated 2015). Psychosocial and environmental pregnancy risks. Retrieved March 2015 from http://emedicine.medscape.com/article/259346-overview.
8. Carson, M. P., Gibson, P. (Updated 2015). Hypertension and pregnancy. Retrieved March 2015 from http://emedicine.medscape.com/article/261435-overview.
9. Yale Medical Group. (Updated 2013). High-risk pregnancy: Maternal and fetal testing. Retrieved March 2015 from http://ymghealthinfo.org/content.asp?pageid=P02469.
10. Yale Medical Group. High-risk pregnancy: Pregnancy and medical conditions. Retrieved March 2015 from http://ymghealthinfo.org/content.asp?pageid=P02483.
11. Yale Medical Group. High-risk pregnancy: Prenatal counseling. Retrieved March 2015 from http://ymghealthinfo.org/content.asp?pageid=P02493.
12. Centers for Disease Control and Prevention. (Updated 2014). STDs and pregnancy. CDC fact sheet. Retrieved March 2015 from http://www.cdc.gov/std/pregnancy/stdfact-pregnancy.htm.
13. U.S. Department of Health and Human Services. (2008, reviewed 2012). HIV during pregnancy, labor and delivery, and after birth. Retrieved March 2015 from http://permanent.access.gpo.gov/lps80129/perinatal_fs_en.pdf.
14. Springhouse Staff. (2008). Complications and high-risk conditions of the prenatal period. *Straight A's in Maternal-Neonatal Nursing*. 2nd ed. Philadelphia, PA: Lippincott Williams & Wilkins.
15. Holloway, B., Moredich, C., Aduddell, K. (2006). *OB Peds Women's Health Notes: Nurse's Clinical Pocket Guide*. Philadelphia, PA: F. A. Davis.
16. RDAs for pregnant women. (2007). *Lippincott Manual of Nursing Practice Pocket Guides: Maternal-Neonatal Nursing*. Philadelphia, PA: Lippincott Williams & Wilkins.
17. Barclay, L., Vega, C. (2009). Severe adverse effects of smoking may be reversible if mothers quit early in pregnancy. Retrieved March 2015 from http://www.medscape.org/viewarticle/590543.
18. National Institute of Child Health and Human Development. (Updated 2014). What can I do to promote a healthy pregnancy? Retrieved March 2015 from http://www.nichd.nih.gov/news/resources/spotlight/040710-pregnancy-healthy-weight.cfm.
19. Yale Medical Group. High-risk pregnancy: Hyperemesis gravidarum. Retrieved March 2015 from http://ymghealthinfo.org/content.asp?pageid=P02457.
20. Centers for Disease Control and Prevention. (2009). Violence and reproductive health. Retrieved March 2015 from www.cdc.gov/reproductivehealth/violence/index.htm.

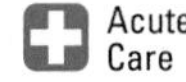

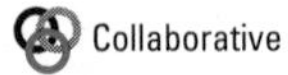

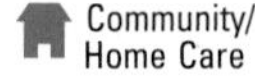

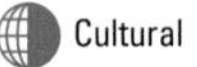

21. Institute of Medicine. (2007). Preterm birth: Causes, consequences, and prevention. Retrieved March 2015 from http://www.ncbi.nlm.nih.gov/books/NBK11362/.
22. Ross, M. G., Eden, R. D. (Updated 2014). Preterm labor. Retrieved March 2015 from http://emedicine.medscape.com/article/260998-overview.
23. Ricci, S. S., Kyle, T. (2008). *Maternity and Pediatric Nursing*. Philadelphia, PA: Lippincott Williams & Wilkins.
24. National Heart, Lung, and Blood Institute. (Updated 2011). What is Rh incompatibility? Retrieved March 2015 from http://www.nhlbi.nih.gov/health/health-topics/topics/rh.
25. Maloni, J. A., Kane, J. H., Suen, L. J., et al. (2002). Dysphoria among high-risk pregnant hospitalized women on bed rest: A longitudinal study. *Nurs Res*, 51(2), 92–99.

impaired Memory

Taxonomy II: Perception/Cognition—Class 4 Cognition (00131) [**Diagnostic Division:** Neurosensory], Submitted 1994

DEFINITION: Inability to remember or recall bits of information or behavioral skills.

RELATED FACTORS

Hypoxia; anemia
Electrolyte imbalance; decrease in cardiac output
Neurological impairment (e.g., positive EEG, head trauma, seizure disorders)
Distractions in the environment
[Substance abuse; effects of medications]
[Age]

DEFINING CHARACTERISTICS

Subjective

Inability to recall events or factual information

Objective

Inability to recall if a behavior was performed; forgets to perform a behavior at a scheduled time
Inability to learn/retain new skills or information
Inability to perform a previously learned skill
Forgetfulness

Sample Clinical Applications: Brain injury, stroke, dementia, Alzheimer's disease, hypoxia (e.g., chronic obstructive pulmonary disease [COPD], anemia, altitude sickness), alcohol intoxication or substance abuse

DESIRED OUTCOMES/EVALUATION CRITERIA

Sample NOC linkages:

Memory: Ability to cognitively retrieve and report previously stored information
Cognition: Ability to execute complex mental processes

Client Will (Include Specific Time Frame)

- Verbalize awareness of memory problems.
- Establish methods to help in remembering essential things when possible.
- Accept limitations of condition and use resources effectively.

(continues on page 530)

impaired Memory (continued)
ACTIONS/INTERVENTIONS

Sample NIC linkages:
Memory Training: Facilitation of memory
Surveillance: Safety: Purposeful and ongoing collection and analysis of information about the patient and the environment for use in promoting and maintaining patient safety

NURSING PRIORITY NO. 1 To assess causative factor(s)/degree of impairment:

- Determine physical, biochemical, and environmental factors (e.g., systemic infections, brain injury, pulmonary disease with hypoxia, use of multiple medications, exposure to toxic substances; use or abuse of alcohol or other drugs, traumatic event, removal from known environment) *that may be related to changes in memory.*
- Note client's age and potential for depression symptoms in elderly. *Depressive disorders are particularly prevalent in older adults (approximately 15%) who report an inability to concentrate and poor memory; however, impairments can occur in depressed persons of any age. While substantial memory loss is not a normal aspect of aging, a number of studies have demonstrated that certain aspects of memory are somehow altered in the aging process and that generally, memory for past occurrences is superior to the retention and recall of more recent information.*[1,2,5–7]
- Note presence of stressful situation(s) and degree of anxiety. *Can increase client's confusion and disorganization and further interfere with attempts at recall. Stress may also speed up memory decline in people whose cognitive function is already impaired.* (Refer to ND Anxiety for additional interventions as indicated.)
- Collaborate with medical and psychiatric providers *to evaluate extent of impairment to orientation, attention span, ability to follow directions, send/receive communication, and appropriateness of response.*
- Assist with or review results of cognitive testing (e.g., Blessed Information-Memory-Concentration test, Clinical Dementia Rating Scale, Mini-Mental State Examination). *Although the etiology for some memory impairments may be obvious or established by client/significant other (SO)/caregiver report, a combination of tests may be needed to demonstrate that the client is below some cut-point on standardized memory tests that represents a significant change from the client's baseline to obtain a complete picture of the client's overall condition and prognosis.*[3,6,7]
- Evaluate skill proficiency levels. *Evaluation may include many self-care activities (e.g., daily grooming, steps in preparing a meal, participating in a lifelong hobby, balancing a checkbook, driving ability) to determine level of independence or needed assistance.*[8]
- Ascertain how client/family views the problem (e.g., practical problems of client being able to take care of physical/grooming/toileting issues; forgetting to turn off the stove when cooking for self; client gets lost when driving, client has role and responsibility impairments related to loss of memory and concentration) *to determine significance and impact of problem and suggest direction of interventions, especially as relates to basic safety issues.*[1,8]

NURSING PRIORITY NO. 2 To maximize level of function:

- Assist with treatment of underlying conditions (e.g., electrolyte imbalances, infection, anemia, drug interactions/reaction to medications, alcohol or other drug intoxication, malnutrition, vitamin deficiencies, pain) *where treatment can improve memory processes.*
- Orient and reorient client, as needed, to environment. Introduce self with each client contact *to meet client's safety and comfort needs.* (Refer to NDs acute/chronic Confusion for additional interventions as appropriate.)
- Implement appropriate memory-retraining techniques (e.g., keeping calendars, writing lists, memory cue games, mnemonic devices, using computers) *to provide restorative or compensatory training for cognitive function. Note: One evidence-based review of clients with memory impairments associated with moderate to severe brain injury showed that "memory retraining programs appear effective, particularly for functional recovery although performance on specific tests of memory may or may not change."*[4,9]

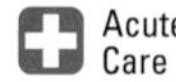

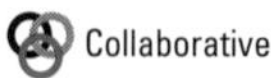

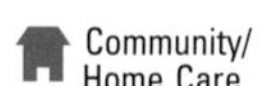

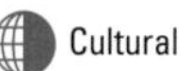

- Assist in and instruct client and family in associate-learning tasks (e.g., practice sessions recalling personal information, reminiscing, locating a geographic location [stimulation therapy]). *Practice may improve performance and integrate new behaviors into the client's coping strategies.*
- Support and reinforce client's efforts to remember information or behavioral skills. *Can decrease anxiety levels and perhaps help with further memory recovery.*
- Encourage ventilation of feelings of frustration and helplessness. Refocus attention to areas of control and progress *to diminish feelings of powerlessness or hopelessness.*
- Provide for and emphasize importance of pacing learning activities and getting sufficient rest *to avoid fatigue and frustration that may further impair cognitive abilities.*[1]
- Monitor client's behavior and assist in use of stress-management techniques (e.g., music therapy, reading, television, games, socialization) *to reduce boredom and enhance enjoyment of life.*
- Structure teaching methods and interventions *to client's level of functioning or potential for improvement.*[5]
- Determine client's response to and effects of medications prescribed to improve attention, concentration, memory processes, and to lift spirits or modify emotional responses. *Medications used for cognitive enhancement can be effective (especially in the case of short-term impairments such as might occur following surgery or when client is being treated for infections or delirium), but long-term use and benefits need to be weighed against whether quality of life is improved when considering side effects and cost of drugs.*[3,6]

NURSING PRIORITY NO. 3 To promote wellness (Teaching/Discharge Considerations):

- Assist client/SO(s) to establish compensation strategies, such as menu planning with a shopping list, timely completion of tasks on a daily planner, and checklists at the front door to ascertain that lights and stove are off before leaving, *to improve functional lifestyle and safety.*[6]
- Teach client and family/caregivers memory involvement tasks, such as reminiscence and memory practice exercises *geared toward improving client's functional ability.*[6]
- Refer to or encourage follow-up with counselors, rehabilitation programs, job coaches, and social or financial support systems *to help deal with persistent or difficult problems.*
- Refer to rehabilitation services *that are matched to the needs, strengths, and capacities of individual and modified as needs change over time.*[4]
- Discuss and encourage safety interventions, as indicated (e.g., assistance with meal preparation, evaluation of driving abilities, cessation of tobacco use or its use only under supervision, removal of guns and other weapons) *to prevent injury to client/others.*
- Identify resources to meet individual needs (e.g., home-care assistant, Meals on Wheels, companion, short-term residential care), *thereby maximizing independence and general well-being.*

DOCUMENTATION FOCUS

Assessment/Reassessment

- Individual findings, testing results, and perceptions of significance of problem.
- Actual impact on lifestyle and independence.

Planning

- Plan of care and who is involved in planning process.
- Teaching plan.

Implementation/Evaluation

- Responses to interventions, teaching, and actions performed.
- Attainment or progress toward desired outcome(s).
- Modifications to plan of care.

Discharge Planning

- Long-term needs and who is responsible for actions to be taken.
- Specific referrals made.

References

1. Luo, L. (2008). Aging and memory: A cognitive approach. *Can J Psychiatry*, 53(6), 346–353.
2. Roussel, L. A. (1999). The aging neurological system. In Stanley, M., Beare, P. G. (eds). *Gerontological Nursing: A Health Promotion/Protection Approach.* 2nd ed. Philadelphia: F. A. Davis.
3. Alzheimer's Association. (Healthcare Professionals and Alzheimer's (various pages). (2015). Retrieved November 2015 from http://www.alz.org/health-care-professionals/health-care-clinical-medical-resources.asp.
4. NIH Consensus Panel. (1999). Rehabilitation of persons with traumatic brain injury. *JAMA*, 8(10), 974–983.
5. Mayo Clinic Staff. (Updated 2012). Mild cognitive impairments (MCI). Retrieved November 2015 from http://www.mayoclinic.org/diseases-conditions/mild-cognitive-impairment/basics/definition/con-20026392.
6. Kirshner, H. S. (2015). Confusional states and acute memory disorders. Retrieved November 2015 from http://misc.medscape.com/pi/iphone/medscapeapp/html/A1135767-business.html.
7. Anderson, H. S. (Updated 2014). Mild cognitive impairment. Retrieved November 2015 from http://emedicine.medscape.com/article/1136393-overview.
8. Family Caregiver Alliance: National Center on Caregiving. (No date). Caring for adults with cognitive and memory impairments. Retrieved November 2015 from http://www.caregiver.org/caring-adults-cognitive-and-memory-impairment.
9. Teasell, R., Marshall, S., Cullen, N., et al. (2013). Evidence-based review of moderate to severe acquired brain injury. The National Center for Evidence-Based Practice in Communication Disorders. Retrieved November 2015 from http://www.abiebr.com/executiveSummary.pdf.

impaired bed Mobility

Taxonomy II: Activity/Rest—Class 2 Activity/Exercise (00091) [**Diagnostic Division:** Safety], Submitted 1998; Revised 2006

DEFINITION: Limitation of independent movement from one bed position to another.

RELATED FACTORS

Neuromuscular or musculoskeletal impairment
Insufficient muscle strength; physical deconditioning; obesity
Environmental barrier (e.g., bed size or type, equipment, restraints)
Pain; pharmaceutical agent
Insufficient knowledge of mobility strategies
Alteration in cognitive functioning

DEFINING CHARACTERISTICS

Objective

Impaired ability to: reposition self in bed, turn from side to side
Impaired ability to move between: prone and supine positions, sitting/long sitting and supine positions

Sample Clinical Applications: Paralysis (e.g., spinal cord injury [SCI], stroke), traumatic brain injury, neuromuscular disorders (e.g., amyotrophic lateral sclerosis [ALS]), major chest or back surgery, severe depression, dementia, catatonic schizophrenia

DESIRED OUTCOMES/EVALUATION CRITERIA

Sample NOC linkages:

Body Positioning: Self-Initiated: Ability to change own body position independently with or without assistive device

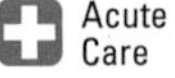

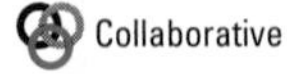

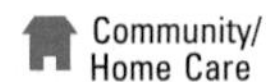

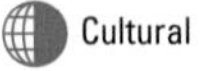

Coordinated Movement: Adequacy of muscles to work together voluntarily for purposeful movement
Immobility Consequences: Physiological: Severity of compromise in physiological functioning due to impaired physical mobility

---

Client/Caregiver Will (Include Specific Time Frame)

- Verbalize willingness to and participates in repositioning program.
- Verbalize understanding of situation or risk factors, individual therapeutic regimen, and safety measures.
- Demonstrate techniques or behaviors that enable safe repositioning.
- Maintain position of function and skin integrity as evidenced by absence of contractures, foot drop, decubitus, and other skin disorders.
- Maintain or increase strength and function of affected and/or compensatory body part.

ACTIONS/INTERVENTIONS

Sample NIC linkages:
Bed Rest Care: Promotion of comfort and safety and prevention of complications for a patient unable to get out of bed
Positioning: Deliberative placement of the patient or a body part to promote physiological and/or psychological well-being
Teaching: Prescribed Activity/Exercise: Preparing a patient to achieve and/or maintain a prescribed level of activity

NURSING PRIORITY NO. 1 To identify causative/contributing factors:

- Determine diagnoses that contribute to current immobility (e.g., multiple sclerosis, arthritis, Parkinson's disease, hemi-/para- or tetraplegia; fractures [especially hip joint and long bone fractures], multiple trauma, head injury, burns) *to identify interventions specific to client's mobility impairment and needs.*
- Note individual factors (e.g., surgery, casts, amputation, traction, pain, advanced age, general weakness or debilitation, severe depression, dementia) *that can contribute to problems related to bedrest.*
- Determine degree of perceptual or cognitive impairment or ability to follow directions. *Impairments related to age, acute or chronic conditions (including severe depression, dementia), trauma, surgery, or medications require alternative interventions or changes in plan of care. Note: Studies have shown that cognitive abilities are crucial to ongoing planning, decision making, and monitoring of one's own movements necessary for successful mobility.*[1,3,9]
- Review results of testing (e.g., Lower Extremity Functional Scale, Harris Hip Score; the self-paced walk, timed up-and-go tests) *to determine limitations in body activity, function, and structure.*[8]

NURSING PRIORITY NO. 2 To assess functional ability:

- Determine functional level classification 0 to 4 *(level 0 is full self-care, level I requires use of equipment or device, level II requires assistance or supervision of another person, level III requires assistance or supervision of another person and equipment or device, level IV is dependent and does not participate).*[12]
- Note emotional and behavioral responses to problems of immobility. *Can negatively affect self-concept and self-esteem, autonomy, and independence. Feelings of frustration and powerlessness may impede attainment of goals. Social, occupational, and relationship roles can change, leading to isolation, depression, and economic consequences.*[4,5]
- Note presence of complications related to immobility. *The effects of immobility are rarely confined to one body system and can include muscle wasting, contractures, pressure sores, constipation, aspiration pneumonia, etc. Studies have shown that as much as 5.5% of muscle strength can be lost each day of rest and immobility.*[1] *Other complications include changes in circulation and impairments of organ function affecting the*

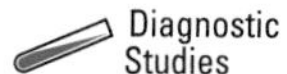
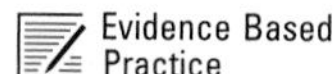
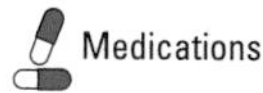

whole person (e.g., cognition, immune system function, emotional state). (Refer to ND risk for Disuse Syndrome for additional interventions.)

NURSING PRIORITY NO. 3 To promote optimal level of function and prevent complications:

- Assist with treatment of underlying condition(s) *to maximize potential for mobility and optimal function.*
- Ascertain that dependent client is placed in best bed for situation (e.g., properly functioning equipment, correct size and support surface) *to promote environmental, client, and caregiver safety.*[6]
- Instruct client/caregiver in bed capabilities (e.g., mobility functions and set positions), encouraging client to participate as much as possible, even if only to move head or run bed controls. *Promotes independence and purposeful movement.*
- Change client's position frequently, moving individual parts of the body (e.g., legs, arms, head), using appropriate support and proper body alignment. Encourage periodic changes in head of bed (if not contraindicated by conditions such as acute SCI), with client in supine and prone positions at intervals *to improve circulation and reduce tightening of muscles and joints, normalizing body tone and more closely simulating body positions individual would normally use.*[2]
- Instruct caregivers in methods of moving client relative to specific situations (e.g., turning side to side, or prone or sitting) *to provide support for the client's body and to prevent injury to the lifter. Note: Positioning instructions and detailed sketches are available (e.g., Ossman)*[7] *on proper positions for certain conditions (e.g., paralyzed client) as well as the safe movement and positioning of body parts (e.g., rolling, bridging, scooting, sitting), which should become well known to caregivers in order to prevent injury to both the client and the caregivers.*
- Place client in upright position at intervals, or out of bed into upright chair, if condition allows. *Being vertical has been shown to reduce the work of heart, improve circulation and lung ventilation, and may improve cognition and awareness.*[3]
- Use pressure-relieving devices (e.g., egg crate, alternating air pressure, or water mattress) and padding and positioning devices (e.g., foam wedge, pillows, hand rolls, etc., for bony prominences, feet, hands, elbows, head) *to prevent dermal injury or stress on tissues and reduce potential for disuse complications.*[3,6] Refer to ND risk for peripheral neurovascular Dysfunction for additional interventions.
- Perform and encourage regular skin examination for reddened or excoriated areas. Use a pressure risk assessment scale (e.g., Braden, Norton) as appropriate. *A review of 33 studies revealed no decrease in pressure ulcer incidence which might be attributed to use of an assessment scale. However, the use of scales increased the intensity and effectiveness of prevention interventions.*[10]
- Provide frequent skin care (e.g., cleansing, moisturizing, gentle massage) *to reduce pressure on sensitive areas and prevent development of problems with skin or tissue integrity.* Refer to NDs impaired Skin Integrity; impaired Tissue Integrity.
- Provide or assist with daily range-of-motion interventions (active and passive) *to maintain joint mobility, improve circulation, and prevent contractures. Note: A random clinical trial found that regular exercising of joints prevented stiffness of knee tendons and improved joint function in clients on bedrest.*[11]
- Collaborate with rehabilitation team and physical or occupational therapists to create exercise and adaptive program designed specifically for client and to identify assistive devices (e.g., splints, braces, boots) and equipment (e.g., transfer board, sling, trapeze, hydraulic lift, specialty beds).
- Assist with activities of hygiene, feeding, and toileting, as indicated. Assist on and off bedpan and into sitting position (or use cardioposition bed or foot-egress bed) to facilitate elimination.
- Note change in strength to do more or less self-care (e.g., hygiene, feeding, toileting) *to promote psychological and physical benefits of self-care and to adjust level of assistance as indicated.*
- Administer medication before activity as needed for pain relief *to permit maximal effort and involvement in activity.*
- Provide diversional activities (e.g., television, books, music, games, visiting) as appropriate *to decrease boredom and potential for depression.*

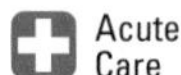
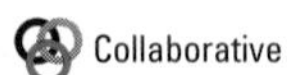
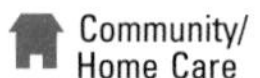
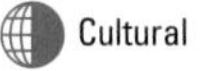

- Ensure telephone or call bell is within reach and client is able to activate surveillance alarm if provided. *Provides individually appropriate methods for client to communicate needs for assistance.*
- Refer to NDs Activity Intolerance, impaired physical Mobility, impaired wheelchair Mobility, risk for Disuse Syndrome, impaired Transfer Ability, and impaired Walking for additional interventions.

NURSING PRIORITY NO. 4 To promote wellness (Teaching/Discharge Considerations):

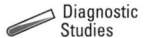

- Involve client/significant other in determining activity schedule. *Promotes commitment to plan, maximizing outcomes.*
- Instruct all caregivers in safety concerns regarding body mechanics, as well as client's required positions and exercises, *to prevent injury to both and to minimize potential for preventable complications.*
- Encourage continuation of regular exercise program *to maintain or enhance gains in strength and muscle control.*
- Obtain or identify sources for assistive devices. Demonstrate safe use and proper maintenance. *Promotes independence and enhances safety.*

DOCUMENTATION FOCUS

Assessment/Reassessment

- Individual findings, including level of function and ability to participate in specific or desired activities.

Planning

- Plan of care and who is involved in the planning.
- Teaching plan.

Implementation/Evaluation

- Responses to interventions, teaching, and actions performed.
- Attainment or progress toward desired outcome(s).
- Modification to plan of care.

Discharge Planning

- Discharge and long-range needs, noting who is responsible for each action to be taken.
- Specific referrals made.
- Sources of and maintenance for assistive devices.

References

1. Stanley, M. (1999). The aging musculoskeletal system. In Stanley, M., Beare, P. G. (eds). *Gerontological Nursing: A Health Promotion/Protection Approach.* 2nd ed. Philadelphia, PA: F. A. Davis.
2. Kumagai, K. A. S. (1998). Physical management of the neurologically involved client: Techniques for bed mobility and transfers. In Chin, P. A., Finocchiaro, D., et al. (eds). *Rehabilitation Nursing Practice.* New York, NY: McGraw-Hill.
3. Buchman, A. S., Boyle, P. A., Leurgans, S. E., et al. (2011). Cognitive function is associated with the development of mobility impairments in community-dwelling elders. *Am J Geriatr Psychiatry*, 19(6), 571–580.
4. Mass, M. L. (1989). Impaired physical mobility. Unpublished manuscript. Cited in research article for National Institutes for Health.
5. Hogue, C. C. (1984). Falls and mobility late in life: An ecological model. *J Am Geriatr Soc*, 32, 858–861.
6. Dionne, M. (2005). This bed is just right. *Rehabil Manage*, 18(1), 32–39.
7. Ossman, N., Campbell, M. (1995). *Adult Positions, Transitions, and Transfers: Reproducible Instruction Cards for Caregivers.* Tuscon, AZ: Communication Skill Builders/Therapy Skill Builders.
8. Cibulka, N. T., White, D. M., Woehrle, J., et al. (2009). Hip pain and mobility deficits—Hip osteoarthritis: Clinical practice guidelines linked to the International Classification of Functioning Disability, and Health from the Orthopaedic Section of the American Physical Therapy Association. *J Orthop Sports Phys Ther*, 39(4), A1–A25.

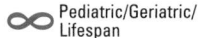

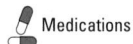

9. Bakker, M., De Lange, F. P., Helmich, R. C., et al. (2006). Cerebral correlates of motor imagery of normal and precision gait. *Neuroimage*, 41, 998–1010.
10. Pancorbo-Hidalgo, P. L., Garcia-Fernandez, F. P., Lopez-Medina, I. M. (2006). Risk assessment scales for pressure ulcers prevention: A systematic review. *J Adv Nurs*, 54(1), 94–110.
11. Kubo, K., Akima, H., Ushiyama, J., et al. (2004). Effects of resistance training during bed rest on the viscoelastic properties of tendon structures of tendon structures in the lower limb. *Scand J Med Sci Sports*, 14(5), 296–302.
12. Gordon, M. (2010). Functional levels code. *Manual of Nursing Diagnosis*. 12th ed. Sudbury, MA: Jones and Bartlett.

impaired physical Mobility

Taxonomy II: Activity/Rest—Class 2 Activity/Exercise (00085) [**Diagnostic Division:** Safety], Submitted 1973; Revised 1998, 2013

DEFINITION: Limitation in independent, purposeful physical movement of the body or of one or more extremities.

RELATED FACTORS

Activity intolerance; decrease in endurance; physical deconditioning; sedentary lifestyle
Alteration in bone structure integrity; neuromuscular, musculoskeletal, or sensorioperceptual impairment; disuse
Alteration in cognitive functioning; developmental delay
Alteration in metabolism; body mass index above 75th age-appropriate percentile; malnutrition
Anxiety; depression
Cultural belief regarding appropriate activity
Decrease in muscle mass, control or strength; joint stiffness; contractures
Insufficient environmental support (e.g., physical, social)
Insufficient knowledge of value of physical activity
Pain
Pharmaceutical agent
Prescribed movement restrictions; reluctance to initiate movement

DEFINING CHARACTERISTICS

Subjective

Discomfort; [reluctance/unwillingness to move]

Objective

Alteration in gait; postural instability
Decrease in fine or gross motor skills; movement-induced tremor
Decrease in range of motion; difficulty turning
Decrease in reaction time; slowed or spastic movement; uncoordinated movement
Engages in substitutions for movement (e.g., attention to other's activities, controlling behavior, focus on pre-illness activity)
Exertional dyspnea

Sample Clinical Applications: Neuromuscular disorders (e.g., multiple sclerosis [MS], amyotrophic lateral sclerosis [ALS], Parkinson's disease), traumatic injuries (e.g., fractures, spinal cord or brain injuries), osteoarthritis, rheumatoid arthritis, severe depression

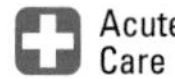

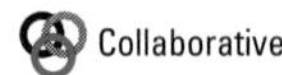

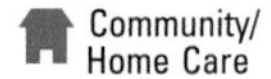

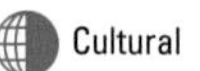

SUGGESTED FUNCTIONAL LEVEL CLASSIFICATION

0—Full self-care
I—Requires use of equipment or device
II—Requires assistance or supervision of another person
III—Requires assistance or supervision of another person and equipment or device
IV—Is dependent and does not participate[12]

DESIRED OUTCOMES/EVALUATION CRITERIA

Sample NOC linkages:
Mobility: Ability to move purposefully in own environment independently with or without assistive device
Immobility Consequences: Physiological: Severity of compromise in physiological functioning due to impaired physical mobility
Knowledge: Prescribed Activity: Extent of understanding conveyed about prescribed activity and exercise

Client Will (Include Specific Time Frame)
- Verbalize understanding of situation and individual treatment regimen and safety measures.
- Demonstrate techniques or behaviors that enable resumption of activities.
- Participate in activities of daily living (ADLs) and desired activities.
- Maintain position of function and skin integrity as evidenced by absence of contractures, footdrop, decubitus, etc.
- Maintain or increase strength and function of affected or compensatory body part.

ACTIONS/INTERVENTIONS

Sample NIC linkages:
Exercise Therapy: Joint Mobility/Muscle Control: Use of active or passive body movement to maintain or restore flexibility/use of specific activity or exercise protocols to enhance or restore controlled body movement, etc.
Pain Management: Alleviation of pain or a reduction in pain to a level of comfort that is acceptable to the patient
Traction/Immobilization Care: Management of a patient who has traction and/or a stabilizing device to immobilize and stabilize a body part

NURSING PRIORITY NO. 1 To identify causative/contributing factors:

- Determine diagnosis that contributes to immobility (e.g., MS, arthritis, Parkinson's disease, cardiopulmonary disorders, hemi/paraplegia, depression, developmental delays). *These conditions can cause physiological and psychological problems that can seriously impact physical, social, and economic well-being.*[1]
- Note factors affecting current situation (e.g., surgery, fractures, amputation, tubings [chest tube, Foley catheter, IVs, pumps], and potential time involved [e.g., few hours in bed after surgery versus serious trauma requiring long-term bedrest or debilitating disease limiting movement]). *Identifies potential impairments and determines type of interventions needed to provide for client's safety.*
- Assess client's developmental level, motor skills, ease and capability of movement, and posture and gait *to determine presence of characteristics of client's unique impairment and to guide choice of interventions.*[8]
- Note older client's general health status. *Hogue identified mobility as the most important functional ability that determines the degree of independence and healthcare needs among older persons.*[2] *While aging does not cause impaired mobility, per se, several predisposing factors in addition to age-related changes can lead to immobility (e.g., diminished body reserves of musculoskeletal system, chronic diseases, sedentary*

lifestyle, decreased ability to quickly and adequately correct movements affecting center of gravity). Thus, falls are a major source of morbidity and mortality for older persons.[3,6,8]

- Evaluate for presence and degree of pain, listening to client's description about manner in which pain limits mobility *to determine if pain management can improve mobility.*[4]
- Ascertain client's perception of activity and exercise needs and impact of current situation. Identify cultural beliefs and expectations affecting recovery or response to long-term limitations. *Helps to determine client's expectations and beliefs related to activity and potential long-term effect of current immobility. Also identifies barriers that may be addressed (e.g., lack of safe place to exercise, focus on pre-illness or disability activity, controlling behavior, depression, cultural expectations, distorted body image).*[5]
- Assess nutritional status and client's report of energy level. *Deficiencies in nutrients and water, electrolytes, and minerals can negatively affect energy and activity tolerance.*
- Determine history of falls and relatedness to current situation. *Client may be restricting activity because of weakness or debilitation, actual injury during a fall, or from psychological distress (i.e., fear and anxiety) that can persist after a fall.*[6–8]

NURSING PRIORITY NO. 2 To assess functional ability:

- Determine degree of immobility in relation to 0–4 scale, noting muscle strength and tone, joint mobility, cardiovascular status, balance, and endurance. *Identifies strengths and deficits (e.g., ability to ambulate with or without assistive devices, inability to transfer safely from bed to wheelchair) and may provide information regarding potential for recovery (e.g., client with severe brain injury may have permanent limitations because of impaired cognition affecting memory, judgment, problem solving, and motor planning, requiring more intensive inpatient and long-term care).*[1,6]
- Determine degree of perceptual or cognitive impairment and ability to follow directions. *Impairments related to age, chronic or acute disease condition, trauma, surgery, or medications require alternative interventions or changes in plan of care.*[3]
- Observe movement when client is unaware of observation *to note any incongruency with reports of abilities.*
- Note emotional or behavioral responses to problems of immobility. *Can negatively affect self-concept and self-esteem, autonomy, and independence. Feelings of frustration and powerlessness may impede attainment of goals. Social, occupational, and relationship roles can change, leading to isolation, depression, and economic consequences.*[1,2]
- Determine presence of complications related to immobility. *The effects of immobility are rarely confined to one body system and can include muscle wasting, contractures, pressure sores, constipation, aspiration pneumonia, etc. Studies have shown that healthy individuals who were subjected to immobility experienced a 1.3% to 3% loss in muscle strength per day, and overall postural muscle strength decreased by 10% during 1 wk of bed rest.*[5,7] *Other complications include changes in circulation and impairments of organ function affecting the whole person (e.g., cognition, bone demineralization, venous pooling, thromboembolic phenomena, weakened immune system function).* (Refer to ND risk for Disuse Syndrome.)

NURSING PRIORITY NO. 3 To promote optimal level of function and prevent complications:

- Assist with treatment of underlying condition(s) *to maximize potential for mobility and optimal function.*
- Discuss discrepancies in movement with client aware and unaware of observation and methods for dealing with identified problems. *May be necessary when client is using avoidance or controlling behavior or is not aware of own abilities due to anxiety or fear.*
- Assist with or encourage client to reposition self on a regular schedule as dictated by individual situation (including frequent shifting of weight when client is wheelchair-bound) *to enhance circulation to tissues and reduce risk of tissue ischemia.*
- Review and encourage use of proper body mechanics *to prevent injury to client and caregiver.*
- Demonstrate and assist with use of siderails, overhead trapeze, roller pads, and hydraulic lifts or chairs *for position changes and transfers.* Instruct in safe use of walker or cane *to facilitate safe ambulation.*

Acute Care

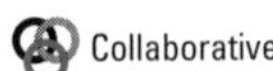
Collaborative

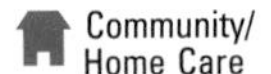
Community/ Home Care

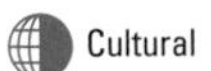
Cultural

- Support affected body parts and joints using pillows or rolls, foot supports, shoes, gel pads, etc., *to maintain position of function and reduce risk of pressure ulcers.*
- Provide or recommend pressure-reducing mattress, such as egg crate, or pressure-relieving mattress, such as alternating air pressure or water. *Reduces tissue pressure and aids in maximizing cellular perfusion to prevent dermal injury.*
- Use padding and positioning devices (e.g., foam wedge, pillows, hand rolls) for bony prominences, feet, hands, elbows, head) *to prevent stress on tissues and reduce potential for disuse complications.*
- Collaborate with physical medicine specialist and occupational or physical therapists in providing range-of-motion exercise (active or passive), isotonic muscle contractions (e.g., flexion of ankles, push and pull exercises), assistive devices, and activities (e.g., early ambulation, transfers, stairs) *to limit or reduce effects and complications of immobility (e.g., contracture deformities, deep vein thromboses). Techniques such as gait training, strength training, and exercise to improve balance and coordination can be helpful in preventing complications and in rehabilitating client.*[11]
- Encourage client's participation in self-care activities and physical or occupational therapies as well as diversional and recreational activities. *Reduces sensory deprivation, enhances self-concept and sense of independence, and improves body strength and function.*
- Provide client with ample time to perform mobility-related tasks. Schedule activities with adequate rest periods during the day *to reduce fatigue and improve endurance and strength.*
- Avoid routinely assisting or doing for client those activities that client can do for self. *Caregivers can contribute to impaired mobility by being overprotective or helping too much.*
- Identify and encourage energy-conserving techniques for ADLs. *Limits fatigue, maximizing participation.*
- Provide for safety measures as indicated by individual situation, including environmental management and fall prevention. (Refer to ND risk for Falls.)
- Note change in strength to do more or less self-care (e.g., hygiene, feeding, toileting, therapies) *to promote psychological and physical benefits of self-care and to adjust level of assistance as indicated.*
- Administer medications before activity as needed for pain relief *to permit maximal effort and involvement in activity.*
- Perform and encourage regular skin examination and care *to reduce pressure on sensitive areas and to prevent development of problems with skin integrity.* (Refer to NDs risk for impaired Skin Integrity and risk for impaired Tissue Integrity for additional interventions.)
- Encourage adequate intake of fluids and nutritious foods. *Promotes well-being and maximizes energy production.*
- Refer to NDs Activity Intolerance, risk for Falls, impaired bed Mobility, impaired wheelchair Mobility, impaired Transfer Ability, impaired Sitting, impaired Standing, or impaired Walking for additional interventions.

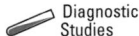

NURSING PRIORITY NO. 4 To promote wellness (Teaching/Discharge Considerations):

- Encourage client's/significant other's (SO's) involvement in decision making as much as possible. *Enhances commitment to plan, optimizing outcomes.*
- Review importance and purpose of exercise *(e.g., increased cardiovascular and respiratory tolerance; improved flexibility, balance, and muscle strength and tone; enhanced sense of well-being).*
- Discuss safe ways that client can exercise. *Multiple options provide client choices and variety (e.g., walking around the block with companion or in a mall during bad air days, participating in a water aerobics class, attending regular rehab sessions).*
- Assist client/SO to learn safety measures as individually indicated. *May need instruction and to give return demonstration (e.g., use of heating pads, locking wheelchair before transfers, removal or securing of scatter or area rugs, judicious and accurate use of medications, supervised exercise).*
- Involve client and SO(s) in care, assisting them to learn ways of managing problems of immobility, especially when impairment is expected to be long term. *May need referral for support and community services to provide care, supervision, companionship, respite services, nutritional and ADL assistance, adaptive devices or changes to living environment, financial assistance, etc.*[8]

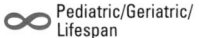

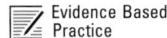

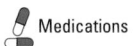

- Demonstrate use of standing aids and mobility devices (e.g., walkers, strollers, scooters, braces, prosthetics) and have client/care provider demonstrate knowledge about and safe use of device. Identify appropriate resources for obtaining and maintaining appliances or equipment. *Safe use of mobility aids promotes client's independence and enhances quality of life and safety for client and caregiver.*[9,10]

DOCUMENTATION FOCUS

Assessment/Reassessment
- Individual findings, including level of function and ability to participate in specific or desired activities.
- Use of assistive devices.

Planning
- Plan of care and who is involved in the planning.
- Teaching plan.

Implementation/Evaluation
- Responses to interventions, teaching, and actions performed.
- Attainment or progress toward desired outcome(s).
- Modifications to plan of care.

Discharge Planning
- Discharge and long-term needs, noting who is responsible for each action to be taken.
- Specific referrals made.
- Sources of and maintenance for assistive devices.

References

1. Mass, M. L. (1989). Impaired physical mobility. Unpublished manuscript. Cited in research article for National Institutes for Health.
2. Hogue, C. C. (1984). Falls and mobility late in life: An ecological model. *J Am Geriatr Soc*, 32, 858–861.
3. Rowe, J. W., Kahn, R. L. (1987). Human aging: Usual and successful. *Science*, 237, 143–149.
4. McCaffrey, M., Pasero, C. (1999). *Pain: Clinical Manual.* 2nd ed. St. Louis, MO: Mosby.
5. Pattillo, M. A., Stanley, M. (1999). The aging musculoskeletal system. In Stanley, M., Beare, P. G. (eds). *Gerontological Nursing: A Health Promotion/Protection Approach.* 2nd ed. Philadelphia, PA: F. A. Davis.
6. Tinetti, M. E., Williams, T. F., Mayewski, R. (1986). Fall risk index for elderly patients based on number of chronic disabilities. *Am J Med*, 80, 429–434.
7. Hopkins, R., Spuhler, V., Thomsen, G., et al. (2007). Transforming ICU culture to facilitate early mobility. *Crit Care Clin*, 23(1), 81–96.
8. Michael, K. M., Allen, J. K., Macko, R. F. (2006). Fatigue after stroke: Relationship to mobility, fitness, ambulatory activity, social support, and falls efficiency. *Rehabil Nurs*, 31(5), 210–217.
9. Becker, B. (2005). To stand or not to stand. *Rehabil Manage*, 18(2), 28–34.
10. Dworak, P. A., Levy, A. (2005). Strolling along. *Rehabil Manage*, 18(9), 26–31.
11. Ship, K. M. (2010). Gait disturbances in older age: The reasons are many and varied, but researchers agree that identifying the source and preserving mobility are primary concerns. *Duke Med Health News*, 16(8), 3–4.
12. Gordon, M. (2010). Functional levels code. *Manual of Nursing Diagnosis.* 12th ed. Sudbury, MA: Jones and Bartlett.

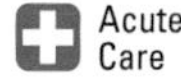

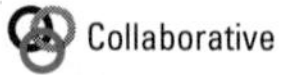

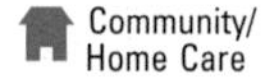

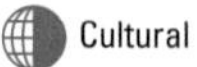

impaired wheelchair Mobility

Taxonomy II: Activity/Rest—Class 2 Activity/Exercise (00089) [**Diagnostic Division:** Safety], Submitted 1998; Revised 2006

DEFINITION: Limitation of independent operation of wheelchair within environment.

RELATED FACTORS

Neuromuscular or musculoskeletal impairments
Insufficient muscle strength; decrease in endurance; physical deconditioning; obesity
Impaired vision
Pain
Alteration in mood; alteration in cognitive functioning
Insufficient knowledge of wheelchair use
Environmental barrier (e.g., stairs, inclines, uneven surfaces, obstacles, distance)

DEFINING CHARACTERISTICS

Objective

Impaired ability to operate manual or power wheelchair on even/uneven surface, an incline/ decline, on curbs
[**Note:** Specify level of independence using a standardized functional scale, refer to ND impaired physical Mobility]

Sample Clinical Applications: Neuromuscular disorders (e.g., multiple sclerosis [MS], amyotrophic lateral sclerosis [ALS]), paralysis (e.g., brain injury/stroke, spinal cord injury [SCI]), muscular dystrophy, cerebral palsy, fractures

DESIRED OUTCOMES/EVALUATION CRITERIA

Sample NOC linkage:

Ambulation: Wheelchair: Ability to move from place to place in a wheelchair
Coordinated Movement: Ability of muscles to work together voluntarily for purposeful movement

Client Will (Include Specific Time Frame)

- Move safely within environment, maximizing independence.
- Identify and use resources appropriately.

Sample NOC linkages:

Fall Prevention Behavior: Personal or family caregiver actions to minimize risk factors that might precipitate falls in the personal environment

Caregiver Will (Include Specific Time Frame)

- Provide safe mobility within environment and community

ACTIONS/INTERVENTIONS

Sample NIC linkages:

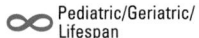

Positioning: Wheelchair: Placement of a patient in a properly selected wheelchair to enhance comfort, promote skin integrity, and foster independence
Exercise Therapy: Muscle Control: Use of specific activity or exercise protocols to enhance or restore controlled body movement
Self-Care Assistance: Transfer: Assisting a patient with limitation of independent movement to learn to change body location

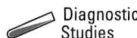

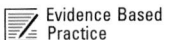

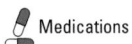

NURSING PRIORITY NO. 1 To identify causative/contributing factors:

- Determine diagnosis that contributes to immobility (e.g., ALS, SCI, spastic cerebral palsy, brain injury) and client's functional level and individual abilities (e.g., 0–4 scale; see ND impaired physical Mobility).
- Identify factors in environments frequented by the client that contribute to inaccessibility (e.g., uneven floors or surfaces, lack of ramps, steep incline or decline, narrow doorways or spaces).
- Ascertain access to and appropriateness of public and/or private transportation.

NURSING PRIORITY NO. 2 To promote optimal level of function and prevent complications:

- Determine that client's underlying physical, cognitive, and emotional impairment(s) (e.g., brain or spinal cord injury, fractures or other trauma; pain, depression, vision deficits) are treated or being managed *to maximize ability, desire, and motivation to participate in wheelchair activities.*[6]
- Collaborate with physical medicine or physical or occupational therapists in planning activities to improve client's ability to independently operate wheelchair within limits of tolerance and adjustment to various environments. *May require individual instruction and encouragement, strengthening exercises, assistance with various tasks, and close supervision.*
- Ascertain that wheelchair provides the base mobility to maximize function. *Wheelchairs must be matched with client's age and size/body type; developmental level and diagnosis or reason to use wheelchair; desired activities; and unique functional needs (e.g., proper seating and support for people in wheelchairs is critical to their ability to travel, work, participate in sports, learn at school, play, and interact socially). If a spouse or family member will be assisting the person using the wheelchair their needs may also need to be considered in the wheelchair selection.*[1,10] *Correct seating is essential for prevention, correction, and compensation for postural changes in order to maintain client's comfort and function. Chair should provide for maximum reach, maneuverability, function, and center of gravity positioning and propulsion; should recline to change back contours, hip angles, and pelvic restrictions; should have back adjustment for changing trunk stability requirements; and should tilt for reposition, pressure relief, and comfort.*[1,2,7,8]
- Perform periodic assessments of client and wheelchair to monitor chair usage and function as well as changes in client's postural, behavioral, and functional status. *Helps to identify problems (e.g., abnormal wear patterns on the chair requiring mechanical adjustments/repair; loss of client's strength where power add-ons to the chair would improve mobility; or alternate methods of mobility that might be needed).*[2]
- Provide for or instruct client in safety while in a wheelchair (e.g., cushions, supports for all body parts, repositioning and transfer assistive devices, position and pressure relief products, feet and leg support, armrest choices, back and height adjustment).[2,7]
- Note surfaces client needs to negotiate and refer to appropriate sources for modifications (e.g., replacing carpet with tile; revising ramps that are too steep, narrow, or slippery). Clear pathways of obstructions.[2,10]
- Recommend and arrange for modifications to home, work, school, or recreational settings frequented by client. *Although most public buildings have certain adaptations in rooms and accesses, they are not always well constructed or in good working order. The client may need assistance in these settings and with requesting that appropriate alterations be carried out.*[9]
- Determine need for and capabilities of assistive persons. Provide training and support, as indicated. *Enhances safety for both client and caregiver.*
- Monitor client's use of joystick, sip and puff, sensitive mechanical switches, etc., *to provide necessary equipment if condition or capabilities change.*
- Monitor client for adverse effects of immobility (e.g., contractures, muscle atrophy, deep venous thrombosis, pressure ulcers). (Refer to NDs Disuse Syndrome and risk for peripheral neurovascular Dysfunction for additional interventions.)

NURSING PRIORITY NO. 3 To promote wellness (Teaching/Discharge Considerations):

- Identify and refer to medical equipment suppliers *to customize client's wheelchair for size, proper seating angle, positioning aids, incline or decline stability, accessories (e.g., side guards, headrests, heel loops, brake extensions, tool packs), and electronics suited to client's ability (e.g., sip and puff, head movement, sensitive switches).*[6,8]

- Encourage client's/significant others' (SOs') involvement in decision making as much as possible. *Enhances sense of control and commitment to plan, thereby optimizing outcomes.*
- Involve client/SO(s) in care, assisting them in managing immobility problems. *Promotes independence in self-evaluation and self-care, including managing the type of wheelchair and other assistive devices best for client, how the user's needs and abilities change over time, and modifications that might be made (e.g., number and placement of ramps around the home; modifications to rooms, doors, and vehicles).*[3]
- Demonstrate, discuss, and provide information regarding wheelchair safety as individually appropriate, including safe transfers, dealing with uneven surfaces, ramps, and curbs; programming speed on power chairs; etc. Include information and refer for wheelchair preventative maintenance measures (e.g., for wheelchair locks, tires, axles, casters, metal parts, batteries) as indicated. *Wheelchair safety involves people and equipment and is a daily factor in the life of the client and caregivers. This includes not only acquiring the best chair, but also maintenance of the chair and provision for obtaining relief when chair malfunctions. Many states have enacted wheelchair lemon laws that "mandate warranties to maintain assistive technology in proper working condition, to assure availability of appropriate loaner replacement chairs during repair time, and to encourage manufacturers and dealers to cooperatively pool assistive technology resources for loaner purposes to assure availability without undue burden."*[4]
- Refer to support groups relative to specific medical condition/disability and geared toward client's independence. Suggest involvement in political action group, as indicated. *Provides role modeling, assistance with problem solving, and social change.*
- Identify community resources to provide ongoing support. *The current societal view (that persons with disabilities have the right to be self-determining and to make their own choices about their lives and to achieve the quality of life each believes is personal best) places as much emphasis on community regarding integration as on physical rehabilitation and functional capabilities.*[5]

DOCUMENTATION FOCUS

Assessment/Reassessment

- Individual findings, including level of function/ability to participate in specific/desired activities.
- Type of wheelchair and equipment needs.
- Environmental factors and problems.

Planning

- Plan of care and who is involved in the planning.
- Teaching plan.

Implementation/Evaluation

- Responses to interventions, teaching, and actions performed.

Discharge Planning

- Discharge and long-term needs, noting who is responsible for each action to be taken.
- Specific referrals made.
- Sources of and maintenance for assistive devices.

References

1. Rodby-Bousquet, E., Hagglund, C. (2010). Use of manual and powered wheelchair in children with cerebral palsy: A cross-sectional study. BMC Pediatrics, 10:59. Retrieved October 2015 from http://www.biomedcentral.com/1471-2431/10/59.
2. Rader, J., Jones, D., Miller, L. Individualizing wheelchair seating: For older adults. Part 1: A guide for caregivers. Benedictine Institute for Long Term Care. Retrieved November 2015 from http://primaris.org/sites/default/files/resources/Restraints%20and%20Falls/A%20Guide%20for%20Caregivers_Individualized%20Wheelchair%20Seating.pdf.
3. Lathrop, D. (2000). Making mobility ramps work for you. Retrieved November 2015 from http://www.mobility-advisor.com/mobility-ramps.html.
4. Concerning Self-Sufficiency for Persons with Disabilities by Assuring Reliable Assistive Technology. Denver, CO. Colorado House Bill 97-1194 Bill signed into law April 30, 1997.
5. Scherer, M. (2002). *The Importance of Assistive Technology Outcomes*. Washington, DC: Institute for Matching Person & Technology.
6. Cohen, D. (2005). Optional but necessary. *Rehabil Manage*, 18(10), 26–29.
7. Rosen, L. (2005). Sit on it. *Rehabil Manage*, 18(2), 36–41.
8. Waugh, K. G. (2005). Measuring the right angle. *Rehabil Manage*, 18(1), 40–49.
9. McCullagh, M. C. (2006). Home modification. *Am J Nurs*, 106(10), 54–63.
10. Department of Rehabilitation Science and Technology. (2006). Wheelchair selection: How to choose a new wheelchair. Fact sheet from WheelchairNet. Retrieved November 2015 from http://www.wheelchairnet.org/wcn_prodserv/consumers/selectwc.html.

impaired Mood Regulation

Taxonomy II: Coping/Stress Tolerance—Class 2 Coping Responses (00241) [**Diagnostic Division:** Ego Integrity], Submitted 2013

DEFINITION: A mental state characterized by shifts in mood or affect and which is comprised of a constellation of affective, cognitive, somatic and/or physiological manifestations varying from mild to severe.

RELATED FACTORS

Appetite or weight change; alteration in sleep pattern
Chronic illness; pain; functional impairment
Loneliness; impaired social functioning; social isolation
Recurrent thoughts of death or suicide
Anxiety; hypervigilance; psychosis
Substance misuse

DEFINING CHARACTERISTICS

Subjective

Excessive self-awareness, guilt, self-blame
Hopelessness

Objective

Sad affect, withdrawal
Irritability; impaired concentration
Psychomotor agitation, retardation
Changes in verbal behavior; flight of thoughts; dysphoria; disinhibition
Influenced self-esteem

Sample Clinical Applications: depression, bipolar disorder, anxiety states, autism spectrum disorder

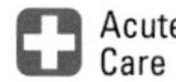

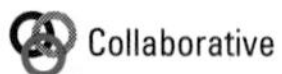

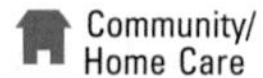

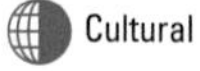

DESIRED OUTCOMES/EVALUATION CRITERIA

Sample NOC linkage:
Mood Equilibrium: Appropriate adjustment of prevailing emotional tone in response to circumstances

Client Will (Include Specific Time Frame)
- Acknowledge reality of mood problems/needs.
- Identify areas of concern.
- Participate in treatment program or therapy regimen.
- Maintain physical health as evidenced by adequate nutrition, weight within normal limits, and good sleep habits.

ACTIONS/INTERVENTIONS

Sample NIC linkage:
Mood Management: Providing for safety, stabilization, recovery, and maintenance of a person who is experiencing dysfunctionally depressed or elevated mood

NURSING PRIORITY NO. 1 To assess causative/contributing factors:

- Determine specific reasons for client's mood swings/difficulties. (Refer to Related Factors and Defining Characteristics.) *Allows for accurate planning of care for individual.*[1]
- Assess ability to understand current situation. *Mood disturbances are prevalent in many disorders and may affect individual's cognitive functioning and understanding of events.*[1]
- Review history and evaluate for underlying neurological disorders. *Presence of traumatic brain injuries, tumors, stroke, and autism may result in variations of mood and emotional processing deficits.*[1]
- Ascertain degree of depression individual is experiencing. *Impaired mood regulation is known to be a factor in vulnerability to depression.*[5]
- Identify behaviors that interfere with person's daily activities. *Being aware of behaviors, such as sleep or appetite disturbances, altered social activity, irritability, and impaired concentration, facilitates identification of treatment options for change.*[2]
- Determine availability and use of resources.

NURSING PRIORITY NO. 2 To assist client to regulate mood changes more effectively:

- Discuss how client perceives the current situation and how it is affecting emotions. *A negative outlook is associated with difficulty in cognitive control and emotional regulation strategies.*[5]
- Determine extent of rumination and reappraisal and expressive suppression. *As the individual goes over and over the negative thoughts, it is more difficult to effect cognitive control and depression can worsen.*[5]
- Encourage client to pay attention to emotional states and feelings and identify when they occur and record in a journal or notebook. *Awareness of one's emotions helps the individual to deal appropriately with them.*[3]
- Clarify meanings of feelings by checking meaning with client and providing feedback. *Validates and ensures accuracy of meaning of the communication.*[6]
- Discuss how negative thinking and rumination intensify depression. *It appears individual differences can affect the strategies the person uses to recover from a negative mood.*[5]
- Provide information regarding use of electroconvulsive therapy (ECT) as indicated. *It is not known exactly how this treatment helps; it is thought to alter brain chemistry and function that relieves depression in 80% to 90% of clients.*[8] *The client with severe depression that does not respond to medication may benefit from ECT along with psychotherapy.*[7]

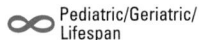

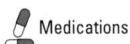

NURSING PRIORITY NO. 3 To promote wellness (Teaching/Discharge Considerations):

- Involve client in cognitive/behavioral, mindfulness-based, or individual psychotherapy. *Having the client identify thinking patterns that result in depression allows the individual to recognize and avoid them, improving the ability to recover.*[5]
- Discuss the use of and administer medications as indicated. *Antidepressants can be useful in mood disorders and along with psychotherapy can help the client maintain usual activities.*[7]
- Involve client in group therapy. *Group discussions promote awareness of others who are experiencing similar difficulties and promotes new ideas for dealing with own concerns.*[4]
- Encourage client to become involved in community activities. *Provides opportunity to develop social skills and interests outside of own concerns.*[5]

DOCUMENTATION FOCUS

Assessment/Reassessment
- Individual findings, including client's specific situation and impact on functioning/life.
- Description of negative thinking patterns.

Planning
- Treatment plan and individual responsibility for activities.
- Teaching plan.

Implementation/Evaluation
- Client involvement and response to interventions, teaching and actions performed.
- Attainment or progress toward desired outcomes.
- Modification to plan of care.

Discharge Planning

Specific referrals made and follow-up plan.

References

1. Brockmeyer, T. et al. (2012). Mood Regulation Expectancies and Emotion Avoidance in Depression Vulnerability. Elsevier. Retrieved January 2015 from http://www.sciencedirect.com/science/article/pii/S0191886912001353.
2. Malefsky, C., et al. (2013). The role of emotion regulation in autism spectrum disorder. Journal of the American Academy of Child & Adolescent Psychiatry. Retrieved January 2015 from http://www.sciencedirect.com/science/article/pii/S0890856713003080.
3. Eijndhover, P., et al. (2013). Paralimbic cortical thickness in first-episode depression: Evidence for trait-related differences in mood regulation. Am J Psych. Retrieved January 2015 from http://www.mdlinx.com/psychiatry/news-article.cfm/4987221/depressive-disorders-mood-major-depressive-disorder.
4. Hoppes, K. (2006). The application of mindfulness-based cognitive interventions in the treatment of co-occurring addictive and mood disorders. CNS Spectrums. Retrieved January 2015 from http://www.cnsspectrums.com/aspx/article_pf.aspx?articleid=790.
5. Joorman, J., and Gottlieb, I. (2010). Emotion regulation in depression: Relation to cognitive inhibition. NIH. Retrieved January 2015 from http://www.ncbi.nlm.nih.gov/pmc/articles/PMC2839199.
6. Burns, D. D. (1999). *Feeling Good: The New Mood Therapy*. New York, NY, Avon.
7. Cherie, M., and Paradisio, S. (2008). Cognitive and neurological impairment in mood disorders. NIH Public Access. Retrieved January 2015 from http://www.ncbi.nlm.nih.gov/pmc/articles/PMC2570029/.
8. Miller, M.C. (medical editor) (2013) Understanding depression: Special health report. Harvard Health Pub. Retrieved January 2015 from www.health.harvard.edu.

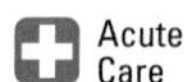

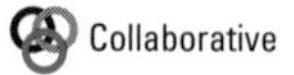

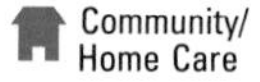

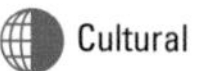

Moral Distress

Taxonomy II: Life Principles—Class 3 Value/Belief/Action Congruence (00175) [**Diagnostic Division:** Ego Integrity], Submitted 2006

DEFINITION: Response to the inability to carry out one's chosen ethical/moral decision/action.

RELATED FACTORS

Conflict among decision makers [e.g., client/family, healthcare providers, insurance payers, regulatory agencies]
Conflicting information available for moral or ethical decision making; cultural incongruences
Treatment decision; end-of-life decisions; loss of autonomy
Time constraint for decision making; physical distance of decision maker

DEFINING CHARACTERISTICS

Subjective

Anguish about acting on one's moral choice (e.g., powerlessness, anxiety, fear)

DESIRED OUTCOMES/EVALUATION CRITERIA

Sample NOC linkages:
Decision-Making: Ability to make judgments and choose between two or more alternatives
Client Satisfaction: Protection of Rights: Extent of positive perception of a patient's legal and moral rights provided by nursing staff
Participation in Health-Care Decision: Personal involvement in selecting and evaluating healthcare options to achieve desired outcome

Client Will (Include Specific Time Frame)

- Verbalize understanding of causes for conflict in own situation.
- Be aware of own moral values conflicting with desired or required course of action.
- Identify positive ways or actions necessary to deal with own self and situation.
- Express sense of satisfaction with or acceptance of resolution.

ACTIONS/INTERVENTIONS

Sample NIC linkages:
Values Clarification: Assisting another to clarify her or his own values in order to facilitate effective decision making
Decision-Making Support: Providing information and support for a patient who is making a decision regarding healthcare
Mutual Goal-Setting: Collaborating with a patient to identify and prioritize care goals, then developing a plan of care for achieving those goals

NURSING PRIORITY NO. 1 To identify cause/situation in which moral distress is occurring:

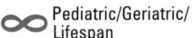

- Note situations or individuals at high risk for conflict. *For example, family members not agreeing on proper course of action for comatose loved one, parents faced with expectation of taking ventilator-dependent child home and effect on family as a whole,*[8] *and care providers discontinuing life support measures for preterm infant are likely to encounter some degree of distress with decision making but may be silent about their dis-*

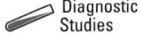

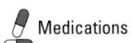

comfort. Recognizing potential for moral distress allows for timely intervention and support for involved parties.

- Determine client's perceptions and specific factors resulting in a sense of distress and all parties involved in situation. *Conflict may be personal or job related. Moral conflict centers around lessening the amount of harm suffered, with the involved individuals usually struggling with decisions such as what "can be done" to prevent, improve, or cure a medical condition or what "ought to be done" in a specific situation, often within financial constraints or scarcity of resources.*[6]
- Note use of sarcasm, avoidance, apathy, crying, reports of depression, or loss of meaning. *Individuals may not understand their feelings of uneasiness or distress or know that the emotional basis for moral distress is anger.*[4]
- Ascertain response of family/significant others (SOs) to client's situation/healthcare choices. *May provide clues to emotional or conflictual problems individual is experiencing.*
- Identify healthcare goals and expectations. *New treatment options and technology can prolong life or postpone death based on the individual's personal viewpoint, increasing the possibility of conflict with others, including healthcare providers.*[2]
- Ascertain cultural beliefs and values and degree of importance to client. *Cultural diversity may lead to disparate views and expectations between client, SO/family members, and healthcare providers. When tensions between conflicting values cannot be resolved, persons experience moral distress.*[2]
- Note attitudes and expressions of dissatisfaction of caregivers/staff. *Client may feel pressure or disapproval if own views are not congruent with expectations of those perceived to be more knowledgeable or in "authority." Furthermore, healthcare providers may themselves feel moral distress in carrying out or refraining from performing requested interventions.*[7]
- Determine degree of emotional and physical distress (e.g., fatigue, headaches, forgetfulness, anger, guilt, resentment) individual(s) are experiencing and impact on ability to function. *Moral distress can be very destructive, affecting one's ability to carry out daily tasks and care for self or others, and may lead to a crisis of faith.*[5]
- Assess sleep habits of involved parties. *Evidence suggests that sleep deprivation can harm a person's physical and emotional well-being, hindering the ability to integrate emotion and cognition to guide moral judgment.*[5]
- Perform or review results of moral distress test, such as the Moral Distress Assessment Questionnaire or the Moral Distress Scale, *to help measure degree of involvement and identify possible actions to improve situation.*[3,10]
- Note availability of family/friends/coworkers. *Provides support and encouragement for difficult situation.*[4]

NURSING PRIORITY NO. 2 To assist client/involved individuals to develop/effectively use problem-solving skills:

- Encourage involved individuals to recognize and name the experience, resulting in moral sensitivity. *Brings concerns out in the open so they can be dealt with.*[1]
- Provide time for nonjudgmental discussion of philosophical issues or questions about impact of conflict leading to moral questioning of current situation. *Moral issues have been discussed and studied for many years (e.g., philosophers, such as Piaget [1932] with his early work in developmental moral psychology, discussed what is the basis for moral reasoning). It is not possible to accurately read another's mind, and open discussion helps those involved in conflict to better understand the situation and begin to look at options.*[9]
- Use skills such as active listening, "I" messages, and problem solving *to clarify feelings of anxiety and conflict. Helps to understand what the ethical dilemmas are that lead to moral distress (e.g., family members ignoring advanced directives of loved one, providing lifesaving care to a death row inmate, terminally ill individual requesting assistance to die, families living with the moral experience of caring for a ventilator-assisted child in the home).*[8]
- Provide privacy when discussing sensitive personal issues. *Shows regard and concern for individual's self-worth.*[2]

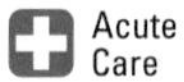

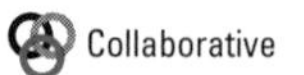

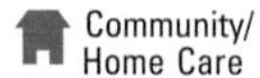

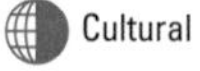

- Ascertain coping behaviors client has used successfully in the past that may be used in the current situation. *When encouraged, individuals can recall past situations where they had a positive experience and used successful coping skills.*[4]
- Identify role models (e.g., other individuals who have experienced similar problems in their lives). *Sharing of experiences and identifying options can be helpful to deal with current situation.*[1]
- Involve facility or local ethics committee or ethicist as appropriate *to educate, make recommendations, and facilitate mediation or resolution of conflicts.*[3]

NURSING PRIORITY NO. 3 To promote wellness (Teaching/Discharge Considerations):

- Engage all parties, as appropriate, in developing plan to address conflict. *Resolving one's moral distress requires making changes or compromises while preserving one's integrity and authenticity.*[4]
- Incorporate identified familial, religious, and cultural factors that have meaning for client. *Can provide comfort for the person.*[7]
- Refer to appropriate resources for support/guidance (e.g., pastoral care, counseling, organized support groups, classes) as indicated. *These resources can help client as they pursue the search for moral resolution.*[8]
- Assist individual to recognize that if she or he follows their moral decisions, they may clash with the legal system, and refer to appropriate resource for legal opinion/options.[3]
- Encourage the work organization to provide better support resources and structures. Discuss changes in the healthcare system that have resulted in more complex healthcare decisions. *The complexity of healthcare choices, expectations of clients/families, increasing costs or limitations in resources has resulted in increased pressures on healthcare providers and has led to ethics becoming a required component of clinical practice. Acknowledging reality of potential areas of conflict and providing proactive discussions for staff as well as support for involved individuals when making difficult decisions can decrease moral distress for staff and families.*[2,8]

DOCUMENTATION FOCUS

Assessment/Reassessment

- Individual findings, including nature of moral conflict, individuals involved in conflict.
- Physical and emotional responses to conflict.
- Individual cultural or religious beliefs and values, healthcare goals.
- Responses and involvement of family/SOs or coworkers.

Planning

- Plan of care and who is involved in planning.
- Teaching plan.

Implementation/Evaluation

- Responses to interventions and teaching.
- Effects of participation in classes or mediation activities.
- Attainment or progress toward desired outcome(s).
- Modifications to plan of care.

Discharge Planning

- Long-term needs and who is responsible for actions to be taken.
- Available resources.
- Specific referrals made.

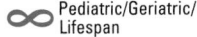

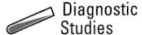

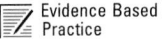

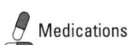

References

1. Elpern, E. H., Covert, B., Kleinpell, R. (2005). Moral distress of staff nurses in a medical intensive care unit. *Am J Crit Care*, 14, 523–539.
2. Kalvemark, S., Hogland, A. T., Hansson, M. G., et al. (2004). Living with conflicts—Ethical dilemmas and moral distress in the health care system. *Soc Sci Med*, 58(6), 1075–1084. Department of Public Health and Caring Sciences, Uppsala University, Uppsala, Sweden.
3. Hanna, D. R. (2005). The lived experience of moral distress: Nurses who assisted with elective abortions. *Res Theory Nurs Pract*, 19(1), 95–124.
4. Cheshire, W. P. (2007). Grey matters when eloquence is inarticulate. The Center for Bioethics and Human Dignity. Retrieved November 2015 from http://cbhd.org/content/grey-matters-when-eloquence-inarticulate.
5. Kilgore, W. D., Kilgore, D. B., Day, L. M., et al. (2006). The effects of 53 hours of sleep deprivation on moral judgment. *Sleep*, 30(3), 345–352.
6. Kopala, B., Burkhart, L. (2005). Ethical dilemma and moral distress: Proposed new NANDA diagnoses. *Int J Nurs Terminol Classif*, 16(1), 3–13.
7. Nichols, S. (2002). Mindreading and the core architecture of moral psychology. *Cognition*, 84, 221–236.
8. Carnevale, F. A., Alexander, E., Renneck, J. (2006). Daily living with distress and enrichment: The moral experience of families with ventilator-assisted children at home. *Pediatrics*, 117(1), e48–e60.
9. Piaget, J. (1932). In Gabain, M. (ed). *The Psychology of Moral Development: The Nature and Validity of Moral Stages*. (Translation published 1965). New York, NY: Free Press.
10. Corley, M. (1993). Moral distress of critical care nurses. *Am J Crit Care Nurs*, 4(4), 280–285.

impaired oral Mucous Membrane

Taxonomy II: Safety/Protection—Class 2 Physical Injury (00045) [**Diagnostic Division:** Food/Fluid], Submitted 1982; Revised 1998, 2013

DEFINITION: Injury to the lips, soft tissue, buccal cavity, and/or oropharynx.

RELATED FACTORS

Alcohol consumption; smoking
Allergy; stressors
Alteration in cognitive functioning
Autoimmune disease; immunodeficiency; immunosuppression; infection
Autosomal disorder; syndrome (e.g., Sjögren's)
Barrier to dental care or oral self-care; insufficient oral hygiene; insufficient knowledge of oral hygiene
Behavior disorder (e.g., attention deficit, oppositional defiant); depression
Chemical injury agent (e.g., burn, capsaicin, methylene chloride, mustard agent)
Cleft lip or palate; loss of oral support structure
Decrease in hormone level in women
Decrease in platelets; treatment regimen
Decrease in salivation; dehydration; malnutrition
Mechanical factor (e.g., ill-fitting dentures, braces, endotracheal/nasogastric tube, oral surgery) oral trauma
Mouth breathing; nil per os (NPO) > 24 hours

DEFINING CHARACTERISTICS

Subjective

Xerostomia [dry mouth]
Oral pain or discomfort
Bad taste in mouth; decrease in taste sensation; difficulty eating or swallowing
Exposure to pathogen

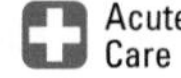

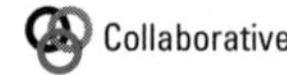

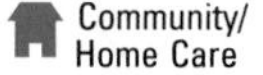

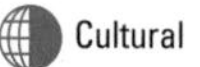

Objective

Coated tongue; smooth atrophic; geographic tongue
Gingival or mucosal pallor
Stomatitis; hyperemia; ; macroplasia; vesicles; nodules; papules
White patches or plaques, spongy patches; white curdlike exudate
Oral lesions or ulcers; fissures; bleeding; cheilitis; desquamation; mucosal denudation
Purulent oral-nasal drainage or exudates; enlarged tonsils
Oral edema
Halitosis
Gingival hyperplasia or recession, pocketing deeper than 4 mm; [carious teeth]
Presence of mass (e.g., hemangiomas)
Difficulty speaking

Sample Clinical Applications: Oral trauma, cancer, chemo/radiation therapy, malnutrition, infection, oral surgery, cleft lip/palate, conditions requiring endotracheal (ET) intubation (e.g., brain injury, stroke, spinal cord injury [SCI], chronic obstructive pulmonary disease [COPD], acute respiratory distress syndrome, amyotrophic lateral sclerosis [ALS])

DESIRED OUTCOMES/EVALUATION CRITERIA

Sample NOC linkages:

Self-Care: Oral Hygiene: Ability to care for own mouth and teeth independently with or without assistive device

Tissue Integrity: Skin & Mucous Membranes: Structural intactness and normal physiological function of skin and mucous membranes

Client/Caregiver Will (Include Specific Time Frame)

- Verbalize understanding of causative factors.
- Identify specific interventions to promote healthy oral mucosa.
- Demonstrate techniques to restore and maintain integrity of oral mucosa.

Sample NOC linkages:

Oral Hygiene: Condition of the mouth, teeth, gums, and tongue

Client Will (Include Specific Time Frame)

- Report or demonstrate a decrease in signs/symptoms as noted in Defining Characteristics.

ACTIONS/INTERVENTIONS

Sample NIC linkages:

Oral Health Restoration: Promotion of healing for a patient who has an oral mucosa or dental lesion

Oral Health Maintenance: Maintenance and promotion of oral hygiene and dental health for the patient at risk for developing oral or dental lesions

Oral Health Promotion: Promotion of oral hygiene and dental care for a patient with normal oral and dental health

NURSING PRIORITY NO. 1 To identify causative/contributing factors affecting oral health:

- ✚ Perform oral screening or comprehensive assessment upon admission to facility using tool (e.g., Oral Health Assessment Tool for Long-Term Care), as indicated. *Use of standardized tool is beneficial in evaluating health of entire mouth including lips, tongue, gums, and other soft tissues, as well as condition of natural teeth or dentures, and status of oral hygiene.*[18]

- Note presence of systemic or local conditions (e.g., oral infections; dehydration, malnutrition, facial fractures, head or neck cancers or treatment including chemotherapy or radiation; AIDS, systemic lupus erythematosus, rheumatoid arthritis, Sjögren syndrome, scleroderma, sarcoidosis, amyloidosis, hypothyroidism, diabetes) *that can affect health of buccal tissues. Note: Oral mucositis is a major complication of chemotherapy and/or radiation therapy.*[10,12,16]
- Note client's age and functional status upon admission to facility. *The very young, elderly, or any client with functional deficits (e.g., age-related dependency needs, cognitive or physical impairments, trauma, complex treatments) may require daily assistance with oral care.*[17]
- Determine if client is resistant to oral care. *Client with behavioral and/or communication difficulties (e.g., dementia, won't open mouth or is agitated or lethargic, doesn't understand instructions) may require special equipment, timing of efforts, and/or referral for professional services.*[17]
- Investigate reports of oral pain to determine possible source (e.g., oral lesion, gum disease, tooth abscess, ill-fitting dentures) *to identify needed interventions and reduce risk of complications such as systemic infection.*[1]
- Obtain history of client's medications *to identify those medications that can impact health of buccal tissues or cause immunosuppression which can impact oral health. Note: Many drugs (e.g., anticholinergics, antidepressants, anti-Parkinson drugs, antihistamines or decongestants, urinary antispastics, antipsychotics, diuretics, hypnotics, systemic bronchodilators, muscle relaxants, reserpine, laxatives, beta blockers, narcotics) can impair salivary function and promote xerostomia.*[3,8]
- Observe for abnormal lesions of mouth, tongue, and cheeks (e.g., white or red patches, ulcers). *White ulcerated spots may be canker sores, especially in children; white curd patches (thrush) are common in infants. Reddened, swollen bleeding gums may indicate infection, poor nutrition, or poor oral hygiene. A red tongue may be related to vitamin deficiencies.*[2,14] *Malignant lesions are more common in elderly than younger persons (especially if there is a history of smoking or alcohol use) or in persons who rarely visit a dentist.*[3,15]
- Note use of tobacco (including smokeless) and alcohol/other drugs [e.g., methamphetamines], *which may predispose gums and mucosa to effects of nutritional deficiencies, infection, cell damage, and cancer.*[10,12]
- Observe for chipped, sharp-edged teeth, or malpositioned teeth. Note fit of dentures or other prosthetic appliances when used. *Factors that increase the risk of injury to delicate tissues.*
- Determine problems with food and fluid intake (e.g., avoiding eating, reports change in taste, chews painstakingly, swallows numerous times for even small bites; insufficient fluid intake/dehydration; unexplained weight loss). *Malnutrition and dehydration are associated with problems with oral mucous membranes.*[6]
- Determine allergies to foods, drugs, or other substances *that may result in irritation of oral mucosa.*
- Review oral hygiene practices, noting frequency and type (e.g., brushing, flossing, water appliances). Inquire about client's professional dental care, regularity, and date of last dental examination.
- Evaluate client's ability to provide self-care and availability of necessary equipment and assistance. *Client's age (very young or elderly) impacts client's habits and lifestyle and ability to provide self-care, as well as current health issues (e.g., disease condition or treatment, weakness).*[4]

NURSING PRIORITY NO. 2 To correct identified/developing problems:

- Collaborate in treatment of underlying conditions (e.g., structural defects, infections) *that may correct or limit problem with oral tissues.*
- Inspect oral cavity routinely and recommend that client establish regular schedule of self-inspection, such as when performing oral care activities. *Can help with early identification and management of mucous membrane concerns.*
- Adjust medication regimen *to reduce use of drugs with potential for causing or exacerbating painful dry mouth.*
- Administer medications, as indicated (e.g., antibiotics, antifungal agents, including antimicrobial mouth rinse or spray) *to treat oral infections or reduce potential for bacterial overgrowth.*[8–10]
- Provide anesthetic lozenges or analgesics such as Stanford solution, viscous lidocaine (Xylocaine), mouthwash containing lidocaine, and sulfacrate slurry, as indicated *to provide protection and reduce oral dis-*

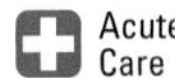

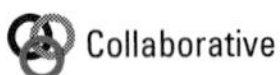

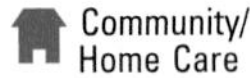

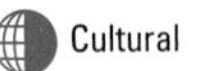

comfort or pain. Note: Pain of mucositis associated with anticancer therapies has been found to be controlled by mouthwashes containing lidocaine to coat the oral cavity.[10,16]

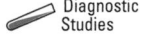

- Discuss safe use of products used to treat xerostomia. *Artificial salivas mimic natural saliva to relieve soft tissue discomfort and are more effective and longer lasting than simple rinses but do not stimulate natural salivary gland production; cholinergic agonist preparations [e.g., pilocarpine, cevimeline] do stimulate saliva production). Note: Little research has been done regarding the causes for xerostomia, but one recent study showed that medication exposure was strongly associated with the incidence of the condition, with recent exposure to diuretics or daily aspirin strongly predicting it.*[13]
- Encourage use of tart, sour foods and drinks and chewing sugar-free gum or sucking hard candy to *stimulate saliva.*[11] Use citrus foods and liquids with caution *as they may irritate mucosa and increase pain.*
- Provide or encourage regular oral care (e.g., after meals and at bedtime, frequently for critically ill client). *Note: Oral care has been determined to be a nursing intervention that decreases colonization of oropharynx and saliva, thereby reducing the incidence of ventilator-associated pneumonia (VAP) in the critically ill client:*[19]

  Use water; bland rinses or sodium bicarbonate solutions; and mucosal coating agents, lubricating agents, and topical anesthetics *for oral hydration or irrigation and treatment of mouth, gums, and mucous membrane surfaces.*[6,10,20]

  Avoid mouthwashes containing alcohol *(drying effect)* or hydrogen peroxide *(drying and foul tasting).*[5,13]

  Use soft-bristle brush or sponge/cotton-tip applicators to cleanse teeth and tongue. *Brushing the teeth is the most effective way to reduce plaque and manage periodontal disease.*[6]

  Floss gently or use a Waterpik® *to remove food particles that promote bacterial growth and gum disease.*

  Use foam sticks where indicated *to swab mouth, tongue, and gums when client is intubated or has no teeth. Note: Chlorhexidine is also used in some critical care areas to decrease risk of VAP.*[21,22]

  Use lemon/glycerin swabs with caution. *Note: Although some end-of-life care discussions mention use of glycerin swabs, the issue appears to be controversial, with some sources stating that glycerin should not be used as it absorbs water and actually dries the oral cavity and can result in decreased salivary amylase, as well as erosion of tooth enamel.*[6,9,13]

  Provide or assist with denture care, as needed. *Evidence-based protocol for denture care states that dentures are to be removed and washed at least once daily, removed and rinsed after every meal, and kept in an appropriate solution at night.*[7]
- Change position of ET tube or airway every 8 hr and as needed when client is on a ventilator *to minimize pressure on fragile tissues and improve access to all areas of oral cavity.*
- Suction oral cavity *if client cannot swallow secretions. Note: Saliva contains digestive enzymes that may be erosive to exposed tissues (such as might occur because of heavy drooling following radical neck surgery).*
- Use gentle low-intensity suctioning *to reduce risk of aspiration in intubated clients or those with decreased gag or swallow reflexes.*[8]
- Lubricate lips and provide commercially prepared oral lubricant solution, when indicated. Encourage use of chewing gum, hard candy, etc., *to stimulate flow of saliva to neutralize acids and limit bacterial growth.*[10]
- Encourage adequate fluids *to prevent dehydration and oral dryness and limit bacterial overgrowth.*[8]
- Suggest use of vaporizer or room humidifier *to increase humidity if client is mouth breather or ambient humidity is low.*[13]
- Implement diet modifications, as indicated:[10]

  Offer foods with adequate nutrients and vitamins to promote healing *when deficits are impairing health of oral tissues.*

  Avoid sharp, hard, coarse, spicy, salty, and acidic foods *that can irritate or damage fragile mucosa and existing ulcers.*

  Include bland, low-acid, high-protein foods (e.g., milkshakes, bananas, applesauce, mashed potatoes, cooked cereals, soft-boiled or scrambled eggs, cottage cheese, macaroni and cheese, pudding, custard, gelatin) *that are nutrient-dense and easy to eat.*

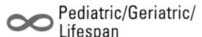

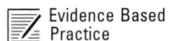

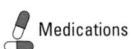

Provide moderate-temperature foods and fluids, soft or pureed foods, popsicles, frozen yogurt or ice cream *that may be soothing to sensitive mucosa.*

Drink liquids with meals and use gravies and sauces *to make food easier to swallow.*

Avoid dry foods, such as crackers, cookies, and toast, or soften them with liquids before eating.[13]

NURSING PRIORITY NO. 3 To promote wellness (Teaching/Discharge Considerations) :

- Recommend regular dental checkups and care, and episodic evaluation of oral health prior to certain medical treatments (e.g., chemotherapy, radiation) *to maintain oral health and reduce risks associated with impaired tissues.*[8]
- Review current oral hygiene concerns and provide informational resources including reliable Web sites about oral health *to reinforce learning and encourage proper care.*
- Promote general health and mental health habits *to prevent negative effects that altered immune response and/or neglect can exert on oral mucosa.*
- Provide nutritional information *to correct deficiencies, reduce mucosal inflammation or gum disease, and prevent dental caries.*
- Instruct parents in oral hygiene techniques and proper dental care for infants/children (e.g., safe use of pacifier, brushing of teeth and gums, avoidance of sweet drinks and candy, recognition and treatment of thrush). *Encourages early initiation of good oral health practices and timely intervention for treatable problems.*
- Discuss special mouth care required during and after illness or trauma or following surgical repair (e.g., cleft lip/palate, facial fractures, jaw surgery) *to facilitate healing.*
- Discuss and instruct caregiver(s) in special mouth care required during end-of-life care/hospice *to promote optimal comfort in client who has stopped eating or drinking, who has dry mouth, and may not have sensation of thirst.*[23]
- Recommend avoiding alcohol and smoking or chewing tobacco, *which can contribute to mucosal inflammation and gum disease.*
- Discuss need for and demonstrate use of special appliances (e.g., power toothbrushes, dental water jets, flossing instruments, applicators) if indicated. *Enhances independence in self-care.*
- Identify community resources (e.g., low-cost dental clinics, smoking-cessation resources, cancer information services or support group, Meals on Wheels, supplemental nutrition program, home-care aide) *to meet individual needs.*

DOCUMENTATION FOCUS

Assessment/Reassessment

- Condition of oral mucous membranes, routine oral care habits and interferences.
- Availability of oral care equipment and products.
- Knowledge of proper oral hygiene and care.
- Availability and use of resources.

Planning

- Plan of care and who is involved in planning.
- Teaching plan.

Implementation/Evaluation

- Responses to interventions, teaching, and actions performed.
- Attainment or progress toward desired outcome(s).
- Modifications to plan of care.

Discharge Planning

- Long-term needs and who is responsible for actions to be taken.
- Specific referrals made, resources for special appliances.

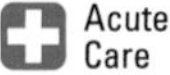

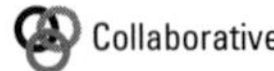

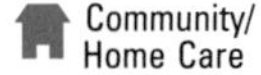

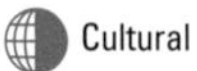

References

1. Carl, W., Havens, J. (2000). The cancer patient with severe mucositis. *Cur Rev Pain*, 4(3), 197–202.
2. Engel, J. (2002). *Pocket Guide to Pediatric Assessment*. 4th ed. St. Louis, MO: Mosby.
3. Aubertin, M. A. (1997). Oral cancer screening in the elderly: The home healthcare nurse's role. *Home Healthcare Nurse*, 15(9), 594–604.
4. White, R. (2000). Nurse assessment of oral health: A review of practice and education. *Br J Nurs*, 9(5), 260–266.
5. Winslow, E. H. (1994). Don't use H_2O_2 for oral care. *Am J Nurse*, 94(3), 19.
6. Stiefel, K. A., Damron, S., Sowers, N. J., et al. (2000). Improving oral hygiene for the seriously ill patient: Implementing research-based practice. *Medsurg Nurs*, 9(1), 40–46.
7. Curzio, J., McCowan, M. (2000). Getting research into practice: Developing oral hygiene standards. *Br J Nurs*, 9(7), 434–438.
8. Trieger, N. (2004). Oral care in the intensive care unit. *Am J Crit Care*, 13(1), 24.
9. Munro, C., Grap, M. J. (2004). Oral health and care in the intensive care unit: State of science. *Am J Crit Care*, 13(1), 25–33.
10. National Cancer Institute. (2014). Oral complications of chemotherapy and head/neck radiation: Various sections. Retrieved July 2014 from http://www.cancer.gov/cancertopics/pdq/supportivecare/oralcomplications/HealthProfessional/page1/AllPages.
11. Stegeman, C. A. (2005). Oral manifestations of diabetes. *Home Healthcare Nurse*, 23(4), 233–240.
12. National Library of Medicine. (2013). Oral cancer. Retrieved July 2014 from http://www.ncbi.nlm.nih.gov/pubmedhealth/PMH0002030/.
13. Murray, T. W., Chalmers, J. M., Spenser, J. A. (2006). A longitudinal study of medication exposure and xerostomia among older people. *Gerodontology*, 23(4), 205–213.
14. Ranney, R. (1993). Classification of periodontal diseases. *Periodontology*, 2(1), 13–25.
15. HealthPartners Dental Group and Clinics. (2011). Guidelines for the diagnosis and treatment of periodontal diseases. Retrieved December 2014 from http://www.guideline.gov/content.aspx?id=35130.
16. Li, E., Trovato, J. A. (2012). New developments in management of oral mucositis in patients with head and neck cancer or receiving targeted anticancer therapies. *Am J Health-Syst Pharm*, 69(12), 1031–1037.
17. Johnson, V. B., Chalmers, J. (2012). Oral hygiene care for functionally dependent and cognitively impaired older adults. *J Gerontol Nurs*, 38(11), 11–19.
18. University of Iowa College of Nursing, John A. Hartford Foundation Center of Geriatric Nursing Excellence - Academic Institution. (2011). Oral hygiene care for functionally dependent and cognitively impaired older adults. Revised guideline. Retrieved November 2014 from http://www.guideline.gov/content.aspx?id=34447.
19. Cutler, C., Davis, N. (2005). Improving oral care in patients receiving mechanical ventilation. *Am J Crit Care*, 14(5), 389–394.
20. Farris, C., McEnroe Petitte, D. (2013). Head, neck, and cancer update. *Home Healthcare Nurs*, 31(6), 322–328.
21. Feider, L. L., Mitchell, P., Bridges, E. (2010). Oral care practices for orally intubated critically ill adults. *Am J Crit Care*, 19(2), 175–183.
22. WebMD Drugs & Medications. (No date). Chlorhexidine gluconate mouth and throat. Retrieved November 2014 from http://www.webmd.com/drugs/2/drug-5356/chlorhexidine-gluconate-mucous-membrane/details#uses.
23. Schwarz, J. K. (2014). Hospice care for patients who choose to hasten death by voluntarily stopping eating and drinking. *J Hospice & Palliative Nursing*, 16(3), 126–131.

risk for impaired oral Mucous Membrane

Taxonomy II: Safety/Protection—Class 2 Physical Injury (00247) [**Diagnostic Division:** Food/Fluid], Submitted 2013

DEFINITION: Vulnerable to Injury to the lips, soft tissue, buccal cavity, and/or oropharynx, which may compromise health.

RISK FACTORS

Alcohol consumption; smoking
Allergy; stressors
Alteration in cognitive functioning
Autoimmune disease; immunodeficiency; immunosuppression; infection
Autosomal disorder; syndrome (e.g., Sjögren's)
Barrier to dental care or oral self-care
Behavior disorder (e.g., attention deficit, oppositional defiant); depression
Chemotherapy; radiation therapy
Economically disadvantaged
Decrease in hormone level in women
Inadequate nutrition
Insufficient oral hygiene; insufficient knowledge of oral hygiene
Mechanical factor (e.g., orthodontic appliance, device for ventilation or food, ill-fitting dentures)
Surgical procedure; trauma
Note: A risk diagnosis is not evidenced by signs and symptoms, as the problem has not occurred; rather, nursing interventions are directed at prevention.

DESIRED OUTCOMES/EVALUATION CRITERIA

Sample NOC linkages:
Self-Care: Oral Hygiene: Ability to care for own mouth and teeth independently with or without assistive device
Tissue Integrity: Skin & Mucous Membranes: Structural intactness and normal physiological function of skin and mucous membranes

Client/Caregiver Will (Include Specific Time Frame)
- Verbalize understanding of causative factors.
- Identify specific interventions to promote healthy oral mucosa.
- Demonstrate techniques to maintain integrity of oral mucosa.

Sample NOC linkages:
- Client will be free of signs of mucosal irritation/injury.

Oral Hygiene: Condition of the mouth, teeth, gums, and tongue

ACTIONS/INTERVENTIONS

Sample NIC linkages:
Oral Health Maintenance: Maintenance and promotion of oral hygiene and dental health for the patient at risk for developing oral or dental lesions
Oral Health Promotion: Promotion of oral hygiene and dental care for a patient with normal oral and dental health

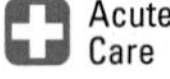
Acute Care
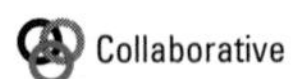
Collaborative
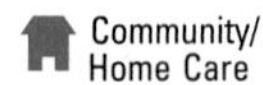
Community/ Home Care
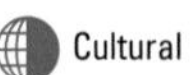
Cultural

NURSING PRIORITY NO. 1 To identify factors/conditions that can affect oral health:

- Note presence of systemic or local conditions (e.g., oral infections; dehydration, malnutrition, facial fractures, head or neck cancers or treatment including chemotherapy or radiation; AIDS, systemic lupus erythematosus, rheumatoid arthritis, Sjögren syndrome, scleroderma, sarcoidosis, amyloidosis, hypothyroidism, diabetes) *that can affect health of oral tissues. Note: Oral mucositis is a major complication of chemotherapy and/or radiation therapy.*[1,2,3]
- Note client's age and functional status. *The very young, the elderly client, or any client with functional deficits (e.g., age-related dependency needs, cognitive or physical impairments, trauma, complex treatments) may require daily assistance with oral care.*[4]
- Determine if client is resistant to oral care. *Client with behavioral and/or communication difficulties (e.g., dementia, won't open mouth or is agitated or lethargic, doesn't understand instructions) may require special equipment, timing of efforts, and/or referral for professional services.*[4]
- Obtain history of client's medications *to identify those medications that can impact health of buccal tissues or cause immunosuppression, which can impact oral health. Note: Many drugs (e.g., anticholinergics, antidepressants, anti-Parkinson drugs, antihistamines or decongestants, urinary antispastics, antipsychotics, diuretics, hypnotics, systemic bronchodilators, muscle relaxants, reserpine, laxatives, beta blockers, narcotics) can impair salivary function and promote xerostomia.*[5,6]
- Note use of tobacco (including smokeless) and alcohol/other drugs [e.g., methaphetamines], *which may predispose gums and mucosa to effects of nutritional deficiencies, infection, cell damage, and cancer.*[1,2]
- Observe for chipped, sharp-edged teeth, or malpositioned teeth. Note fit of dentures or other prosthetic appliances when used. *Factors that increase the risk of injury to delicate tissues.*
- Determine problems with food and fluid intake (e.g., avoiding eating, reports change in taste, chews painstakingly, swallows numerous times for even small bites; insufficient fluid intake/dehydration; unexplained weight loss). *Malnutrition and dehydration are associated with problems with oral mucous membranes.*[7]
- Determine allergies to foods, drugs, or other substances *that may result in irritation of oral mucosa.*
- Evaluate client's ability to provide self-care and availability of necessary equipment and assistance. *Client's age (very young or elderly) impacts client's habits and lifestyle, ability to provide self-care, and current health issues (e.g., disease condition or treatment, weakness).*[8]

NURSING PRIORITY NO. 2 To correct developing/potential problems:

- Collaborate in treatment of underlying conditions (e.g., structural defects, cancer, surgical/traumatic injuries) *that may impact oral tissues.*
- Inspect oral cavity routinely and recommend that client establish regular schedule of self-inspection, such as when performing oral care activities. *Can help with early identification and management of mucous membrane concerns.*
- **Refer to ND impaired oral Mucous Membrane, Nursing Priority No. 2 for interventions related to best practice nursing care to prevent oral complications.**

NURSING PRIORITY NO. 3 To promote wellness (Teaching/Discharge Considerations):[6–8]

- Recommend regular dental checkups and care and episodic evaluation of oral health prior to certain medical treatments (e.g., chemotherapy, radiation, total joint replacement) *to maintain oral health and reduce risks associated with impaired tissues.*
- Review current oral hygiene concerns and provide informational resources including reliable Web sites about oral health *to reinforce learning and encourage proper care.*
- Promote general health and mental health habits *to prevent negative effects that altered immune response and/or neglect can exert on oral mucosa.*
- Provide nutritional information *to correct deficiencies, reduce mucosal inflammation or gum disease, and prevent dental caries.*

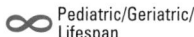

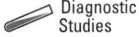

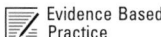

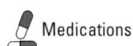

- ∞ Instruct parents in oral hygiene techniques and proper dental care for infants/children (e.g., safe use of pacifier, brushing of teeth and gums, avoidance of sweet drinks and candy, recognition and treatment of thrush). *Encourages early initiation of good oral health practices and timely intervention for treatable problems.*
- Discuss need for and demonstrate use of special appliances (e.g., power toothbrushes, dental water jets, flossing instruments, applicators), if indicated. *Enhances independence and excellence in oral self-care.*
- Discuss special mouth care required during and after illness or trauma or following surgical repair (e.g., cleft lip/palate, facial fractures, jaw surgery) *to facilitate healing.*
- Recommend avoiding alcohol and smoking or chewing tobacco, *which can contribute to mucosal inflammation and gum disease.*
- Identify community resources (e.g., low-cost dental clinics, smoking-cessation resources, cancer information services or support group, Meals on Wheels, nutritional assistance program, home-care aide) *to meet individual needs.*

DOCUMENTATION FOCUS

Assessment/Reassessment

- Condition of oral mucous membranes, routine oral care habits and interferences.
- Availability of oral care equipment and products.
- Knowledge of proper oral hygiene and care.
- Availability and use of resources.

Planning

- Plan of care and who is involved in planning.
- Teaching plan.

Implementation/Evaluation

- Responses to interventions, teaching, and actions performed.
- Attainment or progress toward desired outcome(s).
- Modifications to plan of care.

Discharge Planning

- Long-term needs and who is responsible for actions to be taken.
- Specific referrals made, resources for special appliances.

References

1. National Cancer Institute. (2014). Oral complications of chemotherapy and head/neck radiation: Various sections. Retrieved July 2014 from http://www.cancer.gov/cancertopics/pdq/supportivecare/oralcomplications/HealthProfessional/page1/AllPages.
2. National Library of Medicine. (2013). Oral cancer. Retrieved July 2014 from http://www.ncbi.nlm.nih.gov/pubmedhealth/PMH0002030/.
3. Li, E., Trovato, J. A. (2012). New developments in management of oral mucositis in patients with head and neck cancer or receiving targeted anticancer therapies. *Am J Health-Syst Pharm*, 69(12), 1031–1037.
4. Johnson, V. B., Chalmers, J. (2012). Oral hygiene care for functionally dependent and cognitively impaired older adults. *J Gerontol Nurs*, 38(11), 11–19.
5. Aubertin, M. A. (1997). Oral cancer screening in the elderly: The home healthcare nurse's role. *Home Healthcare Nurse*, 15(9), 594–604.
6. Trieger, N. (2004). Oral care in the intensive care unit. *Am J Crit Care*, 13(1), 24.
7. Stiefel, K. A., Damron, S., Sowers, N. J., et al. (2000). Improving oral hygiene for the seriously ill patient: Implementing research-based practice. *Medsurg Nurs*, 9(1), 40–46.
8. White, R. (2000). Nurse assessment of oral health: A review of practice and education. *Br J Nurs*, 9(5), 260–266.

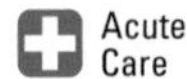

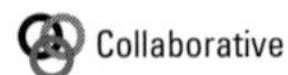

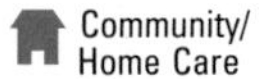

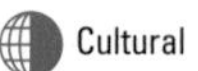

Nausea

Taxonomy II: Comfort—Class 1 Physical Comfort (00134) [**Diagnostic Division:** Food/Fluid], Submitted 1998; Revised 2002, 2010

DEFINITION: A subjective phenomenon of an unpleasant feeling in the back of the throat and stomach, which may or may not result in vomiting.

RELATED FACTORS

Biophysical

Biochemical disfunction (e.g., uremia, diabetic ketoacidosis); pregnancy
Localized tumor (e.g., acoustic neuroma, brain tumor, bone metastasis); intra-abdominal tumors
Exposure to toxins
Esophageal or pancreatic disease; liver or splenetic capsule stretch
Gastric distention; gastrointestinal (GI) irritation
Motion sickness; Ménière's disease; labyrinthitis
Increase in intracranial pressure; meningitis
Treatment regimen

Situational

Noxious taste
Unpleasant visual stimuli; noxious environmental stimuli
Anxiety; fear; psychological disorder

DEFINING CHARACTERISTICS

Subjective

Nausea; sour taste

Objective

Aversion toward food
Increase in salivation
Increase in swallowing; gagging sensation
Sample Clinical Applications: Surgery, anesthesia, cancer, pregnancy, AIDS, gastritis, peptic ulcer disease, renal failure, brain injury, meningitis, panic disorders, phobias

DESIRED OUTCOMES/EVALUATION CRITERIA

Sample NOC linkages:

Nausea & Vomiting Severity: Severity of nausea, retching, and vomiting symptoms
Nausea & Vomiting Control: Personal actions to control nausea, retching, and vomiting symptoms
Appetite: Desire to eat when ill or receiving treatment

Client Will (Include Specific Time Frame)

- Be free of nausea.
- Manage chronic nausea, as evidenced by acceptable level of dietary intake.
- Maintain or regain weight, as appropriate.

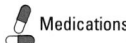

(continues on page 560)

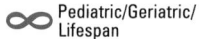

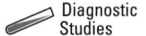

Nausea (continued)
ACTIONS/INTERVENTIONS

Sample NIC linkages:
Nausea Management: Prevention and alleviation of nausea
Vomiting Management: Prevention and alleviation of vomiting
Fluid Management: Promotion of fluid balance and prevention of complications resulting from abnormal or undesired fluid levels

NURSING PRIORITY NO. 1 To determine causative/contributing factors:

- Assess for presence of conditions of the GI tract (e.g., peptic ulcer disease, bleeding into the stomach; cholecystitis, appendicitis, gastritis, constipation, intestinal blockage, ingestion of "problem" foods; food poisoning; excessive alcohol intake) *that may cause or exacerbate nausea.*
- Note systemic conditions that may result in nausea (e.g., pregnancy, cancer treatment, myocardial infarction, hepatitis, acid-base and metabolic disturbances, systemic infections; toxins, drug toxicity, migraine headache, presence of neurogenic causes—stimulation of the vestibular system, concussion, central nervous system trauma/tumor). *Helpful in determining appropriate interventions/need for treatment of underlying conditions.*
- Identify situations that client perceives as anxiety inducing, threatening, or distasteful (e.g., "this is nauseating") such as might occur if client is having multiple diagnostic studies or is facing surgery or other stressful situations.
- Note psychological factors, including those that are culturally determined (e.g., eating certain foods considered repulsive in one's culture, seeing or smelling something "gross"; anorexia and bulemia).
- Determine if nausea is potentially self-limiting and/or mild (e.g., first trimester of pregnancy, 24-hr GI tract viral infection) or is severe and prolonged (e.g., advanced cancer with multiple medications accompanied by anorexia, constipation, imbalances of calcium/other electrolytes; certain cancer treatments; hyperemesis gravidarum). *Indicates potential degree of effect on fluid/electrolyte balance and nutritional status and determines type and intensity of interventions.*[3]
- Record food intake and changes in symptoms *to help identify food intolerances when nausea is chronic.*
- Note client age and developmental level. *Vomiting may occur along with nausea, especially in children (usually part of a short-lived viral infection). Nausea can occur with food intolerances, inner ear problems, pain, or medication reactions in any age client. Nausea in the elderly (in the absence of acute disease condition) may be associated with GI motility dysfunction or medications, pain, or end-or-life issues. Nausea in a female of childbearing age may indicate pregnancy or hormonal influences associated with menstruation, anorexia, or migraine headaches.*[5]
- Review medication regimen, especially in elderly client on multiple drugs. *Polypharmacy with drug interactions and side effects may cause or exacerbate nausea.*
- Review results of diagnostic studies. *Various studies may be done depending on the clinical suspicion of cause, such as blood tests (to check electrolytes, blood cell count), urinalysis (to check for dehydration and infection), and x-rays or computed tomography scan (may help identify or localize cause).*

NURSING PRIORITY NO. 2 To promote comfort and enhance intake:

- Collaborate with physician to treat underlying medical condition *when cause of nausea is known (e.g., infection, adverse side effect of medications, recent anesthesia, food allergies, GI reflux).*
- Administer and monitor response to medications used to treat underlying type of nausea (e.g., vestibular, bowel obstruction, dysmotility of gut, infection or inflammation, toxins) *to determine effectiveness of treatment. Note: Targeting antiemetics to specific receptors associated with a certain type of nausea can optimize treatment. For example, receptors causing nausea in vestibular disorders and infection are cholinergic and histaminic. A targeted antiemetic drug class could be anticholinergic or antihistaminic such as promethazine [Phergan]. Antiemetics must also be monitored for adverse side effects, such as oversedation with risk of aspiration.*[4,7]

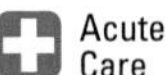

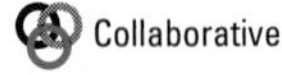

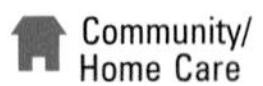

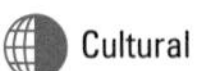

- Select route of medication administration best suited to client's needs (i.e., oral, sublingual, injectable, rectal, transdermal).[6]
- Administer antiemetic on regular schedule before, during, and after administration of antineoplastic agents or radiation therapy as indicated. *Antiemetic agents may be administered prophylactically to prevent or limit severity of nausea and vomiting.*
- Administer analgesics and/or antiemetics as scheduled *when postoperative pain is a factor in nausea and vomiting.*[1]
- Review pain control regimen for client experiencing nausea. *Converting to long-acting opioids or combination drugs may decrease stimulation of the chemotactic trigger zone, reducing the occurrence of narcotic-related nausea.*[4,7]
- Manage food and fluids:

  Have client try dry foods such as toast, crackers, or dry cereal before arising *when nausea occurs in the morning or throughout the day.*[7]

  Encourage client to begin with ice chips or sips/small amounts of fluids—4 to 8 oz for adult, 1 oz or less for child.[5]

  Advise client to drink liquids 30 min before or after meals instead of with meals.[7]

  Suggest sipping fluids slowly and using cool, clear liquids (e.g., water, ginger ale or lemon-lime soda, electrolyte drinks).

  Recommend avoiding milk and other dairy products (especially during acute episodes); overly sweet, fried, or fatty foods; and gas-forming vegetables (e.g., broccoli, cauliflower, cucumbers) *that may increase nausea and be more difficult to digest.*[3,5,7]

  Provide soft-bland diet and snacks high in carbohydrates with substitutions of preferred foods (including skinless chicken, rice, toast, pasta, potatoes) and fluids (including caffeine-free nondiet carbonated beverages, clear soup broth, nonacidic fruit juice, gelatin, sherbet, ices) *to reduce gastric acidity and improve nutrient intake.*[3,5,7]

  Instruct client to eat small meals spaced throughout the day rather than large meals *so stomach does not feel too full.*[3,7]

  Instruct client to eat and drink slowly, chewing food well *for easier digestion.*[7]

  Advise client to suck on ice cubes or tart or hard candies. *Keeps mucous membranes moist and can provide some fluid and nutrient intake.*

  Time chemotherapy doses *for least interference with food intake.*

  Monitor infusion rate of tube feeding, if present, *to prevent rapid administration that can cause gastric distention and produce nausea.*
- Manage environment *to reduce risk of nausea caused by noxious sights or smells:*

  Elevate head of bed or have client sit upright after meals *to promote digestion by gravity and eliminate feeling of fullness when that is causing nausea.*[7]

  Apply cool cloth to face and neck.

  Provide clean, pleasant-smelling, quiet environment and fresh air with fan or open window.

  Avoid offending odors (e.g., cooking smells, smoke, perfumes, mechanical emissions).[6,7]
- Implement nonpharmacological measures:

  Encourage slow, deep breathing *to promote relaxation.*

  Use such distraction techniques as guided imagery, music therapy, chatting with family/friends, and watching television *to refocus attention away from unpleasant sensations.*

  Provide frequent oral care *to cleanse mouth and minimize "bad tastes."*

  Avoid sudden changes in position or excessive motion; move to aisle seat on plane or front seat of car. Focus on distance and face forward when riding *to prevent or limit severity of nausea associated with motion sickness.*[5]
- Investigate use of electrical nerve stimulation or acupressure point therapy (e.g., elastic band worn around wrist with small, hard bump that presses against acupressure point). *Some individuals with chronic nausea or history of motion sickness report this to be helpful and without the sedative effect of medication.*[2]

NURSING PRIORITY NO. 3 To promote wellness (Teaching/Discharge Considerations):

- Review individual factors or triggers causing nausea and ways to avoid problem (e.g., identifying offending medications or foods). *Provides necessary information for client to manage own care. Note: Some individuals develop anticipatory nausea (a conditioned reflex) that recurs each time he or she encounters the situation that triggers the reflex.*[7]
- Instruct in proper use, side effects, and adverse reactions of antiemetic medications. *Enhances client safety and effective management of condition.*
- Discuss appropriate use of over-the-counter medications and herbal products (e.g., Dramamine, antacids, antiflatulents, ginger) or the use of THC (Marinol).[5,7]
- Encourage use of nonpharmacological interventions. *Activities such as self-hypnosis, progressive muscle relaxation, biofeedback, guided imagery, and systemic desensitization promote relaxation, refocus client's attention, increase sense of control, and decrease feelings of helplessness.*[6]
- Advise client/significant other to prepare and freeze meals in advance, have someone else cook, or use microwave or oven instead of stove-top cooking for days when nausea is severe or cooking is impossible, as with chemotherapy/radiation therapy.[7]
- Suggest wearing loose-fitting clothing *to reduce pressure on abdomen if that is causing or exacerbating nausea.*[7]
- Recommend recording weight weekly, if appropriate, *to help monitor fluid and nutritional status.*
- Identify signs requiring immediate notification of healthcare provider (e.g., emesis appears bloody, black, or like coffee grounds; feeling faint) *to facilitate timely evaluation and intervention.*[7]
- Review signs of dehydration and emphasize importance of replacing fluids and/or electrolytes (with products such as Gatorade for adults or Pedialyte for children) if vomiting occurs, especially in young children or frail elderly. *Increases likelihood of preventing potentially serious complications.*[5]

DOCUMENTATION FOCUS

Assessment/Reassessment
- Individual findings, including individual factors causing nausea.
- Baseline periodic weight, vital signs.
- Specific client preferences for nutritional intake.

Planning
- Plan of care and who is involved in planning.
- Teaching plan.

Implementation/Evaluation
- Response to interventions, teaching, and actions performed.
- Response to medication.
- Attainment or progress toward desired outcome(s).
- Modifications to plan of care.

Discharge Planning
- Individual long-term needs, noting who is responsible for actions to be taken.
- Specific referrals made.

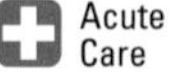

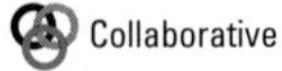

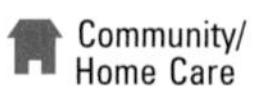

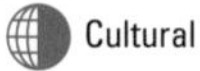

References

1. McCaffrey, R. (2007). Make POVN prevention a priority. *OR Nurse 2012*, 1(2), 39–45.
2. Mann, E. (1999). Using acupuncture and acupressure to treat postoperative emesis. *Prof Nurs*, 14(10), 691–694.
3. The American Gastroenterological Association medical position statement: Nausea and vomiting. (2001). *Gastroenterology*, 120(1), 261–262.
4. Hallenbeck, J. (2003). Treatment of nausea and vomiting. *Palliative Care Perspectives*. New York: Oxford University Press.
5. Cunha, J. P. (2011). Vomiting and nausea. Retrieved February 2014 from http://www.emedicinehealth.com/vomiting_and_nausea/article_em.htm.
6. National Cancer Institute. (Updated 2015). Nausea and vomiting (PDQ®) summary. Retrieved November 2015 from http://www.cancer.gov/about-cancer/treatment/side-effects/nausea/nausea-pdq.
7. World Health Organization. (2004). Palliative care & symptom management: Nausea & vomiting. Retrieved February 2014 from http://www.who.int/hiv/pub/imai/genericpalliativecare082004.pdf.

Noncompliance [ineffective Adherence] [specify]

Taxonomy II: Life Principles—Class 3 Value/Belief/Action Congruence (00079) [**Diagnostic Division:** Teaching/Learning], Submitted 1973; Revised 1996, 1998

DEFINITION: Behavior of person and/or caregiver that fails to coincide with a health-promoting or therapeutic plan agreed on by the person (and/or family and/or community) and healthcare professional. In the presence of an agreed-upon health-promoting or therapeutic plan, the person's or caregiver's behavior is fully or partially nonadherent and may lead to clinically ineffective or partially effective outcomes. [Author Note: When the plan of care is reviewed with client/significant other (SO), use of the term *noncompliance* may create a negative response and sense of conflict between healthcare providers and client. Labeling the client noncompliant may also lead to problems with third-party reimbursement. Where possible, use of the ND ineffective Health Management is recommended.]

RELATED FACTORS

Healthcare Plan

Lengthy duration or intensity of regimen; complex treatment regimen

Financial barriers; high-cost regimen

Individual Factors

Insufficient knowledge about the regimen; insufficient skills to perform regimen; expectations incongruent with developmental phase

Health beliefs, values, or spiritual values incongruent with plan; cultural incongruence

Insufficient motivation; insufficient social support

[Denial; issues of secondary gain]

Health System

Insufficient health insurance coverage; insufficient provider reimbursement

Perceived low credibility of provider; difficulty in client-provider relationship; provider discontinuity; insufficient follow-up with provider; ineffective communication or insufficient teaching skills of the provider

Inadequate access or inconvenience of care; low satisfaction with care

Network

Insufficient involvement of members in plan; low social value attributed to plan

Perception that beliefs of significant other differ from plan

(continues on page 564)

Noncompliance (continued)

DEFINING CHARACTERISTICS

Subjective

[Does not believe in efficacy of therapy, unwilling to follow treatment regimen]

Objective

Nonadherence behavior

Failure to progress; exacerbation of symptoms; development-related complication

Failure to meet outcomes; missing of appointments

Sample Clinical Applications: Any new diagnosis, chronic conditions, or situations requiring undesired or major lifestyle changes

DESIRED OUTCOMES/EVALUATION CRITERIA

Sample NOC linkages:

Compliance Behavior: Personal actions to promote wellness, recovery, and rehabilitation recommended by a health professional

Participation in Healthcare Decisions: Personal involvement in selecting and evaluating healthcare options to achieve desired outcome

Treatment Behavior: Illness or Injury: Personal actions to palliate or eliminate pathology

Client Will (Include Specific Time Frame)

- Verbalize accurate knowledge of condition and understanding of treatment regimen.
- Make choices at level of readiness based on accurate information.
- Verbalize commitment to mutually agreed-upon goals and treatment plan.
- Access resources appropriately.
- Demonstrate progress toward desired outcomes or goals.

ACTIONS/INTERVENTIONS

Sample NIC linkages:

Mutual Goal-Setting: Collaborating with patient to identify and prioritize care goals, then developing a plan for achieving those goals

Self-Modification Assistance: Reinforcement of self-directed change initiated by the patient to achieve personally important goals

Values Clarification: Assisting another to clarify her/his own values in order to facilitate effective decision making

NURSING PRIORITY NO. 1 To determine reason for alteration/disregard of therapeutic regimen/instructions:

- Determine client/SO(s) perception and understanding of the situation (illness, treatment). *Basic information needed to understand client's/SO's position and possible conflicts in order to develop plan of care.*[2]
- Active listen to client's complaints and comments. *Conveys confidence in individual's ability to understand and manage own care.*[1] *Helps to identify client's thinking about the treatment regimen (e.g., may be concerned about side effects of medications or success of procedures or transplantation).*[11]
- Note language spoken, read, and understood. *Lack of understanding of words that are used in explanations may result in client lack of cooperation with therapeutic regimen.*[2,10]
- Identify developmental level as well as chronological age of client. *Determines how to interact with client on appropriate level to enhance relationship and ability to discuss lack of cooperation with medical regimen.*[2]
- Assess level of anxiety, locus of control, sense of powerlessness, etc. *Presence of these factors will affect how client is managing illness or situation and therapeutic regimen.*[1,11]

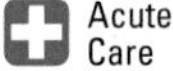

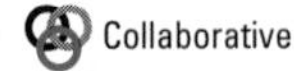

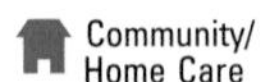

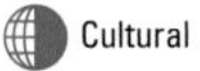

- Note length of illness. *People tend to become passive and dependent in long-term, debilitating illnesses and find it difficult to expend energy to follow through with therapeutic regimen.*[6]
- Clarify value system; e.g., cultural or religious values and health and illness beliefs and practices of the client/SO(s). *These factors will influence individual's view of the therapeutic regimen and willingness to follow through on some interventions; for instance, Hispanics may believe the future is in God's hands and women may delay Pap smears and mammograms because of modesty.*[10]
- Determine social characteristics and demographic and educational factors, as well as personality of the client. *Educated individuals may be more oriented to health promotion and disease prevention, while lower-socioeconomic individuals may be focused on the basics of living and may not pay attention to or follow healthcare recommendations. Personality characteristics such as suspiciousness and obsessive features may affect how client views medical regimen.*[9]
- Verify psychological meaning of the behavior (e.g., may be in denial). Note issues of secondary gain. *Family dynamics, school or workplace issues, and involvement in legal system may unconsciously affect client's decision regarding care and necessary follow-through.*[3]
- Assess availability and use of support systems and resources. *Failure to follow through with recommended therapies may be due to lack of or incorrect usage of support that is available.*[9]
- Be aware of nurses'/healthcare providers' attitudes and behaviors toward the client. Do they have an investment in the client's compliance or recovery? What is the behavior of the client and healthcare provider when client is labeled "noncompliant"? *Some care providers may be enabling client, whereas others' judgmental attitudes may impede treatment progress.*[1]
- Determine who (e.g., client, SO, other) manages the medication regimen and whether individual knows what the medications are and why they are prescribed. *Assures that medications are given accurately and safely:*[1]

  Ascertain how client remembers to take medications and how many doses have been missed in the last 72 hours, last week, last 2 weeks, and last month. *While clients claiming to take their medication often do not, self-reported nonadherence is likely to be accurate and should be taken seriously.*[13]

  Identify factors that interfere with taking medications or lead to lack of adherence (e.g., depression, active alcohol or other drug use, low literacy, lack of support, lack of belief in treatment efficacy). *Forgetfulness is the most common reason given for not complying with the treatment plan.*[12]

NURSING PRIORITY NO. 2 To assist client/SO(s) to develop strategies for dealing effectively with the situation:

- Develop therapeutic nurse-client relationship. *Promotes trust and provides atmosphere in which client/SO(s) can freely express views or concerns and explore reasons for lack of compliance with therapeutic regimen. Adherence assessment is most successful when conducted in a positive, nonjudgmental atmosphere.*[1]
- Explore client involvement in or lack of mutual goal setting. *Client will be more likely to follow through on goals he or she participated in developing.*[5,8]
- Review treatment strategies. Identify which interventions in the plan of care are most important in meeting therapeutic goals and which are least amenable to cooperation. *Sets priorities and encourages problem solving areas of conflict, enabling client to make decisions related to choices of care.*[7]
- Contract with the client for participation in care. *Enhances commitment to follow-through.*
- Encourage client to maintain self-care, providing for assistance when necessary. Accept client's evaluation of own strengths and limitations while working with client to improve abilities. *Promotes self-esteem, enabling client to have a sense of control over illness and treatment regimen.*[7]
- Provide for continuity of care in and out of the hospital or care setting, including long-range plans. *Supports trust and facilitates progress toward goals as client illness is dealt with over time.*[6,14]
- Provide information and help client to know where and how to find it on own. *Promotes independence and encourages informed decision making and control over illness, enhancing compliance with therapeutic regimen.*[4]
- Present information in manageable amounts, using verbal, written, and audiovisual modes at level of client's ability. *Individuals learn in many ways, and using different modes at client's own pace facilitates learning and enhances assimilation of the information.*

- Have client/SO paraphrase instructions and information heard. *Validates understanding and reveals misconceptions so that corrections can be made and appropriate questions can be asked and answered.*[4]
- Accept the client's choice or point of view, even if it appears to be self-destructive. Avoid confrontation regarding beliefs. *Maintaining open communication is important to continuing to provide correct information and therapeutic relationship with the client/SO(s). If illness is terminal, accept client's wishes regarding continued care or treatments whenever possible.*[1]
- Establish graduated goals or modified regimen as necessary. *Client with chronic obstructive pulmonary disease who smokes a pack of cigarettes a day may be willing to reduce that amount but not give up smoking altogether. This choice may improve quality of life, and success with this goal may encourage progression to more advanced goals.*

NURSING PRIORITY NO. 3 To promote wellness (Teaching/Discharge Considerations):

- Emphasize importance of the client's knowledge and understanding of the need for treatment or medication, as well as consequences of actions and choices. *Client who is not adhering to the treatment regimen may not have complete information or may not understand the reasons for the recommendations. With full understanding, client can make a more informed decision about care.*[1,11,14]
- Develop a system for self-monitoring. *Provides a sense of control and enables the client to follow own progress, seek timely evaluation/intervention by healthcare provider, and assist with making choices.*[7]
- Suggest using a medication reminder system. *These have been shown to improve client adherence by a significant percentage.*
- Provide support systems to reinforce negotiated behaviors. Encourage client to continue positive behaviors, especially if client is beginning to see benefit. *Individuals who feel alone and do not hear any positive reinforcement for changes that have been made will have difficulty maintaining the changes. When clients do hear positive comments and see the results for themselves, they are more apt to be willing to continue treatment regimen.*[7,8]
- Refer to counseling or therapy or other appropriate resources. *May need additional assistance to resolve situation and enable client to progress as desired.*[1]
- Refer to NDs Anxiety, compromised family Coping, ineffective Coping, deficient Knowledge (specify), and ineffective Health Management.

DOCUMENTATION FOCUS

Assessment/Reassessment

- Individual findings, deviation from prescribed treatment plan, and client's reasons in own words.
- Cultural or religious values, beliefs, and expectations.
- Availability and use of resources.
- Involvement of SO/family.
- Consequences of actions to date.

Planning

- Plan of care and who is involved in planning.
- Teaching plan.

Implementation/Evaluation

- Response to interventions, teaching, and actions performed.
- Attainment or progress toward desired outcome(s).
- Modifications to plan of care.

Discharge Planning

- Long-term needs and who is responsible for actions to be taken.
- Specific referrals made.

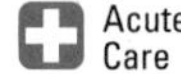

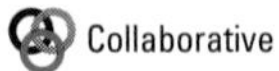

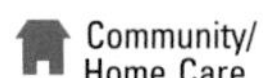

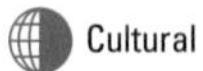

References

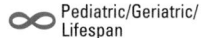

1. Azlin, B., Hatta, S., Norzila, Z., et al. (2007). Health locus of control among non-compliant hypertensive patients undergoing pharmacotherapy. *Malaysian J Psychiatry*, 16(1), 20–29.
2. Locher, J., Burgio, K. L., Goode, P. S., et al. (2002). Effects of age and casual attribution to aging on health-related behaviors associated with urinary incontinence in older women. *Gerontologist*, 42(4), 515–521.
3. Fishbain, D. A., Cole, B., Cutler, R. B., et al. (2003). A structured evidenced-based review on the meaning of non-organic physical signs: Waddell's signs. *Pain Med*, 4(2), 141–181.
4. Pozza, A. M., Windle, M. L., Chrousos, G. P. (Updated 2014). Pediatric type 2 diabetes mellitus. Medscape Reference. Retrieved November 2015 from http://emedicine.medscape.com/article/925700-overview.
5. Deckelbaum, R. J., Williams, C. L. (2001). Childhood obesity: The health issue. *Obes Res*, 9(4 Suppl), 239s–243s.
6. Smith, J. S. (2006). The psychology of burns. *J Trauma Nurs*, 13(3), 105–106.
7. Adcock, G. (2004). Highlights of the 2004 National Clinical Symposium of the American College of Nurse Practitioners. [T Bartol lecture about noncompliance.]. Retrieved November 2015 from http://www.medscape.com/viewarticle/493600_4.
8. Turnbull, G. B. (2002). The importance of coordinating ostomy care and teaching across settings. Ostomy Wound Management. Retrieved November 2015 from http://www.o-wm.com/content/the-importance-coordinating-ostomy-care-and-teaching-across-settings.
9. American Society of Pain Management Nurses. (2002). Position paper on pain management in patients with addictive disease. Pensacola, FL.
10. Kotelnikov, V. Personal beliefs, values and basic assumptions and attitudes—Understanding what drives you and others. E-Coach. Retrieved November 2015 from http://www.1000ventures.com/business_guide/crosscuttings/character_beliefs-values.html.
11. Sherry, D. C., Simmons, B., Wung, S-F., et al. (2003). Noncompliance in heart transplantation: A role for advanced practice nurses. Medscape Nurses. Retrieved November 2015 from http://www.medscape.com/viewarticle/459038.
12. Hassan, N. B., Hasanah, C. I., Foong, K., et al. (2006). Identification of psychosocial factors in noncompliance in hypertensive patients. *J Human Hypertension*, 20(1), 23–29.
13. Martin, L. R., Williams, S. L., Haskard, K. B., et al. (2005). The challenge of patient adherence. *Ther Clin Risk Manag*, 1(3), 189–199.
14. Laws, M. B., Wilson, I., Lee, Y., et al. (2012). Lecture or listen: When patients waver on meds. Retrieved November 2015 from https://news.brown.edu/articles/2012-02/aids.

imbalanced Nutrition: less than body requirements

Taxonomy II: Nutrition—Class 1 Ingestion (00002) [**Diagnostic Division:** Food/Fluid], Submitted 1975; Revised 2000

DEFINITION: Intake of nutrients insufficient to meet metabolic needs.

RELATED FACTORS

Insufficient dietary intake
Inability to ingest or digest food; inability to absorb nutrients
Biological factors; psychological disorder
Economically disadvantaged
[Increased metabolic demands, such as with burns]

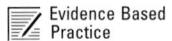

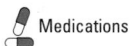

(continues on page 568)

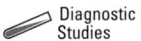

imbalanced Nutrition: less than body requirements (continued)

DEFINING CHARACTERISTICS

Subjective

Insufficient interest in food; food aversion; alteration in taste sensation; perceived inability to digest food
Satiety immediately upon ingesting food
Abdominal pain or cramping; sore buccal cavity
Insufficient information; misinformation; misconception

Objective

Body weight 20% or more below ideal weight range; [decreased subcutaneous fat or muscle mass]
Weight loss with adequate food intake
Food intake less than recommended daily allowances
Hyperactive bowel sounds; diarrhea; steatorrhea
Weakness of muscles required for mastication or swallowing; insufficient muscle tone
Pale mucous membranes; capillary fragility
Excessive hair loss [or increased growth of hair on body (lanugo)]; [cessation of menses]
[Abnormal laboratory studies (e.g., decreased albumin, total proteins; iron deficiency; electrolyte imbalances)]

Sample Clinical Applications: Cancer, AIDS, anorexia or bulimia nervosa, burns, facial trauma, brain injury, coma, stroke, Parkinson's disease, cleft lip/palate, anemia, dementia, Alzheimer's disease, major depression, schizophrenia

DESIRED OUTCOMES/EVALUATION CRITERIA

Sample NOC linkages:

Nutritional Status: Extent to which nutrients are available to meet metabolic needs
Knowledge: Diet: Extent of understanding conveyed about recommended diet
Weight Gain Behavior: Personal actions to gain weight following voluntary or involuntary significant weight loss

Client Will (Include Specific Time Frame)

- Demonstrate progressive weight gain toward goal.
- Display normalization of laboratory values and be free of signs of malnutrition as reflected in Defining Characteristics.
- Verbalize understanding of causative factors when known and necessary interventions.
- Demonstrate behaviors and lifestyle changes to regain or maintain appropriate weight.

ACTIONS/INTERVENTIONS

Sample NIC linkages:

Nutrition Management: Assisting with or providing a balanced dietary intake of foods and fluids
Weight-Gain Assistance: Facilitating gain of body weight
Eating Disorders Management: Prevention and treatment of severe diet restrictions and overexercising or binging and purging of foods and fluids

NURSING PRIORITY NO. 1 To assess causative/contributing factors:

- Identify client at risk for malnutrition (e.g., institutionalized elderly; client with chronic illness; child or adult living in poverty/low-income area; client with facial injuries or deformities; restrictive weight-loss program or surgical intervention; prolonged time of restricted intake, prior nutritional deficiencies; hypermetabolic states [e.g., hyperthyroidism, burns]; malabsorption syndromes).[2,9,10]

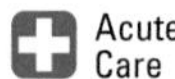

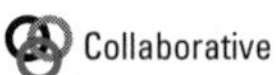

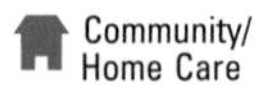

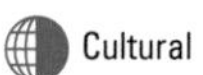

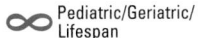

- Obtain dietary history *to determine chronic problems and ongoing needs, such as:*
  Increased caloric requirements with difficulty ingesting sufficient calories (e.g., cancer, burns).
  Maturational or developmental issues (e.g., premature baby with sucking difficulties, child with lack of emotional stimulation, frail elderly living alone).
  Swallowing difficulties (e.g., stroke, Parkinson's disease, cerebral palsy, other neuromuscular disorders).[2]
  Poor dentition (damaged or missing teeth, ill-fitting dentures, gum disease).
  Decreased absorption (e.g., lactose intolerance, Crohn's disease).
  Diminished desire or refusal to eat (e.g., anorexia nervosa, cirrhosis, pancreatitis, alcoholism, bipolar disorder, chronic fatigue).[2,6]
  Treatment-related issues (e.g., chemotherapy, radiation, stomatitis, facial surgery, wired jaw).
  Personal or situational factors (e.g., inability to procure or prepare food, social isolation, grief, loss).[8]
- Assess pediatric concerns (e.g., changes in nutritional needs related to growth phase; congenital anomalies, including tracheoesophageal fistula, cleft lip/palate; metabolic or malabsorption problems, such as diabetes, phenylketonuria, cerebral palsy; chronic infections).[4]
- Determine lifestyle factors that may affect weight. *Socioeconomic resources, amount of money available for purchasing food, proximity of grocery store, and available storage space for food are all factors that may impact food choices and intake.*
- Evaluate impact of cultural, ethnic, and religious influences. *The nutritional balance of a diet is recognized by most cultures, with distinct theories of nutritional practices for health promotion and disease prevention. Foods are used for prevention or treatment of disease (e.g., client may believe in use of "hot" or "cold" foods to treat certain conditions or use low-fat, low-sodium foods to prevent heart disease). Certain foods may be thought to cause a disease condition (e.g., upset stomach caused from eating too many cold foods). Special diets or food preparation may be cultural or religious based (e.g., kosher preparation for Jewish client or eating no meat or meat by-products for vegetarian).*[1]
- Explore specific eating habits, the meaning of food to client (e.g., never eats breakfast, snacks throughout entire day, fasts for weight control, no time to eat properly), and individual food preferences and intolerances/aversions. *Identifies eating practices that may need to be corrected and provides insight into dietary interventions that may appeal to client.*
- Obtain history or review diary of daily portion (or calorie) intake and patterns and times of eating *to reveal recent changes in client's weight or appetite and to identify strengths and weaknesses in client's dietary habits.*[2]
- Assess client's knowledge of nutritional needs and ways client is meeting these needs. *Identifies teaching needs and/or helps guide choice of interventions.*[2]
- Note availability and use of financial resources and support systems. *These factors affect or determine ability to acquire, prepare, and store food. Lack of support or socialization may impact client's desire to eat.*
- Assess medication regimen, noting possible drug side effects or interactions, allergies, use of laxatives, and diuretics. *These factors may be affecting appetite, food intake, or absorption.*[2,8]
- Note client's ability to feed self or presence of interfering factors. *Difficulties such as paralysis, tremor, or injury to hands or arms with inability to grasp or lift utensils to mouth; cognitive impairments affecting coordination or remembering to eat; age; and/or developmental issues may require input of multiple providers and therapists to develop individualized plan of care.*[2]
- Auscultate for presence and character of bowel sounds *to determine ability and readiness of intestinal tract to handle digestive processes (e.g., hypermotility accompanies vomiting or diarrhea, while absence of bowel sounds may indicate bowel obstruction).*
- Determine psychological factors that may affect food choices. Perform psychological assessment as indicated *to assess body image and congruency with reality or to identify factors (e.g., dementia, severe depression) that may be interfering with client's appetite and food intake.*[2]
- Note occurrence of amenorrhea, tooth decay, swollen salivary glands, or report of constant sore throat. *May be signs of eating disorder, such as bulimia, affecting eating patterns and requiring additional evaluation.*[5,6]

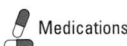

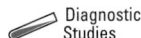

- Review usual activities and exercise program, noting repetitive activities (e.g., constant pacing) or inappropriate exercise (e.g., prolonged jogging). *Individuals with dementia may pace or be in constant motion, increasing energy needs. Clients who have eating disorders, such as anorexia or bulimia, may use obsessive activities as weight-control measures.*[6]

NURSING PRIORITY NO. 2 To evaluate degree of deficit:

- Assess current weight, compared to usual weight and norms for age and body size *to identify changes (e.g., sudden loss related to medical illness versus ongoing chronic depression with anorexia and weight loss; toddler with failure to meet growth expectations) that affect choice of intervention and help clarify expectations.*
- Obtain weights using same scale, same time of day, and same clothing as much as possible *to provide for accurate comparison to evaluate effectiveness of therapeutic regimen.*[2]
- Calculate growth percentiles in infants/children using growth chart *to identify deviations from the norm.*[4]
- Measure or calculate body fat, body water, and muscle mass (via triceps skinfold or other anthropometric measurements) or calculate body mass index (BMI) *to establish baseline parameters and assist in determining therapeutic goals. Note: BMI = weight (lb)/height (inches squared) × 704. Desirable BMI is 23 to 25, with less than 19 being severely underweight.*[2,8]
- Observe for absence of subcutaneous fat or muscle wasting, loss of hair, fissuring of nails, delayed healing, gum bleeding, swollen abdomen, etc., that indicate protein-energy malnutrition.[9]
- Perform or review results of nutritional assessment using screening tools such as the Malnutrition Universal Screening Tool, the Veterans Affairs Nutrition Status Classification system, the screening tool developed by Brugler et al., or the Mini Nutritional Assessment (MNA). *Note: In 2006, Guigoz reported that the MNA had been used in 36 studies to assess the nutritional status of 8,596 hospitalized older adults worldwide; of these, 50% to 80% were classified as either at risk for malnourishment or malnourished.*[11,12,13]
- Review laboratory studies (e.g., serum albumin, prealbumin, transferrin, amino acid profile, iron, blood urea nitrogen, nitrogen balance studies, glucose, liver function, electrolytes, total lymphocyte count, indirect calorimetry). *Baseline screening may be done to determine whether more in-depth evaluation is needed. Note: Brugler et al. found that the characteristics that correlated best with malnutrition-related complications were occurrence of a wound, poor oral intake, malnutrition-related admission diagnosis, serum albumin value, hemoglobin value, and total lymphocyte count.*[2,14]

NURSING PRIORITY NO. 3 To establish a nutritional plan that meets individual needs:

- Collaborate with interdisciplinary team *to set nutritional goals when client has specific dietary needs, malnutrition is profound, or long-term feeding problems exist.*[2,7,9]
- Calculate client's energy and protein requirements using basal energy expenditure and the Harris-Benedict (or similar) formula. *The essential nutritional requirements include the needs for energy, protein, and hydration, along with vitamins and electrolytes. Various factors may be considered in choosing a useful formula, including age, sex, disease state, stress associated with current illness, body size (e.g., obesity), and activity (e.g., bedbound versus out of bed).*[15]
- Establish ongoing method of evaluating intake (e.g., calories/day, percent of food consumed at each feeding) *to assist in determining both amount of food taken and what food groups are consumed or left uneaten, to identify nutritional deficits.*[2]
- Discuss with client/significant other (SO) aspects of diet that can remain unchanged *to preserve those that are valuable or meaningful to individual, and enhance sense of control.* Negotiate with client aspects of diet that need to be changed, especially if eating or psychiatric disorder is limiting food intake.

NURSING PRIORITY NO. 4 To address specific underlying condition/treatment needs:

- Assist in treatments to correct or control underlying causative factors *to improve intake and utilization of nutrients:*[2,7]
  - Administer oral antifungal agent *to treat cutaneous lesions of the mouth (e.g., candidiasis) that limit client's ability or desire for food.*
  - Medicate for pain or nausea and manage drug side effects *to increase physical comfort and appetite.*
  - Provide pureed foods, formula tube feedings, or parenteral nutrition infusions when indicated by client's condition (e.g., wired jaws or paralysis following stroke) and degree of malnutrition. *Enteral route is preferred when oral feeding is not appropriate; however, parenteral nutrition is recommended if client is not able to tolerate at least 50% of the goal rate of enteral feedings.*[7]
  - Consult occupational therapist *to identify appropriate assistive devices to facilitate independence in feeding and self-esteem.*
  - Consult speech therapist *to develop specific exercises or activities to address swallowing difficulties related to neurological problems (e.g., stroke, amyotrophic lateral sclerosis).* (Refer to ND impaired Swallowing for additional interventions.)
  - Refer for dental care *to correct missing teeth or poorly fitting dentures that affect client's ability to chew food or enjoy process of eating.*
  - Develop or refer client to structured (behavioral modification) program for nutrition therapy, which may include documenting time/length of eating period, putting food in a blender, and tube feeding food not eaten. *These programs are used to change the maladaptive eating behaviors of clients with anorexia and bulimia and ensure adequate caloric intake. Because "control" is central to the etiology of these disorders, it is important to ensure that the client is perceived to be "in control."*[6]
  - Recommend or support hospitalization for controlled environment, as indicated, in severe malnutrition or life-threatening situations.

NURSING PRIORITY NO. 5 To enhance dietary intake:

- Avoid or limit withholding of food (e.g., prolonged NPO for surgery) as much as possible and reinstitute oral feedings as early as possible *to reduce adverse effects of malnutrition.*
- Increase specific nutrients (e.g., protein, carbohydrates, fats, calories) as needed, providing client with preferred food and seasoning choices where possible *to enhance intake.*[9]
- Determine when client prefers or tolerates largest meal of the day. Maintain flexibility in timing of food intake *to promote sense of control and give client opportunity to eat when feeling more rested, less pain or nausea, family coming at mealtime, etc.*[2]
- Provide numerous small feedings as indicated; supplement with easily digested snacks *to reduce feeling of fullness that can accompany larger meals and to improve chances of increasing the amount of nutrients taken over 24-hr period.*[5]
- Promote adequate and timely fluid intake. *Fluid is essential to the digestive process and is often taken with meals. Fluids may need to be withheld before meals or with meals if interfering with food intake.*
- Encourage variety in food choices, varying textures and taste sensations (e.g., sweet, salty, fresh, methods of cooking) *to enhance food satisfaction and stimulate appetite.*[2]
- Offer and keep available to client finger foods and snacks *that are easy to self-feed.*
- Provide oral care before and after meals. *Reduces discomfort associated with nausea, vomiting, oral lesions, mucosal dryness, and halitosis, making eating easier or food more palatable.*
- Encourage use of lozenges, gum, hard candy, and beverages *to stimulate salivation when dryness is a factor.*
- Use alternative flavoring agents (e.g., lemon and herbs) *to enhance taste of foods, especially if salt is restricted.*
- Add nonfat milk powder to foods with a high liquid content (e.g., gravy, puddings, cooked cereal) and sugar or honey in beverages if carbohydrates are tolerated *to increase caloric value.*[2]

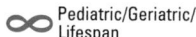

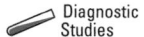

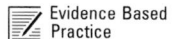

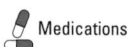

- Avoid foods that cause intolerances or increase gastric motility (e.g., gas-forming foods, hot or cold, spicy, caffeinated beverages, milk products, etc.) *to reduce postprandial discomfort that may discourage client from eating.*[3]
- Limit high-fat foods or fiber and bulk if indicated *because they may lead to early satiety.*
- Offer supplement drinks (or dispense in 2- to 4-oz portions several times/day). *Client may view this as a "medication" and thus will drink it, improving intake and energy level.*[2]
- Promote pleasant, relaxing environment, including socialization when possible. *Promotes focus on activity of eating, enhancing intake.*[2]
- Prevent or minimize unpleasant odors and sights or cooking odors. *Often have a negative effect on appetite or activate gag reflex.*
- Administer pharmaceutical agents as indicated. *Appetite stimulants and dietary supplements and digestive drugs or enzymes, vitamins and minerals (e.g., iron), antacids, anticholinergics, antiemetics, antidiarrheals, etc., may be used to enhance intake, improve digestion, and correct nutritional deficiencies.*[2]

NURSING PRIORITY NO. 6 To promote wellness (Teaching/Discharge Considerations):

- Discuss myths client/SO(s) may have about weight and weight gain *to address misconceptions and perhaps improve motivation for needed behavior changes.*
- Emphasize importance of well-balanced, nutritious intake. Provide nutritional information as indicated, taking into account client's age and developmental stage (e.g., toddler, teenager, pregnant woman, elderly person with chronic disease), physical health and activity tolerance, financial and socioeconomic factors, and client's/SO's potential for management of underlying conditions. *For example, older adults need same nutrients as younger adults but in smaller amounts and with attention to certain components, such as calcium, fiber, vitamins, protein, and water.*[3] *Infants/children require small meals and constant attention to needed nutrients for proper growth and development while dealing with child's food preferences and eating habits.*[4]
- Address financial issues and identify ways to meet dietary needs using nutrient-dense, low-budget foods.
- Involve SO(s) in treatment plan as much as possible *to provide ongoing support and increase likelihood of accomplishing dietary goals.*
- Consult with dietitian/nutritional support team as necessary *for long-term needs.*
- Involve client in developing behavior modification program appropriate to specific needs based on consistent, realistic weight gain goal. *Enhances commitment to change and likelihood of accomplishing desired outcomes.*[5,6]
- Provide positive regard, love, and acknowledgment of "voice within" guiding client with eating disorder. *These efforts encourage the client to recognize maladaptive eating patterns as defense mechanisms to ease the emotional pain and begin to resolve underlying issues and develop more adaptive coping strategies for dealing with stressful situations.*[6]
- Weigh as needed/prescribed and document results *to monitor effectiveness of dietary plan.*
- Develop regular exercise and stress-reduction programs. *Enhances general well-being, improves organ function/muscle tone, and increases appetite.*
- Review medical regimen and provide information or assistance as necessary. Discuss drug side effects and potential interactions with other medications and over-the-counter drugs.
- Assist client to identify and access community resources such as nutrition assistance program, budget counseling, Meals on Wheels, community food banks, or other appropriate assistance programs.
- Refer for dental hygiene and professional care, counseling or psychiatric care, and family therapy as indicated.
- Provide and reinforce client teaching regarding preoperative and postoperative dietary needs when surgery is planned.
- Assist client/SO(s) to learn how to blenderize food or perform tube feeding when indicated. *Promotes independence in self-care and sense of some degree of control in a difficult situation.*
- Refer to home health resources *for initiation and supervision of home nutrition therapy when used.*

Acute Care 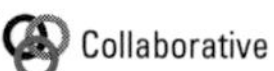 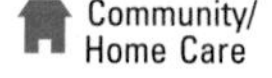 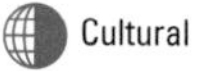

DOCUMENTATION FOCUS

Assessment/Reassessment

- Baseline and subsequent assessment findings to include signs/symptoms and laboratory diagnostic findings.
- Caloric and nutrient intake.
- Individual cultural or religious restrictions, personal preferences.
- Availability and use of resources.
- Personal understanding and perception of problem.

Planning

- Plan of care and who is involved in planning.
- Teaching plan.

Implementation/Evaluation

- Client's responses to interventions, teaching, and actions performed.
- Results of periodic weigh-in.
- Attainment or progress toward desired outcome(s).
- Modifications to plan of care.

Discharge Planning

- Long-term needs and who is responsible for actions to be taken.
- Specific referrals made.

References

1. Purnell, L. D. (2011). *Guide to Culturally Competent Health Care.* 2nd ed. Philadelphia, PA: F. A. Davis.
2. Sloane, P. D., Ivey, J., Helton, M., et al. (2001). Nutritional issues in long term care. *JAMDA*, 9(7), 476–485.
3. American Dietetic Association. (2005). Nutrition across the spectrum of aging. *J Am Diet Assoc*, 105(4), 616–633.
4. Engel, J. (2002). *Pocket Guide to Pediatric Assessment.* 4th ed. St. Louis, MO: Mosby.
5. Smith, M., Robinson, L., Segal, J. (2015). Retrieved November 2015 from http://www.helpguide..org/articles/eating-disorders/helping-someone-with-an-eating-disorder.htm.
6. Townsend, M. C. (2011). *Psychiatric Mental Health Nursing Concepts of Care in Evidence-Based Practice.* 7th ed. Philadelphia, PA: F. A. Davis.
7. Jacobs, D. G., Jacobs, D. O., Kudsk, K. A. (2004). Practice management guidelines for nutritional support of the trauma patient. *J Trauma*, 57(3), 660–678.
8. Nursing Standard of Practice Protocol: Assessment and management of mealtime difficulties. (2014). Geriatric Nursing Resources for Care of Older Adults. Retrieved November 2015 from http://consultgerirn.org/topics/mealtime_difficulties/want_to_know_more.
9. Scheinfeld, N. S., Lin, A., Mokashi, A. (2014). Protein-energy malnutrition. Retrieved November 2015 from http://emedicine.medscape.com/article/1104623-overview.
10. Sullivan, C. S., Logan, J., Kolasa, K. M. (2006). Medical nutrition therapy for the bariatric patient. *Nutr Today*, 41(5), 207–212.
11. DiMaria, R. A., Amelia, E. (2005). Nutrition in older adults: Intervention and assessment can curb the growing threat of malnutrition. *Am J Nurs*, 105(3), 40–50.
12. Guigoz, Y. (2006). The Mini Nutritional Assessment (MNA) review of the literature—What does it tell us? *J Nutr Health Aging*, 10(6), 466–485.
13. Malnutrition Advisory Group. (No date). Malnutrition Universal Screening Tool (MUST). Retrieved November 2015 from http://www.bapen.org.uk/pdfs/must/must_full.pdf.
14. Brugler, L., Stankovic, A. K., Scheifer, M., et al. (2005). A simplified nutrition screen for hospitalized patients using readily available laboratory and patient information. *Nutrition*, 21(6), 650–658.
15. Dawodu, S. T., Scott, D. D., Chase, M. (2015). Nutritional management in the rehabilitation setting. Retrieved November 2015 from http://emedicine.medscape.com/article/318180-overview#a1.

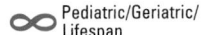

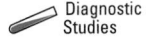

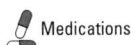

readiness for enhanced Nutrition

Taxonomy II: Nutrition—Class 4 Metabolism (00163) [**Diagnostic Division:** Food/Fluid], Submitted 2002; Revised 2013

DEFINITION: A pattern of nutrient intake, which can be strengthened.

DEFINING CHARACTERISTICS

Subjective

Expresses desire to enhance nutrition

Sample Clinical Applications: As a health-seeking behavior the client may be healthy or this diagnosis can occur in any clinical condition

DESIRED OUTCOMES/EVALUATION CRITERIA

Sample NOC linkages:

Nutritional Status: Extent to which nutrients are available to meet metabolic needs
Knowledge: Diet: Extent of understanding conveyed about recommended diet
Weight Maintenance Behavior: Personal actions to maintain optimum body weight

Client Will (Include Specific Time Frame)

- Demonstrate behaviors to attain or maintain appropriate weight.
- Be free of signs of malnutrition.
- Be able to safely prepare and store foods.

ACTIONS/INTERVENTIONS

Sample NIC linkages:

Nutritional Counseling: Use of an interactive helping process focusing on the need for diet modification
Teaching: Prescribed Diet: Preparing a patient to correctly follow a prescribed diet
Weight Management: Facilitating maintenance of optimal body weight and percent body fat

NURSING PRIORITY NO. 1 To determine current nutritional status and eating patterns:

- Assess client's knowledge of current nutritional needs and ways client is meeting these needs. *Provides baseline for further teaching or interventions.*
- Assess eating patterns and food and fluid choices in relation to any health-risk factors and health goals. *Helps to identify specific strengths and weaknesses that can be addressed.*
- Verify that age-related and developmental needs are met. *These factors are constantly present throughout the life span, although differing for each age group. For example, older adults need the same nutrients as younger adults, but in smaller amounts and with attention to certain components, such as calcium, fiber, vitamins, protein, and water.*[1] *Infants/children require small meals and constant attention to needed nutrients for proper growth and development while dealing with child's food preferences and eating habits.*[2]
- Evaluate influence of cultural and religious factors *to determine what client considers to be normal dietary practice as well as to identify food preferences and restrictions and eating patterns that can be strengthened or altered if indicated.*[3]
- Assess how client perceives food, food preparation, and the act of eating *to determine client's feeling and emotions regarding food (including the use of food for celebrations or as a reward) and self-image.*
- Ascertain occurrence of or potential for negative feedback from significant others (SOs). *May reveal control issues that could impact client's motivation for and commitment to change.*

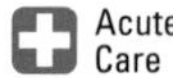

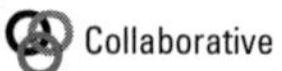

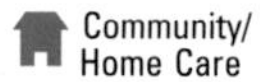

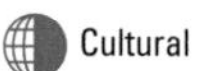

- Determine patterns of hunger and satiety. *Helps identify strengths and weaknesses in eating patterns and potential for change (e.g., person predisposed to weight gain may need a different time for a big meal than evening or may need teaching as to what foods reinforce feelings of satisfaction).*
- Assess client's ability to shop for, safely store, and prepare foods *to determine if health information or financial resources might be needed.*

NURSING PRIORITY NO. 2 To assist client/SO(s) to develop plan to meet individual needs:

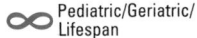

- Determine motivation and expectation for change. *Motivation to improve and high expectations can encourage client to make changes that will improve his or her life. However, presence of unrealistic expectations may hamper efforts. Client may actually be satisfied with current nutritional state and eating behaviors or may be changing some aspect of food intake or preparation in response to new dietary information or change in health status.*
- Assist in obtaining or review results of individual testing (e.g., weight and height, body fat percent, lipids, glucose, complete blood count, total protein) *to determine that client is healthy and/or identify dietary changes that may be helpful in attaining health goals.*[5]
- Encourage client's beneficial eating patterns and habits (e.g., controlling portion size; eating regular meals; reducing high-fat, high-sugar, or fast-food intake; following specific dietary program; drinking water and healthy beverages). *Provides reinforcement and supports client's efforts to incorporate changes into lifestyle habits and continue with new behaviors.*[6]
- Provide instruction and reinforce information regarding special needs. *Client/SO may benefit from or desire assistance in learning new eating habits or following medically prescribed diets (e.g., very low-calorie diet, tube feedings, diabetic or renal dialysis diet).*[4]
- Encourage the client to carefully read food labels, instructing in meaning of labeling, as indicated, *to assist client/SO in making healthful choices.*[6]
- Consult with or refer to nutritionist/physician, as indicated. *Client/SO may benefit from advice regarding specific nutrition or dietary issues or may require regular follow-up to determine that needs are being met when following a medically prescribed program.*
- Develop a system for self-monitoring *to provide a sense of control and enable the client to track own progress as well as to assist in making informed choices.*

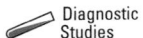

NURSING PRIORITY NO. 3 To promote optimum wellness (Teaching/Discharge Considerations):

- Review individual risk factors and provide additional information or response to concerns. *Assists the client with motivation and decision making.*
- Provide bibliotherapy and help client/SO(s) identify and evaluate resources he or she can access. *Reinforces learning, allows client to progress at own pace, and encourages client to be responsible for own learning. When referencing the Internet and nontraditional or unproven resources, the individual must exercise some restraint and determine the reliability of the source and information before acting on it.*
- Encourage variety and moderation in dietary plan *to decrease boredom and encourage client in efforts to make healthy choices about eating and food.*
- Discuss use of nutritional supplements and over-the-counter and herbal products. *Confusion may exist regarding the need for and use of these products in a balanced dietary regimen.*
- Assist client to identify and access community resources when indicated. *May benefit from assistance, such as nutritional assistance program, budget counseling, Meals on Wheels, community food banks, and other assistance programs.*

DOCUMENTATION FOCUS

Assessment/Reassessment

- Baseline information, client's perception of need.
- Nutritional intake and metabolic needs.
- Motivation and expectations for change.

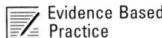

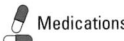

Planning
- Plan of care, specific interventions, and who is involved in planning.
- Teaching plan.

Implementation/Evaluation
- Client's responses to interventions, teaching, and actions performed.
- Attainment or progress toward desired outcome(s).
- Modifications to plan of care.

Discharge Planning
- Long-term needs and actions to be taken.
- Support systems available, specific referrals made, and who is responsible for actions to be taken.

References

1. American Dietetic Association. (2005). Nutrition across the spectrum of aging. *J Am Diet Assoc*, 105(4), 616–633.
2. Caprio, S., Daniels, S. R., Drewnowski, A., et al. (2008). Influence of race, ethnicity, and culture on childhood obesity: Implications for prevention and treatment: A consensus statement of Shaping America's Health and the Obesity Society. *Diabetes Care*, 31(11), 2211–2221.
3. Purnell, L. D. (2011). *Guide to Culturally Competent Health Care*. 2nd ed. Philadelphia: F. A. Davis.
4. Pignone, M. P. (2003). Counseling to promote a healthy diet in adults: A summary of the evidence for the U.S. Preventive Services Task Force. *Am J Prev Med*, 24(1), 75–92.
5. Vogelzang, J. L. (2003). Making nutrition sense from OASIS. *Home Healthcare Nurse*, 21(9), 592–600.
6. U.S. Department of Health and Human Services, Department of Agriculture. *Dietary Guidelines for Americans*, 2010. Various parts. Retrieved November 2015 from http://www.cnpp.usda.gov/DietaryGuidelines.htm.

Obesity

Taxonomy II: Nutrition—Class 1 Ingestion (00232) [**Diagnostic Division:** Food/Fluid], Submitted 2013

DEFINITION: A condition in which an individual accumulates abnormal or excessive fat for age and gender that exceeds overweight.

RELATED FACTORS

Average daily physical activity is less than recommended for gender and age; energy expenditure below energy intake based on standard assessment (e.g., WAVE [weight, activity, variety in diet, excess] assessment)

Consumption of sugar-sweetened beverages; frequent snacking; high frequency of restaurant or fried food; portion sizes larger than recommended

Disordered eating behaviors or perceptions; fear regarding lack of food supply; high disinhibition and restraint eating behavior score

Economically disadvantaged

Formula- or mixed-fed infants; overweight in infancy; low dietary calcium intake in children

Genetic disorder; heritability of interrelated factors (e.g., adipose tissue distribution, energy expenditure, lipid synthesis, lipolysis

Maternal diabetes mellitus, smoking; parental obesity

Sample Clinical Applications: Bulimia nervosa, morbid obesity, diseases requiring long-term steroid use (e.g., chronic obstructive pulmonary disease [COPD]), conditions associated with immobility (e.g., stroke/paralysis, multiple sclerosis [MS], amputation), Alzheimer's disease, depression, developmental delay

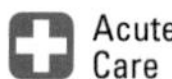

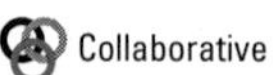

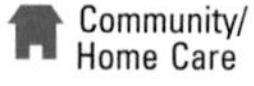

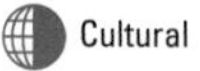

DEFINING CHARACTERISTICS

Objective

ADULT: BMI of >30 kg/m^2

CHILD <2 years: Term not used with children this age

CHILD 2–18 years: BMI of >30 kg/m^2 or >95th percentile for age and gender

DESIRED OUTCOMES/EVALUATION CRITERIA

Sample NOC linkages:

Weight Loss Behavior: Personal actions to lose weight through diet, exercise, and behavior modification

Knowledge: Diet: Extent of understanding conveyed about recommended diet

Nutritional Status: Extent to which nutrients are available to meet metabolic needs

Weight: Body Mass: Extent to which body weight, muscle, and fat are congruent to height, frame, gender, and age

Client Will (Include Specific Time Frame)

- Verbalize a realistic self-concept or body image (congruent mental and physical picture of self).
- Participate in development of, and commit to, a personal weight loss program.
- Demonstrate appropriate changes in lifestyle and behaviors, including eating patterns, food quantity/quality, and exercise program.
- Attain desirable body weight with optimal maintenance of health.

ACTIONS/INTERVENTIONS

Sample NIC linkages:

Weight-Reduction Assistance: Facilitating loss of weight and/or body fat

Nutrition Management: Assisting with or providing a balanced dietary intake of foods and fluids

Nutritional Counseling: Use of an interactive helping process focusing on the need for diet modification

NURSING PRIORITY NO. 1 To identify contributing factors/health status:

- Obtain weight history, noting if client has weight gain out of character for self or family, is or was obese child, or used to be much more physically active than is now *to identify trends. Note: Obesity is now the most prevalent nutritional disorder among children and adolescents in the United States (approximately 21% to 24% of American children and adolescents are overweight, and another 16% to 18% are obese).*[1] *Being overweight during older childhood is highly predictive of adult obesity, especially if a parent is also obese.*[2]
- Assess risk and presence of factors or conditions associated with obesity (e.g., familial pattern of obesity; genetic disorders in children [e.g., Prader-Willi syndrome, Laurence-Moon-Biedl syndrome]; hypothyroidism; type 2 diabetes; reproductive dysfunction; menopause; chronic disorders, such as heart disease, kidney disease, chronic pain; food or other substance addictions; stressful or sedentary lifestyle; depression; use of certain medications such as steroids, birth control pills; physical disabilities or limitations; lack of socioeconomic resources for obtaining or preparing healthy foods) *to determine treatments and interventions that may be indicated in addition to weight management.*[2,3]
- Ascertain current and previous dieting history. *Client may report normal or excessive intake of food, but calories and intake of certain food groups (e.g., sweets and fats) are often underestimated. Client may report experimentation with numerous types of diets, repeated dieting efforts ("yo-yo" dieting) with varying results, or may never have attempted a weight-management program.*
- Assess client's knowledge of own body weight and nutritional needs and determine cultural expectations regarding size. *Although nutritional needs are not always understood, being overweight or*

having large body size may not be viewed negatively by individual because it is considered within relationship to family eating patterns and peer and cultural influences.[2] *Ethnicity factors may influence the age of onset and the rapidity of weight gain. African American women and Hispanic women tend to experience weight gain earlier in life than Caucasians and Asians. Hispanic men tend to develop obesity earlier than African American and Caucasian men.*[3,4] *Note: In 2010, a Centers for Disease Control and Prevention (CDC) report noted that in the United States (in most states examined) blacks had the highest prevalence of obesity, followed by Hispanics, and then whites. Greater prevalences of obesity for non-Hispanic blacks and whites were found in the Midwest and South. Among Hispanics, a lower prevalence was observed in the Northeast compared to other regions.*[5]

- Identify familial and cultural influences regarding food. *People of many cultures place high importance on food and food-related events, while some cultures routinely observe fasting days (e.g., Arab, Greek, Irish, Jewish) that may be done for health or religious purposes.*[4]
- Ascertain how client perceives food and the act of eating. *Individual beliefs, values, and types of foods available influence what people eat, avoid, or alter. Client may be eating to satisfy an emotional need rather than physiological hunger, not only because food plays a significant role in socialization, but also because food can offer comfort, sense of security, and acceptance.*[3,4]
- Assess dietary practices by means of diary covering 3 to 7 days. *Recall of foods and fluids ingested; times, patterns, and place of eating; whether alone or with other(s); and feelings before, during, and after eating can increase client's understanding of eating behavior and serve as the basis for dietary modifications.*[6,7]
- Identify problems with energy balance. *Few people can accurately estimate the number of calories they should consume in a day for a person their age, height, weight, and physical activity.*[8] *Note: Eating and physical activity patterns that are focused on consuming fewer calories, making informed food choices, and being physically active can help people attain and maintain a healthy weight, reduce their risk of chronic disease, and promote overall health. Note: For people who are overweight or obese, this will mean consuming fewer calories from both foods and beverages.*[9]
- Review daily activity and regular exercise program *for comparative baseline and to identify areas for modification. Note: The 2008 National Health Interview Survey showed that only 33% of American adults participated in leisure-time physical activity on a regular basis.*[9]
- Obtain anthropometric measurements *to determine presence and severity of obesity:*

  Calculate body mass index (BMI) *to estimate percentage of body fat. Note: The CDC has standardized BMI calculations, removing age and sex differences for adults with obesity being defined as 30 and above. Morbid obesity is defined as BMI equal to or greater than 40.*[13] *The CDC has recommended that children (over age 2) and adolescents be considered obese if their BMI exceeds the 95th percentile on growth curves or exceeds 30 kg/m at any age. Note: Normal BMI in children changes as age and growth occurs and is also different between the sexes.*[14]

  Refer to ND Overweight for additional diagnostic studies information.
- Collaborate in assessment and interventions for client with disordered eating habits or eating perceptions:

  Obtain a comparative body drawing, having client draw self on wall with chalk and then standing against it and having actual body outline drawn to note difference between the two. *Determines whether client's view of self-body image is congruent with reality.*

  Ascertain occurrence of negative feedback from significant others (SOs). *May reveal control issues and impact motivation for change.*

  Identify unhelpful eating behaviors (e.g., eating over sink; "gobbling, nibbling, or grazing") and address kinds of activities associated with eating (e.g., watching television or reading, being unmindful of eating or food) *that result in taking in too many calories as well as eliminating the joy of food because of failure to notice flavors or sensation of fullness or satiety.*[2]

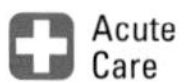
Acute Care
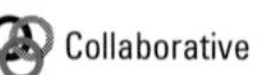
Collaborative
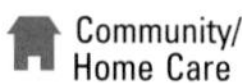
Community/ Home Care
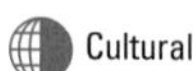
Cultural

NURSING PRIORITY NO. 2 To establish weight-reduction program:

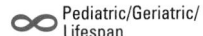

- **Refer to ND Overweight, Nursing Priority 2 for interventions common to weight-loss programs.**
- Collaborate with nutritionist in addressing/implementing client's specific needs (e.g., what foods to incorporate or limit, how to identify nutrient dense-foods and beverages). *A healthy eating pattern limits intake of sodium, solid fats, added sugars, and refined grains and emphasizes nutrient-dense foods and beverages (e.g., vegetables, fruits, whole grains, fat-free or low-fat milk and milk products), seafood, lean meats and poultry, eggs, beans and peas, and nuts and seeds.*[9]
- Assist client in using technology to manage food choices. *Technology offers applications that can assist in monitoring dietary intake and food choices. Some calculate calories, providing immediate feedback and generating individualized reminders. The best applications include (1) a large database of foods with nutritional information for various serving sizes, (2) a bar scanner that allows users to add information about prepared foods to their database, (3) a calorie tracker that is easy to use, and (4) the ability to track other nutrients (e.g., carbohydrates, protein, calcium).*[6]
- Engage client and family in structured weight loss programs, as indicated. *Approaches to the treatment of severely obese individuals may include lifestyle modifications, physical activity, very controlled diets, and intensive psychiatric interventions, including individual, group, and family therapy.*[2] *Note: DeBar et al. recently reported that an intensive, group therapy approach was superior to standard, family-based therapy in achieving lifestyle changes (e.g., less consumption of fast foods) and in reducing the BMI of overweight adolescents.*[15]
- Refer to bariatric physician/surgeon, as indicated. *Evaluation for special measures may be needed (e.g., supervised fasting or bariatric surgery) for obese persons with comorbidities and for morbidly obese persons with BMI greater than 40. Currently there are several bariatric surgical procedures (e.g., gastric bypass [Roux-en-Y], laparoscopic adjustable gastric banding, biliopancreatic diversion [rare], vertical banded gastroplasty). At present, gastric bypass is the most successful procedure.*[16]

NURSING PRIORITY NO. 3 To promote wellness (Teaching/Discharge Considerations):

- **Refer to ND Overweight for related interventions.**

DOCUMENTATION FOCUS

Assessment/Reassessment

- Individual findings, including current weight, dietary pattern; perceptions of self, food, and eating; motivation for loss, support or feedback from SO(s).
- Results of laboratory and diagnostic testing.

Planning

- Plan of care, specific interventions, and who is involved in planning.
- Teaching plan.

Implementation/Evaluation

- Responses to interventions and actions performed.
- Attainment or progress toward desired outcome(s).
- Modifications to plan of care.

Discharge Planning

- Long-term needs and who is responsible for actions to be taken.
- Specific referrals made.

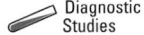

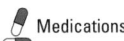

References

1. Ogden, C. L., Yanovski, S. Z., Carroll, M. D., et al. (2007). The epidemiology of obesity. *Gastroenterology*, 132(6), 2087–2103.
2. Schwarz, S. M. (Updated 2014). Obesity in children. Retrieved January 2015 from http://emedicine.medscape.com/article/985333-overview.
3. Caprio, S., Daniels, S. R., Drewnowski, A., et al. (2008). Influence of race, ethnicity, and culture on childhood obesity: Implications for prevention and treatment: A consensus statement of Shaping America's Health and the Obesity Society. *Diabetes Care*, 31(11), 2211–2221.
4. Purnell, L. D., Paulanka, B. J. (1998). *Transcultural Health Care: A Culturally Competent Approach.* Philadelphia: F. A. Davis, 22.
5. Centers for Disease Control and Prevention. (2010). Compared with whites, Blacks had 51% higher and Hispanics had 21% higher obesity rates. Data & Statistics. Retrieved January 2015 from http://www.cdc.gov/features/dsobesityadults/.
6. Budd, G. M., Peterson, J. A. (2015). The obesity epidemic, Part 2: Nursing assessment and intervention. *Am J Nurs*, 115(1), 38–46.
7. Fleury, J. (1991). Empowering potential: A theory of wellness motivation. *Nurs Res*, 40(5), 286–291.
8. International Food Information Council. (2010). Consumer attitudes towards food safety, nutrition, & health. 2010 Food & Health Survey. Retrieved January 2015 from http://www.foodinsight.org/2012_Food_Health_Survey_Consumer_Attitudes_toward_Food_Safety_Nutrition_and_Health.
9. 2010 Dietary Guidelines Advisory Committee. (2010). Dietary guidelines for Americans. Retrieved January 2015 from http://www.health.gov/dietaryguidelines/dga2010/DietaryGuidelines2010.pdf.
10. American Medical Directors Association. (2001, updated 2010). Altered nutritional status in the long term care setting. Retrieved January 2015 from http://www.guideline.gov/content.aspx?id=15590.
11. Lab test: Insulin. (2014). Lab Tests Online. Retrieved January 2015 from http://labtestsonline.org/understanding/analytes/insulin/tab/test/.
12. Perry, B., Wang, Y. (2012). Appetite regulation and weight control: The role of gut hormones. *Nutr Diabetes*, 2(1), e26.
13. Centers for Disease Control and Prevention. (2014). About BMI for adults. Retrieved January 2015 from http://www.cdc.gov/healthyweight/assessing/bmi/adult_bmi/index.html.
14. Centers for Disease Control and Prevention. (2014). About BMI for children and teens. Retrieved January 2015 from http://www.cdc.gov/healthyweight/assessing/bmi/childrens_bmi/about_childrens_bmi.html.
15. DeBarr, L. L., Stevens, V. J., Perrin, N., et al. (2012). A primary care-based, multicomponent lifestyle intervention for overweight adolescent females. *Pediatrics*, 129(3), e611–e620.
16. Saber, A., Hale, K. L. (2014). Surgery in the treatment of obesity. Retrieved January 2015 from http://www.emedicinehealth.com/surgery_in_the_treatment_of_obesity/page5_em.htm#operative_procedures.

Overweight

Taxonomy II: Nutrition—Class 1 Ingestion (00233) [**Diagnostic Division:** Food/Fluid], Submitted 2013

DEFINITION: A condition in which an individual accumulates abnormal or excessive fat for age and gender.

RELATED FACTORS

Average daily physical activity is less than recommended for gender and age; sedentary behavior occurring for >2 hours/day; energy expenditure below energy intake based on standard assessment (e.g., WAVE [weight, activity, variety in diet, excess] assessment)

Consumption of sugar-sweetened beverages; frequent snacking; high frequency of restaurant or fried food; portion sizes larger than recommended

Disordered eating behaviors or perceptions; fear regarding lack of food supply; high disinhibition and restraint eating behavior score

Economically disadvantaged

Genetic disorder; heritability of interrelated factors (e.g., adipose tissue distribution, energy expenditure, lipid synthesis, lipolysis)

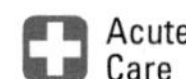

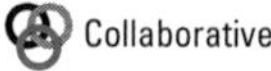

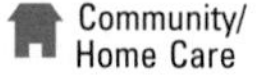

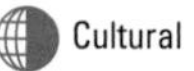

Maternal diabetes mellitus; maternal smoking; parental obesity
Rapid weight gain during infancy, including first week, first 4 months, and first year; solid foods as major food source at <5 months of age
Rapid weight gain during childhood, obesity in childhood; low dietary calcium intake in children; premature pubarche
Shortened sleep time; sleep disorder
Sample Clinical Applications: Bulimia nervosa, morbid obesity, diseases requiring long-term steroid use (e.g., chronic obstructive pulmonary disease [COPD]), conditions associated with immobility (e.g., stroke/paralysis, multiple sclerosis [MS], amputation), depression, developmental delay

DEFINING CHARACTERISTICS

Objective
ADULT: BMI of $>25 kg/m^2$
CHILD <2 years: Weight-for-length > 95th percentile
CHILD 2–18 years: BMI >25 kg/m^2 or > 85th but <95th percentile (whichever is smaller)

DESIRED OUTCOMES/EVALUATION CRITERIA

Sample NOC linkages:
Weight Loss Behavior: Personal actions to lose weight through diet, exercise, and behavior modification
Knowledge: Diet: Extent of understanding conveyed about recommended diet
Nutritional Status: Extent to which nutrients are available to meet metabolic needs
Weight: Body Mass: Extent to which body weight, muscle, and fat are congruent to height, frame, gender, and age

Client Will (Include Specific Time Frame)
- Verbalize a realistic self-concept or body image (congruent mental and physical picture of self).
- Participate in development of, and commit to, a personal weight-loss program.
- Demonstrate appropriate changes in lifestyle and behaviors, including eating patterns, food quantity/quality, and exercise program.
- Attain desirable body weight with optimal maintenance of health.

ACTIONS/INTERVENTIONS

Sample NIC linkages:
Weight-Reduction Assistance: Facilitating loss of weight and/or body fat
Nutrition Management: Assisting with or providing a balanced dietary intake of foods and fluids
Nutritional Counseling: Use of an interactive process focusing on the need for diet modification

NURSING PRIORITY NO. 1 To identify contributing factors/health status:

- Obtain weight history, noting if client has weight gain out of character for self or family, is or was obese child, or used to be much more physically active than is now *to identify trends. Note: Unchecked weight gain can lead to obesity, which is now the most prevalent nutritional disorder among children and adolescents in the United States (approximately 21% to 24% of American children and adolescents are overweight, and another 16% to 18% are obese).*[18] *Being overweight during older childhood is highly predictive of adult obesity, especially if a parent is also obese.*[1]
- Assess risk and presence of factors or conditions associated with obesity (e.g., familial pattern of obesity; decreased basal metabolic rate or hypothyroidism; type 2 diabetes; reproductive dysfunction; menopause; chronic disorders, such as heart disease, kidney disease, chronic pain; food or other substance addictions;

stressful or sedentary lifestyle; depression; use of certain medications such as steroids, birth control pills; physical disabilities or limitations; lack of socioeconomic resources for obtaining or preparing healthy foods) *to determine treatments and interventions that may be indicated in addition to weight management.*[1,3]

- Assess client's knowledge of own body weight and nutritional needs and determine cultural expectations regarding size. *Although nutritional needs are not always understood, being overweight or having large body size may not be viewed negatively by individual because it is considered within relationship to family eating patterns and peer and cultural influences.*[1] *Ethnicity factors may influence the age of onset and the rapidity of weight gain. African American women and Hispanic women tend to experience weight gain earlier in life than Caucasians and Asians. Hispanic men tend to develop obesity earlier than African American and Caucasian men. Some cultures place importance on large body size.*[2,3]
- Identify familial and cultural influences regarding food. *People of many cultures place high importance on food and food-related events, while some cultures routinely observe fasting days (e.g., Arab, Greek, Irish, Jewish) that may be done for health or religious purposes.*[2]
- Ascertain how client perceives food and the act of eating. *Individual beliefs, values, and types of foods available influence what people eat, avoid, or alter. Client may be eating to satisfy an emotional need rather than physiological hunger, not only because food plays a significant role in socialization, but also because food can offer comfort, sense of security, and acceptance.*[2,3]
- Evaluate client's routine medications. *Some medications can contribute to weight gain (e.g., cortisol and other glucocorticoids; sulfonylureas, tricyclic antidepressants, monoamine oxidase inhibitors; oral contraceptives; insulin [in excessive doses]; risperidone).*[6]
- Assess dietary practices by means of diary covering 3 to 7 days. *Recall of foods and fluids ingested; times, patterns, and place of eating; whether alone or with other(s); and feelings before, during, and after eating can increase client's understanding of eating behavior and serve as the basis for dietary modifications. Note: Few people can accurately estimate the number of calories they should consume in a day for a person their age, height, weight, and physical activity.*[4,7,19]
- Ascertain previous dieting history. *Client may report normal or excessive intake of food, but calories and intake of certain food groups (e.g., sweets and fats) are often underestimated. Client may report experimentation with numerous types of diets, repeated dieting efforts ("yo-yo" dieting) with varying results, or may never have attempted a weight-management program.*
- Collaborate in assessment and interventions for client with disordered eating habits or eating perceptions:
  Obtain a comparative body drawing, having client draw self on wall with chalk and then standing against it and having actual body outline drawn to note difference between the two. *Determines whether client's view of self-body image is congruent with reality.*
  Ascertain occurrence of negative feedback from significant others (SOs). *May reveal control issues and impact motivation for change.*[1]
- Review daily activity and regular exercise program *for comparative baseline and to identify areas for modification. Note: The 2008 National Health Interview Survey showed that only 33% of American adults participated in leisure-time physical activity on a regular basis.*[20]
- Review laboratory test results (e.g., complete blood count with differential, full lipid panel, fasting glucose, A_1C, insulin levels; thyroid, leptins; proteins, Mini-Nutritional Assessment) *that may reveal medical conditions associated with obesity and identify problems that may be treated with alterations in diet or medications.*[5,10,21]

NURSING PRIORITY NO. 2 To determine weight-loss goals:

- Obtain anthropometric measurements *to determine presence and severity of obesity:*
  Calculate body mass index (BMI) *to estimate percentage of body fat. Note: The Centers for Disease Control and Prevention (CDC) has standardized BMI calculations, removing age and sex differences for adults with obesity being defined as 25 to 29.9 kg/m² overweight.*[16,22] *The CDC has recommended that children*

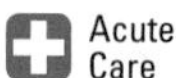

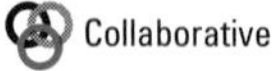

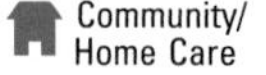

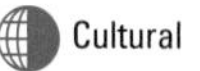

(over age 2) and adolescents be considered overweight if the BMI exceeds the 85th percentile (and is less than the 95th percentile) on growth curves or exceeds 25 kg/m² at any age. Note: Normal BMI in children changes as age and growth occurs and is also different between the sexes.[23]

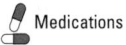

Determine waist circumference (WC), if indicated. *Some studies support that WC is more closely linked to cardiovascular risk factors than BMI alone because a high WC can occur in persons with normal or near normal BMIs. These sources indicate high risk if WC is greater than 35 inches (for women) and greater than 40 inches (for men), even if BMI is greater than 25 but is accompanied by family history of cardiovascular disease or diabetes or exists in conjunction with two or more chronic health conditions.*[9]

Evaluate body fat, body water, and muscle mass via scale skin caliper measurements and scale weight (*direct* measurement), bioelectric impedance analysis, dual-energy x-ray absorptiometry, and hydrostatic weighing (*indirect* measurement) per facility protocol. *Note: The CDC does not recommend these methods of measuring body weight (over BMI) because "they are not always readily available, and they are either expensive or need highly trained personnel. Furthermore, many of these methods can be difficult to standardize across observers or machines, complicating comparisons across studies and time periods."*[9,22]

- Determine client's motivation for weight loss (e.g., for own satisfaction or self-esteem, to improve health status, to gain approval from another person). *Client is more likely to succeed and maintain desired weight when change is for self (e.g., acceptance of self "as is," general well-being) rather than to please others.*
- Discuss myths client/SO may have about weight and weight loss *to address misconceptions and possibly enhance motivation for needed behavior changes.*

NURSING PRIORITY NO. 3 To establish weight-reduction program:

- Obtain commitment or contract for weight loss. *Verbal agreement to goals or written contract formalizes the plan and may enhance efforts and maximize outcomes.*
- Involve SO(s) in treatment plan as much as possible *to provide ongoing support and increase likelihood of success.*
- Set realistic goals (short and long term) for weight loss. *Reasonable weight loss (1 to 2 lb/wk) has been shown to have more lasting effects than rapid weight loss, although sustaining motivation for small losses often makes it difficult for client to stick with a program. Note: A loss of 5% to 20% of total body weight can reduce many of the health risks associated with obesity in adults.*[1,12,13]
- Collaborate with physician and nutritionist *to develop and implement comprehensive weight-loss program that includes food, activity, behavior alteration, and support.*
- Calculate calorie requirements based on physical factors and activity. *While many weight-reduction programs focus on portion size and food components (e.g., low-fat, high-protein, low-glycemic foods), reducing calorie intake is essential for weight loss. Note: Decreasing calories by 500/day or expending 500 calories/day through exercise results in a weight loss of about 1 lb/wk.*[6]
- Provide information regarding specific nutritional needs. *Individual may be deficient in needed nutrients (e.g., proteins, vitamins, or minerals) or may eat too much of one food group (e.g., fats or carbohydrates) and not enough of another food group (e.g., vegetables).*[11,12] *Note: A recent CDC report revealed that between 2007 and 2010, children did not meet recommendations for the amount of fruit and vegetables they should eat, although fruit intake did increase with fresh fruit replacing juices.*[24]
- Discuss modifications to achieve healthy body weight:[8,12–16,19]

  Eat from each food group (fruits, vegetables, whole grains, lean meats, low-fat dairy, oils).

  Start with small changes, such as adding one more vegetable/day or introducing healthier versions of favorite foods.

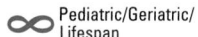

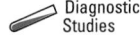

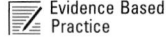

Choose "nutrient-dense" forms of foods that provide substantial amounts of fiber, vitamins, electrolytes, and minerals.

Avoid saturated fats, trans fats, cholesterol, salt (sodium), and added sugars.

Focus on portion sizes: calorie-dense foods (high in fat and/or sugar) should be eaten in smaller quantities, whereas high-fiber foods can be eaten in larger quantities.

Discuss smart snacks (e.g., low-fat yogurt with fruit, nuts, apple slices with peanut butter, low-fat string cheese).

Emphasize need for adequate fluid intake and taking fluids between meals rather than with meals to provide fluid while leaving more room for food intake at meals *to assist in digestive process and to quench thirst, which is often mistakenly identified as hunger.*

- Encourage involvement in planned activity program of client's choice and within physical abilities. Refer to formal exercise program, if desired. *Moderately increased physical activity for 30 to 45 min for 5 days/wk can expend an additional 1,500 to 2,000 calories/wk, supporting both loss of pounds and maintenance of lower weight.*[12,14] *Children should participate in vigorous physical activity throughout adolescence and limit time spent watching television and playing computer games to facilitate weight control.*[1]
- Recommend weighing only once/week, at the same time and wearing the same clothes, and graph it on chart. Measure and monitor body fat when possible *to track progress while focusing more on the idea of being health conscious and responsible than what scale may reveal.*
- Provide positive reinforcement and encouragement for efforts as well as actual weight loss. *Enhances commitment to program and enhances person's sense of self-worth.*
- Refer to bariatric physician/surgeon when indicated. *Evaluation for special measures may be needed (e.g., supervised fasting or bariatric surgery) for morbidly obese persons with BMI greater than 40.* Refer to ND Obesity for related interventions.

NURSING PRIORITY NO. 4 To promote wellness (Teaching/Discharge Considerations):

- Assist in and encourage periodic evaluation of nutritional status and alteration of dietary plan. *May be desired or needed for addressing special needs (e.g., diabetes mellitus, age considerations, very low calorie or fasting) and monitoring health status.*[17]
- Emphasize importance of avoiding fad diets *that may be harmful to health and often do not produce long-term positive results.*
- Identify and encourage finding ways to reduce tension when eating. *Promotes relaxation to permit focus on act of eating and awareness of satiety.*
- Identify unhelpful eating behaviors (e.g., eating over sink; "gobbling, nibbling, or grazing") and address kinds of activities associated with eating (e.g., watching television or reading, being unmindful of eating or food) *that result in taking in too many calories as well as eliminating the joy of food because of failure to notice flavors or sensation of fullness or satiety.*
- Review and discuss strategies to deal appropriately with stressful events *to avoid overeating as a means of coping.*
- Discuss importance of an occasional treat by planning for inclusion in diet *to avoid feelings of deprivation arising from self-denial.*
- Advise planning for special occasions (birthday or holidays) by reducing intake before event and/or eating "smart" *to redistribute or reduce calories and allow for participation in food events.*
- Discuss normalcy of ups and downs of weight loss: plateau, set point (at which weight is not being lost), hormonal influences, etc. *Prevents discouragement when progress stalls.*

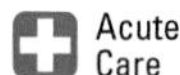

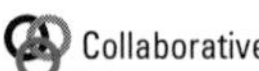

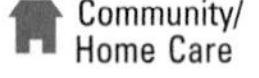

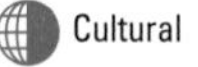

- Encourage buying personal items and clothing *as reward for weight loss or other accomplishments*. Suggest disposing of "fat clothes" *to encourage positive attitude of permanent change and remove "safety valve" of having wardrobe available "just in case" weight is regained.*
- Review prescribed drug regimen (e.g., appetite suppressants, hormone therapy, vitamin and mineral supplements) *for benefits or adverse side effects and drug interactions.*
- Recommend reading labels of nonprescription diet aids if used. *Herbals containing diuretics or ma huang (product similar to ephedrine) may cause adverse side effects in vulnerable persons.*
- Encourage parents and school dieticians to model and offer good nutritional choices (e.g., offer vegetables, fruits, and lower-fat foods in daily meals and snacks) *to assist child in accepting healthy eating styles. Note: Studies have shown a high correlation between parents and children regarding patterns of food intake and food choices. Conversely, adult intake of fat has been shown to be higher when children under 17 are in the home (more pizza, cheese, processed food, junk food and fast food).*[1,15]
- Refer to community support groups or psychotherapy, as indicated, *to provide role models and address issues of body image or self-worth.*
- Provide contact number for dietitian/nutritionist and/or audiovisual materials, bibliography, and reliable Internet sites for resources *to address ongoing nutrition needs and dietary changes.*
- Refer to NDs disturbed Body Image, ineffective Coping, and Obesity for additional interventions, as appropriate.

DOCUMENTATION FOCUS

Assessment/Reassessment

- Individual findings, including current weight, dietary pattern; perceptions of self, food, and eating; motivation for loss, support or feedback from SO(s).
- Results of laboratory and diagnostic testing.
- Results of interval weigh-ins.

Planning

- Plan of care, specific interventions, and who is involved in planning.
- Teaching plan.

Implementation/Evaluation

- Responses to interventions, weekly weight, and actions performed.
- Attainment or progress toward desired outcome(s).
- Modifications to plan of care.

Discharge Planning

- Long-term needs and who is responsible for actions to be taken.
- Specific referrals made.

References

1. Schwarz, S. M. (2012, updated 2014). Obesity in children. Retrieved January 2015 from http://emedicine.medscape.com/article/985333-overview.
2. Purnell, L. D., Paulanka, B. J. (1998). *Transcultural Health Care: A Culturally Competent Approach.* Philadelphia: F. A. Davis, 22.
3. Caprio, S., Daniels, S. R., Drewnowski, A., et al. (2008). Influence of race, ethnicity, and culture on childhood obesity: Implications for prevention and treatment: A consensus statement of Shaping America's Health and the Obesity Society. *Diabetes Care*, 31(11), 2211–2221.
4. Fleury, J. (1991). Empowering potential: A theory of wellness motivation. *Nurs Res*, 40, 286–291.
5. American Medical Directors Association. (2001, updated 2010). Altered nutritional status in the long term care setting. Retrieved January 2015 from http://www.guideline.gov/content.aspx?id=15590.
6. Galletta, G. M. (2014). Obesity. Retrieved January 2015 from http://www.emedicinehealth.com/obesity/page9_em.htm#surgery_for_obesity.
7. Lutz, C. A., Przytulski, K. R. (2010). *Nutrition and Diet Therapy*. 5th ed. Philadelphia: F. A. Davis.
8. U.S. Department of Health and Human Services, Department of Agriculture. The Dietary Guidelines for Americans, 2010. Various parts. Retrieved January 2015 from http://www.health.gov/dietaryguidelines/dga2010/DietaryGuidelines2010.pdf.
9. Zhu, S., Wang, Z., Heska, S. (2002). Waist circumference and obesity-associated risk factors among whites in the third National Health and Nutrition Examination Survey: clinical action thresholds. *Am J Clin Nutr*, 75(4), 743–749.
10. Lab test: Insulin. (2014). Lab Tests Online. Retrieved January 2015 from http://labtestsonline.org/understanding/analytes/insulin/tab/test/.
11. Rippe, J. M., Hess, S. (1998). The role of physical activity in the prevention and management of obesity. *J Am Diet Assoc*, 10 (suppl 2), S31–S38.
12. Miller, C. K., Ulbrecht, J. S., Lyons, J., et al. (2007). A reduced-carbohydrate diet improves outcomes in patients with metabolic syndrome: A transitional study. *Top Clin Nutr*, 22(1), 82–91.
13. Wing, R., Phelan, S. (2005). Long-term weight loss maintenance. *Am J Clin Nutr*, 82(1 suppl), 222S–225S.
14. Meadows, M. (2008). Nutrition: Healthy eating. Retrieved January 2015 from http://www.medicinenet.com/script/main/art.asp?articlekey=61982.
15. Laroche, H. H., Hofer, T. P., Davis, M. M. (2007). Adult fat intake associated with the presence of children in households: Findings from NHANES III. *J Am Board Fam Med*, 20(1), 9–15.
16. Hamdy, O., Uwaifo, G. I., Oral, E. A., et al. (2012, updated 2014). Obesity. Retrieved January 2015 from http://emedicine.medscape.com/article/123702-overview.
17. Flegal, K. M., Ogden, C. L., Wei, R., et al. (2001). Prevalence of overweight in U.S. children: Comparison of U.S. growth charts from the Centers for Disease Control and Prevention with other reference values for body mass index. *Am J Clin Nutr*, 73(6), 1086–1093.
18. Ogden, C. L., Yanovski, S. Z., Carroll, M. D., et al. (2007). The epidemiology of obesity. *Gastroenterology*, 132(6), 2087–2102.
19. Budd, G. M., Peterson, J. A. (2015). The obesity epidemic, Part 2: Nursing assessment and intervention. *Am J Nurs*, 115(1), 38–46.
20. 2010 Dietary Guidelines Advisory Committee. Dietary guidelines for Americans. Retrieved January 2015 from http://www.health.gov/dietaryguidelines/dga2010/DietaryGuidelines2010.pdf.
21. Perry, B., Wang, Y. (2012). Appetite regulation and weight control: The role of gut hormones. *Nutr Diabetes*, 2(1), e26.
22. Centers for Disease Control and Prevention. (2014). About BMI for adults. Retrieved January 2015 from http://www.cdc.gov/healthyweight/assessing/bmi/adult_bmi/index.html.
23. Centers for Disease Control and Prevention. (2014). About BMI for children and teens. Retrieved January 2015 from http://www.cdc.gov/healthyweight/assessing/bmi/childrens_bmi/about_childrens_bmi.html.
24. Centers for Disease Control and Prevention. (2014). Progress on children eating more fruit, not vegetables. CDC Vital Signs. Retrieved January 2015 from http://www.cdc.gov/vitalsigns/pdf/2014-08-vitalsigns.pdf.

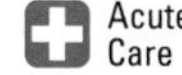

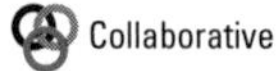

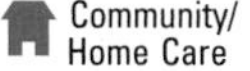

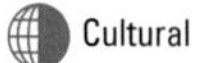

risk for Overweight

Taxonomy II: Nutrition—Class 1 Ingestion (00234) [**Diagnostic Division:** Food/Fluid], Submitted 2013

DEFINITION: Vulnerable abnormal or excessive fat accumulation for age and gender, which may compromise health.

RISK FACTORS

ADULT: BMI approaching 25kg/m^2
CHILD <2 years: Watch for weight-for-length approaching 95th percentile
CHILD 2–18 years: BMI approaching 25 kg/m^2, or 85th percentile (whichever is smaller)
Children with high BMI percentiles, or who are crossing BMI percentiles upward
Consumption of sugar-sweetened beverages; high frequency of restaurant or fried food; portion sizes larger than recommended
Disordered eating behaviors (e.g., binge eating, extreme weight control); disordered eating perceptions; fear regarding lack of food supply; high disinhibition and restraint eating behavior score
Eating in response to external cues (e.g., time of day, social situations); eating in response to internal cues other than hunger (e.g., anxiety); frequent snacking
Economically disadvantaged
Energy expenditure below energy intake based on standard assessment (e.g., WAVE [weight, activity, variety in diet, excess] assessment); sedentary behavior occurring for >2 hours/day
Excessive alcohol consumption
Formula- or mixed-fed infants
Genetic disorder; heritability of interrelated factors (e.g., adipose tissue distribution, energy expenditure, lipid synthesis, lipolysis)
Higher baseline weight at beginning of each pregnancy; maternal diabetes, maternal smoking
Low dietary calcium intake in children
Rapid weight gain during infancy, including first week, first 4 months, and first year; solid foods as major food source at <5 months of age
Rapid weight gain in childhood; obesity in childhood; premature pubarche; parental obesity
Shortened sleep time; sleep disorder
Note: A risk diagnosis is not evidenced by signs and symptoms, as the problem has not occurred; rather, nursing interventions are directed at prevention.
Sample Clinical Applications: Bulimia nervosa, diseases requiring long-term steroid use (e.g., chronic obstructive pulmonary disease [COPD]), conditions associated with immobility (e.g., stroke, paralysis, multiple sclerosis [MS], amputation), Alzheimer's disease, depression, developmental delay

DESIRED OUTCOMES/EVALUATION CRITERIA

Sample NOC linkages:
Weight Maintenance Behavior: Personal actions to maintain optimum body weight
Knowledge: Diet: Extent of understanding conveyed about recommended diet
Nutritional Status: Nutrient Intake: Nutrient intake to meet metabolic needs

Client/Caregiver Will (Include Specific Time Frame)

- Verbalize understanding of body and energy needs.
- Identify lifestyle and cultural factors that predispose to obesity.
- Demonstrate behaviors and lifestyle changes to reduce risk factors.
- Acknowledge responsibility for own actions and need to "act, not react" to stressful situations.

(continues on page 588)

risk for Overweight (continued)

Sample NOC linkages:

Weight: Body Mass: Extent to which body weight, muscle, and fat are congruent to height, frame, gender, and age

Client Will (Include Specific Time Frame)

- Maintain weight at a satisfactory level for height, body build, age, and gender.

ACTIONS/INTERVENTIONS

Sample NIC linkages:

Weight Management: Facilitating maintenance of optimal body weight and percent body fat
Nutritional Counseling: Use of an interactive helping process focusing on the need for diet modification
Nutrition Management: Assisting with or providing a balanced dietary intake of foods and fluids

NURSING PRIORITY NO. 1 To assess potential factors for undesired weight gain:

- Note presence of factors or conditions that can contribute to weight gain or obesity (e.g., familial pattern of obesity; hypothyroidism; type 2 diabetes; pregnancy; menopause; chronic disorders [e.g., heart, kidney disease, chronic pain]; food, alcohol/other substance addictions; stressful and/or sedentary lifestyle; depression; use of certain medications [e.g., steroids, birth control pills, antipsychotics]; physical disabilities or limitations; lack of socioeconomic resources for obtaining or preparing healthy foods) *to determine treatment needs and possible behavioral changes for weight management.*[1]
- Note client's particular situation and number/seriousness of risk factors *to help determine level of concern. For example, a high correlation exists between obesity in parents and children, which may reflect (in part) family patterns of food intake, exercise, selection of leisure activity (e.g., amount of television watching), family and cultural patterns of food selection. Also, family studies (e.g., twin and adoption) suggest genetic factors.*[2,3]
- Evaluate familial and cultural influences *that often place high importance on food and food-related events or groups that place importance on large body size or frame of reference for "normal body weight" is higher than standard indicators (e.g., athletes such as football players or wrestlers).*[2–4]
- Note client's age and activity level and exercise patterns *to identify areas where changes might be useful to prevent obesity and promote health. For example, older adults need same nutrients as younger adults but in smaller amounts and with attention to certain components, such as calcium, fiber, vitamins, protein, and water.*[5] *Infants/children require small meals and constant attention to needed nutrients for proper growth and development while dealing with child's food preferences and eating habits.*[6]
- Calculate growth percentiles in infants/children using growth chart specific to child's age and gender or BMI-for-age calculator if child is greater than 2 years old *to identify deviations from the norm.*[2,7]
- Review laboratory test results (e.g., complete blood count with differential, full lipid panel, fasting glucose, A_1C, insulin levels; thyroid, leptins; proteins, Mini-Nutritional Assessment) *that may reveal medical conditions associated with obesity and identify problems that may be treated with alterations in diet or medications.*[8–10]
- Assess eating patterns in relation to risk for obesity and disease conditions. *Food choices and amounts of certain food groups are known to impact health (in both children and adults) and cause or exacerbate disease conditions (e.g., heart disease, diabetes, hypertension, gallstones, colon cancer).*[1,11]
- Determine patterns of hunger and satiety. *Eating patterns often differ in those who are predisposed to weight gain and may include such factors as skipping meals (decreases the metabolic rate), fasting and binging (causes wide fluctuations in glucose and insulin), and eating or overeating in response to emotions (e.g., loneliness, anger, happiness).*
- Note history of dieting and kinds of diets used. *Client may have tried multiple diets with varying degrees of success in the past, but often has history of regaining weight ("yo-yo" dieting) or finding that diets are not desirable.*

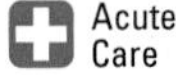

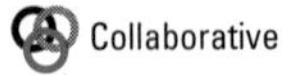

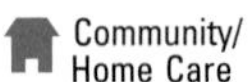

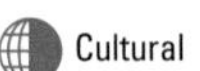

- Determine whether binging or purging (bulimia) is a factor *to identify potential for eating disorder requiring in-depth intervention.*
- Identify personality characteristics (e.g., rigid thinking patterns, external locus of control, negative body image or self-concept, negative monologues [self-talk], dissatisfaction with life) *that are often associated with obesity and can impact choice and/or success of interventions.*
- Determine psychological significance of food to the client (e.g., derives love and comfort from food, uses food to escape deep unhappiness, eats when stressed or anxious).
- Listen to concerns and assess motivation to prevent weight gain. *If client's concerns regarding weight control are motivated for reasons other than personal well-being (e.g., partner's expectations or demands), the likelihood of success is decreased.*

NURSING PRIORITY NO. 2 To assist client to develop preventive program to avoid weight gain:

- Assess client's knowledge of nutritional needs and ways client is meeting these needs. *Provides baseline for further teaching and/or interventions.*
- Provide information, as indicated, on nutrition, taking into account client's age and developmental stage (e.g., toddler, teenager, pregnant woman, elderly person with chronic disease), physical health and activity tolerance, financial and socioeconomic factors, and client's/significant other's (SO's) potential for management of risk factors.
- Review and encourage client/caregiver to implement guidelines for achieving and maintaining healthy body weight:[2,12]

  Eat from each food group (fruits, vegetables, whole grains, lean meats, low-fat dairy, oils).

  Start with small changes, such as adding one more vegetable/day or introducing healthier versions of favorite foods.

  Choose "nutrient-dense" forms of foods that provide substantial amounts of fiber, vitamins, electrolytes, and minerals.

  Avoid saturated fats, trans fats, cholesterol, salt (sodium), and added sugars.

  Focus on portion sizes: calorie-dense foods (high in fat and/or sugar) should be eaten in smaller quantities, whereas high-fiber foods can be eaten in larger quantities.

  Discuss smart snacks (e.g., low-fat yogurt with fruit, nuts, apple slices with peanut butter, low-fat string cheese).

  Review healthy eating patterns or habits (e.g., eating slowly and only when hungry, stopping when full, avoiding skipping meals, eating foods from every food group, using smaller plates, chewing food thoroughly, making healthy food choices even when eating fast food).

  Encourage involvement in planned exercises of client's choice and within physical abilities. Refer to formal exercise program, if desired.

NURSING PRIORITY NO. 3 To promote wellness (Teaching/Discharge Considerations):

- Provide information about individual risk factors *to enhance decision making and support motivation.*
- Consult with nutritionist *to address client-specific issues (e.g., how to use food groups, how to read food labels and apply to self, how to help child avoid junk food, dietary restrictions that might be needed for certain chronic diseases such as kidney disease or diabetes).*
- Provide information to new mothers about nutrition for developing babies *to reduce potential for childhood obesity related to lack of knowledge.*
- Encourage parents and school dietitians to model and offer good nutritional choices (e.g., offer vegetables, fruits, and lower-fat foods in daily meals and snacks) *to assist child in accepting healthy food styles.*[2,12]
- Encourage the client to make a commitment to lead an active life, to manage food habits, and to develop a system for self-monitoring *to provide a sense of control and assist with making choices.*
- Provide bibliography including reliable Internet sites for resources *to reinforce learning, address ongoing nutrition needs, support informed decision making.*

- Refer to support groups and appropriate community resources for such things as food-buying assistance, cooking and food safety courses, and behavior modification as indicated. *Provides role models and assistance for making lifestyle changes.*

DOCUMENTATION FOCUS

Assessment/Reassessment

- Findings related to individual situation, risk factors, current caloric intake and dietary pattern; activity level.
- Baseline height and weight, growth percentile.
- Results of laboratory tests.
- Motivation to reduce risks or prevent weight problems.

Planning

- Plan of care and who is involved in the planning.
- Teaching plan.

Implementation/Evaluation

- Response to interventions, teaching, and actions performed.
- Attainment or progress toward desired outcome(s).
- Modifications to plan of care.

Discharge Planning

- Long-term needs, noting who is responsible for actions to be taken.
- Specific referrals made.

References

1. Galletta, G. M. (2014). Obesity. Retrieved January 2015 from http://www.emedicinehealth.com/obesity/page9_em.htm#surgery_for_obesity.
2. Schwarz, S. M. (2012, updated 2014). Obesity in children. Retrieved January 2015 from http://emedicine.medscape.com/article/985333-overview.
3. Purnell, L. D., Paulanka, B. J. (1998). *Transcultural Health Care: A Culturally Competent Approach.* Philadelphia: F. A. Davis.
4. Caprio, S., Daniels, S. R., Drewnowski, A., et al. (2008). Influence of race, ethnicity, and culture on childhood obesity: Implications for prevention and treatment: A consensus statement of Shaping America's Health and the Obesity Society. *Diabetes Care*, 31(11), 2211–2221.
5. American Dietetic Association. (2005). Nutrition across the spectrum of aging. *J Am Diet Assoc*, 105(4), 616s–633s.
6. Engel, J. (2006). *Mosby's Pocket Guide to Pediatric Assessment, 5th ed.* St. Louis, MO: Mosby.
7. Centers for Disease Control and Prevention. (2014). About BMI for children and teens. Retrieved January 2015 from http://www.cdc.gov/healthyweight/assessing/bmi/childrens_bmi/about_childrens_bmi.html.
8. American Medical Directors Association. (2001, updated 2010). Altered nutritional status in the long term care setting. Retrieved January 2015 from http://www.guideline.gov/content.aspx?id=15590.
9. Lab test: Insulin. (2014). Lab Tests Online. Retrieved January 2015 from http://labtestsonline.org/understanding/analytes/insulin/tab/test/.
10. Perry, B., Wang, Y. (2012). Appetite regulation and weight control: The role of gut hormones. *Nutr Diabetes*, 2(1), e26.
11. Laroche, H. H., Hofer, T. P., Davis, M. M. (2007). Adult fat intake associated with the presence of children in households: Findings from NHANES IIIs. *J Am Board Fam Med*, 20(1), 9–15.
12. 2010 Dietary Guidelines Advisory Committee. Dietary guidelines for Americans. Retrieved January 2015 from http://www.health.gov/dietaryguidelines/dga2010/DietaryGuidelines2010.pdf.

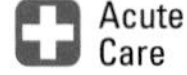
Acute Care
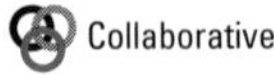
Collaborative
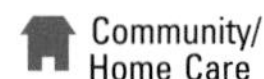
Community/ Home Care
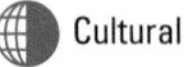
Cultural

acute Pain

Taxonomy II: Comfort—Class 1 Physical Comfort (00132) [**Diagnostic Division:** Pain/Discomfort], Submitted 1986; Revised 2013

DEFINITION: An unpleasant sensory and emotional experience associated with actual or potential tissue damage or described in terms of such damage (International Association for the Study of Pain); sudden or slow onset of any intensity, from mild to severe, with an anticipated or predictable end.

RELATED FACTORS

Biological injury agent (e.g., infection, ischemia, neoplasm)
Chemical injury agent (e.g., burn, capsaicin, methylene chloride, mustard agent)
Physical injury agent (e.g., abscess, amputation, burn, cut, heavy lifting, operative procedure, trauma, overtraining)

DEFINING CHARACTERISTICS

Subjective

Self-report of intensity using standardized pain scale (e.g., Wong-Baker FACES scale, visual analogue scale, numeric rating scale)
Self-report of pain characteristics using standardized pain instrument (e.g., McGill Pain Questionnaire, Brief Pain Inventory)
Appetite change; hopelessness
Proxy report of pain behavior activity changes (e.g., family member, caregiver)

Objective

Guarding behavior; protective behavior; positioning to ease pain
Facial expression of pain (e.g., eyes lack luster, beaten look, fixed or scattered movement, grimace)
Expressive behavior (e.g., restlessness, crying)
Distraction behavior
Diaphoresis; changes in physiological parameter (e.g., blood pressure, heart rate, respiratory rate, oxygen saturation, and end-tidal volume); pupil dilation
Self-focused; narrowed focus (e.g., time perception, thought process, interaction with people and environment)
Evidence of pain using standard pain behavior checklist for those unable to communicate verbally (e.g., Neonatal Infant Pain Scale, Pain Assessment Checklist for Seniors with Limited Ability to Communicate)
Sample Clinical Applications: Traumatic injuries, surgical procedures, infections, cancer, burns, skin lesions, gangrene, thrombophlebitis, pulmonary embolus, neuralgia

DESIRED OUTCOMES/EVALUATION CRITERIA

Sample NOC linkages:

Pain Level: Severity of observed or reported pain
Pain Control: Personal actions to control pain
Pain: Adverse Psychological Response: Severity of observed or reported adverse cognitive and emotional responses to physical pain

Client Will (Include Specific Time Frame)

- Report pain is relieved or controlled.
- Follow prescribed pharmacological regimen.
- Verbalize methods that provide relief.

(continues on page 592)

acute Pain (continued)
- Demonstrate use of relaxation skills and diversional activities as indicated for individual situation.
- Verbalize sense of control of response to acute situation and positive outlook for the future.

ACTIONS/INTERVENTIONS

Sample NIC linkages:
Pain Management: Alleviation of pain or a reduction in pain to a level of comfort that is acceptable to the patient
Analgesic Administration: Use of pharmacological agents to reduce or eliminate pain
Environmental Management: Comfort: Manipulation of the patient's surroundings for promotion of optimal comfort

NURSING PRIORITY NO. 1 To assess etiology/precipitating contributory factors:

- Note possible pathophysiological and psychological causes of pain (e.g., inflammation, tissue trauma, burns, fractures, surgery; infections, heart attack, angina; abdominal conditions [e.g., appendicitis, cholecystitis], grief, fear, anxiety, depression, personality disorders). *Acute pain is that which follows an injury, trauma, or procedure such as surgery or occurs suddenly with the onset of a painful condition (e.g., herniated disk, migraine headache, pancreatitis).*[11]
- Note client's age, developmental level, and current condition (e.g., infant/child; critically ill; ventilated, sedated, or cognitively impaired client) *affecting ability to report pain parameters.*[9,10]
- Determine history or presence of chronic conditions (e.g., multiple sclerosis, stroke, diabetes, depression) *that may also cause pain, be associated with an exacerbation of pain symptoms, or interfere with accurate assessment of acute pain.*[3]
- Note anatomical location of surgical incisions or procedures. *This can influence the amount of postoperative pain experienced; for example, vertical or diagonal incisions are more painful than transverse or S-shaped. Presence of known and unknown complication(s) may make the pain more severe than anticipated.*[2,3]
- Assess client's perceptions of pain, along with behaviors and cultural expectations regarding pain. *Client's perception of and expression of pain is influenced by age, developmental stage, underlying problem causing pain, cognitive, and behavioral and sociocultural factors.*[6]
- Note client's attitude toward pain and use of specific pain medications, including any history of substance abuse. *Client may have beliefs restricting use of medications, may have a high tolerance for drugs because of recent or current use, or may not be able to take pain medications at all if participating in a substance abuse recovery program.*
- Note client's locus of control (internal or external). *Individuals with external locus of control may take little or no responsibility for pain management.*
- Determine medications (e.g., skeletal muscle relaxants, antibiotics, antidepressants, anticoagulants), alcohol or other drugs currently being used, and any medication allergies *that may affect choice of analgesics.*[2,3]
- Collaborate with medical providers in pain assessment, including neurological and psychological factors (pain inventory, psychological interview) as appropriate when pain persists.
- Assist with and review results of laboratory tests and diagnostic studies depending on results of history and physical examination.

NURSING PRIORITY NO. 2 To evaluate client's response to pain:

- Obtain client's/ significant other's (SO's) assessment of pain to include location, characteristics, onset, duration, frequency, quality, and intensity. Identify precipitating or aggravating and relieving factors *in order to fully understand client's pain symptoms. Note: Experts agree that attempts should always be made to obtain self-reports of pain. When that is not possible, credible information can be received from another person who knows the client well (e.g., parent, spouse, caregiver).*[14] *Numerous studies have revealed that physicians and nurses need to be aware of their tendency to underestimate client's pain in early postoperative days.*[16]

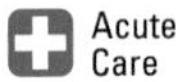 Acute Care 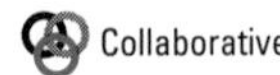 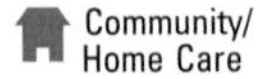 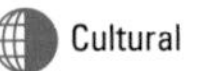

- Perform pain assessment each time pain occurs. Document and investigate changes from previous reports and evaluate results of pain interventions *to demonstrate improvement in status or to identify worsening of underlying condition/developing complications.*[4,12]
- Accept client's description of pain. Be aware of the terminology client uses for pain experience (e.g., young child may say "owie" or "hurt"; elderly may say "it aches so bad"). *Pain is a subjective experience and cannot be felt by others.*[3] *Note: Some elderly clients experience a reduction in perception of pain or have difficulty localizing or describing pain, and pain may be manifested as a change in behavior (e.g., restlessness, loss of appetite, increased confusion or wandering, acting out, change in functional abilities).*[15]
- Note cultural influences affecting pain response. *Verbal or behavioral cues may have no direct relationship to the degree of pain perceived (e.g., client may deny pain even when feeling uncomfortable, reactions can be stoic or exaggerated, reflecting cultural and familial norms). These factors affect client's and caregiver's attitudes and beliefs regarding the pain experience, expressions of pain, and expectations regarding pain management.*[6,10]
- Observe nonverbal cues (e.g., how client walks, holds body, guarding behaviors; sleeplessness; grimacing facial expressions; distraction behaviors, narrowed focus; crying, poor feeding, lethargy in infants). Ask others who know client well (e.g., spouse, parent) to identify behaviors that may indicate pain in persons who cannot communicate verbally. *Helpful in recognizing presence of pain; however, cues not congruent with verbal reports indicate need for further evaluation.*[1–4,6]
- Assess for referred pain, as appropriate, *to help determine possibility of underlying condition or organ dysfunction causing pain to be perceived in area other than site of the problem.*
- Monitor vital signs during episodes of pain. *Blood pressure, respiratory and heart rate are usually altered in acute pain.*[1–3]
- Ascertain client's knowledge of and expectations about pain management. *Provides baseline for interventions and teaching, provides opportunity to allay common fears and misconceptions (e.g., fears about addiction to opiates, belief that complete pain relief is possible in every situation) or to address expected side effects of analgesics (e.g., constipation).*
- Review client's previous experiences with pain and methods found either helpful or unhelpful for pain control in the past. *Useful in determining appropriate interventions.*
- Be aware of client's "Right to Treatment" *that includes prevention of or adequate relief from pain*[5] *and that failure to meet the standard of assessing for pain can be considered negligence. This means that the nurse is obligated to do everything within his/her professional capacity to relieve the pain when the client requests pain relief. Furthermore, professional standards require that nurses assess pain and reassess pain even when the client has not made a specific request.*[17]

NURSING PRIORITY NO. 3 To assist client to explore methods for alleviation/control of pain:

- Determine client's acceptable level of pain and pain control goal. *Client may not be 100% pain free but may feel that a "3" is a manageable level of discomfort, while another may require medication for pain at the same level because the experience is subjective.*[1–4,6]
- Determine factors in client's lifestyle (e.g., alcohol or other drug use or abuse) that can affect responses to analgesics and/or choice of interventions for pain management.[10]
- Note when pain occurs (e.g., only with ambulation, every night) *to medicate prophylactically as appropriate.*
- Collaborate in treatment of underlying condition or disease processes causing pain and proactive management of pain (e.g., epidural analgesia, nerve blockade for postoperative pain, surgical plication of a nerve, implantation of nerve stimulator).
- Work with client *to prevent rather than "chase" pain.* Use flow sheet to document pain, therapeutic interventions, response, and length of time before pain recurs. Instruct client to report pain as soon as it begins, *because timely intervention is more likely to be successful in alleviating pain.*[7]
- Encourage verbalization of feelings about the pain such as concern about tolerating pain, anxiety, and pessimistic thoughts *to evaluate coping abilities and to identify areas of additional concern.*[1,7]

- Review procedures and expectations and inform client when treatments will hurt. Discuss pain management methods that will be used *to reduce concerns of the unknown and muscle tension associated with anxiety or fear.*
- Use puppets or dolls for explanations and teaching, when indicated, *to demonstrate procedures for child and enhance understanding to reduce level of anxiety or fear.*
- Provide or promote nonpharmacological pain management, such as:
  a quiet environment and calm activities;
  comfort measures (e.g., back rub, change of position, use of heat or cold compresses);
  use of relaxation exercises (e.g., focused breathing, visualization, guided imagery);
  diversional or distraction activities, such as television and radio, socialization with others, and commercial or individualized tapes (e.g., "white" noise, music, instructional);
  presence of parent during painful procedures *to comfort child;*
  identification of ways to avoid or minimize pain *(e.g., splinting incision during cough, keeping body in good alignment and using proper body mechanics, and resting between activities can reduce occurrence of muscle tension or spasms or undue stress on incision).*
- Establish collaborative approach for pain management based on client's understanding about and acceptance of available treatment options. *Pharmacological management is based on client's symptomatology and mechanism of pain as well as tolerance for pain and for the various analgesics. Pain medications may include pills, liquids, or suckers to take by mouth, skin patch, or suppository forms and injections, IV dosing, or patient-controlled analgesia (PCA) or regional analgesia (e.g., epidural and spinal blocking).*[3,7,10,12]
- Administer analgesics to maximal dosage as needed *to maintain "acceptable" level of comfort. The type of medication(s) ordered depends on the type and severity of pain (e.g., acetaminophen and NSAIDs are commonly used to treat mild to moderate pain, while opiates [e.g., morphine, oxycodone, fentanyl] are used to treat moderate to severe pain). Note: Combinations of medications may be used at prescribed intervals.*[3,8]
- Notify physician/healthcare provider if regimen is inadequate to meet pain control goal. Assist client to prevent (rather than treat pain) and alter drug regimen based on individual needs. *Once established, pain is more difficult to suppress. Increasing dosage, changing medication, or using a stepped program (e.g., switching from injection to oral route, or lengthening time interval between doses) helps in self-management of pain.*[2,5]
- Evaluate and document client's response to analgesics and assist in transitioning or altering drug regimen based on individual needs and planned interventions *to limit adverse effects and barriers to adequate use of analgesics.*
- Evaluate for adverse medication effects (e.g., decrease in mental acuity, change in thought processes, confusion or delirium, urinary retention, severe nausea, vomiting, pruritus). *Intolerable symptoms that usually require change of medication(s).*[3,7,8]
- Demonstrate and monitor use of self-administration/PCA that involves client in plan *to administer own IV pain medication or bolus additional dose when on continual basis drip.*[3,7,8]
- Provide information and monitor use of site-specific medications (e.g., spinal, epidural, regional anesthesia) *that might be used for certain procedures such as back surgery, amputation, or labor and delivery.*[2,7,8]
- Instruct client in use of transcutaneous electrical stimulation unit when ordered.

NURSING PRIORITY NO. 4 To promote wellness (Teaching/Discharge Considerations):

- Acknowledge the pain experience and convey acceptance of client's response to pain. *Reduces defensive responses, promotes trust, and enhances cooperation with regimen.*
- Encourage adequate rest periods *to prevent fatigue that can impair ability to manage or cope with pain.*
- Review nonpharmacological measures for lessening pain. *Relaxation skills and techniques such as self-hypnosis, biofeedback, and therapeutic touch have no detrimental side effects.*
- Provide information and discuss pain management before planned procedures. *The primary concern of most clients/families is pain and discomfort following surgery or invasive procedure.*

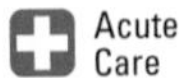

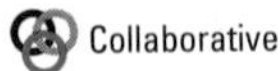

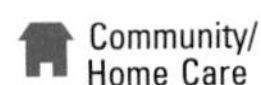

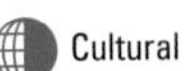

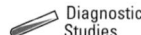

- Encourage performance of individualized physical therapy/exercise program. *Promotes active role in preventing muscle spasms or contractures and enhances sense of control.*
- Discuss ways SO(s) can assist client with pain management. *Family members/SOs may provide assistance by transporting client to prevent walking long distances or by taking on client's strenuous chores, supporting timely pain control, encouraging eating nutritious meals to enhance wellness, and providing gentle massage to reduce muscle tension.*
- Identify specific signs/symptoms and changes in pain requiring evaluation by healthcare provider.

DOCUMENTATION FOCUS

Assessment/Reassessment

- Individual assessment findings, including client's description of response to pain, specifics of pain inventory, expectations of pain management, and acceptable level of pain.
- Locus of control and cultural beliefs affecting response to pain.
- Prior medication use; substance abuse.

Planning

- Plan of care and who is involved in planning.
- Teaching plan.

Implementation/Evaluation

- Response to interventions, teaching, and actions performed.
- Attainment or progress toward desired outcome(s).
- Modifications to plan of care.

Discharge Planning

- Long-term needs, noting who is responsible for actions to be taken.
- Specific referrals made.

References

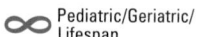

1. Engel, J. (2002). *Pocket Guide to Pediatric Assessment.* 4th ed. St. Louis, MO: Mosby.
2. Department of Defense, Veterans Health Administration. (Updated 2002). Clinical practice guideline for the management of postoperative pain (version 1.2). Washington, DC. Retrieved March 2015 from http://www.healthquality.va.gov/guidelines/Pain/pop/pop_fulltext.pdf.
3. Ameres, M. J., Yeh, B. (Reviewed 2014). Pain after surgery. Retrieved March 2015 from http://www.emedicinehealth.com/pain_after_surgery/page2_em.htm.
4. Smith, R., Curci, M., Silverman, A. (2002). Pain management: The global connection. *Nurs Manage*, 33(6), 26–29.
5. Agency for Health Care Policy and Research, Public Health Service, U.S. Department of Health and Human Services. (1992). Acute pain management: Operative or medical procedures and trauma: Clinical Practice Guideline. *Clin Pharm*, 11(5), 391–414.
6. Narayan, M. C. (2010). Culture's effects on pain assessment and management. *Am J Nurs*, 110(4), 38–48.
7. Institute for Clinical Systems Improvement. (Revised 2012). Low back pain: Adult acute and subacute. Retrieved March 2015 from https://www.icsi.org/guidelines__more/catalog_guidelines_and_more/catalog_guidelines/catalog_musculoskeletal_guidelines/low_back_pain/.
8. Cluett, J. (Updated 2014). Types of pain medicine. Retrieved March 2015 from http://orthopedics.about.com/od/medicati3/p/medications.htm.
9. Pasero, C., McCaffrey, M. (2005). No self-report means no pain-intensity rating. *Am J Nurs*, 105(10), 50–53.
10. Mann, A. R. (2006). Manage the power of pain. *Men in Nursing*, 1(4), 20–28.
11. D'Arcy, Y. (2007). Managing pain in a patient who's drug-dependent. *Nursing*, 37(3), 36–40.
12. Wheeler, M. S. (2006). Pain assessment and management in the patient with mild to moderate cognitive impairment. *Home Healthcare Nurse*, 24(6), 354–359.
13. Zwakhalen, S. M. G., Hamers, J. P. H., Abu-Saad, H. H., et al. (2006). Pain in elderly people with severe dementia: A systematic review of behavioural pain assessment tools. *BMC Geriatrics*, 6(3), 1–37.

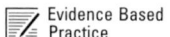

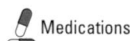

14. Herr, K., Coyne, P. J., Key, T., et al. (2006). Pain assessment in the nonverbal patient: Position statement with clinical practice recommendations. *Pain Manag Nurs*, 7(2), 44–52.
15. Kamel, H. K., Phlavan, M., Malekqoudarzi, B., et al. (2001). Utilizing pain assessment scales increases the frequency of diagnosing pain among elderly nursing home residents. *J Pain Symptom Manage*, 21(6), 450–455.
16. Rosenberger, P. H., Jokl, P., Cameron, A., et al. (2001). Shared decision making, preoperative expectations, and postoperative reality: Differences in physician and patient predictions and ratings of knee surgery outcomes. *Arthroscopy*, 21(5), 562–569.
17. O'Malley, P. (2005). The undertreatment of pain: Ethical and legal implications for the clinical nurse specialist. *Clin Nurs Spec*, 19(5), 236–237.

chronic Pain and chronic Pain Syndrome [CPS]

Taxonomy II: Comfort—Class 1 Physical Comfort (00133) [**Diagnostic Division:** Pain/Discomfort], Submitted 1986; Revised 1996, 2013

DEFINITION: chronic Pain: Unpleasant sensory and emotional experience arising from actual or potential tissue damage or described in terms of such damage (International Association for the Study of Pain); sudden or slow onset of any intensity, from mild to severe, constant or recurring without an anticipated or predictable end and a duration of greater than three (>3) months.

Taxonomy II: Comfort—Class 1 Physical Comfort (0000255) [**Diagnostic Division:** Pain/Discomfort], Submitted 2013

DEFINITION: chronic Pain Syndrome: Recurrent or persistent pain that has lasted at least three months, and that significantly affects daily functioning or well-being.
[Author Note: Pain is a signal that something is wrong. Chronic pain may be recurrent and periodically disabling (e.g., migraine headaches, kidney stones, prostatitis) or may be unremitting. It is a complex entity, combining elements from many other NDs, such as risk for Disuse Syndrome; deficient Diversional Activity; disturbed Body Image; compromised family Coping; interrupted Family Processes; Powerlessness; Self-Care Deficit (specify); sexual Dysfunction; Social Isolation]. The nurse is encouraged to refer to other NDs as indicated

RELATED FACTORS (chronic Pain)
[Author Note: A syndrome diagnosis does not have Related Factors.]
Age >50 years; female gender; genetic disorder
Alteration in sleep pattern
Anorexia; emotional distress; fatigue; prolonged increase in cortisol level; whole body vibration; chronic musculoskeletal condition; muscle injury; damage to the nervous system; imbalance of neurotransmitters, neuromodulators, and receptors; nerve compression; ischemic condition; spinal cord injury; tumor infiltration
Contusion; crush injury; fracture; injury agent; post-trauma related condition (e.g., infection, inflammation)
History of abuse (e.g., physical, psychological, sexual; history of genital mutilation; history of substance abuse
History of overindebtedness
History of static work postures; prolonged computer use (>20 hours/week); repeated handling of heavy loads
Immune disorder (e.g., HIV-associated neuropathy, varicella-zoster virus; impaired metabolic functioning)
Increase in body mass index; malnutrition
Ineffective sexuality pattern; social isolation

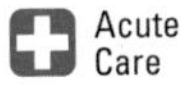

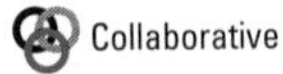

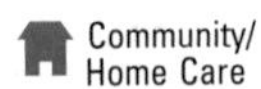

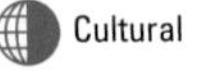

DEFINING CHARACTERISTICS

Subjective (chronic Pain)

Self-report of intensity using standardized pain scale (e.g., Wong-Baker FACES scale, visual analogue scale, numeric rating scale)
Self-report of pain characteristics using standardized pain instrument (e.g., McGill Pain Questionnaire, Brief Pain Inventory)
Alteration in ability to continue previous activities
Alteration in sleep pattern; anorexia
[Preoccupation with pain]
[Desperately seeks alternative solutions or therapies for relief or control of pain]

Subjective (chronic Pain Syndrome)

Anxiety, fear; stress overload
Constipation
Disturbed sleep pattern, fatigue; insomnia

Objective (chronic Pain)

Evidence of pain using standardized pain behavior checklist for those unable to communicate verbally (e.g., Neonatal Infant Pain Scale, Pain Assessment Checklist for Seniors with Limited Ability to Communicate)
Facial expression of pain (e.g., eyes lack luster, beaten look, fixed or scattered movement, grimace); self-focused
Proxy report of pain behavior/activity changes (e.g., family member, caregiver)

Objective (chronic Pain Syndrome)

Deficient knowledge
Impaired mood regulation; social isolation
Impaired physical mobility
Obesity
Sample Clinical Applications: Traumatic injuries, migraines, repetitive motion injury (carpal or cubital tunnel syndrome), osteoarthritis, rheumatoid arthritis; peripheral neuropathies in diabetes or AIDS, cancer, burns, endometriosis, neuralgia, gangrene

DESIRED OUTCOMES/EVALUATION CRITERIA

Sample NOC linkages:

Pain Control: Personal actions to control pain
Pain: Disruptive Effects: Severity of observed or reported disruptive effects of chronic pain on daily functioning
Pain: Adverse Psychological Response: Severity of observed or reported adverse cognitive and emotional responses to physical pain

Client Will (Include Specific Time Frame)

- Verbalize and demonstrate (nonverbal cues) relief or control of pain or discomfort.
- Verbalize recognition of interpersonal and family dynamics, and reactions that affect the pain problem.
- Demonstrate or initiate behavioral modifications of lifestyle and appropriate use of therapeutic interventions.
- Verbalize increased sense of control and enhanced enjoyment of life.

Sample NOC linkage:

- **Family Coping:** Family actions to manage stressors that tax family resources

Family/SO(s) Will (Include Specific Time Frame)

- Cooperate in pain management and rehabilitation programs. (Refer to ND readiness for enhanced family Coping.)

(continues on page 598)

chronic Pain and chronic Pain Syndrome [CPS] (continued)
ACTIONS/INTERVENTIONS

Sample NIC linkages:
Pain Management: Alleviation of pain or a reduction in pain to a level of comfort that is acceptable to the patient
Medication Management: Facilitation of safe and effective use of prescription and over-the-counter drugs
Relaxation Therapy: Use of techniques to encourage and elicit relaxation for the purpose of decreasing undesirable signs and symptoms such as pain, muscle tension, or anxiety

NURSING PRIORITY NO. 1 To assess etiology/precipitating factors:

- Identify contributing physical factors where known. *These factors associated with chronic pain and CPS appear to include (1) musculoskeletal disorders such as osteoarthritis, rheumatoid arthritis, and fibromyalgia; (2) back pain from various causes such as disc herniation, vertebral fractures, muscular strains/sprains, overuse syndromes such as tendonitis, and bursitis, as well as pelvic disorders; (3) neurological disorders, such as spinal/other conditions causing nerve impingement, and radiculopathies and neuropathies with direct or referred pain; (4) urologic disorders such as bladder neoplasms, chronic urinary tract infections or stones, testicular torsion, prostatitis; (5) gastrointestinal disorders such as colitis, gastroesophageal reflux, inflammatory bowel disease, and pancreatitis; (6) reproductive/gynecological disorders including endometriosis, disorders of ovaries, prolapse, intrauterine contraceptive devices, etc.; and (7) miscellaneous/other causes including cardiovascular disease, peripheral vascular disease, and complications of medical treatments such as chemotherapy, radiation, or surgery.*[2,8]
- Evaluate for presence of/suspected psychological disorders. *Psychological factors may include (but are not limited to) depression, anxiety, somatization, and bipolar personality disorders. Testing may be indicated if organic cause of pain cannot be found, when psychological factors are known to exist, or when pain problems are prolonged and/or life-limiting.*[12]
- Assist in and/or review diagnostic testing, including physical (e.g., selected tests for identifying and/or monitoring suspected for known disease states; urine or blood toxicology for drug detoxification or therapy; imaging studies), neurological, and psychological evaluations (e.g., Minnesota Multiphasic Personality Inventory, pain inventory, psychological interview). *Note: While additional diagnostic studies may be indicated when advanced treatment of the client with CPS is initiated, care should be exercised in avoiding duplication of tests. This prevents unnecessary costs, as well as inadvertent reinforcement of client's psychological need for "something to be physically wrong."*[2]
- Evaluate emotional/psychological components of individual situation. *Individuals with certain psychological syndromes (e.g., major depression, somatization disorder, hypochondriasis) are prone to develop CPS. Note: Research suggests that 35% to 50% of people with chronic pain have depression.*[2,6,12]
- Determine if client has history of physical or sexual abuse as a child. *A review of the literature shows that abuse in childhood is a strong predictor of depression and physical complaints, both expanded and unexplained, in adulthood.*[13]
- Evaluate client's pattern of coping and locus of control (internal or external). *Passive and avoidant behavioral patterns or lack of active engagement in self-management activities can contribute to diminished activity and perpetuation of chronic pain. Individuals with external locus of control may take little or no responsibility for pain management.*[13]
- Determine relevant cultural and spirituality factors affecting pain response. *Pain is accepted and expressed in different ways (e.g., moaning aloud or enduring in stoic silence); some may magnify symptoms to convince others of reality of pain or believe that suffering in silence helps atone for past wrongdoing.*[3] *A person with chronic pain who identifies himself or herself as a spiritual being may report the link to divine help as empowering him/her to use strategies for healing.*[14]
- Note gender and age of client. *There may be differences between women and men as to how they perceive and/or respond to pain. Pain in children, ethnic minorities, or cognitively impaired persons is often*

Acute Care 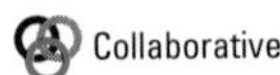 Collaborative 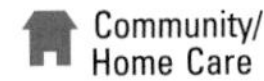 Community/ Home Care 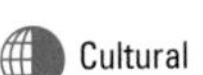 Cultural

underestimated and undertreated. Recent studies are revealing large numbers of pediatric clients with chronic pain issues affecting academic attendance and function.[11] *While the prevalence of chronically painful conditions (e.g., arthritis) and illnesses (e.g., cancers) is common in the elderly, they may be reluctant to report pain.*[4]
- Evaluate current and past analgesic or narcotic drug use and nonprescription drug use (including alcohol). *Provides clues to options to try or avoid and identifies need for changes in medication regimen, as well as possible need for detoxification program.*

NURSING PRIORITY NO. 2 To determine client response to chronic pain situation:

- Evaluate pain behavior, noting past and current pain experience, using pain rating scale or diary, and including functional effects and psychological factors. *Pain behaviors can include the same ones present in acute pain (e.g., crying, grimacing, withdrawal, narrowed focus), but may also include other behaviors (e.g., dramatization of complaints, depression, drug misuse). Pain complaints may be exaggerated because of client's perception that pain reports are not believed or because client believes caregivers are discounting reports of pain.*[12]
- Provide comprehensive assessment of pain problem, noting its duration, who has been consulted, and what therapies (including alternative/complementary) have been used. *The pathophysiology of chronic pain is multifactorial. If the condition causing the persistent pain is physiological and noncurable (e.g., terminal cancer), all diagnostics and treatments may have been exhausted and pain management becomes the primary goal. If medical treatments are ongoing for painful conditions (e.g., spinal stenosis, pancreatitis, endometriosis, arthritis), consultations with specialists may be helpful in finding curative or palliative treatments. If pain is present without a clear etiology or continues unabated, complex rehabilitation techniques may be required, incorporating physical, occupational, psychological, and recreational therapies.*[1,2,12]
- Note lifestyle effects of pain. *Major effects of chronic pain on the client's life can include depressed mood, fatigue, weight loss or gain, sleep disturbances, reduced activity and libido, excessive use of drugs and alcohol, dependent behavior, and disability seemingly out of proportion to impairment.*[2,4,12]
- Assess degree of personal maladjustment of the client such as isolationism, anger, irritability, loss of work time or employment, and school absenteeism. *Chronic pain reduces client's coping abilities and psychological well-being, often resulting in problems with relationships and life functioning.*[11,12]
- Determine issues of secondary gain for the client/SO(s), such as financial or insurance compensation pending, legal or marital or family concerns, and school or work issues, *which may be present if there is marked discrepancy between claimed distress and objective findings or there is a lack of cooperation during evaluation and in complying with prescribed treatment.*[5]
- Note codependent components and enabling behaviors of caregivers/family members *that support continuation of the status quo and may interfere with progress in pain management or resolution of situation.*
- Note availability and use of personal and community resources. *Client/SO may need many things (e.g., equipment, financial resources, vocational training, respite services, placement in rehabilitation facility) in order to manage painful conditions and/or concerns or difficulties associated with condition.*
- Make home visit when indicated, observing such factors as client's safety, equipment, adequate lighting, or family interactions, *to note impact of home environment on the client and to determine changes that might be useful in improving client's life (e.g., grab bars in bathrooms and hallways, wider doors, ramps, assistance with activities of daily living, housekeeping, yard work).*
- Acknowledge and assess pain matter-of-factly, avoiding undue expressions of concern, as well as expressions of disbelief about client's suffering. *Conveying an attitude of empathic understanding of client's disabling distress can have a beneficial impact on client's perception of health.*

NURSING PRIORITY NO. 3 To assist client to deal with pain:

- Encourage participation in multidisciplinary pain management plan. *Comprehensive team may include physical medicine specialist; physical, occupational, recreational, and vocational therapists; and emotional or behavioral therapists to address complex issues of unresolved pain issues, to set goals for pain relief, and to develop an individualized treatment and evaluation plan. Treatments could involve extended-relief oral pain medications or dermal patches, nerve-blocking injections or an implanted pump, and massage and other hands-on therapies, as well as counseling and home exercise programs.*[8]

- Discuss pain management goals and review client expectations versus reality *because it may be that while pain cannot be completely resolved, it can be significantly reduced or managed to the degree that client can participate in desired or needed life activities, thus improving quality of life.*[8]
- Discuss the physiological dynamics of tension and anxiety and how this affects pain.
- Administer or encourage client use of analgesics, as indicated. *Medications may be available in pills, liquids, or suckers to take by mouth, and in injection, skin patch, and suppository forms. Different medications or combinations of drugs may be used such as opioids/narcotics, nonopioids, and adjuvant medications (e.g., muscle relaxants, anticonvulsants, antidepressants, serotonin and norepinephrine reuptake inhibitors) to manage persistent pain so that client may find relief and increase level of function.*[2,8,12] *Note: Studies support that people with intense pain can take very high doses of opioids without experiencing side effects. "Some people with intense pain receive such high doses that the same dose would be fatal if taken by someone who was not suffering from pain. In chronic pain that same high dose can control pain and still allow the person to be wide awake enough to do his or her activities of daily living."*[1]
- Provide consistent and sufficient medication for pain relief, tailored to the individual, especially in those who tend to be undermedicated (e.g., elderly, cognitively impaired, person with lifelong pain, those with terminal cancer). *Medications may need to be scheduled around the clock (not just administered "as needed"), doses titrated either up or down, and dose maximized to optimize pain relief while managing side effects.*[7]
- Recommend or employ nonpharmacological interventions, methods of pain control (e.g., heat or cold applications, progressive muscle relaxation, biofeedback, deep breathing, meditation, visualization or guided imagery, posture correction and muscle strengthening exercises, water therapy, electrical stimulation, massage, acupuncture, therapeutic touch) *to obtain comfort, improve healing, and decrease dependency on analgesics.*[9]
- Address medication misuse with client/SO and refer for appropriate counseling or interventions *when addiction is known or suspected to be interfering with client's well-being. Most people (if they don't already have a substance [drug or alcohol] abuse problem) don't become addicted to pain medications even when used on a long-term basis. These individuals will take the pain medications in order to go about the business of their lives. Addicts may misrepresent their pain levels and their activities in order to obtain pain medications or progressively higher doses of medications, and they require specialized evaluation and interventions.*[1,2,5]
- Assist family in developing a program of coping strategies (e.g., staying active even when modified activities are required, living a healthy lifestyle). *Positive reinforcement and encouraging client to use own control can aid in focusing energies on more productive activities.*[10]
- Encourage limiting attention to pain behaviors when appropriate (e.g., discussing pain for only a specified time; acknowledging "I'm sorry your pain returned today, but you need to go to school"; actively practicing relaxation or coping skills). *Reduces focus on pain, especially if client is highly dependent on pain for secondary gain issues or is addicted to medications.*[6]
- Encourage client to use positive affirmations (e.g., "I am healing," "I am relaxed," "I love this life"). Have client be aware of internal-external dialogue. Say "cancel" when negative thoughts develop. *Negative thinking can exacerbate feelings of hopelessness, and replacing those thoughts with positive ones can be helpful to pain management.*
- Encourage right-brain stimulation with activities such as love, laughter, and music. *These actions can release endorphins, enhancing sense of well-being.*
- Encourage use of subliminal tapes *to bypass logical part of the brain by reinforcing "I am becoming a more relaxed person" and "It is all right for me to relax."*

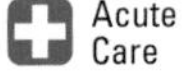

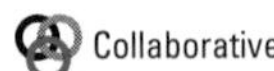

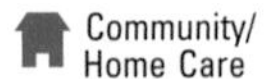

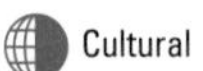

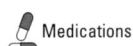

- Use tranquilizers, narcotics, and analgesics sparingly. *These drugs are physically and psychologically addicting and promote sleep disturbances, especially interference with deep rapid eye movement sleep. Client may need to be detoxified if many medications are currently used.*
- Be alert to changes in pain characteristics*that may indicate a new physical problem or developing complication.*

NURSING PRIORITY NO. 4 To promote wellness (Teaching/Discharge Considerations):

- Provide anticipatory guidance to client with condition in which pain is common and educate about when, where, and how to seek intervention or treatments.
- Discuss potential for developmental delays in child with chronic pain. Identify current level of function and review appropriate expectations for individual child.
- Instruct client/SO in medication administration, including use of patient-controlled analgesia pumps, as indicated. Review safe use of analgesics, including side effects requiring home management (e.g., constipation) or adverse effects requiring medical intervention (e.g., possible drug reactions). *Appropriate instruction in home management increases the accuracy and safety of medication administration.*
- Encourage and assist family member/SO(s) to learn home-care interventions. *Massage and other nonpharmacological pain management techniques benefit the client through reduction of pain level and sense that client is not alone/has support of SO.*
- Incorporate desired folk healthcare practices and beliefs into regimen whenever possible. *Has been shown to increase compliance with pain management treatment plan.*[12]
- Identify and discuss potential hazards of unproved or nonmedical therapies or remedies.
- Assist client and SO(s) to learn how to heal *by developing sense of internal control, by being responsible for own treatment, and by obtaining the information and tools to accomplish this.*
- Recommend that client and SO(s) take time for themselves. *Provides opportunity to reenergize and refocus on living/tasks at hand.*
- Address client's preferences and wishes for incurable pain or end-of-life pain management via advance directives *in order to assist family/SO in attending to client's needs.*[7]
- Identify community support groups and resources to meet individual needs (e.g., yard care, home maintenance, transportation). *Proper use of resources may reduce negative pattern of "overdoing" heavy activities and then spending several days in bed recuperating.*
- Refer for counseling (e.g., individual, family, marital therapy, parent effectiveness classes) as needed. *Presence of chronic pain affects all relationships and family dynamics.*
- Refer to NDs compromised family Coping and ineffective Coping.

DOCUMENTATION FOCUS

Assessment/Reassessment

- Individual findings, including duration of problem, specific contributing factors, previously and currently used interventions.
- Perception of pain, effects on lifestyle, and expectations of therapeutic regimen.
- Locus of control and cultural beliefs affecting response to pain.
- Family's/SO's response to client and support for change.
- Availability and use of resources.

Planning

- Plan of care and who is involved in planning.
- Teaching plan.

Implementation/Evaluation

- Responses to interventions, teaching, and actions performed.
- Attainment or progress toward desired outcome(s).
- Modifications to plan of care.

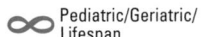

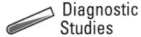

Discharge Planning

- Long-term needs and who is responsible for actions to be taken.
- Specific referrals made.

References

1. Stoppler, M. C. (Updated 2014). Chronic pain. Retrieved November 2015 from http://www.emedicinehealth.com/chronic_pain/page10_em.htm.
2. Singh, M. K., Patel, J., Gallagher, R. M. (2012, updated 2014). Chronic pain syndrome. Retrieved November 2014 from http://emedicine.medscape.com/article/310834-overview.
3. Narayan, M. C. (2010). Culture's effects on pain assessment and management. *Am J Nurs*, 110(4), 38–48.
4. AGS Panel on Persistent Pain in Older Persons. The management of persistent pain in older persons. (2002). *J Am Geriatr Soc*, 50(6 suppl), S205–S224.
5. Bienenfeld, D. (2010, updated 2013). Malingering. Retrieved January 2015 from http://emedicine.medscape.com/article/293206-overview.
6. Spratt, E. G., Ibeziako, P. I., DeMaso, D. (2012, updated 2014). Somatoform disorder. Retrieved January 2015 from http://emedicine.medscape.com/article/918628-overview.
7. American Medical Directors Association. (2009, updated 2012). Pain management in the long-term care setting. Retrieved January 2015 from http://www.guideline.gov/content.aspx?id=45524.
8. D'Arcy, Y. (2005). Conquering PAIN: Have you tried these new techniques? *Nursing*, 35(3), 36–41.
9. Lark, S. (2005). The 21-day arthritis and pain miracle. Lark Letter: A Woman's Guide to Optimal Health and Balance, Special Report.
10. Warms, C. A., Marshal, J. M., Hoffman, A. J. (2006). There are a few things you did not ask about my pain: Writing in the margins of a survey questionnaire. *Rehabil Nurs*, 30(6), 248–256.
11. Parkins, J. M., Gfrorer, S. D. (2009). Chronic pain: The impact on academic, social, and emotional functioning. *National Association of School Psychologists: Communique*, 38(1), 24–25.
12. Institutes for Clinical Systems Improvement. (2009, updated 2013). Assessment and management of chronic pain. Retrieved January 2015 from https://www.icsi.org/_asset/bw798b/ChronicPain.pdf.
13. Arnow, B. A. (2004). Relationships between childhood maltreatment, adult health and psychiatric outcomes, and medical utilization. *J Clin Psychiatry*, 65(12 Suppl), s10–s15.
14. Bordreaux, E. D., O'Hea, E., Chasuk, R. (2002). Spiritual role in healing, an alternative way of thinking. *Prim Care Clin Office Pract*, 29(2), 439–454.

labor Pain

Taxonomy II: Comfort—Class 1 Physical Comfort (00256) [**Diagnostic Division:** Pain/Discomfort], Submitted: 2013

DEFINITION: Sensory and emotional experience that varies from pleasant to unpleasant, associated with labor and childbirth.

RELATED FACTORS

Cervical dilation
Fetal expulsion

DEFINING CHARACTERISTICS

Subjective

Pain; unterine contraction; perineal pressure
Increase or decrease in appetite; nausea; vomiting
Alteration in urinary functioning, sleep pattern

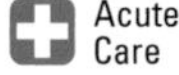

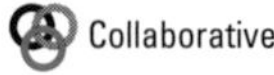

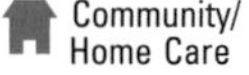

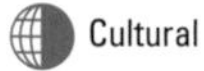

Objective

Alteration in blood pressure/heart rate/respiratory rate
Distraction/expressive behavior; protective behavior; positioning to ease pain
Alteration in muscle tension; diaphoresis
Alteration in neuroendocrine functioning
Narrowed focus; self-focused; pupil dilation
Facial expression of pain (e.g., eyes lack luster, beaten look, fixed or scattered movement, grimace)

DESIRED OUTCOMES/EVALUATION CRITERIA

Sample NOC linkages:

Pain Control: Personal actions to control pain
Client Satisfaction: Pain Management: Extent of positive perception of nursing care to relieve pain

Client Will (Include Specific Time Frame)

- Participate in decision making for pain management plan to include personal preferences and cultural beliefs.
- Engage in nonpharmacological measures to reduce discomfort/pain.
- Report pain at manageable level.

Partner Will (Include Specific Time Frame)
Participate in labor process, providing client's desired level of support.

ACTIONS/INTERVENTIONS

Sample NIC linkages:

Intrapartal Care: Monitoring and management of stages one and two of the birth process
Analgesic Administration: Intraspinal: Administration of pharmacologic agents into the epidural or intrathecal space to reduce or eliminate pain

NURSING PRIORITY NO. 1 To determine client's individual needs:

- Assess stage of labor; perform vaginal exam, noting nature and amount of vaginal show, cervical dilation, effacement, fetal station, and fetal descent. *Choice and timing of medication is affected by degree of dilation and contractile pattern.*[11]
- Note timing of prenatal care and participation in childbirth education classes. *Economic, emotional, and cultural concerns can limit the mother's access or involvement in preparation for labor, increasing her need for information and support during the labor and delivery process.*[1] *Also, research suggests classes and prenatal preparation may help decrease client's perception of pain.*[2]
- Evaluate degree of discomfort through verbal and nonverbal cues; note cultural influences on pain response. *Attitudes and reactions to pain are individual and based on past experiences, understanding of physiological changes, and familial/cultural expectations.*[9,11]
- Ascertain presence of a birth plan, individual expectations, and cultural or religious beliefs affecting the labor and delivery process. *Birth plan provides information about client's childbirth preferences. Cultural influences may include how the laboring mother views pain management, as well as who attends the mother during the birth process (e.g., Hispanic and Asian women often prefer that their mothers be present, in Arab cultures the mother or sister of the baby's father may be preferred). If cultural/religious preferences are not elicited, clients may not have the ability to follow their traditional practices, negatively impacting the birthing experience.*[9,11,12]

- Determine availability and preparation of support person(s). *Presence of a supportive partner, family/friend, or a doula can provide emotional support and enhance level of comfort, reducing analgesia. A doula provides labor coaching and support throughout the birthing process to both the mother and her partner.*[1,6]

NURSING PRIORITY NO. 2 To engage client in nonpharmacological pain management techniques:

- Provide/encourage use of comfort measures (e.g., back/leg rubs, sacral pressure, back rest, mouth care, repositioning; cool, moist cloths to face and neck, hot compresses to perineum, abdomen; perineal care, linen changes). *Promotes relaxation and hygiene, enhancing feeling of well-being, and may reduce the need for analgesia or anesthesia. Position changes can also enhance circulation and reduce muscle tension.*[11]
- Assess client's desire for physical touch during contractions. *Touch may serve as a distraction, reduce anxiety, and provide encouragement, aiding in maintaining sense of control and reducing pain. Note: Remain respectful of client's preferences regarding touch.*[2]
- Coach use of appropriate breathing/relaxation techniques and abdominal effleurage based on stage of labor. *May block pain impulses within the cerebral cortex through conditioned responses and cutaneous stimulation and gives client a means of coping with and controlling the level of discomfort.*[11]
- Recommend client void every 1 to 2 hr. *Reduces bladder distention, which can increase discomfort and prolong labor.*[11]
- Review birth plan. Provide information about stage of labor and projected delivery, available analgesics, usual responses/side effects (client and fetal), and duration of analgesic effect in light of current situation. *Empowers client to make informed choice about means of pain control. Client may not be able to anticipate the degree of labor pain she will experience and may need to reevaluate her options as labor progresses. Note: Being able to move about and change positions at will can be important for some clients and impact their pain management choices.*[6,8]
- Assist with complementary therapies as indicated (e.g., acupressure/acupuncture, hypnosis, yoga). *Some clients and healthcare providers may prefer a trial of therapies theorized to stimulate/regulate contractions, reduce muscle tension, and mediate perception of pain before pursuing pharmacological interventions. For example, hypnosis may reduce fear, tension, and raise pain threshold, reducing need for analgesia. Research suggests acupressure may shorten labor time in addition to diminishing pain level.*[10] *Note: Differences in cultural and regional acceptance of these options as well as provider technique can impact the effectiveness of these interventions.*[1,2]
- Provide for a quiet environment that is adequately ventilated, dimly lit, and free of unnecessary personnel. Offer soothing music as appropriate. *Nondistracting environment provides optimal opportunity for rest and relaxation between contractions. Music may also reduce stress/anxiety, lift client's spirits, and decrease perception of pain.*[2]
- Discuss appropriateness/timing of hydrotherapy (shower, hot tub) as client desires. *Warm water during the first stage of labor stimulates the release of endorphins and relaxes muscles, enhancing circulation and tissue oxygenation with reduction in use of analgesia.*[1–3]
- Offer encouragement, provide information about labor progress, and provide positive reinforcement for client's/couple's efforts. *Provides emotional support, which can reduce fear, lower anxiety levels, and help minimize pain.*[11]

NURSING PRIORITY NO. 3 To provide more intensive pain management measures:

- Time and record the frequency, intensity, and duration of uterine contractile pattern per protocol. *Information necessary for choosing appropriate interventions and preventing or limiting undesired side effects of medication.*[11]
- Review birth plan, provide positive feedback for efforts to date, and be supportive of client's decisions regarding pain management. *Each labor and delivery experience is different and can challenge prenatal expectations. Changes in stated pain management preferences (e.g., unmedicated to medicated birth) can lead to client feeling disappointed or a failure at a life process. Acceptance and support from the nurse can enhance coping and promote a more positive birth experience.*[7]

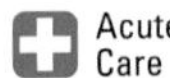

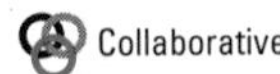

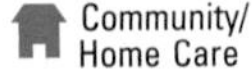

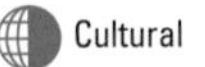

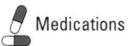

- Administer analgesic, such as butorphanol tartrate (Stadol) or meperidine hydrochloride (Demerol), by IV during contractions or deep intramuscular (IM) if indicated during active phase of stage I labor. *IV route provides more rapid and equal absorption of analgesic, and IM route may require up to 45 min to reach adequate plasma levels. Patient-controlled IV remifentanil provides better analgesia and patient satisfaction during the first and second stages of labor than other opioids but can cause serious maternal side effects. Effectiveness of opioids may be limited with the primary affect being sedation. Note: Administering IV drug during uterine contraction decreases amount of medication that immediately reaches fetus.*[2,3,4]
- Monitor maternal vital signs and fetal heart rate (FHR) variability after drug administration. Note drug's effectiveness and the physiological response. *Narcotics can have a depressant effect on fetus, particularly when administered 2 to 3 hr before delivery.*[11]
- Provide safety measures (e.g., encourage client to move slowly, bed in low position, raise side rails) as indicated post medication administration. *Regional block anesthesia produces vasomotor paralysis, so sudden movement may precipitate hypotension and risk for fall.*[11]
- Assist with neuraxial anesthesia (i.e., epidural, spinal, combined spinal epidural, continuous epidural infusion, intermittent epidural bolus, client-controlled infusion epidural) using an indwelling catheter. *Research supports this method is the most effective in obtaining maternal pain relief once active labor is established. Note: Use of ultra-low-dose epidural is being promoted to achieve pain control without negative effect on client's ability to sense contractions and push effectively.*[2,5,11]
- Monitor FHR electronically and note decreased variability or bradycardia. *Decreased FHR variability is a common side effect of many anesthetics/analgesics. These side effects can begin 2 to 10 min after administration of anesthetic and may last for 5 to 10 min on occasion.*[11]
- Monitor level of block per protocol. *Migration of decreased sensation from belly button (dermatome T-10) to tip of breastbone (approximately T-6) increases risk of respiratory depression and profound hypotension.*[11]
- Turn client side to side periodically during continuous infusions. *Promotes even distribution of drug to prevent "one-sided" or unilateral block.*
- Inform client of onset of contractions as appropriate. *Client may "sleep" and/or encounter partial amnesia between contractions, impairing her ability to recognize contractions as they begin and her ability to initiate pain management techniques.*[11]
- Provide information about type of regional analgesia/anesthesia available at stage II specific to the delivery setting (e.g., local, pudendal block, lumbar epidural reinforcement, spinal block). *Although client is stressed, she still needs to be in control and make informed decisions regarding anesthesia.*

NURSING PRIORITY NO. 4 To support delivery process:

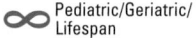

- Note perineal bulging or vaginal show. *Discomfort levels increase as cervix dilates, fetus descends, and small blood vessels rupture.*[11]
- Assist client in assuming optimal position for bearing down (e.g., squatting or lateral recumbent). *Proper positioning with relaxation of perineal tissue optimizes bearing-down efforts and facilitates labor progress, reducing discomfort.*[11]
- Assist with reinforcement of medication via indwelling lumbar epidural catheter when caput is visible. *Reduces discomfort associated with episiotomy, forceps application if needed, and fetal expulsion.*[11]
- Assist as needed with administration of local anesthetic just before episiotomy if performed. *Anesthetizes perineum tissue for incision/repair purposes.*[11]

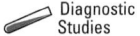

DOCUMENTATION FOCUS

Assessment/Reassessment

- Stages of labor, results of vaginal exam, status of fetus/fetal monitoring.
- Client's degree of preparation and expectations for labor process.
- Choice of support person(s).

Planning
- Specifics of birth plan.
- Plan of care and who is involved in planning.

Implementation/Evaluation
- Response to actions and interventions performed.
- Attainment or progress toward desired outcomes.

Discharge Planning
- Postpartal pain management choices.

References

1. Arendt, K. W., Tessmer-Tuck, J. A. (2013). Nonpharmacologic labor analgesia. *Clin Perinatol*, 40(3), 351–371.
2. Tournaire, M., Theau-Yonneau, A. (2007). Complementary and alternative approaches to pain relief during labor. *Evid Based Complement Alternat Med*, 4(4), 409–417.
3. Rooks, J. P. (2012). Labor pain management other than neuraxial: What do we know and where do we go next? *Birth*, 39(4), 318–322.
4. Tveit, T. O., Halvorsen, A., Seiler, S., et al. (2013). Efficacy and side effects of intravenous remifentanil patient-controlled analgesia used in a stepwise approach for labour: An observational study. *Int J Obstet Anesth*, 22(1), 19–25.
5. Gizzo, S., Noventa, M., Fagherazzi, S., et al. (2014). Update on best available options in obstetrics anaesthesia: Perinatal outcomes, side effects and maternal satisfaction. *Arch Gynecol Obstet*, 290(1), 21–34.
6. Hardin, A. M., Buckner, E. B. (2004). Characteristics of a positive experience for women who have unmedicated childbirth. *J Perinat Educ*, 13(4), 10–16.
7. Carlton, T., Callister, L. C., Stoneman, E. (2005). Decision making in laboring women: Ethical issues for perinatal nurses. *J Perinat Neonatal Nurs*, 19(2), 145–154.
8. Lally, J. E., Thomson, R. G., MacPhail, S., et al. (2014). Pain relief in labour: A qualitative study to determine how to support women to make decisions about pain relief in labour. *BMC Pregnancy and Childbirth*, 14(6). Retrieved April 2015 from http://www.biomedcentral.com/content/pdf/1471-2393-14-6.pdf.
9. Greene, M. J. (2007). Strategies for incorporating cultural competence into childbirth education curriculum. *J Perinat Educ*, 16(2), 33–37.
10. Akbarzadeh, M., Masoudi, Z., Hadianfard, M. J., et al. (2014). Comparison of the effects of maternal supportive care and acupressure (BL32 Acupoint) on pregnant women's pain intensity and delivery outcome. *J Pregnancy*. Retrieved April 2015 from http://dx.doi.org/10.1155/2014/129208.
11. Lowdermilk, D. L., Perry, S. E., Cashion, K. (2013). *Maternity Nursing*. 8th ed. Maryland Heights, MO: Mosby.
12. Ottani, P. A. (2002). When childbirth preparation isn't a cultural norm. *Int J Childbirth Educ*, 17(2), 12–16.

Acute Care

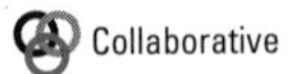

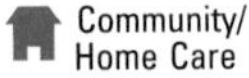

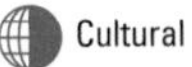

impaired Parenting

Taxonomy II: Role Relationships—Class 1 Caregiving Roles (00056) [**Diagnostic Division:** Social Interaction], Submitted 1998; Revised 1998

DEFINITION: Inability of the primary caretaker to create, maintain, or regain an environment that promotes the optimum growth and development of the child.

RELATED FACTORS

Infant or child
Prematurity; multiple births; gender other than desired
Chronic illness; parent-child separation
Difficult temperament; temperament conflicts with parental expectations
Disabling condition; developmental delay; alteration in perceptual abilities; behavior disorder (e.g., attention deficit, oppositional defiant)
Knowledge
Insufficient knowledge about child development or health maintenance, parenting skills
Insufficient response to infant cues
Unrealistic expectations
Low educational level; alteration in cognitive functioning; insufficient cognitive readiness for parenting
Ineffective communication skills
Preference for physical punishment
Physiological
Physical illness
Psychological
Young parental age
Insufficient prenatal care; difficult birthing process; high number of or closely spaced pregnancies
Alteration in sleep pattern; sleep deprivation; depression
History of mental illness or substance abuse
Disabling condition
Social
Stressors; work difficulty; unemployment; relocation; compromised home environment
Low self-esteem
Insufficient family cohesiveness; conflict between partners; change in family unit; inadequate child-care arrangements
Single parent; father or mother of child not involved
Insufficient parental role model; insufficient valuing of parenthood; inability to put child's needs before own
Unplanned or unwanted pregnancy
Economically disadvantaged; insufficient resources (e.g., financial, social, knowledge); insufficient transportation
Insufficient problem-solving skills; ineffective coping strategies
Insufficient social support; social isolation
History of abuse (e.g., physical, psychological, sexual), being abusive; legal difficulty

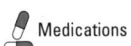

(continues on page 608)

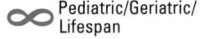

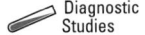

impaired Parenting (continued)
DEFINING CHARACTERISTICS

Subjective
Parental: Perceived inability to meet child's needs
Speaks negatively about child
Frustration with child; perceived role inadequacy

Objective
Infant or child
Frequent accidents or illness; failure to thrive
Low academic performance; delay in cognitive development
Impaired social functioning; behavior disorder (e.g., attention deficit, oppositional defiant)
History of trauma/abuse (e.g., physical, psychological, sexual)
Insufficient attachment behavior; diminished separation anxiety; runaway
Parental
Deficient parent-child interaction; decrease in cuddling
Inadequate child health maintenance; unsafe home environment; inappropriate child-care arrangements; inappropriate stimulation (e.g., visual, tactile, auditory)
Inappropriate care-taking skills; inconsistent care or behavior management
Inflexibility in meeting needs of child
Punitive; rejection of child; hostility; history of child abuse (e.g., physical, psychological, sexual); neglects needs of child; abandonment
Sample Clinical Applications: Prematurity, multiple births, genetic or congenital defects, chronic illness (parent/child), substance abuse, physical or psychological abuse, major depression, developmental delay, schizophrenia

DESIRED OUTCOMES/EVALUATION CRITERIA

Sample NOC linkages:
Knowledge: Parenting: Extent of understanding conveyed about provision of a nurturing and constructive environment for a child from 1 year through 17 years of age
Parenting Performance: Parental actions to provide a child with a nurturing and constructive physical, emotional, and social environment
Child Development: [specify age]: Milestones of physical, cognitive, and psychosocial progression by [specific age]

Parent Will (Include Specific Time Frame)
- Verbalize realistic information and expectations of parenting role.
- Verbalize acceptance of the individual situation.
- Participate in appropriate classes, such as a parenting class.
- Identify own strengths, individual needs, and methods or resources to meet them.
- Demonstrate appropriate parenting behaviors.

ACTIONS/INTERVENTIONS

Sample NIC linkages:
Parenting Promotion: Providing parenting information, support, and coordination of comprehensive services to high-risk families
Family Integrity Promotion: Childbearing Family: Facilitation of the growth of individuals or families who are adding an infant to the family unit
Developmental Enhancement: Child [or] Adolescent: Facilitating or teaching parents/caregivers to facilitate the optimal gross motor, fine motor, language, cognitive, social, and emotional growth of preschool and

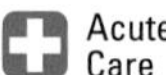

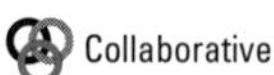

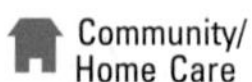

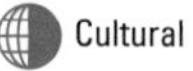

school-age children. Facilitating optimal physical, cognitive, social, and emotional growth of individuals during the transition from childhood to adulthood

NURSING PRIORITY NO. 1 To assess causative/contributing factors:

- Note family constellation: two-parent, single, extended family, or child living with other relative such as grandparent/sibling. *Helps identify problem areas and strengths to formulate plans to change situation that is currently creating difficulties for the parents.*[3]
- Review type, severity, duration of problem and contribution of, as well as impact on, individual family members. *Affects choice of interventions; for example, when abuse is the problem, it is an act of commission, whereas neglect is considered an act of omission. These behaviors indicate the presence of problems with relationships and/or parenting skills and individual problems such as inability to deal with stressors, substance abuse, mental illness, cognitive limitations, or criminality.*[1]
- Note negative statements about child, signs of trauma/failure to thrive, and history of recurring accidents/illness. *May reflect physical or psychological abuse or neglect necessitating appropriate actions as legally and professionally indicated if child's safety is a concern. Note: Safety of child is paramount and needs to be dealt with immediately.*[5]
- Determine developmental stage of the family (e.g., new child, adolescent, child leaving or returning home). *These maturational crises bring changes in the family that can be stressful to parents and the family. Provides direction for improving parenting skills and family interactions.*[1]
- Assess family relationships among individual members and with others, family boundaries, and needs of individual members. *These factors are critical to understanding individual family dynamics and developing strategies for change.*[3]
- Assess parenting skill level, taking into account the individual's intellectual, emotional, and physical strengths and weaknesses. *Parents with significant impairments may need more education or support. Ineffective parenting and unrealistic expectations contribute to problems of abuse and neglect. Understanding normal responses and progression of developmental milestones can help parents understand and cope with changes.*[1]
- Observe attachment behaviors between parental figure and child, recognizing cultural background. *Failure to bond effectively is thought to affect subsequent parent-child interaction. Behaviors such as eye-to-eye contact, use of en face position, and talking to the infant in a high-pitched voice are indicative of attachment behaviors in American culture but may not be appropriate in another culture.*[1,4]
- Note presence of factors in the child (e.g., birth defects, hyperactivity) that may be related to difficulties of parenting. *Unanticipated needs of the child may affect attachment and caretaking needs. Parents have an ideal of what is expected in a child, and when circumstances dictate otherwise, they may experience feelings of sadness and anger.*[1] Refer to ND complicated Grieving.
- Evaluate physical challenges or limitations of parent. *Presence of complicating factors (e.g., visual or hearing impairment, quadriplegia, severe depression, mental illness) may affect ability to care for a child and indicate need for additional planning to assist the parent.*[1]
- Determine presence and effectiveness of support systems, role models, extended family, and community resources available to the parent(s). *Lack of or ineffective use of support systems increases risk of continued inability to parent effectively.*[5]
- Note absence from home setting or lack of child supervision by parent. *Demands of working long hours, out of town, and multiple responsibilities such as working and attending educational classes will affect relationship between parent and child and ability to provide the care and nurturing necessary for children to grow and prosper.*[7]

NURSING PRIORITY NO. 2 To foster development of parenting skills:

- Create an environment in which relationships can be developed and needs of each individual met. *Learning is more effective when individuals feel safe and free to express feelings and concerns without fear of judgment.*[6,7]

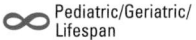

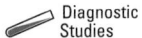

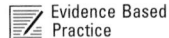

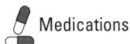

- Make time for listening to concerns of the parent(s). *Listening conveys respect and acceptance, enabling parent(s) to openly discuss needs and desires regarding the situation and future plans.*[2]
- Emphasize positive aspects of the situation. *Maintaining a hopeful attitude toward the parent's capabilities and potential for improving the situation will help the parent to manage what is happening more effectively.*[1]
- Note staff attitudes toward parent/child and specific problem or disability. *The need for disabled parents to be seen as individuals and evaluated apart from a stereotype are crucial to helping individuals to cope with a difficult situation. Negative attitudes are detrimental to promoting positive outcomes.*[3]
- Encourage expression of feelings, such as helplessness, anger, and frustration. Set limits on unacceptable behaviors. *When feelings are expressed openly, they can be acknowledged and dealt with, enabling parent(s) to move forward in dealing with illness or situation. Individual may express anger by acting-out behaviors, which need to be restrained before damage is done to self, self-esteem, others, or environment.*[5,6]
- Acknowledge difficulty of situation and normalcy of feelings. *Individuals feel validated when difficulty is recognized, enhancing feelings of acceptance.*[1]
- Recognize stages of grieving process when the child is disabled or other than anticipated. *Expectation of a "normal" or desired child (e.g., having a girl instead of boy, child with a prominent birthmark or birth defect such as cleft palate) results in grieving for the loss of that expectation.*[1,8]
- Allow time for parents to express feelings and deal with the "loss." *Each person grieves at own pace, and allowing this time facilitates the process.*[8]
- Encourage attendance at skill classes, such as parent effectiveness. *Helps parents to develop communication and problem-solving techniques that promote positive relationships between parent and child.*[6,7]
- Emphasize parenting functions rather than mothering/fathering skills. *By virtue of gender, each person brings something to the parenting role; however, nurturing tasks can be done by both parents.*[1]

NURSING PRIORITY NO. 3 To promote wellness (Teaching/Discharge Considerations):

- Involve all available members of the family in learning. *Promotes understanding and effective communication when each individual has the same information and is able to ask questions and clarify what has been heard.*[2,5]
- Provide information appropriate to the situation, including time management, limit setting, and stress-reduction techniques. *Facilitates satisfactory implementation of plan and new behaviors.*[5]
- Discuss parental beliefs about child-rearing, punishment, and rewards. *Identifying these beliefs allows opportunity to provide new information regarding effective alternatives to spanking and/or yelling and what actions can be substituted for more effective parenting.*
- Develop support systems appropriate to the situation. *Extended family, friends, social worker, home-care services may be needed to help parents cope positively with what is happening.*[3]
- Assist parent to plan time and conserve energy in positive ways. *Enables individual to cope more effectively with difficulties as they arise.*[3]
- Encourage parents to identify positive outlets for meeting their own needs. *Going out for dinner or dating and making time for their own interests and each other promotes general well-being and helps reduce burnout.*[3,9]
- Refer to appropriate support or therapy groups as indicated. *Underlying issues may interfere with adaptation to situation, and additional support may help individuals to deal more effectively with them.*[5]
- Identify community resources (e.g., child-care services). *Will assist with individual needs to provide respite and support.*[2]
- Report and take necessary actions, as legally and professionally indicated, if child's safety is a concern. *Parents may believe corporal punishment is the best way to have children behave but may lead to abuse.*[5]
- Refer to NDs ineffective Coping, compromised family Coping, risk for Violence [specify], Self-Esteem [specify], and interrupted Family Processes for additional interventions as appropriate.

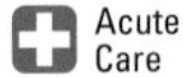

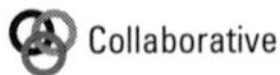

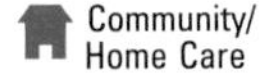

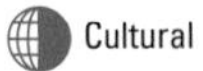

DOCUMENTATION FOCUS

Assessment/Reassessment

- Individual findings, including parenting skill level, deviations from normal parenting expectations.
- Family makeup and developmental stages.
- Interactions between parent and child.
- Availability and use of support systems and community resources.

Planning

- Plan of care and who is involved in planning.
- Teaching plan.

Implementation/Evaluation

- Parent(s')/child's responses to interventions, teaching, and actions performed.
- Attainment or progress toward desired outcome(s).
- Modification to plan of care.

Discharge Planning

- Long-term needs and who is responsible for actions to be taken.
- Specific referrals made.

References

1. Johnson, J. G., Cohen, P., Chen, H., et al. (2006). Parenting behaviors associated with risk for personality disorder during adulthood. *Arch Gen Psychiatry*, 63(5), 579–587.
2. Gordon, T. Origins of the Gordon model. Gordon Training International. Retrieved March 2015 from http://www.gordontraining.com/thomas-gordon/origins-of-the-gordon-model/.
3. Mandie, T. (2011). How parenting styles affect our children's development. Retrieved March 2015 from http://yourkidsed.com.au/info/how-parenting-styles-influence-our-childrens-development.
4. Ho, J., Birnham, C. (2010). Acculturation gaps in Vietnamese immigrant families: Impact on family relationships. *Int J Intercult Relat*, 34(1), 22–23.
5. Child Welfare Information Gateway. (Updated 2013). Long term consequences of child abuse and neglect. U.S. Department of Health and Human Services. Retrieved March 2015 from https://www.childwelfare.gov/pubpdfs/long_term_consequences.pdf.
6. Brhel, R. (2008). The age of gentle discipline. The Attached Family. Retrieved March 2015 from http://theattachedfamily.com/membersonly/?p=177.
7. Oswalt, A. (2008). Urie Bronfenbrenner and child development. Retrieved March 2015 from https://www.mentalhelp.net/articles/urie-bronfenbrenner-and-child-development/.
8. Neeld, E. H. (2003). *Seven Choices: Finding Daylight After Loss Shatters Your Life*. New York: Grand Central.
9. Adams, L. (2011). The language of love. Gordon Training International. Retrieved March 2015 from http://www.gordontraining.com/free-parenting-articles/the-language-of-love/.

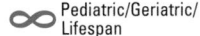

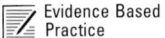

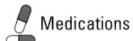

readiness for enhanced Parenting

Taxonomy II: Role Relationships—Class 1 Caregiving Roles (00164) [**Diagnostic Division:** Social Interaction], Submitted 2002; Revised 2013

DEFINITION: A pattern of providing an environment for children or other dependent person(s) to nurture growth and development, which can be strengthened.

DEFINING CHARACTERISTICS

Subjective

Expresses desire to enhance parenting

Parent expresses desire to enhance emotional support of children/other dependent person

Children express desire to enhance home environment

Sample Clinical Applications: As a health-seeking behavior, the client/family may be healthy or this diagnosis can be associated with any clinical condition

DESIRED OUTCOMES/EVALUATION CRITERIA

Sample NOC linkages:

Parenting Performance: Parental actions to provide a child with a nurturing and constructive physical, emotional, and social environment

Knowledge: Parenting: Extent of understanding conveyed about provision of a nurturing and constructive environment for a child from 1 year through 17 years of age

Parenting: Psychosocial Safety: Parental actions to protect a child from social contacts that might cause harm or injury

Client Will (Include Specific Time Frame)

- Verbalize realistic information and expectations of parenting role.
- Identify own strengths, individual needs, and methods or resources to meet them.
- Participate in activities to enhance parenting skills.
- Demonstrate improved parenting behaviors.

ACTIONS/INTERVENTIONS

Sample NIC linkages:

Parent Education: Childrearing Family: Assisting parents to understand and promote the physical, psychological, and social growth and development of their toddler, preschool, or school-age child/children

Parent Education: Adolescent: Assisting parents to understand and help their adolescent children

Parenting Promotion: Providing parenting information, support, and coordination of comprehensive services to high-risk families

NURSING PRIORITY NO. 1 To determine need/motivation for improvement:

- Ascertain motivation and expectations for change. *Motivation to improve and high expectations can encourage client to make changes that will improve skills. However, unrealistic expectations may hamper efforts.*
- Note family constellation, such as two-parent, single, extended family, or child living with other relative such as a grandparent/sibling, or relationship of dependent person (e.g., foster family). *Understanding makeup of the family provides information about needs to assist them in improving their family connections.*[1]
- ∞ Determine developmental stage of the family (e.g., new child, adolescent, child leaving or returning home, retirement). *These maturational crises bring changes in the family that can provide opportunity for enhancing parenting skills and improving family interactions.*[1]

Acute Care 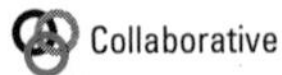 Collaborative 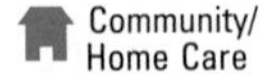 Community/Home Care 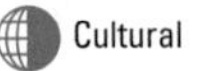 Cultural

- Assess family relationships and identify needs of individual members, noting any special concerns that exist, such as birth defects, illness, and hyperactivity. *The family is a system, and when members make decisions to improve parenting skills, the changes affect all parts of the system. Identifying needs, special situations, and relationships can help to develop plans to bring about effective change.*[1]
- Assess parenting skill level, taking into account the individual's intellectual, emotional, and physical strengths and weaknesses. *Identifies areas of need for education, skill training, and information on which to base plan for enhancing parenting skills.*[2,4]
- Observe attachment behaviors among parent(s) and child(ren), recognizing cultural background, which may influence expected behaviors. *Behaviors such as eye-to-eye contact, use of en face position, and talking to infant in high-pitched voice are indicative of attachment behaviors in American culture but may not be appropriate in another culture. Failure to bond is thought to affect subsequent parent-child interactions.*[3,4]
- Determine presence and effectiveness of support systems, role models, extended family, and community resources available to the parent(s). *Parents desiring to enhance abilities and improve family life can benefit by role models that help them strengthen own style of parenting.*[2,3]
- Note cultural or religious influences on parenting, expectations of self/child, and sense of success or failure. *Expectations may vary with different cultures. Beliefs may interfere with ability to improve parenting skills when there is conflict.*[3,4]

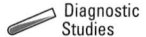

NURSING PRIORITY NO. 2 To foster development of parenting skills:

- Create an environment in which relationships can be strengthened and needs of each individual family member can be met. *A safe environment in which individuals can freely express their thoughts and feelings optimizes learning and positive interactions among family members, enhancing relationships.*[2,5]
- Make time for listening to concerns of the parent(s). *Promotes sense of importance and of being heard and identifies accurate information regarding needs of the family for enhancing relationships.*[2]
- Encourage expression of feelings, such as frustration and anger while setting limits on unacceptable behaviors. *Identification of feelings promotes understanding of self and enhances connections with others in the family. Unacceptable behaviors result in feelings of anger and diminished self-esteem and can lead to problems in family relationships.*[3]
- Emphasize parenting functions rather than mothering/fathering skills. *By virtue of gender, each person brings something to the parenting role; however, nurturing tasks can be done by both parents, enhancing family relationships.*[5]
- Encourage attendance at skill classes, such as parent effectiveness training. *Assists in developing communication skills of active listening, "I" messages, and problem-solving techniques to improve family relationships and promote a win-win environment.*[2]

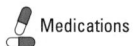

NURSING PRIORITY NO. 3 To promote optimum parenting skills/wellness:

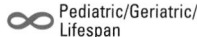

- Involve all members of the family in learning. *The family system benefits from all members participating in learning new skills to enhance family relationships.*[1]
- Encourage parents to identify positive outlets for meeting their own needs. *Activities such as going out for dinner/dating and making time for their own interests and each other promotes general well-being, enhances family relationships, and improves family functioning.*[2]
- Provide information as indicated, including time management and stress-reduction techniques. *Learning about positive parenting skills and understanding growth and developmental expectations and ways to reduce stress and anxiety promotes individual's ability to deal with problems that may arise in the course of family relationships.*[1,6]
- Discuss current "family rules," identifying areas of needed change. *Rules may be imposed by adults rather than through a democratic process, involving all family members, leading to conflict and angry confronta-*

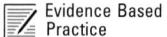

tions. Setting positive family rules with all family members participating can promote an effective, functional family.[2,6]

- Discuss need for long-term planning and ways in which family can maintain desired positive relationships. *Each stage of life brings its own challenges, and understanding and preparing for each stage enables family members to move through them in positive ways, promoting family unity and resolving inevitable conflicts with win-win solutions.*[6]

DOCUMENTATION FOCUS

Assessment/Reassessment

- Individual findings, including parenting skill level, parenting expectations, family makeup, and developmental stages.
- Availability and use of support systems and community resources.
- Motivation and expectations for change.

Planning

- Plan for enhancement, who is involved in planning.

Implementation/Evaluation

- Family members' responses to interventions, teaching, and actions performed.
- Attainment or progress toward desired outcome(s).
- Modifications to plan.

Discharge Planning

- Long-term needs and who is responsible for actions to be taken.
- Modification to plan.

References

1. O'Brien, T. (2008). Parent empowerment program (PEP). Retrieved November 2015 from http://www.tim-obrien.com/empowerment.php?doc=details.
2. Riesch, S. K., Anderson, L. S., Pridham, K. A., et al. (2010). Furthering the understanding of parent-child relationships: A nursing scholarship review series, Part 5: Parent-adolescent and teen parent-child relationships. *J Spec Pediatr Nurs*, 15(3), 182–201.
3. Watson, S. Understanding inappropriate behavior. Retrieved November 2015 from http://specialed.about.com/od/behavioremotional/a/behavsupport.htm.
4. Institute of Public Care. (2008). What works in promoting good outcomes for children in need through enhanced parenting skills? *Social Services Improvement Agency, Wales*. Retrieved November 2015 from http://ipc.brookes.ac.uk/publications/pdf/What_Works_in_Promoting_Good_Outcomes_for_CIN_through_Parenting.pdf.
5. Bronte-Tinkew, J., Burkhauser, M., Metz, A. (2008). Elements of promising practice in teen fatherhood programs: Evidence-based and evidence-informed research findings on what works. *National Fatherhood Responsible Clearing House*. Retrieved November 2015 from http://www.lacdcfs.org/katiea/docs/EPP.pdf.
6. Duncan, L. G., Coatsworth, J. D., Greenberg, M. T. (2009). Pilot study to gauge acceptability of a mindfulness based, family-focused preventive intervention. *J Prim Prev*, 30(5), 605–618.

Acute Care
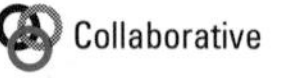
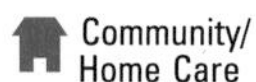
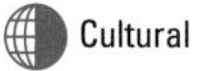

risk for impaired Parenting

Taxonomy II: Role Relationships—Class 1 Caregiving Roles (00057) [**Diagnostic Division:** Social Interaction], Submitted 1978; Revised 1998; 2013

DEFINITION: Vulnerable to inability of the primary caretaker to create, maintain, or regain an environment that promotes the optimum growth and development of the child, which may compromise the well-being of the child.

RISK FACTORS

Infant or child

Alteration in perceptual abilities; behavior disorder (e.g., attention deficit, oppositional defiant)
Difficult temperament; temperamental conflicts with parental expectations
Prematurity; multiple births; gender other than desired
Disabling condition; developmental delay
Illness; prolonged separation from parent

Knowledge

Unrealistic expectations; insufficient knowledge about child development or health maintenance, parenting skills
Low educational level; insufficient cognitive readiness for parenting; alteration in cognitive functioning
Ineffective communication skills
Insufficient response to infant cues
Preference for physical punishment

Physiological

Physical illness

Psychological

Young parental age
Closely spaced pregnancies; high number of pregnancies; difficult birthing process
Nonrestorative sleep pattern (i.e., due to caregiver responsibilities, parenting practices, sleep partner); sleep deprivation
Depression; history of mental illness or substance abuse
Disabling condition

Social

Stressors; work difficulty; unemployment; economically disadvantaged; compromised home environment; relocation
Low self-esteem
Insufficient family cohesiveness; conflict between partners; change in family unit; inadequate child care arrangements
Role strain; single parent; father/mother of child not involved; parent-child separation
Insufficient parental role model; insufficient valuing of parenthood
Unplanned or unwanted pregnancy; insufficient or late-term prenatal care
Insufficient resources (e.g., financial, social, knowledge) or access to resources; insufficient transportation
Insufficient problem-solving skills; ineffective coping strategies
Insufficient social support; social isolation
History of abuse (e.g., physical, psychological, sexual) or being abusive; legal difficulty

Note: A risk diagnosis is not evidenced by signs and symptoms, as the problem has not occurred; rather, nursing interventions are directed at prevention.

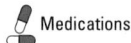

(continues on page 616)

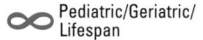

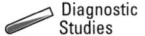

risk for impaired Parenting (continued)
Sample Clinical Applications: Prematurity, multiple births, genetic or congenital defects, chronic illness (parent/child), substance abuse, physical or psychological abuse, major depression, developmental delay, schizophrenia

DESIRED OUTCOMES/EVALUATION CRITERIA

Sample NOC linkages:
Parenting Performance: Parental actions to provide a child a nurturing and constructive physical, emotional, and social environment
Knowledge: Parenting: Extent of understanding conveyed about provision of a nurturing and constructive environment for a child from 1 year to 17 years of age
Social Support: Reliable assistance from others

Client Will (Include Specific Time Frame)
- Verbalize awareness of individual risk factors.
- Identify own strengths, individual needs, and methods or resources to meet them.
- Demonstrate behavior or lifestyle changes to reduce potential for development of problem or reduce or eliminate effects of risk factors.
- Participate in activities, classes to promote growth.

ACTIONS/INTERVENTIONS

Sample NIC linkages:
Parenting Promotion: Providing parenting information, support, and coordination of comprehensive services to high-risk families
Parent Education: Childbearing Family: Assisting parents to understand and promote the physical, psychological, and social growth and development of their toddler, preschool, or school-aged child/children
Family Integrity Promotion: Promotion of family cohesion and unity

Refer to ND impaired Parenting for Actions/Interventions and Documentation Focus.

disturbed Personal Identity

Taxonomy II: Self-Perception—Class 1 Self-Concept (00121) [**Diagnostic Division:** Ego Integrity], Submitted 1978; Revised 2008

DEFINITION: Inability to maintain an integrated and complete perception of self.

RELATED FACTORS

Low self-esteem; dysfunctional family processes
Situational crisis; stages of growth; developmental transition; alteration in social role
Exposure to toxic chemical; pharmaceutical agent
Cultural incongruency; discrimination; perceived prejudice
Manic states; psychiatric disorder; dissociative identity disorder); organic brain disorder
Cult indoctrination

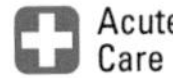

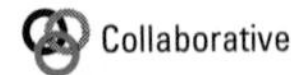

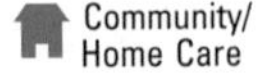

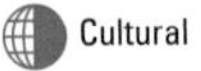

DEFINING CHARACTERISTICS

Subjective

Alteration in body image; delusional description of self
Fluctuating feeling about self; feelings of strangeness or emptiness
Confusion about goals, cultural values, or ideological values
Gender confusion
Inability to distinguish between internal and external stimuli

Objective

Inconsistent behavior
Ineffective relationships
Ineffective coping or role performance

Sample Clinical Applications: Schizophrenia, dissociative disorders, borderline personality disorder, developmental delay, autism, gender identity conflict, dementia, traumatic injury (e.g., amputation, spinal cord injury [SCI], brain injury)

DESIRED OUTCOMES/EVALUATION CRITERIA

Sample NOC linkages:

Identity: Distinguish between self and non-self and characterize one's essence

Distorted Thought Self-Control: Self-restraint of disruption in perception, thought processes, and thought content

Anxiety Self-Control: Personal actions to eliminate or reduce feelings of apprehension, tension, or uneasiness from an unidentifiable source

Client Will (Include Specific Time Frame)

- Acknowledge threat to personal identity.
- Integrate threat in a healthy, positive manner (e.g., state anxiety is reduced, make plans for the future).
- Verbalize acceptance of changes that have occurred.
- State ability to identify and accept self (long-term outcome).

ACTIONS/INTERVENTIONS

Sample NIC linkages:

Self-Esteem Enhancement: Assisting a patient to increase his/her personal judgment of self-worth

Self-Awareness Enhancement: Assisting a patient to explore and understand his/her thoughts, feelings, motivations, and behaviors

Mood Management: Providing for safety, stabilization, recovery, and maintenance of a patient who is experiencing dysfunctionally depressed or elevated mood

NURSING PRIORITY NO. 1 To assess causative/contributing factors:

- Ascertain client's perception of the extent of the threat to self and how client is handling the situation. *Many factors can affect an individual's self-image: illness (chronic or terminal), injuries, changes in body structure (amputation, spinal cord damage, burns), and client's view of what has happened will affect development of plan of care and interventions to be used.*[1,6]
- Determine speed of occurrence of threat. *An event (such as an accident or sudden diagnosis of diabetes or cancer) that has happened quickly may be more threatening.*[7]
- Ask client to define own body image. *Body image is the basis of personal identity, and client's perception will affect how changes are viewed, may prevent achievement of ideals and expectations, and have a negative effect.*[1]

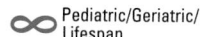

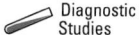

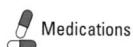

- ∞ Note age of client. *An adolescent may struggle with the developmental task of personal/sexual identity, whereas an older person may have more difficulty accepting or dealing with a threat to identity, such as progressive loss of memory or aging body changes.*[3]
- Assess availability and use of support systems. Note response of family/significant others (SOs). *During stressful situations, support is essential for client to cope with changes that are occurring. Engaging family in choosing supportive interventions will help client and family members deal with situation or illness.*[3]
- ∞ Note withdrawn or automatic behavior, regression to earlier developmental stage, general behavioral disorganization, or display of self-mutilation behaviors in adolescent or adult and delayed development, preference for solitary play, and unusual display of self-stimulation in child. *Indicators of poor coping skills and need for specific interventions to help client develop sense of self and identity. Inability to identify self interferes with interactions with others.*[3]
- Be aware of physical signs of panic state. *Presence of severe anxiety state may progress to panic when concerns seem overwhelming to client.* (Refer to ND Anxiety.)
- Determine presence of hallucinations or delusions or distortions of reality. *Indicators of presence of psychosis and need for immediate interventions to deal with inability to distinguish between self and nonself.*[1,3]

NURSING PRIORITY NO. 2 To assist client to manage/deal with threat:

- Make time to listen to client, encouraging appropriate expression of feelings, including anger and hostility. *Conveys a sense of confidence in client's ability to identify extent of threat, how it is affecting sense of identity, and how to deal with feelings in acceptable ways.*[7,8]
- Note use of alcohol or other drugs. *Individual may turn to these substances to relieve painful feelings, especially in the presence of fearful diagnoses (e.g., cancer, multiple sclerosis).*[8]
- Provide a calm environment. *Feelings of anxiety are contagious, and calm surroundings can help client to relax, maintain control, and be able to think more clearly about how illness or situation can be managed effectively.*[9]
- Use crisis intervention principles when indicated. *May be necessary to help client restore equilibrium when situation escalates.*[1]
- Discuss client's commitment to an identity. *Those who have made a strong commitment to an identity tend to be more comfortable with self and happier than those who have not.*[3]
- Assist client to develop strategies to cope with threat to identity. *Reduces anxiety, promotes self-awareness, and enhances self-esteem, enabling client to deal with threat more realistically.*[10]
- Engage client in activities appropriate to individual situation. *Using activities such as a mirror for visual feedback and tactile stimulation to reconnect with parts of the body (amputation, unilateral neglect) can help to identify self as an individual.*[2]
- Provide for simple decisions, concrete tasks, and calming activities. *Promotes sense of control and positive expectations to enable client to regain sense of self.*[3]
- Allow client to deal with situation in small steps. *May have difficulty coping with larger picture when in stress overload. Taking small steps promotes feelings of success and ability to manage illness or situation.*[9]
- Encourage client to develop and participate in an individualized exercise program. *While walking is an excellent beginning program, it is helpful to choose activities that client enjoys. Exercise releases endorphins, thereby reducing stress and anxiety, promoting a sense of well-being.*[1]
- Provide concrete assistance as needed. *Until basic-level needs, such as activities of daily living and food, are met, individual is unable to deal with higher-level needs. Once these needs are met, client can begin to deal with threat to identity.*[1]
- Take advantage of opportunities to promote growth. Realize that client will have difficulty learning while in a dissociative state. *Alterations in mental status can interfere with ability to process information, and new information can increase confusion and disorientation.*[3]
- Maintain reality orientation without confronting client's irrational beliefs. *Client may become defensive, blocking opportunity to look at other possibilities. Arguing does not change the perceptions and can interfere with or damage nurse-client relationship.*[1]

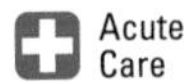

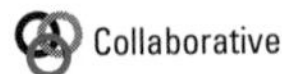

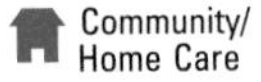

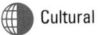

- Use humor judiciously when appropriate. *While humor can lift spirits and provide a moment of levity, it is important to note the mood or receptiveness of the client before using it.*[3]
- Discuss options for dealing with issues of gender identity. *Identification of client's concerns about role dysfunction or conflicting feelings about sexual identity will indicate need for therapies, possible gender-change surgery when client is a transsexual, or other available choices.*[2]
- Refer to NDs disturbed Body Image, Self-Esteem [specify], and Spiritual Distress.

NURSING PRIORITY NO. 3 To promote wellness (Teaching/Discharge Considerations):

- Provide accurate information about threat to and potential consequences for individual in current situation. *Fear and anxiety regarding the threat represented by the illness or situation can be potentiated by lack of knowledge, unknown consequences, and inaccurate beliefs. Accurate information can help client incorporate new knowledge into changed self-concept.*[7]
- Assist client and SO(s) to acknowledge and integrate threat into future planning. *A diagnosis, accident, etc., can require major life changes, such as wearing identification bracelet when prone to mental confusion, a new lifestyle to accommodate change of gender for transsexual client, or a diet and medication routine with the diagnosis of diabetes mellitus. Planning can help the client to make the changes required to move forward with new life.*[4,5]
- Refer to appropriate support groups. *May need additional assistance, such as day-care program, counseling or psychotherapy, gender identity, family or marriage counseling, or parenting classes.*[2]

DOCUMENTATION FOCUS

Assessment/Reassessment

- Findings, noting degree of impairment.
- Nature of and client's perception of the threat.

Planning

- Plan of care and who is involved in the planning.
- Teaching plan.

Implementation/Evaluation

- Client's response to interventions, teaching, and actions performed.
- Attainment or progress toward desired outcome(s).
- Modifications to plan of care.

Discharge Planning

- Long-term needs and who is responsible for actions to be taken.
- Specific referrals made.

References

1. Newell, R. (2002). Terminal illness and body image. *Nursing Times*, 98(14), 36–37.
2. Gillig, P. M. (2009). Dissociative identity disorder—A controversial diagnosis. *Psychiatry (Edgmont)*, 6(3), 24–29. Retrieved March 2015 from http://www.ncbi.nlm.nih.gov/pmc/articles/PMC2719457/.
3. Shaw, G. (2011). Coping with a life threatening illness—Palliative care: Improving life for patients and caregivers. WebMD. Retrieved March 2015 from http://www.webmd.com/palliative-care/coping-with-a-life-threatening-illness.
4. Pinhas-Hamiel, O., Dolan, L. M., Daniels, S. R., et al. (1996). Increased incidence of non-insulin-dependent diabetes mellitus among adolescents. *J Pediatr*, 128(8), 608–615.
5. Deckelbaum, R. J., Williams, C. L. (2001). Childhood obesity: The health issue. *Obesity Res*, 9(5), 239s–243s.
6. Badger, J. M. (2001). Burns: The psychological aspect. *Am J Nurs*, 101(11), 38–41.
7. Bartol, T. (2002). Putting a patient with diabetes in the driver's seat. *Nursing*, 32(2), 53–55.

8. Bruera, E., Moyano, J., Seifert, L., et al. (1995). The frequency of alcoholism among patients with pain due to terminal cancer. *J Pain Symptom Manage*, 10(8), 599–603.
9. Paice, J. (2002). Managing psychological conditions in palliative care. *Am J Nurs*, 102(11), 36–43.
10. Ghosh, S. (2015). Gender identity. Retrieved February 2015 from http://emedicine.medscape.com/article/917990-overview.

risk for disturbed Personal Identity

Taxonomy II: Self-Perception—Class 1 Self-Concept (00225) [**Diagnostic Division:** Ego Identity], Submitted 2010; Revised 2013

DEFINITION: Vulnerable to the inability to maintain an integrated and complete perception of self, which may compromise health.

RISK FACTORS

Low self-esteem; dysfunctional family processes
Situational crisis; stages of growth; developmental transition; alteration in social role
Exposure to toxic chemical; pharmaceutical agent
Cultural incongruency; discrimination; perceived prejudice
Manic states; psychiatric disorder; dissociative identity disorder; organic brain disorder
Cult indoctrination
Note: A risk diagnosis is not evidenced by signs and symptoms as the problem has not occurred, rather, nursing actions are directed at prevention.
Sample Clinical Applications: Traumatic injury (e.g., amputation, spinal cord injury, traumatic brain injury), substance abuse, dementia, schizophrenia, borderline personality disorders, dissociative disorders, developmental delay, autism, gender identity conflict

DESIRED OUTCOMES/EVALUATION CRITERIA

Sample NOC linkages:
Identity: Distinguish between self and non-self and characterize one's essence
Distorted Thought Self-Control: Self-restraint of disruption in perception, thought processes, and thought control
Anxiety Self-Control: Personal actions to eliminate or reduce feelings of apprehension, tension, or uneasiness from an unidentifiable source

Client Will (Include Specific Time Frame)
- Acknowledge concern about potential threat to identity.
- Exhibit reality-based thinking with appropriate thought content.
- Integrate perceived threat in a healthy manner (e.g., accept self in current situation, look to the future).
- Use effective coping strategies to deal with situation/stressors.

ACTIONS/INTERVENTIONS

Sample NIC linkages:
Self-Awareness Enhancement: Assisting a patient to explore and understand his/her thoughts, feelings, motivations, and behaviors
Self-Esteem Enhancement: Assisting a patient to increase his/her personal judgment of self-worth

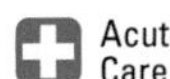
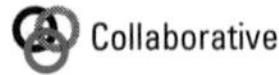
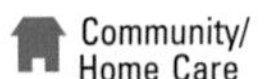
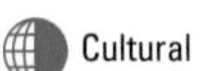

Coping Enhancement: Assisting a patient to adapt to perceived stressors, changes, or threats that interfere with meeting life demands and roles

NURSING PRIORITY NO. 1 To assess risk/contributing factors:

- Ascertain client's perception of threat to self and how it is being dealt with. *Many factors can impinge on client's life and cause concern about possibility of changes that will make life different.*[1,5,12,13,15]
- Ask client to define own body image. *The basis of personal identity is body image, and perception of changes may affect client's view in a negative or positive manner.*[1,6,12,18]
- Determine whether issues of gender identity are a concern. *Client may have conflicting feelings about how to deal with realization he or she is homosexual or transsexual.*[10,12]
- Note age of individual. *Changes affect persons differently depending on their stage of life. The maturational changes of adolescence may generally be viewed as positive, while the older person may view aging changes in a negative way.*[2,12,13,15,17]
- Identify cultural affiliations/discontinuity. *Individuals belonging to subcultures or cults tend to come into conflict with the greater societal views affecting one's perception of self and perception of reality, often resulting in isolation from outside support groups and reluctance to engage in therapeutic interventions.*[12,19–21]
- Determine type and speed of changes that are imminent. *The diagnosis of a chronic illness, such as diabetes versus a terminal illness or a traumatic injury or disfiguring surgery that will change how life is lived, may be threatening, as the thought of how different life will be affects the individual.*[1,6,12,14,15]
- Note availability and use of support systems, including attitude of family/significant others. *Having a positive support system can help individual get through difficult situations/illness.*[3,4,6,14]
- Assess behaviors such as withdrawal, general behavioral disorganization, and delayed development. *Poor coping skills will affect how client deals with possibility of disturbance in personal identity by changes occurring in life.*[2,6,11,13]
- Discuss use of alcohol and other drugs. *Individuals often use these substances to avoid painful stressors.*[2,15]
- Note signs of anxiety. *Use of inadequate coping strategies to deal with changes affecting lifestyle may result in exacerbation of symptoms in anxious person. (Refer to ND Anxiety.)*
- Determine distortions of reality/symptoms of mental illness. *Requires more in-depth psychological counseling/medication to help client distinguish between self and nonself.*[2,11,12,15,18]

NURSING PRIORITY NO. 2 To assist client to manage/deal with stressors:

- Listen/active-listen, making time to encourage client to express feelings, including anger and hostility. *Possibility of changes in life may affect sense of self and identity.*[6,7,9]
- Discuss client's concerns without confronting unreal ideas. *Irrational beliefs may interfere with ability to manage situation and maintain reality-based perception of self.*[2,6]
- Encourage client and family to maintain a calm environment and positive attitude. *Anxiety is contagious and can interfere with client's efforts to maintain control and deal with the situation.*[8,16]
- Help client to identify strategies to cope with current situation/possibility of threat. *Having a plan can reduce anxiety and promote self-esteem.*[2,3,14]
- Use humor when appropriate. *In an established nurse-client relationship, humor can be useful to help client look at reality of situation.*[16]
- Provide activities applicable for client's situation. *For example, viewing body part/using a mirror for visual feedback or tactile stimulation to reconnect with parts of the body (i.e., amputation) or participation in monitored social interactions helps client to confront fear and see self as an individual who is still worthwhile.*[1,18]
- Support client in making decisions and plans for the future. *Provides opportunity for client to feel in control and promotes positive expectations.*[3,14]
- Develop an individualized exercise program. *Releases endorphins, reducing stress and promoting a sense of well-being.*[5,22]

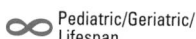

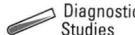

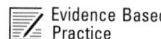

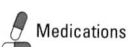

- Refer to NDs disturbed Body Image, Self-Esteem (specify), and Spiritual Distress for additional interventions as appropriate.

NURSING PRIORITY NO. 3 To promote wellness (Teaching/Discharge Considerations):

- Provide accurate information/resources for issues client is concerned about. *Worrying about what might happen is counterproductive to dealing with reality, and information can help to lessen anxiety, allowing individual to deal with current situation.*[3,4,7,18]
- Discuss potential changes in lifestyle that may occur with major diagnosis/accident. *Planning for these possibilities can enhance self-confidence and allow client to move forward with life.*[1,5,7,8]
- Refer to appropriate support groups. *Sharing concerns with others in group settings may help client to be realistic regarding concerns about effects of anticipated changes/life challenges.*[3,4,8,18]
- Explore community resources as appropriate. *Additional assistance such as day programs, individual/family-counseling, and drug/alcohol-cessation programs can strengthen client's coping abilities and sense of control.*[4,12,23,24]

DOCUMENTATION FOCUS

Assessment/Reassessment

- Findings, noting concerns about possible changes in lifestyle, future expectations
- Reality of potential threat

Planning

- Plan of care and who is involved in the planning
- Teaching plan

Implementation/Evaluation

- Client's response to interventions, teaching, and actions performed

Discharge Planning

- Long-term needs, and who is responsible for actions to be taken
- Specific referrals made

References

1. Newell, R. (2002). Terminal illness and body image. *Nursing Times*, 98(14), 36.
2. Gillig, P. M. (2009). Dissociative identity disorder—A controversial diagnosis. *Psychiatry (Edgmont)*, 6(3), 24–29.
3. Shaw, G. (2011). Coping with a life threatening illness. Palliative care: Improving life for patients and caregivers. Retrieved March 2015 from http://www.webmd.com/palliative-care/coping-with-a-life-threatening-illness.
4. Wheeler, S. K., Foster, J. (Updated 2014). Holistic healing: Putting patients in the driver's seat. *Minority Nurse*. Retrieved March 2015 from http://www.minoritynurse.com/holistic-healing-putting-patients-driver%E2%80%99s-seat.
5. Deckelbaum, R. J., Williams, C. L. (2001). Childhood obesity: The health issue. *Obesity Res*, 9(5), S239–S243.
6. Smith, J. S., Smith, K. R., Rainey, S. L. (2006). The psychology of burn care. *J Trauma Nurs*, 13(3), 105–106.
7. Ulene, V. (May 23, 2011). Why are unhealthy people so reluctant to change their lifestyles? *LA Times*. Retrieved March 2015 from http://articles.latimes.com/2011/may/23/health/la-he-the-md-change-illness-20110523.
8. Marshal, C. (2012). Lifestyle changes due to chronic illness and how to deal with it. Retrieved March 2015 from https://msmeans.wordpress.com/2012/01/22/lifestyle-changes-due-to-chronic-illness-and-how-to-deal-with-it/.
9. Active listening: Hear what people are really saying. Mind Tools. Retrieved March 2015 from http://www.mindtools.com/CommSkll/ActiveListening.htm.

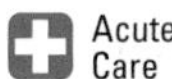

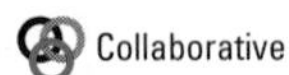

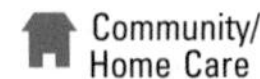

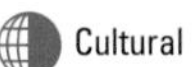

10. Ghosh, S. (2015). Gender identity. Retrieved February 2015 from http://emedicine.medscape.com/article/917990-overview.
11. Willkinson-Ryan, T., Westen, D. (2000). Identity disturbance in borderline personality disorder: An empirical investigation. *Am J Psychiatry*, 157(4), 528–541.
12. Daniels, R. (2003). Nursing Fundamentals: Caring & Clinical Decision Making—Summary Chapter 43: Self-Concept. Retrieved March 2015 from http://www.delmarlearning.com/companions/content/0766838366/students/ch43/summary.asp.
13. Boeree, G. (1997, 2006). Personality theories: Karen Horney. Retrieved March 2015 from webspace.ship.edu/cgboer/horney.html.
14. Breitenbach, M. (2006). Coping with serious illness: Letting change into your life. Retrieved March 2015 from ezinearticles.com/?coping-with-serious-illness-Letting-Change-into-your-Life&id=150109.
15. Gronley, M. (2010). What is depression. Retrieved March 2015 from http://psychiatristscottsdale.com/what-is-depression/.
16. Gronley, M. (2010). Health benefits of laughter. Retrieved March 2015 from http://psychiatristscottsdale.com/health-benefits-of-laughter/.
17. Berger, K. S. (2008). *The Developing Person Through the Life Span*. New York: Worth, 288–290.
18. Newell, R. (2002). The fear-avoidance model: Helping patients to cope with disfigurement. *Nursing Times*, 98(16), 38–39.
19. Langone, M. (No date). Cults: Questions and answers. International Cultic Studies Association. Retrieved March 2015 from http://www.csj.org/studyindex/studycult/cultqa.htm.
20. Lalich, J., Langone, M. (2006). Characteristics associated with cult groups. In Lalich, J., Tobias, M. (eds). *Take Back Your Life: Recovering from Cults and Abusive Relationships*. 2nd ed., revised and expanded Berkeley, CA: Bay Tree, 327–328.
21. Vedantam, S. (June 26, 2005). Patients' diversity is often discounted: Alternatives to mainstream medical treatment call for recognizing ethnic, social differences. *Washington Post*. Retrieved March 2015 from http://vedantam.com/culture1-06-2005.html.
22. Gronley, M. (2010). Effects of exercise on depression. Retrieved March 2015 from http://psychiatristscottsdale.com/effects-of-exercise-on-depression/.
23. Mays, G. P., Smith, S. A. (2011). Evidence links increases in public health spending to decline in preventable deaths. *Health Affairs*, 30(8), 1585–1593.
24. Griswold, K. S. (2012). Communities of solution: The Folsom Report revisited. *Ann Family Med*, 10(3), 250–260.

risk for Poisoning

Taxonomy II: Safety/Protection—Class 4 Environmental Hazards (00037) [**Diagnostic Division:** Safety], Submitted 1980; Revised 2006, 2013

DEFINITION: Vulnerable to accidental exposure to, or ingestion of, drugs or dangerous products in sufficient doses, that may compromise health.

RISK FACTORS

Internal

Alteration in cognitive functioning
Emotional disturbance
Inadequate precautions against poisoning; inadequate knowledge of poisoning prevention
Inadequate knowledge of pharmacological agents; [narrow therapeutic margin of safety of specific pharmaceutical agents (e.g., therapeutic versus toxic level, half-life, method of uptake and degradation in body, adequacy of organ function)]
Occupational setting without adequate safegaurds
Reduced vision
[Cultural or religious beliefs or practices]

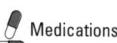

(continues on page 624)

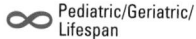

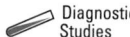

risk for Poisoning (continued)

External

Access to dangerous product

Access to pharmaceutical agent; access to large supply of pharmaceutical agents in house

Access to illicit drugs potentially contaminated by poisonous additives

[Use of multiple herbal supplements or megadosing]

Note: A risk diagnosis is not evidenced by signs and symptoms, as the problem has not occurred; rather, nursing interventions are directed at prevention.

Sample Clinical Applications: Substance abuse, dementia, cataracts, glaucoma, hepatitis, cirrhosis, renal failure, depression, suicidal ideation, developmental delay

DESIRED OUTCOMES/EVALUATION CRITERIA

Sample NOC linkages:

Risk Control: Drug Use: Personal actions to prevent, eliminate, or reduce drug use that poses a threat to health

Knowledge: Medication: Extent of understanding conveyed about the safe use of medication

Safe Home Environment: Physical arrangements to minimize environmental factors that might cause physical harm or injury in the home

Client/Caregiver Will (Include Specific Time Frame)

- Verbalize understanding of dangers of poisoning.
- Identify hazards that could lead to accidental poisoning.
- Correct external hazards as identified.
- Demonstrate necessary actions or lifestyle changes to promote safe environment.

ACTIONS/INTERVENTIONS

Sample NIC linkages:

Medication Management: Facilitation of safe and effective use of prescription and over-the-counter (OTC) drugs

Environmental Management: Safety: Manipulation of the patient's surroundings for therapeutic benefit

Surveillance: Safety: Purposeful and ongoing collection and analysis of information about the patient and the environment for use in promoting and maintaining patient safety

NURSING PRIORITY NO. 1 To assess causative/contributing factors:

- Identify internal and external risk factors in client's environment, including presence of infants, young children, or frail elderly *(who are at risk for accidental poisoning)* and teenagers or young adults *(who are at risk for medication experimentation);* confused or chronically ill person on multiple medications; person with potential for suicidal action; person who partakes in illicit drug use/dealing (e.g., marijuana, cocaine, heroin); and person who manufactures drugs in home (e.g., methamphetamines).
- Note age and cognitive status of client and care providers *to identify individuals who could be at higher risk for accidental poisoning. Babies, toddlers, and preschoolers are at risk because they are curious, like to put things into their mouths, and aren't aware of what's safe to eat. Certain medications (e.g., calcium channel blockers, sulfonylureas, opiates, amphetamines, sodium channel blockers, and tricyclic antidepressants; drugs of abuse that are potentially fatal include opiates and all amphetamines [including methamphetamine and MDMA]) can kill a toddler with a single dose. While school-age children can recognize danger and*

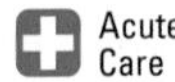

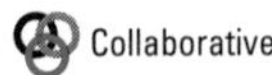

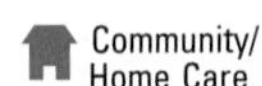

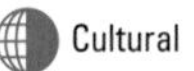

are at lower risk of unintentional poisoning, they are at risk for inadvertent overdose when taking medications without adequate supervision or when taking medications belonging to another. Adolescents are at higher risk for experimentation due to natural inclination to take risks, peer pressure, and easy access to drugs. They are also at risk for suicide attempts (with overdose of medications, from illicit drug overdose or adverse reactions, alcohol toxicity).[1,8,10] *Note: A recent (2013) U.S. study revealed that 67,000 children (most between the ages of 2 and 5 years) were treated in emergency departments for accidental ingestion of OTC or adult prescription drugs found in the home. This represents a 30% increase over the last 10 years.*[2] *Elderly persons are at risk because of the higher number of prescription and OTC medications they consume (polypharmacy) and because of visual and cognitive impairments, which can cause them to forget what medications have been consumed and in what amounts they were taken. Elderly persons are also likely to share medications. In addition, the presence of nutritional deficits and renal or hepatic degeneration can reduce ability to detoxify drugs. Note: One large study showed that certain medication classes such as analgesics, anticoagulants, anticonvulsants, asthma therapies, psychotherapeutics, and some cardiovascular agents were associated with high hazard factors.*[3,4]

- Assess mood, coping abilities, and personality styles (e.g., temperament, impulsive behavior, level of self-esteem) *that may result in carelessness and increased risk taking without consideration of consequences or suicidal actions.* (Refer to ND risk for Suicide.)
- Determine client's allergies to medications and foods *in order to avoid exposure to substances causing potentially lethal reaction.*
- Ascertain client's knowledge and use of medications. *People may believe "if a little is good, a lot is better," placing them at risk for overdose and adverse drug effects or interactions. This belief pattern may also be responsible for client's use of multiple drugs at the same time (polypharmacy), which also can occur when multiple prescribers are unaware of each other or the client has multiple medical conditions requiring medications. Knowledge and use also affect the client's storage (e.g., may/may not use labeled bottles) and/or taking of medications that look alike (potentiating risk of overdose or adverse drug interactions). The elderly may unintentionally take the wrong medication at the wrong time or "double up," forgetting that they already took their daily dose of a prescription medicine.*[14]
- Determine specific drug hazards:

  Use of prescription, OTC medications, and culturally based home remedies. *These have potential for intentional and accidental overdose, as well as dangerous interactions. Drugs that are therapeutic in small doses may be deadly when taken in excess (e.g., beta blockers, warfarin, digoxin). One of the most common problems is inadvertent overdosage of acetaminophen (Tylenol), either by increased dosing or by taking it with a combination product also containing acetaminophen. In children, the most serious accidental poisonings occur with iron, methadone, and tricyclic antidepressants.*[4,11]

  Availability or regular use of vitamins and mineral and herbal supplements. *Vitamins (especially A and D) are toxic in large doses, and iron is especially harmful to children.*[11] *Herbal drugs can be a source of poisoning (usually when taken long term) due to toxicity of individual ingredients or from contaminants (e.g., mercury, lead, arsenic).*

  Abuse of alcohol or other drugs (e.g., cocaine, methamphetamine, lysergic acid diethylamide, methadone). *Those who abuse street drugs are at high risk for overdose because the purity of these drugs is largely unknown. A person may be trying to get high but unwittingly take more drugs than his/her body can handle. These substances have potential for adverse reactions, cumulative effects with other substances, and risk for intentional and accidental overdose. Note: As little as 1 oz of alcohol or a single dose of many drugs of abuse can cause serious injury/death in a small child.*[9,11]

- Identify environmental hazards:

  Storage of household chemicals (e.g., oven, toilet bowl, or drain cleaners; dishwasher products; bleach; hydrogen peroxide; fluoride preparations; essential oils; furniture polish; lighter fluid; lamp oil; kerosene; paints; turpentine; rust remover; lubricant oils; bug sprays or powders; fertilizers) *are readily available toxins in various forms that are often improperly stored.*[5–9]

Review client's home, employment, or work environment *for exposure to chemicals, including vapors and fumes.*
Refer to ND risk for Contamination for environmental issues.

- Review results of laboratory tests and toxicology screening, as indicated. *Guides treatment when overdose or accidental poisoning is known or suspected.*

NURSING PRIORITY NO. 2 To assist in correcting factors that can lead to accidental poisoning:

- Discuss medication safety with client/significant other (SO) according to individual needs:

Prevent accidental ingestion:[3–7,11]
Emphasize importance of supervising infant/child, frail elderly, or individuals with cognitive limitations.
Keep medicines and vitamins out of sight and reach of children or cognitively impaired persons.
Use child-resistant or tamper-resistant caps and lock medication cabinets.
Recap medication containers immediately after obtaining current dosage. Do not leave open container behind. *Note: Many accidental poisonings occur when parent/caregiver steps away for a moment and child gets into product that was left out.*
Code medicines for the visually impaired.
Tell client to turn on light if the room is dark and to put on glasses (if visually impaired) before taking or giving medications.
Refer to/administer children's medications as drugs, not candy, *to prevent confusion.*
Emphasize environmental safety regarding medications for all situations in which young child may be exposed (e.g., all rooms of the home, grandparents' home, day care, preschool).[8]
Discuss vitamin use (especially those containing iron) *that can be poisonous to children if taken in large doses or in small doses over time.*[8–10]

Prevent duplication/possible overdose:[3–7]
Review analgesic safety (e.g., acetaminophen is an ingredient in many OTC medications, and unintentional overdose can occur).[12]
Keep updated list of all medications (prescription, OTC, herbals, supplements) and review with healthcare providers when medications are changed, new ones are added, or new healthcare providers are consulted.
Keep prescription medication in original bottle with label. Do not mix with other medication or place in unmarked containers.
Have responsible SO(s)/home health nurse supervise medication regimen/prepare medications for the cognitively or visually impaired, or obtain prefilled medicine boxes from pharmacy.
Take prescription medications and OTC drugs as prescribed on label.
Do not adjust medication dosage.
Retain and read safety information that accompanies prescriptions about expected effects, nuisance side effects, reportable and adverse affects, and how to manage forgotten dose.

Prevent taking medications that interact with one another or OTC/herbals/other supplements in an undesired or dangerous manner:[3–7]
Keep list of and reveal medication allergies, including type of reaction, to healthcare providers/pharmacist.
Wear medical alert bracelet or necklace, as appropriate.
Do not take outdated or expired medications. Do not save partial prescriptions to use another time.
Encourage discarding outdated or unused drug safely (disposing in hazardous waste collection areas, not down drain or toilet).
Do not take medications prescribed for another person.
Avoid mixing alcohol with medications *(potentiates effects of many drugs).*
Coordinate care when multiple healthcare providers are involved *to limit number of prescriptions and dosage levels.*

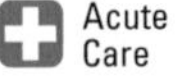

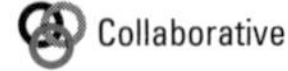

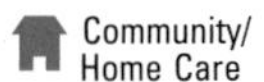

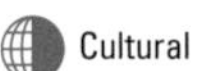

NURSING PRIORITY NO. 3 To promote wellness (Teaching/Discharge Considerations):

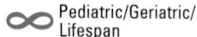

- Discuss general poison-prevention measures:[3–7]
  - Encourage parent/caregiver to place safety stickers on dangerous products (drugs and chemicals) *to warn children of harmful contents.*
  - Teach children about hazards of poisonous substances and to "ask first" before eating or drinking anything.
  - Review drug side effects, potential interactions, and possibilities of misuse or overdosing (as with vitamin megadosing, etc.).[9]
  - Discuss issues regarding drug use in home (e.g., alcohol, marijuana, heroin) *to provide opportunity to address potential for client's/SO's accidental overdose or accidental ingestion by children when drugs or drug paraphernalia are in the home.*[10]
- Provide list of emergency numbers (i.e., local or national poison control numbers, physician's office) to be placed by telephone *for use if poisoning occurs.*
- Instruct caregiver in event of poisoning, to have product container on hand when contacting emergency provider.
- Discuss use of ipecac syrup in home. *The use of ipecac is controversial, as it may delay appropriate medical treatment (e.g., reduce the effectiveness of activated charcoal or oral antidotes) or be used inappropriately with adverse effects. Therefore, use in the home without direct advisement from poison control professionals is not recommended.*[13] *Note: The American Academy of Pediatrics and the American Association of Poison Control Centers no longer recommend that ipecac syrup be stocked at home.*[15]
- Encourage client to obtain regular screening tests at prescribed intervals (e.g., prothrombin time/international normalized ratio for Coumadin; drug levels for Dilantin, digoxin; liver function studies when lipid-lowering agents [statins] are prescribed; renal and thyroid function and serum glucose levels for antimanics [lithium] use) *to ascertain that circulating blood levels are within therapeutic range and absence of adverse effects.*
- Ask healthcare provider/pharmacist about any considered medications if pregnant, nursing, or planning to become pregnant, *as some drugs are dangerous to fetus or nursing infant.*
- Refer substance abuser to detoxification programs, inpatient/outpatient rehabilitation, counseling, support groups, and psychotherapy.
- Encourage participation in community awareness and education programs (e.g., cardiopulmonary resuscitation and first aid class, home and workplace safety, hazardous materials disposal, access emergency medical personnel) *to assist individuals to identify and correct risk factors in environment and be prepared for emergency situation.*

DOCUMENTATION FOCUS

Assessment/Reassessment

- Identified risk factors noting internal and external concerns.
- Drug allergies or sensitivities.
- Current medications prescribed or available to individual, use of OTC medications, herbals or supplements, illicit drug use.

Planning

- Plan of care and who is involved in the planning.
- Teaching plan.

Implementation/Evaluation

- Response to interventions, teaching, and actions performed.
- Attainment or progress toward desired outcome(s).
- Modification to plan of care.

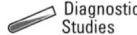

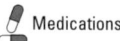

Discharge Planning

- Long-term needs and who is responsible for actions to be taken.
- Specific referrals made.

References

1. Food and Drug Administration. (Updated 2013). FDA committed to addressing growing national overdose problem; various pages. Retrieved March 2015 from hhttp://www.fda.gov/NewsEvents/Newsroom/PressAnnouncements/ucm204962.htm.
2. SafeKids Worldwide. (2013). An in-depth look at keeping young children safe around medications. Retrieved March 2015 from http://issuu.com/safekids/docs/2013-medication-safety-report/1?e=4874392/2095890.
3. Manno, M. S. (2006). Preventing adverse drug events. *Nursing*, 36(3), 56–61.
4. Hayes, B. D., Klein-Schwartz, W., Gonzales, L. F. (2009). Causes of therapeutic errors in older adults: Evaluation of National Poison Center data. *J Am Geriatr Soc*, 57(4), 653–658.
5. Stoppler, M. C. (Updated 2014). Poison proofing your home. Retrieved March 2015 from http://www.emedicinehealth.com/poison_proofing_your_home/article_em.htm.
6. Advance for Nurses. Patient Handouts. Keeping your children safe from accidental poisoning. Retrieved March 2015 from http://nursing.advanceweb.com/article/keeping-your-children-safe-from-accidental-poisoning-html-2.aspx.
7. American Society of Health-System Pharmacists. Preventing accidental poisoning. Retrieved March 2015 from http://www.safemedication.com/safemed/MedicationTipsTools/WhatYouShouldKnow/PreventingAccidentalPoisoning.aspx.
8. Lee, L. Home is where the hurt is? Child proofing your house. Retrieved March 2015 from hhttp://childrenshospitalblog.org/home-is-where-the-hurt-is-tips-for-baby-proofing-your-house/.
9. Hingley, A. T. (2000). Preventing childhood poisoning. Retrieved March 2015 from http://www.kidsource.com/kidsource/content3/fda.poisoning.all.safety.html.
10. Gresham, C., Buller, S. J. (2014). Pediatric single-dose fatal ingestions. Retrieved March 2015 from http://emedicine.medscape.com/article/1011108-overview.
11. National Women's Health Resource Center. (No date). Medication safety (various pages). Retrieved March 2015 from http://www.healthywomen.org/content/article/facts-know-about-medication-safety.
12. Smith, D. H. (2007). Managing acute acetaminophen toxicity. *Nursing*, 37(1), 58–63.
13. Manoguerra, A. S., Cobaugh, D. J. (2005). Guideline on the use of ipecac syrup in the out-of-hospital management of ingested poisons. *Clin Toxicol*, 43(1), 1–10.
14. Zurakowski, T. (2009). The practicalities and pitfalls of polypharmacy. *Nurse Pract*, 34(4), 36–41.
15. National Capital Poison Control Center. (Web site updated 2015). What is ipecac syrup? Retrieved March 2015 from http://www.poison.org/prepared/ipecac.asp.

risk for perioperative Positioning Injury

Taxonomy II: Safety/Protection—Class 2 Physical Injury (00087) [**Diagnostic Division:** Safety], Submitted 1994; Revised 2006, 2013

DEFINITION: Vulnerable to inadvertent anatomical and physical changes as a result of posture or equipment used during an invasive/surgical procedure, which may compromise health.

RISK FACTORS

Disorientation; sensory/perceptual disturbances from anesthesia

Immobilization; muscle weakness; [preexisting musculoskeletal conditions]

Obesity; emaciation; edema

Note: A risk diagnosis is not evidenced by signs and symptoms, as the problem has not occurred; rather, nursing interventions are directed at prevention.

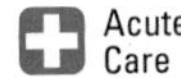

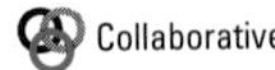

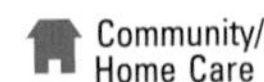

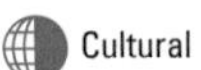

Sample Clinical Applications: Operative procedures, arthritis, obesity, malnutrition, peripheral vascular disease

DESIRED OUTCOMES/EVALUATION CRITERIA

Sample NOC linkages:

Physical Injury Severity: Severity of injuries from accidents and trauma
Risk Control: Personal actions to prevent, eliminate, or reduce modifiable health threats
Tissue Perfusion: Peripheral: Adequacy of blood flow through the small vessels of the extremities to maintain tissue function

Client Will (Include Specific Time Frame)

- Be free of injury related to perioperative disorientation or altered consciousness.
- Be free of untoward skin and tissue injury or changes lasting beyond 24 to 48 hr postprocedure.

ACTIONS/INTERVENTIONS

Sample NIC linkages:

Positioning: Intraoperative: Moving the patient or body part to promote surgical exposure while reducing the risk of discomfort and complications
Skin Surveillance: Collection and analysis of patient data to maintain skin and mucous membrane integrity
Circulatory Precautions: Protection of a localized area with limited perfusion

NURSING PRIORITY NO. 1 To identify individual risk factors/needs:

- Consider anticipated type and length of procedure, type of anesthesia to be used, and customary required position (e.g., supine, lithotomy, prone, lateral, sitting) *to increase awareness of potential postoperative complications. Studies show consensus of clinical opinion that perioperative nerve injury is a significant issue and that safe and correct positioning is crucial to avoid causing peripheral neuropathy during the anesthetic and/or surgical episode. Coppieters et al. (2002) suggest that there is evidence of several identifiable mechanisms that contribute to perioperative positioning injuries. These include stretch, traction, compression, generalized vascular ischemia, and metabolic derangement (e.g., diabetes and atherosclerosis).*[1,2,6,9,12]
- Review client's history, noting age, weight, height, nutritional status, physical limitations (e.g., prostheses, implants, range-of-motion restrictions) and preexisting conditions (vascular, respiratory, circulatory, neurological, immunocompromise). *These factors affect choice of position for the procedure (e.g., elderly person with no subcutaneous padding or severe arthritis). Presence of certain conditions can cause the risk of skin and tissue integrity problems during surgery (e.g., diabetes mellitus, hypertension and hypotension, tobacco use, obesity, presence of peripheral vascular disease, level of hydration, temperature of extremities).*[1,2,8,10,12]
- Evaluate and document client's preoperative reports of neurological, sensory, or motor deficits *for comparative baseline of perioperative and postoperative sensations.*
- Assess the individual's responses to preoperative sedation and medication, noting level of sedation or adverse effects (e.g., drop in blood pressure) and report to surgeon as indicated. *Hypotension is a common factor associated with nerve ischemia.*[3,12]
- Evaluate environmental conditions/safety issues surrounding the sedated client (e.g., client alone in holding area, side rails up on bed and cart, use of tourniquets and arm boards, need for local injections) *that predispose client to potential tissue injury.*[1,3,7,8]

NURSING PRIORITY NO. 2 To position client to provide protection for anatomical structures and to prevent injury:

- Stabilize and lock transport cart or bed when transferring client to and from operating room table. Provide body and limb support for client during transfers, using adequate numbers of personnel *to prevent client fall or shear and friction injuries, as well as to prevent injury to personnel.*[3,8,11]
- Position client, using sufficient staff, appropriate positioning equipment or devices, and padding *to provide protection for anatomic structures and to prevent injury:*[1–3,11]
  - Keep head in neutral position (when client in supine position) and arm boards at less than a 90-degree angle and level with floor *to prevent neural injuries.*
  - Maintain neck alignment and provide protection or padding for forehead, eyes, nose, chin, breasts, genitalia, knees, and feet *when client is in prone position.*
  - Protect bony prominences and pressure points on dependent side (e.g., axillary roll for dependent axilla; lower leg flexed at hip, upper leg straight; padding between knees, ankles, and feet) *when client is in lateral position.*
  - Place legs in stirrups simultaneously, adjusting stirrup height to client's legs, maintaining symmetrical position, and pad popliteal space as indicated *to reduce risk of peroneal and tibial nerve damage, prevent muscle strain, and reduce risk of hip dislocation when lithotomy position is used.*
- Check that positioning equipment is correct size for client, is firm and stable, and is adjusted accordingly.[2,11]
- Use gel pads or similar devices over the operating room bed. *Decreases pressure at any given point by redistributing overall pressure across a larger surface area.*[2,6]
- Limit use of pillows, blankets, molded foam devices, towels, and sheet rolls, *which may produce only a minimum of pressure reduction or contribute to friction injuries.*[2]
- Place safety straps strategically *to secure client for specific procedure.* Avoid pressure on extremities when securing straps *to limit possibility of compromising circulation and pressure injuries.*[11]
- Realign or maintain body alignment during procedure as needed. *Changes in position may expose or damage otherwise protected body tissue. The position change may be planned or imperceptible and may result from adding or deleting positioning devices, adjusting the procedure bed in some manner, or moving the client on the procedure bed.*[2,11]
- Apply and periodically reposition padding of pressure points/bony prominences (e.g., arms, shoulders, ankles) and neurovascular pressure points (e.g., breasts, knees, ears) *to maintain position of safety and prevent injury from prolonged pressure.*
- Protect body from contact with metal parts of the operating table, *which could produce electrical injury or burns.*[1,4]
- Position extremities to facilitate periodic evaluation of hands, fingers, and toes. *Prevents accidental trauma from moving table attachments and allows for repositioning of extremities to prevent neurovascular injuries from prolonged pressure. Extremities should not extend beyond the end of operating table to reduce risk of compression or stretch injury.*[8,11]
- Check peripheral pulses and skin color and temperature periodically *to monitor circulation.*
- Ascertain that eyelids are closed and secured *to prevent corneal abrasions.*
- Prevent pooling of prep and irrigating solutions and body fluids. *Pooling of liquids in areas of high pressure under client increases risk of pressure ulcer development and presents electrical hazard.*[5,6]
- Reposition slowly at transfer and in bed (especially halothane-anesthetized client) *to prevent severe drop in blood pressure, dizziness, or unsafe transfer.*
- Position client following extubation *to protect airway and facilitate respiratory effort.*
- Determine specific postoperative positioning guidelines (e.g., head of bed slightly elevated following spinal anesthesia *to prevent headache,* turn to unoperated side following pneumonectomy *to facilitate maximal respiratory effort*).[1]

NURSING PRIORITY NO. 3 To promote wellness (Teaching/Discharge Considerations):

- Maintain equipment in good working order *to identify potential hazards in the surgical suite and implement corrections as appropriate.*[6]
- Provide perioperative teaching relative to client safety issues (including not crossing legs during procedures performed under local or light anesthesia, postoperative needs or limitations, signs/symptoms requiring medical evaluation) *to reduce incidence of preventable complications.*
- Inform client and postoperative caregivers of expected or transient reactions (e.g., low backache, localized numbness, and reddening or skin indentations, which should quickly resolve) *to help them identify problems or concerns that require follow-up.*
- Assist with therapies and perform nursing actions, including skin care measures, application of elastic stockings, early mobilization *to enhance circulation and venous return, and to promote skin and tissue integrity.*
- Encourage and assist with frequent range-of-motion exercises *to prevent or reduce joint stiffness.*
- Refer to appropriate resources, as needed.

DOCUMENTATION FOCUS

Assessment/Reassessment

- Findings, including individual risk factors for problems in the perioperative setting and need to modify routine activities or positions.
- Periodic evaluation of monitoring activities.

Planning

- Plan of care and who is involved in planning.
- Teaching plan.

Implementation/Evaluation

- Response to interventions and actions performed.
- Attainment or progress toward desired outcome(s).
- Modifications to plan of care.

Discharge Planning

- Long-term needs and who is responsible for actions to be taken.

References

1. Doenges, M. E., Moorhouse, M. F., Murr, A. C. (2010). Surgical intervention. *Nursing Care Plans: Guidelines for Individualizing Client Care Across the Life Span.* 8th ed. Philadelphia, PA: F. A. Davis.
2. Association of Perioperative Registered Nurses. (2001). *AORN Standards and Recommended Practices for Perioperative Nursing.* Denver, CO: AORN.
3. Knight, D. J. W., Mahajan, R. P. (2004). Patient positioning in anaesthesia. *Contin Educ Anaesth Crit Care Pain,* 4(5), 160–163.
4. Rothrock, J. (1996). *Perioperative Nursing Care Planning.* St. Louis, MO: Mosby.
5. Meeker, M., Rothrock, J. (1999). *Alexander's Care of the Patient in Surgery.* 11th ed. St. Louis, MO: Mosby.
6. Dagi, T. F., Schecter, W. (2008). Preparation of the operating room. ACS Surgery: Principles and Practice Online. Retrieved March 2015 from http://www.acssurgery.com/acs/chapters/ch0108.htm.
7. Dunn, D. (2005). Preventing perioperative complications in special populations. *Nursing,* 35(11), 36–43.
8. Dunn, D. (2006). Age-smart care: Preventing perioperative complications in older adults. *Nursing,* 4(3), 30–39.
9. Coppieters, M. W., van de Velde, M., Sappaerts, K. H. (2002). Positioning in anaesthesiology: Toward a better understanding of stretch-induced perioperative neuropathies. *Anesthesiology,* 97, 75–81.

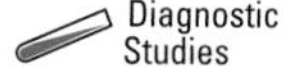
Diagnostic Studies
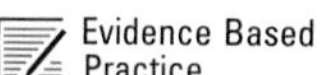
Evidence Based Practice
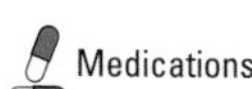
Medications
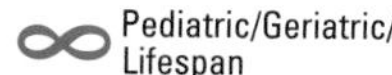
Pediatric/Geriatric/Lifespan

10. Bale, E., Berrecloth, R. (2010). The obese patient. Anaesthetic issues: Airway and positioning. *J Periop Pract*, 8, 294–299.
11. Pirie, S. (2010). Patient care in the preoperative environment. *J Periop Pract*, 8, 294–299.
12. Welch, M. B., Brummett, C. M., Welch, T. D., et al. (2009). Preoperative peripheral nerve injuries: A retrospective study of 380,680 cases during a 10-year period at a single institution. *Anesthesiology*, 111(3), 490–497.

Post-Trauma Syndrome

Taxonomy II: Coping/Stress Tolerance—Class 1 Post-Trauma Responses (00141) [**Diagnostic Division:** Ego Integrity], Submitted 1986; Revised 1998, 2010

DEFINITION: Sustained maladaptive response to a traumatic, overwhelming event.

RELATED FACTORS

Exposure to disaster (natural or man-made); destruction of one's home
Event outside the range of usual human experience; exposure to event involving multiple deaths
Exposure to war; history of being a prisoner of war
History of abuse (e.g., physical, psychological, sexual); history of criminal victimization; history of torture; witnessing mutilation or violent death
Self-injurious behavior
Serious accident (e.g., industrial, motor vehicle); serious injury to loved one
Serious threat to self or loved one

DEFINING CHARACTERISTICS

Subjective

Intrusive thoughts or dreams; nightmares; flashbacks; [repeated verbalization of the traumatic event]
Heart palpitations; headache [loss of interest in usual activities, loss of feeling of intimacy or sexuality]
Hopelessness; shame; guilt; [verbalization of survival guilt or guilt about behavior required for survival]
Anxiety; fear; grieving; depression; horror
Reports feeling numb
Gastrointestinal irritation; [change in appetite]
Alteration in concentration
[Change in sleep; fatigue]

Objective

Alteration in mood; [poor impulse control or explosiveness]; panic attacks
Hypervigilance; exaggerated startle response; irritability; neurosensory irritability
Anger; rage; aggression
Avoidance behaviors; denial; repression; alienation
History of detachment; dissociative amnesia
Substance abuse; compulsive behavior
Enuresis
[Difficulty with interpersonal relationships; dependence on others; work or school failure]
[Stages:
Acute Subtype: Begins within 6 months and does not last longer than 6 months
Chronic Subtype: Lasts more than 6 months
Delayed Subtype: Period of latency of 6 months or more before onset of symptoms]
Sample Clinical Applications: Traumatic injuries, physical/psychological abuse, dissociative disorder

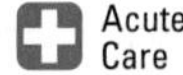

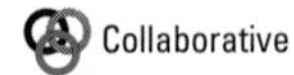

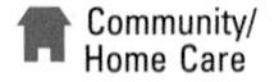

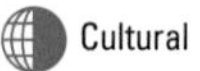

DESIRED OUTCOMES/EVALUATION CRITERIA

Sample NOC linkages:

Comfort Status: Psychospiritual: Psychospiritual ease related to self-concept, emotional well-being, source of inspiration, and meaning and purpose in one's life

Fear Self-Control: Personal actions to eliminate or reduce disabling feelings of apprehension or uneasiness from an identifiable source

Abuse Recovery: Emotional [or] Physical: Extent of healing of psychological/physical injuries due to abuse

Client Will (Include Specific Time Frame)

- Express own feelings and reactions, avoiding projection.
- Verbalize a positive self-image.
- Report reduced anxiety or fear when memories occur.
- Demonstrate ability to deal with emotional reactions in an individually appropriate manner.
- Demonstrate appropriate changes in behavior or lifestyle (e.g., share experiences with others, seek and get support from significant others [SOs] as needed, change in job or residence).
- Report absence of physical manifestations (e.g., pain, chronic fatigue).

ACTIONS/INTERVENTIONS

Sample NIC linkages:

Support System Enhancement: Facilitation of support to patient by family, friends, and community

Counseling: Use of an interactive helping process focusing on the needs, problems, or feelings of the patient and significant others to enhance or support coping, problem solving, and interpersonal relationships

Anxiety Reduction: Minimizing apprehension, dread, foreboding, or uneasiness related to an unidentified source or anticipated danger

NURSING PRIORITY NO. 1 To assess causative factor(s) and individual reaction:

ACUTE

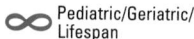

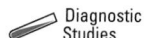

- Observe for and elicit information about physical or psychological injury and note associated stress-related-symptoms (e.g., numbness, headache, tightness in chest, nausea, pounding heart). *Anxiety is viewed as a normal reaction to a realistic danger or threat, and noting these factors can identify the severity of the anxiety the client is experiencing in the circumstances. In posttraumatic stress disorder (PTSD), this reaction is changed or damaged. People who have PTSD may feel stressed or frightened even when they're no longer in danger. Some factors that appear to increase the risk of PTSD are assaultive trauma or trauma that occurs at an early age.*[2,12]
- Identify such psychological responses as anger, shock, acute anxiety, confusion, and denial. Note laughter, crying, calm or agitated, excited (hysterical) behavior, as well as expressions of disbelief, guilt and/or self-blame, and labile emotions. *Indicators of severe response to trauma that client has experienced and need for specific interventions.*[7]
- Assess client's knowledge of and anxiety related to the situation. Note ongoing threat to self (e.g., contact with perpetrator and/or associates) or perception of others as threatening. *Client may be aware but speak as though the incident is related to someone else. Flashbacks may occur with the individual reliving the incident/event.*[7]
- Note occupation (e.g., police, fire, rescue, emergency department staff, corrections officer, mental health worker, disaster responders, soldier or support personnel in combat zone, as well as family members). *These occupations carry a high risk for constantly being involved in traumatic events and the potential for exacerbation of stress response and block to recovery. In addition, family members are subjected to the same trauma*

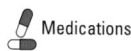

because they see the same events repeated on TV news channels and hear stories repeated by their loved one(s) who were directly involved.[12]

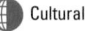

- Identify social aspects of trauma or incident (e.g., disfigurement, chronic conditions or permanent disabilities, loss of home or community) *that affect ability to return to normal involvement in activities and work.*[7]
- Ascertain ethnic background, cultural and religious perceptions, and beliefs about the occurrence. *Client (or significant others) may believe occurrence is retribution from God or result of some indiscretion on client's part; client may in some way also blame self for the incident or occurrence. Individual's view of how he or she is coping may be influenced by cultural and community background, religious beliefs, and family influence.*[3,7]
- Determine degree of disorganization (e.g., task-oriented activity is not goal directed, organized, or effective; individual is overwhelmed by emotion much of the time). *Presence of persistent frightening thoughts and memories, reliving the event, feeling emotionally numb and unable to be close to friends and family members, and suffering from sleep and eating problems interfere with ability to manage daily living, work, and relationships with others.*[7,11]
- Identify whether incident has reactivated preexisting or co-existing situations (physical or psychological). *Traumas or difficulties in client's life and how they were dealt with will affect how the client views the current trauma.*[5]
- Determine disruptions in relationships (e.g., family, friends, coworkers, SOs). *Support persons may not know how to deal with client/situation and may be oversolicitous or withdraw; either of these actions will be counterproductive to client's ability to cope with situation.*[7]
- Note withdrawn behavior, use of denial, and use of chemical substances or impulsive behaviors (e.g., chain smoking, overeating). *Indicators of severity of anxiety and client's difficulty dealing with PTSD and need for interventions to address these behaviors.*[7]
- Be aware of signs of increasing anxiety (e.g., silence, stuttering, inability to sit still). *Increasing anxiety may indicate risk for violence or need for medication or other measures to decrease anxiety and help client manage feelings.*[7]
- Note verbal and nonverbal expressions of guilt or self-blame when client has survived trauma in which others died. Validate congruency of observations with verbalizations. *Sense of own responsibility (blame) and guilt about not having done something to prevent incident or not having been "good enough" to deserve survival are strong beliefs, especially in individuals who are influenced by background, religious, and cultural factors.*[1]
- Assess signs and stage of grieving for self and others. *Identification and understanding of stages of grief assist with choice of interventions, plan of care, and movement toward resolution.*[1]
- Identify development of phobic reactions to ordinary articles (e.g., knives) and situations (e.g., walking in groups of people, strangers ringing doorbell). *These may trigger feelings from original trauma and need to be dealt with sensitively, accepting reality of feelings and stressing ability of client to deal with them.*[1]

CHRONIC (in addition to previous assessment)

- Evaluate continued somatic complaints. Investigate reports of new or changes in symptoms. *Reports of physical symptoms, such as gastric irritation, anorexia, insomnia, muscle tension, and headache may accompany disorganization and need further evaluation and interventions.*[1]
- Note manifestations of chronic pain or pain symptoms in excess of degree of physical injury. *Psychological responses may magnify or exacerbate physical symptoms, indicating need for interventions to help client deal with pain.*[5]
- Be aware of signs of severe or prolonged depression and note presence of flashbacks, intrusive memories, nightmares, panic attacks, and poor impulse control; problems with memory or concentration; thoughts and perceptions; and conflict, aggression, or rage. *Symptoms are not uncommon following a trauma of such magnitude, although client may feel that he or she is "going crazy."*[2,10]
- Assess degree of dysfunctional coping (including substance use or abuse, suicidal ideation) and consequences. *Identifies needs and depth of interventions required. Individuals display different levels of dysfunctional be-*

havior in response to stress, and often the choice of chemical substances or substance abuse is a way of deadening the psychic pain.[1]

NURSING PRIORITY NO. 2 To assist client to deal with situation that exists:

ACUTE

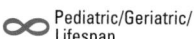

- Allow the client to work through own kind of adjustment. If the client is withdrawn or unwilling to talk, do not force the issue. *Each person is an individual and has own ways of coping. Being there and allowing client to choose own path conveys sense of confidence in ability to deal with situation.*
- Listen for expressions of fear of crowds or people. *May indicate continuing anxiety and difficulty reentering normal activities.*[7]
- Ascertain or monitor sleep pattern of children as well as adults. *Sleep disturbances or nightmares may develop, delaying resolution, impairing coping abilities, and interfering with return to desired lifestyle.*[5]
- Be aware of and assist client to use ego strengths in a positive way by acknowledging ability to handle what is happening. *Enhances self-concept and reduces sense of helplessness and powerlessness, thus enabling client to move on with life.*
- Encourage client to learn stress-management techniques, such as deep breathing, meditation, relaxation, and exercise. *Reduces stress, enhancing coping skills and helping to resolve situation.*[8]
- Assist in dealing with practical concerns and effects of the incident, such as court appearances, altered relationships with SO(s), and employment problems. *In the period immediately following the traumatic incident, individual is in a state of numbness and shock. Thinking becomes difficult, and assistance with practical matters will help manage necessary activities for the person to move through this time.*
- Identify employment and community resource groups. *Provides opportunity for ongoing support to deal with recurrent stressors as individual regroups and moves forward.*[9]
- Administer anti-anxiety or sedative and hypnotic medications with caution.

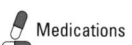

CHRONIC

- Continue listening to expressions of concern. *May have recurring symptoms, thus necessitating the need to continue talking about the incident.*[7]
- Permit free expression of feelings (may continue from the crisis phase). Do not rush client through expressions of feelings too quickly and refrain from providing false reassurances. *Client may believe pain or anguish is misunderstood and may be depressed. Statements such as "You don't understand" or "You weren't there" are a defense—a way of pushing others away—and need to be responded to with empathy and concern.*
- Encourage client to talk out experience when ready, expressing feelings of fear, anger, loss, or grief. (Refer to NDs Grieving and complicated Grieving.) *Client may need to repeat story over and over and needs to be accepted and assured that feelings are normal for the unusual event experienced.*[7]
- Note whether feelings expressed appear congruent with events the client experienced. *Expressing feelings helps client recognize and identify them to enhance coping. Incongruency may indicate deeper conflict that can impede resolution.*[8]
- Encourage client to become aware and accepting of own feelings and reactions as being normal reactions in an abnormal situation. *There are no "bad" feelings, and awareness and acceptance enable client to deal with feelings once identified and move forward in recovery from traumatic event.*[4,11]
- Acknowledge reality of loss of self that existed before the incident. Assist client to move toward an acceptance of the potential for growth that exists within client. *Recognition that individual can never go back to being the person he or she was before the incident allows progress toward life as a different person.*[8]
- Continue to allow client to progress at own pace. *Taking own time to talk about what has happened and allowing feelings to be fully expressed aids in the healing process. If rushed, client may believe he or she is not accepted or understood.*[1]
- Give "permission" to express and deal with anger at the assailant or situation in acceptable ways. *Being free to express anger appropriately allows it to be dissipated so underlying feelings can be identified and dealt with, thus strengthening coping skills.*[1]

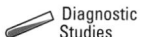

- Avoid prompting discussion of issues that cannot be resolved. Keep discussion on practical and emotional level rather than intellectualizing the experience. *When feelings (the experience) are intellectualized, uncomfortable insights and/or awareness are avoided by the use of rationalization, blocking resolution of feelings and impairing coping abilities.*[1]
- Provide for sensitive, trained counselors/therapists and engage in therapies, such as psychotherapy in conjunction with medications, implosive therapy (flooding), hypnosis, relaxation, Rolfing, memory work, cognitive restructuring, eye movement desensitization and reprocessing, and physical and occupational therapies. *Although it is not necessary for the helping person to have experienced the same kind of trauma as the client, sensitivity and listening skills are important to helping the client confront fears and learn new ways to cope with what has happened. Therapeutic use of desensitization techniques (flooding, implosive therapy) provides for extinction through exposure to the fear. Body work can alleviate muscle tension. Some techniques (Rolfing) help to bring blocked emotions to awareness as sensations of the traumatic event are reexperienced.*[7]
- Discuss use of psychotropic medication. *May be used to decrease anxiety, lift mood, aid in management of behavior, and ensure rest until client regains control of own self. Lithium may be used to reduce explosiveness; low-dose psychotropics may be used when loss of contact with reality is a problem.*[6]

NURSING PRIORITY NO. 3 To promote wellness (Teaching/Discharge Considerations):

- Assist client to identify and monitor feelings while therapy is occurring. *Promotes awareness and helps client know that control of feelings as they arise will help move beyond traumatic episode.*[7]
- Provide information about what reactions client may expect during each phase. Let client know these are common reactions and phrase in neutral terms of "You may or may not. . . ." *Knowledge of what may be experienced helps reduce fear of the unknown, thereby enabling client to manage reactions if they occur. Use of neutral terms lets client understand that not all reactions may occur in own situation.*
- Assist client to identify factors that may have created a vulnerable situation and that he or she may have power to change to protect self in the future. *While client is not responsible for event, may have unknowingly contributed to occurrence by his or her actions. Identifying those actions that are within client's power to change provides sense of control over seemingly uncontrollable situations.*[7]
- Avoid making value judgments. *Client may be judging self and caregiver needs to convey nonjudgmental stance to allow individual to deal with feelings of guilt and recrimination, accepting fact that he or she did the best client was capable of in the circumstances.*
- Discuss lifestyle changes client is contemplating and how they may contribute to recovery. *Client needs to evaluate appropriateness of plans and look at long-range consequences (e.g., moving away from effective support group) to make the best choice for the future.*[2]
- Assist with learning stress-management techniques. *Deep breathing, counting to 10, reviewing the situation, and reframing skills assist client in developing constructive ways to cope with feelings of powerlessness and to regain control of self. Reframing stressors or situation in other words or positive ideas can help client recognize and consider alternatives.*[2]
- Discuss drug regimen, potential side effects of prescribed medications, and necessity of prompt reporting of untoward effects.
- Discuss recognition of and ways to manage "anniversary reactions," reinforcing normalcy of recurrence of thoughts and feelings at this time. *Understanding that these feelings are to be expected and planning for them help client get through the anniversary of the event with the least difficulty.*
- Suggest support group for SO(s). *Family members may not understand client's reactions and need help with understanding them and learning how to deal with client in the most helpful manner.*[1]
- Encourage psychiatric consultation. *May need additional therapy if client is unable to maintain control, is violent or inconsolable, or does not seem to be making an adjustment. Participation in a group may be helpful.*[1]
- Refer for long-term family/marital counseling, if indicated. *Additional and ongoing support or therapy may be needed to help family resolve crisis and look at potential for growth. Client problems affect family*

Acute Care

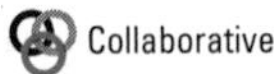
Collaborative

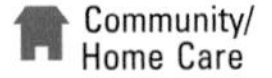
Community/ Home Care

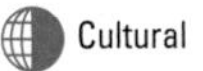
Cultural

members and other relationships, and further counseling may help resolve issues of enabling behavior and communication problems.[9]
- Refer to NDs ineffective Coping, Grieving, complicated Grieving and Powerlessness.

DOCUMENTATION FOCUS

Assessment/Reassessment
- Individual findings, noting current dysfunction and behavioral or emotional responses to the incident.
- Specifics of traumatic event.
- Reactions of family/SO(s).
- Cultural or religious beliefs and expectations.
- Availability and use of resources.

Planning
- Plan of care and who is involved in the planning.
- Teaching plan.

Implementation/Evaluation
- Responses to interventions, teaching, and actions performed.
- Emotional changes.
- Attainment or progress toward desired outcome(s).
- Modifications to plan of care.

Discharge Planning
- Long-term needs and who is responsible for actions to be taken.
- Specific referrals made.

References

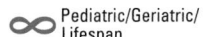

1. Doenges, M., Townsend, M., Moorhouse, M. (1998). *Psychiatric Care Plans: Guidelines for Individualizing Care*. 3rd ed. Philadelphia, PA: F. A. Davis.
2. Townsend, M. (2003). *Psychiatric Mental Health Nursing: Concepts of Care*. 4th ed. Philadelphia, PA: F. A. Davis.
3. Purnell, L. D. (2009). *Guide to Culturally Competent Health Care*. 2nd ed. Philadelphia, PA: F. A. Davis.
4. Stuart, G. W. (2001). Anxiety responses and anxiety disorders. In Stuart, G. W., Laraia, M. T. (eds). *Principles and Practice of Psychiatric Nursing*. 7th ed. St. Louis, MO: Mosby.
5. Porth, C. M., Kunert, P. K. (2002). *Pathophysiology: Concepts of Altered Health States*. Philadelphia, PA: J. B. Lippincott.
6. Townsend, M. (2001). *Nursing Diagnoses in Psychiatric Nursing: Care Plans and Psychotropic Medications*. 5th ed. Philadelphia, PA: F. A. Davis.
7. National Institute of Mental Health. (2009). Anxiety disorders. NIH Publication No. 00-3879. Retrieved April 2015 from http://www.nimh.nih.gov/health/publications/anxiety-disorders/index.shtml?rf=53414.
8. Posttraumatic stress disorder—Part I. (June 1996). *Harvard Mental Health Letter*.
9. Posttraumatic stress disorder—Part II. (July 1996). *Harvard Mental Health Letter*.
10. Gore, T. A., Lucas, J. Z. (Updated 2014). Posttraumatic stress disorder: Treatment and management. Retrieved April 2015 from http://emedicine.medscape.com/article/288154-treatment.
11. Lubit, R. (Updated 2014). Acute treatment of disaster survivors. Retrieved April 2015 from http://emedicine.medscape.com/article/2192581-overview.
12. Breslau, N. (2009). The epidemiology of trauma, PTSD, and other posttrauma disorders. *Trauma Violence Abuse*, 10(3), 198–210.

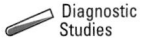

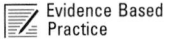

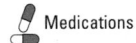

risk for Post-Trauma Syndrome

Taxonomy II: Coping/Stress Tolerance—Class 1 Post-Trauma Responses (00145) [**Diagnostic Division:** Ego Integrity], Submitted 1986; Revised 1998, 2013

DEFINITION: Vulnerable to sustained maladaptive response to a traumatic, overwhelming event, which may compromise health.

RISK FACTORS

Diminished ego strength; environment not conducive to needs; insufficient social support
Displacement from home
Duration of traumatic event; perceives event as traumatic; survival role
Exaggerated sense of responsibility
Human service occupations (e.g., police, fire, rescue, corrections, emergency room, mental health)
Note: A risk diagnosis is not evidenced by signs and symptoms, as the problem has not occurred; rather, nursing interventions are directed at prevention.
Sample Clinical Applications: Traumatic injuries, physical/psychological abuse, dissociative disorder

DESIRED OUTCOMES/EVALUATION CRITERIA

Sample NOC linkages:
Fear Level: Severity of manifested apprehension, tension, or uneasiness arising from an identifiable source
Fear Self-Control: Personal actions to eliminate or reduce disabling feelings of apprehension and tension from an identifiable source
Grief Resolution: Adjustment to actual or impending loss

Client Will (Include Specific Time Frame)

- Verbalize absence of disabling apprehension.
- Demonstrate ability to deal with emotional reactions in an individually appropriate manner.
- Deal with practical aspects of situation (e.g., court appearances, temporary housing, funeral services, rebuilding life).
- Report relief or absence of physical manifestations (pain, nightmares, flashbacks, fatigue) associated with event.

ACTIONS/INTERVENTIONS

Sample NIC linkages:
Crisis Intervention: Use of short-term counseling to help the patient cope with a crisis and resume a state of functioning comparable to or better than the precrisis state
Coping Enhancement: Assisting a patient to adapt to perceived stressors, changes, or threats which interfere with meeting life demands and roles
Support System Enhancement: Facilitation of support to patient by family, friends, and community

NURSING PRIORITY NO. 1 To assess contributing factors and individual reaction:

- Identify client who survived or witnessed traumatic event (e.g., airplane or motor vehicle crash, mass shooting, fire destroying home and lands, robbery at gunpoint, other violent act) *to recognize individual at high risk for posttrauma syndrome.*
- Note occupation (e.g., police, fire, emergency services personnel, rescue workers, disaster responders, soldiers and support personnel in combat areas, and family members). *Studies reveal a moderate to high percentage of*

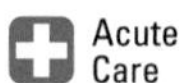

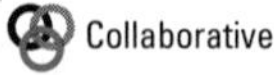

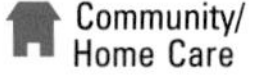

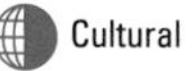

posttraumatic stress disorder (PTSD) cases develop in these populations when they have been exposed to one or more traumatic incidents and their exposure lasts over longer periods of time (e.g., working a bomb site or plane crash).[10] *In addition, family members are also at risk because they are subjected to the same trauma as they see the events repeated on TV news channels/hear stories repeated by their loved one(s) who were directly involved.*

- Assess client risk for developing PTSD using screening tool (e.g., Breslau Short Screening Scale or similar) should client report experiencing a traumatic event. *Short self-report questionnaire or other screening tool with simple "yes" or "no" responses may help with early identification of client at risk for posttrauma response. Recognizing symptoms and providing immediate treatment may prevent the development of PTSD.*[12]
- Assess client's knowledge of and anxiety related to potential for work-related trauma incident (e.g., shooting in line of duty or viewing body of murdered child); and number, duration, and intensity of recurring situations (e.g., emergency medical technician exposed to numerous on-the-job traumatic incidents; rescuers searching for victims of natural or man-made disasters). *Having information about these situations enables individuals to think about and plan for eventualities so anxiety can be dealt with in a positive manner.*[6]
- Ascertain ethnic background and cultural or religious perceptions and beliefs about the occurrence. *Client may believe occurrence is retribution from God, the result of some indiscretion on his or her part, or in some way blame self for the incident or occurrence. Individual's view of how he or she is coping may be influenced by cultural background, religious beliefs, and family influence.*[6]
- Identify how client's experiences may affect current situation. *Individual who has had previous experiences with traumatic events (e.g., firefighter who deals with trauma on a regular basis or person who has been involved in a trauma herself or himself) may be more susceptible to PTSD and ineffective coping abilities.*[1]
- Listen for comments of guilt, humiliation, shame, or taking on responsibility (e.g., "I should have been more careful/gone back to get her"; "Don't call me a hero; I couldn't save my partner"; "My kids are the same age as the ones who died"). *Expressing guilt for actions that individual might have taken can lead to ruminations about lack of responsible behavior, leading to anxiety and PTSD.*[7,10,11]
- Note verbal and nonverbal expressions of guilt or self-blame when client has survived trauma in which others died. *Sense of own responsibility (blame) and guilt about not having done something to prevent incident or not having been "good enough" to deserve surviving are strong beliefs, especially in individuals who are influenced by family background, religious, and cultural factors.*[1]
- Evaluate for life factors and stressors currently or recently occurring, such as displacement from home due to catastrophic event (e.g., illness or injury, fire, flood, violent storm, earthquake) happening to individual whose child is dying of cancer or who suffered abuse as a child. *Cumulative effects of multiple events can put the individual at higher risk for developing PTSD (acute added to delayed-onset reactions) and indicates need for preventive measures to be taken.*[3,10]
- Identify client's coping mechanisms. *Resolution of the posttrauma response is largely dependent on the coping skills the client has developed throughout own life and is able to bring to bear on current situation.*[3]
- Determine availability and usefulness of client's support systems, family, social, community, etc., being aware that family members themselves or community in general may also be at risk. *Having an effective available support system and talking with them about what is happening can help client and family members resolve feelings and move on with life in a positive manner.*[8]

NURSING PRIORITY NO. 2 To assist client to deal with situation that exists immediately postincident:

POSTINCIDENT

- Provide a calm, safe environment. *Client can deal with disruption of life more effectively when surrounded by quiet and by knowing he or she is safe.*[9]
- Assist with documentation for police report, as indicated, and stay with the client. *Developing accurate chain of evidence (maintaining sequencing and collection of evidence) and labeling each specimen and storing and packaging it properly provides important evidence for possibility of future prosecution.*[1]

- Listen to and investigate physical complaints. *Physical injuries may have occurred during incident, which may be masked by emotional reactions and limit client's ability to recognize them. These need to be identified and differentiated from anxiety symptoms so appropriate treatment may be instituted.*[1]
- Identify supportive persons (e.g., loved ones, spiritual advisor or pastor). *Having unconditional support from loving and caring others can help the client cope with the situation and move on to live more fully.*[1]
- Remain with client, listen as client recounts incident and concerns—possibly repeatedly. If client does not want to talk, accept silence. *Establishes trust, thus providing psychological support and allowing client opportunity to vent emotions.*[3]
- Encourage expression of feelings and reinforce that feelings and reactions to trauma are common and not indicators of weakness or failure. Note whether feelings expressed appear congruent with events the client experienced. *Expressing feelings helps client recognize and identify them to enhance coping. Incongruency may indicate deeper conflict that can impede resolution.*[6]
- ∞ Help child to express feelings about event using techniques appropriate to developmental level (e.g., play for young child, stories or puppets for preschooler, peer group for adolescent). *Children are more likely to express in play what they may not be able to verbalize directly. Adolescents may benefit from groups, gaining knowledge, support, decreased sense of isolation, and improved coping skills.*[2]
- Assist with practical realities (e.g., temporary housing, money, notifications of family members, other needs). *Dealing with these issues is necessary and helps client remain connected to reality and maintain sense of control over daily living concerns.*[1]

NURSING PRIORITY NO. 3 To assist client to deal with situation that exists:

- Evaluate client's perceptions of events and personal significance (e.g., police officer who is also a parent and is investigating death of a child). *Individuals perceive events depending on their previous experiences, cultural and religious background, and family of origin and will respond to any given trauma based on these factors. Incidents that touch a person's own life will be more difficult to deal with and may have a deeper effect.*[2]
- Provide emotional and physical presence *to strengthen client's coping abilities. Spending time with the client promotes trust and provides an opportunity for client to think about what will help in the current situation.*[3]
- Observe for signs and symptoms of stress responses, such as nightmares, reliving an incident, poor appetite, irritability, numbness and crying, and family and relationship disruption. *These responses are normal in the early postincident time frame. If prolonged and persistent, the client may be experiencing PTSD.*[7]
- Identify and discuss client's strengths (e.g., very supportive family, usually copes well with stress) as well as vulnerabilities (e.g., client tends toward alcohol or other drugs for coping, client has witnessed a murder). *Knowing one's strengths and weaknesses helps client know what actions to take to cope with and prevent anxiety from becoming overwhelming.*[7]
- Discuss how individual coping mechanisms have worked in past traumatic events. *Awareness of previous successful experiences can help client remember coping skills that can be used to deal with current situation in a positive manner.*[3]

NURSING PRIORITY NO. 4 To promote wellness (Teaching/Discharge Considerations):

- Educate high-risk persons and families about signs/symptoms of posttrauma response, especially if it is likely to occur in their occupation or life. *Awareness allows individual to be proactive and seek support and timely intervention as needed.*
- Encourage client to identify and monitor feelings on an ongoing basis. *Promotes awareness of changes in ability to deal with stressors, allowing prompt intervention when necessary.*[4]
- Encourage learning stress-management techniques, such as deep breathing, meditation, relaxation, and exercise. *Reduces stress, enhancing coping skills and helping to resolve situation.*[5]
- Recommend participation in debriefing sessions that may be provided following major events. *Dealing with the stressor promptly may facilitate recovery from event and prevent exacerbation. Debriefing is being used by*

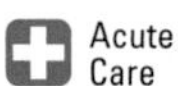
Acute Care
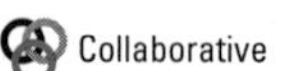
Collaborative
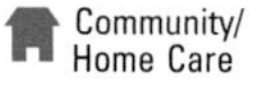
Community/ Home Care
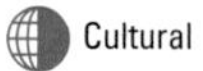
Cultural

many organizations who regularly deal with traumatic events to prevent the development of PTSD, although issues about best timing of debriefing continue to be debated.[3]

- Explain that posttraumatic symptoms can emerge months or sometimes years after a traumatic experience and that help or support can be obtained when needed or desired if client begins to experience intrusive memories or other symptoms.
- Encourage individual to develop a survivor mentality. *People often have it within their means to head off life-threatening situations and even survive the worst when they plan for emergencies and think ahead about ways to survive, such as taking food, water, and protective gear on a day hike in case you get lost, fall and break a bone, or in other ways have to spend more time than anticipated.*[9]
- Identify employment and community resource groups (e.g., Assistance Support and Self Help in Surviving Trauma, employee peer assistance programs, Red Cross or other survivor support services, Compassionate Friends). *Provides opportunity for ongoing support to deal with recurrent stressors as individual moves on with life.*[11]
- Refer for individual or family counseling, as indicated. *May need additional assistance to prevent continuation of anxiety and the onset of PTSD.*[6]

DOCUMENTATION FOCUS

Assessment/Reassessment

- Identified risk factors noting internal and external concerns.
- Client's perception of event and personal significance.
- Cultural or religious beliefs and expectations.

Planning

- Plan of care and who is involved in the planning.
- Teaching plan.

Implementation/Evaluation

- Response to interventions, teaching, and actions performed.
- Attainment or progress toward desired outcome(s).

Discharge Planning

- Long-term needs and who is responsible for actions to be taken.
- Specific referrals made.

References

1. Doenges, M., Townsend, M., Moorhouse, M. (1998). *Psychiatric Care Plans: Guidelines for Individualizing Care.* 3rd ed. Philadelphia, PA: F. A. Davis.
2. American Psychological Association Act Against Violence Project. (No date). *When Children Experience Trauma: A Guide for Parents and Families.* Washington, DC: American Psychological Association.
3. Townsend, M. (2003). *Psychiatric Mental Health Nursing: Concepts of Care.* 4th ed. Philadelphia, PA: F. A. Davis.
4. Stuart, G. W. (2001). Anxiety responses and anxiety disorders. In Stuart, G. W., Laraia, M. T. (eds). *Principles and Practice of Psychiatric Nursing.* 7th ed. St. Louis, MO: Mosby.
5. Porth, C. M., Kunert, P. K. (2002). *Pathophysiology: Concepts of Altered Health States.* Philadelphia, PA: J. B. Lippincott.
6. National Institute of Mental Health. (2009). Anxiety disorders. NIH Publication No. 02-3879. Retrieved April 2015 from http://www.nimh.nih.gov/health/publications/anxiety-disorders/index.shtml?rf=53414.
7. Posttraumatic stress disorder—Part I. (June 1996). *Harvard Mental Health Letter.*
8. Posttraumatic stress disorder—Part II. (July 1996). *Harvard Mental Health Letter.*
9. Kamier, K. (2004). *Surviving the Extremes: A Doctor's Journey to the Limits of Human Endurance.* Boston, MA: St. Martin's.

10. Davis, N. (2002). [Brief summaries from] Multi-Sensory Trauma Processing, A Manual for Understanding and Treating PTSD and Job-Related Trauma. Retrieved April 2015 from http://www.stevedavis.org/sol1art19.html.
11. Galea, S., Nandi, A., Vlahov, D. (2005). The epidemiology of post-traumatic stress disorders after disasters. *Epidemiol Rev*, 27(1), 78–91.
12. Kimerling, R., Ouimette, P., Prins, A., et al. (2006). Brief report: Utility of a short screening scale for DSM-IV PTSD in primary care. *J Gen Intern Med*, 21(1), 65–67.

readiness for enhanced Power

Taxonomy II: Coping/Stress Tolerance—Class 2 Coping Responses (00187) [**Diagnostic Division:** Ego Integrity], Submitted 2006; Revised 2013

DEFINITION: A pattern of participating knowingly in change for well-being, which can be strengthened.

DEFINING CHARACTERISTICS

Subjective

Expresses desire to enhance: power; knowledge for participation in change; awareness of possible changes; identification of choices that can be made for change

Expresses desire to enhance: independence with actions for change; involvement in change; participation in choices for daily living or health

[Note: Even though power (a response) and empowerment (an intervention approach) are different concepts, the literature related to both concepts supports the defining characteristics of this diagnosis.]

Sample Clinical Applications: Any acute or chronic condition, or healthy individual looking to change life/improve well-being

DESIRED OUTCOMES/EVALUATION CRITERIA

Sample NOC linkages:

Personal Autonomy: Personal actions of a competent individual to exercise governance in life decisions

Health Promoting Behavior: Personal actions to sustain or increase wellness

Health Beliefs: Perceived Control: Personal conviction that one can influence a health outcome

Client Will (Include Specific Time Frame)

- Verbalize knowledge of what changes he or she wants to make.
- Express awareness of own ability to be in charge of changes to be made.
- Participate in classes or group activities to learn new skills.
- State readiness to take power over own life.

ACTIONS/INTERVENTIONS

Sample NIC linkages:

Self-Modification Assistance: Reinforcement of self-directed change initiated by the patient to achieve personally important goals

Decision-Making Support: Providing information and support for a person who is making a decision regarding healthcare

Health System Guidance: Facilitating a patient's location and use of appropriate health services

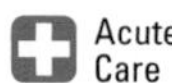

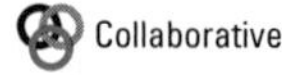

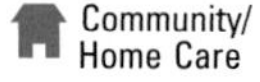

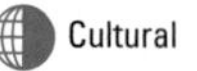

NURSING PRIORITY NO. 1 To determine need/motivation for improvement:

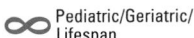

- Determine current situation and circumstances that client is experiencing, leading to desire to improve life. *Provides information to help client with planning for enhancing life.*[8]
- Ascertain motivation and expectations for change. *Motivation to improve and high expectations can encourage client to make changes that will improve his or her life. However, unrealistic expectations or motivation to please someone else may hamper efforts.*[7]
- Identify emotional climate in which client and relationships live and work. *The emotional climate has a great impact between people. When a power differential exists in relationships, the atmosphere is largely determined by the person or people who have the power.*[4]
- Identify client locus of control: internal (expressions of responsibility for self and ability to control outcomes) or external (expressions of lack of control over self and environment). *Understanding locus of control can help client to work toward positive, internal control as he or she develops sense of ability to freely choose own actions.*[9]
- Determine cultural factors or religious beliefs influencing client's self-view. *These factors can be strong determinants in individual's ability to change and view self as powerful and may complicate growth process.*[9]
- Assess degree of mastery client has exhibited in his or her life. *Helps client to understand how he or she has functioned in the past, how that applies to current situation, and what is needed to improve.*[6]
- Note presence of family/significant others that can or do act as support systems for client. *When family understands and supports client's desires and efforts, he or she is more likely to be successful.*[6]
- Determine whether client knows or uses assertiveness skills. *Learning and enhancing these skills will help client to improve ability to take personal responsibility for own self and relationships with others.*[1,3,5,7]

NURSING PRIORITY NO. 2 To assist client to clarify needs relative to ability to improve feelings of power:

- Discuss how client is currently involved in creating change in life. *Provides a baseline to measure growth and suggests possibilities for change.*[8]
- Active listen to client's perceptions and beliefs about the concept of power. *Enables client to identify underlying feelings and thoughts about this issue and how power can be gained in his or her life.*[8]
- Identify strengths, assets, and past coping strategies that were successful. *These strategies can be built on to enhance feelings of control.*[6]
- Discuss the importance of assuming personal responsibility for life and relationships. *This requires one to be open to new ideas and experiences, different values, and beliefs and to be inquisitive.*[7]
- Identify things client can and or cannot control. *Avoids wasting time on things that are not in the control of the client.*[8]
- Treat expressed desires and decisions with respect. Avoid critical parenting expressions. *Individual may express thoughts and opinions that are creative and out of the ordinary, and critical parenting responses such as "That's a dumb idea" can crush person's brainstorming.*[9]

NURSING PRIORITY NO. 3 To promote optimum wellness, enhancing power (Teaching/Discharge Considerations):

- Assist client to set realistic goals for the future. *Even though client is thinking creatively and brainstorming ideas, goals need to be planned step by step to reach the desired outcome.*[6]
- Provide accurate verbal and written information about client's concerns and life situation. *Reinforces learning and promotes self-paced review.*[8]
- Assist client to learn/use assertive communication skills. *These techniques require practice, but as the client becomes more proficient, they will help to develop relationships that are more effective.*[2,3]
- Use "I" messages instead of "You" messages. *"I" messages acknowledge ownership of what is said, whereas "You" messages suggest the other person is wrong or bad, fostering resentment and resistance instead of understanding and cooperation.*[8]

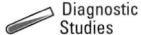

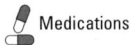

- Discuss importance of client paying attention to nonverbal communication. *Messages are often confusing or misinterpreted when verbal and nonverbal communications are not congruent.*[9]
- Help client learn to problem-solve differences. *Problem-solving process allows for each person involved to have input and promotes win-win solutions.*[8]
- Instruct and encourage use of stress-reduction techniques. *Relaxation helps individual to function more effectively, thus enhancing feelings of power.*[9]
- Refer to support groups or classes, as indicated, assertiveness training, and effectiveness for women to "be your best." *Provides role models and allows individuals to learn from one another, thereby promoting problem solving and enhancing learning.*[7]

DOCUMENTATION FOCUS

Assessment/Reassessment

- Individual findings, noting determination to improve sense of power, locus of control.
- Motivation and expectations for change.
- Cultural or religious beliefs affecting self-view.
- Locus of control.

Planning

- Plan of care, specific interventions, and who is involved in planning.
- Teaching plan.

Implementation/Evaluation

- Client's responses to interventions, teaching, and actions performed.
- Attainment or progress toward desired outcome(s).
- Modifications to plan of care.

Discharge Planning

- Long-term needs and who is responsible for actions to be taken.
- Specific referrals made.

References

1. Lifestrong Contributor. (No date). Improving assertive behavior. Retrieved November 2015 from http://www.livestrong.com/article/14699-improving-assertive-behavior/.
2. Hopkins, L. (2005). Assertive communication: 6 Tips for effective use. Retrieved November 2015 from http://ezinearticles.com/?Assertive-Communication---6-Tips-For-Effective-Use&id=10259.
3. Dombeck, M., Wells-Morgan, J. (Updated 2006). Setting boundaries appropriately: Assertiveness training. Retrieved November 2015 from http://www.mentalhelp.net/articles/setting-boundaries-appropriately-assertiveness-training/.
4. Adams, L. (2011). Climate—The emotional one, that is. Retrieved November 2015 from http://www.gordontraining.com/free-workplace-articles/climate-the-emotional-one-that-is/.
5. Adams, L. (2011). Being a leader doesn't make you one. Retrieved November 2015 from http://www.gordontraining.com/free-workplace-articles/being-a-leader-doesnt-make-you-one/.
6. (No author listed). Assertiveness: What is assertiveness? Retrieved November 2015 from http://www.mtstcil.org/skills/assert-2.html.
7. Gordon, T. (2011). Families need rules. Retrieved November 2015 from http://www.gordontraining.com/free-parenting-articles/families-need-rules/.
8. Clinebell, H. J. (1981). Growth resources in transactional analysis. *In Contemporary Growth Therapies.* Nashville, TN: Abingdon Press.
9. Thompson-Tormaschy, T. (Retrieved 2013). What's the big deal about "I"-Messages? Retrieved November 2015 from http://psychcentral.com/lib/2007/whats-the-big-deal-about-i-messages/.

Powerlessness

Taxonomy II: Coping/Stress Tolerance—Class 2 Coping Responses (00125) [**Diagnostic Division:** Ego Integrity], Submitted 1982; Revised 2010

DEFINITION: The lived experience of lack of control over a situation, including a perception that one's own actions do not significantly affect an outcome.

RELATED FACTORS

Dysfunctional institutional environment
Insufficient interpersonal interactions
Complex treatment regimen

DEFINING CHARACTERISTICS

Subjective

Alienation; shame
Depression
Doubt about inability to perform previous activities; insufficient sense of control

Objective

Dependency
Inadequate participation in care

Sample Clinical Applications: Chronic or debilitating conditions (e.g., chronic obstructive pulmonary disease [COPD], multiple sclerosis [MS]), cancer, spinal cord injury [SCI], major depressive disorder, somatization disorders; post-traumatic stress; sexual assault

DESIRED OUTCOMES/EVALUATION CRITERIA

Sample NOC linkages:

Personal Autonomy: Personal actions of a competent individual to exercise governance in life decisions
Health Beliefs: Perceived Control: Personal conviction that one can influence a health outcome
Participation in Health Care Decisions: Personal involvement in selecting and evaluating healthcare options to achieve desired outcomes

Client Will (Include Specific Time Frame)

- Express sense of control over the present situation and hopefulness about future outcome.
- Verbalize positive self-appraisal in current situation.
- Make choices related to and be involved in care.
- Identify areas over which individual has control.
- Acknowledge reality that some areas are beyond individual's control.

ACTIONS/INTERVENTIONS

Sample NIC linkages:

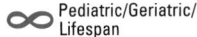

Self-Responsibility Facilitation: Encouraging a patient to assume more responsibility for own behavior
Health System Guidance: Facilitating a patient's location and use of appropriate health services
Decision-Making Support: Providing information and support for a person who is making a decision regarding healthcare

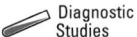

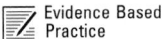

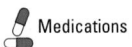

NURSING PRIORITY NO. 1 To assess causative/contributing factors:

- Identify situational circumstances (e.g., strange environment, immobility, diagnosis of terminal or chronic illness, lack of support system(s), lack of knowledge about situation) affecting the client at this time. *Knowing the specific situation of the client is essential to planning care and empowering the individual.*[4]
- Determine client's perception and knowledge of condition and treatment plan. *Identifying how client views and understands what is happening and what the plan of care entails is essential to begin to help client feel empowered.*[2]
- Ascertain client response to treatment regimen. Does client see reason(s) for and understand it is in the client's interest or is client compliant and helpless? *The manner in which the individual responds to the treatment indicates the depth of feelings of powerlessness and may interfere with progress.*[4]
- Identify client locus of control—internal (expressions of responsibility for self and ability to control outcomes—"I didn't quit smoking") or external (expressions of lack of control over self and environment—"Nothing ever works out"; "What bad luck to get lung cancer"). *Locus of control is a term used in reference to an individual's sense of mastery or control over events. Individuals view life change and stressful events differently. Those with internal locus of control tend to be more optimistic about their ability to deal with adversity even in the face of current difficulties. Individuals with external locus of control may attribute feelings of powerlessness to an external source perceiving it as beyond his or her control and will look to others to solve problems and take care of them.*[4,9]
- Note cultural or religious factors that may contribute to how client views self and is handling current situation. *One's values and beliefs may dictate gender roles and the individual's expectations of control, influencing the client's belief in ability to manage situation, participate in decision making, and direct own life.*[9,11]
- Assess degree of mastery client has exhibited in life. *How this individual has dealt with problems throughout life will help to understand feelings of powerlessness client is feeling during this crisis.*[4,5]
- Determine if there has been a change in relationships with significant others (SOs). *Conflict in relationships may be contributing to sense of powerlessness. Domestic violence situations often leave the individuals involved feeling powerless to change what is happening.*[4]
- Note availability/use of resources. *Client who has few options for assistance or who is not knowledgeable about how to use resources needs to be given information and assistance to know how and where to seek help.*[3]
- Investigate healthcare providers and personal caregiver practices to determine if they support client control and responsibility. *Caregivers who do for the client what he or she is able to do for own self diminish client's sense of control. When client is given as much control over self as possible, sense of power is regained.*[3]

NURSING PRIORITY NO. 2 To assess degree of powerlessness experienced by the client:

- Listen to statements client makes, such as "They don't care," "It won't make any difference," and "Are you kidding?" [2]
- Note expressions that indicate "giving up," such as "It won't do any good." *May indicate suicidal intent, indicating need for immediate evaluation and intervention.*[6]
- Note behavioral responses (verbal and nonverbal), including expressions of fear, interest or apathy, agitation, and withdrawal. *These responses can show depth of anxiety, feelings of powerlessness over what is happening, and indicate need for intervention to help client begin to look at situation with some sense of hope.*[6]
- Note lack of communication, flat affect, and lack of eye contact. *May indicate more severe state of mind, such as a psychotic episode, and need for immediate evaluation and treatment.*[4]
- Identify the use of manipulative behavior and reactions of client and caregivers. *Manipulation is used for management of powerlessness because of distrust of others, fear of intimacy, search for approval, and validation of sexuality.*[1,9]

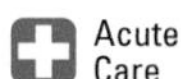
Acute Care
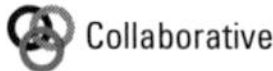
Collaborative
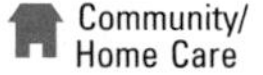
Community/ Home Care
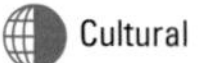
Cultural

NURSING PRIORITY NO. 3 To assist client to clarify needs relative to ability to meet them:

- Show concern for client as a person. *Communicates value of the individual, enhancing self-esteem.*[8]
- Active-listen to client's perceptions and concerns and encourage questions. *Provides time for client to explore views and understand what is happening in order to come to some decisions about situation, enhancing sense of control.*[8,10]
- Accept expressions of feelings, including anger and hopelessness. *Communicates empathy and understanding of reality of those feelings and provides a point of discussion to move toward sense of control.*[4]
- Avoid arguing or using logic with hopeless client. *Client will not accept that anything can make a difference. Arguing denies client's reality and may impede client-nurse relationship.*[2]
- Deal with manipulative behavior by being straightforward and honest with your communication and letting client know that this is a better way to get needs met. *When client makes a commitment to stop using manipulation in life, steps can be taken to recognize the behaviors and feelings and begin to change them. Keeping a journal can help to identify these issues.*[9]
- Express hope for the client. *Although client may not accept expressions of hope, there is always hope of something, and when options are explored, client may begin to see there is hope.*[8]
- Identify strengths, assets, and past coping strategies that were successful. *Helps client to recognize own ability to deal with difficult situation, providing sense of power.*[5]
- Assist client to identify what he or she can do for self. Identify things the client can and cannot control. *Accomplishing something can provide a sense of control and helps client understand that there are things he or she can manage. Accepting that some things cannot be controlled helps client to stop wasting efforts and refocus energy.*[1]
- Encourage client to maintain a sense of perspective about the situation. *Discussing ways client can look at options and make decisions based on which ones will be best leads to the most effective solutions for situation.*[6]

NURSING PRIORITY NO. 4 To promote independence:

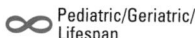

- Use client's locus of control to develop individual plan of care. *Tailoring care to the individual's ability will maximize effectiveness. For instance, client with internal control can take control of own care, and client with external control may need to begin with small tasks and add as tolerated, moving toward learning to take more control of care.*[6]
- Develop contract with client specifying goals agreed on. *When client is involved in planning, commitment to plan is enhanced, optimizing outcomes.*[2]
- Treat expressed decisions and desires with respect. Avoid critical parenting behaviors. *Listening to client and accepting what is said, no matter what the content, helps client hear own words and begin to process information and feelings. Comments that are heard as critical or condescending will block communication and growth.*[1,10]
- Provide client opportunities to control as many events as energy and restrictions of care permit. *Promotes sense of control over situation and helps client begin to feel more confident about own ability to manage what is happening.*[6,7]
- Discuss needs openly with client and set up agreed-on routines for meeting identified needs. *Minimizes use of manipulation. Manipulative behavior is often used to influence others to do what the person thinks he or she should do. Usually this results in defensiveness or outright rebellion against what is suggested, resulting in lack of trust and withdrawal on the part of the person being manipulated.*[9]
- Minimize rules and limit continuous observation to the degree that safety permits. *Provides sense of control for the client while maintaining a safe environment for the client.*[6]
- Support client efforts to develop realistic steps to put plan into action, reach goals, and maintain expectations. *Noting progress that is being made can provide a sense of control and diminish sense of powerlessness.*[6]
- Provide positive reinforcement for desired behaviors. *In behavioral therapy, the belief that when a behavior reinforces another behavior, the second behavior will recur is called a "positive reinforcer," and the function is called "positive reinforcement." By providing this reinforcement, the desired behaviors are more likely to continue.*[4]

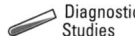

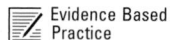

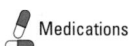

- Direct client's thoughts beyond present state to future when appropriate. *Focusing on possibilities in small steps can help the client see that there can be hope in small things each day.*[1,8]
- Schedule frequent and regular contacts to check on client, deal with client needs, and let client know someone is available. *Communicates caring and concern for client and needs, reinforcing sense of worthiness.*[1]
- Involve SO(s) in client care as desired or appropriate. *Personal involvement by supportive family members can help client see the possibilities for resolving problems related to feelings of powerlessness.*[6]

NURSING PRIORITY NO. 5 To promote wellness (Teaching/Discharge Considerations):

- Instruct in and encourage use of anxiety- and stress-reduction techniques. *Most individuals react to stress in predictable physiological and psychological ways. Feelings of powerlessness related to client's situation can be relieved by use of these techniques.*[5]
- Provide accurate verbal and written information about what is happening and discuss with client/SO(s). Repeat as often as necessary. *Providing information in different modalities allows better access and opportunity for increased understanding. People do not always hear every piece of information the first time it is presented because of anxiety and inattention, so repetition helps to fill in the missed information.*[6]
- Assist client to set realistic goals for the future. *Provides opportunity for client to decide what direction is desired and to gain confidence from completion of each goal.*[10]
- Assist client to learn and use assertive communication skills. *Practicing a new way of expressing thoughts and requests provides the client with a skill to achieve desires and improve relationships.*[10]
- Facilitate return to a productive role in whatever capacity possible for the individual. Refer to occupational therapist or vocational counselor as indicated. *Feelings of powerlessness may result from inability to engage in or resume previous activities, and learning new ways to be productive enhances self-esteem and reduces feelings of powerlessness.*[6]
- Encourage client to think productively and positively and take responsibility for choosing own thoughts. *Negative thinking can result in feelings of powerlessness, and learning to use positive thinking can reverse this pattern, promoting feelings of control and self-worth.*[6]
- Model problem-solving process with client/SO(s). *Learning a problem-solving method that results in a win-win solution improves family relationships and promotes feelings of self-worth in those involved.*[10]
- Suggest client periodically review own needs and goals. *It is easy to become discouraged as time goes on, and reviewing, thinking about needs, and how previously set goals are relevant in the present helps to either renew those goals or develop new goals to meet current situation.*[6,8]
- Refer to support groups, counseling or therapy, etc., as indicated. *May need additional assistance to resolve current problems, long-standing issues, or troubled relationships.*[4]

DOCUMENTATION FOCUS

Assessment/Reassessment

- Individual findings, noting degree of powerlessness, locus of control, individual's perception of the situation.
- Specific cultural or religious factors.
- Availability and use of support system and resources.

Planning

- Plan of care and who is involved in the planning.
- Teaching plan.

Implementation/Evaluation

- Responses to interventions, teaching, and actions performed.
- Specific goals and expectations.
- Attainment or progress toward desired outcome(s).
- Modifications to plan of care.

Discharge Planning

- Long-term needs and who is responsible for actions to be taken.
- Specific referrals made.

References

1. Jordon, D. (2009). "We were powerless over our addiction": Why the first step is so controversial. Retrieved April 2015 from http://www.sunshinecoasthealthcentre.ca/2009/08/powerlessness-addiction/.
2. Bradford Health. (No date). The power of admitting powerlessness. Retrieved April 2015 from https://bradfordhealth.com/power-admitting-powerlessness/.
3. Messina, J. J. (2008). Enabling personality. Retrieved April 2015 from http://www.livestrong.com/article/14675-enabling-personality/.
4. Blackwell, A. (2009). Five powerful ways to regain control of your life. Retrieved April 2015 from http://www.thebridgemaker.com/five-powerful-ways-to-regain-control-of-your-life-now/.
5. Messina, J. J. (2011). Accepting powerlessness. Retrieved April 2015 from http://www.jamesjmessina.com/toolsforcontrolissues/acceptpowerlessness.html.
6. Beaumont, L. R. (2009). Developing the essential social skills to recognize, interpret and respond constructively to yourself and others. Retrieved April 2015 from http://emotionalcompetency.com/.
7. National Institute of Mental Health. (2002). Generalized anxiety disorder (GAD). Retrieved April 2015 from http://www.nimh.nih.gov/health/topics/generalized-anxiety-disorder-gad/index.shtml.
8. Neeld, E. H. (2003). Finding daylight after loss shatters your world. *Seven Choices*. New York, NY: Grand Central Publishing.
9. Messina, J. J. (2010). Eliminating manipulation: Tools for handling control issues. Retrieved April 2015 from http://jamesjmessina.com/toolsforcontrolissues/eliminatemanipulation.html.
10. Bolstadt, R., Hamblett, M. (1997). Win-win. Retrieved April 2015 from http://www.nlpca.com/DCweb/winwin.html.
11. Purnell, L. D. (2011). *Guide to Culturally Competent Health Care*. 2nd ed. Philadelphia, PA: F. A. Davis.

risk for Powerlessness

Taxonomy II: Coping/Stress Tolerance—Class 2 Coping Responses (00125) [**Diagnostic Division:** Ego Integrity], Submitted 2000; Revised 2010; 2013

DEFINITION: Vulnerable to the lived experience of lack of control over a situation, including a perception that one's actions do not significantly affect an outcome, which may compromise health.

RISK FACTORS

Anxiety; ineffective coping strategies; low self-esteem
Caregiver role
Economically disadvantaged
Illness; progressive illness; unpredictability of illness trajectory; pain
Insufficient knowledge to manage a situation
Insufficient social support; social marginalization; stigmatization
Note: A risk diagnosis is not evidenced by signs and symptoms, as the problem has not occurred; rather, nursing interventions are directed at prevention.

Sample Clinical Applications: New or unexpected diagnoses, chronic or debilitating conditions (e.g., chronic obstructive pulmonary disease [COPD], MS), cancer, SCI, major depressive disorder, somatization disorders

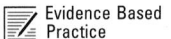

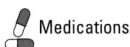

(continues on page 650)

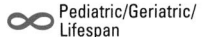

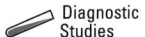

risk for Powerlessness (continued)

DESIRED OUTCOMES/EVALUATION CRITERIA

Sample NOC linkages:

Personal Autonomy: Personal actions of a competent individual to exercise governance in life decisions
Health Beliefs: Perceived Control: Personal conviction that one can influence a health outcome
Participation in Health Care Decisions: Personal involvement in selecting and evaluating healthcare options to achieve desired outcome

Client Will (Include Specific Time Frame)

- Express sense of control over the present situation and hopefulness about future outcomes.
- Verbalize positive self-appraisal in current situation.
- Make choices related to and be involved in care.
- Identify areas over which individual has control.
- Acknowledge reality that some areas are beyond individual's control.

ACTIONS/INTERVENTIONS

Sample NIC linkages:

Self-Responsibility Facilitation: Encouraging a patient to assume more responsibility for own behavior
Health System Guidance: Facilitating a patient's location and use of appropriate health services
Decision-Making Support: Providing information and support for a person who is making a decision regarding healthcare

NURSING PRIORITY NO. 1 To assess causative/contributing risk factors:

- Identify situational circumstances (e.g., acute illness, sudden hospitalization, diagnosis of terminal or debilitating or chronic illness, very young or aging with decreased physical strength and mobility, lack of knowledge about illness, healthcare system). *Necessary information to develop individualized plan of care for client.*[1]
- Determine client's perception and knowledge of condition and proposed treatment plan. *Identifying how client views and understands what is happening and what the plan of care entails is essential to help client feel empowered.*[7]
- Identify client's locus of control—internal (expressions of responsibility for self and ability to control outcomes—"I didn't quit smoking") or external (expressions of lack of control over self and environment—"Nothing ever works out," "What bad luck to get lung cancer"). *Locus of control is a term used in reference to an individual's sense of mastery or control over events. Individuals view life change and stressful events differently. Those with internal locus of control tend to be more optimistic about their ability to deal with adversity even in the face of current difficulties. Individuals with external locus of control may attribute feelings of powerlessness to an external source, perceiving it as beyond his or her control, and will look to others to solve problems and take care of them.*[4,10]
- Note cultural or religious factors that may contribute to how client views self and is handling current situation. *One's values and beliefs may dictate gender roles and the individual's expectations of control, influencing the client's belief in ability to manage situation, participate in decision making, and direct own life.*[9,10]
- Assess client's self-esteem and degree of mastery client has exhibited in life situations. *Provides clues to client's ability to see self as in control and deal with current situation.*[7]
- Note availability and use of resources, relationship with significant other (SO)/family and degree of support provided to client. *Presence of support system and ability to use resources appropriately facilitates problem solving, enhancing sense of control. Client who has few options for assistance or who is not knowledgeable about how to use resources needs to be given information and assistance to know how and where to seek help.*[3]

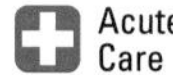

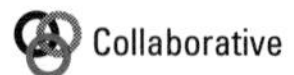

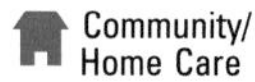

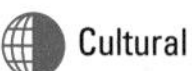

- Listen to statements client makes that might indicate feelings of possibility of loss of control (e.g., "They don't care," "It won't make a difference," "It won't do any good"). *Indicators of sense of powerlessness and hopelessness and need for specific interventions to provide sense of control over what is happening.*[4]
- Determine congruency of responses (verbal and nonverbal) and note expressions of fear, disinterest or apathy, or withdrawal. *These responses can show depth of anxiety over what is happening and indicate need for intervention to help client begin to look at situation with sense of hope.*[5]
- Be alert for signs of manipulative behavior and note reactions of client and caregivers. *Manipulation may be used for management of powerlessness because of fear and distrust.*[4,10]

NURSING PRIORITY NO. 2 To assist client to clarify needs and ability to meet them:

- Show concern for client as a person. Encourage questions. *Communicates value of the individual, enhancing self-esteem. Questions may reveal lack of information or concerns client may have.*[8]
- Make time to listen to client's perceptions of the situation as well as concerns. *Provides time for client to explore views and understand what is happening to come to some decisions about situation, enhancing sense of control.*[5]
- Accept expressions of feelings, including anger and reluctance to try to work things out. *Communicates unconditional regard for the client and encourages individual to think about options even though situation may be difficult.*[5]
- Express hope for client and encourage review of past experiences with successful strategies. *Provides an opportunity for person to remember and accept that he or she has managed difficult situations before and can apply these strategies in current situation.*[4]
- Assist client to identify what he or she can do to help self and what situations cannot be controlled. *Accomplishing something can provide a sense of control and helps client understand that there are things he or she can manage. Accepting that some things cannot be controlled helps client to stop wasting efforts and refocus energy.*[1,2]

NURSING PRIORITY NO. 3 To promote wellness (Teaching/Discharge Considerations):

- Encourage client to be active in own healthcare management and to take responsibility for choosing own actions and reactions. *Discussing ways client can look at options and make decisions based on which ones will be best leads to the most effective solutions for situation.*[6,7]
- Involve client/SO(s) in planning process, using client's locus of control. *Tailoring care to the individual's ability will maximize effectiveness. For instance, client with internal control can take control of own care, and client with external control may need to begin with small tasks and add as tolerated, moving toward learning to take more control of care.*[6]
- Model problem-solving process with client and SOs. *Learning a problem-solving method that results in a win-win solution improves family relationships and promotes feelings of self-worth in those involved.*[8]
- Support client efforts to develop realistic steps to put plan into action, reach goals, and maintain expectations. *Noting progress that is being made can enhance sense of control.*[6]
- Provide accurate instructions in various modalities (e.g., verbal, written, audiovisual, Web sites) about what is happening and what realistically might happen. *Providing information in different formats allows better access and opportunity for increased understanding to support decision-making process.*[6]
- Identify resource books or classes for assertiveness training and stress reduction, as appropriate. *Reinforces learning and promotes self-paced review.*[8]
- Suggest client periodically review own needs and goals. *Reviewing needs and how previously set goals are relevant in the present helps to either renew those goals or develop new goals to meet current situation.*[5]
- Refer to support groups for chronic conditions or disability (e.g., Multiple Sclerosis Society, Easter Seals, Alzheimer's, Al-Anon) or counseling or therapy, as appropriate. *May need additional assistance to manage difficulties of current situation.*[4]

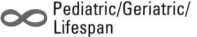

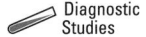

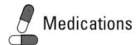

DOCUMENTATION FOCUS

Assessment/Reassessment

- Individual findings, noting potential for powerlessness, locus of control, individual's perception of the situation.
- Cultural values or religious beliefs.
- Locus of control.
- SO/family involvement and support.
- Availability and use of resources.

Planning

- Plan of care and who is involved in the planning.
- Teaching plan.

Implementation/Evaluation

- Responses to interventions, teaching, and actions performed.
- Specific goals and expectations.
- Attainment or progress toward desired outcomes.
- Modifications to plan of care.

Discharge Planning

- Long-term needs and who is responsible for actions to be taken.
- Specific referrals made.

References

1. Sandman, P. (October-November 1987). Explaining risks to non-experts: A communications challenge. *Emergency Preparedness Digest*, 25–29.
2. Herbert, W. (2009). Try a little powerlessness: The pitfalls of self control. *Sci Am Mind*. Retrieved April 2015 from http://www.scientificamerican.com/article.cfm?id=try-a-little-powerlessness.
3. Reilly, P., DiGiovanna, J. J. (2004). Retinoid prevention in high-risk skin cancer patients: Coping with cancer. Retrieved April 2015 from http://www.medscape.com/viewarticle/474868_2.
4. Messina, J. J. (2008). Letting go uncontrollables and unchangables. Retrieved April 2015 from http://www.livestrong.com/article/14701-letting-go-uncontrollables-and-unchangables/.
5. Olson, K. A (Reviewed 2013). Children and a natural disaster: From fear to hope. Retrieved April 2015 from http://www.extension.umn.edu/family/tough-times/disaster-recovery/from-fear-to-hope.html.
6. Kartha, D. (Updated 2012). 6 Steps to decision-making. Retrieved April 2015 from http://www.buzzle.com/articles/6-steps-to-decision-making-process.html.
7. National Institute of Mental Health. Anxiety disorders. (2009). Retrieved April 2015 from http://www.nimh.nih.gov/health/topics/anxiety-disorders/index.shtml.
8. Matta, C. (2012). *The Stress Response: How Dialectical Behavior Therapy Can Free You from Needless Anxiety, Worry, Anger & Other Symptoms of Stress*. Oakland, CA: New Harbinger Publications, Inc.
9. Minority Nurse Staff. (Updated 2013). Culture, grief and bereavement: Applications for clinical practice. *Minority Nurse*. Retrieved April 2015 from http://www.minoritynurse.com/culture-grief-and-bereavement-applications-clinical-practice.
10. Messina, J. J. (no date). Eliminating manipulation: Tools for handling control issues. Retrieved April 2015 from http://jamesjmessina.com/toolsforcontrolissues/eliminatemanipulation.html.

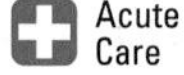

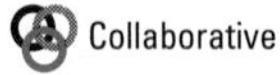

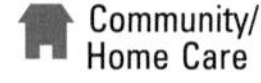

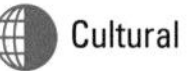

risk for Pressure Ulcer

Taxonomy II: Safety/Protection—Physical Injury 00249) [**Diagnostic Division:** Safety], Submitted 2013

DEFINITION: Vulnerable to localized injury to the skin and/or underlying tissue usually over a bony prominence as a result of pressure, or pressure in combination with shear (National Pressure Ulcer Advisory Panel [NPUAP, 2007]).

RISK FACTORS

ADULT: Braden scale score of <18
CHILD: Braden scale score of ≤ 16
American Society of Anesthesiologists (ASA) Physical Status classification sore ≥ 2
Low score on Risk Assessment Pressure Sore (RAPS) scale
Alteration in cognitive functioning
Alteration in sensation; decrease in mobility; extended period of immobility on hard surface (e.g., surgical procedure ≥ 2 hours)
Anemia; decrease in tissue oxygenation or perfusion; impaired circulation; lymphopenia
Cardiovascular disease; history of cerebral vascular accident
Dehydration; dry or scaly skin; skin moisture; edema
Elevated skin temperature by 1–2°C; hyperthermia
Extremes of age or weight
Female gender
Hip fracture; history of trauma; physical immobilization
History of pressure ulcer
Inadequate nutrition; reduced triceps skin fold thickness; decrease in serum albumin
Incontinence
Insufficient caregiver knowledge of pressure ulcer prevention
Nonblanchable erythema; pressure over bony prominence
Pharmaceutical agents (e.g., vasopressors, antidepressnt, norepinephrine)
Self-care deficit
Shearing forces; friction
Use of linen with insufficient moisture wicking property
Smoking
NOTE: A risk diagnosis is not evidenced by signs and symptoms, as the problem has not occurred; rather, nursing interventions are directed at prevention.
Sample Clinical Applications: Para/quadriplegia; diabetes mellitus; obesity; CVA, coma, dementia; amputation; burns; peripheral vascular disease, thrombophlebitis

DESIRED OUTCOMES/EVALUATION CRITERIA

Sample NOC linkages:
Tissue Integrity: Skin and Mucous Membranes: Structural intactness and normal physiological function of skin and mucous membranes
Risk Control: Personal actions to prevent, eliminate, or reduce modifiable health threats
Immobility Consequences: Physiological: Severity of compromise in physiological functioning due to impaired physical mobility

Client Will (Include Specific Time Frame)

- Display and maintain healthy skin in risk areas (e.g., bony prominences, skin folds) during time in care facility.

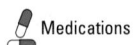

(continues on page 654)

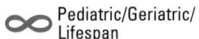

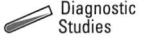

risk for Pressure Ulcer (continued)

- Participate in prevention measures and treatment program.
- Verbalize understanding of risk factors and when to contact healthcare provider.
- Demonstrate behaviors or lifestyle changes to improve circulation (e.g., engage in regular exercise, cessation of smoking, weight reduction, disease management).

Client/Caregiver Will (Include Specific Time Frame)

- Participate in prevention measures.

ACTIONS/INTERVENTIONS

Sample NIC linkages:

Skin Surveillance: Collection and analysis of patient data to maintain skin and mucous membrane integrity

Pressure Management: Minimizing pressure to body parts

Pressure Ulcer Prevention: Prevention of pressure ulcers for a patient at high risk for developing them

NURSING PRIORITY NO. 1 To assess risk and contributing factors:

- Identify presence of underlying condition that increases risk of pressure ulcer. *Skin integrity problems can be the result of (1) disease processes that affect circulation and perfusion of tissues (e.g., arteriosclerosis, venous insufficiency, hypertension, obesity, diabetes, malignant neoplasms), (2) medications (e.g., vasopressors, antidepressants; anticoagulants, corticosteroids, immunosuppressives, antineoplastics) that adversely affect or impair healing, (3) burns or radiation (can break down internal tissues as well as skin), and (4) nutrition and hydration (e.g., malnutrition deprives the body of protein and calories required for cell growth and repair, dehydration impairs transport of oxygen and nutrients).*[1–3]
- Evaluate client's risk for developing pressure ulcer upon admission to care, using Braden risk scale (or similar scale per facility policy) as listed above. *Using susceptibility factors of sensory perception, skin moisture, activity, mobility, nutritional status, friction, and shear potential, the client's risk can be quickly determined. Note: Research is ongoing (and unclear) as to whether use of these scales is validated (i.e., whether scales predict outcomes better than clinician's clinical judgment) and whether incidence of pressure ulcers is reduced given the results obtained from scales.*[9–11]
- Determine client's age and developmental factors affecting skin/tissue health. *One of the structural differences in an infant's skin is that the skin cells are smaller and thinner than an adult's skin, which can result in a weakened barrier to the environment. Infants are also predisposed to a dry, flaky, and impaired skin barrier.*[12] *However, studies have shown that similar to adult patients, acutely ill infants and children are at risk for pressure ulcers. The negative effect of immobility and physiological instability on a patient's skin does not discriminate on age or developmental level.*[13] *In older adults, there are often comorbid conditions (e.g., end-stage renal disease, diabetes, peripheral vascular impairment), as well as decreased epidermal regeneration; fewer sweat glands; and less subcutaneous fat, elastin, and collagen, causing skin to become thinner, drier, and less responsive to pain sensations.*[1,3–5]
- Note skin color discoloration (e.g., nonblanchable erythema; persistent red, blue, or purple hues) in pressure areas *suggestive of impaired tissue health. Note: It may be necessary in a darker-skinned individual to focus more on other evidence of pressure ulcer development, such as bogginess, induration, coolness, or increased warmth, as well as signs of skin discoloration.*[5]
- Note presence of compromised mobility, sensation, vision, hearing, or speech *that may impact client's self-care as relates to skin and pressure area care.*[3]
- Ascertain current medication regimen. *Individual may be receiving medications that affect wound healing (e.g., vasopressors, anticoagulants, immunosuppressives, antineoplastics) and that can adversely affect the skin.*
- Review laboratory results (e.g., hemoglobin/hematocrit, blood glucose, blood and/or wound culture and sensitivities for infectious agents [viral, bacterial, fungal], albumin, prealbumin, transferrin, protein) *to evaluate for potential risk factors or ability to heal. Note: Albumin less than 3.5 correlates to decreased wound healing and increased incidence of pressure ulcers.*[1,6,14]

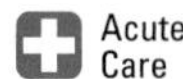

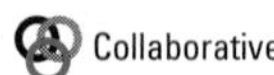

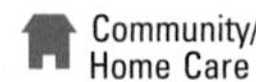

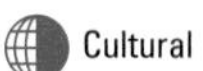

NURSING PRIORITY NO. 2 To maintain optimal skin/tissue integrity :[5,7,8,15]

- Monitor for incontinence, changing diapers, briefs, padding, and bedding as needed. *Maintains skin that is clean, dry, and free of contaminants that can cause/exacerbate skin/tissue breakdown.*
- Develop regularly timed repositioning schedule for client with mobility and sensation impairments; encourage or assist with periodic weight shifts for client in chair *to reduce stress on pressure points and to promote circulation to tissues.*
- Use proper turning and transfer techniques and sufficient personnel when repositioning client. *Avoids movements that cause friction or shearing (e.g., pulling client with parallel force, dragging movements).*
- Use appropriate padding or pressure-reducing devices (e.g., egg crate, gel pads, heel rolls, or foam boots) or pressure-relieving devices (e.g., air or water mattress) when indicated *to reduce pressure on sensitive areas and enhance circulation.*
- Participate in practices that prevent medical device related-pressure ulcers:
  Choose the correct size of medical device(s) (e.g., endotracheal tube [ET], other tubings, anti-embolism stocking, splints) to fit the individual.
  Remove or move the device daily to assess skin.
  Avoid placement of device(s) over sites of prior or existing pressure ulceration.
  Cushion and protect skin with cushioning in high-risk areas (e.g., nasal bridge, ears, sacrum, heels, occipital area of head in infants/small children).
  Educate other care providers about client's devices and interventions for prevention of skin breakdown.
- Provide optimum nutrition (including adequate protein, lipids, calories, trace minerals, and multivitamins [e.g., A, C, D, E]) *to promote skin and tissue health and to maintain general well-being.* Refer to nutritionist as indicated.
- Provide adequate hydration (e.g., oral, tube feeding, IV, ambient room humidity) *to reduce and replenish transepidermal water loss.*

NURSING PRIORITY NO. 3 To promote wellness (Teaching/Discharge Considerations) :

- Encourage regular inspection and monitoring of skin for changes or failure to heal. *Early detection and reporting to healthcare providers promotes timely evaluation and intervention.*
- Encourage good nutrition, adequate hydration, early and ongoing mobility, and range-of-motion and strengthening exercises *to enhance circulation and promote health of skin and other organs.*
- Discuss proper and safe use of equipment or appliances (e.g., heating pad, ostomy appliances, padding straps of braces).
- Encourage abstinence from smoking, *which causes vasoconstriction, impairing circulation.*

DOCUMENTATION FOCUS

Assessment/Reassessment

- Individual findings, including specific risk factors, status of skin, and ability to manage/direct own care.

Planning

- Plan of care and who is involved in planning.
- Teaching plan.

Implementation/Evaluation

- Responses to interventions, teaching, and actions performed.
- Attainment or progress toward desired outcome(s).
- Modifications to plan of care.

Discharge Planning

- Long-term needs and who is responsible for actions to be taken.
- Specific referrals made.

References

1. Llewellyn, S. (2002). *Skin integrity and wound care (lecture materials).* Chapel Hill, NC: Cape Fear Community College Nursing Program.
2. Colburn, L. (2001). Prevention for chronic wounds. In Krasner, D., Rodeheaver, G., et al. (eds). *Chronic Wound Care: A Clinical Source Book for Health-care Professionals.* 2nd ed. Wayne, PA: HMP Communications.
3. LeBlanc, K., Baranoski, S. (2009). Prevention and management of skin tears. *Adv Skin Wound Care,* 22(7), 325–332.
4. Lund, C. H., Osborne, J. W., Culler, J. (2001). Neonatal skin care: Clinical outcomes of the AWHONN/NANN evidence-based clinical practice guideline. *J Neonatal Nurs,* 30(1), 30–40.
5. National Pressure Ulcer Advisory Panel. (2014). Prevention and treatment of pressure ulcers: Clinical practice guideline. Retrieved January 2015 from http://www.npuap.org/resources/educational-and-clinical-resources/prevention-and-treatment-of-pressure-ulcers-clinical-practice-guideline/.
6. Catania, K., Huang, C., James, P., et al. (2007). PUPPI: The pressure ulcer prevention protocol interventions. *Am J Nurs,* 107(4), 44–51.
7. Reddy, M., Gill, S. S., Rochan, P. A. (2006). Preventing pressure ulcers: A systematic review. *JAMA,* 296(8), 974–984.
8. Wadland, D. L. (2010). Maintaining skin integrity in the OR. *OR Nurse 2011,* 4(2), 26–32.
9. Stotts, N. A., Gunningberg, L. (2007). How to try this: Predicting pressure ulcer risk. *Am J Nurs,* 107(11), 40–48.
10. Pancorbo-Hildago, P. L., Garcia-Fernandez, F. P., Lopez-Medina, I. M., et al. (2006). Risk assessment scales for pressure ulcer prevention: A systematic review. *J Adv Nurs,* 54(1), 94–110.
11. Kottner, J., Dassen, T., Lopez-Medina, I. M. (2010). Pressure ulcer risk assessment in critical care: Interrater reliability and validity studies of the Braden and Waterlow scales and subjective ratings in two intensive care units. *Int J Nurs Stud,* 47(6), 671–677.
12. Blume-Peytavi, U., Hauser, M., Pathirana, D, et al. (2012). Skin care practices for newborns and infants: Review of the clinical evidence for best practices. *Pediatric Dermatology,* 29(1), 1–14.
13. Curley, M. A., Razmus, I. S., Roberts, K. E., et al. (2003). Predicting pressure ulcer risk in pediatric patients: The Braden Q Scale. *Nurs Res,* 52(1), 22–33.
14. Kinman, C. N. (2014). Pressure ulcers and wound care. Retrieved January 2015 from http://emedicine.medscape.com/article/190115-overview.
15. Schober-Flores, C. (2012). Pressure ulcers in the pediatric population. *JDNA,* 4(5), 295–306.

ineffective Protection

Taxonomy II: Health Promotion—Class 2 Health Management (00043) [**Diagnostic Division:** Safety], Submitted 1990

DEFINITION: Decrease in the ability to guard self from internal or external threats such as illness or injury.

RELATED FACTORS

Extremes of age
Inadequate nutrition
Substance abuse
Abnormal blood profiles [e.g., leukopenia, thrombocytopenia, anemia]
Pharmaceutical agents [e.g., antineoplastic, corticosteroid, immune, thrombolytic]
Treatment regimen
Cancer; immune disorder (e.g., HIV-associated neuropathy, varicella-zoster virus)

DEFINING CHARACTERISTICS

Subjective

Neurosensory impairment
Chilling
Itching

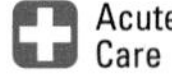 Acute Care 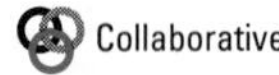 Collaborative 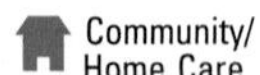 Community/ Home Care 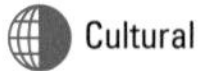 Cultural

Insomnia; fatigue; weakness
Anorexia

Objective
Deficient immunity
Impaired healing; alteration in clotting
Maladaptive stress response
Alteration in perspiration
Dyspnea; coughing
Restlessness; immobility
Disorientation
Pressure ulcer

Sample Clinical Applications: Cancer, AIDS, systemic lupus, substance abuse, tuberculosis, dementia, Alzheimer's disease, anorexia or bulimia nervosa, diabetes mellitus, thrombophlebitis, conditions requiring long-term steroid use (e.g., chronic obstructive pulmonary disease [COPD], asthma, renal failure), major surgery

Author's note: The purpose of this diagnosis seems to combine multiple NDs under a single heading for ease of planning care when a number of variables may be present. It is suggested that the user refer to specific NDs based on identified related factors and individual concerns for this client to find appropriate outcomes and interventions that are specifically tied to individual related factors that are present, such as the following:

Extremes of age: Includes concerns regarding body temperature or thermoregulation; memory or sensory-perceptual alterations; impaired mobility, risk for falls, sedentary lifestyle, or self-care deficits; risk for trauma, suffocation, or poisoning; and risk for skin or tissue integrity and fluid volume imbalances.

Inadequate nutrition: Brings up issues of nutrition and unstable blood glucose; risk for infection and delayed surgical recovery; impaired swallowing; impaired skin or tissue integrity; and trauma, problems with coping, and interrupted family processes.

Substance abuse: May be situational or chronic with problems ranging from impaired respirations, decreased cardiac output, impaired liver function, and fluid volume deficits to nutritional problems, infection, trauma, risk for self- or other-directed violence, and coping or family process difficulties.

Abnormal blood profile: Suggests possibility of fluid volume imbalances, decreased tissue perfusion, problems with oxygenation, activity intolerance, or risk for infection or injury.

Pharmaceutical agents, and treatment-related side effects or concerns: Includes ineffective tissue perfusion and activity intolerance; cardiovascular, respiratory, and elimination concerns; risk for infection, fluid volume imbalances, impaired skin or tissue integrity, and impaired liver function; pain, nutritional problems, fatigue, sleep difficulties, and ineffective health management; and emotional responses (e.g., anxiety, sorrow, grief, coping).

Sample NOC linkages:
Symptom Control: Personal actions to minimize perceived adverse changes in physical and emotional functioning
Blood coagulation: Extent to which blood clots within normal period of time
Immune Status: Natural and acquired appropriately targeted resistance to internal and external antigens

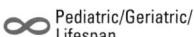

Sample NIC linkages:
Postanesthesia Care: Monitoring and management of the patient who has recently undergone general or regional anesthesia
Bleeding Precautions: Reduction of stimuli that may induce bleeding or hemorrhage in at-risk patients
Infection Protection: Prevention and early detection of infection in a patient at risk
Surveillance: Safety: Purposeful and ongoing collection and analysis of information about the patient and the environment for use in promoting and maintaining patient safety

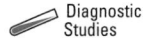

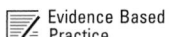

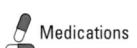

Rape-Trauma Syndrome

Taxonomy II: Coping/Stress Tolerance—Class 1 Post-Trauma Responses (000142) [**Diagnostic Division:** Ego Integrity], Submitted 1980; Revised 1998

DEFINITION: Sustained maladaptive response to a forced, violent, sexual penetration against the victim's will and consent. [Rape is not a sexual crime but a crime of violence and is identified as sexual assault. Although attacks are most often directed toward women, men also may be victims.]

RELATED FACTORS

Rape [actual/attempted forced sexual penetration]

DEFINING CHARACTERISTICS

Subjective

Embarrassment; humiliation; shame; guilt; self-blame
Helplessness; powerlessness
Shock; fear; anxiety; anger; thoughts of revenge
Nightmares; alteration in sleep pattern
Change in relationship(s); sexual dysfunction

Objective

Physical trauma; muscle tension/spasm
Confusion; disorganization; impaired decision making
Agitation; hyperalertness; aggression
Mood swings; perceived vulnerability; dependency; low self-esteem; depression
Substance abuse; history of suicide attempts
Denial; phobias; paranoia; dissociative identity disorder

DESIRED OUTCOMES/EVALUATION CRITERIA

Sample NOC linkages:

Abuse Recovery: Physical: Extent of healing of physical injuries due to sexual abuse
Abuse Recovery: Emotional: Extent of healing of psychological injuries due to abuse
Coping: Personal actions to manage stressors that tax an individual's resources

Client Will (Include Specific Time Frame)

- Report absence of physical complications, pain, and discomfort.
- Deal appropriately with emotional reactions as evidenced by behavior and expression of feelings.
- Verbalize a positive self-image.
- Verbalize recognition that incident was not of own doing.
- Identify behaviors or situations within own control that may reduce risk of recurrence.
- Deal with practical aspects (e.g., court appearances).
- Demonstrate appropriate changes in lifestyle (e.g., change in job, residence) that contribute to recovery or seek and obtain support from significant others (SOs), as needed.
- Interact with individuals or groups in desired and acceptable manner.

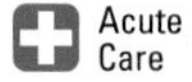

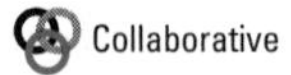

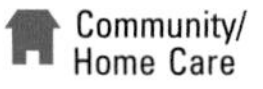

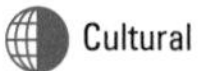

ACTIONS/INTERVENTIONS

Sample NIC linkages:
Rape-Trauma Treatment: Provision of emotional and physical support immediately following a reported rape
Crisis Intervention: Use of short-term counseling to help the patient cope with a crisis and resume a state of functioning comparable to or better than the precrisis state
Counseling: Use of an interactive helping process focusing on the needs, problems, or feelings of the patient and significant others to enhance or support coping, problem solving, and interpersonal relationships

NURSING PRIORITY NO. 1 To assess trauma and individual reaction, noting length of time since occurrence of event:

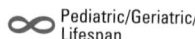

- Observe for and elicit information about physical injury and assess stress-related symptoms such as numbness, headache, tightness in chest, nausea, pounding heart, etc. *Indicators of degree of and reaction to trauma experienced by the client, which may occur immediately and in the days or weeks following the attack.*[4]
- Identify psychological responses such as anger, shock, acute anxiety, confusion, and denial. Note laughter, crying, calm or agitated, excited (hysterical) behavior, and expressions of disbelief or self-blame. *Victim may exhibit expressed response pattern (compound reaction), displaying these feelings openly and freely as manifestations of experiencing the trauma of rape/sexual assault, and the accompanying feelings of fear of death, violation, powerlessness, and helplessness. On the other hand, client may exhibit controlled (silent) response pattern with little or no emotion expressed. Any emotion is appropriate, as each person responds in own individual way; however, inappropriate behaviors or acting out may require intervention.*[3,4] Refer to NDs risk for self-/other-directed Violence.
- Note silence, stuttering, and inability to sit still. *May be signs of increasing anxiety, thus indicating need for further evaluation and intervention. Anxiety is suppressed and client does not talk about the trauma, resulting in an overwhelming emotional burden.*[3,4]
- Determine degree of disorganization. *Initially, the individual may be in shock and disbelief, which is a normal response to the incident. The person may respond by withdrawing and be unable to manage activities of daily living, especially when the incident was particularly brutal, requiring assistance and treatment to enable her or him to recover and move on.*[3,4]
- Identify whether incident has reactivated preexisting or co-existing situations (physical or psychological). *The presence of these factors can affect how the client views the current trauma. Previous traumatic incidents that have not been effectively resolved may compound the current incident.*[1]
- Ascertain cultural values or religious beliefs that may affect how client views incident, self, and expectations of significant other (SO)/family reaction. *Client may believe incident will bring shame on the family, blame self, or believe that family will blame client, thus affecting client's ability to reach out to others for support.*[6]
- Determine sexual orientation of the survivor. *Heterosexual men/boys may believe that they are now gay and need to be assured that is not true. Gay, bisexual, or gay-identified often may be targeted because of this. Healthcare providers may treat these individuals with suspicion, disregard, and disrespect contributing to the survivor's sense of shame and guilt and making it more difficult to seek help.*[5]
- Determine disruptions in relationships with men and with others (e.g., family, friends, coworkers, SO[s]). *Many women find that they react to men in general in a different way, seeing them as reminders of the assault. Male survivors may withdraw entirely from sexual relations.*[5,7]
- Identify development of phobic reactions to ordinary articles (e.g., knives) and situations (e.g., walking in groups of people, strangers ringing doorbell). *These are manifestations of extreme anxiety, and client may need treatment to learn how to manage feelings.*[3,4]
- Note degree of intrusive repetitive thoughts, sleep disturbances. *Survivor may notice disruptions in activities of daily living, reliving the attack, thoughts of recrimination, self-blame ("Why didn't I . . . ?"), and nightmares. Although these factors are distressing and upsetting, they are part of the normal healing process.*[3,4]

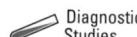

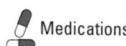

- Assess degree of dysfunctional coping. *Client may turn to use of alcohol or other drugs, have suicidal or homicidal ideation, or display marked change in sexual behavior* in an attempt to cope with traumatic event.[4]

NURSING PRIORITY NO. 2 To assist client to deal with situation that exists:

- Explore own feelings regarding rape/incest issue prior to interacting with the client. *Since the feelings related to these incidents are so pervasive, the individual involved in caregiving needs to recognize own biases to prevent imposing them on the client.*[1]

ACUTE PHASE/IMMEDIATE CARE

- Stay with the client—do not leave child unattended. Listen but do not probe. Tell client you are sorry this has happened and that she or he is safe now. *During this phase, the client experiences a complete disruption of life as she or he has known it, and presence of caregiver may provide reassurance and sense of safety.*[2,4]
- Involve rape or sexual assault response team or sexual assault nurse examiner when available. Provide a same-sex examiner when appropriate. *Presence of the response team trained to collect evidence appropriately and sensitively provides assurance to the survivor that she or he is being taken care of. Client may react to someone who is the sex of the attacker, and use of a same-sex examiner communicates sensitivity to her or his feelings at this difficult time.*[11]
- Be sensitive to cultural factors that may affect specifics of examination process. *For example, in some cultures, women cannot be examined without a male family member present. These issues need to be considered when treating the survivor.*[6]
- Evaluate client as dictated by age, gender, and developmental level. *Age of the survivor is an important consideration in deciding plan of care and appropriate interventions. Note: While underreported, it is believed that 1 in 10 men are sexually assaulted and 1 in 6 boys will be sexually assaulted or abused before the age of 18.*[5,8]
- Assist with documentation of incident for law-enforcement officers and child-protective services reports, explaining each step of the procedure. Maintain sequencing and collection of evidence (chain of evidence), label each specimen, and store and package properly. *It is crucial to provide accurate information to law enforcement for potential legal proceedings when perpetrator is charged.* Be careful to use nonjudgmental language. *Words can carry legal implications that may affect subsequent proceedings.*[1]
- Provide environment in which client can talk freely about feelings and fears. *Client needs to talk about the incident and concerns, such as issues of relationship with or response of SO(s), pregnancy, and sexually transmitted infections (STIs), so they may be dealt with in a positive manner.*[10]
- Provide information about emergency birth control and prophylactic treatment for STIs and assist with finding resources for follow-through. *Promotes client's peace of mind and opportunity to prevent these conditions.*[10]
- Provide psychological support by listening and remaining with client. If client does not want to talk, accept silence. *May indicate silent reaction or controlled style of dealing with the occurrence in which the individual contains his or her emotions, using all his or her energy to maintain composure.*[4]
- Listen to and investigate physical complaints. Assist with medical treatments, as indicated. *Emotional reactions may limit client's ability to recognize physical injury.*[4]
- Assist with practical realities. *Client may be so emotionally distraught that she or he may not be able to attend to needs for such things as safe, temporary housing, money, or other issues that may need to be addressed. Assistance helps individual maintain contact with reality.*
- Determine client's ego strengths and help him or her use them in a positive way by acknowledging client's ability to handle what is happening. *Validation of belief that person can deal with what has happened and move forward with life promotes self-acceptance and helps client begin this process.*[6,9]
- Identify supportive persons for this individual. *Client needs to know she or he can go to a strong system of friends, family, or advocate who will respond with empathy.*[7]

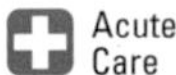
Acute Care
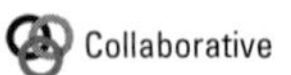
Collaborative
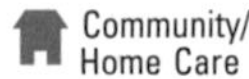
Community/ Home Care
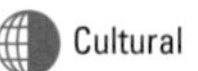
Cultural

POSTACUTE PHASE

- Allow the client to work through own kind of adjustment. Do not force issue if client is withdrawn or unwilling to talk (Silent Reaction). *Individuals react in many ways to the traumatic event of rape, and no response is abnormal. Factors that influence how the survivor deals with the situation are personality, support system, existing life problems and prior sexual victimization, relationship with the offender, degree of violence used, social and cultural influences, and ability to cope with stress.*[2,4]
- Listen for expressions of fear (e.g., of perpetrator returning, of being in crowds or being alone, etc.). *May reveal developing phobias needing evaluation and appropriate interventions and ongoing therapy.*[2,4]
- Discuss specific concerns and fears. Identify appropriate actions and provide information as indicated. *May need diagnostic testing for pregnancy, STIs, or other resources. Meeting these needs and providing information will help client begin the process of recovery.*[10]
- Include written instructions that are concise and clear regarding medical treatments, crisis support services, etc. Encourage return for follow-up. *Reinforces teaching and provides opportunity to deal with information at own pace. Follow-up appointment provides opportunity for determining how client is managing feelings and what needs may not have been met.*[10]

LONG-TERM PHASE

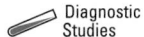

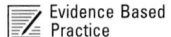

- Continue listening to expressions of concern. Note persistence of somatic complaints (e.g., nausea, anorexia, insomnia, muscle tension, headache). *May need to continue to talk about the assault. Repeating the story helps client to move on, but continued somatic concerns may indicate developing posttraumatic stress disorder.*[6,8]
- Permit free expression of feelings (may continue from the crisis phase). Refrain from rushing client through expressions of feelings too quickly and avoid reassuring inappropriately. *Client may believe pain and/or anguish is misunderstood and depression may limit responses.*[1,6]
- Acknowledge reality of loss of self that existed before the incident. Assist client to move toward an acceptance of the potential for growth that exists within individual. *Following this traumatic event, the individual will not be able to go back to the person he or she was before. Life will always have the memory of what happened, and client needs to accept that reality and move on in the best way possible.*[2]
- Continue to allow client to progress at own pace. *The process of grieving is a very individual one, and each person needs to know that she or he can take whatever time needed to resolve feelings and move on with life.*[4] (Refer to ND Grieving for additional interventions.)
- Give "permission" to express and deal with anger at the perpetrator and situation in acceptable ways. Set limits on destructive behaviors. *Facilitates resolution of feelings without diminishing self-concept.*[6]
- Keep discussion on practical and emotional level rather than intellectualizing the experience. *When the person talks about the incident intellectually, instead of identifying and talking about feelings, client avoids dealing with the feelings, thus inhibiting recovery.*[1]
- Assist in dealing with ongoing concerns about and effects of the incident, such as court appearance, STI, relationship with SO(s), etc. *Depending on degree of disorganization, client will need help to deal with these practical and emotional issues.*
- Provide for sensitive, trained counselors, considering individual needs. *Male/female counselors may be best determined on an individual basis, as counselor's gender may be an issue for some clients, affecting ability to disclose and deal with feelings.*[1]

NURSING PRIORITY NO. 3 To promote wellness (Teaching/Discharge Considerations):

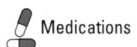

- Provide information about what reactions client may expect during each phase. Let client know these are common reactions and phrase in neutral terms of "You may or may not. . . ." *Such information helps client anticipate and deal with reactions if they are experienced. Note: Be aware that although male rape perpetrators are usually heterosexual, the male victim may be concerned about his own sexuality and may exhibit a homophobic response.*[1]

- Assist client to identify factors that may have created a vulnerable situation and that she or he may have power to change to protect self in the future. *While client needs to be assured that she or he is not to blame for incident, the circumstances of the incident need to be assessed to identify factors that are within the individual's control to avoid a similar incident occurring.*[6]
- Avoid making value judgments. *The survivor often blames self about the incident and agonizes over the circumstances; therefore, nonjudgmental language is very important to help the person accept that the fault is not hers or his.*[1,6]
- Discuss lifestyle changes client is contemplating and how they will contribute to recovery. *Helps client evaluate appropriateness of plans. In the anxiety of the moment, the individual may believe that changing residence, job, or other aspects of her or his environment will be healing. In reality, while this response is normal and represents an attempt to regain control over own life, these changes may not help and may make matters worse.*[4]
- Encourage psychiatric consultation if client is violent, inconsolable, or does not seem to be making an adjustment. Participation in a group may be helpful. *May need intensive professional help to come to terms with the assault.*[1,6]
- Refer to family or marital counseling, as indicated. *When relationships with family members are affected by the incident, counseling may be needed to resolve the issues.*[1,9]
- Refer to NDs Anxiety, ineffective Coping, Fear, Grieving, complicated Grieving, and Powerlessness, as appropriate.

DOCUMENTATION FOCUS

Assessment/Reassessment

- Individual findings, including nature of incident, individual reactions and fears, degree of trauma (physical and emotional), effects on lifestyle.
- Cultural or religious factors.
- Reactions of family/SO(s).
- Samples gathered for evidence and disposition or storage (chain of evidence).

Planning

- Plan of action and who is involved in planning.
- Teaching plan.

Implementation/Evaluation

- Responses to interventions, teaching, and actions performed.
- Attainment or progress toward desired outcome(s).
- Modifications to plan of care.

Discharge Planning

- Long-term needs and who is responsible for actions to be taken.
- Specific referrals made.

References

1. Townsend, M. C. (2010). *Essentials of Psychiatric Mental Health Nursing: Concepts of Care in Evidence-Based Practice*. 5th ed. Philadelphia, PA: F. A. Davis.
2. Rape Crisis Staff. Phases of recovery. Retrieved November 2015 from http://rapecrisis.org.za/information-for-survivors/phases-of-recovery/.
3. Burgess, A. W., Holstrom, L. L. (2003). Dancing in the darkness. Retrieved November 2015 from http://www.dancinginthedarkness.com/articles.php?show=11&arc=83.
4. Rape Victim Advocates. (2008). Rape trauma syndrome. Retrieved November 2015 from http://www.rapevictimadvocates.org/trauma.asp.
5. Rape Victim Advocates. (2008). When the survivor is male. Rape Victim Advocate. Retrieved November 2015 from http://www.rapevictimadvocates.org/male.asp.

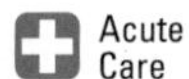
Acute Care
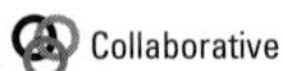
Collaborative
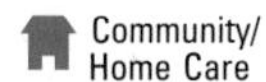
Community/ Home Care
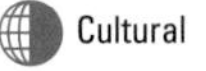
Cultural

6. Hensley, L. G. (2002). Treatment for survivors of rape: Issues and interventions. *J Mental Health Counseling*, 24(4), 330–347.
7. Menna, A. (2004). Rape trauma syndrome: The journey to healing belongs to everyone. Retrieved November 2015 from www.giftfromwithin.org/html/journey.html.
8. Rape, Abuse, & Incest National Network. (2009). Ways to reduce your risk of sexual assault (various pages). Retrieved November 2015 from http://www.rainn.org/get-information/sexual-assault-prevention.
9. Lauer, T. M. (2006). Rape trauma syndrome in intimate relationships. *Family Therapy Magazine*, 5(1), 36–41.
10. Larson, N. (2011). After rape, getting a medical exam is essential. Retrieved November 2015 from http://womenshealth.about.com/lw/Health-Medicine/Womens-Health/After-Rape-Getting-a-Medical-nbsp-Exam-is-Essential.htm.
11. The Advocates for Human Rights. (Updated 2009). Sexual assault response teams. Retrieved November 2015 from http://www.stopvaw.org/sexual_assault_response_teams.html.

risk for adverse Reaction to Iodinated Contrast Media

Taxonomy II: Safety/Protection—Class 5 Defensive Processes (00218) [**Diagnostic Division:** Safety], Submitted 2010, revised 2013

DEFINITION: Vulnerable to noxious or unintended reaction associated with the use of iodinated contrast media that can occur within seven days after contrast agent injection, which may compromise health.

RISK FACTORS

Anxiety
Chronic illness
Concurrent use of pharmaceutical agents (e.g., beta-blockers, interleukin-2, metformin, nephrotoxins)
Contrast media precipitates adverse event (e.g., iodine concentration, viscosity, high osmolality, iron toxicity)
Dehydration
Extremes of age, generalized debilitation
Fragile veins (e.g., chemotherapy or radiation in limb to be injected; indwelling line in place for more than 24 hours; axillary lymph node dissection in limb to be injected; distal intravenous access site)
History of allergies, or previous adverse effect from iodinated contrast media [ICM]
Unconsciousness
NOTE: A risk diagnosis is not evidenced by signs and symptoms, as the problem has not occurred; rather, nursing interventions are directed at prevention.
Sample Clinical Applications: Any condition requiring the use of contrast media for diagnosis or treatment

DESIRED OUTCOMES/EVALUATION CRITERIA

Sample NOC linkages:
Allergic Response: Systemic: Severity of hypersensitive immune response to a specific environmental (exogenous) antigen
Risk Control: Personal actions to prevent, eliminate, or reduce modifiable health threats

Client Will (Include Specific Time Frame)
- Experience no adverse reaction from iodinated contrast media.
- Verbalize understanding of individual risks and responsibilities to avoid exposure.
- Recognize need for/seek assistance to limit allergic response/complications.

(continues on page 664)

risk for adverse Reaction to Iodinated Contrast Media (continued)
ACTIONS/INTERVENTIONS

Sample NIC linkages:
Allergy Management: Identification, treatment, and prevention of allergic responses to food, medications, insect bites, contrast material, blood, and other substances

NURSING PRIORITY NO. 1 To identify causative/precipitating factors related to risk:

- Identify the client at risk for adverse reaction prior to procedures. *A history of allergies; asthma; diabetes; renal insufficiency, including solitary kidney with elevated creatinine; thyroid dysfunction; hypertension; heart failure; current or recent use of nephrotoxic medications; or reaction to previous ICM administration places individual at increased risk.*[1,2]
- Ascertain type of reaction client experienced when there is a history of past reaction. *There are two types of reactions, both of which could change decisions about using ICM for diagnostic purposes. (1) Idiosyncratic reaction typically begins within 20 min of ICM injection. The symptoms are similar to anaphylactic reactions and can be mild (e.g., cough, itching, nasal congestion), moderate (e.g., dyspnea, wheezing), or severe (e.g., respiratory distress, arrhythmias such as bradycardia, seizures, shock, cardiopulmonary arrest). (2) Nonidiosyncratic reaction includes bradycardia, hypotension, and vasovagal reactions; neuropathy; extravasation; sensations of warmth; a metallic taste in the mouth; nausea and vomiting; and delayed reactions.*[1,3]

NURSING PRIORITY NO. 2 To assist client/caregiver to reduce or correct individual risk factors:

- Administer infusions using the "6 rights" system (right client, right medication, right route, right dose, right time, right documentation) *to prevent client from receiving improper contrast agent or dosage. Note: Clients undergoing more than one procedure at a time (such as cardiac angiography and angioplasty) receive a higher dose and are at greater risk for renal insufficiency reactions.*
- Perform imaging tests that do not require contrast media where possible *when client is at high risk for reaction.*
- Administer intravenous fluids as appropriate *to reduce incidence of contrast induced nephropathy by supporting intravascular volume, diluting contrast media, and promoting its elimination.*[4,5]
- Administer medications (e.g., prednisone [Deltasone], Benadryl) before, during, and after injection or procedures *to reduce risk or severity of reaction.*[3]
- Observe intravenous injection site frequently *to ascertain that no extravasation of contrast solution is occurring.*
- Halt infusion immediately to prevent tissue damage from contrast agent if client reports site discomfort or *redness or swelling is noted.*
- Monitor results of lab studies (e.g., creatinine clearance) *to ascertain status of kidney function.*

NURSING PRIORITY NO. 3 To promote wellness (Teaching/Discharge Criteria):

- Instruct client regarding signs and symptoms that should be reported to physician after procedures. *Weight gain, shortness of breath, decreased urination, or new or worsening edema could indicate renal insufficiency. Any delayed signs of reaction should be reported to physician immediately for possible intervention.*
- Instruct client/care provider about puncture sites and to report redness, soreness, or pain *to reduce risk of complications associated with extravasation.*
- Encourage client use of medical alert bracelet/necklace where indicated *to alert healthcare providers of prior reaction to contrast media.*

DOCUMENTATION FOCUS

Assessment/Reassessment

- Individual risk factors identified.
- Client concerns or difficulty making and following through with plan.

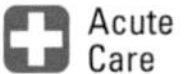

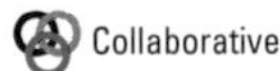

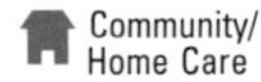

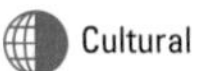

Planning
- Plan of care and who is involved in planning.
- Teaching plan.

Implementation/Evaluation
- Response to interventions, teaching, and actions performed.
- Attainment or progress toward outcomes.

Discharge Planning
- Referrals to other resources.
- Long-term need and who is responsible for actions.

References

1. Siddiqi, N. H. (Updated 2014). Contrast medium reactions. Retrieved March 2015 from http://emedicine.medscape.com/article/422855-overview#a1.
2. Keller, D. M. (2011). Iodinated contrast media raises risk for thyroid dysfunction. *Ann Intern Med*, 172, 153–159.
3. Ilaslan, H. Radiation and imaging. Monograph from the online Merck Manual for Health Care Professionals. Retrieved March 2015 from http://www.merckmanuals.com/professional/special_subjects/principles_of_radiologic_imaging/radiation_and_imaging.html.
4. Kohtz, C., Thompson, M. (2007). Preventing contrast medium-induced nephropathy. *Am J Nurs*, 107(9), 40–49.
5. Bashmore, T. M., Bates, E. R., Berger, P. B., et al. (2001). American College of Cardiology/Society for Cardiac Angiography and Interventions Clinical Expert Consensus Document on cardiac characterizations laboratory standards. A report of the American Cardiology Task Force on Clinical Expert Consensus Documents. *Am Coll Cardiol*, 37(8), 2170–2214.

ineffective Relationship

Taxonomy II: Role Relationships—Class 3 Role Performance (00223) [**Diagnostic Division:** Ego Integrity], Submitted 2010

DEFINITION: A pattern of mutual partnership that is insufficient to provide for each other's needs.

RELATED FACTORS

Stressors; developmental crisis
Substance abuse
Unrealistic expectations
Ineffective communication skills
History of domestic violence
Alteration in cognitive functioning in one partner
Incarceration of one partner

DEFINING CHARACTERISTICS

Subjective
Dissatisfaction with complementary relation between partners
Dissatisfaction with physical or emotional need fulfillment between partners
Dissatisfaction with information or idea sharing between partners

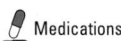

(continues on page 666)

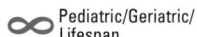

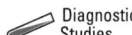

ineffective Relationship (continued)

Objective
Unsatisfactory communication between partner
Insufficient balance in autonomy or collaboration between partners
Insufficient mutual respect between partners
Insufficient mutual support in daily activities between partners
Inadequate understanding of partner's compromised functioning (e.g., physical, social, psychological)
Delay in meeting of developmental goals appropriate for family life-cycle stage
Partner not identified as support person

Sample Clinical Applications: Chronic conditions (e.g., MS, spinal cord injury, gastric bypass surgery, mental health problems, depression, anxiety, bipolar disorder, substance abuse, dementia), domestic violence

DESIRED OUTCOMES/EVALUATION CRITERIA

Sample NOC linkages:

Social Interaction Skills: Personal behaviors that promote effective relationships
Role Performance: Congruence of an individual's role behavior with role expectations
Social Involvement: Social interactions with persons, groups, or communities

Client Will (Include Specific Time Frame)

- Verbalize a desire to improve relationship with partner.
- Acknowledge worth and value of partner as a key person.
- Seek information regarding physical and emotional needs of partner.
- Engage in effective communication skills for both partners.
- Participate in marital therapy sessions to learn ways to develop a satisfactory relationship.

ACTIONS/INTERVENTIONS

Sample NIC linkages:

Conflict Mediation: Facilitation of a constructive dialogue between opposing parties with a goal of resolving disputes in a mutually acceptable manner
Role Enhancement: Assisting a patient, significant other, and/or family to improve relationships by clarifying and supplementing specific role behaviors
Socialization Enhancement: Facilitation of another person's ability to interact with others

NURSING PRIORITY NO. 1 To assess current situation and determine needs:

- Determine makeup of family, length of relationship, and financial situation—parents/children, older/younger, and other members of household. *Stressors of family relationships within a household, difficulties with child-rearing, older adult needing care, and financial difficulties can strain the relationship between partners.*[2,3,7,8]
- Discuss individual's perception of own and other's needs and how partner sees own needs. *Identifies how each person sees situation and areas of agreement and disagreement, providing a basis for beginning plan of care.*[3,6]
- Determine each person's self-image and locus of control. *View of self as a positive or negative individual who is in control or controlled by others influences behavior and how partners react to each other.*[3,4,7,12]
- Assess emotional intelligence skills of each individual. *This is the ability to recognize and control one's own emotions and recognize the emotions of the other.*[1,7]
- Investigate cultural factors that may be affecting relationship and contributing to conflict. *Roles from family of origin for each person may promote conflict when beliefs clash and neither is willing to change or even discuss thinking.*[3,4,12]

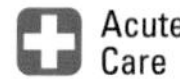
Acute Care
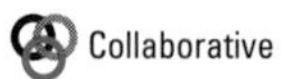
Collaborative
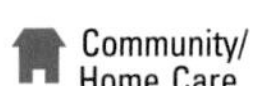
Community/ Home Care
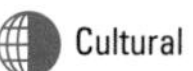
Cultural

- Determine style of communication used by partners. *Poor communication is unclear and indirect leading to conflict, ineffective problem solving, and poor emotional bonding in families with problems.*[1,3]
- Determine how family as a whole functions. *Personal and family history affects relationships between family members and situational dynamics can create conflict as individuals take sides in disagreements, escalating the situation.*[3,4,7]
- Ascertain ways in which family members deal with conflict. *Conflict is inevitable in relationships and partners need to identify whether how they deal with it is effective or ineffective.*[1,2,8]
- Identify concerns about sexual aspects of relationship from both partners' viewpoints. *Intimacy is an important part of a relationship, and if both individuals are avoiding that activity they will need to discuss specific ways to resolve these problems.*[1,4,6,9]
- Note medical problems that may be affecting sexual relationship. *Conditions such as hysterectomy, prostatitis, breast cancer, and erectile dysfunction may cause partners to withdraw from one another.*[8,10]

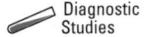

NURSING PRIORITY NO. 2 To assist partners to resolve existing conflict:

- Maintain positive attitude toward partners and family members. *A safe environment allows individuals to speak freely, knowing they will not be judged for comments and opinions, so couple can get to the deeper roots of current situation.*[1,6,7]
- Discuss surface symptoms of dysfunctional relationships and the fact that these are not the problems that need to be dealt with. *Individuals are often not aware of underlying emotions that are influencing their behavior and continue to focus on surface issues.*[6]
- Explore each partner's emotional needs. *Unconscious desires to gain acceptance, recognition, and a sense of being cared about or valued are often motivators for relationships.*[6,7]
- Discuss and clarify nonverbal communication. *Partners need to be aware of and ask about the meaning of body language, tone of voice, and subtle movements that convey positive or negative messages. When these cues are misinterpreted, they can lead to misunderstandings.*[1,6]
- Assist partners/family to learn effective conflict resolution skills such as the win-win method. *Individuals have traditionally used ineffective means of solving conflict or avoided it altogether. Resolving to listen to each other's needs and agree on a mutually acceptable solution provides new ways to resolve problems and enhances relationship.*[5,11]
- Provide information about the active-listening technique. *Avoids giving advice and encourages other person to find own solution, enhancing self-esteem.*[5]
- Have partners identify thoughts and feelings when starting a discussion with each other. *A system of thinking (a paradigm) forms the basis for how we look at and experience life and determines how we perceive our world, forming the basis for our reality, and exists below our level of conscience.*[11,12]
- Recommend individuals verify what they believe the other has said. *Allows speaker to correct misperception and respond more effectively.*[1,5,11,12]
- Have partners role-play a specific conflict that is a frequent issue. *Practicing how to defuse arguments and repair hurt feelings helps to identify other's feelings and use new skills for resolution.*[11]
- Encourage partners to maintain a calm demeanor. *Regardless of circumstances, staying focused enables individuals to think more rationally and come to a desired solution.*[5]
- Discuss sexual concerns and provide opportunity for questions. *Conflict in the relationship inevitability affects these concerns and providing information and discussing them can enhance intimacy.*[1,9]
- Promote nonblameful self-disclosure when having a discussion. *Not placing blame results in a more considerate and respectful resolution.*[7,11]

NURSING PRIORITY NO. 3 To promote optimal functioning (Teaching/Discharge Considerations):

- Have partners acknowledge beliefs they have become aware of during therapy. *Unconscious thinking influences each person's view of the world in negative or positive ways.*[1,11]
- Encourage use of relaxation and mindfulness techniques. *Helps individuals to ease anxiety and learn to relate to each other in a calm manner.*[7]

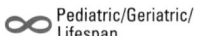

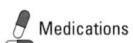

- Discuss the use of humor and laughter in daily lives. *Helps to lighten difficult moments and provide opportunities to share fun moments.*[6]
- Recommend books and Web sites to provide additional information. *Encourages partners to seek and learn new ways to improve relationship.*[3]
- Refer to support groups and classes as indicated. *Parenting, assertiveness, and financial assistance will help partners learn new skills as needed.*[2,3,8,11]
- Include all family members in discussions, as indicated. *Promotes involvement, provides opportunities for communication and clarification of family dynamics, and enhances commitment to achieving goals.*[1,3,7]
- Refer to other physical/psychological resources, as needed. *May need further treatment to address pathology and help partners understand other's needs.*[2,6,8]

DOCUMENTATION FOCUS

Assessment/Reassessment

- Individual's perception of situation and self.
- Partner's views and expectations.
- How partners communicate and deal with conflict.

Planning

- Plan of care and who is involved in planning.
- Teaching plan.

Implementation/Evaluation

- Response of partners to plan, interventions, and actions performed.
- Attainment or progress toward desired outcomes.

Discharge Planning

- Long-range plan and who is responsible for actions to be taken.
- Referrals made.

References

1. Peterson, R. (2009). Families first: Keys to successful family functioning: Communication. Virginia Cooperative Extension. Retrieved April 2015 from http://www.pubs.ext.vt.edu/350/350-092/350-092.html.
2. O'Brien, T. (2008). Parent Empowerment Program (PEP) (various pages). Retrieved April 2015 from http://www.tim-obrien.com/empowerment.php?doc=details.
3. Riesch, S. K., Anderson, L. S., Pridham, K. A., et al. (2010). Furthering the understanding of parent-child relationships: A nursing scholarship review series. Part 5: Parent-adolescent and teen parent-child relationships. *J Spec Pediatr Nurs*, 15(3), 182–201.
4. Fincham, F. D., Bradbury, T. N. (Eds.) (1990). *The Psychology of Marriage: Basic Issues & Applications.* New York: Guilford Press.
5. Scott, E. (Updated 2014). Conflict resolution skills for healthy relationships. Retrieved April 2015 from http://stress.about.com/od/relationships/a/conflict_res.htm.
6. Smith, M., Segal, J. (Updated 2015). Advice for building relationships that are healthy, happy and satisfying. Retrieved April 2015 from http://www.helpguide.org/articles/relationships/relationship-help.htm.
7. Duncan, L. G., Coatsworth, J. D., Greenberg, M. T. (2009). Pilot study to gauge acceptability of a mindfulness based, family-focused preventive intervention. *J Prim Prev*, 30(5), 605–618.
8. Stewart, C. (2008). Common traits of a dysfunctional family. Retrieved April 2015 from http://www.lifescript.com/well-being/articles/c/.
9. Nusbaum, M. R. H., Gamble, G., Skinner, B., et al. (2000). The high prevalence of concerns among women seeking routine gynecological care. *J Fam Pract*, 49(3), 229–232.
10. Vorvick, L. J. (2010). Sexual problems overview. Retrieved April 2015 from http://www.uichildrens.org/Adam/?/HIE%20Multimedia/1/001951.
11. Davidson, J., Wood, C. (Winter 2004). A conflict resolution model. *Theory Into Practice*, 43(1), 6–13.
12. Yolles, M. (1996). The systems paradigm. Retrieved April 2015 from http://www.academia.edu/175318/The_Systems_Paradigm_Paradigm.

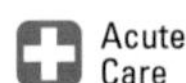

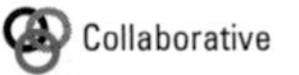

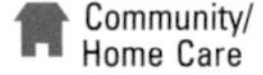

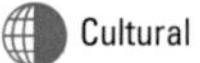

readiness for enhanced Relationship

Taxonomy II: Role Relationships—Class 3 Role Performance (00207) [**Diagnostic Division:** Ego Integrity], Submitted 2006; Revised 2013

DEFINITION: A pattern of mutual partnership to provide for each other's needs, which can be strengthened.

DEFINING CHARACTERISTICS

Subjective

Expresses desire to enhance:

Communication between partners

Satisfaction with information/idea sharing between partners

Emotional need fulfillment for each partner

Satisfaction with physical or emotional need fulfillment for each partner

Satisfaction with complementary relation between partners

Mutual respect between partners

Autonomy or collaboration between partners

Understanding of partners' functional deficit (e.g., physical, social, psychological)

Sample Clinical Applications: Applicable in any setting, not dependent on presence of pathology although may be useful in chronic physical conditions or mental health challenges

DESIRED OUTCOMES/EVALUATION CRITERIA

Sample NOC linkages:

Social Interaction Skills: Personal behaviors that promote effective relationships

Role Performance: Congruence of an individual's role behavior with role expectations

Social Involvement: Social interactions with persons, groups, or organizations

Client Will (Include Specific Time Frames)

- Verbalize a desire to learn more effective communication skills.
- Verbalize understanding of current relationship with partner.
- Seek information to improve emotional and physical needs of both partners.
- Talk with partner about circumstances that can be improved.
- Develop realistic plans to strengthen relationship.

ACTIONS/INTERVENTIONS

Sample NIC linkages:

Role Enhancement: Assisting a patient, significant other, and/or family to improve relationships by clarifying and supplementing specific role behaviors

Socialization Enhancement: Facilitation of another person's ability to interact with others

NURSING PRIORITY NO. 1 To assess current situation and determine needs:

- ∞ Determine makeup of family: parents/children, older/younger. *Life changes, such as developmental, situational, and health-illness, can affect the relationship between partners and require readjustment and thinking of ways to enhance situation.*[1]
- Discuss client's perception of needs and how partner sees desire to improve relationship. *Identifies thinking and whether both partners see the situation in the same way and individual expectations for change.*[4]

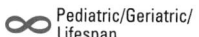

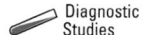

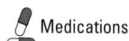

- Identify use of effective communication skills. *May need to improve understanding of words partners use in discussion of sensitive subjects.*[4]
- Help client to identify thoughts and feelings when starting a discussion with partner. *A system of thinking (referred to as a paradigm) forms the basis for how we look at and experience life and determines how we perceive our world, forms the basis for our reality, and exists below our level of conscience.*[4]
- Ask partners how they deal with conflict. *Since conflict is a normal, natural, and inevitable part of life, this needs to be acknowledged, and individuals need to learn how to deal with it effectively.*[4]
- Ascertain client's view of sexual aspects of relationship. *Changes that occur with aging or medical conditions, such as hysterectomy or erectile dysfunction, can affect the relationship and need specific interventions to resolve.*[2]
- Identify cultural factors relating to individual's view of role in relationship.
- Discuss how family as a whole functions. *Interrelationships with members of the family, personal and family history, and situational dynamics can impact the functioning of the whole family.*[2]

NURSING PRIORITY NO. 2 To assist the client to enhance existing relationship:

- Maintain positive attitude toward client. *Promotes safe relationship in which client can feel free to speak openly and plan for a positive future.*[1]
- Have couple discuss paradigms that they have become aware of in own thinking that interfere with relationship. *These beliefs exist below our conscious mind, influencing our behavior and whether we see the world in negative or positive ways.*[4]
- Determine how each person views himself of herself as a positive or negative person. *One's self-image influences behavior and how he or she relates to others. When emotional needs are met, individuals relate to others in positive ways, while unmet needs result in low self-image and insecurity.*[5]
- Discuss the skills of emotional intelligence, which are important for maintaining positive relationships. *This is the ability to recognize and effectively control our own emotions and to recognize the emotions of others.*[6]
- Help couple to recognize that surface symptoms of dysfunctional relationships are not the problems that need to be dealt with. *Underlying emotions influence our behaviors and individuals often are not aware of them and continue to deal with the superficial conflicts.*[6]
- Explore individual's emotional needs. *Relationships are often motivated by unconscious desires to gain acceptance, recognition, and a sense of being cared about or valued.*[5]
- Note client's awareness of nonverbal communications. *Body language, tone of voice, a roll of the eyes, or subtle movements convey strong messages, positive or negative, that need to be discussed and clarified.*[6]
- Discuss effective conflict-resolution skills. *People tend to be afraid of conflict because effective ways to deal with it have not been learned, and it often ends in a lose-lose situation.*[4]
- Encourage client to remain calm and focused regardless of circumstances. *Maintaining a calm demeanor helps individual to be able to think more clearly and be more rational in dealing with situation.*[6]
- Recommend cross-checking or verifying what listener believes speaker said. *Clarifies communication and allows speaker to respond or correct perception of listener as needed.*[5]
- Help partners to learn the win-win method of conflict resolution. *Although conflict can damage a relationship, learning to listen to each other's needs can assist partners to arrive at mutually acceptable solutions.*[4]
- Role-play ways to defuse arguments and repair injured feelings. *Provides a realistic situation wherein each person can identify own and partner's view and practice new ways of interacting.*[6]
- Provide open environment for partners to discuss sexual concerns and questions. *Problems may arise out of lack of information about these issues, and when individuals are comfortable with this knowledge, the relationship can be improved.*[2]
- Discuss nonblameful self-disclosure when having a dialogue. *Partners take turns talking about own needs and feelings without blaming the other, resulting in being able to find a solution in a climate of mutual consideration and respect.*[4]

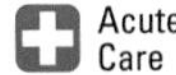

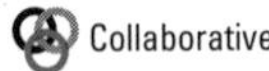

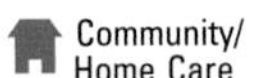

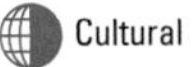

NURSING PRIORITY NO. 3 To promote optimal relationship (Teaching/Discharge Considerations):

- Provide information for partners, using bibliotherapy and appropriate Web sites. *Promotes continuation of learning about how to enhance relationship.*[3]
- Encourage couple to use humor and playfulness in their relationship. *Sharing laughter and enjoying life helps to weather difficult times that may occur.*[6]
- Discuss the importance of being an empathic, understanding, and nonjudgmental listener when either partner has a problem. *The expectation that the partner will be willing to help by listening eases the anxiety of talking about major problems.*[5]
- Encourage use of the active-listening technique. *This avoids giving advice and helps other person to find own solution, enhancing self-esteem.*[4]
- Refer to support groups and classes on assertiveness and parenting, as indicated by individual needs.[3]
- Include family members in discussions as needed. *Knowing how the family relates as a whole will help improve relationships of partners as well as the other family members.*[3]
- Refer for care as indicated by psychological or physical problems of either individual. *May need further treatment and explanation to help partner understand these situations.*[1]

DOCUMENTATION FOCUS

Assessment/Reassessment
- Baseline information, individual's perception of situation and self.
- Reasons for desire to improve relationship and expectations for change.

Planning
- Plan of care and who is involved in planning.
- Teaching plan.

Implementation/Evaluation
- Response of partners to plan, interventions, and actions performed.
- Attainment or progress toward desired outcomes(s).

Discharge Planning
- Long-term plan and who is responsible for actions to be taken.

References

1. Perrone, L. M., Webb, L. K., Jackson, Z. V. (2007). Relationships between parental attachment, work and family roles and life satisfaction. *Career Dev Quart*, 55(3), 237–248.
2. Denberg, D. (1999). Factors that influence a couple's relationship. *Couple Therapy: An Information Guide*. Toronto, CA: The Centre for Addiction and Mental Health.
3. Glass, J. S., Mann, M. A. (2004). Harmonious families: Using family counseling and adventure based learning opportunities to enhance growth. Retrieved November 2015 from http://www.shsu.edu/~piic/spring%202006/Glass.html.
4. Wilmot, W. W., Bergstrom, M. J. (2003). Relationship theories—Self-other relationship. *International Encyclopedia of Marriage and Family Therapy*. Retrieved November 2015 from http://family.jrank.org/pages/1373/Relationship-Theories-Self-Other-Relationshiip.html.
5. Hollister, W. G., Edgerton, J. W. (1974). Teaching relationship building skills. *Am J Public Health*, 64(1), 41–46.
6. Smith, M. A., Segal, J. (Updated 2015). Relationship help: Tips for building romantic relationships that last. Retrieved November 2015 from http://www.helpguide.org/articles/relationships/relationship-help.htm.

risk for ineffective Relationship

Taxonomy II: Role Relationships—Class 3 Role Performance (00229) [**Diagnostic Division:** Ego Integrity], Submitted 2010; Revised 2013

DEFINITION: Vulnerable to developing a pattern that is insufficient for providing a mutual partnership to provide for each other's needs.

RISK FACTORS

Stressors; developmental crisis
Substance abuse
Unrealistic expectations
Ineffective communication skills
History of domestic violence; incarceration of one partner
Alteration in cognitive functioning in one partner
Note: A risk diagnosis is not evidenced by signs and symptoms, as the problem has not occurred: rather nursing interventions are directed at prevention
Sample Clinical Applications: Chronic conditions (e.g., MS, spinal cord injury, gastric bypass surgery, mental health problems, depression, anxiety, bipolar disorder, substance abuse, dementia/Alzheimer's), domestic violence

DESIRED OUTCOMES/EVALUATION CRITERIA

Sample NOC linkages:
Social Interaction Skills: Personal behaviors that promote effective relationships
Role Performance: Congruence of an individual's role behavior with role expectations
Social Involvement: Social interactions with persons, groups, or communities

Client Will (Include Specific Time Frames)
- Verbalize desire to make changes to meet each other's needs as appropriate.
- Express a desire to improve communication skills.
- Develop realistic plans to improve relationship.

ACTIONS/INTERVENTIONS

Sample NIC linkages:
Counseling: Use of an interactive helping process focusing on the needs, problems, or feelings of the patient and significant others to enhance or support coping, problem solving, and interpersonal relationships
Role Enhancement: Assisting a patient, significant other, and/or family to improve relationships by clarifying and supplementing specific role behaviors
Socialization Enhancement: Facilitation of another person's ability to interact with others

NURSING PRIORITY NO. 1 To assess current situation and determine needs:

- Determine makeup of family, length of relationship, and specific stressors. *Stressors of family—developmental issues, elderly parents needing assistance, financial difficulties, and domestic violence—strain relationships between partners.*[2,3,7,8]
- Identify how each partner sees own self-image and locus of control. *View of self as a positive or negative person who is in control or controlled by others influences how each relates to the other.*[3,4,7,8,12]

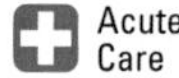
Acute Care
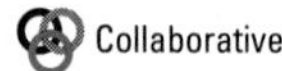
Collaborative
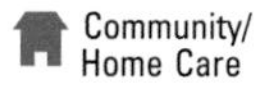
Community/ Home Care
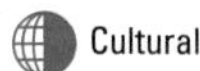
Cultural

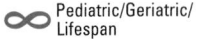

- Discuss needs of each partner and how each views the other's needs. *Identifies misperceptions and areas of disagreement to provide a basis of planning for change.*[1,3]
- Identify style of communication and understanding of nonverbal cues used by family members. *Poor communication and lack of understanding of what the other is saying, or inferring, leads to conflicts and lack of problem solving.*[1,3]
- Determine how partners deal with conflict. *Many individuals try to avoid conflict instead of working to resolve it.*[5,6]
- Identify cultural beliefs that affect how each person deals with daily activities in family. *Family of origin influences how individuals think roles are to be dealt with, and conflict arises if partners are not willing to discuss and change beliefs.*[3,4,12]
- Identify medical problems/sexual concerns that may affect relationship. *Conditions such as prostate problems, breast cancer, hysterectomy, and erectile dysfunction can affect interactions between partners.*[4,8,10]
- Ascertain how couple deals with sexual aspects of their relationship. *When anger and conflict interfere with intimacy, couple may distant themselves from one another.*[1,4,6,9]
- Note how family as a whole functions. *Interactions among family members and situational dynamics provide information about need to improve relationships.*[3,7]

NURSING PRIORITY NO. 2 To assist couple to improve relationship:

- Maintain positive attitude in interactions with individuals. *Provides an environment in which clients feel comfortable and safe discussing problems openly.*[1,6,7]
- Promote discussion of awareness of individuals' beliefs and thoughts that may strain relationship. *Enables individuals to begin to discuss potential problem areas.*[3,6]
- Have client identify thoughts and feelings when starting a conversation with partner. *Individuals have a system of thinking that forms the basis for reality, determines how we see the world, and exists below the level of our consciousness.*[11]
- Discuss the skills of emotional intelligence. *The ability to recognize and control own emotions and recognize emotions of others is important to maintain healthy relationships.*[1,7]
- Explore each person's emotional needs. *Understanding that unconscious needs underlie desire to gain acceptance, recognition, and sense of being cared about or valued help client to deal more openly with these issues.*[6,7]
- Assist partners to understand effects of nonverbal language. *Lack of awareness of body language, tone of voice, and subtle movements can be misinterpreted and need to be discussed and clarified.*[1,6]
- Encourage couple to learn effective conflict-resolution skills. *Family may have used ineffective ways to deal with conflict, resulting in fighting and a lose-lose situation.*[5,11]
- Role-play a specific problem couple argues about, using the win-win method of resolution. *Practicing how to defuse arguments and repair hurt feelings helps to identify other's feelings and use new skills for resolution.*[11]
- Encourage partners to practice remaining calm and focused regardless of circumstances. *When issue has previously resulted in violence, remaining calm can help individuals think more clearly and be more rational in dealing with situation, avoiding further conflict.*[5]
- Have each person verify what he or she heard the other person say. *Provides the opportunity for the speaker to correct or acknowledge what was said.*[1,5,11]
- Discuss issues/provide information about sexual relationship. *Conflict inevitably affects intimacy, and couple may need to resolve issues around this part of their life.*[1,9]
- Discuss use of nonblameful self-disclosure during discussions with partner. *Promotes an atmosphere of respect and mutual consideration in which individuals can talk about feelings and resolve problems.*[7,11]

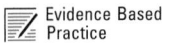

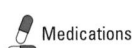

NURSING PRIORITY NO. 3 To promote optimal relationship between couple/family (Teaching/Discharge Considerations):

- Involve all family members in discussions, as indicated. *Encourages input from each member so he/she feels heard and views self as part of the solution.*[1,3,7,11]
- Encourage family members to use active listening. *Avoids giving advice and allows others to find their own solution, enhancing self-esteem.*[1,5,11]
- Discuss appropriate use of humor and playfulness in daily interactions. *Helps family members to enjoy life and makes difficult issues easier to deal with.*[6]
- Encourage use of relaxation, mindfulness techniques. *Promotes calm manner and ability to deal with difficult issues more effectively.*[7]
- Recommend information sources, books, and Web sites as appropriate. *Provides additional resources to access information to assist couple in learning to deal with relationship/family issues.*[3]
- Identify community resources/support groups as appropriate. *Individuals who have successfully dealt with similar issues can provide role model for change and effective use of problem-solving skills.*[2,3,8,11]
- Refer to therapy as indicated. *May need further in-depth care to deal with individual physical/psychological problems.*[2,6,8,11]

DOCUMENTATION FOCUS

Assessment/Reassessment

- Individual's perception of situation and self.
- Partner's views and expectations.
- How partners communicate and deal with conflict.

Planning

- Plan of care and who is involved in planning.
- Teaching plan.

Implementation/Evaluation

- Response of partners to plan, interventions, and actions performed.
- Attainment or progress toward desired outcomes.

Discharge Planning

- Long-range plan and who is responsible for actions to be taken.
- Any referrals made.

References

1. Peterson, R. (2009). Families first: Keys to successful family functioning: Communication. Virginia Cooperative Extension. Retrieved April 2015 from http://www.pubs.ext.vt.edu/350/350-092/350-092.html.
2. O'Brien, T. (2008). Parent Empowerment Program (PEP) (various pages). Retrieved April 2015 from http://www.tim-obrien.com/empowerment.php?doc=details.
3. Riesch, S. K., Anderson, L. S., Pridham, K. A., et al. (2010). Furthering the understanding of parent-child relationships: A nursing scholarship review series. Part 5: Parent-adolescent and teen parent-child relationships. *J Spec Pediatr Nurs*, 15(3), 182–201.
4. Anderson, L. S., Riesch, S. K., Pridham, K. A., et al. (2010). Furthering the understanding of parent-child relationships: A nursing scholarship review series. Part 4: Parent-child relationships at risk. *J Spec Pediatr Nurs*, 15(2), 111–134.
5. Scott, E. (Updated 2014). Conflict resolution skills for healthy relationships. Retrieved April 2015 from http://stress.about.com/od/relationships/a/conflict_res.htm.
6. Smith, M., Segal, J. (Updated 2015). Advice for building relationships that are healthy, happy and satisfying. Retrieved April 2015 from http://www.helpguide.org/articles/relationships/relationship-help.htm.

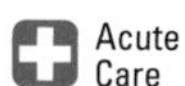

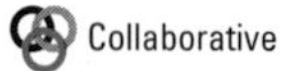

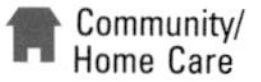

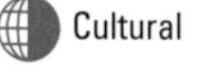

7. Duncan, L. G., Coatsworth, J. D., Greenberg, M. T. (2009). Pilot study to gauge acceptability of a mindfulness based, family-focused preventive intervention. *J Prim Prev*, 30(5), 605–618.
8. Stewart, C. (2008). Common traits of a dysfunctional family. Retrieved April 2015 from http://www.lifescript.com/well-being/articles/c/.
9. Nusbaum, M. R. H., Gamble, G., Skinner, B., et al. (2000). The high prevalence of concerns among women seeking routine gynecological care. *J Fam Pract*, 49(3), 229–232.
10. Vorvick, L. J. (2010). Sexual problems overview. Retrieved April 2015 from http://www.uichildrens.org/Adam/?/HIE%20Multimedia/1/001951.
11. Davidson, J., Wood, C. (Winter 2004). A conflict resolution model. *Theory Into Practice*, 43(1), 6–13.
12. Yolles, M. (1996). The systems paradigm. Retrieved April 2015 from http://www.academia.edu/175318/The_Systems_Paradigm_Paradigm.

impaired Religiosity

Taxonomy II: Life Principles—Class 3 Value/Belief/Action Congruence (00169) [**Diagnostic Division:** Ego Integrity], Submitted 2004

DEFINITION: Impaired ability to exercise reliance on beliefs and/or participate in rituals of a particular faith tradition.

RELATED FACTORS

Developmental and Situational
Life transition; aging; end-stage life crisis
Physical
Illness; pain
Psychological
Ineffective coping strategies or social support
Anxiety; fear of death
Personal crisis; insecurity
History of religious manipulation
Sociocultural
Cultural or environmental barrier to practicing religion
Insufficient social integration or sociocultural interaction
Spiritual
Spiritual crises; suffering

DEFINING CHARACTERISTICS

Subjective
Distress about separation from faith community
Desire to reconnect with previous belief pattern or customs
Questioning of religious belief patterns or customs

(continues on page 676)

impaired Religiosity (continued)

Difficulty adhering to prescribed religious beliefs and rituals (e.g., ceremonies, regulations, clothing, prayer, services, holiday observances)

Sample Clinical Applications: Any acute or chronic condition, palliative care, end-of-life situation

DESIRED OUTCOMES/EVALUATION CRITERIA

Sample NOC linkages:

Spiritual Health: Connectedness with self, others, higher power, all life, nature, and the universe that transcends and empowers the self

Client Will (Include Specific Time Frame)

- Express ability to once again participate in beliefs and rituals of desired religion.
- Discuss beliefs and values about spiritual or religious issues.
- Attend religious or worship services of choice, as desired.
- Verbalize concerns about end-of-life issues and fear of death.

ACTIONS/INTERVENTIONS

Sample NIC linkages:

Spiritual Growth Facilitation: Facilitation of growth in patients' capacity to identify, connect with, and call upon the source of meaning, purpose, comfort, strength, and hope in their lives

Religious Ritual Enhancement: Facilitating participation in religious practices

Spiritual Support: Assisting the patient to feel balance and connection with a greater power

NURSING PRIORITY NO. 1 To assess causative/contributing factors:

- Determine client's usual religious and spiritual beliefs, values, and past spiritual commitment. *Provides a baseline for understanding current problem.*[5]
- Note client's/significant other's (SO's) reports and expressions of anger/concern, alienation from God, and sense of guilt or retribution. *Perception of guilt may cause spiritual crisis and suffering, resulting in rejection of religious beliefs or anger toward God.*[6]
- Determine sense of futility, feelings of hopelessness, and lack of motivation to help self. *Indicators that client may see no, or only limited, options or personal choices, and treatment needs to be directed at finding what happened in client's life to bring about these feelings.*[5]
- Assess extent of depression client may be experiencing. *Some studies suggest that a focus on religion may protect against depression.*[7]
- Note recent changes in negative behaviors (e.g., withdrawal from others or religious activities, dependence on alcohol or medications). *Lack of connectedness with self and others impairs ability to trust others or feel worthy of trust from others or God.*[6,7]
- Identify cultural values and expectations regarding religious beliefs or practices. *Individuals grow up in a family that instills a value system within them. As the person grows up, ideas, values, and expectations may change or be strengthened by new information, different questioning, and alternative viewpoints, which may affect current situation.*[3]
- Note socioeconomic status of individual/family. *Women who are poor may have high levels of personal religiosity yet participate less in organized religion because they may feel stigmatized by their situation (e.g., single mothers, those receiving public assistance, those engaging in a lifestyle that conflicts with church norms).*[2]

NURSING PRIORITY NO. 2 To assist client/SOs to deal with feelings/situation:

- Use therapeutic communication skills of reflection and active listening. *Communicates acceptance and enables client to find own solutions to concerns as situation is discussed and deeper meanings are discovered.*[4]

- Encourage expression of feelings about illness or condition or death. *As people age, they become more concerned about their own mortality, and others often see them as in poor health and as spiritual and religious. If they have been diagnosed with a long-term chronic or terminal illness, they may be feeling more angry and rejecting of God than seeking his help.*[5,8]
- Discuss personal beliefs that may hinder participation in religious activities. *Provides opportunity for self-reflection, such as own worthiness and ability to forgive self for past decisions/life choices.*
- Discuss differences between grief and guilt and help client to identify and deal with each. Point out consequences of actions based on guilt. *Individuals often feel guilty about the "what if's" of life. "If only I had done this!" "If only I had paid more attention!" "If only I had made him go to the doctor!" Most of these guilty feelings are not based on reality and, when they are acted on, the individual does not get the release he or she seeks.*[5]
- Suggest use of journaling and reminiscence. *Promotes life review and can assist in clarifying values and ideas, recognizing and resolving feelings and situation.*[4]
- Encourage client to identify individuals who can provide needed support (e.g., spiritual advisor, parish nurse). *When client is seeking to restore reliance on religious beliefs, these providers can often be helpful.*[6]
- Review client's religious affiliation, associated rituals, and beliefs. *Helps client examine what was important in the past and may trigger some desire to reconnect with these previous beliefs.*[6]
- Provide opportunity for nonjudgmental discussion of philosophical issues related to religious belief patterns and customs. *Open communication can assist client to check reality of perceptions and identify personal options and willingness to resume desired activities.*[1]
- Discuss desire to continue or reconnect with previous belief patterns and customs and perceived barriers. *As client begins to think about current feelings of alienation from previous religious connections, these discussions can help to clarify and allow client to think about how these beliefs can be regained.*[5]
- Identify ways to strengthen spiritual or religious expression. *There are multiple options for enhancing participation in faith community (e.g., joining prayer or study group, volunteering time to community projects, singing in the choir, reading spiritual writings).*
- Involve client in refining healthcare goals and therapeutic regimen as appropriate. *Identifies role illness or condition is playing in current concerns about ability to participate and appropriateness of participating in desired religious activities.*[7]

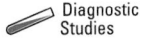

NURSING PRIORITY NO. 3 To promote spiritual wellness (Teaching/Discharge Considerations):

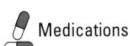

- Assist client to identify spiritual counselor who could be helpful (e.g., minister, priest, spiritual advisor who has qualifications or experience) in dealing with specific concerns of client. *Provides answers to spiritual questions, assists in the journey of self-discovery, and can help client learn to accept and forgive self.*[6]
- Provide privacy for meditation or prayer and performance of rituals, as appropriate. *Many individuals prefer to pray or meditate in private so they can concentrate without interruption or questions from others.*
- Explore alternatives or modifications of ritual based on setting and individual needs and limitations. *Individual may not be able to go to a church or temple, so providing another setting—chapel in the facility or quiet room with appropriate religious artifacts or material—can provide the setting desired.*[6]
- Provide bibliotherapy, including list of relevant resources and Web sites *for later reference, promoting self-paced learning and ongoing support.*[4]

DOCUMENTATION FOCUS

Assessment/Reassessment

- Individual findings, including nature of spiritual conflict, effects of participation in treatment regimen.
- Physical and emotional responses to conflict.

Planning

- Plan of care and who is involved in planning.
- Teaching plan.

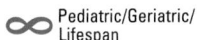

Implementation/Evaluation

- Responses to interventions, teaching, and actions performed.
- Attainment or progress toward desired outcomes(s).
- Modifications to plan of care.

Discharge Planning

- Long-term needs and who is responsible for actions to be taken.
- Available resources, specific referrals made.

References

1. Smith, A. R. (2006). Using the synergy model to provide spiritual nursing care in cardiovascular settings. *Crit Care Nurs*, 26(2), 41–47.
2. Sullivan, S. (Updated 2013). Faith and poverty: Personal religiosity and organized religion in the lives of low-income urban mothers. Retrieved April 2015 from http://www.bc.edu/content/bc/centers/boisi/publicevents/s06/sullivan.html.
3. Ahrold, T. K., Meston, C. (2010). Ethnic differences in sexual attitudes among U.S. college students: Gender, acculturation, and religiosity. *Arch Sex Behav*, 39(1), 190–202.
4. Herbert, R. S., Jenckes, M. W., Ford, D. E., et al. (2001). Patient perspectives on spirituality and the patient-physician relationship. *J Gen Intern Med*, 16(10), 685–692.
5. McNamara, P., Durso, R., Brown, A. (2006). Religiosity in Parkinson's patients. *Neuropsychiatr Dis Treat*, 2(3), 341–348.
6. Ko, B., Khurana, R., Spenser, J., et al. (2007). Religious beliefs and quality of life in an American inner city haemodialysis population. *Nephrol Dial Transplant*, 22(10), 2985–2990.
7. Murray-Swank, A., Luckstead, A., Medoff, D. R., et al. (2006). Religiosity, psychosocial adjustment, and subjective burden of persons who care for those with mental illness. *Psychiatr Serv*, 57(3), 361–365.
8. Mills, J. (1999). The ontology of religiosity: The oceanic feeling and the value of the lived experience. Humanists. Retrieved April 2015 from http://huumanists.org/publications/journal/ontology-religiosity-oceanic-feeling-and-value-lived-experience.

readiness for enhanced Religiosity

Taxonomy II: Life Principles—Class 3 Value/Belief/Action Congruence (00171) [**Diagnostic Division:** Ego Integrity], Submitted 2004; Revised 2013

DEFINITION: A pattern of reliance on religious beliefs and/or participation in rituals of a particular faith tradition, which can be strengthened.

DEFINING CHARACTERISTICS

Subjective

Expresses desire to enhance belief patterns or religious customs used in the past

Expresses desire to enhance participation in religious experiences or practices (e.g., ceremonies, regulations, clothing, prayer, services, holiday observances)

Expresses desire to enhance religious options, use of religious materials

Expresses desire to enhance connection with religious leader

Expresses desire to enhance forgiveness

Sample Clinical Applications: As a health-seeking behavior, the client/family may be healthy, or this diagnosis can be associated with any clinical condition or life process

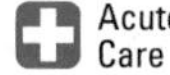

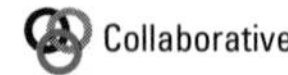

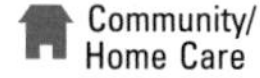

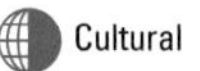

DESIRED OUTCOMES/EVALUATION CRITERIA

Sample NOC linkages:

Spiritual Health: Connectedness with self, others, higher power, all life, nature, and the universe that transcends and empowers the self

Client Will (Include Specific Time Frame)

- Acknowledge need to strengthen religious affiliations and continue or resume previously comforting rituals.
- Verbalize willingness to seek help to enhance desired religious beliefs.
- Become involved in spiritually based programs of own choice.
- Recognize the difference between belief patterns and customs that are helpful and those that may be harmful.

ACTIONS/INTERVENTIONS

Sample NIC linkages:

Spiritual Growth Facilitation: Facilitation of growth in patients' capacity to identify, connect with, and call upon the source of meaning, purpose, comfort, strength, and hope in their lives

Religious Ritual Enhancement: Facilitating participation in religious practices

Spiritual Support: Assisting the patient to feel balance and connection with a greater power

NURSING PRIORITY NO. 1 To determine spiritual state/motivation for growth:

- Determine client's current thinking about desire to learn more about religious beliefs and actions.
- Ascertain religious beliefs or cultural values of family of origin and climate in which client grew up. *Early religious training deeply affects children and is carried on into adulthood. Conflict between family's beliefs and client's current learning may need to be addressed.*[7]
- Identify cultural values and expectations regarding religious beliefs and/or practices. *Individuals grow up in a family that instills a value system within them. As the person grows up, ideas, values, and expectations may change or be strengthened by new information, different questioning, and alternative viewpoints.*[3]
- Note socioeconomic status of individual/family. *Women who are economically disadvantaged may have high levels of personal religiosity, yet participate less in organized religion because they feel stigmatized by their situation (e.g., single mothers, those receiving public assistance, those engaging in a lifestyle that conflicts with church norms).*[2]
- Discuss client's spiritual commitment, beliefs, and values. *Enables examination of these issues and helps client learn more about self and what he or she desires/believes.*[7]
- Explore how spirituality and religious practices have affected client's life. *Some philosophers believe that the value of religiosity is the deepened sense of quality of life associated with practicing one's beliefs or tenets.*[8]
- Ascertain motivation and expectations for change. *The client's motivation needs to be for self and not for others, and client needs to understand own expectations to move forward with desire to improve status.*[4]

NURSING PRIORITY NO. 2 To assist client to integrate values and beliefs to strengthen sense of wholeness and achieve optimum balance in daily living:

- Establish nurse-client relationship in which dialogue can occur. *Client can feel safe in this relationship to say anything and know it will be accepted.*[5]
- Identify barriers and beliefs that may hinder growth or self-discovery. *Provides opportunity for self-reflection such as own worthiness and ability to forgive self for past decisions or life choices. Previous practices and beliefs may need to be considered and accepted or discarded in new search for religious beliefs.*[8]
- Discuss cultural beliefs of family of origin and how they have influenced client's religious practices. *As client expands options for learning new or other religious beliefs and practices, these influences will provide information for comparing and contrasting new information.*[7]
- Explore connection of desire to strengthen belief patterns and customs to daily life. *Becoming aware of how these issues affect the individual's daily life can enhance ability to incorporate them into everything he or she does.*[1]

- Identify ways in which individual can develop a sense of harmony with self and others. *Client may have some new beliefs that may or may not be shared with others, and discussing these can clarify understanding by each individual.*[1]

NURSING PRIORITY NO. 3 To enhance spiritual wellness (Teaching/Discharge Considerations) :

- Encourage client to seek out and experience different religious beliefs, services, and ceremonies, as desired. *Trying out different religions will give client more information to contrast and compare what will fit his or her belief system.*[6]
- Provide bibliotherapy or reading materials pertaining to spiritual issues. *Client may be interested in learning about new spiritual ideas, and finding resources that clarify thinking will help to develop own beliefs.*[4]
- Encourage client to engage in stress-reducing activities, such as meditation, relaxation exercises, or mindfulness (method of being in the moment). *Promotes general well-being and sense of control over self and ability to choose desired religious activities.*[5]
- Encourage participation in religious activities, worship or religious services, and prayer or study groups; volunteering in church choir or other needed duties; and reading/viewing religious materials and media. *Enhances client's knowledge and promotes connectedness with self, others, and/or higher power.*[4]
- Refer to community resources (e.g., parish nurse, religion classes, other support groups).

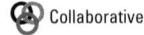

DOCUMENTATION FOCUS

Assessment/Reassessment

- Assessment findings, including client perception of needs and desire for growth.
- Motivation and expectations for change.

Planning

- Plan for growth and who is involved in planning.

Implementation/Evaluation

- Response to activities, learning, and actions performed.
- Attainment or progress toward desired outcome(s).
- Modifications to plan.

Discharge Planning

- Long-term needs, expectations, and plan of action.
- Specific referrals made.

References

1. Burkhardt, L. (2005). A click away: Documenting spiritual care. *J Cardiovasc Nurs*, 22(1), 6–12.
2. Sullivan, S. (Updated 2013). Faith and poverty: Personal religiosity and organized religion in the lives of low-income urban mothers. Retrieved November 2015 from http://www.bc.edu/content/bc/centers/boisi/publicevents/s06/sullivan.html.
3. Lipson, J. G., Dibble, S. L., Minarik, P. A. (1999). *Culture & Nursing Care: A Pocket Guide*. San Francisco, CA: UCSF Nursing Press.
4. Townsend, M. (2006). *Psychiatric Mental Health Nursing Concepts of Care*. 5th ed. Philadelphia, PA: F. A. Davis.
5. Doenges, M., Moorhouse, M., Murr, A. (2006). *Nursing Care Plans: Guidelines for Individualizing Patient Care*. 7th ed. Philadelphia, PA: F. A. Davis.
6. Doenges, M., Moorhouse, M., Murr, A. (2008). *Nurse's Pocket Guide: Diagnoses, Prioritized Interventions, and Rationales*. 11th ed. Philadelphia, PA: F. A. Davis.
7. Murray-Swank, A., Lucksted, A., Medoff, D. R., et al. (2006). Religiosity, psychosocial adjustment, and subjective burden of persons who care for those with mental illness. *Psychiatr Serv*, 57(3), 361–365.
8. Mills, J. (1999). The ontology of religiosity: The oceanic feeling and the value of the lived experience. Humanists. Retrieved November 2015 from http://humanists.org/publications/journal/ontology-religiosity-oceanic-feeling-and-value-lived-experience.

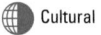

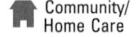

risk for impaired Religiosity

Taxonomy II: Life Principles—Class 3 Value/Belief/Action Congruence (00170) [**Diagnostic Division:** Ego Integrity], Submitted 2004; Revised 2013

DEFINITION: Vulnerable to an impaired ability to exercise reliance on religious beliefs and/or participate in rituals of a particular faith tradition, which may compromise health.

RISK FACTORS

Developmental
Life transition
Environmental
Insufficient transportation
Barrier to practicing religion
Physical
Illness; hospitalization; pain
Psychological
Ineffective coping strategies, or caregiving
Depression
Ineffective security; insufficient social support
Sociocultural
Insufficient social interaction
Cultural barrier to practicing religion
Spiritual
Suffering
Note: A risk diagnosis is not evidenced by signs and symptoms, as the problem has not occurred; rather, nursing interventions are directed at prevention.
Sample Clinical Applications: Any acute or chronic condition, palliative care, end-of-life situation

DESIRED OUTCOMES/EVALUATION CRITERIA

Sample NOC linkages:
Spiritual Health: Connectedness with self, others, higher power, all life, nature, and the universe that transcends and empowers the self

Client Will (Include Specific Time Frame)
- Express understanding of relation of situation or health status to thoughts and feelings of concern about ability to participate in desired religious activities.
- Seek solutions to individual factors that may interfere with reliance on religious beliefs or participation in religious rituals.
- Identify and use resources appropriately.

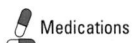

(continues on page 682)

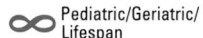

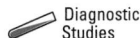

risk for impaired Religiosity (continued)
ACTIONS/INTERVENTIONS

Sample NIC linkages:
Religious Ritual Enhancement: Facilitating participation in religious practices
Spiritual Growth Facilitation: Facilitation of growth in patients' capacity to identify, connect with, and call upon the source of meaning, purpose, comfort, strength, and hope in their lives
Spiritual Support: Assisting the patient to feel balance and connection with a greater power

NURSING PRIORITY NO. 1 To assess causative/contributing factors:

- Ascertain current situation (e.g., illness, hospitalization, prognosis of death, depression, lack of support systems, financial concerns). *Identifies problems client is dealing with in the moment that may be affecting desire to be involved with religious activities.*[1]
- Note client's concerns, expressions of anger, and belief that illness or condition is result of lack of faith. *Individual may blame own self for what has happened and could reject religious beliefs and/or God.*[6]
- Determine client's usual religious or spiritual beliefs and past or current involvement in specific church activities. *Provides an understanding of how client saw religion in own life before current disruption.*[1]
- Identify cultural values and expectations regarding religious beliefs and/or practices. *Individuals grow up in a family that instills a value system within them. As the person grows up, ideas, values, and expectations may change or be strengthened by new information, different questioning, and alternative viewpoints, which may affect current situation.*[3]
- Note quality of relationships with significant others and friends. *Individual may withdraw from others in relation to the stress of illness, pain, and suffering. Others may be encouraging client to rely on religious beliefs at a time when individual is questioning own beliefs in the current situation.*[1]
- Note socioeconomic status of individual/family. *Women who are poor may have high levels of personal religiosity, yet participate less in organized religion because they feel stigmatized by their situation (e.g., single mothers, those receiving public assistance, those engaging in a lifestyle that conflicts with church norms).*[2]
- Assess lack of transportation or environmental barriers to participation in desired religious activities. *These barriers can be realistic in the face of such issues as poor bus systems, inability of individual to get to bus stop (physical problems of walking or distance to the bus stop), or inability to drive a car.*[2]
- Ascertain substance use or abuse. *Individuals often turn to use of various substances in distress, and this can affect the ability to deal with problems in a positive manner.*[7]

NURSING PRIORITY NO. 2 To assist client to deal with feelings/situation:

- Develop nurse-client relationship. *Individual can express feelings and concerns freely when he or she feels safe to do so.*[5]
- Discuss personal beliefs that may hinder participation in religious activities. *Provides opportunity for self-reflection such as own worthiness and ability to forgive self for past decisions or life choices.*[5]
- Use therapeutic communication skills of active listening, reflection, and "I" messages. *Helps client to find own solutions to problems/concerns and promotes sense of control.*[4]
- Have client identify and prioritize current and immediate needs. *Dealing with current needs is easier than trying to predict the future. Also, it is important to take care of basic needs before moving on to higher needs.*[4]
- Provide time for nonjudgmental discussion of individual's spiritual beliefs and fears about impact of current illness and/or treatment regimen. *Helps to clarify thoughts and promote ability to deal with stresses of what is happening.*[6]
- Review with client past difficulties in life and coping skills that were used at that time. *Recalling problems with family, peers, and colleagues or individuals in position of authority can help client to remember how those were handled and how those skills could be used in current situation.*

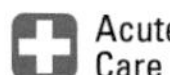

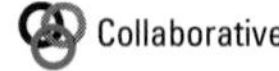

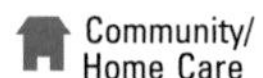

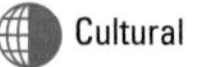

- Encourage client to discuss feelings about death and end-of-life issues when illness or prognosis is grave. *People are often afraid to talk about the possibility of their own death for fear it will bring reality to self and upset family.*[1]

NURSING PRIORITY NO. 3 To promote wellness (Teaching/Discharge Considerations):

- Have client identify support systems available. *Individual will usually know who can provide the best support for him or her in present situation. Family may not be the most supportive if they don't want to accept the reality of client's illness or situation.*[5]
- Help client learn relaxation techniques, meditation, guided imagery, and mindfulness (living in the moment and enjoying it). *Learning to relax can help client to process information and make decisions in a more positive manner.*[4]
- Take the lead from the client in initiating participation in religious activities, prayer, and other activities. *Client may be vulnerable in current situation and needs to be allowed to decide own participation in these actions. Living and participating in desired religious activities will help client to understand the tenets of his or her choice.*[8]
- Refer to appropriate resources such as crisis counselor, governmental agencies, spiritual advisor (who has qualifications or experience dealing with specific problems such as death or dying process, relationship problems, substance abuse, suicide), hospice, psychotherapy, and Alcoholics or Narcotics Anonymous. *May require additional help to deal with current situation.*[4,6,7]

DOCUMENTATION FOCUS

Assessment/Reassessment

- Individual findings, including risk factors, nature of current distress.
- Physical and emotional response to distress.
- Access to and use of resources.

Planning

- Plan of care and who is involved in planning.
- Teaching plan.

Implementation/Evaluation

- Responses to interventions, teaching, and actions performed.
- Attainment or progress toward desired outcome(s).
- Modifications to plan of care.

Discharge Planning

- Long-term needs and who is responsible for actions to be taken.
- Available resources and specific referrals made.

References

1. Burkhardt, L. (2005). A click away: Documenting spiritual care. *J Cardiovasc Nurs*, 22(1), 6–12.
2. Sullivan, S. (Updated 2013). Faith and poverty: Personal religiosity and organized religion in the lives of low-income urban mothers. Retrieved April 2015 from http://www.bc.edu/content/bc/centers/boisi/publicevents/s06/sullivan.html.
3. Herbert, R. S., Jenckes, M. W., Ford, D. E., et al. (2001). Patient perspectives on spirituality and the patient-physician relationship. *J Gen Intern Med*, 16(10), 685–692.
4. Maslow, A. H. (1970). *Religions, Values, and Peak-Experiences*. New York, NY: Penguin Books.
5. Wilkinson, M. L., Tanner, W. C. (1980). The influence of family size, interaction, and religiosity on family affection in a Mormon sample. *J Marriage Family*, 42(2), 297–304.
6. Rowthorn, R. (2011). Religion, fertility and genes: A dual inheritance model. The Royal Society Biological Sciences. Retrieved April 2015 from http://rspb.royalsocietypublishing.org/content/early/2011/01/07/rspb.2010.2504.

7. Murray-Swank, A., Luckstead, A., Wilkinson, M. L., et al. (2006). Religiosity, psychosocial adjustment and subjective burden of persons who care for those with mental illness. *Psychiatr Serv*, 57(3), 361–365.

8. Mills, J. (1999). The ontology of religiosity: The oceanic feeling and the value of the lived experience. Humanists. Retrieved April 2015 from http://huumanists.org/publications/journal/ontology-religiosity-oceanic-feeling-and-value-lived-experience.

Relocation Stress Syndrome

Taxonomy II: Coping/Stress Tolerance—Class 1 Post-Trauma Responses (00114) [**Diagnostic Division:** Ego Integrity], Submitted 1992; Revised 2000

DEFINITION: Physiological and/or psychosocial disturbance following transfer from one environment to another.

RELATED FACTORS

Move from one environment to another
History of loss; powerlessness
Insufficient support system; insufficient predeparture counseling; unpredictability of experience
Social isolation; language barrier
Impaired psychosocial functioning; ineffective coping strategies
Compromised health status

DEFINING CHARACTERISTICS

Subjective

Anxiety (e.g., separation); anger
Insecurity; worry; fear
Loneliness; depression
Unwillingness to move; concern about relocation
Alteration in sleep pattern

Objective

Increase in verbalization of needs
Pessimism; frustration
Increase in physical symptoms or illness
Withdrawal; aloneness; alienation
Loss of identity or self-worth; low self-esteem; dependency
[Increased confusion, cognitive impairment]

Sample Clinical Applications: Chronic conditions (e.g., multiple sclerosis [MS], asthma, cystic fibrosis), brain injury, stroke, dementia, schizophrenia, developmental delay, end-of-life/hospice care

DESIRED OUTCOMES/EVALUATION CRITERIA

Sample NOC linkages:

Psychosocial Adjustment: Life Change: Adaptive psychosocial response of an individual to a significant life change
Quality of Life: Extent of positive perception of current life circumstances
Coping: Personal actions to manage stressors that tax an individual's resources

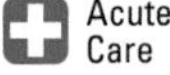

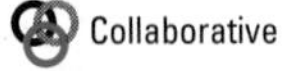

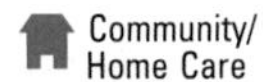

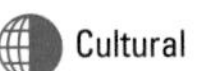

Client Will (Include Specific Time Frame)

- Verbalize understanding of reason(s) for change.
- Demonstrate appropriate range of feelings and reduced fear.
- Participate in routine and special or social events, as able.
- Verbalize acceptance of situation.
- Experience no catastrophic event.

ACTIONS/INTERVENTIONS

Sample NIC linkages:

Relocation Stress Reduction: Assisting the individual to prepare for and cope with movement from one environment to another

Hope Inspiration: Enhancing the belief in one's capacity to initiate and sustain actions

Family Involvement Promotion: Facilitating participation of family members in the emotional and physical care of the patient

NURSING PRIORITY NO. 1 To assess degree of stress as perceived/experienced by client and determine issues of safety:

- Determine situation or cause for relocation (e.g., planned move for new job, change in marital status, deployment or returning from military duty, loss of home or community due to natural or man-made disaster, deterioration in health status or ability to care for self, caregiver burnout, older parent being requested to move closer to adult child). *Although nursing and medical research is early and inconclusive in validating the defining characteristics of relocation stress syndrome as a nursing diagnosis,*[1,7,12,13] *the belief that stress associated with relocation can be extreme is widely accepted in society. The effects of relocation can be minimal and transient or very troubling and persistent.*[14]
- Note client's age, developmental level, and role in family. *Age and position in life cycle make a difference in the impact of issues involved in relocating. For example, children can be traumatized by transfer to new school and loss of friends and familiar surroundings,*[2] *and older persons may be affected by loss of their long-term home with its memories, neighborhood setting, and support persons.*[8]
- Identify cultural or religious concerns that may affect client's coping or impact social interactions and expectations. *Cultural norm may be that elders are cared for by family—not placed in a facility—causing client to feel abandoned, or individual may be required to defer to family decision maker and feel powerless in determining own destiny.*[8]
- Note ethnic ties and primary language spoken and read. *During times of stress, individuals may lapse into language of childhood. This affects healthcare providers who must try to reduce the client's feelings of alienation or confusion while communicating with client of another primary language or client who is displaced from cultural attachments.*[4]
- Ascertain if client participated in the decision to relocate and perceptions about change(s) and expectations for the future. *A forced relocation is much more stressful than one that is desired. Client may be concerned that temporary placement will deplete savings or be fearful of being a burden on family members.*
- Determine involvement of family/significant others (SOs). Note availability and use of support systems and resources. Ascertain presence or absence of comprehensive information and planning (e.g., when and how move took place, if the environment for the client is similar or greatly changed). *These factors can greatly affect client's ability to adjust to change.*
- Note signs of increased stress in recently relocated client. *Client may report or demonstrate irritability, withdrawal, crying, moodiness, problems sleeping, or fatigue; "new" physical discomfort or pain (e.g., stomachaches, headaches, back pain); change in appetite; increased use of alcohol or other drugs; or greater susceptibility to colds.*[3,8]

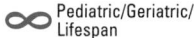

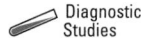

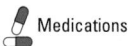

- Observe behavior, noting presence of increasing anxiety, suspiciousness or paranoia, and defensiveness. Compare with SO's/staff's description of customary responses. *Relocation may temporarily exacerbate mental deterioration (cognitive inaccessibility) and impair communication (social inaccessibility).*
- Identify issues of safety that may be involved, such as difficulty adjusting to new environment (e.g., navigating streets or choosing correct bus; locating dining hall or bathroom in facility) or concerns of elopement or running away.

NURSING PRIORITY NO. 2 To assist client to deal with situation/changes:

- Collaborate in treatment of underlying conditions (e.g., chronic confusional states, brain injury, posttrauma rehabilitation) and physical stress symptoms *that are potentially exacerbating relocation stress or that may affect the length of time that relocation is required.*
- Begin relocation planning with client and SOs as early as possible. Provide support and advocate for client who is unable to participate in decisions. *Having a well-organized plan for move with support and advocacy may reduce anxiety.*[15]
- Encourage free expression of feelings about reason for relocation, including venting of anger; grief; loss of personal space, belongings, and friends; financial strains; powerlessness; etc. Acknowledge reality of situation and maintain hopeful attitude regarding move or change. *Bringing feelings out into the open helps clarify emotions and make feelings easier to deal with.*[6,9] Refer to NDs relating to client's particular situation (e.g., ineffective Coping, Grieving) for additional interventions.
- Anticipate variety of emotions and reactions. *May vary from insomnia and loss of appetite to becoming involved with alcohol or other drugs, exacerbation of health problems, onset of serious illness, or behavioral problems.*
- Identify strengths and successful coping behaviors the individual has used previously. *Incorporating these into problem solving builds on past successes.*
- Encourage client to maintain contact with friends (e.g., telephone, letters, e-mail, video/audiotapes, arranged visits) *to reduce sense of isolation.*
- Provide client with information and list of organizations or community services (e.g., Welcome Wagon, senior citizens or teen clubs, churches, singles' groups, sports leagues) *to provide contacts for client to develop new relationships and learn more about the new setting.*[6]
- Obtain interpreter (where language differences exist) *to exchange information with the client/SO regarding residence or relocation wishes and to make helpful referrals.*[4]
- Refer to professionals (e.g., social worker, financial resources, mental healthcare provider, minister or spiritual advisor) if serious difficulties develop (e.g., depression, alcohol or other drug abuse, deteriorating behavior of child) *to assist client with special needs and/or persistent problems with adaptation.*[3,10]
- Take practical steps to alleviate stress for child. Encourage parents to walk with child to school or rehearse boarding the school bus, visit new classroom, contact friends child left behind, drive past places of interest to child, find a safe play place, unpack child's favorite toys, invite neighborhood children to a get-acquainted party, etc. *Helps child to maintain ties and develop new ones, thus reducing sense of loss and shifting focus to the future.*[2]
- Facilitate client's adjustment to new environment or facility:[5,8,11,16]
  - Determine client's usual schedule of activities and incorporate into facility routine, as possible. *Reinforces sense of importance of individual.*
  - Orient to surroundings and schedules and repeat directions, as needed.
  - Introduce to new staff members, roommate, and other residents.
  - Provide clear, honest information about actions and events.
  - Provide consistency in daily routine; maintain same staff with client in new facility, as possible, during adjustment phase.
  - Address ways to preserve lifestyle (e.g., usual bath and bedtimes in new facility, involvement in church activities). *Helps reduce the sense of loss associated with move.*

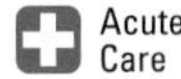
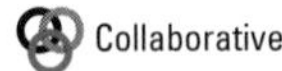
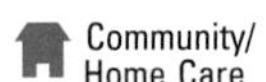
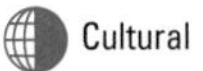

Encourage individual/family to personalize area with pictures, own belongings, etc., as soon as possible. *Enhances sense of belonging, self-expression, and creation of personal space.*

Introduce socialization and diversional activities, such as meals with new acquaintances, art therapy, music, movies, etc. *Involvement increases opportunity to interact with others and form new friendships, thus decreasing isolation and stress reactions.*

Encourage hugging and use of touch unless client prefers to abstain from hugging or is paranoid or agitated at the moment. *Human connection reaffirms acceptance of individual.*

Place in private room, if appropriate, and include SO(s)/family in care activities, mealtime, etc. *Keeping client secluded may be needed under some circumstances (e.g., advanced Alzheimer's disease with fear or aggressive reactions) to decrease the client's stress reactions to new environment.*

Deal with aggressive behavior by imposing calm, firm limits. Control environment and protect others from client's disruptive behavior. *Promotes safety for client/others.*

Remain calm, place in a quiet environment, and provide a time-out *to prevent escalation of disruptive behaviors (e.g., panic state, violence).*

- Anticipate and address feelings of distress and grieving in family/caregivers when placing loved one in a different environment (e.g., nursing home, foster care). *Support and referrals may be needed to help SOs in practical issues and adjustment.*

NURSING PRIORITY NO. 3 To enhance adjustment (Teaching/Discharge Considerations):

- Involve client in formulating goals and plan of care when possible. *Supports independence and commitment to achieving outcomes.*
- Encourage communication between client/family/SO *to provide mutual support and problem-solving opportunities.*[3]
- Discuss benefits of adequate nutrition, rest, and exercise *to maintain physical well-being and reduce adverse effects of stressful situation.*
- Instruct in anxiety- and stress-reduction activities (e.g., meditation, other relaxation techniques, exercise program, group socialization), as able, *to enhance psychological well-being and coping abilities.*
- Encourage participation in activities, hobbies, or personal interactions, as appropriate. *Promotes creative endeavors, stimulating the mind.*
- Identify community support or cultural or ethnic groups client can access.
- Support self-responsibility and coping strategies *to foster sense of control and self-worth.*

DOCUMENTATION FOCUS

Assessment/Reassessment

- Assessment findings, individual's perception of the situation and changes, specific behaviors.
- Cultural or religious concerns.
- Safety issues.

Planning

- Note plan of care, who is involved in planning, and who is responsible for proposed actions.
- Teaching plan.

Implementation/Evaluation

- Response to interventions (especially time-out or seclusion), teaching, and actions performed.
- Sentinel events.
- Attainment or progress toward desired outcome(s).
- Modifications to plan of care.

Discharge Planning

- Long-term needs and who is responsible for actions to be taken.
- Specific referrals made.

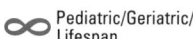

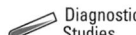

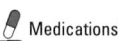

References

1. Mallick, M. J., Whipple, T. W. (2000). Validity of the nursing diagnosis of relocation stress syndrome. *Nurs Res*, 49(2), 97–100.
2. Chiaro, C. (2003). Preventing relocation stress, easing children's transition. Special report. *Colorado Springs Business Journal*.
3. Solomon, A. (2000). Relocation stress: The warning signs. Retrieved April 2015 from http://www.therapyinla.com/psych/psych0100.html.
4. Purnell, L. D., Paulanka, B. J. (1998). Purnell's model for cultural competence. *Transcultural Health Care: A Culturally Competent Approach*. Philadelphia, PA: F. A. Davis, 11–14.
5. Nypaver, J. M., Titus, M., Brugler, C. J. (1996). Patient transfer to rehabilitation: Just another move? Relocation stress syndrome. *Rehabil Nurs*, 21(2), 94–97.
6. Puskar, K. R., Dvorsak, K. G. (1991). Relocation stress in adolescents: Helping teenagers cope with a moving dilemma. *Pediatr Nurs*, 17(3), 295–298.
7. Walker, C. A., Curry, L. C., Hogstel, M. O. (2007). Relocation stress syndrome in older adults transitioning from home to long term care facility: Myth or reality? *J Psychosoc Nurs Ment Health Serv*, 45(1), 38–45.
8. Mintz, T. G. (2005). Relocation stress syndrome in older adults. *Social Work Today*, 5(6), 38–45.
9. Dion, R. (2005). Overcoming relocation stress. Military OneSource, PTSD Support Services. Retrieved April 2015 from http://www.ptsdsupport.net/relocation_stress.html.
10. Murphy, K. (2005). Anxiety: When is it too much? *Nursing Made Incredibly Easy!*, 3(5), 22–31.
11. Munche, J. A., McCarty, S. (Updated 2015). Geriatric rehabilitation. Retrieved April 2015 from http://emedicine.medscape.com/article/318521-overview.
12. Capazuti, E., Boltz, M., Renz, S., et al. (2006). Nursing home involuntary relocation: Clinical outcomes and perceptions of residents and families. *J Am Med Dir Assoc*, 7(8), 486–492.
13. Hodgson, N., Freedman, V. A., Granger, D. A., et al. (2004). Biobehavioral correlates of relocation in the frail elderly: Salivary cortisol, affect, and cognitive function. *J Am Geriatr Soc*, 52(11), 1856–1862.
14. Hertz, J. E., Koren, M. E., Rossetti, J., et al. (2008). Early identification of relocation risk in older adults with critical illness. *Crit Care Quart*, 31(1), 59–64.
15. Talerico, K. A. (2004). Relocation to a long-term care facility: Working with patients and families before, during, and after. *J Psychosoc Nurs*, 42(3), 10–16.
16. Hertz, J. E., Rossetti, J., Koren, M. E., et al. (2007). Evidence-based guideline: Management of relocation in cognitively intact older adults. *J Geront Nurs*, 33(11), 12–18.

risk for Relocation Stress Syndrome

Taxonomy II: Coping/Stress Tolerance—Class 1 Post-Trauma Responses (00149) [**Diagnostic Division:** Ego Integrity], Submitted 2000; Revised 2013

DEFINITION: Vulnerable to physiological and/or psychosocial disturbance following transfer from one environment to another that may compromise health.

RISK FACTORS

Move from one environment to another

History of loss; powerlessness

Insufficient support system; insufficient predeparture counseling; unpredictability of experience

Social isolation; language barrier

Impaired psychosocial functioning; ineffective coping strategies

Compromised health status

Note: A risk diagnosis is not evidenced by signs and symptoms, as the problem has not occurred; rather, nursing interventions are directed at prevention.

Sample Clinical Applications: Chronic conditions (e.g., multiple sclerosis [MS], asthma, cystic fibrosis), brain injury, stroke, dementia, schizophrenia, developmental delay

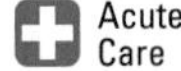

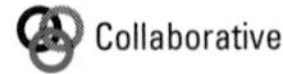

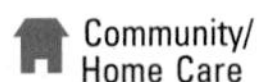

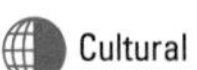

DESIRED OUTCOMES/EVALUATION CRITERIA

Sample NOC linkages:

Psychosocial Adjustment: Life Change: Adaptive psychosocial responses of an individual to a significant life change

Quality of Life: Extent of positive perception of current life circumstances

Grief Resolution: Adjustment to actual or impending loss

Client Will (Include Specific Time Frame)

- Verbalize understanding of reason(s) for change.
- Express feelings and concerns openly and appropriately.
- Experience no catastrophic event.

ACTIONS/INTERVENTIONS

Sample NIC linkages:

Discharge Planning: Preparation for moving a patient from one level of care to another within or outside the current healthcare agency

Relocation Stress Reduction: Assisting the individual to prepare for and cope with movement from one environment to another

Emotional Support: Provision of reassurance, acceptance, and encouragement during times of stress

NURSING PRIORITY NO. 1 To identify risk/contributing factors:

- Determine situation or cause for relocation (e.g., planned move for new job, deployment or returning from military duty, change in marital status, loss of home or community due to natural or man-made disaster, deterioration in health status or ability to care for self, caregiver burnout, older parent being requested to move closer to adult child). *Although nursing research is early and inconclusive in validating the defining characteristics of relocation stress syndrome as a nursing diagnosis,*[1,3,7,8] *the belief that stress associated with relocation can be extreme is widely accepted in society. The effects of relocation can be minimal and transient or very troubling and persistent.*[9]
- Note client's age, developmental level, and role in family. *Age and position in life cycle makes a difference in the impact of issues involved in relocating. For example, children can be traumatized by transfer to new school, loss of friends and familiar surroundings,*[2] *and older persons may be affected by loss of their long-term home with its memories, neighborhood setting, and support persons.*[4]
- Identify cultural and/or religious concerns that may affect client's coping or impact social interactions and expectations. *Cultural norm may be that elders are cared for by family—not placed in a facility—causing client to feel abandoned, or individual may be required to defer to family decision maker and feel powerless in determining own destiny.*[4]
- Note ethnic ties and primary language spoken and read. *During times of stress, individuals may lapse into language of childhood. This affects healthcare providers who must try to reduce client's feelings of alienation while communicating with client of another primary language or client who is displaced from cultural, familial attachments.*[5]
- Ascertain if client has participated in the decision to relocate, perceptions about change(s), and expectations for the future. *Decision may have been made without client's input or understanding of event or consequences, which can impact adjustment. A forced relocation is much more stressful than one that is desired.*[4] *Client may be concerned that temporary placement will deplete savings or may be fearful of being a burden on family members and may have felt pressured to move.*
- Note whether relocation will be temporary (e.g., extended care for rehabilitation therapies, moving in with family while house being repaired after fire) or long term or permanent (e.g., move from home of many years, placement in long-term care facility). *To some degree, a temporary relocation is usually easier to cope with*

than a permanent relocation. However, any anticipated disruption of the client's usual way of living is upsetting, and emotional responses aren't always congruent with the magnitude of the event.

- Determine involvement of family/significant others (SOs). Note availability and use of support systems and resources. Ascertain presence or absence of comprehensive information and planning (e.g., when and how move will take place, if the environment for the client will be similar or greatly changed). *These factors can greatly affect client's ability to cope with change.*

NURSING PRIORITY NO. 2 To prevent/minimize adverse response to change:

- Collaborate in treatment of underlying conditions (e.g., chronic confusional states, brain injury, posttrauma rehabilitation) and physical stress symptoms *that could exacerbate relocation stress or that affect length of time that relocation may be needed.*
- Provide information to client/SO as early in process as possible *to eliminate misconceptions and facilitate decision-making process. This can include obtaining audiovisual materials or Web sites about the new home, city, region, or country.*[5,6]
- Discuss relocation or move with child. *Information for child must be aimed at level of understanding and interest.*[2] *Child lacks ability to put problem into perspective, so minor mishap may seem catastrophic. Also, child is more vulnerable to stress because he or she has less control over environment than most adults.*[6]
- Avoid moving adolescent in middle of school year when possible. *Adolescent is vulnerable to emotional, social, and cognitive dysfunction because of the great importance of peer group and loss of friends and social standing caused by relocation.*[6]
- Involve client in placement choices when possible (e.g., move to nursing home or adult foster care) *to provide client with some control over the situation.*
- Encourage visit to new community, surroundings, or school before transfer when possible. *Provides opportunity to "get acquainted" with new situation, reducing fear of unknown.*
- Suggest contact with someone (friend, family, business associate) who has been to or lived in new area where move is being planned *to absorb some of that person's experience and knowledge.*[5,6]
- Take practical steps to alleviate stress for child. Encourage parents to walk with child to school or rehearse boarding the school bus, visit new classroom, contact friends child left behind, drive past places of interest to child, find a safe play place, unpack child's favorite toys, invite neighborhood children to a get-acquainted party, etc. *Helps child to maintain ties and develop new ones, reducing sense of loss and shifting focus to the future.*[2]
- Encourage free expression of feelings about reason for relocation. Acknowledge reality of situation and maintain hopeful attitude regarding move or change. *Bringing feelings out into the open helps clarify emotion and make feelings easier to deal with.*[6]

NURSING PRIORITY NO. 3 To promote wellness (Teaching/Discharge Considerations):

- Involve client in formulating goals and plan of care when possible. *Fosters sense of control and self-worth, supports independence and commitment to achieving outcomes.*
- Encourage client/SO to accept that relocation is an adjustment and that it takes time to adapt to new circumstances or environment.
- Instruct in anxiety- and stress-reduction activities (e.g., meditation, other relaxation techniques, exercise program, group socialization) as able *to enhance psychological well-being and coping abilities.*
- Provide client with information and list of organizations or community services (e.g., Welcome Wagon, senior citizens or teen clubs, churches, singles' groups, sports leagues) *to provide contacts for client to develop new relationships and learn more about the new setting.*[10]
- Discuss safety issues regarding new environment (e.g., how to navigate streets or choose correct bus, locate dining hall or bathroom in facility) and concerns of elopement or running away. *May help prevent adverse reactions.*

Acute Care 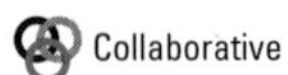 Collaborative 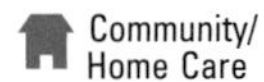 Community/Home Care 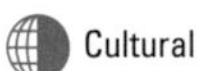 Cultural

- Anticipate variety of emotions and reactions. *May vary from insomnia and loss of appetite to becoming involved with alcohol or other drugs, exacerbation of health problems, onset of serious illness, or behavioral problems. Awareness provides opportunity for timely intervention.*[6]
- Refer to ND Relocation Stress Syndrome for additional interventions.

DOCUMENTATION FOCUS

Assessment/Reassessment

- Assessment findings, individual's perception of the situation/changes, specific behaviors.
- Cultural or religious concerns.
- Safety issues.

Planning

- Note plan of care, who is involved in planning, and who is responsible for proposed actions.
- Teaching plan.

Implementation/Evaluation

- Response to interventions (especially time-out/seclusion), teaching, and actions performed.
- Sentinel events.
- Attainment or progress toward desired outcome(s).
- Modifications to plan of care.

Discharge Planning

- Long-term needs and who is responsible for actions to be taken.
- Specific referrals made.

References

1. Mallick, M. J., Whipple, T. W. (2000). Validity of the nursing diagnosis of relocation stress syndrome. *Nurs Res*, 49(2), 97–100.
2. Chiaro, C. (2003). Preventing relocation stress, easing children's transition. Special report. *Colorado Springs Business Journal.*
3. Walker, C. A., Curry, L. C., Hogstel, M. O. (2007). Relocation stress syndrome in older adults transitioning from home to long term care facility: Myth or reality? *J Psychosoc Nurs Ment Health Serv*, 45(1), 38–45.
4. Mintz, T. G. (2005). Relocation stress syndrome in older adults. *Social Work Today*, 5(6), 38.
5. Solomon, A. (2000). Relocation stress: The warning signs. Retrieved April 2015 from http://www.therapyinla.com/psych/psych0100.html.
6. Dion, R. (2005). Overcoming relocation stress. Military OneSource, PTSD Support Services. Retrieved April 2015 from http://www.ptsdsupport.net/relocation_stress.html.
7. Capazuti, E., Boltz, M., Renz, S., et al. (2006). Nursing home involuntary relocation: Clinical outcomes and perceptions of residents and families. *J Am Med Dir Assoc*, 7(8), 486–492.
8. Hodgson, N., Freedman, V. A., Granger, D. A., et al. (2004). Biobehavioral correlates of relocation in the frail elderly: Salivary cortisol, affect, and cognitive function. *J Am Geriatr Soc*, 52(11), 1856–1862.
9. Hertz, J. E., Koren, M. E., Rossetti, J., et al. (2008). Early identification of relocation risk in older adults with critical illness. *Crit Care Quart*, 31(1), 59–64.
10. Puskar, K. R., Dvorsak, K. G. (1991). Relocation stress in adolescents: Helping teenagers cope with a moving dilemma. *Pediatr Nurs*, 17(3), 295–298.

risk for ineffective Renal Perfusion

Taxonomy II: Activity/Rest—Class 4 Cardiovascular/Pulmonary Responses (00203) [**Diagnostic Division:** Circulatory], Submitted 2008; Revised 2013

DEFINITION: Vulnerable to a decrease in blood circulation to the kidney, which may compromise health.

RISK FACTORS

Alteration in metabolism; diabetes mellitus
Renal disease (e.g., polycystic kidney, renal artery stenosis, failure); bilateral cortical necrosis; exposure to nephrotoxin; glomerulonephritis; interstitial nephritis; polynephritis
Burns; infection; systemic inflammatory response syndrome (SIRS)
Cardiac surgery; vascular embolism; vasculitis
Abdominal compartment syndrome
Extremes of age; female gender
Hypertension; malignant hypertension; hypovolemia; hypoxema
Malignancy
Smoking; substance abuse
Trauma; treatment regimen
NOTE: A risk diagnosis is not evidenced by signs and symptoms, as the problem has not occurred; rather, nursing interventions are directed at prevention.
Sample Clinical Applications: Diabetes mellitus, hypertension, atherosclerosis, atrial fibrillation, sickle cell anemia, heat stroke, aortic aneurysm, shock states

DESIRED OUTCOMES/EVALUATION CRITERIA

Sample NOC linkages:
Kidney Function: Filtration of blood and elimination of metabolic waste products through the formation of urine
Knowledge: Disease Process: Extent of understanding conveyed about a specific disease process and prevention of complications

Client Will (Include Specific Time Frame)

- Demonstrate adequate renal perfusion as evidenced by urine output appropriate for individual, balanced intake and output, absence of edema formation, or inappropriate weight gain.
- Verbalize understanding of condition, therapy regimen, side effects of medication, and when to contact healthcare provider.
- Engage in behaviors or lifestyle changes to improve circulation (e.g., smoking cessation, diabetic glucose control, medication management).

ACTIONS/INTERVENTIONS

Sample NIC linkages:
Fluid/Electrolyte Management: Regulation and prevention of complications from altered fluid and/or electrolyte levels

NURSING PRIORITY NO. 1 To assess causative/contributing factors:

- Determine history or presence of severe hypotension and hypoxemia; cardiogenic, hypovolemia, or obstructive or septic shock; blunt or penetrating trauma with internal hemorrhage; and surgery with excess bleeding or

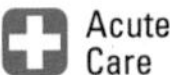
Acute Care
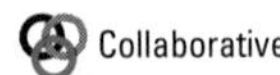
Collaborative
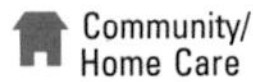
Community/ Home Care
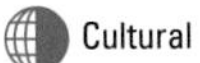
Cultural

fluid loss, prolonged dehydration, poorly controlled dehydration, etc. *These conditions are associated with decreased circulation and kidney ischemia.*[1,2]

- Note history or presence of abrupt onset or severe hypertension, persistent hypertension (greater than 160/100 mmHg) over time, or hypertension resistant to appropriately dosed multidrug antihypertensive therapy, *any of which places client at high risk for kidney damage associated with renovascular hypertension.*[3,4]
- Assess hydration status. *Dehydration reduces glomerular filtration rate.*[5]
- Auscultate for bruit over each renal artery in the abdomen at the midclavicular line. *Bruit suggests renal artery stenosis, which is associated with renal insufficiency.*[3,5]
- Determine usual voiding pattern and investigate reported deviations, such as low output or need for diuretics. *May indicate problems with kidney perfusion associated with conditions such as hypovolemia, obstructive problem in urinary tract, shock states, and heart failure, requiring further evaluation.*
- Note urine color—pale (dilute), dark (concentrated)—and measure specific gravity, as indicated, *to evaluate hydration status and ability of kidneys to concentrate the urine. Note: In a recent descriptive correlational design study, urine color was significantly correlated with urine specific gravity and osmolality.*[6]
- Monitor fluid intake, urine output, and weight on a regular schedule. *Changes in weight and fluid intake, especially when calculated against output on a regular basis (e.g., 24 hr), can provide noninvasive assessment of cardiovascular and renal function.*
- Monitor for edema. *Edema may be present with increased fluid retention due to impaired renal function related to decreased renal perfusion.*[12]
- Note mentation and behavior. *Adverse changes may be the consequence of fluid shifts, accumulation of toxins, acidosis, electrolyte imbalances, and/or azotemia when kidney dysfunction is occurring.*[5]
- Review laboratory studies (e.g., complete blood count, blood urea nitrogen/creatinine levels, protein, specific gravity, 24-hr creatinine clearance, glucose, electrolytes) *to assess status of renal function and evaluate progression of renal dysfunction or failure and effects on body and organ function.*
- Review diagnostic studies, as indicated, including Doppler ultrasonography, computed tomography, renogram, intravenous pyelogram, and contrast or magnetic resonance angiography, *to evaluate kidney size, perfusion, and function.*
- Review medication regimen, observing for certain antimicrobials, antivirals, chemotherapy agents, analgesics, immunosuppressives, herbals, and diagnostic agents. Monitor peak and trough blood levels when client receiving nephrotoxic agents such as aminoglycocides (e.g., vancomycin) *known for potential side or toxic effects that may substantially alter kidney perfusion. Note: The list of commonly nephrotoxic agents is sizable, and risk must be evaluated for individual when drugs are prescribed.*[11]
- Discuss client's history of and current alcohol and illicit substance use/abuse. *Most street drugs, including heroin, cocaine, and ecstasy can cause high blood pressure, a risk factor for impaired renal function. Alcohol (when used heavily), cocaine, heroin, and amphetamines also can cause kidney damage.*[13]

NURSING PRIORITY NO. 2 To reduce or correct individual risk factors:

- Collaborate in treatment of underlying conditions (e.g., angioplasty with stent placement, surgical revascularization procedures, fluids, electrolytes, nutrients, antibiotics, thrombolytics, oxygen) *to improve tissue perfusion/organ function.*
- Administer medications (e.g., vasoactive medications, including antihypertensive agents, diuretics, steroids, insulin) as indicated *to treat underlying condition and improve renal blood flow and function.*
- Exercise caution when administering nephrotoxic agents, particularly when dehydration is present, *to reduce risk for acute or chronic renal failure.*[5]
- Provide for fluid and diet restrictions, as indicated, while providing adequate calories and hydration *to meet the body's needs without overtaxing kidney function.*
- Refer to NDs deficient or excess Fluid Volume and impaired Urinary Elimination for additional interventions.

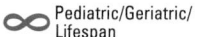

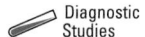

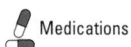

NURSING PRIORITY NO. 3 To promote optimal renal function (Teaching/Discharge Considerations):

- Discuss individual risk factors (e.g., family history, obesity, age, smoking, hypertension, diabetes, clotting disorders) and potential outcomes of atherosclerosis such as systemic and peripheral vascular disease. *Information can assist client to make informed choices about remedial risk factors and needed lifestyle changes to prevent onset of complications or manage symptoms when condition is present.*[7,8]
- Identify necessary changes in lifestyle and assist client to incorporate disease management into activities of daily living. *Promotes independence and enhances self-concept regarding ability to deal with change and manage own needs.*
- Emphasize need to manage blood pressure when client is hypertensive. Instruct about individual's antihypertensive medications (e.g., angiotensin-converting enzyme [ACE] inhibitors, diuretics, beta-blockers) and necessity for taking them as prescribed and with physician follow-up *to reduce cardiovascular complications and inhibit progression of renal dysfunction.*[5]
- Instruct in home blood pressure monitoring, advise purchase of appropriate equipment, and refer to community resources as indicated. *Facilitates management of hypertension, which is a major risk factor for damage to blood vessels and organ function.*[5,9]
- Encourage client to quit smoking and join Smoke-out or other smoking-cessation programs. *Smoking causes vasoconstriction, potentially compromising renal perfusion.*
- Review specific fluid and dietary requirements with client/SO (e.g., reduction of cholesterol, carbohydrates, or sodium) as indicated by individual situation *to promote circulatory health and kidney function.*
- Establish regular exercise program *to enhance circulation and promote general well-being.*[10]
- Encourage periodic medical and laboratory follow-up *to provide monitoring and earlier intervention for underlying conditions and evaluate effectiveness of therapeutic interventions.*
- Refer to specific support groups and counseling as appropriate *to assist with problem solving, provide role model, and enhance coping ability.*

DOCUMENTATION FOCUS

Assessment/Reassessment

- Individual physical findings; identified risk factors.
- Baseline kidney function.
- Intake and output, and weight as indicated.

Planning

- Plan of care and who is involved in planning.
- Teaching plan.

Implementation/Evaluation

- Response to interventions, teaching, and actions performed.
- Attainment or progress toward desired outcome(s).
- Modifications to plan of care.

Discharge Planning

- Long-term needs and who is responsible for actions to be taken.
- Available resources, specific referrals made.

References

1. Kanaparthi, L. K., Lessnau,, K. D., Peralta, R. (Updated 2013). Distributive shock. Retrieved April 2015 from http://emedicine.medscape.com/article/168689-overview.
2. Editorial staff. (2006). Renal system. *Pathophysiology Made Incredibly Easy!*. 3rd ed. Philadelphia, PA: Lippincott Williams & Wilkins.

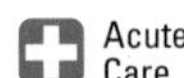

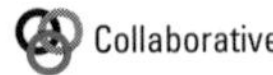

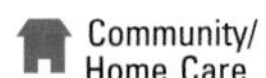

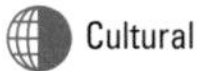

3. Spinowitz, B. S., Rodriguez, J. (Updated 2013). Renal artery stenosis. Retrieved April 2015 from http://emedicine.medscape.com/article/245023-overview.
4. Schmidt, R. J., Mustafa, M. R. (Updated 2015). Renovascular hypertension. Retrieved April 2015 from http://emedicine.medscape.com/article/245140-overview.
5. Winkleman, C. (2006). Assessment of the renal/urinary system. In Ignatavicius, N. N., Workman, M. L. (eds.) (eds). *Medical-Surgical Nursing: Critical Thinking for Collaborative Care*. 5th ed. St. Louis, MO: Elsevier Saunders.
6. Mentes, J. C., Wakefield, B., Culp, K. (2006). Use of a urine color chart to monitor hydration status in nursing home residents. *Biol Res Nurs*, 7(3), 197–203.
7. Seiggreen, M. Y. (2006). Getting a leg up on managing venous ulcers. *Nursing Made Incredibly Easy!*, 4(6), 52–60.
8. Baldwin, K. M. (2006). Stroke: It's a knock-out punch. *Nursing Made Incredibly Easy!*, 4(2), 10–23.
9. Sauerbeck, L. R. (2006). Primary stroke prevention. *Am J Nurs*, 106(11), 40–49.
10. Frost, K. L., Topp, R. (2006). A physical activity Rx for the hypertensive patient. *Nurse Pract*, 31(4), 29–37.
11. Parazella, M. A. (2009). Renal vulnerability to drug toxicity: Drug table. *CJASN*, 4(7), 1275–1283.
12. Broscious, S. K., Castagnola, J. (2006). Chronic kidney disease: Acute manifestations and role of critical care nurses. *Crit Care Nurse*, 26(4), 17–27.
13. Crowe, A. V., Howse, M., Bell, G. M., et al. (2000). Substance abuse and the kidney. *QJM*, 93(3), 147–153.

impaired Resilience

Taxonomy II: Coping/Stress Tolerance—Class 2 Coping Responses (00210) [**Diagnostic Division:** Ego Integrity], Submitted 2008; Revised 2013

DEFINITION: Decreased ability to sustain a pattern of positive responses to an adverse situation or crisis.

RELATED FACTORS

Community violence; exposure to violence
Demographics that increase changes of maladjustment; ethnic minority status
Economically disadvantaged; perceived vulnerability
Female gender; large family size
Inconsistent parenting; parental mental illness; psychological disorder
Low intellectual ability; low maternal educational level
Insufficient impulse control; substance abuse

DEFINING CHARACTERISTICS

Subjective

Depression; guilt; shame
Impaired health status
Renewed elevation of distress
Decreased interest in academic or vocational activities

Objective

Ineffective coping skills; social isolation; low self-esteem

Sample Clinical Applications: Substance abuse, mental health issues—depression, phobia, bipolar disorder, schizophrenia; chronic illness—renal failure, heart failure, cancer; debilitating conditions—multiple sclerosis (MS), Parkinson's disease, obesity; domestic abuse or violence

(continues on page 696)

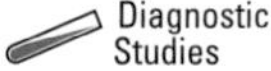
Diagnostic Studies
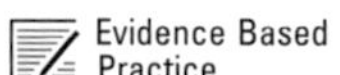
Evidence Based Practice
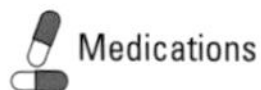
Medications
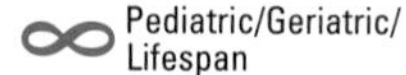
Pediatric/Geriatric/Lifespan

impaired Resilience (continued)
DESIRED OUTCOMES/EVALUATION CRITERIA

Sample NOC linkages:
Personal Resiliency: Positive adaptation and function of an individual following significant adversity or crisis
Hope: Optimism that is personally satisfying and life supporting
Family Resiliency: Positive adaptation and function of the family system following significant adversity or crisis

Client Will (Include Specific Time Frame)
Acknowledge reality of current situation or crisis.
Express positive feelings about self and situation.
Seek appropriate resources to change circumstances that affect adaptation and resilience.
Be involved in programs to address problems presenting in life (e.g., substance abuse, low self-esteem, poverty).

ACTIONS/INTERVENTIONS

Sample NIC linkages:
Resiliency Promotion: Assisting individuals, families, and communities in development, use, and strengthening of factors to be used in coping with environmental and societal stressors
Hope Inspiration: Enhancing the belief in one's capacity to initiate and sustain actions
Family Mobilization: Utilization of family strengths to influence patient's health in a positive direction

NURSING PRIORITY NO. 1 To assess causative/contributing factors:

- Determine individuals involved, family, children, ages, and current circumstances. *Understanding the family makeup provides information that will guide choice of interventions.*[1]
- Note underlying stressors, health concerns, debilitating conditions, and mental health or behavioral issues, such as unemployment, poverty, diabetes, obesity, chronic obstructive pulmonary disease, Alzheimer's disease, and parental mental illness. *Provides information about situation to plan appropriate care.*[1,5]
- Identify locus of control. *Individuals with external locus of control are less likely to feel in control or rely on their own abilities or judgment to manage a situation.*[1,2,6]
- Determine client's education level, family dynamics, and parenting styles if relevant. *Drug use, violence, and poor impulse control affect ability of individual to develop resilience to adverse situations or crisis and may result in individual viewing self as a victim rather than a survivor.*[1,3]
- Note communication patterns within the family. *Skills learned within the family can make the difference between whether the individual develops low self-esteem or has positive feelings about self.*
- Identify maladaptive coping skills used by individual and in the family. *The use of food or drugs to deal with feelings, acting-out behaviors or violence, devaluing education or importance of learning new skills, and focusing on the negative in situations lead to members learning these methods of dealing with problems and difficulties that arise, resulting in lack of ability to adjust positively and learn attributes of resiliency.*[3]
- Note parental status including age and maturity. *Young parents may lack ability to deal with family responsibilities, financial concerns, and low socioeconomic factors.*[2,10]
- Ascertain stability of relationship, presence of separation or divorce. *Family members are vulnerable to breakup of the family unit and, depending on perception and circumstances, see it as causing long-term liability.*[4]
- Determine availability and use of resources, family, support groups, and financial. *Appropriate use can help individuals overcome and manage problems in their lives.*
- (Cultural) Discuss religious and cultural beliefs held by the individual and family. *Including the members of the family in this discussion promotes the idea that they are partners in their healthcare and enables them to*

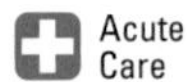

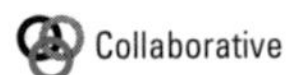

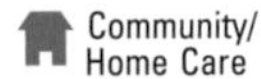

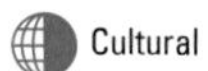

learn and have input into how these beliefs affect what they do. Knowing the role of the elements of culture in shaping and defining health behavior helps the family understand how this is important to them.[5]

NURSING PRIORITY NO. 2 To assist client to improve skills to deal with adverse situations or crises:

- Encourage free expressions of feelings, including feelings of anger and hostility, setting limits on unacceptable behavior. *When feelings are verbalized, client begins to identify them and recognize how they affect personal behavior. Unacceptable behavior leads to feelings of shame and guilt if it is not controlled.*[1,2]
- Listen to client's concerns and acknowledge difficulty of adversity and making changes in situation. *Often, individuals who are feeling that life is difficult begin to doubt their ability to deal with circumstances and are not able to see positive outcomes. Being listened to provides opportunity for client to feel valued, capable, and like a survivor rather than a victim.*[3]
- Help client to assume responsibility for own life, to look at situation as a challenge rather than an obstacle, and to refrain from viewing crisis as insurmountable. *Resilience is not something that people have or do not have; it is learned and developed in people as they deal with adversities of life. Taking care of oneself keeps the mind ready to deal with adverse situations.*[3,6,9]
- Provide information at client's level of comprehension, being honest in explanations. *Provides data to assist in decision-making process and enhances client's cooperation in change process.*[1]
- Have client paraphrase information provided during teaching session. *Assures client's understanding and provides opportunity to correct misunderstandings.*[1]
- Promote parent involvement in developing a positive mind-set for fostering resilience in their children. *Parents are concerned that their children grow up to be competent adults. They can learn the parenting skills that promote optimal growth and resilience in their children for the problems they will face as grown-ups*[3,9]
- Facilitate communication skills between client and family. *Sometimes, individuals who find themselves in difficult situations withdraw because they do not know what to do or say. Helping the client to learn new ways to interact will not only help him or her but also family members learn effective ways of communicating.*[2,3,7]
- Focus on strengths of the individual as problems are being assessed and diagnosed. *Improving the future for the client is based on developing the capacity to deal successfully with the obstacles he or she meets in life.*[3]
- Encourage client/parents to model empathy with family members. *Empathy is an important interpersonal skill and a cornerstone of emotional intelligence.*[8] *Children learn empathy when parents are empathic with them.*[2,6]
- Discuss individual issues, such as obesity, substance use, poor impulse control, or violent behavior, providing information about the risks and helping client/parent understand how he or she can help family members develop habits that will promote physical and mental well-being. *For example, recent studies suggest that encouraging children to reduce sedentary behavior (e.g., watching TV, playing video games) can promote weight loss and reduce the intake of calorie-dense foods. Choosing enjoyable exercise and video games that provide for movement helps to improve feelings of satisfaction and sense of control.*[3,9]

NURSING PRIORITY NO. 3 To promote resilience (Teaching/Discharge Considerations):

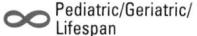

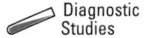

- Reinforce that client is responsible for self, for choices made, and actions taken. *The road to resilience is developed by the individual accepting that change is a part of living and beginning to live life more fully.*[3,9]
- Provide or identify learning opportunities specific to individual needs. *Activities such as assertiveness, regular exercise, and parenting classes can enhance knowledge and help develop a resilience mind-set.*[1,2,6]
- Discuss use of the problem-solving method to set mutually agreed-on goals. *As family accepts solutions that are acceptable to each member, their self-esteem is enhanced and individuals are more apt to follow through on decisions.*[2,3,10]
- Provide anticipatory guidance relevant to current situation and long-term expectations. *Client may have many issues to resolve, and planning ahead can help client make changes, have hope for the future, and have a sense of control over his or her life.*
- Encourage client/parents to take time for themselves. *They may believe they need to devote all their time to the family and feel guilty if they take time for themselves. This provides an opportunity for personal growth,*

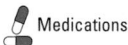

and respite allows individuals to pursue own interests and return to tasks of life or parenting with renewed vigor.[2]

- Refer to community resources as appropriate, such as social services, financial, domestic violence or elder abuse program, family therapy, divorce counseling, and special needs support services. *Appropriate support enhances ability to develop resilience in challenges client is dealing with.*[10]

DOCUMENTATION FOCUS

Assessment/Reassessment

- Findings, including specifics of individual situations or parental concerns, perceptions, expectations.
- Locus of control and cultural beliefs.

Planning

- Plan of care and who is involved in the planning.
- Teaching plan.

Implementation/Evaluation

- Response to interventions, teaching, and actions performed.
- Attainment or progress toward desired outcome(s).
- Modifications to plan of care.

Discharge Planning

- Long-term needs and who is responsible for actions to be taken.
- Specific referrals made.

References

1. Zandonella, C. (2006). Resilience in children. The New York Academy of Sciences. Retrieved April 2015 from http://www.nyas.org/Publications/Ebriefings/Detail.aspx?cid=25e9b1f7-2dc4-4c3e-bd63-440afcb8441d.
2. Patten, M. (Updated 2008). Are you resilient? Retrieved April 2015 from http://ezinearticles.com/?Are-You-Resilient?.
3. Comas-Diaz, M., Luthar, S. S., Maddi, S. R. (No date). The road to resilience. American Psychological Association Brochure. Retrieved April 2015 from http://www.apa.org/helpcenter/road-resilience.aspx.
4. Eldar-Avidan, D., Haj-Yahia, M., Greenbaum, C. (2009). Divorce is a part of my life . . . resilience, survival, and vulnerability: Young adults' perception of the implications of parental divorce. *J Marital Fam Ther*, 35(1), 30–46.
5. Calamaro, C., Waite, R. (2008). Cultural proficiency, research, and evidence-based practice: Implications for the nurse practitioner. *J Pediatr Health Care*, 23(1), 69–72.
6. Adams, L. (2011). How do you deal with adversity? Gordon Training International. Retrieved April 2015 from http://www.gordontraining.com/free-workplace-articles/how-do-you-deal-with-adversity/.
7. Brooks, R. L., Goldstein, S. (2006). Risk, resilience and futurists: Changing the lives of our children. *Education Horizons*, 9(3), 14–15.
8. National Institute for Mental Health Promotion and Youth Violence Prevention. Social and Emotional Learning and Bullying Prevention. Retrieved April 2015 from http://www.promoteprevent.org/sites/www.promoteprevent.org/files/resources/SELBullying(1).pdf.
9. Adams, L. (2011). Taking personal responsibility. Gordon Training International. Retrieved April 2015 from http://www.gordontraining.com/free-workplace-articles/taking-personal-responsibility/.
10. Bonanno, G., Galea, S., Buchiarelli, A., et al. (2007). What predicts psychological resilience after disaster? The role of demographics, resources, and life stress. *J Consult Clin Psychol*, 75(5), 671–682.

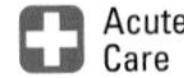
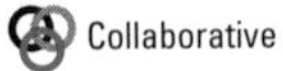
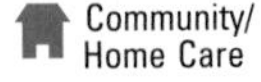
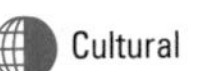

readiness for enhanced Resilience

Taxonomy II: Coping/Stress Tolerance—Class 2 Coping Responses (00212) [**Diagnostic Division:** Ego Integrity], Submitted 2008; Revised 2013

DEFINITION: A pattern of positive responses to an adverse situation or crisis, which can be strengthened.

DEFINING CHARACTERISTICS

Subjective

Expresses desire to enhance: communication skills, relationships with others
Expresses desire to enhance use of: coping skills, conflict management strategies
Expresses desire to enhance: resilience, self-esteem
Expresses desire to enhance: involvement in activities, own responsibility for action, sense of control
Expresses desire to enhance: goal-setting, progress toward goal
Expresses desire to enhance: support system, available resources, use of resources
Expresses desire to enhance: environmental safety

Objective

Demonstrates positive outlook
Exposure to crisis

Sample Clinical Applications: Chronic health conditions (e.g., asthma, diabetes mellitus, arthritis, systemic lupus, multiple sclerosis [MS], AIDS); mental health concerns (e.g., depression, anxiety, bipolar disorder, attention deficit-hyperactivity disorder)

DESIRED OUTCOMES/EVALUATION CRITERIA

Sample NOC linkages:

Personal Resiliency: Positive adaptation and function of an individual following significant adversity or crisis
Hope: Optimism that is personally satisfying and life supporting
Family Resiliency: Positive adaptation and function of the family system following significant adversity or crisis

Client Will (Include Specific Time Frame)

- Describe current situation accurately.
- Identify positive responses currently being used.
- Verbalize feelings congruent with behavior.
- Express desire to strengthen ability to deal with current situation or crisis.

ACTIONS/INTERVENTIONS

Sample NIC linkages:

Resiliency Promotion: Assisting individuals, families, and communities in development, use, and strengthening of factors to be used in coping with environmental and societal stressors
Hope Inspiration: Enhancing the belief in one's capacity to initiate and sustain actions
Family Mobilization: Utilization of family strengths to influence patient's health in a positive direction

NURSING PRIORITY NO. 1 To determine needs and desires for improvement:

- Evaluate client's perception and ability to provide a realistic view of the situation. *Provides information about how the client views the situation and specific expectations to aid in formulating plan of care.*[5]

- Determine client's coping abilities in current situation and expectations for change. *Client may be stressed to the point of having difficulty coping, recognizing need to improve ability to manage.*[4,6] *Motivation to improve and high expectations can encourage client to make changes that will improve his or her life. However, unrealistic expectations may hamper efforts.*
- Note client's verbal expressions indicating belief that he or she owns the responsibility for how to deal with adverse situation. *When client has internal locus of control, he or she accepts that life has its adversities and one needs to deal with them.*[3]
- Discuss religious and cultural beliefs held by the individual. *Knowing the role of the elements of culture and religion in shaping and defining health behaviors and expectations of client helps determine individual needs and possible options.*[1]
- Identify support systems available to client. *Having family and friends who are willing to listen as client works through problems can help to resolve them.*[5]

NURSING PRIORITY NO. 2 To assist client to enhance resilience to adverse situation:

- Active-listen and identify client's concerns about situation. *Reflecting client's statements helps to clarify what he or she is thinking and promotes accurate interpretation of reality.*[2]
- Determine previous methods of dealing with adversity. *Helps client to remember successful skills used in the past and see what might be helpful in current situation.*[3]
- Discuss desire to improve ability to handle adverse situations that arise throughout life. *The willingness to be open to change requires curiosity, listening to other's ideas and beliefs, and looking at new ways to do things.*[3]
- Discuss concept of what can be changed versus what cannot be changed. *Understanding that some things cannot be changed helps client to focus energies on those things that can be changed.*[2]
- Determine how client is dealing with activities of daily living. *While client may have some transient problems with sleeping or managing daily affairs, most people have the ability to function in a healthy manner over time.*[6]
- Help client to learn how to empathize with others. *Understanding own emotions as well as feelings of others enhances one's resiliency during stressful times.*[4]

NURSING PRIORITY NO. 3 To promote optimum growth and resiliency:

- Provide factual information and anticipatory guidance relevant to current situation and long-term expectations. *Planning ahead allows for problem solving and review of options in a relaxed atmosphere, reinforcing sense of control and hope for the future.*[3]
- Review factors that might impact individual's response to stress. *Genetic influences, past experiences, and existing conditions can determine whether the client's response is adaptive or maladaptive and help individual to be resilient.*[3]
- Encourage client to maintain or establish good relationships with family and friends. *These connections are important, and accepting help and support from others enhances own coping and strengthens resilience.*[7]
- Help client to avoid seeing situation as insurmountable. *Catastrophic thinking locks individual into believing he or she has no control over outcome. While one cannot change the fact of the circumstances, how individual interprets and responds is within his or her control.*[7]
- Recommend setting realistic goals and doing something regularly, even if it is small. *Moving toward goals encourages a feeling of accomplishment and self-esteem.*[7]
- Encourage client to maintain a hopeful outlook, nurture a positive view of self, and take care of self. *Keeping a long-term perspective and paying attention to own needs helps maintain and build resilience.*[7]
- Refer to classes and/or reading materials as appropriate. *Learning skills of meditation and assertiveness and engaging in enjoyable exercises helps to foster resilience.*[3,7]

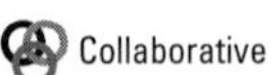
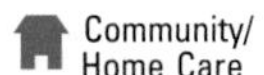
 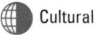

DOCUMENTATION FOCUS

Assessment/Reassessment

- Baseline information, including client's perception of situation, view of own ability to be resilient, and support systems available.
- Ways of dealing with previous life problems.
- Motivation and expectations for change.
- Cultural or religious influences.

Planning

- Plan of care and who is involved in planning.
- Teaching plan.

Implementation/Evaluation

- Responses to interventions, teaching, and actions performed.
- Attainment or progress toward desired outcomes(s).
- Modifications to plan.

Discharge Planning

- Long-term needs and who is responsible for actions to be taken.
- Specific referrals made.

References

1. Calamaro, C., Waite, R. (2008). Cultural proficiency, research, and evidence-based practice: Implications for the nurse practitioner. *J Pediatr Health Care*, 23(1), 69–72.
2. Adams, L. (2011). How do you deal with adversity? Retrieved November 2015 from http://www.gordontraining.com/free-workplace-articles/how-do-you-deal-with-adversity/.
3. Brooks, R. (2003). The power to change your life: Ten keys to resilient living. Retrieved November 2015 from http://www.drrobertbrooks.com/wp/wp-content/uploads/2003/10/The-Power-to-Change-Your-Life-Ten-Keys-to-Resilient-Living.pdf.
4. Comas-Diaz, L., Luthar, S. S., Maddi, S. R. (2011). The road to resilience. Retrieved June 2012 from http://www.apa.org/helpcenter/road-resilience.aspx.
5. Eldar-Avidan, D., Haj-Yahia, M., Greenbaum, C. (2009). Divorce is a part of my life . . . resilience, survival and vulnerability: Young adults' perception of the implications of parental divorce. *J Marital Fam Ther*, 35(1), 30–46.
6. McKeever, M. (2011). The brain and emotional intelligence: An interview with Daniel Goleman. Trycycle Blog. Retrieved November 2015 from http://www.tricycle.com/blog/brain-and-emotional-intelligence-interview-daniel-goleman.
7. Adams, L. (2011). Taking personal responsibility. Retrieved November 2015 from http://www.gordontraining.com/free-workplace-articles/taking-personal-responsibility/.

risk for impaired Resilience

Taxonomy II: Coping/Stress Tolerance—Class 2 Coping Responses (00211) [**Diagnostic Division:** Ego Integrity], Submitted 2008; Revised 2013

DEFINITION: Vulnerable to decreased ability to sustain a pattern of positive responses to an adverse situation or crisis, which may compromise health.

RISK FACTORS

Chronicity of existing crisis
Multiple coexisting adverse situations
New crisis (e.g., unplanned pregnancy, loss of housing, death of family member)
Note: A risk diagnosis is not evidenced by signs and symptoms, as the problem has not occurred; rather, nursing interventions are directed at prevention.
Sample Clinical Applications: Chronic or debilitating illness (e.g., Alzheimer's disease, multiple sclerosis [MS], Parkinson's disease, Crohn's disease, diabetes, heart failure, cancer, renal failure); mental health issues (e.g., depression, anxiety)

DESIRED OUTCOMES/EVALUATION CRITERIA

Sample NOC linkages:
Personal Resiliency: Positive adaptation and function of an individual following significant adversity or crisis
Hope: Optimism that is personally satisfying and life supporting
Family Resiliency: Positive adaptation and function of the family system following significant adversity or crisis

Client Will (Include Specific Time Frame)
- Acknowledge reality of individual situation or crisis.
- Verbalize feelings associated with chronic situation.
- Verbalize awareness of own ability to deal with problems.
- Identify resources for assisting with chronic and new adverse occurrence.

ACTIONS/INTERVENTIONS

Sample NIC linkages:
Resiliency Promotion: Assisting individuals, families, and communities in development, use, and strengthening of factors to be used in coping with environmental and societal stressors
Hope Inspiration: Enhancing the belief in one's capacity to initiate and sustain actions
Family Mobilization: Utilization of family strengths to influence patient's health in a positive direction

NURSING PRIORITY NO. 1 To determine individual stressors/potential challenges:

- Note underlying stressors, health concerns, debilitating conditions, and mental health or behavioral issues, such as unemployment, pregnancy, diabetes, Alzheimer's disease, and anxiety disorder. *Provides information about situation to plan appropriate care.*[5]
- Determine alcohol or other drug use, smoking, sleeping, and eating habits. *Affects ability to cope with added stress of crises effectively and in a healthy manner.*[5]
- Assess functional capacity and how it affects client's ability to manage daily needs. *Presence of physical impairments may bring additional stress to adverse situation and unplanned new crisis.*[5]
- Evaluate client's ability to verbalize and understand current situation and impact of new crisis. *Informed choice cannot be made without a good understanding of reality of situation.*[5]

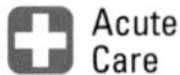

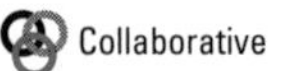

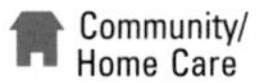

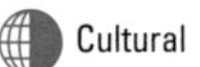

- Note speech and communication patterns. *Provides information about level of education and ability to understand situation and relate problems to caregiver(s).*[5]
- Determine locus of control. *Individuals with external locus of control are less likely to feel in control or rely on their own abilities or judgment to manage a situation and may wait for someone else, or luck, to change the circumstances and make life better.*[2,4,5]
- Evaluate client's current decision-making ability. *Crises affect individual's ability to think clearly and trust own ability to deal with situation.*[3]
- Ascertain stability of relationship, presence of separation or divorce, deteriorating health, or recent death of family member. *Family members are vulnerable to breakup of the family unit and, depending on perception and circumstances, may see it as causing long-term liability.*[3]

NURSING PRIORITY NO. 2 To assess coping skills and degree of resilience:

- Active listen and identify client's perceptions of what has occurred as well as previous concerns. *Helps client to reflect back reality and distinguish between perceptions and actual events.*[2]
- Determine how adverse situation is affecting client's ability to deal with what is happening now. *When an unplanned situation occurs in addition to existing problems, it often results in decreased ability to maintain optimism.*[3,5,8]
- Determine how individual has dealt with problems in the past. *Having client remember these skills helps client to recognize what can be used to enhance current response or address future challenges.*[3,7]
- Note cultural factors and religious beliefs that may affect situation. *Knowing how these factors shape and define health behavior and expectations of client/significant other (SO) helps determine individual needs and possible options.*[1]
- Determine availability and use of resources, family, support groups, and financial. *Appropriate use can help individuals continue to manage problems in their lives and plan for future needs.*

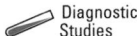

NURSING PRIORITY NO. 3 To assist client to deal with current/future situation:

- Ask client what name he or she prefers. *Acknowledging how client wants to be addressed provides sense of self, promoting esteem.*[5]
- Encourage free expressions of feelings, including feelings of anger and hostility, setting limits on unacceptable behavior. *When feelings are verbalized, client begins to identify them and recognize how they affect personal behavior. Unacceptable behavior leads to feelings of shame and guilt if it is not controlled.*[2,5]
- Allow client to react in own way without judgment by caregivers. Provide support and diversion as indicated. *Unconditional positive regard and support promote acceptance and help client to realize own ability to deal with situation.*[6]
- Listen to client's concerns and acknowledge difficulty of adversity and possible need to make changes. *Often, individuals who are feeling that life is difficult begin to doubt their ability to deal with circumstances. Being listened to provides opportunity for client to feel valued, capable, and like a survivor rather than a victim.*[8]
- Encourage communication with caregivers and SO(s). *Promotes effective interactions and common understanding of what is being said.*
- Provide reality orientation when necessary. *Depending on nature of crises, client may be disoriented by change in environment, serious diagnosis/treatment regimen, death of family member.*[5]
- Provide client with factual information and expected course of situation or crisis if known. *Knowledge helps to allay anxiety, enabling client to manage more effectively and begin to consider the possible resolution of the current situation.*[7]
- Focus on strengths of the individual as the problems are being assessed and diagnosed. *Treatment or intervention has often been based on a deficit model rather than a wellness approach. Improving the future for the client is based on strengthening the capacity to deal successfully with the obstacles he or she meets in life.*[6]

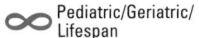

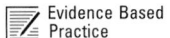

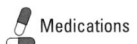

NURSING PRIORITY NO. 4 To promote optimum resiliency (Teaching/Discharge Considerations):

- Provide or identify learning opportunities specific to individual needs. *Referral to activities such as assertiveness training, regular exercise, parenting classes, can enhance knowledge and help develop a resilient mind-set.*[2,3,5]
- Encourage an attitude of realistic hope. *Client can accept that change is a part of living, and while some goals cannot be attained because of crisis or new circumstances, new goals can be developed and life can move forward.*[7]
- Support client in evaluating current lifestyle and changes that will need to be made. *Helps to put things in perspective and develop new plans gradually to avoid undue anxiety.*[9]
- Provide anticipatory guidance relevant to current situation and long-term expectations. *Client may have many issues to resolve, and planning ahead can help client make changes, have hope for the future, and have a sense of control over his or her life.*[3]
- Determine need or desire for religious, spiritual counselor and make arrangements for visit. *Spiritual needs are part of being human, and providing the client an opportunity to discuss concerns about what has happened helps to build resilience to face future stressors.*[5]
- Reinforce importance of clients/SO(s) taking time for themselves. *They may believe they need to devote all their time to the family and feel guilty if they take time for themselves. This provides an opportunity for personal growth; respite allows individuals to pursue own interests and return to tasks of life with renewed vigor.*[2,9]
- Refer to community resources as appropriate. *May need professional counseling, assistance with financial concerns, special needs support services, and child or parenting care in order to sustain move forward.*[2,5]

DOCUMENTATION FOCUS

Assessment/Reassessment

- Assessment findings, including details of this client's situation or crisis, expectations.
- Client's degree of resiliency.

Planning

- Plan of care, and who is involved in planning.
- Teaching plan.

Implementation/Evaluation

- Response to interventions, teaching, and actions performed.
- Attainment or progress toward desired outcome(s).
- Modifications to plan of care.

Discharge Planning

- Long-term needs and who is responsible for actions to be taken.
- Support systems available, specific referrals made.

References

1. Calamaro, C., Waite, R. (2008). Cultural proficiency, research, and evidence-based practice: Implications for the nurse practitioner. *J Pediatr Health Care*, 23(1), 69–72.
2. Gordon, T. (1970). Origins of the Gordon model. Retrieved April 2015 from http://www.gordontraining.com/thomas-gordon/origins-of-the-gordon-model/.

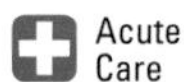

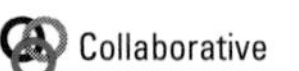

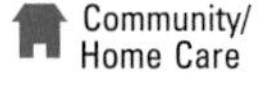

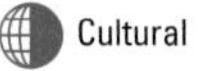

3. Eldar-Avidan, D., Haj-Yahia, M., Greenbaum, C. (2009). Divorce is a part of my life . . . resilience, survival, and vulnerability: Young adults' perception of the implications of parental divorce. *J Marital Fam Ther*, 35(1), 30–46.
4. Adams, L. (2011). How do you deal with adversity? Gordon Training International. Retrieved April 2015 from http://www.gordontraining.com/free-workplace-articles/how-do-you-deal-with-adversity/.
5. Brooks, R., Goldstein, S. (2006). Risk, resilience and futurists: Changing the lives of our children. *Education Horizons*, 9(3), 14–15.
6. Zandonella, C. (2006). Resilience in children. New York Academy of Sciences. Retrieved April 2015 from http://www.nyas.org/Publications/Ebriefings/Detail.aspx?cid=25e9b1f7-2dc4-4c3e-bd63-440afcb8441d.
7. Patten, M. (Updated 2008). Are you resilient? Retrieved April 2015 from http://ezinearticles.com/?Are-You-Resilient?.
8. Graham, L. (Updated 2015). Resilience. Sources for Recovering Resilience. Retrieved April 2015 from http://lindagraham-mft.net/resources/published-articles/resilience/.
9. Mills, H., Dombeck, M. (2005). Resilience: Underlying attitudes and skills. Mentalhelp.net. Retrieved April 2015 from http://www.mhcmc.org/298-emotional-resilience/article/5786-resilience-underlying-attitudes-and-skills.

parental Role Conflict

Taxonomy II: Role Relationships—Class 1 Role Performance (00064) [**Diagnostic Division:** Social Interaction], Submitted 1988

DEFINITION: Parental experience of role confusion and conflict in response to crisis.

RELATED FACTORS

Parent-child separation
Intimidation by invasive modalities (e.g., intubation); by restrictive modalities (e.g., isolation)
Home care of a child with special needs
Living in nontraditional setting (e.g., foster, group or institutional care)
Change in marital status; [conflicts of the role of single parent]
Interruptions in family life due to home-care regimen (e.g., treatments, caregivers, lack of respite)

DEFINING CHARACTERISTICS

Subjective

Perceived inadequacy to provide for child's needs (e.g., physical, emotional)
Concern about change in parental role; concern about family (e.g., functioning, communication, health)
Perceived loss of control over decisions relating to child
Guilt; frustration; anxiety; fear

Objective

Disruption in caregiver routines
Reluctance to participate in usual caregiver activities

Sample Clinical Applications: Prematurity, genetic or congenital conditions, chronic illness (parent/child)

(continues on page 706)

parental Role Conflict (continued)

DESIRED OUTCOMES/EVALUATION CRITERIA

Sample NOC linkages:

Parenting Performance: Parental actions to provide a child nurturing and constructive physical, emotional, and social environment

Role Performance: Congruence of an individual's role behavior with role expectations

Caregiver Lifestyle Disruption: Severity of disturbances in the lifestyle of a family member due to caregiving

Parent(s) Will (Include Specific Time Frame)

- Verbalize understanding of situation and expected parent's/child's role.
- Express feelings about child's illness or situation and effect on family life.
- Demonstrate appropriate behaviors concerning parenting role.
- Assume caretaking activities, as appropriate.
- Handle family disruptions effectively.

ACTIONS/INTERVENTIONS

Sample NIC linkages:

Parenting Promotion: Providing parenting information, support, and coordination of comprehensive services to high-risk families

Role Enhancement: Assisting a patient, significant other, or family to improve relationships by clarifying and supplementing specific role behaviors

Caregiver Support: Provision of the necessary information, advocacy, and support to facilitate primary patient care by someone other than a healthcare professional

NURSING PRIORITY NO. 1 To assess causative/contributory factors:

- Assess individual situation and parent's perception of and concern about what is happening and expectations of self as caregiver. *Identifies needs of the family to deal realistically with the current situation and what interventions are necessary to work toward identified goals.*[5]
- Note parental status, including age and maturity, stability of relationship, single parent, and other responsibilities. *Young parents may lack the necessary maturity to deal with unexpected illness of infant or child. Single parent may feel overwhelmed in trying to balance work and caretaking responsibilities. Increasing numbers of elderly individuals who were expecting retirement and a simpler life are providing full-time care for young grandchildren whose parents are unavailable or unable to provide care.*[1]
- Ascertain parent's understanding of child's developmental stage and expectations for the future to identify misconceptions and strengths. *Parents often have no information regarding developmental stages and have unrealistic expectation of abilities of the child. Identifying what the parents know and providing information can help them deal more realistically with the situation.*[1]
- Note coping skills currently used by each individual as well as how problems have been dealt with in the past. *Provides basis for comparison and reference for client's coping abilities in current situation.*[1]
- Determine use of substances (e.g., alcohol, other drugs, including prescription medications). *May interfere with individual's ability to cope/problem solve and manage current illness/situation and indicates need for additional interventions.*[8]
- Determine availability and use of resources, including extended family, support groups, and financial. *Factors that may affect ability to manage illness, unexpected expenses, caregiving activities, etc.*[1]
- Perform testing such as Parent-Child Relationship Inventory for further evaluation as indicated. *Provides information on which to develop plan of care and appropriate interventions.*[1]

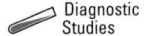

- Determine cultural or religious influences on parenting expectations of self and child and sense of success or failure. *Parenting is one of the most important jobs individuals will have and one for which they are least prepared. Family of origin practices and beliefs will influence parents in how they parent, and this information is crucial to developing a plan of care that meets their needs.*[4]

NURSING PRIORITY NO. 2 To assist parents to deal with current crisis:

- Encourage free verbal expression of feelings (including negative feelings of anger and hostility), setting limits on inappropriate behavior. *Verbalization of feelings enables parent(s) to sift through situation and begin to deal with reality of what is happening. Inappropriate behavior is not helpful for dealing with the situation and will lead to feelings of guilt and low self-worth.*[2]
- Acknowledge difficulty of situation and normalcy of feeling overwhelmed and helpless. Encourage contact with parents who experienced similar situation with child and had positive outcome. *Parents feel listened to when feelings are acknowledged, and hearing how other parents have dealt with situation can give them hope.*[2]
- Provide information in an honest and forthright manner at level of understanding of the client, including technical information when appropriate. *Helping client understand what is happening corrects misconceptions and helps to make decisions that meet individual needs.*[3,12]
- Promote parental involvement in decision making and care as much as possible or desired. *When family members are involved in the process, it enhances their sense of control, and they are more likely to follow through on plans that are made.*[2]
- Encourage interaction and facilitate communication between parent(s) and child. *Sometimes people who find themselves in difficult or distressful situations tend to withdraw because they do not know what to do. Encouraging these interactions enables them to connect with one another to facilitate dealing with situation.*[2]
- Discuss problems of attachment disorder when diagnosed in an adopted child. *Children who have been adopted often suffer from problems of believing they will not be loved, and parents need to learn reasons behind problems as well as skills to deal with them.*[9,10]
- Promote use of assertiveness and relaxation skills. *Providing information and helping individuals learn these skills will help them to deal more effectively with situation or crisis.*[6]
- Instruct parent in proper administration of medications and treatments as indicated. *May need to be involved in care, and knowing how to do these activities enhances their sense of control and comfort in their ability to handle situation.*[5]
- Provide for and encourage use of respite care and parent time off. *Parents may believe they are being "selfish" if they take time out for themselves and that they have to remain with the child. However, parents are important, children are important, and the family is important, and when parents take time for themselves, it enhances their emotional well-being and promotes ability to deal with ongoing situation.*[7,11]
- Help single parent distinguish between parental love and partner love. *New focus of parent's attention or love may result in neglect of relationship with child. Attention needs to be given to both individuals for the relationships to flourish.*[9]

NURSING PRIORITY NO. 3 To promote wellness (Teaching/Discharge Considerations):

- Provide anticipatory guidance relevant to the situation and long-term expectations of the illness. *Encourages making plans for future needs, provides feelings of hope, and promotes sense of control over difficult situation.*[12]
- Encourage parents to set realistic and mutually agreed-on goals. *As family members work together, they can feel empowered and more apt to follow through on decisions that they are involved in making.*[2]
- Discuss infant attachment behaviors such as breastfeeding on cue, cosleeping, and babywearing (carrying baby around on chest or back), as appropriate. *Dealing with ill child and home-care pressures can strain the bond between parent/child. Activities such as these encourage secure relationships.*

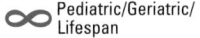

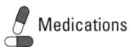

- Provide and identify learning opportunities specific to needs. *Activities such as parenting classes, information about equipment use, and methods of troubleshooting can enhance knowledge and ability to deal with situation.*[3,12]
- Refer to community resources, as appropriate (e.g., visiting nurse, respite care, social services, psychiatric care or family therapy, well-baby clinics, special needs support services). *Provides additional assistance as needed to handle individual situation or illness.*[5]
- Refer to ND impaired Parenting for additional interventions.

DOCUMENTATION FOCUS

Assessment/Reassessment

- Findings, including specifics of individual situation, parental concerns, perceptions, expectations.

Planning

- Plan of care and who is involved in the planning.
- Teaching plan.

Implementation/Evaluation

- Parent's responses to interventions, teaching, and actions performed.
- Attainment or progress toward desired outcome(s).
- Modifications to plan of care.

Discharge Planning

- Long-term needs and who is responsible for each action to be taken.
- Specific referrals made.

References

1. Scott, E. (Updated 2013). Coping skills for parents and kids. Retrieved November 2015 from http://stress.about.com/od/parentingskills/a/coping_skills.htm.
2. McIntyre, L. L. (2008). Parent training for young children with developmental disabilities: Randomized control trial. *Am J Ment Retard*, 113(5), 356–368.
3. Harbaugh, B. L. (2005). Correlates of family-nurse boundary ambiguity in parents of hospitalized children. Retrieved November 2015 from http://www.nursinglibrary.org/vhl/handle/10755/147936.
4. Purnell, L. D. (2011). *Guide to Culturally Competent Health Care*. 2nd ed. Philadelphia, PA: F. A. Davis.
5. Power, N., Franck, L. (2008). Parent participation in the care of hospitalized children: A systematic review. *J Adv Nurs*, 62(6), 622–641.
6. Assertiveness skills. (1998). Brain Injury Resource Center. Retrieved November 2015 from http://www.headinjury.com/assertskills.html.
7. Major, D. A. (2001). Utilizing role theory to help employed parents cope with children's chronic illness. *Health Research Education*, 18(1), 45–57.
8. CRC Health Group. (No date). Using parent effectiveness training to help families in crisis. Retrieved November 2015 from http://www.adolescent-substance-abuse.com/substance-abuse/using-parent-effectiveness-training-to-help-families-in-crisis.htm.
9. Pickhardt, C. (2002). Role conflict of the single parent. Retrieved November 2015 from http://www.carlpickhardt.com/page48.html.
10. Breazeale, T. (2007). Attachment parenting: A practical approach for the reduction of attachment disorders and the promotion of emotionally secure children. Retrieved November 2015 from http://www.visi.com/~jlb/thesis/ch1.html.
11. Walant, K. (2000). When the going gets tough: A little self-care goes a long way. Attachment Parenting International News. Retrieved November 2015 from http://www.attachmentparenting.org/support/articles/artselfcare.php.
12. Berge, J. M., Holm, K. E. (2007). Boundary ambiguity in parents with chronically ill children: Integrating theory and research. *Family Relations*, 56(2), 123–134.

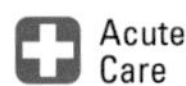

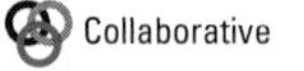

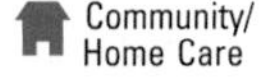

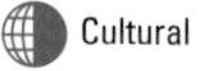

ineffective Role Performance

Taxonomy II: Role Relationships—Class 3 Role Performance (00055) [**Diagnostic Division:** Social Interaction], Submitted 1978; Revised 1996, 1998

DEFINITION: A pattern of behavior and self-expression that does not match the environmental context, norms, and expectations.
[Note: There is a typology of roles, including sociopersonal (friendship, family, marital, parenting, community); home management; intimacy (sexuality, relationship building); leisure, exercise, and recreation; self-management; socialization (developmental transitions); community contributor; and religious, that can help to understand ineffective Role Performance.]

RELATED FACTORS

Knowledge
Insufficient role model
Insufficient role preparation (e.g., role transition, skill rehearsal, validation)
Low educational level
Unrealistic role expectations
Physiological
Alteration in body image ; neurological deficit; physical illness; low self-esteem
Mental health issue (e.g., depression, psychosis, personality disorder, substance abuse)
Fatigue; pain
Social
Insufficient role socialization
Young age; developmental level inappropriate for role expectation
Insufficient resources (e.g., financial, social, knowledge); economically disadvantaged
Stressors; conflict; high demands of job schedule
[Family conflict]; domestic violence
Insufficient support system; insufficient rewards
Inappropriate linkage with the healthcare system

DEFINING CHARACTERISTICS

Subjective
Alteration in role perception; change in self-/other's perception of role
Change in usual pattern of responsibility or in capacity to resume role
Insufficient opportunity for role enactment
Role dissatisfaction; role denial
Discrimination; powerlessness

Objective
Insufficient knowledge of role requirements
Ineffective adaptation to change; inappropriate developmental expectations
Insufficient confidence, motivation, self-management, or skills
Ineffective coping strategies; ineffective role performance
Inadequate external support for role enactment

(continues on page 710)

ineffective Role Performance (continued)
Role strain, conflict, confusion, or ambivalence; [failure to assume role]
Uncertainty; anxiety; depression; pessimism
Domestic violence; harassment; system conflict
Sample Clinical Applications: Chronic conditions (e.g., multiple sclerosis [MS], pain, chronic fatigue syndrome [CFS]), cancer, substance abuse, brain or spinal cord injury (SCI), major surgery, major depression, bipolar disorder, borderline personality disorder, schizophrenia

DESIRED OUTCOMES/EVALUATION CRITERIA

Sample NOC linkages:
Role Performance: Congruence of an individual's role behavior with role expectations
Coping: Personal actions to manage stressors that tax an individual's resources
Psychosocial Adjustment: Life Change: Adaptive psychosocial response of an individual to a significant life change

Client Will (Include Specific Time Frame)
- Verbalize realistic perception and acceptance of self in changed role.
- Verbalize understanding of role expectations or obligations.
- Talk with family/significant others (SOs) about situation and changes that have occurred and limitations imposed.
- Develop realistic plans for adapting to new role or role changes.

ACTIONS/INTERVENTIONS

Sample NIC linkages:
Role Enhancement: Assisting a patient, significant other, and/or family to improve relationships by clarifying and supplementing specific role behaviors
Normalization Promotion: Assisting parents and other family members of children with chronic diseases or disabilities in providing normal life experiences for their children and families
Values Clarification: Assisting another to clarify her/his own values in order to facilitate effective decision making

NURSING PRIORITY NO. 1 To assess causative/contributing factors:

- Identify type of role dysfunction. *Life changes such as developmental (adolescent to adult), situational (husband to father, change in employment status, gender identity), and health-illness transitions can affect how client functions in usual role. This information is important to developing a plan of care and appropriate interventions and goals.*[1]
- Determine client role in family constellation. *How client has functioned in the past (i.e., husband/father, wife/mother) provides a beginning point of reference for understanding changes that have occurred due to health alterations (mental or physical), lack of knowledge about role or role skills, lack of role model, or what other situation has occurred to bring about a role change.*[1]
- Identify how client sees self as a man/woman in usual lifestyle and role functioning. *Each person has a perception of self that is important to know to understand changes that may be occurring.*[1]
- Ascertain client's view of sexual functioning. *Changes (e.g., loss of childbearing ability following hysterectomy, erectile dysfunction following prostate surgery) can affect how client views self in role as male or female and may need specific interventions to resolve feelings of loss.*[1]
- Identify cultural factors relating to individual's gender roles. *Varies with the culture; for instance, for American Indians who are in matrilineal clans or band, women may make important decisions and male roles*

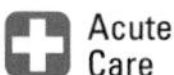

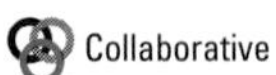

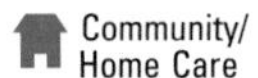

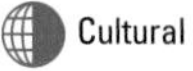

include rituals to protect family and community well-being. In Arab American families, men are expected to be responsible for financial affairs and women typically assume subservient and caregiving roles.[4]

- Determine client's perceptions and concerns about current situation. *May believe current role is more appropriate for the opposite sex (e.g., passive role of the "client" may be somewhat less threatening for women).*[2]
- Interview SO(s) regarding their perceptions and expectations. *The beliefs of the individuals who will be directly involved with the client and the situation (e.g., parents bringing a new baby home from the hospital, adult child assuming responsibility for elder parent) are important to understanding the new roles the individuals are undertaking. Conflicts can arise when expectations vary from individual to individual.*[5]
- Determine client's socioeconomic status and linkage to the healthcare system. *People who are poor may not have healthcare insurance or access to care and perceive themselves as unworthy.*[1]
- Identify availability and use of resources. *Individual may be unaware or have difficulty accessing community support or assistance programs.*
- Investigate history of incidents of domestic violence in the family. *Neither individual in this situation sees self as worthy and both have poor self-esteem. The perpetrator does not get what he or she wants through the use of violence, and the survivor (the battered person) often believes she or he deserves this treatment. The roles of perpetrator and survivor are difficult to alter without intensive therapy as well as support for other family members/children.*[1,7]

NURSING PRIORITY NO. 2 To assist client to deal with existing situation:

- Discuss perceptions and significance of the situation as seen by client. *Provides opportunity to clarify any misperceptions and discuss changes client may have to make in regard to what has happened (e.g., loss of a limb, disfiguring surgery).*
- Maintain positive attitude toward the client. *Promotes safe relationship in which client can discuss changes that are occurring and plan for a positive future.*[1]
- Provide opportunities for client to exercise control over as much of situation as possible. *Enhances self-concept and promotes commitment to goals.*[1]
- Offer realistic assessment of situation and communicate hope. *Client may or may not accept reality, but opportunity to discuss issues and have a sense of hope can help client begin to accept reality.*[6]
- Discuss and assist the client/SO(s) to develop strategies for dealing with changes in role related to past transitions, cultural expectations, and value or belief challenges. *Helps those involved deal with differences between individuals (e.g., adolescent task of separation in which parents clash with child's choices).*[4,8]
- Acknowledge reality of situation related to role change and help client to express feelings of anger, sadness, grief, and depression. Encourage celebration of positive aspects of change and expressions of feelings. *Changes in role necessitated by illness, trauma, changes in family structure (new baby, child leaving home for college, elderly parent needing care), or any other circumstance result in a sense of loss and need to deal with the feelings that accompany the change.*[1,5]
- Provide open environment for client to discuss concerns about sexuality. *Embarrassment can block discussion of sensitive subject and potentially impede progress.* (Refer to NDs Sexual Dysfunction and ineffective Sexuality Pattern.)[7]
- Educate about role expectations using written and audiovisual materials. *Using different modalities enables client to review material at leisure and begin to incorporate information into own thinking.*
- Identify role model for the client. *Offers opportunity for client to observe how someone else functions in a role that is new to him or her.*[3]
- Use techniques of role rehearsal to practice new role. *Provides opportunity for the client to try and develop new skills to cope with anticipated changes.*[7]

NURSING PRIORITY NO. 3 To promote role enhancement (Teaching/Discharge Considerations):

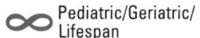

- Make information available (including bibliotherapy, appropriate Web sites) for client to learn about role expectations and demands that may occur. *Provides opportunity to be proactive in dealing with changes, such as*

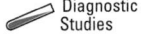

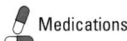

classes to help new parent(s) learn about new roles and credible Web sites for additional information regarding individual's specific concerns.[4]
- Discuss use of medication as appropriate. *Client may benefit from antidepressants to combat depression, or psychotropic medications may be required to address other mental health issues.*[1,7]
- Accept client in changed role. Encourage and give positive feedback for changes and goals achieved. *Provides reinforcement and facilitates continuation of efforts.*
- Refer to support groups, employment counselors, parent effectiveness classes, and counseling or psychotherapy, as indicated by individual need(s). *Provides ongoing support to sustain progress.*[6]
- Refer to NDs impaired Parenting and Self-Esteem [specify] as appropriate.

DOCUMENTATION FOCUS

Assessment/Reassessment
- Individual findings, including specifics of predisposing crises or situation, perception of role change.
- Cultural or religious factors.
- Expectations of SO(s).
- Availability and use of resources.

Planning
- Plan of care and who is involved in planning.
- Teaching plan.

Implementation/Evaluation
- Responses to interventions, teaching, and actions performed.
- Attainment or progress toward desired outcome(s).
- Modifications of plan of care.

Discharge Planning
- Long-term needs and who is responsible for actions to be taken.
- Specific referrals made.

References

1. Karola, K. M. (1998). Family roles, alcoholism, and family dysfunction. *J Mental Health Counseling*, 20(3), 250–260.
2. Santuzzi, A. M., Metzger, P. L., Ruscher, J. B. (2006). Body image and expected future interactions. *Curr Res Soc Psychol*, 11(11), 153–171.
3. O'Hara, V. Stress and the role of perception. Retrieved November 2015 from http://stresscourse.tripod.com/id100.html.
4. Rideway, C. S., Correll, S. (2004). Unpacking the gender system: A theoretical perspective on gender beliefs and social relations. *Gender and Society*, 18(4), 510–531.
5. Gjerdingen, D., Center, B. A. (2003). First time parents prenatal to postnatal changes in health and the relation of postpartum health to work and partner relationships. *J Am Board Fam Med*, 16(4), 304–311.
6. Rice, J., Hicks, P. B., Wiche, V. (2000). Life care planning: A role for social workers. *Soc Work Health Care*, 31(1), 85–94.
7. Collinson, T. Domestic violence and self-esteem: Low self-esteem linked to domestic violence. Retrieved November 2015 from http://womensissues.about.com/od/domesticviolence/a/DomesticViolenceSelfEsteem.htm.
8. McLeod, S. (2008). The self-concept in psychology. *Simply Psychology*. Retrieved November 2015 from http://www.simplypsychology.org/self-concept.html.

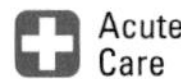

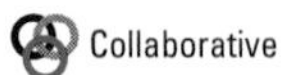

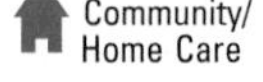

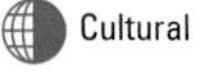

caregiver Role Strain

Taxonomy II: Role Relationships—Class 1 Caregiving Roles (00061) [**Diagnostic Division:** Social Interaction], Submitted 1992; Revised 1998, 2000

DEFINITION: Difficulty in performing family/significant other caregiver role.

RELATED FACTORS

Care Receiver Health Status

Alteration in cognitive functioning

Chronic illness; illness severity; increase in care needs; unpredictability of illness trajectory; unstable health condition

Codependency; dependency; substance abuse

Problematic behavior; psychiatric disorder

Caregiver Health Status

Alteration in cognitive functioning; physical conditions

Codependency; substance abuse

Ineffective coping strategies; insufficient fulfillment of others' or self-expectations; unrealistic care receiver expectations

Caregiver–Care Receiver Relationship

Abusive or violent relationship; pattern of ineffective relationships

Care receiver's condition inhibits conversation; unrealistic care receiver expectations

Caregiving Activities

Around-the-clock care responsibilities; change in nature or complexity of care activities

Duration of caregiving; unpredictably of care situation

Excessive caregiving activities; recent discharge home with significant care needs

Family Processes

Pattern of ineffective family coping or family dysfunction

Resources

Caregiver is not developmentally ready for caregiver role; insufficient time

Difficulty accessing assistance, support, or community resources; insufficient knowledge about community resources; insufficient community services (e.g., respite , recreation, social support); insufficient transportation

Financial crisis (e.g., debt, insufficient finances)

Insufficient emotional resilience, social support, time, or energy

Insufficient physical environment or equipment for providing care

Socioeconomic

Alienation or social isolation

Competing role commitments

Insufficient recreation

(continues on page 714)

caregiver Role Strain (continued)

DEFINING CHARACTERISTICS

Subjective

Caregiving Activities:
Apprehensiveness about: future ability to provide care or well-being of care receiver if unable to provide care; apprehensiveness about future health or institutionalization of care receiver
Caregiver Health Status: Physiological:
Fatigue; gastrointestinal distress; headache, rash, weight change
Hypertension; cardiovascular disease; diabetes
Caregiver Health Status: Emotional:
Alteration in sleep pattern
Anger, emotional vacillation; depression; frustration, impatience; nervousness
Insufficient time to meet personal needs; stressors
Caregiver Health Status: Socioeconomic: Change in leisure activities; low work productivity; refuses career advancement
Caregiver-Care Receiver Relationship:
Difficulty watching care receiver with illness
Grieving changes or uncertainty in relationship with care receiver
Family Processes: Concern about family members; family conflict

Objective

Caregiving Activities:
Difficulty performing or completing required tasks
Dysfunctional change in caregiving activities
Preoccupation with care routine
Caregiver Health Status: Physiological:
Cardiovascular disease; diabetes mellitus
Hypertension; weight change; rash
Caregiver Health Status: Emotional:
Anger, emotional vacillation; depression; frustration, impatience; nervousness
Ineffective coping strategies
Somatization
Caregiver Health Status: Socioeconomic: Low work productivity, refusal of career advancement; social isolation
Family Processes: Family conflict
[Note: The presence of this problem may encompass other numerous problems/high-risk concerns, such as deficient Diversional Activity, Insomnia, Fatigue, Anxiety, ineffective Coping, compromised family Coping or disabled family Coping, Decisional Conflict, ineffective Denial, Grieving, Hopelessness, Powerlessness, Spiritual Distress, ineffective Health Maintenance, impaired Home Maintenance, Sexual Dysfunction or ineffective Sexuality Pattern, readiness for enhanced family Coping, interrupted Family Processes, and Social Isolation. Careful attention to data gathering will identify and clarify the client's specific needs, which can then be coordinated under this single diagnostic label.]

Sample Clinical Applications:
Chronic conditions (e.g., severe brain injury, spinal cord injury [SCI], severe developmental delay), progressive debilitating conditions (e.g., muscular dystrophy, multiple sclerosis [MS], dementia or Alzheimer's disease, end-stage chronic obstructive pulmonary disease [COPD], renal failure, renal dialysis), substance abuse, end-of-life care, psychiatric conditions (e.g., schizophrenia, personality disorders).

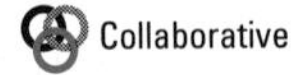

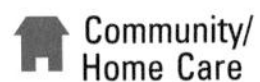

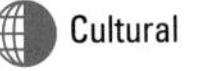

DESIRED OUTCOMES/EVALUATION CRITERIA

Sample NOC linkages:

Caregiver Role Endurance: Factors that promote family care provider's capacity to sustain caregiving over an extended period of time

Caregiver Stressors: Severity of biopsychosocial pressure on a family care provider caring for another over an extended period of time

Caregiver Well-Being: Extent of positive perception of primary care provider's health status

Caregiver Will (Include Specific Time Frame)

- Identify resources within self to deal with situation.
- Provide opportunity for care receiver to deal with situation in own way.
- Express more realistic understanding and expectations of the care receiver.
- Demonstrate behavior or lifestyle changes to cope with or resolve problematic factors.
- Report improved general well-being, ability to deal with situation.

ACTIONS/INTERVENTIONS

Sample NIC linkages:

Caregiver Support: Provision of the necessary information, advocacy, and support to facilitate primary patient care by someone other than a healthcare professional

Family Involvement Promotion: Facilitating participation of family members in the emotional and physical care of the patient

Parenting Promotion: Providing parenting information, support, and coordination of comprehensive services to high-risk families

NURSING PRIORITY NO. 1 To assess degree of impaired function:

- Inquire about and observe physical condition of care receiver and surroundings as appropriate. *Important to determine factors that may indicate problems that can interfere with ability to continue caregiving.*[4]
- Assess caregiver's current state of health and functioning (e.g., caregiver has multiple medical issues; is unable to get enough sleep, has poor nutritional intake, personal appearance and demeanor are indicating stress). *Provides basis for determining needs that indicate caregiver is having difficulty dealing with role.*[4]
- Determine use of prescription, over-the-counter, or illicit drugs and/or alcohol. *Caregiver may turn to using these substances to deal with situation.*[1]
- Identify safety issues concerning caregiver and receiver. *The stress and anxiety of caregiving situations can lead to inattention, and by identifying these issues, an opportunity is provided to correct problems before injury occurs.*[1]
- Assess current actions of caregiver and how they are received by care receiver. *Caregiver may be trying to be helpful but is not perceived as helpful; may be too protective or may have unrealistic expectations of care receiver's abilities, which can lead to misunderstanding and conflict.*[4]
- Note choice and frequency of social involvement and recreational activities. *Caregiver needs to take time away from situation to maintain own sense of self and ability to continue in role.*[1]
- Determine use and effectiveness of resources and support systems. *May not be aware of what is available or may need help in using them to the best advantage.*[4]

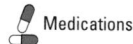

NURSING PRIORITY NO. 2 To identify the causative/contributing factors relating to the impairment:

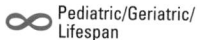

- Note presence of high-risk situations (e.g., elderly client with total care dependence on spouse; or caregiver with several small children, with one child requiring extensive assistance due to physical condition or developmental delays). *Such situations result in added stress (e.g., imposing unwanted role reversal, placing excessive demands on parenting skills).*[4]

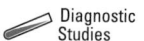

- Determine current knowledge of the situation, noting misconceptions and lack of information. *May interfere with caregiver/care receiver's response to situation.*
- Identify relationship of caregiver to care receiver (e.g., spouse/lover, parent/child, sibling, friend). *Close relationships may make it more difficult to remain separate when caring for care receiver. Note: Younger-aged family caregivers are at increased risk for lower levels of hope and higher levels of caregiver strain.*[6]
- Determine quality of couple's relationship/presence of intimacy issues. *Disease/condition, caregiving activities, and possible change in role responsibilities may strain relationship, adding to sense of loss and unmet needs.*[3]
- Ascertain proximity of caregiver to care receiver. *Caregiver could be living in the home of care receiver (e.g., spouse or parent of disabled child) or could be adult child stopping by to check on elderly parent each day, providing support, food preparation, shopping, and assistance in emergencies. Note: There is added stress in maintaining own life and responsibilities when caregiver has to travel some distance to provide care.*[4,10]
- Note care receiver's physical and mental condition, as well as the complexity of therapeutic regimen. *Caregiving activities can be complex, requiring hands-on care, problem-solving skills, clinical judgment, and organizational and communication skills that can tax the caregiver, increasing likelihood of burnout.*[7,10]
- Determine caregiver's level of involvement in and preparedness for the responsibilities of caring for the client and anticipated length of care. *Information needed to develop plan of care that takes into consideration who will provide care, timing, and any other factors to maintain coverage for situation.*[4]
- Ascertain physical and emotional health, developmental level and abilities, and additional responsibilities of caregiver (e.g., job, raising family). *Provides clues to potential stressors and possible supportive interventions.*[10,11]
- Assess caregiver as appropriate, using tool such as Burden Interview, Herth Hope Index, Caregiver Reaction Assessment, or Caregiver Strain Index *to further determine caregiver's stressors and abilities, providing additional information to aid in planning.*[17,18]
- Identify individual cultural factors and impact on caregiver. *Helps clarify expectations of caregiver and receiver, family, and community. Many cultures may believe strongly in keeping care receivers in the home and caring for them.*[5]
- Identify presence and degree of conflict between caregiver/care receiver/family. *Stressful situations can exacerbate underlying feelings of anger and resentment, resulting in difficulty managing caregiving needs.*[1]
- Determine pre-illness and current behaviors that may be interfering with the care or recovery of the care receiver. *Underlying personality of care receiver may create situation in which old conflicts interfere with current treatment regimen.*[1]
- Note codependency needs and enabling behaviors of caregiver. *These behaviors can interfere with competent caregiving and contribute to caregiver burnout.*[2]

NURSING PRIORITY NO. 3 To assist caregiver to identify feelings and begin to deal with problems:

- Establish a therapeutic relationship, conveying empathy and unconditional positive regard. *A compassionate approach blending the nurse's expertise in healthcare with the caregiver's firsthand knowledge of the care receiver can provide encouragement, especially in a long-term difficult situation.*[10,12]
- Acknowledge difficulty of the situation for the caregiver/family. *Research shows that the two greatest predictors of caregiver strain are poor health and the feeling that there is no choice but to take on additional responsibilities.*[10]
- Discuss caregiver's view of and concerns about situation. *Important to identify issues so planning and solutions can be developed.*[7]
- Encourage caregiver to acknowledge and express negative feelings. Discuss normalcy of the reactions without using false reassurance. *Individual needs to understand that all feelings are acceptable to be expressed and dealt with, but not acted on in the situation.*[1]

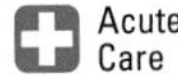

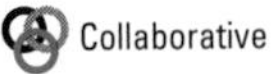

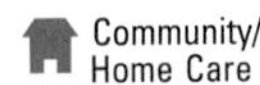

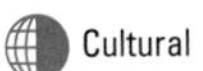

- Discuss caregiver's life goals, perceptions, and expectations of self. *Clarifies unrealistic thinking and identifies potential areas of flexibility or compromise.*[4]
- Discuss caregiver's perception of impact of and ability to handle role changes necessitated by situation. *May not initially realize the changes that will be encountered as situation develops, and it helps to identify and plan for changes before they arise.*

NURSING PRIORITY NO. 4 To enhance caregiver's ability to deal with current situation:

- Identify strengths of caregiver and care receiver. *Bringing these to the individual's awareness promotes positive thinking and helps with problem solving to deal more effectively with circumstances.*[4]
- Discuss strategies to coordinate caregiving tasks and other responsibilities (e.g., employment, care of children/other dependents, housekeeping activities). *Managing these tasks will reduce the stress associated with performing the activities of daily living.*[1]
- Facilitate family conference to share information and develop plan for involvement in care activities as appropriate. *Involving everyone promotes sense of control and ownership of plan and willingness to follow through on responsibilities.*
- Identify classes or needed specialists (e.g., first aid and cardiopulmonary resuscitation classes, enterostomal specialist, physical therapist). *Provides information needed to manage tasks of caregiving more effectively, giving individuals more sense of control.*
- Determine need for and sources of additional resources (e.g., financial, legal, respite care, educational, social, spiritual). *Can help to resolve problems that arise in the course of caregiving that are out of the knowledge or abilities of the individual. Solving these issues can relieve caregiver of anxiety and concern.*[4,13]
- Provide information or demonstrate techniques for dealing with acting out, violent, or disoriented behavior. *Presence of dementia necessitates learning these techniques or skills to enhance safety of caregiver and receiver.*[1]
- Identify equipment needs and resources and appropriate adaptive aids. *Enhances the independence and safety of the care receiver and makes the task of caregiving easier.*
- Provide contact person or case manager to partner with care provider(s) in coordinating care, providing physical and social support, and to assist with problem solving as needed or desired. *As care receiver's condition declines or caregiving activities are prolonged/intensify, caregiver strain may escalate and psychological well-being of caregiver may decline. Ongoing support by health and social services promotes more effective caregiving and thereby lessens strain on caregiver.*[2,10,14]

NURSING PRIORITY NO. 5 To promote wellness (Teaching/Discharge Considerations):

- Advocate for and assist caregiver to plan for and implement changes that may be necessary (e.g., home-care providers, adult day care, eventual placement in long-term care facility). *As caregiving tasks become more difficult, other options need to be considered, and planning ahead can promote acceptance of necessary changes.*[8,11,15]
- Encourage attention to own needs (e.g., eating and sleeping regularly, setting realistic goals, talking with trusted friend, periodic respite from caregiving), accepting own feelings, acknowledging frustrations and limitations, and being realistic about loved one's condition. *Supports and enhances caregiver's general well-being and coping ability.*[15,16]
- Review signs of burnout (e.g., emotional or physical exhaustion, changes in appetite and sleep, withdrawal from friends/family or life interests). *Recognition of developing problem allows for timely intervention.*
- Discuss and demonstrate stress management techniques and importance of self-nurturing (e.g., pursuing self-development interests, hobbies, social activities, spiritual enrichment). *Being involved in activities such as these can prevent caregiver burnout.*[4,15]
- Encourage involvement in caregiver support group. *Having others to share concerns and fears is therapeutic and provides ideas for different ways to manage problems, helping caregivers deal more effectively with the situation.*[1]

- Refer to classes or other therapies as indicated. *Provides additional information as needed.*
- Identify an available 12-step program when indicated *to provide tools to deal with enabling or codependent behaviors that impair level of function. Provides a more structured environment to learn how to deal with problems of caregiving situation.*[1]
- Refer to counseling or psychotherapy as needed. *Intensive treatment may be needed in highly stressful situations.*
- Provide bibliotherapy of appropriate references and Web sites for self-paced learning and updated information and contact with other caregivers. *Further information can help individuals understand what is happening and manage more effectively.*[9]

DOCUMENTATION FOCUS

Assessment/Reassessment

- Assessment findings, functional level and degree of impairment, caregiver's understanding and perception of situation.
- Identified risk factors.

Planning

- Plan of care and individual responsibility for specific activities.
- Identification of inner resources, behavior or lifestyle changes to be made.
- Needed resources, including type and source of assistive devices and durable equipment.
- Teaching plan.

Implementation/Evaluation

- Caregiver's/receiver's response to interventions, teaching, and actions performed.
- Attainment or progress toward desired outcome(s).
- Modifications to plan of care.

Discharge Planning

- Plan for continuation or follow-through of needed changes.
- Referrals for assistance and evaluation.

References

1. Townsend, M. C. (2011). *Psychiatric Mental Health Nursing: Concepts of Care in Evidence-Based Practice*. 7th ed. Philadelphia: F. A. Davis.
2. Peters, M., Fitzpatrick, R., Doll, H., et al. (2012). The impact of perceived lack of support provided by health and social care services to caregivers of people with motor neuron disease. *Amyotroph Lateral Scler*, 13(2), 223–228.
3. Harris, S. M., Adams, M. S., Zubatsky, M., et al. (2011). A caregiver perspective of how Alzheimer's disease and related disorders affect couple intimacy. *Aging Mental Health*, 15(8), 950–960.
4. Newfield, S. A., Hinz, M. D., Tilley, D. S., et al. (2007). *Cox's Clinical Applications of Nursing Diagnosis: Adult, Child, Women's, Psychiatric, Gerontic, and Home Health Considerations*. 5th ed. Philadelphia: F. A. Davis.
5. Purnell, L. D., Paulanka, B. J. (2008). *Transcultural Health Care—A Culturally Competent Approach*. 3rd ed. Philadelphia: F. A. Davis.
6. Lohve, V., Miaskowski, C., Rusteen, T. (2011). The relationship between hope and caregiver strain in family caregivers of parents with advanced cancer. *Cancer Nurs*, 35(2), 99–105.
7. Hareven, T. K. (ed). (1995). *Aging and Generational Relations over the Life Course: A Historical and Cross-Cultural Perspective*. New York: Walter De Gruyter.
8. Liken, M. A. (2001). Caregivers in crisis: Moving a relative with Alzheimer's to assisted living. *Clin Nurs Res*, 10(1), 53–69.
9. Liken, M. A. (2001). Experiences of family caregivers of a relative with Alzheimer's disease. *J Psychosoc Nurs*, 39(12), 32–37.
10. Schumacher, K., Beck, C. A., Marren, J. M. (2006). Family caregivers: Caring for older adults, working with their families. *Am J Nurs*, 106(8), 40–49.
11. Weiss, B. (2005). When a family member requires your care. *RN*, 68(4), 63–65.

12. Raina, P., O'Donnell, M., Rosenbaum, P., et al. (2005). The health and well-being of caregivers of children with cerebral palsy. *Pediatrics*, 115(6), e626–e636.
13. Spurlock, W. R. (2005). Spiritual well-being and caregiver burden in Alzheimer's caregivers. *Geriatr Nurs*, 26(3), 154–161.
14. Haigler, D. H., Bauer, L. J., Travis, S. S. (2006). "Caring for you, caring for me": A ten-year caregiver educational initiative of the Rosalynn Carter Institute for Human Development. *Health Soc Work*, 31(2), 149–152.
15. Beckerman, J. (2015). Heart failure and caregiver burnout. Retrieved March 2015 from http://www.webmd.com/heart-disease/heart-failure/heart-failure-recognizing-burnout-caregiver.
16. Boyles, S. (2005). Spouse caregivers most likely to be abusive. Retrieved March 2015 from http://www.webmd.com/balance/news/20050211/spouse-caregivers-most-likely-to-be-abusive.
17. Given, C. W., Given, B., Stommel, M., et al. (1992). The caregiver reaction assessment (CRA) for caregivers to persons with chronic physical and mental impairments. *Res Nurs Health*, 15, 271–283.
18. Zarit, S. H., Todd, P. A., Zarit, J. M. (1986). Subjective burden of husbands and wives as caregivers: A longitudinal study. *Gerontologist*, 26, 260–266.

risk for caregiver Role Strain

Taxonomy II: Role Relationships—Class 1 Caregiving Roles (00062) [**Diagnostic Division:** Social Interaction], Submitted 1992; Revised 2010, 2013

DEFINITION: Vulnerable to difficulty in performing the family/significant other caregiver role, which may compromise health.

RISK FACTORS

Illness severity of the care receiver; alteration in cognitive functioning in care receiver; psychological disorder in care receiver; care receiver exhibits bizarre or deviant behavior
Care receiver discharged home with significant needs; prematurity; congenital disorder; developmental delay
Unpredictable illness trajectory; instability in care receiver's health
Substance abuse; codependency
Extended duration of caregiving required; inexperience with caregiving; caregiving task complexity; excessive caregiving activities
Caregiver health impairment; psychological disorder in caregiver
Partner is caregiver, female
Caregiver not developmentally ready for caregiver role [e.g., a young adult needing to provide care for middle-aged parent]; developmental delay of caregiver
Stressors; caregiver's competing role commitments
Inadequate physical environment for providing care
Family or caregiver isolation
Insufficient caregiver respite or recreation
Ineffective family adaptation; pattern of family dysfunction prior to the caregiving situation
Ineffective caregiver coping pattern
Pattern of ineffective relationship between caregiver and care receiver
Exposure to violence; presence of abuse (e.g., physical, psychological, sexual)
Note: A risk diagnosis is not evidenced by signs and symptoms, as the problem has not occurred; rather, nursing interventions are directed at prevention.

(continues on page 720)

risk for caregiver Role Strain (continued)

Sample Clinical Applications: Chronic conditions (e.g., severe brain injury, spinal cord injury [SCI], severe developmental delay), progressive debilitating conditions (e.g., muscular dystrophy, multiple sclerosis [MS], dementia/Alzheimer's disease, end-stage chronic obstructive pulmonary disease [COPD], renal failure, renal dialysis), substance abuse, end-of-life care, psychiatric conditions (e.g., schizophrenia, personality disorders)

DESIRED OUTCOMES/EVALUATION CRITERIA

Sample NOC linkages:

Caregiver Home Care Readiness: Preparedness of a caregiver to assume responsibility for the healthcare of a family member in the home

Caregiver Stressors: Severity of biopsychosocial pressure on a family care provider caring for another over an extended period of time

Family Resiliency: Positive adaptation and function of the family system following significant adversity or crisis

Caregiver Will (Include Specific Time Frame)

- Identify individual risk factors and appropriate interventions.
- Demonstrate or initiate behaviors or lifestyle changes to prevent development of impaired function.
- Use available resources appropriately.
- Report satisfaction with current situation.

ACTIONS/INTERVENTIONS

Sample NIC linkages:

Caregiver Support: Provision of the necessary information, advocacy, and support to facilitate primary patient care by someone other than a healthcare professional

Family Support: Promotion of family values, interests, and goals

Parenting Promotion: Providing parenting information, support, and coordination of comprehensive services to high-risk families

NURSING PRIORITY NO. 1 To assess factors affecting current situation:

- Note presence of high-risk situations (e.g., elderly client with total self-care dependence; having several small children, with one child requiring extensive assistance due to physical condition or developmental delays). *May necessitate role reversal resulting in added stress or places excessive demands on parenting skills. Identification of high-risk situations can help in planning and resolving problems before they can become unmanageable.*[4]
- Identify relationship and proximity of caregiver to care receiver (e.g., spouse/lover, parent/child, friend). *There is added stress in maintaining own life and responsibilities when caregiver has to travel some distance to provide care.*[11] *Close relationships may create problems of codependency and identification that can be counterproductive to caregiving. Note: Younger-aged family caregivers are at increased risk for lower levels of hope and higher levels of caregiver strain.*[2]
- Determine current knowledge of the situation, noting misconceptions and lack of information. *May interfere with caregiver/care receiver's response to situation.*
- Compare caregiver's and receiver's views of situation. *Different views need to be openly expressed so each person understands how other sees situation.*[1,3]
- Note complexity of therapeutic regimen and physical and mental status of care receiver to ascertain potential areas of need (e.g., teaching, direct care support, respite). *Knowledge of these factors is necessary for planning adequate care for the individual. Plans for additional help may be necessary to prevent caregiver role strain.*[1]

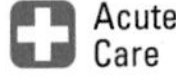

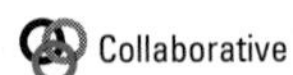

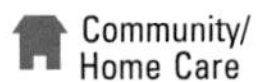

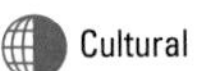

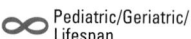

- Determine caregiver's level of responsibility, involvement in care, and anticipated length of care. *Information that may indicate level of stress that could be anticipated for the situation. Progressive debilitation taxes caregiver and may alter ability to meet client's and own needs.*[4]
- Identify individual cultural factors and impact on caregiver. *Helps clarify expectations of caregiver/receiver, family, and community. Many cultures may believe strongly in keeping care receiver in the home and caring for them.*[5]
- Ascertain caregiver's physical and emotional health, developmental level and abilities, and additional responsibilities of caregiver (e.g., job, raising family). *Provides information indicative of ability of the individual to take on the task of caregiver, as well as clues to potential stressors and possible supportive interventions.*[11,12]
- Assess caregiver as appropriate, using tool such as Burden Interview, Herth Hope Index, Caregiver Reaction Assessment, or Caregiver Strain Index *to further determine caregiver's stressors and abilities providing additional information to aid in planning.*[6,7,9]
- Identify strengths and weaknesses of caregiver and care receiver. *Caregiver may not be aware of demands that will be expected. Knowing these factors helps to determine how to use them to advantage in planning and delivering care.*[9]
- Note any codependency needs of caregiver and plan for dealing appropriately with them. *Can contribute to burnout unless identified and dealt with.*[15]
- Verify safety of caregiver/receiver. *Identifying and correcting unsafe situations is crucial so both individuals can be assured of safety in dealing with difficult situation.*[1,9]
- Determine available supports and resources currently used. *Helpful to identify if they are being used effectively.*[4]

NURSING PRIORITY NO. 2 To enhance caregiver's ability to deal with current situation:

- Establish a therapeutic relationship, conveying empathy and unconditional positive regard. *Promotes positive environment in which needs and concerns can be discussed and proactive solutions identified.*
- Discuss strategies to coordinate care and other responsibilities (e.g., employment, care of children/dependents, housekeeping activities). *Such planning can prevent chaos and resultant burnout.*[8]
- Facilitate family conference as appropriate to share information and develop plan for involvement in care activities. *When everyone is involved and listened to, each person is more likely to carry out his or her responsibilities.*[4]
- Refer to classes and/or specialists (e.g., first-aid and cardiopulmonary resuscitation classes, enterostomal specialist, physical therapist) for special training as indicated. *Additional information that can help individuals involved feel more competent and able to deal with situation more effectively.*[3]
- Identify additional resources, including financial, legal, and respite care. *Can help to resolve problems that arise in the course of caregiving that are outside of the knowledge or abilities of the individual. Solving these issues can relieve caregiver of associated anxiety and concern.*[1]
- Identify equipment needs and resources, and appropriate adaptive aids. *Enhances the independence and safety of the care receiver and reduces chances for untoward incidents.*[14]
- Identify contact person or case manager as needed to coordinate care, provide support, and assist with problem solving. *Assistance with planning minimizes problems that could arise.*[10]
- Provide information or demonstrate techniques for dealing with acting out, violent, or disoriented behavior. *Planning ways to deal with these behaviors before they occur promotes safety and enhances positive outcomes.*[4]
- Assist caregiver to recognize codependent behaviors (i.e., doing things for others that others are able to do for themselves) and how these behaviors affect the situation. *Provides options for changing behaviors in ways that enhance the caregiving situation.*[15]

NURSING PRIORITY NO. 3 To promote wellness (Teaching/Discharge Considerations):

- Review signs of burnout (e.g., emotional or physical exhaustion, changes in appetite and sleep, withdrawal from friends/family or life interests). *Recognition of developing problem allows for timely intervention.*[13]

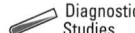

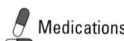

- Discuss and demonstrate stress management techniques and importance of self-nurturing (e.g., meeting personal needs, pursuing self-development interests, hobbies, social activities, spiritual enrichment). *Improves or maintains quality of life for caregiver and may provide caregiver with options to protect self.*[6,13,14]
- Encourage involvement in caregiver or other specific support group(s). *Opportunity to be with others in similar situations and discussing different ways to handle problems help caregiver deal with difficult role in positive ways.*[1]
- Provide bibliotherapy of appropriate references and Web sites and encourage discussion of information. *Promotes retention of new information that can help caregiver manage more effectively.*[1]
- Advocate for and assist caregiver to plan for and implement changes that may become helpful or necessary for the care receiver. *Getting information and thinking about possibilities will help with decision making. These may include transportation, meal delivery, home health care services, home modification, and legal and financial counseling, as well as eventual placement in a long-term care facility and use of palliative or hospice services. As caregiving tasks at home become more difficult, other options need to be considered, and planning ahead can promote acceptance of necessary changes.*[8,12,13]
- Identify an available 12-step program when indicated to provide tools *to deal with codependent behaviors that impair level of function. Provides a more structured environment to learn how to deal with problems of caregiving situation in positive ways.*[3]
- Refer to counseling or psychotherapy as needed. *May need additional help to resolve issues that are interfering with caregiving responsibilities.*

DOCUMENTATION FOCUS

Assessment/Reassessment

- Identified risk factors and caregiver perceptions of situation.
- Reactions of care receiver/family.

Planning

- Treatment plan and individual responsibility for specific activities.
- Teaching plan.

Implementation/Evaluation

- Caregiver/receiver response to interventions, teaching, and actions performed.
- Attainment or progress toward desired outcome(s).
- Modifications to plan of care.

Discharge Planning

- Long-term needs and who is responsible for actions to be taken.
- Specific referrals provided for assistance and evaluation.

References

1. National Center on Elder Abuse. (2002). Preventing elder abuse by family caregivers. Retrieved November 2015 from http://www.ncea.aoa.gov/Resources/Publication/docs/caregiver.pdf.
2. Lohve, V., Miaskowski, C., Rusteen, T. (2011). The relationship between hope and caregiver strain in family caregivers of parents with advanced cancer. *Cancer Nurs*, 35(2), 99–105.
3. Townsend, M. C. (2011). *Psychiatric Mental Health Nursing: Concepts of Care in Evidence-Based Practice*. 6th ed. Philadelphia: F. A. Davis.
4. Newfield, S. A., Hinz, C., Tilley, D. S., et al. (2007). *Cox's Clinical Applications of Nursing Diagnosis: Adult, Child, Women's, Psychiatric, Gerontic, and Home Health Considerations*. 5th ed. Philadelphia: F. A. Davis.

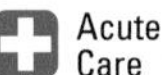

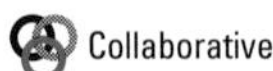

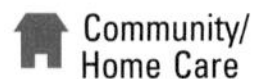

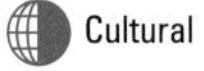

5. Purnell, L. D., Paulanka, B. J. (2008). *Transcultural Health Care—A Culturally Competent Approach.* 3rd ed. Philadelphia: F. A. Davis.
6. Given, C. W., Given, B., Stommel, M., et al. (1992). The caregiver reaction assessment (CRA) for caregivers to persons with chronic physical and mental impairments. *Res Nurs Health*, 15(4), 271–283.
7. Zarit, S. H., Todd, P. A., Zarit, J. M. (1986). Subjective burden of husbands and wives as caregivers: A longitudinal study. *Gerontologist*, 26(3), 260–266.
8. Liken, M. A. (2001). Caregivers in crisis: Moving a relative with Alzheimer's to assisted living. *Clin Nurs Res*, 10(1), 53–69.
9. Liken, M. A. (2001). (Not) a Hallmark holiday: Experiences of family caregivers of a relative with Alzheimer's disease. *J Psychosoc Nurs Ment Health Serv*, 39(12), 33–37.
10. Halper, J., Harris, C. J. (2003). *Multiple Sclerosis: Best Practices in Nursing Care*. Hackensack, NJ: International Organization of Multiple Sclerosis Nursing.
11. Schumacher, K., Beck, C. A., Marren, J. M. (2006). Family caregivers: Caring for older adults, working with their families. *Am J Nurs*, 106(8), 40–49.
12. Weiss, B. (2005). When a family member requires your care. *RN*, 68(4), 63–65.
13. Beckerman, J. (2015). Heart failure and caregiver burnout. Retrieved March 2015 from http://www.webmd.com/heart-disease/heart-failure/heart-failure-recognizing-burnout-caregiver.
14. Greene, R. C. (2012). Caregiver stress fact sheet. Retrieved March 2015 from http://www.womenshealth.gov/publications/our-publications/fact-sheet/caregiver-stress.html?from=AtoZ.
15. O'Regan, M. K. (2007). When caring becomes caretaking. Retrieved March 2015 from http://ezinearticles.com/?When-Caring-Becomes-Caretaking&id=774141.

Self-Care Deficit: bathing, dressing, feeding, toileting

Taxonomy II: Activity/Rest—Class 5 Self-Care (Bathing 00108, Dressing 00109, Feeding 00102, Toileting 00110) [**Diagnostic Division:** Hygiene], Submitted 1980; Nursing Diagnosis Extension and Classification Revision 1998, Bathing/Dressing/Toileting 2008

DEFINITION: Impaired ability to perform or complete bathing, dressing, feeding, or toileting activities for self [on a temporary, permanent, or progressing basis].
[Note: Self-Care also may be expanded to include the practices used by the client to promote health, the individual responsibility for self, and a way of thinking. Refer to NDs ineffective Health Maintenance and impaired Home Maintenance.]

RELATED FACTORS

Alteration in cognitive functioning; perceptual impairment
Weakness; fatigue; decrease in motivation; anxiety
Neuromuscular or musculoskeletal impairment
Environmental barrier; [mechanical restrictions such as cast, splint, traction, ventilator]
Pain, discomfort
Inability to perceive body part or spatial relationship [bathing]
Impaired mobility or transfer ability [toileting]

DEFINING CHARACTERISTICS

bathing Self-Care Deficit
Impaired ability to: access bathroom [tub], gather bathing supplies, access water, regulate bath water, wash or dry body

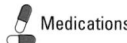

(continues on page 724)

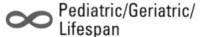

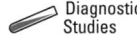

Self-Care Deficit: bathing, dressing, feeding, toileting (continued)

dressing Self-Care Deficit

Impaired ability to: choose clothing, gather clothing, pick up clothing, put clothing on upper or lower body, fasten clothing

Impaired ability to: put on/remove various items of clothing (e.g., shirt, socks, shoes)

Impaired ability to: use zipper or assistive device, maintain appearance

feeding Self-Care Deficit

Impaired ability to: prepare food, open containers

Impaired ability to: handle utensils, get food onto utensil, bring food to the mouth, use assistive device, pick up cup

Impaired ability to: manipulate food in mouth, chew food, swallow food or swallow sufficient amount of food, self-feed a complete meal or in an acceptable manner

toileting Self-Care Deficit

Impaired ability to: reach toilet, manipulate clothing for toileting, sit on or rise from toilet, complete toilet hygiene, flush toilet

Sample Clinical Applications: Arthritis, neuromuscular impairment (e.g., multiple sclerosis [MS], brain injury, stroke, Parkinson's disease, spinal cord injury [SCI]), chronic pain, chronic fatigue syndrome [CFS], depression, dementia, autism, developmental delay, end-of-life/hospice care

DESIRED OUTCOMES/EVALUATION CRITERIA

Sample NOC linkages:

Self-Care Status: Ability to perform basic personal care activities and instrumental activities of daily living

Self-Care: Bathing: Ability to cleanse own body independently with or without assistive device

Self-Care: Dressing: Ability to dress self independently with or without assistive device

Self-Care: Eating: Ability to prepare and ingest food and fluid independently with or without assistive device

Self-Care: Toileting: Ability to toilet self independently with or without assistive device

Client Will (Include Specific Time Frame)

- Identify individual areas of weakness and needs.
- Verbalize knowledge of healthcare practices.
- Demonstrate techniques or lifestyle changes to meet self-care needs.
- Perform self-care activities within level of own ability.
- Identify personal and community resources that can provide assistance.

ACTIONS/INTERVENTIONS

Sample NIC linkages:

Self-Care Assistance: Assisting another to perform activities of daily living

Bathing: Cleaning of the body for the purpose of relaxation, cleanliness, and healing

Dressing: Choosing, putting on, and removing clothes for a person who cannot do this for self

Hair Care [or] Nail Care: Promotion of neat, clean, attractive hair/nails and prevention of skin lesions related to improper care of nails

Feeding: Providing nutritional intake for patient who is unable to feed self

Bowel [or] Urinary Elimination Management: Establishment and maintenance of a regular pattern of bowel elimination/maintenance of an optimum urinary elimination pattern

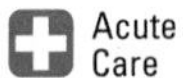

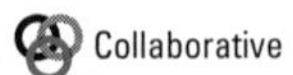

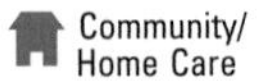

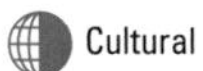

NURSING PRIORITY NO. 1 To identify causative/contributing factors:

- Determine age or developmental issues and existing conditions (e.g., heart or renal failure, SCI, malnutrition, pain, trauma, surgery) and cognitive or psychological factors (e.g., mental illness, brain injury, cerebrovascular accident, MS, Alzheimer's disease) *affecting ability of individual to care for own needs. Assists in setting realistic goals and creates baseline for evaluating effectiveness of interventions.*[1,8]
- Identify other etiological factors present, including language barriers, speech impairment, visual acuity, loss of visual or spatial orientation, hearing problem, and emotional instability or lability *that can both affect and be affected by self-care needs and deficits.* Refer to NDs impaired verbal Communication, Unilateral Neglect, and [disturbed Sensory Perception (specify)] for related interventions.
- Review medication regimen *for possible effects on alertness and mentation, energy level, balance, and perception. Note: All prescribed and over-the-counter medications have the potential for side effects, adverse effects, and interactions that may be harmful to the client or affect client's ability to provide self-care.*
- Assess barriers to participation in regimen *that can limit use of resources or choice of options (e.g., lack of information, insufficient time for discussion, psychological or intimate family problems that may be difficult to share, fear of appearing stupid or ignorant, social or economic limitations, work or home environment problems).*

NURSING PRIORITY NO. 2 To assess degree of disability:

- Identify degree of individual impairment and functional level according to a functional scale as below:[16]
  0—Completely independent
  1—Requires use of equipment or device
  2—Requires help from another person for assistance, supervision, or teaching
  3—Requires help from another person and equipment device
  4—Dependent, does not participate in activity
- *Many instruments have been developed to assess client's functional status. In the community healthcare setting, a more complex assessment may be used (e.g., Lawton and Brody's scale of Instrumental Activities of Daily Living) to determine client's self-care abilities (e.g., to communicate by phone, drive, cook, shop, balance a checkbook, manage medical appointments or medications, etc.). In an acute or long-term care setting, the assessment may be confined to personal care (e.g., Katz Activities of Daily Living Scale). These instruments are used (1) to determine client's safety issues and care needs upon admission and (2) to ascertain changes in functional abilities as a result of client's condition and treatment.*[15]
- Note anticipated duration of disruption and intensity of care required. *A wide variety of factors can impact self-care, some of which may be (1) invariable or permanent (e.g., quadriplegia or advanced dementia), (2) temporary (e.g., fractures requiring immobilization, mild stroke with potential for good recovery), and (3) variable (e.g., person having episode of severe depression or episodes of relapsing-remitting–type MS).*
- Assess cognitive functioning (e.g., memory, intelligence, concentration, ability to attend to task) *to determine client's ability to participate in care and potential to return to normal functioning or to learn/relearn tasks.*
- Determine individual strengths and skills of the client *to incorporate into plan of care enhancing likelihood of achieving outcomes.*

NURSING PRIORITY NO. 3 To assist in correcting/dealing with deficit(s) in general:

- Collaborate in treatment of underlying conditions *to enhance client's capabilities and maximize rehabilitation potential.*
- Promote communication among all those involved in caring for or assisting the client. *Enhances coordination and continuity of care.*
- Active-listen client's/significant other's (SO's) concerns. *Exhibits regard for client's values and beliefs, clarifies barriers to participation in self-care, provides opportunity to work on problem-solving solutions, and provides encouragement and support.*[8,10]

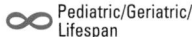

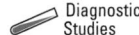

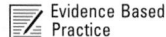

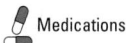

- Provide accurate and relevant information regarding current and future needs *so that client can incorporate into self-care plans while minimizing problems (e.g., heightened anxiety, depression, resistance) often associated with change.*[9]
- Promote client/SO participation in problem identification and desired outcomes. *Can ease frustration of current loss of independence, enhancing recovery, optimizing outcomes, and supporting health promotion.*[10]
- Establish "contractual" partnership with client/SO(s) if appropriate or indicated for motivation or behavioral modification.
- Practice and promote short-term goal setting and achievement *to recognize that today's success is as important as any long-term goal, accept ability to do one thing at a time, and conceptualize self-care in a broader sense.*
- Instruct in or review appropriate skills necessary for self-care, using terms understandable to client (e.g., child, adult, cognitively impaired person) and with sensitivity to developmental needs for practice, repetition, or reluctance. *Individualized teaching best affords reinforcement of learning. Sensitivity to special needs attaches value to the client's needs.*[1]
- Encourage client to use vision and hearing aids as appropriate. *Improves reception and interpretation of sensory input to facilitate self-care.*
- Perform or assist with meeting client's needs when he or she is unable to meet own needs *(e.g., personal care assistance is part of nursing care and should not be neglected while promoting and integrating self-care independence).*
- Anticipate needs and begin with familiar, easily accomplished tasks *to encourage client and build on successes.*
- Cue client, as indicated. *A cognitively impaired or forgetful client can often successfully participate in many activities with cueing, which can enhance self-esteem and potentiate learning or relearning of self-care tasks.*[1]
- Maintain a supportive attitude and allow sufficient time for client *to accomplish tasks to fullest extent of ability.*
- Refrain from unnecessary conversation or interruptions *that divert focus from the task at hand and can contribute to client's level of frustration.*
- Avoid doing things for client that client can do for self, but provide assistance as needed. *Client may be fearful or dependent, and although assistance is helpful in preventing frustration (and sometimes easier for the caregivers in terms of their time), it is important for client to do as much as possible for self to regain or maintain self-esteem, reduce helplessness, and promote optimal recovery.*
- Review coping skills (e.g., assertiveness, interpersonal relations, decision making, problem solving, stigma management, time management) *that are useful in managing a wide range of stressful conditions.* Encourage client to ask for assistance as needed or desired.[9]
- Schedule activities *to conform to client's normal schedule as much as possible (e.g., bathing at a relaxing time for client, rather than on a set routine).*
- Plan activities to prevent or accommodate fatigue and/or exacerbation of pain *to conserve energy and promote maximum participation in self-care.*
- Identify energy-saving behaviors *(e.g., sitting instead of standing when possible, organizing needs before beginning tasks).* Refer to NDs Activity Intolerance and Fatigue for additional interventions.
- Review medication needs (e.g., vitamins, nutritional supplements, pain reliever, antidepressants) *that may improve general well-being and ability to participate in self-care.*
- Arrange for home visit, as indicated, *to assess environmental concerns that can impact client's abilities to care for self in home. If necessary modifications are not feasible or cannot be made, client may require temporary or long-term relocation or regular home-care assistance.*
- Consult with rehabilitation professionals to identify and obtain assistive devices (e.g., modified eating utensils, modified clothing), mobility aids (e.g., rolling commode, shower chair), and home modification as necessary (e.g., adequate lighting; cutout under kitchen and bathroom sink; lowering cabinets and closet rods; handheld shower, raised toilet seat, grab bars for bathroom) *to optimize self-care efforts.*[1,8,10]

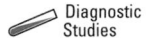

- Note availability and use of resources and supportive person(s) *to ascertain that client has means for sharing common concerns, needs, and wishes, as well as access to social support and approval (e.g., support group participants, family members, professionals).*[9]

NURSING PRIORITY NO. 4 To meet specific self-care needs:

BATHING DEFICIT

- Ask client/SO for input on bathing habits or cultural bathing preferences. *Creates opportunities for client to (1) keep long-standing routines (e.g., bathing at bedtime to improve sleep) and (2) exercise control over situation. This enhances self-esteem, while respecting personal and cultural preferences.*[3]
- Bathe or assist client in bathing, providing for any or all hygiene needs as indicated. *Type of bath (e.g., bed bath, towel bath, tub bath, shower) and purpose (e.g., cleansing, removing odor, simply soothing agitation) is determined by individual need. Note: Bathing is a healing rite and should be a comforting experience that focuses on the client's needs, rather than being a routinely scheduled task.*[11]
- Obtain hygiene supplies (e.g., soap, toothpaste, toothbrush, mouthwash, lotion, shampoo, razor, towels) for specific activity to be performed and place in client's easy reach *to provide visual cues and facilitate completion of activity.*
- Ascertain that all safety equipment is in place and properly installed (e.g., grab bars, antislip strips, shower chair, hydraulic lift) and that client/caregiver(s) can safely operate equipment *to prevent injury to client and caregivers.*[4]
- Instruct client to request assistance when needed and place call device within easy reach *so client can summon help if bathing alone* or stay with client *as dictated by safety needs.*
- Provide for adequate warmth (e.g., covering client during bed bath or warming bathroom). *Certain individuals (especially infants, the elderly, very thin or debilitated persons) are prone to hypothermia and can experience evaporative cooling during and after bathing.*[5]
- Determine that client can perceive water temperature and adjust water temperature safely or that water is correct temperature for client's bath or shower *to prevent chilling or burns. This step requires that client is cognitively and physically able to perceive hot and cold and to adjust faucets safely; otherwise, adequate supervision must be provided at all times.*[5]
- Assist client in and out of shower or tub as indicated. *Needs are variable (e.g., client may need to get into tub before running water, may require a shower chair, may be independent with one fixture and not another), requiring assessment of individual situations.*
- Assist with or cue client to complete hygiene steps (e.g., oral care, lotion application, applying deodorant, washing and styling hair). *These steps may be completed at same or different time as bathing, but are usually part of a regular routine that is necessary for client's physical well-being and emotional or social comfort.*

DRESSING DEFICIT

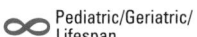

- Ascertain that appropriate clothing is available. *Client may not have sufficient clothing, clothing may be inadequate for situation or weather conditions, or clothing may need to be modified for client's particular medical condition or physical limitations.*
- Assist client in choosing clothing or lay out clothing as indicated. *May be needed when client has cognitive, physical, or psychiatric conditions affecting ability to choose appropriate pieces of clothing or to maintain a satisfactory appearance.*[1]
- Dress client or assist with dressing, as indicated. *Client may need assistance in putting on or taking off items of clothing (e.g., shoes and socks, over-the-head shirt) or may require partial or complete assistance with fasteners (e.g., buttons, snaps, zippers, shoelaces).*
- Allow sufficient time for dressing and undressing *because tasks may be tiring, painful, and difficult to complete. Dressing may be done from seated position if balance is impaired.*
- Use adaptive clothing as indicated (e.g., clothing with front closure, wide sleeves and pant legs, Velcro or zipper closures). *These may be helpful for client with limited arm or leg movement or impaired fine motor*

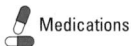

skills or for cognitively impaired person who desires to dress self but cannot do so with regular clothing fasteners.[12]

- Teach client to dress affected side first and then unaffected side (when client has paralysis or injury to one side of body) *to allow for easier manipulation of clothing.*[12]

FEEDING DEFICIT

- Assess client's need and ability to prepare food as indicated (including shopping, cooking, cutting food, opening containers, etc.). *Identifies specific assistance required.*
- Encourage food and fluid choices reflecting individual likes and abilities and that meet nutritional needs *to maximize food intake.*[2]
- Ascertain that client can swallow safely, checking gag and swallow reflexes, as indicated. Refer to ND impaired Swallowing for related interventions.
- Provide food and fluid of appropriate consistency *to facilitate swallowing.* Cut food into bite-size pieces *to prevent overfilling mouth and reduce risk of choking.*
- Assist client to handle utensils or in guiding utensils to mouth. *May require specialized equipment (e.g., rocker knife, plate guard, built-up handles) to increase independence or assistance with movement of arms and hands.*[1]
- Assist client with small cup, glass, or bottle for liquids, using straw or adaptive lids as indicated, *to enhance fluid intake while reducing spills.*
- Allow client time for intake of sufficient food *for feeling satisfied or completing a meal.*
- Assist client with social graces when eating with others; provide privacy *when manners might be offensive to others or client could be embarrassed.*
- Collaborate with nutritionist, speech-language pathologist, occupational therapist, or physician *for special diets or feeding methods necessary to provide adequate nutrition.*[13]
- Feed client, allowing adequate time for chewing and swallowing, *when client is not able to obtain nutrition by self-feeding.* Avoid providing fluids until client has swallowed food and mouth is clear. *Prevents "washing down" foods, reducing risk of choking.*

TOILETING DEFICIT

- Provide mobility assistance to bathroom or commode or place on bedpan or offer urinal, as indicated. *Client might be impaired because of age, cognitive problems, weakness, or acute injury or illness, requiring a range of interventions from complete care to help with walking.*
- Direct or accompany cognitively impaired client to bathroom, as needed. *May need directions to the facilities or reminders to use the bathroom, etc.*[6]
- Observe for behaviors such as pacing, fidgeting, and holding crotch *that may be indicative of need for prompt toileting.*
- Provide privacy *to enhance self-esteem and improve ability to urinate or defecate.*[1]
- Assist with manipulation of clothing if needed, *to decrease incidence of functional incontinence caused by difficulty removing clothing/underwear.*[7]
- Observe need for and assist in obtaining modified clothing or fasteners *to assist client in manipulation of clothing, fostering independence in self-toileting.*
- Provide or assist with use of assistive equipment (e.g., raised toilet seat, support rails, spill-proof urinals, fracture pans, bedside commode) *to promote independence and safety in sitting down or arising from toilet or for aiding elimination when client unable to go to bathroom.*[14]
- Keep toilet paper or wipes and hand-washing items within client's easy reach *to enhance self-cleansing efforts.*
- Implement bowel or bladder training/retraining programs as indicated. *This may include developing a schedule for toileting and other interventions as seen in NDs bowel Incontinence, Constipation, urinary Incontinence [specify], and impaired Urinary Elimination.*

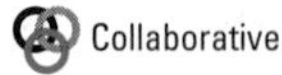

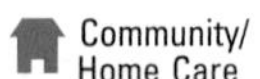

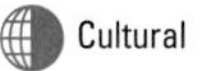

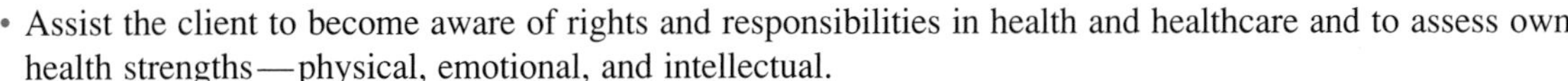

NURSING PRIORITY NO. 5 To promote optimal independence (Teaching/Discharge Considerations):

- Assist the client to become aware of rights and responsibilities in health and healthcare and to assess own health strengths—physical, emotional, and intellectual.
- Support client in making health-related decisions and assist in developing self-care practices and goals that promote health.
- Instruct in relaxation techniques (e.g., deep breathing, meditation, music, yoga) *to reduce frustration and enhance coping.*
- Provide for ongoing evaluation of self-care program *to note progress and identify changes in needs.*
- Modify program periodically *to accommodate changes in client's abilities. Assists client to adhere to plan of care to fullest extent.*
- Encourage keeping a journal *to note progress and identify factors affecting ability to perform self-care activities and to foster self-care and self-determination.*[9]
- Review safety concerns. Modify activities and environment *to reduce risk of injury and promote successful community functioning.*
- Refer to home-care provider, social services, physical or occupational therapy, speech-language pathologist, and rehabilitation and counseling resources as indicated.
- Arrange consult with community resources (e.g., Meals on Wheels, home care or visiting nurse service, senior services, nutritionist) *to provide long-term support and additional forms of assistance that may improve client's independence and self-care.*[1]
- Review instructions from other members of the healthcare team and provide written copy. *Provides clarification and reinforcement and opportunities for periodic review by client/caregivers.*
- Discuss respite or other care options with family. *Allows them free time away from the care situation to renew themselves and enhances coping abilities.* Refer to ND Caregiver Role Strain for related interventions.
- Assist or support family with alternative placements as necessary. *Enhances likelihood of finding individually appropriate situation to meet client's needs.*
- Be available for discussion of feelings (e.g., grieving, anger, frustration). *Provides opportunity for client/family to get feelings out in the open, realize the feelings are normal, and begin to problem solve solutions as indicated.*
- Refer to NDs ineffective Coping, compromised family Coping, risk for Disuse Syndrome, risk for Falls/Injury/Trauma, impaired physical Mobility, Powerlessness, and situational low Self-Esteem, as appropriate.

DOCUMENTATION FOCUS

Assessment/Reassessment

- Individual findings, functional level, and specifics of limitation(s).
- Needed resources and adaptive devices.
- Availability and use of community resources.
- Who is involved in care and provides assistance.

Planning

- Plan of care and who is involved in planning.
- Teaching plan.

Implementation/Evaluation

- Response to interventions, teaching, and actions performed.
- Attainment or progress toward desired outcome(s).
- Modifications of plan of care.

Discharge Planning

- Long-term needs and who is responsible for actions to be taken.
- Type of and source for assistive devices.
- Specific referrals made.

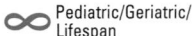

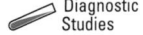

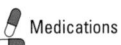

References

1. Newfield, S. A., Hinz, M. D., Tilley, D. S., et al. (2007). ND: Self Care Deficit (feeding, bathing-hygiene, dressing-grooming, toileting). *Cox's Clinical Applications of Nursing Diagnosis: Adult, Child, Women's, Psychiatric, Gerontic, and Home Health Considerations*. 5th ed. Philadelphia: F. A. Davis.
2. Kayser-Jones, J., Schell, E. (1997). The mealtime experience of a cognitively impaired elder: Ineffective and effective strategies. *J Gerontol Nurs*, 23(7), 33.
3. Freeman, E. (1997). International perspectives on bathing. *J Gerontol Nurs*, 22(1), 40–44.
4. Schemm, R. L., Gitlin, L. N. (1998). How occupational therapists teach older patients to use bathing and dressing devices in rehabilitation. *Am J Occup Ther*, 52(4), 276–282.
5. Miller, M. (1997). Physically aggressive resident behavior during hygienic care. *J Gerontol Nurs*, 23(5), 24–39.
6. Sloane, P. (1995). Bathing the Alzheimer's patient in long term care: Results and recommendation from three studies. *Am J Alzheimer's Dis*, 10(4), 3–11.
7. Penn, C. (1996). Assessment of urinary incontinence. *J Gerontol Nurs*, 22, 8–19.
8. Baldwin, K. M. (2006). Stroke: It's a knock-out punch. *Nursing Made Incredibly Easy!*, 4(2), 10–23.
9. Livneh, H., Antonak, R. F. (2005). Psychosocial adaptation to chronic illness and disability: A primer for counselors. *J Couns Dev*, 83(1), 12–20.
10. Singleton, J. K. (2000). Nurses' perspectives of encouraging client's care-of-self in a short-term rehabilitation unit within a long-term care facility. *Rehab Nurse*, 21(1), 23–30, 35.
11. Rasin, J., Barrick, A. L. (2004). Bathing persons with dementia. *Am J Nurs*, 104(3), 30–34.
12. Swann, J. (2008). Managing dressing problems in older adults in long-term care. *Nurs Resident Care*, 10(11), 564–567.
13. McCullough, K., Estes, J., McCullough, G., et al. (2008). RN compliance with SLP dysphagia recommendations in acute care. *Top Geriatr Rehabil*, 23(4), 330–340.
14. Cohen, D. (2008). Providing an assist. *Rehab Manag*, 21(8), 16–19.
15. Graf, C. (2008). The Lawton Instrumental Activities of Daily Living Scale. *Am J Nurs*, 108(4), 52–62.
16. Gordon, M. (2010). Functional levels code. *Manual of Nursing Diagnosis*. 12th ed. Sudbury, MA: Jones and Bartlett.

readiness for enhanced Self-Care

Taxonomy II: Activity/Rest—Class 5 Self-Care (00182) [**Diagnostic Division:** Teaching/Learning], Submitted 2006; Revised 2013

DEFINITION: A pattern of performing activities for oneself to meet health-related goals, which can be strengthened.

DEFINING CHARACTERISTICS

Subjective

Expresses desire to enhance independence with life, health, personal development, or well-being
Expresses desire to enhance knowledge of self-care strategies
Expresses desire to enhance self-care
[Note: Based on the definition and defining characteristics of this ND, the focus appears to be broader than simply meeting routine basic activities of daily living (ADLs) and addresses independence in maintaining overall health, personal development, and general well-being.]

Sample Clinical Applications: Presence of chronic physical or psychological conditions, or any individual seeking improved well-being or independence in meeting own needs

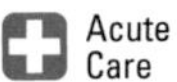

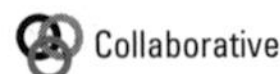

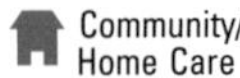

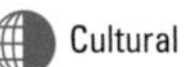

DESIRED OUTCOMES/EVALUATION CRITERIA

Sample NOC linkages:

Self-Care Status: Ability to perform basic personal care activities and instrumental activities of daily living

Self-Care: Instrumental Activities of Daily Living (IADL): Ability to perform activities needed to function in the home or community independently with or without assistive device

Self-Direction of Care: Care recipient actions taken to direct others who assist with or perform physical tasks and personal healthcare

Client Will (Include Specific Time Frame)

- Maintain responsibility for planning and achieving self-care goals and general well-being.
- Demonstrate proactive management of chronic conditions, potential complications, or changes in capabilities.
- Identify and use resources appropriately.
- Remain free of preventable complications.

ACTIONS/INTERVENTIONS

Sample NIC linkages:

Self-Care Assistance: IADL: Assisting and instructing a person to perform instrumental activities of daily living (IADL) needed to function in the home or community

Self-Modification Assistance: Reinforcement of self-directed change initiated by the patient to achieve personally important goals

Self-Efficacy Enhancement: Strengthening an individual's confidence in his/her ability to perform a health behavior

NURSING PRIORITY NO. 1 To determine current self-care status and motivation for improvement:

- Determine individual strengths and skills of the client *to incorporate into plan of care, enhancing likelihood of achieving outcomes. Note: Assessment might include use of an instrument to evaluate client's current functional status, in addition to client's self-report. In the community healthcare setting, a complex assessment tool may be used (e.g., Lawton and Brody's scale of IADL to determine client's self-care abilities (e.g., to communicate by phone, drive, cook, shop, balance a checkbook, manage medical appointments or medications, etc.). In an acute-care (or emergent) setting, the assessment may be confined to personal care (e.g., Katz Activities of Daily Living Scale). These instruments are used to determine (1) client's safety issues and care needs upon entry into acute care and (2) to ascertain changes in functional abilities as a result of client's condition and treatment.*[4]
- Ascertain motivation and expectations for change. *Motivation to improve and high expectations can encourage client to make changes that will improve his or her life. However, unrealistic expectations may hamper efforts.*
- Note availability and use of resources and supportive person(s) *to ascertain that client has means for sharing common concerns, needs, and wishes, as well as has access to social support and approval (e.g., support group participants, family members, professionals).*[2]
- ∞ Determine age, developmental issues, and presence of medical conditions resulting in specific deficits (e.g., loss of visual or spatial orientation affecting driving, muscular weakness affecting fine motor coordination, peripheral neuropathy impairing sensory interpretation, fractured ankle affecting ability to transfer or ambulate) *that could impact potential for growth or interrupt client's ability to meet own needs.*[2,3]
- Assess for potential challenges to enhanced participation in self-care (e.g., language barrier with healthcare providers, lack of information, insufficient time for discussion; sudden or progressive change in health status, catastrophic events).

NURSING PRIORITY NO. 2 To assist client/significant other (SO) plan to meet individual needs:

- Discuss client's understanding of current situation *to determine areas that can be clarified or strengthened. When health changes occur, the ability to make necessary adaptations is influenced by a wide range of variables that include understanding the changes necessary, the readiness and motivation to change, and the motor and sensory abilities to execute those activities.*[5]
- Provide accurate and relevant information regarding current and future needs *so that client can incorporate into self-care plans while minimizing problems (e.g., stress, resistance) often associated with change.*[1]
- Promote client/SO participation in problem identification and decision making. *Optimizes outcomes and supports health promotion.*[3]
- Review coping skills (e.g., assertiveness, interpersonal relations, decision making, problem solving, stigma management, time management) *that are useful in managing a wide range of stressful conditions.* Encourage client to ask for assistance, as needed or desired.[1]
- Active listen to client's/SO's concerns. *Exhibits regard for client's values and beliefs and provides opportunity to support positive responses and address questions or concerns.*[2]
- Encourage communication among those who are involved in the client's health promotion. *Periodic review provides clarification of issues, reinforcement of successful interventions, and possibility for early intervention, where needed, to manage chronic conditions.*

NURSING PRIORITY NO. 3 To promote optimum functioning (Teaching/Discharge Considerations):

- Assist client to set realistic goals for the future. *Enhances likelihood of success and commitment to behavioral changes.*
- Support client in making health-related decisions and pursuit of self-care practices that promote health *to foster self-esteem and support positive self-concept.*
- Identify reliable reference sources (including Web sites) regarding individual needs and strategies for self-care. *Reinforces learning and promotes self-paced review.*
- Provide for ongoing evaluation of self-care program *to identify progress and needed changes for continuation of health and adaptation in management of limiting conditions.*
- Review safety concerns and modification of medical therapies or activities and environment, as needed, *to prevent injury and enhance successful functioning.*
- Refer to home-care provider, social services, physical or occupational therapy, speech-language pathologist, rehabilitation, and counseling resources, as indicated or requested, *for education, assistance, and adaptive devices and modifications that may be desired.*
- Identify additional community resources (e.g., senior services, handicap transportation van for appointments, accessible and safe locations for social or sports activities, Meals on Wheels) *to obtain additional forms of assistance that may improve client's independence and self-care.*

DOCUMENTATION FOCUS

Assessment/Reassessment

- Individual findings, including strengths, health status, and any limitation(s).
- Availability and use of resources, support person(s), assistive devices.
- Motivation and expectations for change.

Planning

- Plan of care, specific interventions, and who is involved in planning.
- Teaching plan.

Implementation/Evaluation

- Client's responses to interventions, teaching, and actions performed.
- Attainment or progress toward desired outcome(s).
- Modifications to plan.

Discharge Planning

- Long-term needs and who is responsible for actions to be taken.
- Type of and source for assistive devices.
- Specific referrals made.

References:

1. Livneh, H., Antonak, R. F. (2005). Psychosocial adaptation to chronic illness and disability: A primer for counselors. *J Couns Dev*, 83(1), 12–20.
2. Baldwin, K. M. (2006). Stroke: It's a knock-out punch. *Nursing Made Incredibly Easy!*, 4(2), 10–23.
3. Singleton, J. K. (2000). Nurses' perspectives of encouraging client's care-of-self in a short-term rehabilitation unit within a long-term care facility. *Rehab Nurse*, 21(1), 23–30, 35.
4. McCullough, K., Estes, J., McCullough, G., et al. (2008). RN compliance with SLP dysphagia recommendations in acute care. *Top Geriatr Rehabil*, 23(4), 330–340.
5. Kresevic, D. M. (Updated 2012). Nursing standard of practice protocol: Assessment of function in acute care. Retrieved November 2015 from http://consultgerirn.org/topics/function/want_to_know_more.

readiness for enhanced Self-Concept

Taxonomy II: Self-Perception—Class 1 Self-Concept (00167) [**Diagnostic Division:** Ego Integrity], Submitted 2002

DEFINITION: A pattern of perceptions or ideas about the self, which can be strengthened.

DEFINING CHARACTERISTICS

Subjective

Expresses desire to enhance self-concept, role performance
Acceptance of strengths, limitations
Confidence in abilities
Satisfaction with thoughts about self, sense of worth
Satisfaction with body image, personal identity

Objective

Actions congruent with verbal expressions

Sample Clinical Applications: As a health-seeking behavior, the client may be healthy or this diagnosis can occur in any clinical condition or life process

DESIRED OUTCOMES/EVALUATION CRITERIA

Sample NOC linkages:

Self-Esteem: Personal judgment of self-worth
Hope: Optimism that is personally satisfying and life supporting
Personal Autonomy: Personal actions of a competent individual to exercise governance in life decisions

Client Will (Include Specific Time Frame)

- Verbalize understanding of own sense of self-worth.
- Participate in programs and activities to enhance self-esteem.
- Demonstrate behaviors or lifestyle changes to promote positive self-esteem.
- Participate in family, group, or community activities to enhance self-concept.

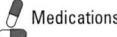

(continues on page 734)

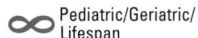

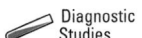

readiness for enhanced Self-Concept (continued)
ACTIONS/INTERVENTIONS

Sample NIC linkages:
Self-Modification Assistance: Reinforcement of self-directed change initiated by the patient to achieve personally important goals
Self-Awareness Enhancement: Assisting a patient to explore and understand his/her thoughts, feelings, motivations, and behaviors
Self-Esteem Enhancement: Assisting a patient to increase his/her personal judgment of self-worth

NURSING PRIORITY NO. 1 To assess current situation and desire to enhance self-concept:

- Determine current status of individual's belief about self. *Self-concept consists of the physical self (body image), personal self (identity), and self-esteem, and information about client's current thinking about self provides a beginning for making changes to improve self.*[1,2]
- Determine availability and quality of family/significant other (SO) support. *Presence of supportive people who reflect positive attitudes regarding the individual promotes a positive sense of self.*[1]
- Identify family dynamics, both present and past. *Self-esteem begins in early childhood and is influenced by the perceptions of how the individual is viewed by significant others. Provides information about family functioning that will help to develop plan of care for enhancing client's self-concept.*[1,2]
- Note willingness to seek assistance and motivation for change. *Individuals who have a sense of their own self-image and are willing to look at themselves realistically will be better able to achieve desired growth.*[1]
- Determine client's concept of self in relation to cultural or religious ideals and beliefs. *Culture and religion play a major role in view individual has of self in relation to self-worth.*[9]
- Observe nonverbal behaviors and note congruence with verbal expressions. Discuss cultural meanings of nonverbal communication. *Incongruence between verbal and nonverbal communication requires clarification. Interpretation of nonverbal expressions is culturally determined and needs to be identified to avoid misinterpretation.*[1,9]

NURSING PRIORITY NO. 2 To promote client sense of self-esteem:

- Develop therapeutic relationship. Be attentive, validate client's communication, maintain open communication, and use skills of active listening and "I" messages. *Promotes trusting situation in which client is free to be open and honest with self and others.*[2–4]
- Accept client's perceptions and view of current status. *Avoids threatening existing self-esteem and provides opportunity for client to develop realistic plan for improving self-concept.*[3]
- Be aware that people are not programmed to be rational. *Individuals must seek information—choosing to learn and to think rather than merely accepting/reacting—in order to have respect for self, facts, and honesty and to develop positive self-regard.*[7]
- Discuss client perception of self, confronting misconceptions and identifying negative self-talk. Address distortions in thinking, such as self-referencing (beliefs that others are focusing on individuals' weaknesses or limitations), filtering (focusing on negative and ignoring positive), and catastrophizing (expecting the worst outcomes). *Addressing these issues openly allows client to identify things that may negatively affect self-concept and provides an opportunity for change.*[7,8]
- Have client list current and past successes and strengths. *Emphasizes fact that client is and has been successful in many actions taken.*[1,8]
- Use positive "I" messages rather than praise. *Praise is a form of external control, coming from outside sources, whereas "I" messages allow the client to develop internal sense of self-worth.*[4,5]
- Discuss what behavior does for client (positive intention). Ask what options are available to the client/SO(s). *Encourages thinking about what inner motivations are and what actions can be taken to enhance self-esteem.*[3]
- Provide reinforcement for progress noted. *Positive words of encouragement support development of effective coping behaviors and promotes continuation of efforts and personal growth.*[6]

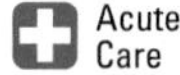
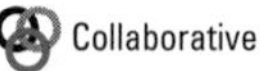
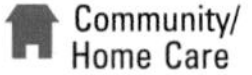
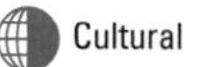

- Allow client to progress at own rate. *Adaptation to a change in self-concept depends on its significance to the individual and disruption to lifestyle.*[3]
- Involve in activities or exercise program of choice and promote socialization. *Enhances sense of well-being and can help to energize client.*[6,8]

NURSING PRIORITY NO. 3 To promote enhanced sense of personal worth (Teaching/Discharge Considerations):

- Assist client to identify personally achievable goals. Provide positive feedback for verbal and behavioral indications of improved self-view. *Increases likelihood of success and commitment to change.*[3,6]
- Refer to vocational or employment counselor and educational resources, as appropriate. *Assists with improving development of social or vocational skills.*[3]
- Encourage participation in classes, activities, or hobbies that client enjoys or would like to experience. *Provides opportunity for learning new information or skills that can enhance feelings of success, improving self-concept.*[5]
- Reinforce that current decision to improve self-concept is ongoing. *Continued work and support are necessary to sustain behavior changes and personal growth.*[3,5]
- Discuss ways to develop optimism. *Optimism is a key ingredient in happiness and can be learned.*[7]
- Suggest enrolling in assertiveness training classes. *Promotes learning to assist with developing new skills of voice control, posture, eye contact, or expression of feelings in an assertive, rather than aggressive or passive, manner to promote self-esteem.*[3]
- Emphasize importance of grooming and personal hygiene and assist in developing skills to improve appearance and dress for success. *Looking your best improves sense of self-worth, and presenting a positive appearance enhances how others see you. While these things are important, having an adequate foundation for the experience of competence and worth is essential to maintaining one's self-concept.*[1,6]

DOCUMENTATION FOCUS

Assessment/Reassessment

- Individual findings, including evaluations of self and others, current and past successes.
- Interactions with others, family dynamics, lifestyle.
- Cultural or religious influences.
- Motivation for and willingness to change.

Planning

- Plan of care and who is involved in planning.
- Educational plan.

Implementation/Evaluation

- Responses to interventions, teaching, and actions performed.
- Attainment or progress toward desired outcome(s).
- Modifications to plan of care.

Discharge Planning

- Long-term needs and who is responsible for actions to be taken.
- Specific referrals made.

References

1. Purkey, W. W. (1988). An overview of self-concept theory for counselors. Retrieved November 2015 from http://www.ericdigests.org/pre-9211/self.htm.
2. Rohany, N., Ahmad, Z. Z., Rozainee, K., et al. (2011). Family functioning, self esteem, self concept and cognitive distortion among juvenile delinquents. *The Social Sciences*, 6(3), 155–163.
3. Top, B. L., Chadwick, B. S., McClendon, R. J. (2010). Spirituality and self-worth. *The role of religion in shaping teens' self-image. The Religious Educator*, 4(2), 77–93.
4. Rogers, C., Farson, R. E. (Updated 2012). Active listening. Gordon Training International. Retrieved November 2015 from http://www.gordontraining.com/free-workplace-articles/active-listening/.
5. Gordon, T. (2011). The power of the language of acceptance. Natural Child Project. Retrieved November 2015 from http://www.gordontraining.com/free-parenting-articles/the-power-of-the-language-of-acceptance/.
6. Branden, N. (2010). Self esteem FAQ. National Association of Self-Esteem. Retrieved November 2015 from http://www.self-esteem-nase.org/faq.php.
7. Beattie, L. (No date). Optimism and the power of positive thinking: Change your thoughts, change your life! Retrieved November 2015 from http://www.sparkpeople.com/resource/wellness_articles.asp?id=835.
8. Beland, N. (2010). How to be happy. *Women's Health.* Retrieved November 2015 from http://www.womenshealthmag.com/health/be-happy-happily-ever-after.
9. Purnell, J. D. (2011). *Guide to Culturally Competent Health Care*. 2nd ed. Philadelphia: F. A. Davis.

chronic low Self-Esteem

Taxonomy II: Self-Perception—Class 2 Self-Esteem (00119) [**Diagnostic Division:** Ego Integrity], Submitted 1988; Revised 1996, 2008

DEFINITION: Long-standing negative self-evaluation/feelings about self or self-capabilities.

RELATED FACTORS

Repeated negative reinforcement or failures
Receiving insufficient affection, approval from others
Inadequate belonging; insufficient group membership
Inadequate respect from others
Cultural or spiritual incongruence
Exposure to traumatic situation
Ineffective coping with loss
Psychiatric disorder

DEFINING CHARACTERISTICS

Subjective

Shame; guilt
Underestimates ability to deal with situation
Rejection of positive feedback

Objective

Hesitant to try new experiences
Repeatedly unsuccessful in life events
Exaggerates negative feedback about self
Overly conforming; dependent on others' opinions
Poor eye contact
Nonassertive or indecisive behavior; passivity

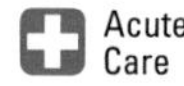

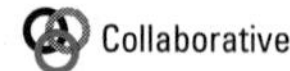

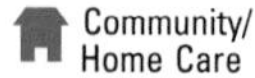

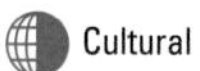

Excessive seeking of reassurance
Sample Clinical Applications: Chronic health conditions, degenerative diseases, eating disorders, substance abuse, depressive disorders, personality disorders, pervasive developmental disorders

DESIRED OUTCOMES/EVALUATION CRITERIA

Sample NOC linkages:
Self-Esteem: Personal judgment of self-worth
Personal Autonomy: Personal actions of a competent individual to exercise governance in life decisions
Hope: Optimism that is personally satisfying and life supporting

Client Will (Include Specific Time Frame)
- Verbalize understanding of negative evaluation of self and reasons for this problem.
- Participate in treatment program to promote change in self-evaluation.
- Demonstrate behaviors or lifestyle changes to promote positive self-image.
- Verbalize increased sense of self-worth in relation to current situation.
- Participate in family, group, or community activities to enhance change.

ACTIONS/INTERVENTIONS

Sample NIC linkages:
Self-Esteem Enhancement: Assisting a patient to increase his/her personal judgment of self-worth
Self-Awareness Enhancement: Assisting a patient to explore and understand his/her thoughts, feelings, motivations, and behaviors
Body Image Enhancement: Improving a patient's conscious and unconscious perceptions and attitudes toward his/her body

NURSING PRIORITY NO. 1 To assess causative/contributing factors:

- Determine factors in current situation that can exacerbate low self-esteem, noting age and developmental level of individual. *Identifying potentially aggravating occurrences (e.g., family crises, physical disfigurement from an accident or illness, feelings of abandonment by significant other [SO] resulting in social isolation) are important for developing plan of care and choosing appropriate interventions that help client develop a sense of self-worth.*[1]
- Assess content of negative self-talk. Note client's perceptions of how others view him or her. *Constant repetition of negative words and thoughts reinforce idea that individual is worthless and belief that others view him or her in a negative manner. Identifying these negative ruminations and bringing them to the client's awareness enables person to begin to replace them with positive thoughts.*[1]
- Note nonverbal behavior (e.g., nervous movements, lack of eye contact). *Incongruencies between verbal and nonverbal communication require clarification to ensure accuracy of interpretation.*[1,5]
- Determine availability and quality of family/SO(s) support. *Family is an important component of how an individual views self. The development of a positive sense of self depends on how the person relates to members of the family, as they are growing up and in the current situation.*[1,3]
- Identify family dynamics, present and past. *How family members interact affects an individual's development and sense of self-esteem. Whether family members are negative and nonsupportive, or positive and supportive, affects the needs of the client at this time.*[4]
- Be alert to client's concept of self in relation to cultural and religious ideal(s). *Composition and structure of nuclear family influences individual's sense of who they are in relation to others in the family and in society.*[9]

- Determine degree of participation and cooperation with therapeutic regimen. *Maintaining scheduled medications (e.g., antidepressants, antipsychotics) and other aspects of the plan of care requires ongoing evaluation and possible changes in regimen.*[1,2]
- Note willingness to seek assistance and motivation for change. *Determines client's degree of participation in adhering to therapeutic regimen.*[1,10]

NURSING PRIORITY NO. 2 To promote client's sense of self-esteem in dealing with situation:

- Develop therapeutic nurse/client relationship. Be attentive, validate client's communication, provide encouragement for efforts, maintain open communication, and use skills of active listening and "I" messages. *Promotes trusting environment in which client is free to be open and honest with self and therapist so current situation can be dealt with most effectively.*[1,4]
- Collaborate in addressing/presenting medical issues and safety concerns. *Client's self-esteem may be affected by physical changes of current medical situation. Changes in body, such as weight loss or gain, chronic illness, or amputation, will affect how client sees self as a person. Attitude may contribute to feelings of depression and lack of attention to personal safety requiring evaluation and assistance.*[1,3,7]
- Accept client's perceptions or view of situation. Avoid threatening existing self-esteem. *Promotes trust and allows client to begin to look at options for improving self-esteem.*[2,8]
- Be aware that people are not programmed to be rational. *They must seek information—choosing to learn and to think rather than merely accepting or reacting—in order to have respect for self, facts, and honesty and to develop positive self-esteem.*[1,3]
- Discuss client perceptions of self related to what is happening; confront misconceptions and negative self-talk. Address distortions in thinking, such as self-referencing (belief that others are focusing on individual's weaknesses or limitations), filtering (focusing on negative and ignoring positive), and catastrophizing (expecting the worst outcomes). *Addressing these issues openly provides opportunity for change.*[1,3,10]
- Emphasize need to avoid comparing self with others. Encourage client to focus on aspects of self that can be valued. *Changing negative thinking can be effective in developing positive self-talk to enhance self-esteem.*[2,5]
- Have client review current and past successes and strengths. *Often in the depths of despair and sense of failure in current situation, individual forgets positive aspects of his or her life. Bringing them to mind can remind client of these successes, enhancing sense of self-esteem.*[3,4]
- Use positive "I" messages rather than praise. *Praise may be heard as manipulative and insincere and be rejected. Use of positive "I" messages communicates a feeling that is genuine and real and allows client to feel good about himself or herself, developing internal sense of self-esteem.*[4,5]
- Discuss what behavior does for client (positive intention) and what options are available to the client/SO(s). *Helping client begin to look at what rewards are gained from current actions and what actions might be taken to achieve the same rewards in a more positive way can provide a realistic and accurate self-appraisal, enhancing sense of competence and self-worth.*[1,3,10]
- Assist client to deal with sense of powerlessness. Refer to ND Powerlessness.
- Set limits on aggressive or problem behaviors such as acting out, suicide preoccupation, or rumination. Put self in client's place using empathy, not sympathy. *Preventing undesirable behavior prevents feelings of worthlessness. Suicidal thoughts need further evaluation and intervention. Use of empathy helps caregiver to understand client's feelings better.*[1,2]
- Give reinforcement for progress noted. *Positive words of encouragement promote continuation of efforts, supporting development of coping behaviors.*[2,4,10]
- Encourage client to progress at own rate. *Adaptation to a change in self-concept depends on its significance to individual, disruption to lifestyle, and length of crisis or condition.*[1,2,5]
- Assist client to recognize and cope with events, alterations, and sense of loss of control. *Incorporating changes accurately into self-concept enhances sense of self-worth.*[1,2,7]
- Involve in activities/exercise program and promote socialization. *Enhances sense of well-being and can help energize client.*[1,5]

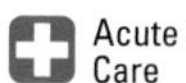

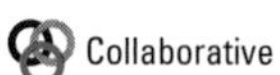

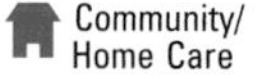

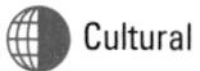

NURSING PRIORITY NO. 3 To promote wellness (Teaching/Discharge Considerations):

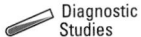

- Discuss inaccuracies in self-perception with client/SO(s). *Enables client and SOs to begin to look at misperceptions and accept reality and look at options for change to improve sense of self-worth.*[1,6,8]
- Model behaviors being taught, involving client in goal setting and decision making. *Facilitates client developing trust in his or her own unique strengths.*
- Prepare client for events or changes that are expected, when possible. *Providing time to adapt to changes allows client to prepare self and feel more confident in ability to manage the changes, enhancing sense of self-worth.*[1,2,7]
- Provide structure in daily routine and care activities. *Knowing what to expect promotes a sense of control and ability to deal with activities as they occur.*[1,2]
- Emphasize importance of grooming and personal hygiene. Assist in developing skills as indicated (e.g., makeup classes, dressing for success). *People feel better about themselves when they present a positive outer appearance.*[1,3,5]
- Assist client to identify goals that are personally achievable. Provide positive feedback for verbal and behavioral indications of improved self-view. *Increases likelihood of success and commitment to change.*[5,11]
- Refer to vocational or employment counselor and educational resources as appropriate. *Assists with development of social or vocational skills, promoting sense of competence and self-responsibility.*[1,2,5]
- Encourage participation in classes, activities, or hobbies that client enjoys or would like to experience. *Meaningful accomplishment, assuming self-responsibility, and participating in new activities engenders one's sense of competence and self-worth.*[8,12]
- Reinforce that this therapy is a brief encounter in overall life of the client/SO(s), with continued work and ongoing support being necessary to sustain behavior changes and personal growth. *Provides individual with information and encouragement to build on for the future.*[1,6,7]
- Refer to classes to assist with learning new skills (e.g., assertiveness training, positive self-image, communication skills). *These skills can help client develop a sense of competence through realistic and accurate self-appraisal promoting self-esteem.*[10]
- Refer to counseling or therapy and mental health or other special needs support groups as indicated. *May need additional intervention to develop needed changes.*[1,10,11]

DOCUMENTATION FOCUS

Assessment/Reassessment

- Individual findings, including early memories of negative evaluations (self and others), subsequent and precipitating failure events.
- Effects on interactions with others, family dynamics, lifestyle.
- Specific medical or safety issues.
- Cultural or religious factors.
- Motivation for and willingness to change.

Planning

- Plan of care and who is involved in planning.
- Teaching plan.

Implementation/Evaluation

- Responses to interventions, teaching, and actions performed.
- Attainment or progress toward desired outcome(s).
- Modifications to plan of care.

Discharge Planning

- Long-term needs and who is responsible for actions to be taken.
- Specific referrals made.

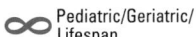

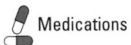

References

1. Townsend, M. C. (2006). *Psychiatric Mental Health Nursing Concepts of Care*. 5th ed. Philadelphia: F. A. Davis.
2. Doenges, M. E., Townsend, M. C., Moorhouse, M. F. (1998). *Psychiatric Care Plans: Guidelines for Individualizing Patient Care*. 3rd ed. Philadelphia: F. A. Davis.
3. Doenges, M. E., Moorhouse, M. F., Geissler-Murr, A. C. (2004). *Nurse's Pocket Guide: Diagnoses, Interventions, and Rationales*. 9th ed. Philadelphia: F. A. Davis.
4. Gordon, T. (2000). *Parent Effectiveness Training*. updated ed. New York: Three River Press.
5. Branden, N. (2010). Self esteem FAQs. National Association of Self-Esteem. Retrieved April 2015 from www.self-esteem-nase.org/faq.php.
6. Vasconcellos, J., Reasoner, R., Borba, M., et al. (No date). In defense of self-esteem. Retrieved April 2015 from http://www.self-esteem-nase.org/amember/newsarticles/InDefenseofSelf-Esteem.pdf.
7. Battle, J. (1990). *Self-Esteem: The New Revolution*. Edmonton, Alberta, Canada: James Battle & Associates.
8. Reasoner, R. (2010). The true meaning of self-esteem. Retrieved April 2015 from http://www.self-esteem-nase.org/what.php.
9. Purnell, J. D. (2011). *Guide to Culturally Competent Health Care*. Philadelphia: F. A. Davis.
10. Peden, A. R., Hall, L. A., Rayens, M. K., et al. (2000). Reducing negative thinking and depressive symptoms in college women. *J Nurs Scholar*, 32(2), 145–151.
11. Seligman, M., Reivich, K., Jaycox, L. H., et al. (1996). *The Optimistic Child*. New York: Houghton Mifflin.
12. Branden, N. (1995). *The Six Pillars of Self-Esteem*. New York: Bantam Book.

risk for chronic low Self-Esteem

Taxonomy II: Self-Perception—Class 2 Self-Esteem (00224) [**Diagnostic Division:** Ego Integrity], Submitted 2010; Revised 2013

DEFINITION: Vulnerable to long-standing negative self-evaluating/feelings about self or self-capabilities, which may compromise health.

RISK FACTORS

Exposure to traumatic situation
Repeated failures/negative reinforcement
Ineffective coping with loss
Inadequate affection received
Insufficient feeling of belonging; inadequate respect from others; inadequate group membership
Cultural or spiritual incongruence
Psychiatric disorder
Sample Clinical Applications: Chronic health conditions, eating disorders, substance abuse, depression, personality/pervasive developmental disorders

DESIRED OUTCOMES/EVALUATION CRITERIA

Sample NOC linkages:
Self-Esteem: Personal judgment of self-worth
Coping: Personal actions to manage stressors that tax an individual's resources
Personal Resiliency: Positive adaptation and function of an individual following significant adversity or crisis

Client Will (Include Specific Time Frame)
- Acknowledge understanding of discrepancy between self and cultural/spiritual norms.
- Participate in therapy program to improve self-esteem.

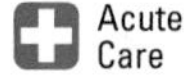

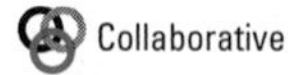

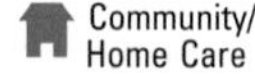

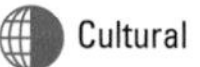

- Demonstrate behaviors to change negative self-evaluation.
- Verbalize understanding of reason for failures and how to make changes for success.
- Participate in family, group, or community activities to enhance change.

ACTIONS/INTERVENTIONS

Sample NIC linkages:
Self-Esteem Enhancement: Assisting a patient to increase his/her personal judgment of self-worth
Coping Enhancement: Assisting a patient to adapt to perceived stressors, changes, or threats that interfere with meeting life demands and roles
Socialization Enhancement: Facilitation of another person's ability to interact with others

NURSING PRIORITY NO. 1 To assess causative/contributing factors:

- Note age and developmental level of client and circumstances surrounding current situation. *Younger people may not have learned skills to deal with negative occurrences and/or rejection from others.*[2,16]
- Elicit client's perceptions of current situation. *Provides understanding of underlying/aggravating occurrences (e.g., family crisis, loss of employment, academic failure, physical disfigurement from an accident or illness, relationship problems/divorce with feelings of abandonment by significant other [SO] resulting in social isolation) necessary for choosing interventions appropriate to assist client to address feelings and develop realistic sense of self-worth.*[1,16]
- Ascertain sense of control client perceives to have over self/situation. *Client's locus of control or the degree of control client believes he or she has may be a critical factor in ability to deal with current situation. Individuals with external locus of control tend to blame others for their problems rather than taking responsibility for their actions. As a result they may feel helpless or powerless and look to others to solve problems and take care of them.*[3,14–16]
- Determine client's awareness of self-destructive behavior, acting out, aggression, and suicidal thoughts. *Choices individual makes result from low self-esteem and pleasing others and lead to feelings of worthlessness.*[1,8]
- Note content of negative self-talk and client's perception of how others see him or her. *As negative thoughts are repeated in one's head, they become the basis for believing that the individual is indeed worthless and others must agree with that conclusion.*[1,3]
- Observe nonverbal behavior (e.g., nervous movements, lack of eye contact) and how it relates to verbal statements. *Incongruencies between verbal and nonverbal need to be clarified to be sure perceived meaning of communication is accurate.*[10]
- Note religious and cultural factors that have influenced client. *Family of origin affects how one views self in relation to family members and others in society.*[5,8]
- Determine family makeup and whether they are available and supportive. *Support of family is essential to client's self-esteem. Predominant world view is determined by the time an individual is 5 years of age.*[3,16]
- Note family dynamics and how client interacts within the family. *Crucial to individual's development and self-esteem in a positive or negative way.*[8,16]
- Evaluate current medication regimen noting client adherence. *Maintaining therapeutic regimen requires ongoing evaluation to determine efficacy or need for change. The client who is asymptomatic or depressed may not feel the need to take prescribed medications. Other factors can also impact client's willingness to follow therapeutic plan (e.g., complexity of regimen, poor quality of the client-provider relationship, issues of access to care).*[13,17]

NURSING PRIORITY NO. 2 To promote client's sense of self-esteem in dealing with changes in life:

- Establish therapeutic nurse/client relationship, maintaining open communication and using active listening and "I" messages. *Promotes a trusting environment in which client is free to talk about potential problems that may arise.*[9]

- Determine willingness to improve attitudes and sense of self. *Negative perceptions, sense of alienation, and lack of involvement in positive activities lead to sense of worthlessness. Making a commitment to change provides an opportunity to learn new ways to interact with others and choose activities that promote individual successes.*[1,8]
- Address possible situations that client may be facing. *Sense of loss, lack of involvement in group, traumatic event, and repeated failures in attempts to change situation may discourage client from wanting to try to make life better.*[1,16]
- Avoid challenging client's perception of events. *May threaten sense of self-esteem, limiting client's ability to check out perceptions and make own corrections.*[11]
- Reinforce that people are not programmed to be rational. *They must seek information, choosing to learn and to think, rather than merely accepting or reacting, in order to have respect for self and develop positive self-esteem.*[1,3,8]
- Discuss misperceptions and negative self-talk as well as distortions in thinking, such as self-referencing (belief that others are focusing on person's weaknesses or limitations), filtering (focusing on negative and ignoring positive), or catastrophizing (believing the worst will happen). *These issues keep individual believing in a negative, worthless view of self and need to be addressed before person can move on and improve life.*[1,3]
- Discuss the problem of comparing self to others. Encourage client to focus on own positive aspects. *These actions will help individual to change negative thinking.*[1,3]
- List current and previous successes. *Focusing on these can help the client realize that failures can be overcome.*[1]
- Provide positive feedback, for verbal and behavioral indications of improved self-view, using "I" messages instead of praise. *Praise can be interpreted as insincere and manipulative and be rejected. Positive "I" messages convey a sense of acceptance and let the individual feel good about self, enhancing self-esteem and encouraging individual to continue efforts.*[9,12]
- Ask client to think about what behavior does (positive intention) in relation to low self-esteem, reluctance to join groups, and seeing self as less than others. *As individual thinks about this aspect of behavior, awareness of having a choice to change life may facilitate positive changes.*[3,8]
- Discuss feelings of powerlessness. *It is important to differentiate between what the client can control or change and what cannot be controlled. Inability of the client to make this distinction can cause client to feel defeated and increase sense of low self-esteem. Understanding that one is incapable of making everything right and perfect with all people, places, and things in life gives the individual the ability to retain the "locus of control."*[15,16] Refer to ND: Powerlessness.
- Contract with client/set limits on acting out and aggressive or self-destructive behaviors. *Aids in preventing negative behaviors that can result in/exacerbate feelings of worthlessness.*[7] Refer to NDs risk for other-/self-directed Violence and risk for Suicide for additional interventions.
- Encourage client to progress at own pace, providing reinforcement as progress is made. *Helps individual to value self and believe life changes can be made.*[1,8]
- Promote socialization and involvement in exercise and activity programs. *Helps individual to realize involvement with others can lead to positive feelings about self.*[4,6]

NURSING PRIORITY NO. 3 To promote wellness (Teaching/Discharge Considerations):

- Involve client in goal setting and decision making. *Facilitates trust and belief that change can be made and life can improve.*[9]
- Encourage client to structure daily activities so routine becomes manageable. *Promotes a sense of control and belief in own abilities.*[6]
- Discuss importance of grooming and personal hygiene, involvement in classes (i.e., Dress for Success). *Others often judge an individual by the outward appearance presented, as well as individual's own positive appraisal and sense of confidence.*[10]
- Refer to educational resources and vocational or employment counselor as indicated. *Promotes future success, reinforcing self-worth.*[4,16]

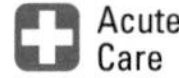
Acute Care
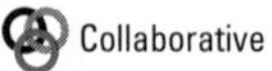
Collaborative
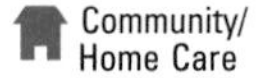
Community/ Home Care
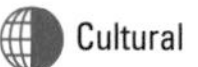
Cultural

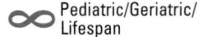

- Identify/refer to support groups and classes, such as assertiveness, communication skills, and parenting as appropriate. *These skills can help client develop or strengthen a sense of competence through realistic and accurate self-appraisal, promoting self-esteem.*[4,6,12,16]
- Review importance of adherence to medication regimen when prescribed. *A number of factors influence client's decisions about taking medications, including awareness of illness, beliefs about treatment, and side effects of medication. While education increases client's understanding of his or her illness/situation and treatment, it does not always improve compliance. Interventions such as individual or group counseling or compliance therapy based on cognitive–behavioral techniques may be useful in supporting personal growth and commitment to change.*[13,17]

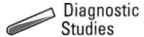

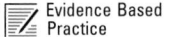

DOCUMENTATION FOCUS

Assessment/Reassessment

- Individual findings, noting risk factors, client's perceptions, interaction with others.
- Cultural values or religious beliefs, locus of control.
- Family support, availability, and use of resources.

Planning

- Plan of care and who is involved in planning.
- Individual teaching plan.

Implementation/Evaluation

- Response to interventions, teaching, actions performed, and changes that may be indicated.
- Attainment or progress toward desired outcomes.
- Modification to plan of care.

Discharge Planning

- Long-term needs and goals and who is responsible for actions to be taken.
- Specific referrals made.

References

1. Mayo Clinic Staff. (Updated 2014). Self-esteem: Take steps to feel better about yourself. Retrieved April 2015 from http://www.mayoclinic.org/healthy-lifestyle/adult-health/in-depth/self-esteem/art-20045374.
2. Watson, S. (No date). Understand inappropriate behavior. Retrieved April 2015 from http://specialed.about.com/od/behavioremotional/a/behavsupport.htm.
3. Selvarajah, A. (2000). Self-esteem: The problem behind all problems. Retrieved April 2015 from http://www.selfgrowth.com/articles/selvarajah13.html.
4. Garcia, J., Beyers, J., Uetrecht, C., et al. (2010). Healthy eating, physical activity, and healthy weights guideline for public health in Ontario. Retrieved April 2015 from https://www.cancercare.on.ca/common/pages/UserFile.aspx?fileId=64413.
5. Alaoui, S. (2011). Women's status in Islam: The line between culture and religion. Retrieved April 2015 from http://prospectjournal.org/2011/02/22/womens-status-in-islam-the-line-between-culture-and-religion/.
6. National Institute for Health and Clinical Excellence. (2009). Occupational therapy interventions and physical activity interventions to promote the mental well being of older people in primary care and residential care. Retrieved April 2015 from http://www.nice.org.uk/guidance/ph16/resources/guidance-occupational-therapy-and-physical-activity-interventions-to-promote-the-mental-wellbeing-of-older-people-in-primary-care-and-residential-care-pdf.
7. Webster, J. (No date). Behavior contracts to support good behavior: Explicit contracts can help students improve problem behavior. Retrieved April 2015 from http://specialed.about.com/od/behavioremotional/a/Behavior-Contracts-To-Support-Good-Behavior.htm.
8. Corey, G., Corey, M. S. (2010). *I Never Knew I Had a Choice—Explorations in Personal Growth.* 9th ed. Belmont, CA: Brooks/Cole.
9. McGreevey, M. (2006). *Patients as Partners: How to Involve Patients and Families in Their Own Care.* Oak Brook, IL: Joint Commission Resources.

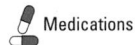

10. Knapp, M. L., Hall, J. A. (2010). *Nonverbal Communication in Human Interaction*. 7th ed. Boston, MA: Wadsworth/Cengage Learning.
11. Taylor, S. E., Brown, J. D. (1988). Illusion and well-being: A social psychological perspective on mental health. *Psychol Bull*, 103(2), 193–210.
12. Bright Horizons Family Resources (No date). Positive Parenting: Encourage vs Praise. Retrieved April 2015 from http://www.brighthorizons.com/family-resources/e-family-news/2012-positive-parenting-encouragement-versus-praise/.
13. Gray, R., Wykes, T., Gournay, K. (2002). From compliance to concordance: A review of the literature on interventions to enhance compliance with antipsychotic medication. *J Psychiatr Ment Health Nurs*, 9(3), 277–284.
14. Judge, T. A. (2009). Core self-evaluations and work success. *Curr Dir Psychol Sci*, 18(1), 58–62.
15. Messina, J. J. (1992). Accepting powerlessness. Tools for Handling Control Issues. Retrieved April 2015 from http://jamesjmessina.com/toolsforcontrolissues/acceptpowerlessness.html.
16. Daniels, R. (2009). Self-concept. *Nursing Fundamentals: Caring & Clinical Decision Making*. 2nd ed. Clifton Park, NY: Delmar Cengage Learning.
17. Ho, P. M., Bryson, C. L., Rumsfield, J. S. (2009). Medication adherence—Its importance in cardiovascular outcomes. *Circulation*, 119(23), 3028–3035.

situational low Self-Esteem

Taxonomy II: Self-Perception—Class 2 Self-Esteem (00120) [**Diagnostic Division:** Ego Integrity], Submitted 1988; Revised 1996, 2000

DEFINITION: Development of a negative perception of self-worth in response to a current situation.

RELATED FACTORS

Developmental transition
Functional impairment; alteration in body image
History of loss
Alteration in social role
Pattern of failure; history of rejection; inadequate recognition
Behavior inconsistent with values

DEFINING CHARACTERISTICS

Subjective

Helplessness; purposelessness
Underestimates ability to deal with situation

Objective

Situational challenge to self-worth
Self-negating verbalizations
Indecisive or nonassertive behavior

Sample Clinical Applications: Traumatic injuries, surgery, pregnancy, newly diagnosed conditions (e.g., diabetes mellitus), adjustment disorders, substance use, stroke, dementia

DESIRED OUTCOMES/EVALUATION CRITERIA

Sample NOC linkages:

Self-Esteem: Personal judgment of self-worth
Psychosocial Adjustment: Life Change: Adaptive psychosocial response of an individual to a significant life change
Personal Resiliency: Positive adaptation and function of an individual following significant adversity or crisis

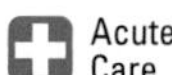
Acute Care
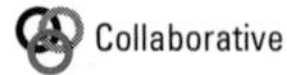
Collaborative
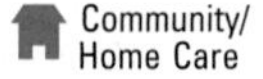
Community/ Home Care
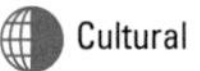
Cultural

Client Will (Include Specific Time Frame)

- Verbalize understanding of individual factors that precipitated current situation.
- Identify feelings and underlying dynamics for negative perception of self.
- Express positive self-appraisal.
- Demonstrate behaviors to restore positive self-image.
- Participate in treatment regimen or activities to correct factors that precipitated crisis.

ACTIONS/INTERVENTIONS

Sample NIC linkages:

Self-Esteem Enhancement: Assisting a patient to increase his/her personal judgment of self-worth

Coping Enhancement: Assisting a patient to adapt to perceived stressors, changes, or threats that interfere with meeting life demands and roles

Support System Enhancement: Facilitation of support to patient by family, friends, and community

NURSING PRIORITY NO. 1 To assess causative/contributing factors:

- Determine individual situation (e.g., family crisis, termination of a relationship, loss of employment, physical disfigurement) related to low self-esteem in the present circumstances. *Many factors are involved in a person's self-esteem, and this information is essential for planning accurate care.*[1]
- Identify basic sense of self-esteem of client; image client has of self—existential, physical, and psychological. *The components of self-concept consist of the physical self or body image, the personal self or personal identity, and the self-esteem. Each aspect plays a role in the client's ability to deal with current situation/crisis.*[1]
- Assess degree of threat and perception of client concerning crisis. *How individuals perceive themselves is based on the self-judgments they make. How the client sees the current situation in relation to ability to cope will affect his or her sense of self-worth and needs to be acknowledged and planned for to help client deal with feelings of low self-esteem.*[1,2]
- Ascertain sense of control client has (or perceives to have) over self and situation. *Client's locus of control or degree of control client believes or perceives he or she has may be a critical factor in ability to deal with current situation or crisis. Individuals with internal locus of control tend to be more optimistic about their ability to deal with adversity even in the face of current difficulties. Individuals with external locus of control will look to others to solve problems and take care of them.*[1–3]
- Determine client's awareness of own responsibility for dealing with situation, personal growth, etc. *These factors enhance the ability of the client to effectively manage situation in a positive manner.*[4]
- Assess family/SO(s) dynamics and support of client. *How family members interact affects an individual's development and sense of self-esteem. Effective interactions among family members usually lead to positive support for the client in current situation. Dysfunctional interactions may be detrimental to client's ability to deal with what is happening.*[2,3]
- Verify client's concept of self in relation to cultural and religious ideals. *Self-esteem is developed by many factors, including genetics and environment. Cultural and religious influences during the individual's life affect beliefs about self, measure of worth, and ability to deal with current situation or crisis.*[1,5] *Note: Recent studies support that self-esteem functions similarly across cultures.*[6]
- Determine past coping skills in relation to current episode. *Trust is built over time, and past experiences with failure or success will affect client's expectations regarding the eventual outcome of dealing with current illness or crisis.*[8,9]
- Assess negative attitudes or self-talk. *An individual who is feeling unimportant, incompetent, and not in control often is unconsciously saying negative things to himself or herself that contribute to a loss of self-esteem and an attitude of despair, affecting current situation.*[1,7]
- Note nonverbal body language. *Incongruencies between verbal or nonverbal communication require clarification to ensure accuracy of interpretation.*[1,2]

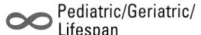

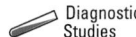

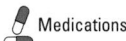

- Assess for self-destructive or suicidal thoughts or behavior. *Client who believes situation is hopeless often begins to consider suicide as an option.* Refer to ND risk for Suicide as appropriate.[1]
- Identify previous adaptations to illness or disruptive events in life. *May be predictive of current ability to deal with situation and suggest eventual outcome.*[1]
- Note availability and use of resources to address specific need (e.g., rehabilitation services, home-care support, job placement). *Individual may be unaware or have difficulty accessing community supports or assistance programs.*

NURSING PRIORITY NO. 2 To assist client to deal with loss/change and recapture sense of positive self-esteem:

- Assist with treatment of underlying condition when possible. *For example, cognitive restructuring and improved concentration in mild brain injury often result in restoration of positive self-esteem.*[1]
- Encourage expression of feelings, anxieties; facilitate grieving the loss. *As client expresses feelings and anxieties, he or she begins to deal with the realities of the current situation and the loss that occurs with the changes of illness.*[1] Refer to ND Grieving as appropriate.
- Active-listen to client's concerns or negative verbalizations without judgment. *Conveys a message of acceptance and confidence in client's ability to deal with whatever occurs.*
- Identify individual strengths, assets, and aspects of self that remain intact and can be valued. Reinforce positive traits, abilities, and self-view. *Client may not see these in the anxiety and hopelessness of the immediate situation, and reminding client of own positive attributes can help him or her recover hope and develop a positive attitude about situation.*[1,7]
- Help client identify own responsibility and control or lack of control in situation. *Accepting responsibility enables client to look realistically at what is under own control and what is not. When client stops expending energy on issues that cannot be controlled, energy is freed up to concentrate on more productive avenues.*[1,8]
- Assist client to problem solve situation, developing a plan of action and setting goals to achieve desired outcome. *Personal involvement enhances commitment to plan, optimizing outcomes.*
- Convey confidence in client's ability to cope with current situation. *Validation helps client accept own ability to deal with what is happening.*[1]
- Mobilize support systems; identify individuals in similar circumstances. *Feeling hopeless and alone lowers client's ability to manage care and concentrate on healing. Support systems can provide role modeling and the help needed to engender hope and enhance self-esteem.*[1,3]
- Provide opportunity for client to practice alternative coping strategies, including progressive socialization opportunities. *Involvement with others provides client with situation in which new actions can be tried out and validated or discarded to enhance feelings of self-worth.*[1,3]
- Encourage use of visualization, guided imagery, and relaxation. *These strategies promote a positive sense of self and general well-being, enhancing client's coping ability.*[1]
- Provide feedback about client's self-negating remarks or behavior, using "I" messages. *Allows client to experience a different view. "I" messages are a nonjudgmental way to let individual understand how behavior is perceived by or affecting others and self.*
- Encourage involvement in decisions about care when possible. *Promotes sense of control over what is happening, enhancing feelings of self-worth.*[1,8]
- Give reinforcement for progress noted. *Positive words of encouragement promote continuation of efforts, supporting development of coping behaviors.*[10]

NURSING PRIORITY NO. 3 To promote wellness (Teaching/Discharge Considerations):

- Assist client to identify personally achievable goals. *Increases likelihood of client's success and commitment to change.*[2,10]
- Encourage client to look to the future and set long-range goals for achieving necessary lifestyle changes. *Supports view that this is an ongoing process, providing client with hope for the future.*[1,3]
- Support independence in activities of daily living and mastery of therapeutic regimen. *Individuals who are confident are more secure and positive in self-appraisal.*[1,2]

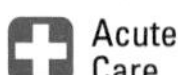

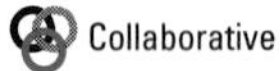

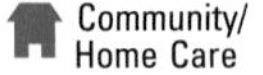

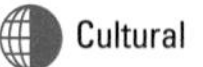

- Promote attendance in therapy or support group as indicated. *Provides opportunity to discuss own situation and hear how others are dealing with similar problems, promoting new ideas about own ability to deal with issues.*[1,9,10]
- Involve extended family/SO(s) in treatment plan as appropriate. *Enhances their understanding of what client wishes to accomplish, increasing likelihood they will provide appropriate support to client.*[1]
- Provide information and bibliotherapy, including reliable Web sites as appropriate. *Reinforces learning, allowing client to progress at own pace. Promotes opportunity for making informed decisions and improving ability to deal with situation.*[1,7]
- Refer to vocational or employment counselor and educational resources, as appropriate. *Assists with development of social or vocational skills, promoting sense of competence and self-responsibility.*[1,2]
- Suggest participation in group or community activities (e.g., assertiveness classes, volunteer work, support groups). *Provides opportunities for learning new information and being appreciated for contributions, enhancing sense of self-worth.*[1,2]
- Refer to counseling or therapy, mental health, or other special-needs support groups, as indicated. *May need additional support to deal with crisis.*[1,10]

DOCUMENTATION FOCUS

Assessment/Reassessment

- Individual findings, noting precipitating crisis, client's perceptions, effects on desired lifestyle/interaction with others.
- Cultural values or religious beliefs, locus of control.
- Family support, availability and use of resources.

Planning

- Plan of care and who is involved in planning.
- Teaching plan.

Implementation/Evaluation

- Responses to interventions, teaching, actions performed, and changes that may be indicated.
- Attainment or progress toward desired outcome(s).
- Modifications to plan of care.

Discharge Planning

- Long-term needs and goals and who is responsible for actions to be taken.
- Specific referrals made.

References

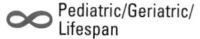

1. Townsend, M. C. (2003). *Psychiatric Mental Health Nursing Concepts of Care*. 4th ed. Philadelphia: F. A. Davis.
2. Reasoner, R. (2010). The true meaning of self-esteem. National Association for Self-Esteem. Retrieved April 2015 from http://www.self-esteem-nase.org/what.php.
3. Murray, E., Murray, C. A., Murray, M. P. (2009). Two experiments examine induced anxiety, depression, anger and assertiveness that are contrasted with the conditions of relaxed music, role playing and silence and indicate their impacts on cognitions and the emotion of anxiety. Retrieved April 2015 from http://www.nssa.us/journals/2009-33-1/2009-33-1-12.htm.
4. Selvarajah, A. (2000). Self-esteem: The problem behind all problems. Retrieved April 2015 from http://www.selfgrowth.com/articles/selvarajah13.html.
5. Purnell, L. D. (2011). *Guide to Culturally Competent Health Care*. 2nd ed. Philadelphia: F. A. Davis.
6. Brown, J. D., Cai, H., Oakes, M. A., et al. (2009). Cultural similarities in self-esteem functioning. *Psychology*, 40(1), 140–157.
7. Peden, A. R., Hall, L. A., Rayens, M. K., et al. (2000). Reducing negative thinking and depressive symptoms in college women. *J Nurs Scholarsh*, 32(2), 145–151.

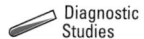

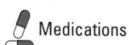

8. Munson, P. J. (1991). Life's decisions—By chance or by choice? *Adapted from Winning Teachers, Teaching Winners*. Santa Cruz, CA: ETR Associates.
9. Stepp, G. (2010). Helping children develop a positive sense of self. Retrieved April 2015 from http://www.vision.org/visionmedia/family-relationships/children-and-self-esteem/34763.aspx.
10. Seligman, M., Reivich, K., Jaycox, L. H., et al. (1996). *The Optimistic Child*. New York: Houghton Mifflin.

risk for situational low Self-Esteem

Taxonomy II: Self-Perception—Class 2 Self-Esteem (00153) [**Diagnostic Division:** Ego Integrity], Submitted 2000; Revised 2013

DEFINITION: Vulnerable to developing a negative perception of self-worth in response to a current situation, which may compromise health.

RISK FACTORS

Alteration in body image; physical illness
Alteration in social role; history of abandonment
Behavior inconsistent with values; unrealistic self-expectations
Decrease in control over environment
Developmental transition; functional impairment
History neglect or rejection; history of abuse (e.g., physical, psychological, sexual)
Inadequate recognition; pattern of failure; pattern of helplessness
Note: A risk diagnosis is not evidenced by signs and symptoms, as the problem has not occurred; rather, nursing interventions are directed at prevention.
Sample Clinical Applications: Traumatic injuries, surgery, pregnancy, newly diagnosed conditions (e.g., diabetes mellitus, hypertension), adjustment disorders, substance use, stroke, dementia

DESIRED OUTCOMES/EVALUATION CRITERIA

Sample NOC linkages:
Self-Esteem: Personal judgment of self-worth
Psychosocial Adjustment: Life Change: Adaptive psychosocial response of an individual to a significant life change
Abuse Recovery: Emotional: Extent of healing of psychological injuries due to abuse

Client Will (Include Specific Time Frame)
- Acknowledge factors that lead to possibility of feelings of low self-esteem.
- Verbalize view of self as a worthwhile, important person who functions well both interpersonally and occupationally.
- Demonstrate self-confidence by setting realistic goals and actively participating in life situation.

ACTIONS/INTERVENTIONS

Sample NIC linkages:
Self-Esteem Enhancement: Assisting a patient to increase his/her personal judgment of self-worth
Coping Enhancement: Assisting a patient to adapt to perceived stressors, changes, or threats that interfere with meeting life demands and roles
Self-Awareness Enhancement: Assisting a patient to explore and understand his/her thoughts, feelings, motivations, and behaviors

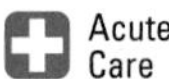
Acute Care
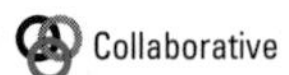
Collaborative
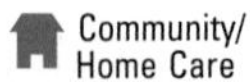
Community/ Home Care
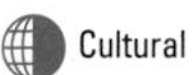
Cultural

NURSING PRIORITY NO. 1 To assess causative/contributing factors:

- Determine individual factors that may contribute to diminished self-esteem. *Proactive information allows identification of appropriate interventions to deal with current situation.*[1,2]
- Identify basic sense of self-worth of client and image client has of self—existential, physical, and psychological. *The components of self-concept consist of the physical self or body image, the personal self or personal identity, and the self-esteem, with each aspect playing a role in the client's ability to deal with anticipated changes.*[1]
- Note client's perception of threat to self in current situation. *Perception is more important than reality of what is happening. Some individuals view a potentially severe situation as something easily handled, while another may view a minor problem with anxiety and catastrophizing.*[2,3]
- Ascertain sense of control client has (or perceives to have) over self and situation. *Individual with internal locus of control tends to perceive self in control of what is happening and will participate more actively in care and feel more sense of self-worth.*[7,8]
- Determine client awareness of own responsibility for dealing with situation, personal growth, etc. *Acceptance of responsibility for self enables client to feel more comfortable with treatment regimen and participate more fully, promoting self-esteem.*[1,9]
- Assess family/SO(s) dynamics and support of client. *How family interacts with one another affects not only the development of self-esteem but also the maintenance of a sense of self-worth when client is facing an illness or crisis. Dysfunctional interactions may be detrimental to client's ability to deal with what is happening.*[1,5]
- Verify client's concept of self in relation to cultural or religious ideals. *Culture and religion play a major role in view individual has of self in relation to self-worth. Illness may interfere with this view.*[4] *Note: Recent studies support that self-esteem functions similarly across cultures.*[10]
- Assess negative attitudes and/or self-talk. *Contributes to view of situation as hopeless and/or difficult.*[3,6]
- Listen for or note self-destructive or suicidal thoughts or behaviors. *Indicates high level of stress and need for further evaluation and referral for mental health services.*[1,6] Refer to ND risk for Suicide as appropriate.
- Note nonverbal body language. *Incongruencies between verbal and nonverbal communications require clarification to ensure accuracy of interpretation.*[1]
- Identify previous adaptations to illness or disruptive events in life. *Provides information about how client handled those situations and may be predictive of current outcome.*[1]
- Determine availability and use of support systems. *Feeling hopeless and alone lowers client ability to manage care and concentrate on healing. Support systems can provide role modeling and the help needed to engender hope and enhance self-esteem.*[1]
- Note availability and use of resources to address specific need (e.g., rehabilitation services, home-care support, job placement). *Individual may be unaware or have difficulty accessing community supports or assistance programs.*

NURSING PRIORITY NO. 2 To assist client to deal with loss/change and maintain sense of positive self-esteem:

- Encourage expression of feelings and anxieties. *Facilitates grieving the loss.*
- Active-listen client's concerns without comment or judgment.
- Help client identify individual strengths and assets, reinforcing positive traits and self-view.
- Assist client to problem solve situation and develop plan of action.
- Convey confidence in client's ability to cope with current situation.
- Mobilize appropriate support systems.

NURSING PRIORITY NO. 3 To promote wellness (Teaching/Discharge Considerations):

- Provide information to assist client in making desired changes. *Appropriate books, DVDs, or Internet resources allows client to learn at own pace.*

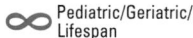

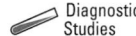

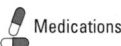

- Suggest participation in group or community activities or volunteer work *that can provide opportunity for success and positive feedback for accomplishments.*
- Involve significant others/extended family in treatment plan. *Increases likelihood they will provide appropriate support to client.*
- Promote attendance in therapy or support groups as indicated.

DOCUMENTATION FOCUS

Assessment/Reassessment

- Individual findings, including individual expressions of lack of self-esteem, effects on interactions with others, lifestyle.
- Underlying dynamics and duration (situational or situational exacerbating chronic).
- Cultural values or religious beliefs, locus of control.
- Family support, availability and use of resources.

Planning

- Plan of care and who is involved in planning.
- Teaching plan.

Implementation/Evaluation

- Responses to interventions, teaching, actions performed, and changes that may be indicated.
- Attainment or progress toward desired outcome(s).
- Modifications to plan of care.

Discharge Planning

- Long-term needs and goals, and who is responsible for actions to be taken.
- Specific referrals made.

References

1. Townsend, M. C. (2003). *Psychiatric Mental Health Nursing Concepts of Care.* 4th ed. Philadelphia: F. A. Davis.
2. Gross, S. J. (Reviewed 2013). How to raise your self esteem. PsychCentral. Retrieved April 2015 http://psychcentral.com/lib/how-to-raise-your-self-esteem/000737.
3. Reasoner, R. (2010). What is self-esteem? National Association for Self Esteem. Retrieved April 2015 from http://www.self-esteem-nase.org/what.php.
4. Purnell, L. D. (2011). *Guide to Culturally Competent Health Care.* 2nd ed. Philadelphia: F. A. Davis.
5. Pearson, A. B. (Updated 2010). Effective communication with children. Retrieved April 2015 from http://www.education.com/reference/article/effective-parent-child-communication/.
6. Adams, L. (2011). Working together with I-messages. Gordon Training International. Retrieved April 2015 from http://www.gordontraining.com/free-workplace-articles/working-together-with-i-messages/.
7. Peden, A. R., Hall, L. A., Ravens, M. K., et al. (2000). Reducing negative thinking and depressive symptoms in college women. *J Nurs Scholarsh,* 32(2), 145–151.
8. Munson, P. J. (1991). Life's decisions—By chance or by choice? *Adapted from Winning Teachers, Teaching Winners.* Santa Cruz, CA: ETR Associates.
9. Vasconcellos, J., Reasoner, R., Borba, M., et al. (No date). In defense of self-esteem. National Association of Self Esteem. Retrieved April 2015 from http://www.self-esteem-nase.org/amember/newsarticles/InDefenseofSelf-Esteem.pdf.
10. Brown, J. D., Cai, H., Oakes, M. A., et al. (2009). Cultural similarities in self-esteem functioning. *Psychology,* 40(1), 140–157.

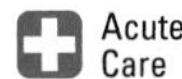

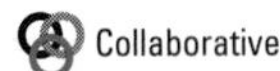

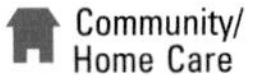

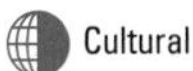

Self-Mutilation

Taxonomy II: Safety/Protection—Class 3 Violence (00151) [**Diagnostic Division:** Safety], Submitted 2000

DEFINITION: Deliberate self-injurious behavior causing tissue damage with the intent of causing nonfatal injury to attain relief of tension.

RELATED FACTORS

Absence of family confidant; disturbance in interpersonal relationships; feeling threatened with loss of significant relationship
Adolescence; ineffective communication between parent and adolescent; eating disorder
Alteration in body image; impaired or low self-esteem
Autism; childhood illness or surgery; developmental delay
Borderline personality or character disorder; depersonalization; dissociation; psychotic disorder; emotional disorder; labile behavior
Family divorce; family history of substance abuse or self-destructive behavior; violence between parental figures
History of childhood abuse (e.g., physical, psychological, sexual)
History of self-directed violence; irresistible urge for self-directed violence or to cut self
Impulsiveness; ineffective coping strategies; inability to express tension verbally; mounting tension that is intolerable; requires rapid stress reduction
Incarceration
Isolation from peers; peers who self-mutilate
Living in nontraditional setting (e.g., foster, group, or institutional care)
Negative feeling (e.g., depression, rejection, self-hatred, separation anxiety, guilt, depersonalization); perfectionism
Pattern of inability to plan solutions or to seen long-term consequences; history of manipulation to obtain nurturing relationship with others
Sexual identity crisis
Substance abuse

DEFINING CHARACTERISTICS

Subjective

Self-inflicted burn
Ingestion or inhalation of harmful substances or objects

Objective

Cuts or scratches on body
Picking at wound
Biting; abrading
Insertion of object(s) into body orifice(s)
Hitting
Severing or constricting a body part

Sample Clinical Applications: Borderline personality, dissociative disorders, bipolar disorder, developmental delay, autism, eating disorders, substance abuse, physical or psychological abuse, gender identity crisis

(continues on page 752)

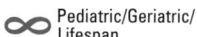

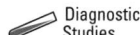

Self-Mutilation (continued)

DESIRED OUTCOMES/EVALUATION CRITERIA

Sample NOC linkages:

Self-Mutilation Restraint: Personal actions to refrain from intentional self-inflicted injury (nonlethal)
Impulse Self-Control: Self-restraint of compulsive or impulsive behaviors
Distorted Thought Self-Control: Self-restraint of disruption in perception, thought processes, and thought content

Client Will (Include Specific Time Frame)

- Verbalize understanding of reasons for occurrence of behavior.
- Identify precipitating factors and awareness of arousal state that occurs prior to incident.
- Express increased self-concept or self-esteem.
- Seeks help when feeling anxious and having thoughts of harming self.

ACTIONS/INTERVENTIONS

Sample NIC linkages:

Behavior Management: Self-Harm: Assisting the patient to decrease or eliminate self-mutilating or self-abusive behavior
Environmental Management: Safety: Monitoring and manipulation of the physical environment to promote safety
Limit Setting: Establishing the parameters of desirable and acceptable patient behavior

NURSING PRIORITY NO. 1 To assess causative/contributing factors:

- Determine underlying dynamics of individual situation as listed in Related Factors. Note previous episodes of self-mutilation behavior. *Although some body piercing (e.g., ears, nose, lip, eyebrow) is generally accepted as decorative, piercing of multiple sites or industrial piercings are often an attempt to establish individuality, addressing issues of separation and belonging, but are not considered self-injury or self-mutilating behaviors.*[1,7]
- Identify previous history of self-mutilative behavior and relationship to stressful events. *Self-injury is considered an attempt to alter a mood state and/or an outlet for negative emotions such as anger and shame. Information about previous behavior and precipitating factors is important to understanding and planning care in current situation.*[1,7,9,11]
- Determine presence of inflexible, maladaptive personality traits that reflect personality or character disorder. *Identification of impulsive, unpredictable, or inappropriate behaviors; intense anger; or lack of control of anger is important for planning appropriate interventions and plan of care. Clients diagnosed as borderline personality disorder are often unstable and prone to self-injury and need a specific treatment plan to diminish these behaviors.*[1,9]
- Evaluate history of mental illness (e.g., borderline personality, identity disorder, bipolar disorder). *These illnesses may be the underlying cause of the self-injurious behavior.*[1,2,10]
- Note beliefs and cultural or religious practices that may be involved in choice of behavior. *Growing up in a family that did not allow feelings to be expressed, individual may believe that feelings are wrong or bad. Family dynamics may come out of religious or cultural expectations that support strict punishment for transgressions. Individuals may believe mental illness is the result of unacceptable actions, and feelings of guilt may lead to anxiety and subsequent self-injurious behaviors.*[4]
- Note use or abuse of addicting substances. *May be indicative of attempt to treat self and needs further evaluation and additional intervention.*[2,6,10]
- Review laboratory findings (e.g., blood alcohol, polydrug screen, glucose, electrolyte levels). *Helpful for identifying drug use or medical problems that may be affecting behavior negatively.*[1]

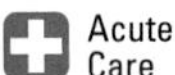

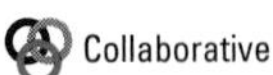

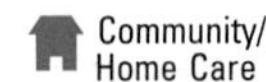

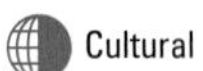

NURSING PRIORITY NO. 2 To structure environment to maintain client safety:

- Assist client to identify feelings leading up to desire for self-mutilation. *Early recognition of recurring feelings provides opportunity to seek other ways of coping.*[5]
- Provide external controls or limit setting. *Reducing opportunities for client to self-mutilate can help client learn to stop the behavior.*[4,8]
- Encourage appropriate expression of feelings. *Helps client to identify feelings and promote understanding of what leads to development of tension and subsequent injurious behavior.*[2]
- Keep client in continuous staff view and do special observation checks during inpatient stay. *Promotes safety by recognizing escalating behaviors and providing timely intervention.*[2,5]
- Structure inpatient milieu to maintain positive, clear, open communication among staff and clients, with an understanding that "secrets are not tolerated" and will be confronted. *Prevents manipulative behavior, so client does not pit one staff member against another to fulfill own desires.*[1,4,5]
- Note feelings of healthcare providers/family, such as frustration, anger, defensiveness, and need to rescue. *Client may be manipulative, evoking defensiveness and conflict. These feelings need to be identified, recognized, and dealt with openly with staff/family and client.*[4]
- Provide care for client's wounds when self-mutilation occurs in a matter-of-fact manner. Refrain from offering sympathy or additional attention. *A matter-of-fact approach can convey empathy and concern but not undue concern that could provide reinforcement for maladaptive behavior and encourage its repetition.*[2]
- Discuss use of medication, such as clozapine. *This medication has been shown to reduce acts of self-injurious behavior and help client maintain a more stable mood.*[3]
- Develop schedule of or refer to alternative healthy, success-oriented activities. *Group or family therapy or groups such as Eating Disorders or a similar 12-step program based on individual needs; self-esteem activities, including positive affirmations; visiting with friends; and exercise helps client to practice new behaviors in a supportive environment.*[7,11]

NURSING PRIORITY NO. 3 To promote movement toward positive changes:

- Encourage client involvement in formulating plan of care and developing goals for preventing undesired behavior. *Being involved in own decisions can help to reestablish ego boundaries and enhance commitment to goals, optimizing outcomes and enhancing self-esteem.*[2,5]
- Develop a contract between client and counselor to enable the client to stay physically safe, such as "I will not cut or harm myself for the next 24 hours." Renew contract on a regular basis and have both parties sign and date each contract. *Making a commitment in writing helps client to think before acting and can prevent new incidents of self-injury.*[4]
- Provide avenues of communication for times when client needs to talk. *Having an opportunity to discuss anxieties helps client to avoid cutting or damaging self.*[4,6]
- Assist client to learn assertive behavior. Include the use of effective communication skills, focusing on developing self-esteem by replacing negative self-talk with positive comments. *Low self-esteem is a factor in this behavior, and by learning new ways of expressing self, client can begin to feel better and deal with anxieties in a more positive manner.*[2,10]
- Choose interventions that help the client to reclaim power in own life (e.g., experiential and cognitive). *Beginning to think in a positive manner and then translating that into action provides reinforcement for using power to stop injurious behaviors and develop a more productive lifestyle.*[2]

NURSING PRIORITY NO. 4 To promote long-term safety (Teaching/Discharge Considerations):

- Discuss commitment to safety and ways in which client will deal with precursors to undesired behavior. *Identifies specific precursors for individual and provides a plan for client to follow when anxiety becomes overwhelming.*[2,8,10]

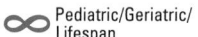

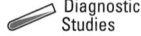

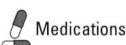

- Promote the use of healthy behaviors, identifying the consequences and outcomes of current actions. *As client develops a more positive attitude and accepts the idea that current actions are being destructive to desired lifestyle, new behaviors can help make needed changes.*[2]
- Identify support systems. *Knowing who client can turn to when anxiety becomes a problem helps to avoid injurious behavior.*[1]
- Discuss living arrangements when client is discharged from inpatient program. *May need assistance with transition to changes required to avoid recurrence of self-mutilating behaviors.*[2,10]
- Involve family/SO(s) in planning for discharge and involve in group therapies as appropriate. *Promotes coordination and continuation of plan and commitment to goals.*[2,6]
- Discuss the role neurotransmitters play in predisposing individual to beginning this behavior. *It is believed that problems in the serotonin system may make the person more aggressive and impulsive, and when combined with a home where they have learned that feelings are bad or wrong, this leads to turning aggression on self.*[8]
- Provide information and discuss the use of medication as appropriate. *Antidepressant medications may be useful, but they need to be weighed against the potential for overdosing.*[1,3]
- Refer to NDs Anxiety, Self-Esteem (specify), and impaired Social Interaction.

DOCUMENTATION FOCUS

Assessment/Reassessment

- Individual findings, including risk factors present, underlying dynamics, prior episodes.
- Cultural or religious practices.
- Laboratory test results.
- Substance use or abuse.

Planning

- Plan of care and who is involved in planning.
- Teaching plan.

Implementation/Evaluation

- Response to interventions, teaching, and actions performed.
- Attainment or progress toward desired outcome(s).
- Modifications to plan of care.

Discharge Planning

- Long-term needs and who is responsible for actions to be taken.
- Community resources, referrals made.

References

1. No surname, Alexandra. (Updated 2014). Self-mutilation: The truth behind the shame. Retrieved April 2015 from http://www.healthyplace.com/eating-disorders/articles/self-mutilation-the-truth-behind-the-shame/.
2. Doenges, M. E., Townsend, M. C., Moorhouse, M. F. (1998). *Psychiatric Care Plans: Guidelines for Individualizing Care.* 3rd ed. Philadelphia: F. A. Davis.
3. Chengappa, K. N. (1999). Clozapine reduces severe self-mutilation and aggression in psychotic patients with borderline personality disorder. *J Clin Psychiatry*, 60(7), 477–484.
4. Clarke, L., Whittaker, M. (1998). Self-mutilation: Culture, contexts, and nursing responses. *J Clin Nurs*, 7(2), 129–137.
5. Dallam, S. J. (1997). The identification and management of self-mutilating patients in primary care. *Nurse Pract*, 22(5), 151–165.
6. Selekman, M. D. (2004). Adolescent self-harm: A growing epidemic. *Family Therapy Magazine*, 1(2), 34–40.
7. Cox, H. C., Sridaromont, K., King, M., et al. (2002). *Clinical Applications of Nursing Diagnosis: Adult, Child, Women's, Psychiatric, Gerontic, and Home Health Considerations.* 4th ed. Philadelphia: F. A. Davis.
8. Martinson, D. (No date). Self-injury. Focus Adolescent Services. Retrieved November 2015 from http://www.psyke.org/history/200003/selfinjury/secretshame03.html.

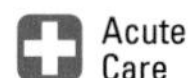

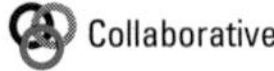

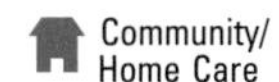

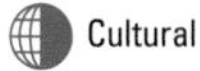

9. Davidson, T., Frey, R. (No date). Self-mutilation. *Gale Encyclopedia of Children's Health: Infancy Through Adolescence*. Retrieved April 2015 from http://www.healthofchildren.com/S/Self-Mutilation.html.
10. Holmes, L. (Updated 2012). Self-injury. About.com Mental Health. Retrieved April 2015 from http://mentalhealth.about.com/cs/familyresources/a/selfinjury.htm.
11. Tamanini, L. (2009). Why do teenagers cut themselves? Examiner.com. Retrieved April 2015 from http://www.examiner.com/kids-mental-health-in-gainesville/why-do-teenagers-cut-themselves.

risk for Self-Mutilation

Taxonomy II: Safety/Protection—Class 3 Violence (00139) [**Diagnostic Division:** Safety], Submitted 1992; Revised 2000, 2013

DEFINITION: Vulnerable to deliberate self-injurious behavior causing tissue damage with the intent of causing nonfatal injury to attain relief of tension.

RISK FACTORS

Adolescence; ineffective communication between parent and adolescent; eating disorder
Alteration in body image; impaired or low self-esteem
Autism; childhood illness or surgery; developmental delay
Borderline personality or character disorder; depersonalization; dissociation; psychotic disorder; emotional disorder
Disturbance in interpersonal relationships; loss of significant relationship(s)
Family divorce; family history of substance abuse or self-destructive behavior; violence between parental figures
History of childhood abuse (e.g., physical, psychological, sexual)
History of self-directed violence; irresistible urge for self-directed violence or to cut self
Impulsiveness; ineffective coping strategies; inability to express tension verbally; mounting tension that is intolerable; requires rapid stress reduction
Incarceration
Isolation from peers; peers who self-mutilate
Living in nontraditional setting (e.g., foster, group, or institutional care)
Negative feeling (e.g., depression, rejection, self-hatred, separation anxiety, guilt, depersonalization); perfectionism
Loss of control over problem-solving situation; pattern of inability to plan solutions or to see long-term consequences; history of manipulation to obtain nurturing relationship with others
Sexual identity crisis
Substance abuse
Note: A risk diagnosis is not evidenced by signs and symptoms, as the problem has not occurred; rather, nursing interventions are directed at prevention.
Sample Clinical Applications: Borderline personality, dissociative disorders, bipolar disorder, developmental delay, autism, eating disorders, substance abuse, physical/psychological abuse, gender identity crisis

DESIRED OUTCOMES/EVALUATION CRITERIA

Sample NOC linkages:
Self-Mutilation Restraint: Personal actions to refrain from intentional self-inflicted injury (nonlethal)
Impulse Self-Control: Self-restraint of compulsive or impulsive behaviors

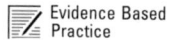

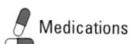

(continues on page 756)

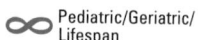

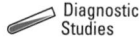

risk for Self-Mutilation (continued)
Distorted Thought Self-Control: Self-restraint of disruption in perception, thought processes, and thought content

Client Will (Include Specific Time Frame)

- Verbalize understanding of reasons for occurrence of behavior.
- Identify precipitating factors and awareness of arousal state that occurs prior to incident.
- Express increased self-concept or self-esteem.
- Demonstrate self-control as evidenced by lessened (or absence of) episodes of self-mutilation.
- Engage in use of alternative methods for managing feelings and individuality.

ACTIONS/INTERVENTIONS

Sample NIC linkages:
Behavior Modification: Promotion of a behavior change
Calming Technique: Reducing anxiety in patient experiencing acute distress
Behavior Management: Self-Harm: Assisting the patient to decrease or eliminate self-mutilating or self-abusive behavior

NURSING PRIORITY NO. 1 To assess causative/contributing factors:

- Determine underlying dynamics of individual situation as listed in Risk Factors. Note the presence of conditions that may interfere with ability to control own behavior (e.g., psychotic state, mental retardation, autism) *and may lead to incidents of self-injury.*[1]
- Assess for inflexible, maladaptive personality traits. *May reflect personality or character disorder (e.g., impulsive, unpredictable, inappropriate behaviors, intense anger or lack of control of anger) that may lead to self-mutilative behaviors.*[1]
- Evaluate history of mental illness (e.g., borderline personality, identity disorder, bipolar disorder). *These illnesses may be the underlying cause of the self-injurious behavior.*[1,2,10]
- Identify previous episodes of self-mutilating behavior (e.g., cutting, scratching, bruising). *Self-injury is considered an attempt to alter a mood state and/or an outlet for negative emotions such as anger and shame. Information about previous behavior and precipitating factors is important to understanding and planning care in current situation.*[1,7–9,11] *Although some body piercing (e.g., ears) is generally accepted as decorative, piercing of multiple sites or industrial piercings are often an attempt to establish individuality, addressing issues of separation and belonging, but are not considered as self-injury or self-mutilating behaviors.*[2]
- Note beliefs and cultural or religious practices that may be involved in choice of behavior. *Growing up in a family that did not allow feelings to be expressed, individual may believe that feelings are wrong or bad. Family dynamics may come out of religious or cultural expectations that support strict punishment for transgressions. Individuals may believe mental illness is the result of unacceptable actions, and feelings of guilt may lead to anxiety and subsequent self-injurious behaviors.*[4]
- Determine use or abuse of addictive substances, including alcohol. *Individuals often use these substances to self-medicate feelings of anxiety and may increase the risk of suicide by sixfold.*[2,8,10]
- Note degree of impairment in social and occupational functioning. *May dictate treatment setting (e.g., specific outpatient program or short-stay inpatient when client is experiencing extreme anxiety).*[1,5,9]
- Review laboratory findings (e.g., blood alcohol, polydrug screen, glucose, electrolyte levels). *Helpful for identifying drug use or medical problems that may be affecting behavior negatively.*[1]

NURSING PRIORITY NO. 2 To structure environment to maintain client safety:

- Assist client to identify feelings and behaviors that precede desire for self-mutilation. *Early recognition of recurring feelings provides client opportunity to seek other ways of coping, including asking for help.*[2,6]

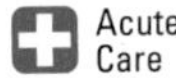

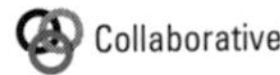

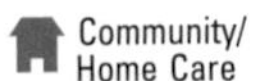

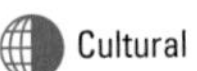

- Provide external controls or limit-setting as indicated. *Decreases the opportunity to injure self and helps client think about reasons for actions and learn different ways to deal with them.*[1]
- Encourage client to recognize and appropriately express feelings verbally. *Learning to express feelings enables client not only to recognize them, but also to begin to find acceptable and appropriate ways to deal with them.*[6,7,11]
- Note feelings of healthcare providers/family, such as frustration, anger, defensiveness, distraction, despair and powerlessness, and need to rescue. *Client may be manipulating or splitting providers/family members, which evokes defensiveness and resultant conflict. These feelings need to be identified, recognized, and dealt with openly with staff/family and client.*[1]
- Refer to alternative healthy, success-oriented activities. *Groups such as Eating Disorders or a similar 12-step program based on individual needs; self-esteem activities, including positive affirmations; visiting with friends; and exercise can help client to practice new behaviors in a supportive environment.*[6]

NURSING PRIORITY NO. 3 To promote movement toward positive actions:

- Encourage client involvement in formulating plan of care and developing goals for preventing undesired behavior. *Being involved in own decisions can help to reestablish ego boundaries and enhance commitment to goals, optimizing outcomes and enhancing self-esteem.*[2,5]
- Develop a contract between client and counselor to enable the client to stay physically safe, such as "I will not cut or harm myself for the next 24 hours." Renew contract on a regular basis, signed and dated by both parties. *Discussing the contract gets issues out in the open and conveys a sense of acceptance of the client, while placing some of the responsibility for safety on the client.*[1,2]
- Provide avenues of communication for times when client needs to talk. *Having an opportunity to discuss anxieties helps client to avoid cutting or damaging self.*[4,6]
- Choose interventions that help the client to reclaim power in own life (e.g., experiential and cognitive). *As client experiences new ways of interacting with others, he or she can begin to think more positively about self-worth and changing behaviors.*[2,10]
- Identify the consequences and outcomes of current actions (e.g., ask "Does this get you what you want?" or "How does this behavior help you achieve your goals?"). *Provides client with opportunity to look at own behaviors in a different way and begin to understand how they are harmful rather than helpful. Contrasting healthy behaviors versus current actions can help client decide to change them. Dialectic behavior therapy is effective in reducing injurious behavior along with the use of medication.*[1,3,6]
- Assist client to learn assertive behavior rather than nonassertive or aggressive behavior. Include use of effective communication skills, focusing on developing self-esteem by replacing negative self-talk with positive comments. *By learning these new skills, client interacts with others and gets needs met in positive, acceptable ways, promoting self-worth and lessening anxiety and risk of injurious actions.*[1,8]
- Discuss with client/family normalcy of adolescent task of separation and ways of achieving. *Helps individual members understand these actions and begin to recognize the normal from the ones that are of concern and need intervention.*[1,6,9]
- Involve client/family in group therapies as appropriate. *Group setting aids in promoting diffusion of anger and provides insight as to how negative, aggressive behavior affects others, making feedback easier to digest and understand.*[2]

NURSING PRIORITY NO. 4 To promote long-term safety (Teaching/Discharge Considerations):

- Discuss commitment to safety and ways in which client will deal with precursors to undesired behavior. *Helps client verbalize anger and anxiety and understand how these feelings lead to desire to injure self and actions that can be taken to prevent this behavior.*[4,6]
- Mobilize support systems. *These individuals often come from abusive families, and unresolved feelings of abandonment remain in adulthood. Positive support by many people in their lives can help them begin to overcome these feelings.*[1,8,9]

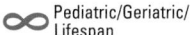

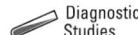

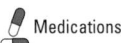

- Arrange for continued involvement in group therapy after discharge from program. *Remaining in this supportive environment can help client maintain new behaviors as he or she begins to increase responsibility for self and own action.*[2,10]
- Discuss and provide information about the use of medication as appropriate. *Antidepressant medications may be useful, but use needs to be weighed against potential for overdosing. (Note: The antidepressant Effexor can cause hostility, suicidal ideas, and self-harm in adolescent or young adults.) Medications that stabilize moods, ease depression, and calm anxiety may be tried to reduce the urge to self-harm.*[1,3]
- Refer to NDs Anxiety, Self-Esteem (specify), and impaired Social Interaction.

DOCUMENTATION FOCUS

Assessment/Reassessment

- Individual findings, including risk factors present, underlying dynamics, prior episodes.
- Cultural or religious practices.
- Laboratory test results.
- Substance use or abuse.

Planning

- Plan of care and who is involved in planning.
- Teaching plan.

Implementation/Evaluation

- Response to interventions, teaching, and actions performed.
- Attainment or progress toward desired outcome(s).
- Modifications to plan of care.

Discharge Planning

- Long-term needs and who is responsible for actions to be taken.
- Community resources, referrals made.

References

1. Townsend, M. C. (2006). *Psychiatric Mental Health Nursing Concepts of Care*. 4th ed. Philadelphia: F. A. Davis.
2. Doenges, M. E., Townsend, M. C., Moorhouse, M. F. (1998). *Psychiatric Care Plans: Guidelines for Individualizing Care*. 3rd ed. Philadelphia: F. A. Davis.
3. Chengappa, K. N., Ebeling, T., Kang, J. S., et al. (1999). Clozapine reduces severe self-mutilation and aggression in psychotic patients with borderline personality disorder. *J Clin Psychiatry*, 60(7), 477–484.
4. Clarke, L., Whittaker, M. (1998). Self-mutilation: Culture, contexts, and nursing responses. *J Clin Nurs*, 7(2), 129–137.
5. Dallam, S. J. (1997). The identification and management of self-mutilating patients in primary care. *Nurse Pract*, 22(5), 151–165.
6. Smith, M., Segal, J. (Updated 2015). Cutting and self-harm. Helpguide.org. Retrieved April 2015 from http://www.helpguide.org/articles/anxiety/cutting-and-self-harm.htm.
7. Selekman, M. D. (2004). Adolescent self-harm: A growing epidemic. *Family Therapy Magazine*, 1(2), 34–40.
8. Davidson, L., Frey, D. (No date). Self-mutilation. *Gale Encyclopedia of Children's Health: Infancy Through Adolescence*. Retrieved April 2015 from http://www.healthofchildren.com/S/Self-Mutilation.html.
9. Estevez, R. (reviewer) (Updated 2011). Self-mutilation. Retrieved April 2015 from http://www.med.nyu.edu/content?ChunkIID=11569.
10. Goldberg, J. (reviewer) (Updated 2014). Mental health and self-injury. WebMD. Retrieved April 2015 from http://www.webmd.com/anxiety-panic/guide/self-injury.
11. Tamanini, K. (2009). Why do teenagers cut themselves? Examiner.com. Retrieved April 2015 from http://www.examiner.com/kids-mental-health-in-gainesville/why-do-teenagers-cut-themselves.

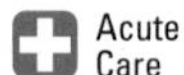

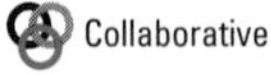

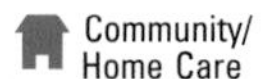

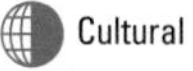

Self-Neglect

Taxonomy II: Activity/Rest—Class 5 Self-Care (00193) [**Diagnostic Division:** Hygiene], Submitted 2008

DEFINITION: A constellation of culturally framed behaviors involving one or more self-care activities in which there is a failure to maintain a socially accepted standard of health and well-being (Gibbons, Lauder, & Ludwick, 2006).

RELATED FACTORS

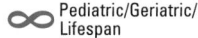

Stressor; psychiatric/psychotic disorder
Frontal lobe dysfunction; deficient executive function; alteration in cognitive functioning; Capgras syndrome
Functional impairment; learning disability
Lifestyle choice; substance abuse; malingering
Inability to maintain control; fear of institutionalization

DEFINING CHARACTERISTICS

Objective

Insufficient personal or environmental hygiene
Nonadherence to health activity

Sample Clinical Applications: Mental illness (as in related factors); terminal illness—cancer, amyotrophic lateral sclerosis (ALS); debilitating conditions—multiple sclerosis (MS), Parkinson's disease; alcohol/drug abuse

DESIRED OUTCOMES/EVALUATION CRITERIA

Sample NOC linkages:

Self-Care Status: Ability to perform basic personal care activities and instrumental activities of daily living (IADLs)

Health Promoting Behavior: Personal actions to sustain or increase wellness

Client Will (Include Specific Time Frame)

- Acknowledge difficulty maintaining hygiene practices.
- Demonstrate ability to manage lifestyle changes and medication regimen.
- Perform ADLs within level of own ability.

Caregiver Will (Include Specific Time Frame)

- Assist individual with personal and environmental hygiene as needed.
- Identify and assist client with medical, dental, and other healthcare appointments as indicated.

ACTIONS/INTERVENTIONS

Sample NIC linkages:

Self-Responsibility Facilitation: Encouraging a patient to assume more responsibility for own behavior

Self-Care Assistance: Assisting another to perform activities of daily living

Cultural Brokerage: The deliberate use of culturally competent strategies to bridge or mediate between the patient's culture and the biomedical healthcare system

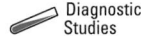

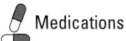

NURSING PRIORITY NO. 1 To identify causative or precipitating factors:

- Determine existing health problems, age, developmental level, and cognitive psychological factors, including presence of delusions affecting ability to care for own needs. Use an appropriate screening instrument, such as the Elder Assessment Instrument. *A wide variety of impairments can cause a person to neglect hygiene needs, particularly aging, homelessness, and dementia. Neglect and elder abuse is underreported, and the use of a good tool can help identify its presence.*[2,3]
- Identify other problems that may interfere with ability to care for self. *A visual or hearing impairment, language barrier, and emotional instability or lability can create difficulties for individual to manage daily tasks.*[2,4]
- Note recent life events or changes in circumstances. *Losses (e.g., loved one, financial security, physical independence) can trigger or exacerbate self-neglect behaviors.*[4]
- Review circumstances of client illness, possible monetary rewards, and sympathy or attention from family. *On occasion, self-neglect may be malingering as an attempt to gain something from others or relinquish unwanted responsibilities.*
- Perform mental status examination. *Mental illness (e.g., psychosis, depression, dementia) can affect individual's ability or desire to maintain self-care activities or care for home surroundings.*[5,11]
- Review studies evaluating frontal lobe dysfunction and possibility of Diogenes syndrome. *These clients present with severe self-neglect and may have coexisting medical and psychiatric conditions.*[10,11]
- Assess economic situation and living arrangements. *May live alone or with family members who are not helpful, may be homeless, and may have little or no financial resources, resulting in inability or lack of concern about personal well-being.*[4]
- Determine availability and use of resources. *Depending on disability of client, agencies can work together to develop a plan to meet needs, noting whether individual is availing self of help.*[6]
- Interview significant other (SO)/family members to determine level of involvement and support. *Client may be exhibiting acting-out or paranoid behaviors, stressing caregivers who may not realize individual is unable to control self because of cognitive impairment.*[3]

NURSING PRIORITY NO. 2 To determine degree of impairment:

- Perform head-to-toe assessment, inspecting scalp and skin; noting personal hygiene, body odor, rashes, bruising, skin tears, lesions, burns, and presence of vermin; and inspecting oral cavity for gum disease, inflammation, lesions, loose or broken teeth, and fit of dentures. *Identifies specific needs and may reveal signs of trauma or abuse.*[1]
- Obtain weight. Perform nutritional assessment as indicated. *Neglecting oneself often includes not eating meals regularly or failing to eat nutritionally balanced foods. When alcoholism or drug abuse is a part of neglect, individual may be severely malnourished.*[1,3]
- Review medication regimen. *In addition to neglecting self-care activities, client will likely not pay attention to taking prescriptions as ordered resulting in exacerbation of medical problem. Note: Some psychotropic medication may cause individual to "feel different" or not in control of self, resulting in reluctance to take drug.*[3]
- Determine willingness to change situation. *Depending on individual's situation (living alone, homeless, mental status), client may have difficulty committing to or be unwilling to change. May see change as a loss of independence.*[3,11]

NURSING PRIORITY NO. 3 To assist in correcting/dealing with situation:

- Develop multidisciplinary team specific to individual needs, such as case manager, physician, dietitian, physical or occupational therapist, rehabilitation specialist, and social worker, *to review assessment data and develop a plan appropriate to the individual situation, making use of client's capabilities and maximizing potential.*[6,11]

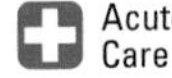
Acute Care
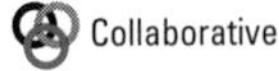
Collaborative
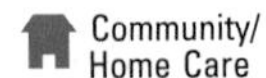
Community/ Home Care
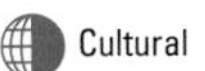
Cultural

- Establish therapeutic relationship with client, as well as family if available and willing to be involved. *Promotes trust and encourages input into planning process.*[7,11]
- Identify specific priorities and goals of client/SOs. *Helps client to look at possibilities for dealing with difficult situation of no longer being able to maintain lifestyle and moving on to a new way of managing.*[6]
- Promote client/SOs participation in problem identification and decision making. *Enhances commitment to plan when individual has input and encourages participation, enhancing outcomes.*[7]
- Evaluate need for safety, balancing client's need for autonomy. *The ethical challenge of providing individual safety within the current laws for client's right to refuse care in face of self-neglect and self-destructive behaviors that can impact others as well as the client is difficult to manage.*[4,9]
- Perform home assessment. *Determines safety issues, cleanliness, compulsive hoarding, and neglected property concerns, so plans can be made to take care of these matters if client is to remain in the home.*[7]
- Instruct in or review skills necessary for caring for self, using terms appropriate to client's level of understanding. *When individual is cognitively impaired or otherwise has difficulty processing information, instructions need to be simplified.*[5]
- Plan time for listening to client's/SOs' concerns. *Provides opportunity to determine whether plan is being followed and what the barriers to participation may be.*[7]
- Refer to NDs Self-Care Deficit [specify], ineffective Health Maintenance, impaired Home Maintenance, and [disturbed Sensory Perception] for additional interventions as appropriate.

NURSING PRIORITY NO. 4 To promote wellness (Discharge/Evaluation Criteria):

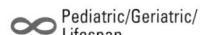

- Establish remotivation or resocialization program when indicated. *Depending on where the client is residing, isolation may become a problem as individual withdraws from contact with others, and these programs may be helpful.*[2]
- Assist with setting up medication regimen. *Client may need help with arranging medications in specific ways to assure correct administration, especially in the presence of cognitive impairment.*[8]
- Discuss dietary needs and client's ability to provide nutritious meals. *May require support such as food stamps, community pantry, senior meal program, and Meals on Wheels.*[1]
- Provide for ongoing evaluation of self-care program. *Helps to identify whether client is managing effectively or whether cognitive functioning is deteriorating and a new plan needs to be developed.*[7]
- Evaluate for appropriateness of providing a companion animal. *Taking responsibility for another life and sharing unconditional love can provide purpose and motivation for client to take more interest in own situation.*[4]
- Refer to support services such as home care, day-care program, social services, food stamps, community clinic, physical or occupational therapy, and senior services as indicated. *Provides for long-term support to facilitate client's independence and general well-being.*[8]
- Investigate alternative placements as indicated. *Client may require group home, assisted living, or long-term care, and it is best to place in least restrictive environment capable of meeting client's needs.*[9]
- Discuss need for respite for family members. *Care of cognitively impaired member can be wearing, and time away allows for renewing oneself and enhancing ability to cope with continued care responsibilities.*[5]
- Refer for counseling as indicated. *Accurate mental health diagnoses may reveal the need for appropriate services, psychiatric, social services, and home care.*[6]

DOCUMENTATION FOCUS

Assessment/Reassessment

- Individual findings, functional level and limitations, mental status.
- Personal safety issues.
- Needed resources, possible need for placement.

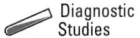

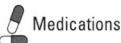

Planning
- Plan of care and who is involved in planning.
- Teaching plan.

Implementation/Evaluation
- Response to interventions, teaching, and actions performed.
- Attainment or progress toward desired outcomes.
- Modifications of plan of care.

Discharge Planning
- Long-term needs and who is responsible for actions to be taken.
- Type of assistance and resources needed.
- Specific referrals made.

References

1. Smith, S. M., Mathews-Oliver, S. A., Zwart, S. R., et al. (2006). Nutritional status is altered in the self-neglecting elderly. *J Nutr*, 136(10), 2534–2541.
2. Abrams, R. C., Lachs, M., McAvay, G., et al. (2002). Predictors of self-neglect in community-dwelling elders. *Am J Psychiatry*, 159(10), 1724–1730.
3. Fulmer, T. (2003). Elder abuse and neglect assessment. *Gerontol Nurs*, 29(1), 8–9.
4. Dong, X., Simon, M., Mendes de Leon, C. (2009). Elder self-neglect and abuse and mortality risk in community dwelling populations. *JAMA*, 302(5), 517–526.
5. Brannon, G. E. (Updated 2013). History and mental status exam. Medscape. Retrieved April 2015 from http://emedicine.medscape.com/article/293402-overview.
6. Lauder, W., Anderson, I., Barclay, A. (2005). A framework for good practice in interagency interventions with cases of self-neglect. *J Psychiatr Ment Health Nurs*, 12(2), 192–198.
7. Lauder, W., Anderson, I., Barclay, A. (2005). Housing and self-neglect: The responses of health, social care and environmental health agencies. *J Interprof Care*, 19(4), 317–325.
8. Tierney, M., Charles, J., Naglie, G. (2004). Risk factors for harm in cognitively impaired seniors who live alone: A prospective study. *J Am Geriatr Soc*, 52(9), 1435–1441.
9. Nusbaum, N. (2004). Safety vs autonomy: Dilemmas and strategies in protection of vulnerable community dwelling elderly. *Ann Long-Term Care*, 12(5), 50–53.
10. Amanullah, S., Oomman, S. K., Datta, S. S. (2009). "Diogenes Sydrome" revisited. Retrieved April 2015 from http://www.gjpsy.uni-goettingen.de/gjp-article-amanullah.pdf.
11. Braye, S., Orr, D., Preston-Shoot, M. (2011). Self-neglect and adult safeguarding: Findings from research. Social Care Institute for Excellence. Retrieved April 2015 from http://www.scie.org.uk/publications/reports/report46.pdf.

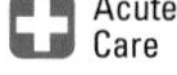

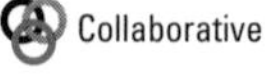

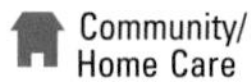

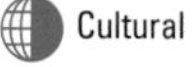

[disturbed Sensory Perception] (specify: visual, auditory, kinesthetic, gustatory, tactile, olfactory)]

Taxonomy II: Perception/Cognition—Class 3 Sensation/Perception (00122) [**Diagnostic Division:** Neurosensory], Submitted 1978; Revised 1980, 1998 (by small group work 1996); Retired 2012

DEFINITION: Change in the amount or patterning of incoming stimuli accompanied by a diminished, exaggerated, distorted, or impaired response to such stimuli.

RELATED FACTORS

Insufficient environmental stimuli: [therapeutically restricted environments (e.g., isolation, intensive care, bedrest, traction, confining illnesses, incubator); socially restricted environment (e.g., institutionalization, homebound, aging, chronic/terminal illness, infant deprivation), stigmatized (e.g., mentally ill/developmentally-delayed/handicapped)]
Excessive environmental stimuli
Altered sensory reception/transmission/integration
Biochemical imbalances [e.g., elevated blood urea nitrogen (BUN), ammonia; hypoxia]; electrolyte imbalance; [drugs, e.g., stimulants or depressants, mind-altering drugs]
Psychological stress; [sleep deprivation]

DEFINING CHARACTERISTICS

Subjective

[Reported] change in sensory acuity [e.g., photosensitivity, hypoesthesias or hyperesthesias, diminished or altered sense of taste, inability to tell position of body parts (proprioception)]
Sensory distortions

Objective

[Measured] change in sensory acuity
Change in usual response to stimuli
Change in behavior pattern; restlessness; irritability
Change in problem-solving abilities; poor concentration
Disorientation; hallucinations; [illusions]
Impaired communication
[Motor incoordination, altered sense of balance, falls (e.g., Ménière's syndrome)]

Sample Clinical Applications: Glaucoma, cataract, brain tumor, stroke, traumatic injury, amputation, surgery, immobility, peripheral neuropathy (e.g., diabetes), substance abuse, schizophrenia, developmental delay

DESIRED OUTCOMES/EVALUATION CRITERIA

Sample NOC linkages:

Sensory Function: Extent to which an individual correctly senses skin stimulation, sounds, proprioception, taste and smell, and visual images

Distorted Thought Self-Control: Self-restraint of disruptions in perception, thought processes, and thought content

Risk Control: Hearing/Visual Impairments: Personal actions to prevent, eliminate, or reduce threats to hearing [or] visual function

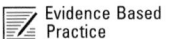

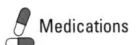

(continues on page 764)

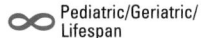

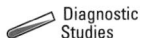

[disturbed Sensory Perception] (continued)

Client Will (Include Specific Time Frame)

- Regain or maintain usual level of cognition.
- Recognize and correct or compensate for sensory impairments.
- Verbalize awareness of sensory needs and presence of overload and/or deprivation.
- Identify and modify external factors that contribute to alterations in sensory or perceptual abilities.
- Use resources effectively and appropriately.
- Be free of injury.

ACTIONS/INTERVENTIONS

Sample NIC linkages:

Communication Enhancement: Hearing [or] Vision Deficit: Assistance in accepting and learning alternative methods for living with diminished hearing [or] vision

Peripheral Sensation Management: Prevention or minimization of injury or discomfort in the patient with altered sensation

Hallucination [or] Delusion Management: Promoting the comfort, safety, and reality orientation of a patient experiencing hallucinations [or] false, fixed beliefs that have little or no basis in reality

Environmental Management: Manipulation of the patient's surroundings for therapeutic benefit, sensory appeal, and psychological well-being

NURSING PRIORITY NO. 1 To assess causative/contributing factors:

- Identify client with condition that can affect sensing, interpreting, and communicating stimuli, as noted in Related Factors. *Specific clinical concerns (e.g., neurological disease or trauma, intensive care unit confinement, surgery, pain, biochemical imbalances, psychosis, substance abuse, toxemia) have the potential for altering one or more of the senses, with resultant change in the reception, sensitivity, or interpretation of sensory input.*[1]
- Be aware of current diagnosis or treatments *(e.g., glaucoma, surgery, immobility, recent stroke, diabetes, mental illness; drug toxicity or side effects [e.g., halos around lights, ringing in ears]; middle-ear disturbances [altered sense of balance]) that can cause or exacerbate sensory problems.*
- Note age and developmental stage. *Problems with sensory perception may be known to client/caregiver (e.g., child wearing hearing aid, elderly adult with known macular degeneration) where compensatory interventions are in place. Screening or evaluation may be required if sensory impairments are suspected but not obvious, as might occur when an infant is not progressing developmentally or an older individual has a gradual loss of sensory discrimination associated with aging, or sensory changes are associated with a sudden neurological event.*[2,3,8]
- Evaluate medication regimen and determine possible use or misuse of drugs (prescription, over the counter, illicit) *to identify effects, side effects, adverse effects, or drug interactions that may be causing or exacerbating sensory or perceptual problems.*
- Review results of sensory and motor neurological testing and laboratory studies (e.g., cognitive testing or laboratory values, such as electrolytes, chemical profile, arterial blood gases, serum drug levels) *to note presence or possible cause of changes in response to sensory stimuli.*

NURSING PRIORITY NO. 2 To determine degree of impairment:

- Assess ability to speak, hear, interpret, and respond to simple commands *to obtain an overview of client's mental and cognitive status and ability to interpret stimuli.*
- Evaluate sensory awareness (e.g., hot and cold, dull or sharp, smell, taste, visual acuity and hearing, gait, mobility, location or function of body parts). *Screening can be done in clinic or facility may identify problems requiring more extensive evaluation.*

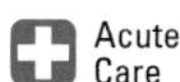
Acute Care
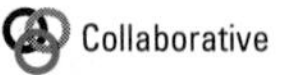
Collaborative
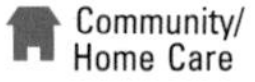
Community/ Home Care
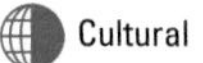
Cultural

- Determine response to touch and painful stimuli *to note whether response is appropriate to stimulus and whether it is immediate or delayed. The sense of touch is usually maintained throughout life and may become more important if other senses are diminished. Different types of touch or contact are associated with different meanings (including communication of ideas, information, emotion).*[3]
- Observe for behavioral responses (e.g., illusions, hallucinations, delusions; withdrawal, hostility, crying, inappropriate affect; confusion or disorientation) *that may indicate mental or emotional problems or chemical toxicity (as might occur with digoxin or other drug overdose or reaction) or be associated with brain or neurological trauma or infection.*
- Note inattention to body parts and segments of environment and lack of recognition of familiar objects or persons. *Loss of comprehension of auditory, visual, or other sensations may be indicative of unilateral neglect or inability to recognize and respond to environmental cues.*[9]
- Ascertain client's perception of problem or changes. Note significant other's (SO's) observations of changes that have occurred and client's responses to changes. *Client may or may not be aware of changes (e.g., diabetic with neuropathy may not realize he or she has lost discrimination for pain in feet, parents may notice child's problem with coordination or difficulty with words).*
- Refer to additional NDs Anxiety, acute/chronic Confusion, and Unilateral Neglect, as appropriate and based on findings.

NURSING PRIORITY NO. 3 To promote normalization of response to stimuli:

GENERAL INTERVENTIONS

- Note degree of alteration or involvement (single or multiple senses) *to determine scope and complexity of condition and needed interventions.*
- Ascertain and validate client's perceptions. Listen to and respect client's expressions of deprivation *to assist in planning of appropriate care, to identify inconsistencies in reception and integration of stimuli, and to provide compassionate regard for client's feelings.*
- Provide means of communication as indicated by client's current situation.
- Document perceptual deficit in chart and code on wall in client's room, if needed, *so caregivers are aware of specific needs or limitations.*
- Avoid isolating client, physically or emotionally, *to prevent sensory deprivation and limit confusion.*
- Address client by name and have personnel wear name tags and reintroduce self, as needed, *to preserve client's sense of identity and orientation.*
- Reorient to time, place, and situation or events, as necessary, *to reduce confusion and provide sense of normalcy to client's daily life.*
- Explain procedures and activities, expected sensations, and outcomes. *Helpful in reducing anxiety associated with altered interpretation of environment.*
- Promote a stable environment with assignment of same personnel as much as possible *to promote continuity of care and limit confusion.*
- Provide appropriate sensory stimulation, including familiar smells and sounds, tactile stimulation with a variety of objects, and changing of light intensity and other cues (e.g., clocks, calendars).
- Eliminate extraneous noise or stimuli, including nonessential equipment, alarms, and audible monitor signals, when possible. *Reduces anxiety and exaggerated emotional responses or confusion associated with sensory overload.*
- Provide feedback *to assist client to separate reality from fantasy and altered perception.*
- Protect from bodily harm (e.g., falls, burns, positioning problems) *as client may not perceive pain or have impaired sense of position, thereby increasing the risk for falls.*
- Provide undisturbed rest and sleep periods *to reduce anxiety, agitation, or psychosis that can accompany sleep deprivation, particularly when client is confined to bed (e.g., intensive care unit).*
- Plan care with client/SO(s), as appropriate. *Enhances commitment to and continuation of plan, thus optimizing outcomes.*

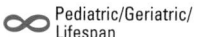

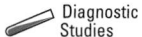

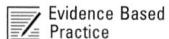

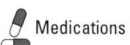

- Encourage SO(s) to bring in familiar objects and to talk with and touch the client. *Client often can experience positive response to loved ones, thus enhancing recovery.*
- Collaborate with other healthcare team members in providing rehabilitative therapies and stimulating modalities (e.g., music therapy, sensory training, remotivation therapy) *to achieve maximal gains in function and psychosocial well-being.*[10]
- Limit and carefully monitor use of sedation, especially in older population *who are more sensitive to side effects.*
- Identify and encourage use of resources and prosthetic devices (e.g., hearing aids, computerized visual aid or glasses with a level plumb line for balance). *Useful for augmenting senses.*

VISUAL DEFICITS

- Note particular vision problem (e.g., loss of visual field, change in depth perception, double vision, blindness) *that affects client's ability to perceive environment and learn or relearn motor skills.*[3]
- Speak to visually impaired or unresponsive client frequently, especially when first entering room or client's presence, *to provide auditory stimulation and prevent startle reflex. Note: A recent study on unconscious patients with brain injury supports the theory that sensory stimulation can enhance brain recovery.*[12]
- Approach from visually intact side, position objects to take advantage of intact visual field, and use eye patch, when needed, *to decrease sensory confusion when client has acute loss of vision or field of vision in one eye.*[3]
- Provide or encourage listening to music, radio, TV, talking books, and use of talking timepieces and computers, as appropriate.
- Supply adequate lighting for reading and activities.
- Place glasses or contacts where they can be easily found and encourage client to wear corrective lenses during waking hours.
- Arrange bed, personal articles, and food trays to take advantage of functional vision. *Enhances independence and safety.*
- Describe food and placement, feeding or assisting client as necessary (e.g., cooking, cutting food, offering finger food, placing food in clock-position on plate) *when vision impairments could hinder nutritional intake or cause social discomfort.*
- Assist client with picking out clothing *if problems with color discrimination cause mismatching.*[3]
- Color-code doors and drawers to assist client with low vision *in locating belongings or a particular site (e.g., bathroom).*

AUDITORY DEFICITS

- Determine if client reads lips and turn toward/face client, making sure you have his/her attention, and enunciating words clearly.
- Encourage client's use of hearing aid when one is available.
- Lower the pitch of the voice and speak in tone that does not include shouting *(which increases the pitch of the voice).*[3]
- Speak slowly and distinctly; use simple sentences. Rephrase sentences rather than repeating them. Avoid asking multiple questions at one time *to enhance client's comprehension and ability to respond.*[13]
- Use touch to get the client's attention, if needed.
- Be aware and careful of facial expressions.
- Pay attention to background noise and reduce it to a minimum when attempting conversation. *Background noise is often amplified, causing misinterpretation of conversation or inability to hear words, and often results in overstimulation of senses.*[3]
- Refer for periodic evaluation by audiologist *to note changes in acuity and determine if client might benefit from a hearing aid.*[3]

KINESTHETIC AND TACTILE DEFICITS

- Encourage proper body positioning and alignment *to prevent muscle strain or injury.*
- Provide firm mattress or chair cushion *to maintain positioning and good posture.*

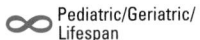

- Assist with or recommend periodic weight shifts *to enhance circulation and relieve tissue pressure, reducing risk of tissue damage.*
- Provide tactile stimulation as care is given and when communicating with or comforting client (respecting cultural and personal preferences). *Communicates presence and connection with other human being because touching is an important part of caring, and the need for touch is a deep psychological need. Note: The meaning people associate with touching is culturally determined to a great degree. Always consider a patient's culturally defined sense of modesty when giving nursing care. A recent research study concludes that nurses touch patients to perform clinical tasks, communicate caring, and ensure comfort. Nurses must exercise clinical judgment in deciding when, where, and how to touch patients. In providing the patient's perspective on intimate touch (e.g., bathing, catheterization, other sensitive procedures), participants said they want to know before intimate touch is provided, why it's necessary, and what it will involve.*[14,15]
- Be aware that older clients may be more interested in touching *because they have lost loved ones, their appearance may not be as attractive as it once was, and the attitude of the public toward older adults does not encourage physical contact with them. Note: A recent study found that comfort touch improved the perceptions of self-esteem, well-being and social processes, health status, life satisfaction and self-actualization, faith or belief, and self-responsibility in institutionalized older female residents.*[3,16]
- Stimulate sense of touch (e.g., give client objects to touch, grasp; have client practice touching walls and other boundaries). *Aids in retraining sensory pathways to integrate reception and interpretation of stimuli.*
- Provide touch, using level of appropriate intensity (e.g., light, moderate, deep, strong), *depending on the need (e.g., light touch to get client's attention, stroking to convey love to infant).*[3,4]
- Teach client/SO to frequently inspect skin and extremities for redness, pressure points, bony deformities, or skin trauma *when client is unable to sense pain and is prone to tissue injury.*[5]

TASTE AND SMELL

- Note taste and smell dysfunction (loss or distortion of function) that may be associated with chronic conditions (e.g., cystic fibrosis, chronic sinusitis, hypothyroidism, multiple sclerosis, Alzheimer's disease, head trauma) or may suggest a new or developing problem (e.g., zinc deficiency, dental conditions, allergies).[6]
- Investigate reports of changes in tastes of foods (foods taste or smell odd), ability to salivate, or loss of appetite. *May reflect loss or distortion of smell and taste functions or side effects or interactions with medications.*[3,6,7]
- Encourage client to chew food well and to experiment with a variety of food colors, textures, and flavor enhancers *to maximize taste sensation.*[3,7]
- Discuss with client how he or she can check with others in observing for offensive or dangerous odors (e.g., body odor, spoiled foods, propane gas or smoke) *if sense of smell is diminished.*[3]
- Remove offensive odors from client's presence, especially *when client is immobile, debilitated, and/or suffering from oversensitivity to odors, nausea, or vomiting.*

NURSING PRIORITY NO. 4 To prevent injury/complications:

- Place call bell or other communication device within reach and verify that client knows where it is and how to use it.
- Provide safety measures (e.g., side rails or grab pole, bed in low position, adequate lighting, use of vision or hearing devices, assistance with walking, providing basic and specific information [e.g., "I am on your right side," "This water is hot," "Swallow now," "Stand up"]) *to protect client from injury or enhance client's ability to interpret stimuli.*[10]
- Monitor use of heating pads or lights and ice packs, the temperature of bath water, etc., *to reduce risk of thermal injury.*
- Position doors, rugs, and furniture so they are out of travel path and ambulate with assistance or strategically place grab bars *to aid in maintaining balance and reducing risk for falls.*

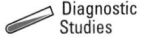

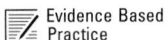

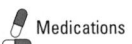

- Refer for evaluation of vocational abilities and driving skills. *Changes in sensory reception or integration may impair ability to perform complicated tasks, putting client and others at risk for injury.*
- Refer to NDs risk for Falls, risk for Thermal Injury, and risk for Trauma.

NURSING PRIORITY NO. 5 To promote optimal functioning (Teaching/Discharge Considerations):

- Provide explanations of and plan care with client, involving SO(s) as much as possible. *Enhances commitment to and continuation of plan, optimizing outcomes.*
- Review ways to prevent or limit exposure to conditions affecting sensory functions (e.g., how exposure to loud noise and toxins can impair hearing; early childhood screening for speech and language disorders; vaccines to prevent measles, mumps, and meningitis, once known to be major causes of hearing loss).[11]
- Assist client/SO(s) *to learn effective ways of coping with and managing sensory disturbances, anticipating safety needs according to client's sensory deficits and developmental level.*
- Demonstrate use and care of sensory prosthetic devices (e.g., assistive vision or hearing devices).
- Review home safety measures pertinent to deficits.
- Identify resources and community programs for acquiring and maintaining assistive devices.
- Discuss need for regular evaluation of drug regimen, noting possible toxic side effects or interactions of both prescription and OTC drugs. *Prompt recognition of side effects allows for timely intervention or change in drug regimen.*
- Promote meaningful socialization and diversional activities as able (e.g., TV/radio, conversation, large print or talking books). Refer to NDs deficient Diversional Activity and Social Isolation for related interventions.
- Refer to helping resources such as Society for the Blind, Self-Help for the Hard of Hearing, or local support groups, screening programs, etc., as indicated.
- Refer to additional NDs Anxiety, acute/chronic Confusion, and Unilateral Neglect as appropriate.

DOCUMENTATION FOCUS

Assessment/Reassessment

- Individual findings, noting specific deficit/associated symptoms, perceptions of client/SO(s).
- Safety issues.
- Assistive device needs.
- Availability and use of resources.

Planning

- Plan of care, including who is involved in planning.
- Teaching plan.

Implementation/Evaluation

- Responses to interventions, teaching, and actions performed.
- Attainment or progress toward desired outcome(s).
- Modifications to plan of care.

Discharge Planning

- Long-term needs and who is responsible for actions to be taken.
- Available resources; specific referrals made.

References

1. Cox, H. C., Hinz, M. D., Lubno, M. A., et al. (2002). ND: Sensory Perception, disturbed. *Clinical Applications of Nursing Diagnosis: Adult, Child, Women's, Psychiatric, Gerontic, and Home Health Considerations*. 4th ed. Philadelphia: F. A. Davis.
2. Engel, J. (2002). *Pocket Guide to Pediatric Assessment*. 4th ed. St. Louis, MO: Mosby.
3. Gallman, L., Elfervig, L. S. (1999). The aging sensory system. In Stanley, M., Beare, P. G. (eds). *Gerontological Nursing: A Health Promotion/Protection Approach*. 2nd ed. Philadelphia: F. A. Davis.

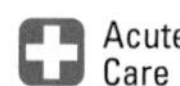
Acute Care
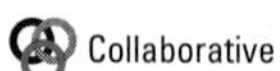
Collaborative
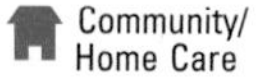
Community/ Home Care
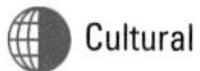
Cultural

4. D'Apolito, K., McGrath, J., O'Brien, A. (2000). Infant and family centered developmental care guidelines. *National Association of Neonatal Nurses Clinical Practice Guidelines*. 3rd ed. Des Plaines, IL: National Association of Neonatal Nurses.
5. American Diabetes Association (2003). Preventative foot care in people with diabetes. *Diabetes Care*, 26(Suppl 1), 578–579.
6. Henkin, R. I. (2000–2014). Taste and Smell Clinic research and clinical overview. Retrieved April 2015 from http://www.tasteandsmell.com/clinical.htm.
7. Leopold, D., Cairns, C. D., Holbrook, E. H. (Updated 2014). Disorders of taste and smell. Retrieved April 2015 from http://emedicine.medscape.com/article/861242-overview.
8. Whiteside, M. M., Wallhagen, M. I., Pettengill, E. (2006). Sensory impairment in older adults: Part 2: Vision loss. *Am J Nurs*, 106(11), 52–61.
9. Baldwin, K. M. (2006). Stroke: It's a knock-out punch. *Nursing Made Incredibly Easy!*, 4(2), 10–23.
10. Muche, J. A., McCarty, S. (Updated 2015). Geriatric rehabilitation. Retrieved April 2015 from http://emedicine.medscape.com/article/318521-overview.
11. National Institute on Deafness and Other Communication Disorders. (2010). Strategic plan: Plain language version FY 2003–2005. Retrieved April 2015 from http://www.nidcd.nih.gov/about/plans/strategic/pages/strategic03-05PL.aspx.
12. Urbenjaphol, P., Jitpanya, C., Khaoropthum, S. (2009). Effects of the sensory stimulation program on recovery in unconscious patients with traumatic brain injury. *J Neurosci Nurs*, 41(3), E10–E16.
13. Bagai, A., Thavendiranathan, P., Detsky, A. S. (2006). Does this patient have hearing impairment? *JAMA*, 295(4), 416–428.
14. No author listed. (2005). Understanding transcultural nursing. *Nurs*, 35(Suppl 14, 16, 18).
15. O'Lynn, C., Krautscheid, L. (2011). How should I touch you? A qualitative study of attitudes on intimate touch in nursing care. *Am J Nurs*, 111(3), 24–31.
16. Butts, J. B. (2001). Outcomes of comfort touch in institutionalized elderly female residents. *Geriatr Nurs*, 22(4), 180–184.

Sexual Dysfunction

Taxonomy II: Sexuality—Class 2 Sexual Function (00059) [**Diagnostic Division:** Sexuality], Submitted 1980; Revised 2006

DEFINITION: A state in which an individual experiences a change in sexual function during the sexual response phases of desire, excitation, and/or orgasm, which is viewed as unsatisfying, unrewarding, or inadequate.

RELATED FACTORS

Inadequate role model; absence of significant other
Absence of privacy
Misinformation or insufficient knowledge about sexual function
Vulnerability
Presence of abuse (e.g., physical, psychological, sexual); psychosocial abuse (e.g., controlling, manipulation, verbal abuse)
Alteration in body function or structure (due to pregnancy, medication, surgery, anomaly, disease, trauma, radiation, etc.)
Value conflict

DEFINING CHARACTERISTICS

Subjective

Change in sexual role
Perceived sexual limitation
Alteration in sexual activity, excitation, or satisfaction; decrease in sexual desire

(continues on page 770)

Sexual Dysfunction (continued)
Undesired change in sexual function
Seeks confirmation of desirability
Change in self-interest/interest toward others
Sample Clinical Applications: Arthritis, cancer, major surgery, heart disease, hypertension, diabetes mellitus, spinal cord injury (SCI), multiple sclerosis (MS), traumatic injury, pregnancy, childbirth, abuse, depression

DESIRED OUTCOMES/EVALUATION CRITERIA

Sample NOC linkages:
Sexual Functioning: Integration of physical, socioemotional, and intellectual aspects of sexual expression and performance
Physical Aging: Normal physical changes that occur with the natural aging process
Abuse Recovery: Sexual: Extent of healing of physical and psychological injuries due to sexual abuse or exploitation

Client Will (Include Specific Time Frame)
- Verbalize understanding of sexual anatomy, function, and alterations that may affect function.
- Verbalize understanding of individual reasons for sexual problems.
- Identify stressors in lifestyle that may contribute to the dysfunction.
- Identify satisfying, acceptable sexual practices and alternative ways of dealing with sexual expression.
- Discuss concerns about body image, sex role, desirability as a sexual partner with partner/significant other (SO).

ACTIONS/INTERVENTIONS

Sample NIC linkages:
Sexual Counseling: Use of an interactive helping process focusing on the need to make adjustments in sexual practice or to enhance coping with a sexual event/disorder
Teaching: Sexuality: Assisting individuals to understand physical and psychosocial dimensions of sexual growth and development
Values Clarification: Assisting another to clarify her/his own values in order to facilitate effective decision making

NURSING PRIORITY NO. 1 To assess causative/contributing factors:

- Perform a complete history and physical, including a sexual history, noting usual pattern of functioning and level of desire and issues of rape or abuse. *Establishes a database from which an individualized plan of care can be formulated.*[15]
- Note vocabulary and style of communication used by the individual/significant other (SO). *Maximizes communication and understanding of words and meaning in an area that individual may find difficult to discuss. Knowing that male and female brains are organized differently may help with recognizing different styles of communication.*[4]
- Have client describe problem in own words. *Sexual dysfunction is divided into four categories—sexual desire (decreased libido), arousal (erectile dysfunction [ED] or aversion or avoidance of sex), orgasm (delay, absence), and sexual pain disorders (dyspareunia, vaginismus).*[13,15] *Client's perception of the problem may differ from the care provider's, and plan of care needs to be based on client's perceptions for maximum effectiveness.*[1,9]
- Be alert to comments of client. *Sexual concerns are often disguised as humor, sarcasm, or off-hand remarks. Many people are uncomfortable talking about sexual issues but want to discuss them with care provider, so*

they use this method to bring up the subject. It is important for the caregiver to recognize and acknowledge client's concern.[2,5]

- Determine importance of sex to individual/partner and client's motivation for change. *Both individuals may have differing levels of desire and expectations that may create conflict in relationship.*[3,15]
- Assess client's/SO's knowledge of sexual anatomy, function, and effects of current situation or condition (e.g., client's concern about penis size, failure with performance). *Basic knowledge is essential for understanding the problem and how it is affecting the individual. Lack of knowledge may impact client's understanding of situation and expectation for return to previous norm or change for the future.*[3,7]
- Determine preexisting problems or conditions (e.g., illness, surgery, trauma) that may affect current situation and perception of individual/SO. *Physical conditions (e.g., arthritis, MS, hypertension, diabetes mellitus, fatigue, presence of a colostomy, urinary incontinence) can directly affect sexual functioning, or individual can believe that condition precludes sexual activity, such as recent myocardial infarction or heart surgery.*[3,6,7,13,16,18]
- Identify stress factors in individual situation (e.g., marital or job stress, role conflicts). *Interpersonal problems (marital and relationship) and lack of trust and open communication between partners can contribute to difficulties. These factors may be producing enough anxiety to cause depression or other psychological reaction(s) that would cause physiological symptoms.*[5,11]
- Observe behavior and stage of grieving when related to body changes, loss of a body part, or change in function (e.g., pregnancy, obesity, amputation, mastectomy, hysterectomy, menopause). *A change in body image can affect how individual views body in many aspects, but particularly in the sensitive area of sexual functioning and indicates need for information and additional support.*[7,18]
- Discuss cultural values or religious beliefs and conflicts present. *Client may feel guilt or shame about sexual desires or difficulties because of family beliefs about sex and genital area of the body and how sexuality was communicated to the client as he or she was growing up or through religious teachings. Note: Research indicates that measurement of acculturation may reveal information about an individual's unique behavioral pattern that is not evident when focusing solely on ethnic group comparisons.*[1,2,17]
- Explore with client the meaning of client's behavior. *Masturbation, for instance, may have many meanings or purposes, such as for relief of anxiety, sexual deprivation, pleasure, a nonverbal expression of need to talk, and a way of alienating.*[3] *Or, client's inhibitions may be diminished by changes in cognition.*[12]
- Review medication regimen and drug use (prescription, over the counter, illegal, alcohol) and cigarette use. *Antihypertensives may cause ED; monoamine oxidase inhibitors and tricyclics can cause erection or ejaculation problems and anorgasmia in women; selective serotonin reuptake inhibitor antidepressants can cause decreased libido or orgasm disorders; antihistamines may cause temporary vaginal dryness (dyspareunia); narcotics and alcohol produce ED and inhibit orgasm; and smoking creates vasoconstriction and may be a factor in ED. Evaluation of drug and individual response is important to determine accurate intervention.*[1,10,13,15]
- Review lab results (e.g., hormone levels, serum glucose, red blood cell count, drug levels). *Testing may reveal undiagnosed conditions, such as diabetes resulting in ED in men or anemia, affecting arousal. Inappropriate drug levels or hormone deficiencies—decreased estrogen in women and decreased testosterone in men and women—may result in decreased libido; and hypothyroidism may impair sexual arousal.*[15]
- Assist with or review diagnostic studies to determine cause of ED. *More than half of the cases have a physical cause such as diabetes, vascular problems, etc.* Monitor penile tumescence during rapid eye movement sleep *to determine physical ability. Men are embarrassed to bring up the subject with their healthcare provider even when they are seeing him or her for other conditions; unless the provider specifically asks, the subject is not addressed.*[6,8,9,13]
- Assist with or review diagnostic studies for female sexual disorders (e.g., vaginal photoplethysmography *to assess vaginal blood flow and engorgement,* vaginal pH *to identify infection or diminished secretions,* and biothesiometer *to test sensitivity of clitoris and labia*).[16]

NURSING PRIORITY NO. 2 To assist client/SO(s) to deal with individual situation:

- Establish therapeutic nurse-client relationship. *Promotes treatment and facilitates sharing of sensitive information and feelings in a safe environment.*[1]
- Avoid making value judgments. *They do not help the client to cope with the situation. Nurse needs to be aware of and be in control of own feelings and response to client expressions and/or concerns. Client needs to be free to express concerns in whatever way is comfortable to individual.*[3] *Even clients with limited cognition have a right to engage in intimate behaviors.*[12]
- Assist with treatment of underlying medical conditions, including changes in medication regimen, weight management, cessation of smoking, etc. *Many conditions (e.g., cardiovascular, diabetes, arthritis) can affect sexual functioning, and medication side effects may affect sexual ability.*[7,13–15]
- Collaborate with physical therapist to identify mechanical aides that may be useful for clients with physical conditions/disabilities.[15]
- Provide factual information about individual condition (e.g., premature ejaculation, female problems of dyspareunia; low sexual desire). *Accurate information helps client make informed decisions about own situation.*[2,8,15]
- Determine what client wants to know to tailor information to client needs. *Providing too much information may be overwhelming and result in client not remembering something that is essential. Information affecting client safety and consequences of actions may need to be reviewed or reinforced.*[1,7,9]
- Encourage and accept expressions of concern, anger, grief, and fear. *Individuals need to be free to express these feelings and be accepted so they can begin to deal with situation and move on in a positive way.*[6,13]
- Assist client to be aware and deal with stages of grieving for loss or change. *Sexual dysfunction is often a result of losses such as breast cancer treatment or prostate surgery and need to be addressed in the context of the whole. Healthcare providers need to be willing to help client understand grieving issues.*[2,7,11]
- Encourage client to share thoughts and concerns with partner and to clarify values or impact of condition on relationship. *Helps to identify issues in the relationship that may be related to the sexual dysfunction.*[3,11,15]
- Provide for or identify ways to obtain privacy to allow for sexual expression for individual or between partners without embarrassment or objections of others. *Often caregivers do not think about the importance of providing this basic need for couples, but in any setting, privacy may be difficult to provide unless it is thought about and planned for.*[6,12]
- Discuss client's rights regarding intimacy in residential or extended care settings with SO/family. Review appropriateness of home visits or provision for privacy for intimate contact. *Family members may not realize that the need for sexual expression is not limited by advancing age, declining cognition, or marital status, and they may be unaware that client has a right to engage in appropriate intimate behaviors.*[12]
- Assist client/SO(s) to problem solve alternative ways of sexual expression. *When an illness or condition, such as arthritis or paraplegia, interfere with a couple's usual sexual activities, the couple needs to learn new ways to achieve satisfaction.*[3]
- Discuss use of medications such as papaverine, sildenafil (Viagra), or vardenafil (Levitra) *for ED,* or lubricating gels, hormone creams, or possibly hormonal replacement therapy *for vaginal dryness and dyspareunia* as appropriate.[15,16]
- Provide information about availability of corrective measures such as reconstructive surgery (e.g., penile or breast implants), Eros Therapy (handheld device used to improve blood flow to clitoris and external labia to increase sensitivity of tissues), or behavioral therapies (e.g., self-stimulation, sensate focus exercises, Masters & Johnson treatment strategies), when indicated. *Sexual problems, such as ED, female orgasmic disorders, and female sexual arousal disorders, may respond to these interventions, providing more satisfactory sexual life.*[8,10,14–16]
- Refer to appropriate resources as need indicates (e.g., healthcare coworker with greater comfort level and/or knowledgeable clinical nurse specialist or professional sex therapist, family counseling). *Not all professionals are knowledgeable or comfortable dealing with sexual issues, and referrals to more appropriate resources can provide client/couple with accurate assistance.*[2,6,12]

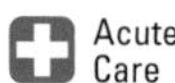

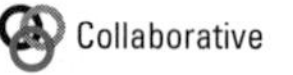

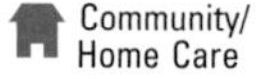

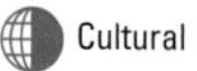

NURSING PRIORITY NO. 3 To promote sexual wellness (Teaching/Discharge Considerations):

- Provide sex education and explanation of normal sexual functioning when necessary. *Many individuals are not knowledgeable about these areas, and often providing accurate information can help assuage anxiety about unknowns, such as normal changes of aging, or provide an accurate basis for understanding problems being experienced.*[6,15,16]
- Provide written material appropriate to individual needs. Include bibliotherapy and reliable Internet resources related to client's concerns. *Provides reinforcement for client to read and access at his or her leisure when ready to deal with sensitive materials.*[3,6,7]
- Encourage ongoing dialogue and take advantage of teachable moments that occur. *Within a therapeutic relationship, comfort is achieved and individual is encouraged to ask questions and be receptive to continuing conversation about sexual issues.*[1,2]
- Demonstrate and assist client to learn relaxation or visualization techniques. *Stress is often a component of sexual dysfunction, and using these skills can help with resolution of problems.*[2,5]
- Identify resources for assistive devices/sexual "aids." *These aids can enhance sex life of couple and prevent or help with problems of dysfunction.*[3,6]
- Emphasize importance of engaging in regular self-examination as indicated (e.g., breast and testicular examinations). *Encourages client to participate in own health prevention activities, become more aware of potential problems, and become more comfortable with sexual self.*[3,5]
- Identify community resources for further assistance, such as Reach for Recovery, CanSurmount, and the Ostomy Association, *to provide role models and to problem solve issues.*
- Refer for further professional assistance concerning relationship difficulties, low sexual desire, and other sexual concerns such as premature ejaculation, vaginismus, and painful intercourse. *May need additional or continuing support to deal with individual situation or associated depression.*[3,15] *Note: Referral to counselor expert in trauma may be preferred to assist sexual abuse survivors to overcome sexual difficulties.*[15]

DOCUMENTATION FOCUS

Assessment/Reassessment

- Individual findings, including nature of dysfunction, predisposing factors, perceived effect on sexuality and relationships.
- Cultural or religious factors, conflicts.
- Response of SO(s).
- Motivation for change.

Planning

- Plan of care and who is involved in planning.
- Teaching plan.

Implementation/Evaluation

- Response to interventions, teaching, and actions performed.
- Attainment or progress toward desired outcome(s).
- Modifications to plan of care.

Discharge Planning

- Long-term needs and who is responsible for actions to be taken.
- Community resources, specific referrals made.

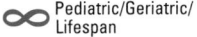

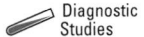

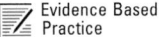

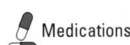

References

1. Townsend, M. C. (2003). *Psychiatric Mental Health Nursing Concepts of Care*. 4th ed. Philadelphia: F. A. Davis.
2. Doenges, M. E., Townsend, M. C., Moorhouse, M. F. (1998). *Psychiatric Care Plans: Guidelines for Individualizing Care*. 3rd ed. Philadelphia: F. A. Davis.
3. Hyde, J., DeLamater, J. (2002). *Understanding Human Sexuality*. 7th ed. New York: McGraw-Hill.
4. Moir, A., Jessel, D. (1991). *Brain Sex: The Real Difference Between Men & Women*. New York: Dell.
5. Boston Women's Health Book Collective. (1998). *Our Bodies, Ourselves for the New Century*. 7th ed. Gloucester, MA: Peter Smith.
6. Harvard Medical School. (2010). *Sexuality in Midlife and Beyond: A Harvard Medical School Special Report*. Cambridge, MA: Harvard Health.
7. Stanley, M., Beare, P. G. (1999). *Gerontological Nursing*. 2nd ed. Philadelphia: F. A. Davis.
8. Carver, C. (1998). Premature ejaculation: A common and treatable concern. *J Am Psy Nurs Assoc*, 4(6), 199–204.
9. McEnany, G. (1998). Sexual dysfunction in the pharmacologic treatment of depression: When "don't ask, don't tell" is an unsuitable approach to care. *J Am Psy Nurs Assoc*, 4(1), 24–29.
10. Phillips, N. A. (2000). Female sexual dysfunction: Evaluation and treatment. *Am Family Phys*, 62(1), 127–136.
11. Phillips, R. L., Slaughter, R. (2000). Depression and sexual desire. *Am Family Phys*, 62(4), 782–786.
12. Sisk, J. (2009). Sexuality in nursing homes: Preserving rights, promoting well-being. Retrieved November 2015 from http://www.todaysgeriatricmedicine.com/news/septstory3.shtml.
13. Dworkin-McDaniel, N. (2013). Beyond Viagra: The hidden roots and risks of erectile dysfunction. Retrieved November 2015 from http://www.lifescript.com/health/centers/cholesterol/articles/.
14. The Turek Clinic Staff. (Updated 2014). Male sexual health issues and treatment. Retrieved November 2015 from http://theturekclinic.com/services/male-mens-sexual-health/.
15. Ballas, P. (reviewer) (2006). Sexual problems overview. Retrieved November 2015 from http://health.nytimes.com/health/guides/specialtopic/sexual-problems-overview/overview.html.
16. Stoppler, M. C. (2015). Female sexual problems. Retrieved November 2015 from http://www.emedicinehealth.com/female_sexual_problems/article_em.htm.
17. Brotto, L., Chik, H. M., Ryder, A. G. (2004). Acculturation and sexual function in Asian women. *Arch Sex Behav*, 34(6), 613–626.
18. Boyles, S. (2012). AHA: Sex safe for most heart patients. Retrieved November 2015 from http://www.webmd.com/heart-disease/news/20120119/aha-sex-safe-most-heart-patients.

ineffective Sexuality Pattern

Taxonomy II: Sexuality—Class 2 Sexual Function (00065) [**Diagnostic Division:** Sexuality], Submitted 1986; Revised 2006

DEFINITION: Expressions of concern regarding own sexuality.

RELATED FACTORS

Insufficient knowledge or skill deficit about alternatives related to sexuality
Absence of privacy
Impaired relationship with a significant other; absence of SO
Inadequate role model
Conflict about sexual orientation or variant preference
Fear of pregnancy or sexually transmitted infection

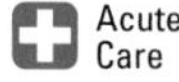

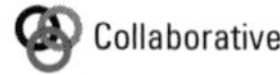

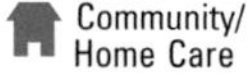

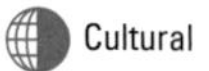

DEFINING CHARACTERISTICS

Subjective

Alteration in relationship with SO

Alteration in/difficulty with sexual activity or behavior

Value conflict

Sample Clinical Applications: Spinal cord injury (SCI), brain injury, stroke, sexually transmitted infection (STI), cancer, mastectomy, hysterectomy, menopause, prostatectomy, gender reassignment

DESIRED OUTCOMES/EVALUATION CRITERIA

Sample NOC linkages:

Sexual Identity: Acknowledgment and acceptance of own sexual identity

Child Development: Adolescence: Milestones of physical, cognitive, and psychosocial progression from 12 years through 17 years of age

Role Performance: Congruence of an individual's role behavior with role expectations

Client Will (Include Specific Time Frame)

- Verbalize understanding of sexual anatomy and function.
- Verbalize knowledge and understanding of sexual limitations, difficulties, or changes that have occurred.
- Verbalize acceptance of self in current (altered) condition.
- Demonstrate improved communication and relationship skills.
- Identify individually appropriate method of contraception.

ACTIONS/INTERVENTIONS

Sample NIC linkages:

Sexual Counseling: Use of an interactive helping process focusing on the need to make adjustments to sexual practice or to enhance coping with a sexual event/disorder

Teaching: Sexuality: Assisting individuals to understand physical and psychosocial dimensions of sexual growth and development

Teaching: Safe Sex: Providing instruction concerning sexual protection during sexual activity

Support System Enhancement: Facilitation of support to patient by family, friends, and community

NURSING PRIORITY NO. 1 To assess causative/contributing factors:

- Obtain complete physical and sexual history, as indicated, including perception of normal function. *Sexuality is multifaceted beginning with one's body, biological sex, and gender (biological, social, and legal status as girl/boy, woman/man).*
- Note use of vocabulary (assessing basic knowledge) and comments or concerns about sexual identity. *Components of sexual identity include one's gender identity (how one feels about his or her gender) as well as one's sexual orientation (straight, lesbian, gay, bisexual, transgendered).*[12]
- Determine importance of sex and a description of the problem in the client's own words. Be alert to comments of client/significant other (SO) (e.g., discount of overt or covert sexual expressions such as "He's just a dirty old man"). *Sexual concerns are often disguised as sarcasm, humor, or off-hand remarks.*[1,2] *Information about client's perception of the problem is essential to planning appropriate care to meet client's needs.*
- Note cultural values or religious beliefs and conflicts that may exist. Elicit impact of perceived problem on SO/family. *Individuals are enculturated as they grow up, and depending on particular family views and taboos, these factors may create conflicts regarding variant sexual practices with resultant feelings of shame and guilt.*[8,14–16]

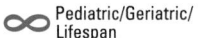

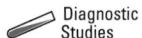

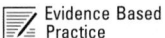

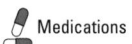

- Assess stress factors in client's environment that might cause anxiety or psychological reactions. *Sexual variant behaviors, power issues involving SO, adult children, aging, employment, and loss of prowess related to illness or condition are often associated with stress in the client's life.*[1,11]
- Explore knowledge of effects of altered body function or limitations precipitated by illness or medical treatment of alternative sexual responses and expressions (e.g., reassignment procedure). *Client needs to understand when conditions, such as undescended testicle in young male, gender change, and mutilating cancer surgery, have an effect on sexuality.*[10]
- Review medication and substance use history (prescription medication, over-the-counter drugs, alcohol, illicit drugs). *Substance or prescription drug use may affect sexual functioning or be used to relieve anxiety of perceived sexually deviant behavior.*[2,17]
- Explore issues and fears associated with sex. *Possibility of pregnancy, acquiring STIs, trust and control issues, inflexible beliefs, preference confusion, and altered performance need to be addressed so they may be understood and resolved.*[3,13]
- Determine client's interpretation of the altered sexual activity or behavior. *May be a way of controlling partner, provide relief of anxiety or pleasure, or reflect a lack of partner. These behaviors, when related to body changes, including pregnancy, weight loss or gain, or loss of body part, may reflect a stage of grieving.*[3,16]
- Assess life-cycle issues, such as adolescence, young adulthood, menopause, and aging. *All people are sexual beings from birth to death. Stage of maturation/transition brings changes that affect sexual self and understanding of the normalcy can help individual grow with them.*[7,16]

NURSING PRIORITY NO. 2 To assist client/SO to deal with individual situation:

- Provide atmosphere in which discussion of sexual problems is permitted and encouraged. *Sense of trust and comfort enhances ability to discuss sensitive matters and begin to resolve issues.*[5]
- Avoid value judgments. *They do not help the client to cope with the situation. Nurse needs to be aware of and in control of own feelings and responses to the client's expressions and/or concerns.*[9]
- Provide information about individual situation, determining client needs and desires. *Lack of knowledge may contribute to current situation, and providing desired information conveys message of importance and self-responsibility.*[3]
- Encourage discussion of individual situation and open expression of feelings without judgment. *Sexuality includes feelings, attitudes, relationships, self-image, ideals, and behaviors, and influences how one experiences the world.*[12] *Talking about sexual practices, concerns about sexual identity, or sexual issues related to illness or condition provides opportunity for resolution.*[1,2]
- Provide specific suggestions about interventions directed toward the identified problems. *Being specific about actions client can take, such as alternate sexual positions when arthritis prevents movement, masturbation when no partner is available, use of condoms when infection is a concern, and positive discussion of normalcy of sexual behavior when identity is being questioned, can lead discussion in appropriate direction to begin to look for options or solutions.*[3,5]
- Identify alternative forms of sexual expression that might be acceptable to both partners. *Being able to communicate satisfactorily with partner and identifying ways to achieve sexual satisfaction for both is important to the relationship.*[1,2]
- Discuss ways to manage individual devices or appliances. *Change in body image or medical condition may require the use of devices, such as an ostomy bag, breast prostheses, or a urinary collection device, that may affect how client views sexual activity. Providing information about ways to deal with these issues helps client to refocus attention on achieving satisfactory sexual experience.*[6,7]
- Discuss use of performance-enhancing medications, such as sildenafil (Viagra), vardenafil (Levitra), and tadalafil (Cialis). *Erectile dysfunction is a common occurrence as men age, and while frequently caused by an underlying physical condition or prescribed medication, psychological issues often accompany this problem. While an accurate diagnosis is necessary, there are many treatments available.*[2,3,17] *Prescription drugs are popular, but the individual needs to feel desire and be sexually stimulated for them to work.*[6]

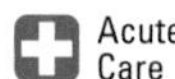

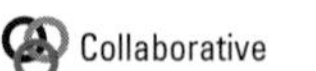

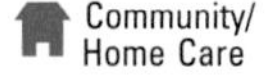

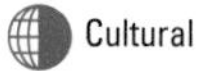

- Determine concerns of older client regarding sexuality. *Myths abound regarding sexual activity as people grow older, and individual may believe he or she is no longer attractive or a satisfying sex life is no longer possible; accurate information can correct misperceptions.*[6,7]
- Provide anticipatory guidance about losses that are to be expected. *Surgical procedures resulting in a major change in body image, whether planned (as in transsexual surgery) or unplanned (as in emergency bowel resection with resultant colostomy or traumatic amputation), result in a loss of known self, which needs specific intervention to integrate change.*[3,9]
- Introduce client to individuals who have successfully managed a similar problem, when possible. *Provides a positive role model and support for problem solving.*[9,18]

NURSING PRIORITY NO. 3 To promote wellness (Teaching/Discharge Considerations):

- Provide factual information about problem(s) as identified by the client. *Specific facts about individual situation will provide client with knowledge needed to deal with what is happening, such as conflict with sexual orientation or variant preferences or impaired relationship with SO.*[9]
- Engage in ongoing dialogue with the client and SO(s) as situation permits. *As communication continues, new insights arise and understanding is enhanced.*[2,4]
- Discuss methods, effectiveness, and side effects of contraceptives if indicated. *Assists individual/couple to make an informed decision on a method that meets own values or religious beliefs and allows client to meet needs and desires to plan for and/or prevent pregnancy.*[1,5]
- Refer to community resources as indicated. *May need additional information and support that can be obtained at resources such as planned parenthood, gender identity clinic, social services, etc.*[9,14,18]
- Refer for intensive individual/group psychotherapy, which may be combined with couple/family and/or sex therapy, as appropriate.[18]
- Refer to NDs disturbed Body Image, Self-Esteem (specify), and Sexual Dysfunction.

DOCUMENTATION FOCUS

Assessment/Reassessment

- Individual findings, including nature of concern, perceived difficulties, limitations or changes; specific needs or desires.
- Cultural or religious beliefs, conflicts.
- Response of SO(s).

Planning

- Plan of care and who is involved in the planning.
- Teaching plan.

Implementation/Evaluation

- Response to interventions, teaching, and actions performed.
- Attainment or progress toward desired outcome(s).
- Modifications to plan of care.

Discharge Planning

- Long-term needs and teaching, and who is responsible for actions to be taken.
- Community resources, specific referrals made.

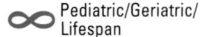

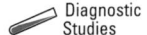

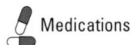

References

1. Townsend, M. C. (2003). *Psychiatric Mental Health Nursing Concepts of Care*. 4th ed. Philadelphia: F. A. Davis.
2. Doenges, M. E., Townsend, M. C., Moorhouse, M. F. (1998). *Psychiatric Care Plans: Guidelines for Individualizing Care*. 3rd ed. Philadelphia: F. A. Davis.
3. Hyde, J., DeLamater, J. (2002). *Understanding Human Sexuality*. 7th ed. New York: McGraw-Hill.
4. Moir, A., Jessel, D. (1991). *Brain Sex: The Real Difference Between Men & Women*. New York: Dell.
5. Mulherin, K. (2009). Sexual dysfunction: Reducing the anxiety. Retrieved November 2015 from http://www.alleviatingstress-anxiety.com/blog/sexual-dysfunction-reducing-the-anxiety/.
6. Harvard Medical School. (2003). *Sexuality in Midlife and Beyond: A Special Health Report from Harvard Medical School*. Cambridge, MA: Harvard Health.
7. Stanley, M., Beare, P. G. (1999). *Gerontological Nursing*. 2nd ed. Philadelphia: F. A. Davis.
8. Johnson, R. (2003). Homosexuality: Nature or nurture. *AllPsych J*. Retrieved June 2012 from http://allpsych.com/journal/homosexuality.html.
9. Becker, J. V., Johnson, B. R. (2004). Sexual and gender identity disorders. In Hales, R. E., Yudofsky, S. C. (eds). *Essentials of Clinical Psychiatry*. 2nd ed. Washington, DC: American Psychiatric Press.
10. Ramirez, M., McMullen, C., Grant, M., et al. (2009). Figuring out sex in a reconfigured body: Experiences of female colorectal cancer survivors with ostomies. *Women's Health*, 49(8), 608–624.
11. Meyer, I. H. (2003). Prejudice, social stress, and mental health in lesbian, gay, and bisexual populations: Conceptual issues and research evidenced. *Psychol Bull*, 129(5), 674–697.
12. Planned Parenthood. (2012). Sex & sexuality. Retrieved November 2015 from http://www.plannedparenthood.org/learn/sexuality.
13. Montgomery, K. A. (2008). Sexual desire disorders. *Psychiatry (Edgmont)*, 5(6), 674–697.
14. Bazemore, P. H., Wilson, W. H., Bigelow, D. A. (2011). Homosexuality. Retrieved April 2012 from http://www.socialvibes.net/socialvi/2012/05/09/homosexualitymedscape/.
15. American Psychological Association. (2009). Resolution on appropriate affirmative responses to sexual orientation distress and change efforts. Retrieved November 2015 from http://www.apa.org/about/governance/council/policy/sexual-orientation.aspx.
16. Johnson, K. (1997). Human sexual motivation. Retrieved November 2015 from http://www.csun.edu/~vcpsy00h/students/sexmotiv.htm.
17. DeBlasio, C. J., Malcolm, J. B., Derweesh, I. H. (2009). Patterns of sexual and erectile dysfunction and response to treatment in patients receiving androgen deprivation therapy in prostate cancer. *BJU Int*, 102(1), 39–42.
18. WebMD staff. (2014). When you don't feel at home with your gender. Retrieved November 2015 from http://www.webmd.com/mental-health/gender-dysphoria.

risk for Shock

Taxonomy II: Safety/Protection—Class 2 Physical Injury (00205) [**Diagnostic Division:** Circulation], Submitted 2008; Revised 2013

DEFINITION: Vulnerable to an inadequate blood flow to the body's tissues that may lead to life-threatening cellular dysfunction, which may compromise health.

RISK FACTORS

Hypotension
Hypovolemia
Hypoxemia, hypoxia
Infection, sepsis; systemic inflammatory response syndrome (SIRS)
Note: A risk diagnosis is not evidenced by signs and symptoms, as the problem has not occurred; rather, nursing interventions are directed at prevention.

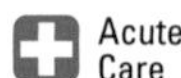

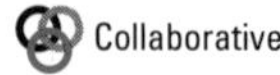

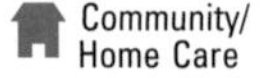

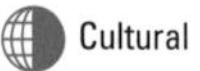

Sample Clinical Applications: Gastrointestinal (GI) bleed, multiple trauma, disseminated intravascular coagulation (DIC); myocardial infarction, cardiomyopathy, malignant hypertension; pulmonary embolus, pneumothorax; spinal cord injury (SCI), anaphylaxis, sepsis

DESIRED OUTCOMES/EVALUATION CRITERIA

Sample NOC linkages:
Circulation Status: Unobstructed, unidirectional blood flow at appropriate pressure through large vessels of the systemic and pulmonary circuits
Blood Loss Severity: Severity of internal or external bleeding/hemorrhage
Infection Severity: Severity of infection and associated symptoms

Client Will (Include Specific Time Frame)

- Display hemodynamic stability as evidenced by vital signs within normal range for client and prompt capillary refill, adequate urinary output with normal specific gravity, and usual level of mentation.
- Verbalize understanding of disease process, risk factors, and treatment plan.
- Be afebrile and free of other signs of infection; achieve timely wound healing.

ACTIONS/INTERVENTIONS

Sample NIC linkages:
Hypovolemia Management: Expansion of intravascular fluid volume in a patient who is volume depleted
Cardiac Care: Limitation of complications resulting from an imbalance between myocardial oxygen supply and demand for a patient with symptoms of impaired cardiac function
Shock Management: Facilitation of the delivery of oxygen and nutrients to systemic tissue with removal of cellular waste products in a patient with severely altered tissue perfusion

NURSING PRIORITY NO. 1 To assess causative/precipitating factors:

- Note possible medical diagnoses or disease processes that can result in one or more types of shock such as major trauma with heavy internal or external bleeding; heart failure; head or spinal cord injury; allergic reactions to insect stings, medications, or foods; pregnancy-related complications; and intra-abdominal infections, ruptured appendix, open wounds, or other conditions associated with sepsis.[1]
- Assess for history or presence of conditions leading to **hypovolemic shock**, such as trauma, surgery, inadequate clotting, and anticoagulant therapy; GI or other organ hemorrhage; prolonged vomiting and diarrhea; diabetes insipidus; and misuse of diuretics. *These conditions deplete the body's circulating blood volume and ability to maintain organ perfusion and function.*[1–3]
- Assess for conditions associated with **cardiogenic shock**, including myocardial infarction, cardiac arrest, lethal ventricular dysrhythmias, severe valvular dysfunction, cardiomyopathies, and malignant hypertension. *These conditions directly impair the heart muscle and its ability to pump.*[1–4,11]
- Assess for conditions associated with **obstructive shock**, including pulmonary embolus, aortic stenosis, cardiac tamponade, and tension pneumothorax. *In these conditions the heart itself may be healthy but cannot pump because of conditions outside the heart that prevent normal filling or adequate outflow.*[1–3]
- Assess for conditions associated with **distributive shock—neural induced**, including pain, anesthesia, and SCI or head injury, or **chemical induced**, including peritonitis, sepsis, burns, anaphylaxis, and hyperglycemia. *These situations result in loss of sympathetic tone, blood vessel dilation, pooling of venous blood, and increased capillary permeability with shifting of fluids.*[2,4]
- Monitor for persistent or heavy fluid loss, including wounds, drains, vomiting, gastrointestinal tube, and chest tube. Check all secretions and excretions for occult blood. Refer to NDs risk for Bleeding and risk for imbalanced Fluid Volume for additional interventions.

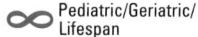

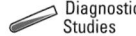

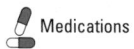

- Inspect skin, noting presence of traumatic or surgical wounds, erythema, edema, tenderness, petechiae, and rashes or hives, *for evidence of hemorrhage, localized infections, or hypersensitivity reaction.*[5,7]
- Investigate reports of increased or sudden pain in wounds or body parts, *which could indicate ischemia or infection.*
- Be aware of invasive devices such as urinary and intravascular catheters, endotracheal tube, and implanted prosthetic devices *that potentiate risk for localized and systemic infections.*
- Assess vital signs and tissue and organ perfusion *for changes associated with shock states:*[1–11]
  Heart rate and rhythm—noting progressive changes in heart rate *(reflecting an attempt to increase cardiac output)* and development of dysrhythmias *suggesting electrolyte imbalances and hypoxia.*
  Respirations—noting rapid, shallow breathing, and use of accessory muscles *(in an attempt to increase vital capacity and compensate for metabolic acidosis associated with poor tissue perfusion and anaerobic metabolism)*, which can progress to respiratory failure.
  Blood pressure—noting hypotension (systolic blood pressure 90 mm Hg [or lower] lasting more than 30 min), postural hypotension, and narrowed pulse pressure. *May indicate hypovolemia and/or failure of cardiac pumping or compensatory mechanisms.*
  Pulses and neck veins—noting rapid, weak, thready peripheral pulses and congested or flat neck veins. *Signs associated with changes in circulating volume, cardiac output, and progressive changes in vascular tone and/or capillary permeability.*
  Temperature—higher than 100.4°F (38°C) or lower than 96.8°F (36°C). *Temperature changes in presence of elevated heart rate and respiratory rate along with mildly elevated white blood cells (WBCs) suggest SIRS, which can manifest in client without a documented infection, requiring prompt intervention to prevent progression to sepsis and septic shock.*[5,6]
  State of consciousness and mentation—noting anxiety, restlessness, confusion, lethargy, or unresponsiveness. *Can occur because of changes in oxygenation, acid-base imbalances, and toxins associated with hypoperfusion. Depressed mentation accompanied by neck stiffness may reflect central nervous system infection.*
  Skin color and moisture—noting overall flushing or pallor, bluish lips and fingernails and slow capillary refill, or cool or clammy skin. *Changes are associated with altered systemic circulation and hypoperfusion.*
  Urine output—noting substantially decreased output. *One of the most sensitive indicators of change in circulating volume or poor perfusion.*
  Urine characteristics—noting color and odor *suggestive of infection source.*
  Bowel sounds—noting diminished or absent bowel sounds or other changes in GI function, such as vomiting, or change in color, amount, or frequency of stools, *reflecting hypoperfusion of GI tract.*
- Measure invasive hemodynamic parameters when available—central venous pressure, mean arterial pressure, and cardiac ouput—*to determine if intravascular fluid deficit or cardiac dysfunction exists.*
- Obtain specimens of wounds, drains, central lines, and blood for culture and sensitivity *to identify offending organisms and to direct antimicrobial therapies.*[8]
- Review lab data such as complete blood count with WBCs and differential; platelet numbers and function; other coagulation factors; tests for cardiac, renal, and hepatic function; pulse oximetry or arterial blood gases, serum lactate, and blood cultures; and urinalysis and urine cultures *to identify potential sources of shock and degree of organ involvement.*
- Review diagnostic studies such as x-ray and electrocardiogram, echocardiogram and angiography with ejection fraction, and computed tomography or magnetic resonance imaging scans and ultrasound *to determine presence of injuries or disorders that could cause or lead to shock conditions.*
- Refer to NDs ineffective peripheral Tissue Perfusion, risk for decreased cardiac Tissue Perfusion, risk for ineffective cerebral Tissue Perfusion, risk for ineffective Gastrointestinal Perfusion, and risk for ineffective Renal Perfusion as indicated.

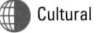

NURSING PRIORITY NO. 2 To prevent/correct potential causes of shock:

- Collaborate in prompt treatment of underlying conditions, such as trauma, heart failure, and infections, and prepare for/assist with medical and surgical interventions *to maximize systemic circulation and tissue and organ perfusion.*
- Administer oxygen by appropriate route (e.g., nasal prongs, mask, ventilator) *to maximize oxygenation of tissues.*
- Administer fluids, electrolytes, colloids, and blood or blood products, as indicated, *to rapidly restore or sustain circulating volume and electrolyte balance and prevent shock states associated with dehydration and hypovolemia.*[3,9]
- Administer medications as indicated (e.g., vasoactive drugs, cardiac glycosides, thrombolytics, anticoagulants, antimicrobials, analgesics) *to treat conditions and maximize organ function.*[4]
- Provide client care with infection-prevention interventions, such as diligent hand hygiene, aseptic wound care or dressing changes, isolation precautions, and early intervention in potential infectious condition *to reduce incidence or progression of infection.*[6,7]
- Provide nutrition by best means—oral, enteral, or parenteral feeding. Refer to nutritionist or dietitian *to provide foods rich in nutrients, vitamins, and minerals needed to promote healing and support immune system health.*

NURSING PRIORITY NO. 3 Promote wellness (Teaching/Discharge Considerations):[1,2,7,9]

- Instruct client/significant other in ways to prevent and/or manage underlying conditions that cause shock, including heart disease, injuries, dehydration, and infection.
- Identify reportable signs and symptoms, including unrelieved pain anywhere in body, unresolved bleeding, excessive fluid loss, persistent fever and chills, and change in skin color accompanied by chest pain, *for timely evaluation and intervention.*
- Emphasize need for recognition of substances that cause hypersensitivity or allergic reactions (e.g., insects, medicines, foods, latex) *to reduce risk of anaphylactic shock state.*
- Teach client purpose, dosage, schedule, precautions, and potential side effects of medications given to treat underlying conditions. *Enhances compliance with drug regimen, reducing individual risk.*
- Instruct in wound and skin care as indicated *to prevent infection and promote healing without complications.*
- Teach client/caregivers importance of good hand hygiene, clean environment, and avoiding crowds when ill, especially if client is immunocompromised.
- Reinforce importance of immunization against infections such as influenza and pneumonia, especially in client with chronic conditions.
- Encourage consumption of healthy diet, participation in regular exercise, and adequate rest *for healing and immune system support.*
- Recommend client at risk for hypersensitivity reactions wear medical alert device and maintain readily accessible emergency medication (e.g., Benadryl and/or Epi-pen).

DOCUMENTATION FOCUS

Assessment/Reassessment

- Individual risk factors such as blood loss, presence of infection.
- Assessment findings, including respiratory rate, character of breath sounds; heart rate and rhythm; temperature; frequency, amount, and appearance of secretions; presence of cyanosis; and mentation level.
- Results of laboratory tests and diagnostic studies.

Planning

- Plan of care, specific interventions, and who is involved in the planning.
- Teaching plan.

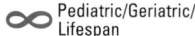

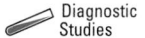

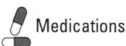

Implementation/Evaluation

- Client's responses to treatment, teaching, and actions performed.
- Attainment or progress toward desired outcome(s).
- Modifications to plan of care.

Discharge Planning

- Long-term needs, identifying who is responsible for actions to be taken.
- Community resources for equipment and supplies postdischarge.
- Specific referrals made.

References

1. Cunha, J. P. (Reviewed 2015). Medical shock. Retrieved April 2015 from http://www.medicinenet.com/shock/article.htm.
2. Workman, M. L. (2006). Interventions for clients with shock. In Inatavicius, D. D., Workman, M. L. (eds). *Medical-Surgical Nursing: Critical Thinking for Collaborative Care*. 5th ed. St. Louis, MO: Elsevier Saunders.
3. Spaniol, J. R., Knight, A. R., Zebley, J. L., et al. (2007). Fluid resuscitation therapy for hemorrhagic shock. *J Trauma Nurs*, 14(13), 152–160.
4. Gorman, D., Calhoun, K., Carassco, M., et al. (2008). Take a rapid treatment approach to cardiogenic shock. *Nurs Crit Care*, 3(4), 18–27.
5. Kalil, A., Bailey, L. L. (Updated 2014). Septic shock. Retrieved April 2015 from http://emedicine.medscape.com/article/168402-overview.
6. Nelson, D. P., LeMaster, T. H., Plost, G. N., et al. (2009). Recognizing sepsis in the adult patient. *Am J Nurs*, 109(3), 40–50.
7. Sommers, M. S., Johnson, S. A., Beery, T. A. (2007). *Diseases and Disorders: A Nursing Therapeutics Manual*. 3rd ed. Philadelphia: F. A. Davis.
8. Dellinger, R. P., Levy, M. M., Carlet, J. M., et al. (2008). Surviving sepsis campaign: Guidelines for management for severe sepsis and septic shock: 2008. *Crit Care Med*, 36(1), 296–327.
9. Maier, R. V. (2005). Approach to the patient with shock. In Kasper, D. L., Harrison, T. R. (eds). *Harrison's Principles of Internal Medicine*. 16th ed. New York: McGraw-Hill.
10. Adams, S. (2003). Shock, systemic inflammatory response and multiple organ dysfunction. In Brooker, C., Nicol, M. (eds). *Nursing Adults: The Practice of Caring*. Edinburgh: Mosby.
11. Ren, X. (Mike), Lenneman, A., Ooi, H. H. (Updated 2014). Cardiogenic shock. Retrieved December 2014 from http://emedicine.medscape.com/article/152191-overview.

impaired Sitting

Taxonomy II: Safety/Protection—Class 2 Activity/Exercise (000237) [**Diagnostic Division:** Safety], Submitted 2013

DEFINITION: Limitation of ability to independently and purposefully attain and/or maintain a rest position that is supported by the buttocks and thighs in which the torso is upright.

RELATED FACTORS

Alteration in cognitive functioning; psychological disorder
Impaired metabolic functioning; malnutrition; sarcopenia
Insufficient endurance
Neurological disorder
Orthopedic surgery
Pain
Prescribed posture; self-imposed relief posture

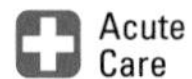

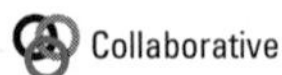

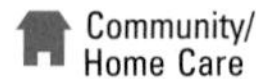

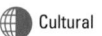

DEFINING CHARACTERISTICS

Objective

Impaired ability to attain or maintain a balanced position of the torso; impaired ability to stress torso with body weight
Impaired ability to adjust position of one or both lower limbs on uneven surface
Impaired ability to flex or move both hips or knees
Insufficient muscle strength
Sample Clinical Applications: Neuromuscular disorders (e.g., multiple sclerosis [MS], amyotrophic lateral sclerosis [ALS], Parkinson's disease), traumatic injuries (e.g., fractures, spinal cord or brain injuries), rheumatoid arthritis, severe depression, dementia

DESIRED OUTCOMES/EVALUATION CRITERIA

Sample NOC linkages:

Knowledge: Body Mechanics: Extent of understanding conveyed about proper body alignment, balance, and coordinated movement
Balance: Ability to maintain body equilibrium
Body Mechanics Performance: Personal actions to maintain proper body alignment and to prevent musculoskeletal strain

Client Will (Include Specific Time Frame)

- Verbalize understanding of individual treatment regimen and safety measures.
- Attain and maintain sitting position that enables activities.
- Participate in activities of daily living (ADLs) and desired activities and prevent complications.

ACTIONS/INTERVENTIONS

Sample NIC linkages:

Positioning: Deliberative placement of the patient or a body part to promote physiological and/or psychological well-being
Exercise Therapy: Muscle Control: Use of specific activity or exercise protocols to enhance or restore controlled body movement
Body Mechanics Promotion: Facilitating the use of position and movement in daily activities to prevent fatigue and musculoskeletal strain or injury

NURSING PRIORITY NO. 1 To identify causative/contributing factors:

- Determine diagnosis that contributes to sitting balance problems, (e.g., MS, arthritis, Parkinson's disease, cardiopulmonary disorders, back pain conditions with client use of compensatory positions to reduce pain; traumatic brain injury, spinal cord injury with hemi/paraplegia; lower-limb injuries or amputations; psychiatric conditions including severe depression, dementias). *These conditions can cause postural impairments, muscular weakness, and inadequate range of motion. Sensory deficits may also be involved (e.g., impaired proprioception and/or visual processing, cognitive impairments). Note: Several studies have shown that sitting balance is a valid predictor for functional outcome in patients with stroke, paraplegia, and brain injury.*[1–6] *Sitting and standing balance are of major concern when assessing amputee's ability to maintain the center of gravity over the base of support. Both balance and coordination are required for weight shifting from one limb to another, thus improving the potential for an optimal gait.*[7]
- Note factors affecting current situation (e.g., surgery, fractures, amputation, tubings [chest tube, indwelling catheter, IVs, pumps]; potential time involved [e.g., few hours in bed after surgery versus serious trauma re-

quiring long-term bedrest or debilitating disease or pain limiting movement]). *Identifies potential impairments and determines type of interventions needed to provide for client's safety.*

- Note older client's general health status. *Hogue identified mobility as the most important functional ability that determines the degree of independence and healthcare needs among older persons.*[8] *While aging does not cause impaired mobility, per se, several aging-related changes can lead to immobility (e.g., sarcopenia with diminished endurance and core strength; impaired vision; loss of balance; decreased ability to quickly and adequately correct movements affecting center of gravity). Thus, falls are a major risk and source of morbidity and mortality.*[9–11]
- Assess nutritional and hydration status and client's report of energy level. *Deficiencies in nutrients and water, as well as electrolytes and minerals, can negatively affect energy and activity tolerance. Note: Research supports that the obese individual shows lower sitting functional reach values when compared to normal and overweight subjects.*[12]

NURSING PRIORITY NO. 2 To assess functional ability:

- Determine functional status using a 0–4 scale, noting muscle strength and tone, joint mobility, cardiovascular status, balance, and endurance. *Identifies strengths and deficits (e.g., inability to sit upright, reach forward, or transfer safely from bed to wheelchair) and may provide information regarding potential for recovery (e.g., client with severe brain injury may have permanent limitations because of impaired cognition affecting memory, judgment, problem solving, and motor planning).*[1,14]
- Determine degree of perceptual or cognitive impairment and ability to follow directions. *Impairments related to age, chronic or acute disease condition, trauma, surgery, or medications require alternative interventions or changes in plan of care.*
- Refer to physician and/or physical therapy specialists for special testing, as indicated. *May include many different functional tests (e.g., function in sitting test, balance performance monitor, Berger Balance Scale) to determine potential for improvement and direction for therapies.*[13]

NURSING PRIORITY NO. 3 To promote optimal level of function and prevent complications:

- Assist with treatment of underlying condition(s) *to maximize potential for optimal function.*
- Encourage client's participation in self-care activities and in physical or occupational therapies. *Improves body strength and function and enhances self-concept and sense of independence. Note: Sitting balance affects ADLs, including feeding, dressing, bathing, transfers, and mobility.*
- Support trunk and extremities when in seated position, using pillows or rolls, braces, shoes, gel pads, etc., *to maintain upright position and optimal internal organ function and to reduce risk of pressure ulcers.*
- Demonstrate and assist with use of assistive devices (e.g., side rails, overhead trapeze, roller pads, safety belt, hydraulic lifts, chairs) *for position changes and safe transfers.*
- Avoid routinely doing for client those activities that client can do for self. *Caregivers can contribute to deficits by being overprotective or helping too much.*
- Provide for safety measures as indicated by individual situation, including environmental management and fall prevention. (Refer to ND risk for Falls.)
- Note changes in ability to do more or less self-care (e.g., hygiene, feeding, toileting, therapies) *to promote psychological and physical benefits of self-care and to adjust level of assistance as indicated.*
- Collaborate with physical medicine specialist and occupational or physical therapists in providing range-of-motion exercise (active or passive), isotonic muscle contractions (e.g., sitting reach, push, and pull exercises), assistive devices, and activities.
- Administer pain medications before activity as needed *to promote maximal effort and involvement in activity.*
- Collaborate with nutritionist in providing nutritious foods and needed feeding assistance, maximizing client's abilities in ingesting and swallowing (upright position) *to optimize available energy for activities.*

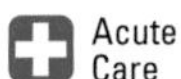

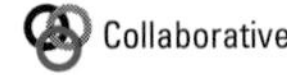

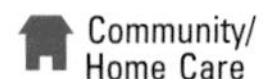

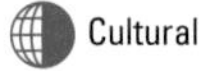

- Refer to NDs Activity Intolerance, impaired bed Mobility, impaired wheelchair Mobility, impaired Transfer Ability, impaired Standing, and impaired Walking for additional interventions.

NURSING PRIORITY NO. 4 To promote wellness (Teaching/Discharge Considerations):

- Encourage client's/significant other's (SO's) involvement in decision making as much as possible. *Enhances commitment to plan, optimizing outcomes.*
- Demonstrate use of mobility devices (e.g., walkers, strollers, scooters, braces, prosthetics) and have client/caregiver demonstrate knowledge about and safe use of device. Identify appropriate resources for obtaining and maintaining appliances or equipment. *Safe use of mobility aides promotes client's independence and enhances quality of life and safety for client and caregiver.*
- Discuss ways that client can exercise safely. *Options may be limited, but attending regular rehab sessions may provide best opportunity for improvement in function, including self-care, social independence, and recreation.*
- Involve client and SO(s) in care, assisting them to learn ways of managing problems of immobility and imbalanced sitting, especially when impairment is expected to be long term. Refer to support and community services as indicated *to provide care, supervision, companionship, respite services, nutritional and ADL assistance, adaptive devices or changes to living environment, financial assistance, etc.*

DOCUMENTATION FOCUS

Assessment/Reassessment
- Individual findings, including level of function and ability to participate in specific or desired activities.

Planning
- Plan of care and who is involved in the planning.
- Teaching plan.

Implementation/Evaluation
- Responses to interventions, teaching, and actions performed.
- Attainment or progress toward desired outcome(s).
- Modifications to plan of care.

Discharge Planning
- Discharge and long-term needs, noting who is responsible for each action to be taken.
- Specific referrals made.
- Sources of and maintenance for assistive devices.

References

1. Black, K., Zafonte, R., Millis, S., et al. (2000). Sitting balance following brain injury (does it predict outcome?). *Brain Inj*, 14(2), 141–152.
2. Wade, D. T., Skilbeck, C. E., Langton, R., et al. (1984). Therapy after stroke: Amounts, determinants and effects. *Int Rehabil Med*, 6(3), 105–110.
3. Nichols, D. S., Miller, L., Colby, L. A., et al. (1996). Sitting balance: Its relation to function in individuals with hemiparesis. *Arch Phys Med Rehabil*, 77(9), 865–869.
4. Juneja, G., Czyrny, J. J., Linn, R. T. (1998). Admission balance and outcomes of patients admitted for acute inpatient rehabilitation. *Arch Phys Med Rehabil*, 77(5), 388–393.
5. Feigen, L., Sharon, B., Czaczkes, B., et al. (1996). Sitting equilibrium 2 weeks after stroke can predict walking ability after six months. *Gerontology*, 42(6), 348–353.
6. Nixon, V. (1985). *Spinal Cord Injury: A Guide to Functional Outcomes in Physical Therapy Management.* Rockville, MD: Aspen.
7. Gaily, R. S., Clark, C. S. (2002). Physical therapy management of adult lower-limb amputees. Atlas of Limb Prosthetics. Online Orthotics and Prosthetics Virtual Library. Retrieved January 2015 from http://www.oandplibrary.org/alp/.
8. Hogue, C. C. (1984). Falls and mobility late in life: An ecological model. *J Am Geriatr Soc*, 32(11), 858–861.

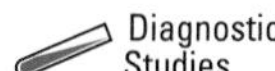

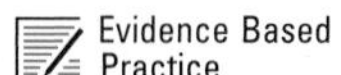

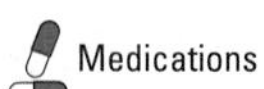

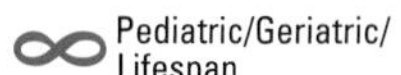

9. Rowe, J. W., Kahn, R. L. (1987). Human aging: Usual and successful. *Science*, 237(4811), 143–149.
10. Tinetti, M. E., Williams, T. F., Mayewski, R. (1986). Fall risk index for elderly patients based on number of chronic disabilities. *Am J Med*, 80(3), 429–434.
11. Michael, K. M., Allen, J. K., Macko, R. F. (2006). Fatigue after stroke: Relationship to mobility, fitness, ambulatory activity, social support, and falls efficiency. *Rehabil Nurs*, 31(5), 210–217.
12. Kumareason, A., Pathrap, S., Anadh, V. (2012). Influence of body mass index on balance in sitting and standing. *International J Current Research Pharmaceutical and Review*, 4(5), 22–27.
13. Gorman, S. L., Rivera, M., McCarthy, L. (2014). Reliability of the function in sitting test (FIST). Rehabilitation Research and Practice. Retrieved January 2015 from http://www.hindawi.com/journals/rerp/2014/593280/.
14. Dworak, P. A., Levy, A. (2005). Strolling along. *Rehabil Manage*, 18(9), 26–31.
15. Gordon, M. (2009). Functional levels code. *Manual of Nursing Diagnosis*. 12th ed. Sudbury, MA: Jones and Bartlett.

impaired Skin Integrity

Taxonomy II: Safety/Protection—Class 2 Physical Injury 00046) [**Diagnostic Division:** Safety], 1975, Revised 1998

DEFINITION: Altered epidermis and/or dermis.

RELATED FACTORS

External

Chemical injury agent (e.g., burn, capsaicin, methylene chloride, mustard agent); radiation therapy
Hypothermia; hyperthermia
Humidity; moisture; [excretions; secretions]
Extremes of age
Mechanical factors (e.g., shearing forces, pressure, physical immobility [restraint]); [trauma: injury, surgery]
Pharmaceutical agent

Internal

Alteration in metabolism; inadequate nutrition [e.g., obesity, emaciation]
Alteration in pigmentation, skin turgor, or sensation (resulting from spinal cord injury, diabetes mellitus, etc.)
Hormonal change
Immunodeficiency; impaired circulation; alteration in fluid volume [including presence of edema]
Pressure over bony prominence
[Psychogenic factor (e.g., obsessive compulsive disorder)]

DEFINING CHARACTERISTICS

Subjective

[Reports of itching, pain, numbness of affected/surrounding area]

Objective

Alteration in skin integrity [i.e., disruption of skin surface (epidermis), destruction of skin layers (dermis)]
Foreign matter piercing skin
[Invasion of body structures]

Sample Clinical Applications: Anemias; arthritis; end-of-life conditions; contagious diseases, coronary artery disease; dementias; burns; diabetes mellitus, obesity; peripheral vascular disease, Raynaud's disease

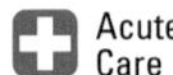

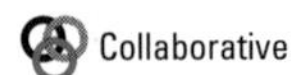

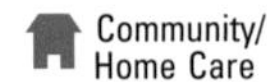

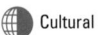

DESIRED OUTCOMES/EVALUATION CRITERIA

Sample NOC linkages:
Tissue Integrity: Skin & Mucous Membranes: Structural intactness and normal physiological function of skin and mucous membranes
Wound Healing: Primary Intention: Extent of regeneration of cells and tissues following intentional closure
Wound Healing: Secondary Intention: Extent of regeneration of cells and tissues in an open wound

Client Will (Include Specific Time Frame)

- Display timely healing of skin lesions, wounds, or pressure sores without complication.
- Maintain optimal nutrition and physical well-being.
- Participate in prevention measures and treatment program.
- Verbalize feelings of increased self-esteem and ability to manage situation.

ACTIONS/INTERVENTIONS

Sample NIC linkages:
Wound Care: Prevention of wound complications and promotion of wound healing
Incision Site Care: Cleansing, monitoring, and promotion of healing in a wound that is closed with sutures, clips, or staples

NURSING PRIORITY NO. 1 To assess causative/contributing factors:

- Identify underlying condition or pathology involved. *Skin integrity problems can be the result of (1) disease processes that affect circulation and perfusion of tissues (e.g., arteriosclerosis, venous insufficiency, hypertension, obesity, diabetes, malignant neoplasms); (2) conditions that can be associated with rashes (e.g., contagious diseases such as measles, chicken pox; infections such as methicillin-resistant* Staphylococcus aureus, *toxic shock syndrome; skin disorders such as exzema; disorders caused by spiders/insects such as lyme disease, lice, bedbugs; contact dermatitis such as occurs with latex allergy, poison ivy; autoimmune disorders such as lupus; internal diseases such as liver disease, celiac disease, kidney failure, iron deficiency anemia, thyroid problems, and cancers, including leukemia and lymphoma); (3) medications that adversely affect skin or impair healing (e.g., anticoagulants, antibiotics, corticosteroids, immunosuppressives, antineoplastics); (4) burns or radiation (can break down internal tissues as well as skin); and (5) nutrition and hydration (e.g., malnutrition deprives the body of protein and calories required for cell growth and repair, dehydration impairs transport of oxygen and nutrients).*[1,2,5,12,19]
- *Note: Disruption in skin integrity can be* ***intentional*** *(e.g., surgical incision) or* ***unintentional*** *(e.g., accidental trauma, drug effect, allergic reaction, rashes) and* ***open*** *(e.g., laceration, skin tears, penetrating wound, ulcerations) or* ***closed*** *(e.g., contusion, abrasion, rash).*
- Evaluate client's health status in general terms. *Many factors (e.g., debilitation; immobility; use of restraints; extremes of age; mental status; dehydration or malnutrition; presence of chronic disease; occupational, treatment, and environmental hazards) can affect the ability of the skin to perform its functions (e.g., protection, sensation, movement and growth, chemical synthesis, immunity, thermoregulation and excretion).*[3,4]
- Determine client's age and developmental factors and ability to care for self. *Newborn/infant's skin is thin, provides ineffective thermal regulation, and nails are thin. Infant skin also has a higher absorption and deabsorption rate as compared with an adult's skin, which predisposes infants to a dry, flaky, and impaired skin barrier.*[9] *Babies and children are prone to skin rashes associated with viral, bacterial, and fungal infections and allergic reactions. In adolescence, hormones stimulate hair growth and sebaceous gland activity.*[1,3,4,6] *In adults, it takes longer to replenish epidermis cells, resulting in increased risk of skin cancers and infection. In older adults, there is decreased epidermal regeneration, fewer sweat glands, less subcutaneous fat, elastin, and collagen, causing skin to become thinner, drier, and less responsive to pain sensations.*[7,12]

- Evaluate client's skin care practices and hygiene issues. *Individual's skin may be oily, dry and scaly, or sensitive and is affected by bathing frequency (or lack of bathing), temperature of water, and types of soap and other cleansing agents. Incontinence (urinary or bowel) and ineffective hygiene can result in serious skin impairment and discomfort.*[17]
- Note presence of compromised mobility, sensation, vision, hearing, or speech *that may impact client's self-care as relates to skin care (e.g., diabetic with impaired vision probably cannot satisfactorily examine own feet).*[10,12]
- Ascertain allergy history. *Individual may be sensitive or allergic to substances (e.g., insects, grasses, medications, lotions, soaps, foods) that can adversely affect the skin.*
- Assess blood supply (e.g., capillary return time, color, warmth) and sensation of skin surfaces and affected area on a regular basis *to provide comparative baseline and opportunity for timely intervention when problems are noted.*[3]
- Note distribution and scarcity of hair *(e.g., loss of hair on lower legs may indicate peripheral vascular disease).* Refer to ND risk for Peripheral Neurovascular Dysfunction for additional interventions.[13]
- Calculate ankle-brachial index *to evaluate actual or potential for impairment of circulation to lower extremities. Result less than 0.9 indicates need for close monitoring or more aggressive intervention (e.g., tighter blood glucose and weight control in diabetic client).*[14]
- Determine treatment-related skin or tissue conditions (e.g., surgical incision, IV/invasive line insertion site, use of restraints). Assess surgical sites *for signs of infection (e.g., swelling, redness, pain);* assess IV site *for infiltration (e.g., swelling, erythema, coolness, pain; failure of infusion) or evidence of extravasation (e.g., blistering, blanching, skin sloughing).*[4] Evaluate skin surrounding restraints for abrasions, contusions, skin breaks, or skin color and temperature changes distal to restraints *suggesting impaired circulation.*
- Review lab results (e.g., hemoglobin/hematocrit, blood glucose, blood and/or wound culture, sensitivities for infectious agents [viral, bacterial, fungal], albumin, protein) *to evaluate causative factors or ability to heal. Note: Albumin less than 3.5 correlates to decreased wound healing and increased incidence of pressure ulcers.*[1,14,15]

NURSING PRIORITY NO. 2 To assess extent of involvement/injury:

- Obtain a complete history of current skin condition(s) (especially in children where recurrent rash or lesions are common), including age at onset, date of first episode, duration, original site, characteristics of lesions, and any changes that have occurred. *Common skin manifestations of sensitivity or allergies are hives, eczema, and contact dermatitis. Contagious rashes include measles, rubella, roseola, chickenpox, and scarlet fever. Bacterial, viral, and fungal infections can also cause skin problems (e.g., impetigo, cellulitis, cold sores, shingles, athlete's foot, candidiasis, diaper rashes).*[5,6,19]
- Perform routine skin inspections describing observed changes. Note color, temperature, surface changes, texture, and contours. Evaluate color changes in areas of least pigmentation (e.g., sclera, conjunctiva, nailbeds, buccal mucosa, tongue, palms, soles of feet). *Systematic inspection can identify improvement or changes for timely intervention.*

GENERAL WOUNDS/LESIONS

- Describe rash or lesion, noting color, location, and significant characteristics (e.g., flat or raised rash, weeping or painful blisters, itching wheal) and surrounding information (e.g., exposure to contagious disease, reaction to medication, recent insect bite, ingrown toenail, sexually transmitted infection) *to assist in diagnosing problem and needed interventions.*
- Determine anatomic location and depth of skin or tissue injury or damage (e.g., epidermis, dermis, underlying issues) and describe (e.g., partial or full-thickness burn) *to provide baseline and document changes.* Use a skin integrity risk assessment tool (e.g., White et al. or Payne-Martin) if available *to classify skin tears.*[3,12]
- Photograph lesion(s) as appropriate *to document status and provide visual baseline for future comparisons.*
- Note character and color of drainage, when present (e.g., blood, bile, pus, stoma effluent), *which can cause or exacerbate skin irritation or excoriation.*

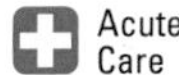

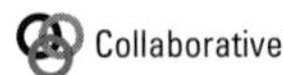

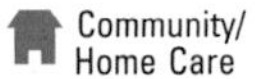

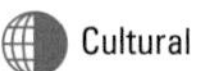

PRESSURE ULCERS/DECUBITUS

- Determine, document, and reassess periodically (1) dimensions and depth in centimeters; (2) exudates—color, odor, and amount; (3) margins—fixed or unfixed; (4) tunneling or tracts; and (5) evidence of necrosis (e.g., color gray to black) or healing (e.g., pink or red granulation tissue) *to establish comparative baseline and evaluate effectiveness of interventions.* Refer to ND risk for Pressure Ulcer for assessments and preventive interventions.[8,12,15]

NURSING PRIORITY NO. 3 To determine impact of condition:

- Determine if wound is acute (e.g., injury from surgery or trauma) or chronic (e.g., venous or arterial insufficiency), *which affects healing time and the client's emotional and physical responses. For example, an acute and noninfected wound can heal in about 4 weeks, while a chronic wound often does not progress through phases of healing in an orderly or timely fashion.*[8]
- Determine client's level of discomfort (e.g., can vary widely from minor itching or aching to deep pain with burns or excoriation associated with drainage) *to clarify intervention needs and priorities.*
- Ascertain attitudes of individual/significant others(s) about condition (e.g., cultural values, stigma). Obtain or review psychological assessment of client's emotional status, noting potential or sexual problems arising from presence of condition. *The healthy wholeness and beauty of skin impacts the client's body image and self-esteem. Lesions or wounds that disfigure can be especially devastating.*

NURSING PRIORITY NO. 4 To assist client with correcting/minimizing condition and achieving optimal healing:

- Practice and instruct client/caregiver(s) in scrupulous hand hygiene and clean or sterile technique *to reduce incidence of contamination or infection.*
- Provide optimum nutrition (including adequate protein, lipids, calories, trace minerals, and multivitamins [e.g., A, C, D, E]) *to promote skin health and healing and to maintain general good health.*
- Provide adequate hydration (e.g., oral, tube feeding, IV, ambient room humidity) *to reduce and replenish transepidermal water loss.*
- **Manage itching conditions:**[5,19,20]
  Cover itchy area, trim nails, and wear gloves at night.
  Apply cool, wet compresses.
  Take a lukewarm bath with baking soda, uncooked oatmeal, or colloidal oatmeal—a finely ground oatmeal made for the bathtub (e.g., Aveeno).
  Choose mild soaps without dyes or perfumes. Rinse the soap completely off body.
  Use a mild, unscented laundry detergent when washing clothes, towels, and bedding.
  Avoid substances that irritate skin or that cause an allergic reaction (e.g., nickel, jewelry, perfume or skin products containing fragrance).
  Encourage use of stress-management techniques (e.g., biofeedback, meditation, yoga).
- Apply high-quality moisturizing cream (e.g., Eurecin) or anti-itch creams (e.g., hydrocortisone cream, menthol, camphor, calamine) or topical anesthetics (e.g., lidocaine or benzocaine), concentrating on the areas where itching is most severe.
- Encourage client to verbalize feelings and discuss how or if condition affects self-concept. (Refer to NDs disturbed Body Image and situational low Self-Esteem.)
- Assist client to work through stages of grief and feelings associated with individual condition.
- Use touch, facial expressions, and tone of voice *to lend psychological support and acceptance of client.*
- Refer for counseling and/or behavior modification therapy, if indicated. *Client may need additional medical/psychological interventions if itching is severe, prolonged, or believed to be psychogenic in origin.*[20]
- **Promote wound healing:**[1,11–13,16]
  Keep surgical area(s) clean and dry, carefully dress wounds, support incision (e.g., use of Steri-Strips, splinting when coughing), and stimulate circulation to surrounding areas *to assist body's natural process of repair.*

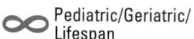

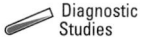

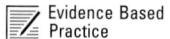

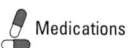

Consult with physician or wound specialist as indicated *to assist with developing plan of care for problematic or potentially serious wounds.*

Assist with débridement or enzymatic therapy as indicated (e.g., burns, skin tears, severe pressure sores) *to remove nonviable, contaminated, or infected tissue.*[12,16]

Use body temperature physiological solutions (e.g., isotonic saline) *to clean or irrigate wounds and prevent washout of electrolytes.*

Cleanse wound with irrigation syringe or gauze squares, avoiding cotton balls or other products *that shed fibers.*

Maintain appropriate moisture environment for particular wound (e.g., expose lesions or ulcer to air and light if excess moisture is impeding healing, use occlusive dressings to maintain a moist environment for autolytic débridement of wound) as indicated.[12,16]

Use appropriate barrier dressings or wound coverings (e.g., semipermeable, occlusive, wet-to-damp, DuoDerm, Tegaderm, hydrocolloid, hydrofiber or gel, hydropolymers), drainage appliances, and skin-protective agents for open or draining wounds and stomas *to protect wound and surrounding tissues from excoriating secretions or drainage and to promote wound healing.*[12,16]

Administer topical or systemic drugs as indicated *for individual situation.*

- **Prevent skin impairment:**[3–5,7,11,13,17,18]

Maintain or instruct in overall skin hygiene (e.g., shower instead of bathe, wash thoroughly, pat dry, gently massage with lotion or appropriate cream) *to provide barrier to infection, reduce risk of dermal trauma, improve circulation, and enhance comfort.*

Cleanse skin after toileting and incontinent or diaphoretic episodes *to restore normal skin pH and flora and limit potential for infection.*

Use proper turning and transfer techniques. Avoid movements *(e.g., pulling client with parallel force, dragging) that cause friction or shearing*

Encourage early ambulation or mobilization. *Reduces risks associated with immobility.*

Develop regularly timed repositioning schedule for client with mobility and sensation impairments, using turn sheet as needed; encourage or assist with periodic weight shifts for client in chair *to reduce stress on pressure points and to promote circulation to tissues.*

Use appropriate padding or pressure-reducing devices (e.g., heel rolls, foam boots, egg crate, gel pads) or pressure-relieving devices (e.g., air or water mattress) when indicated *to reduce pressure on sensitive areas and enhance circulation to compromised tissues.*

Avoid or limit use of plastic material (e.g., rubber sheet, plastic-backed linen savers) and remove wet or wrinkled linens promptly. *Moisture potentiates skin breakdown and increases risk for infection.*

Remove adhesive products with care, removing on horizontal plane, and using mineral oil or Vaseline for softening, if needed, *to prevent abrasions or tearing of skin.*

Secure dressings with tape (e.g., elastic, paper tape, nonadherent dressings) or Montgomery straps when frequent dressing changes are required. Use stockinette, tubular or gauze wrap, or similar product instead of tape to secure dressings and drains *to limit dermal injury.*[12]

Apply hot and cold applications judiciously *to reduce risk of dermal injury in persons with circulatory and neurosensory impairments.*

Avoid use of latex products *when client has known or suspected sensitivity.* Refer to ND Latex Allergy Response.

NURSING PRIORITY NO. 5 To promote wellness (Teaching/Discharge Considerations):

- Discuss importance of skin and measures to maintain proper skin functioning. *The integumentary system is the largest multifunctional organ of the body and thus merits special care.*
- Review benefits of following medical regimen. *Enhances commitment to plan, optimizing outcomes.*
- Encourage regular inspection and monitoring of skin for changes or failure to heal. *Early detection and reporting to healthcare providers promotes timely evaluation and intervention.*
- Identify safety measures for client with persistent sensation impairments. *Proper care of skin and extremities during cold or hot weather (e.g., wearing gloves; clean, dry socks; properly fitting shoes or boots; face protection) reduces risk of injury.*[10,14]

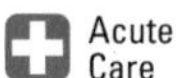

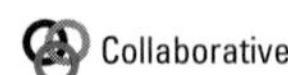

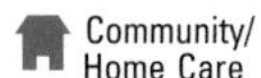

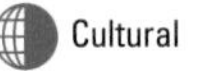

- Encourage continued mobility, activity, and range of motion *to enhance circulation and promote health of skin and other organs.*
- Discuss avoidance of products containing perfumes, dyes, preservatives *(may cause dermatitis reactions)* or alcohol, povidone-iodine, and hydrogen peroxide *(may hinder wound healing).*
- Encourage restriction or abstinence from smoking, *which causes vasoconstriction.*
- Review measures *to avoid spread or reinfection of communicable conditions.*
- Discuss proper and safe use of equipment or appliances (e.g., heating pad, ostomy appliances, padding straps of braces).
- Emphasize wisdom of limiting lengthy or unnecessary sun exposure, using high sun protection factor (SPF) sunblock and avoiding tanning beds.
- Assist client to learn stress reduction and alternate therapy techniques *to control feelings of helplessness and enhance coping ability.*
- Refer to dietitian or certified diabetes educator as appropriate *to manage general well-being, enhance healing, and reduce risk of recurrence of diabetic ulcers.*

DOCUMENTATION FOCUS

Assessment/Reassessment
- Characteristics of lesion(s) or condition, ulcer classification.
- Causative or contributing factors.
- Impact of condition.

Planning
- Plan of care and who is involved in planning.
- Teaching plan.

Implementation/Evaluation
- Responses to interventions, teaching, and actions performed.
- Attainment or progress toward desired outcome(s).
- Modifications to plan of care.

Discharge Planning
- Long-term needs and who is responsible for actions to be taken.
- Specific referrals made.

References

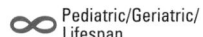

1. Llewellyn, S. (2002). *Skin integrity and wound care (lecture materials).* Chapel Hill, NC: Cape Fear Community College Nursing Program.
2. Colburn, L. (2001). Prevention for chronic wounds. In Krasner, D., Rodeheaver, G., Sibbald, R. G. (eds). *Chronic Wound Care: A Clinical Source Book for Healthcare Professionals.* 2nd ed. Wayne, PA: HMP Communications.
3. Calianno, C. (1999). Patient hygiene: Part 2. Skin care. Keeping the outside healthy. *Nursing*, 29(suppl 1)(12), 1–13.
4. Lund, C. H., Osborne, J. W., Culler, J. (2001). Neonatal skin care: Clinical outcomes of the AWHONN/NANN evidence-based clinical practice guideline. *J Neonatal Nurs*, 30(1), 30–40.
5. WebMD staff. (No date). Skin problems & treatments. Skin Problems & Treatments Health Center (various pages). Retrieved January 2015 from http://www.webmd.com/skin-problems-and-treatments/guide/default.htm.
6. Engel, J. (2002). *Pocket Guide to Pediatric Assessment.* 4th ed. St. Louis, MO: Mosby, 99–112.
7. Wiersema, L. A., Stanley, M. (1999). The aging integumentary system. In Stanley, M., Beare, P. G. (eds). *Gerontological Nursing: A Health Promotion/Protection Approach.* 2nd ed. Philadelphia: F. A. Davis.
8. Krasner, D., Rodeheaver, G., Sibbald, R. G. (2001). Advanced wound caring for a new millennium. In Krasner, D., Rodeheaver, G., Sibbald, R. G. (eds).

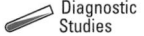

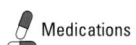

Chronic Wound Care: A Clinical Source Book for Healthcare Professionals. 2nd ed. Wayne, PA: HMP Communications.
9. Blume-Peytavi, U., Hauser, M., Stamatas, G. N. (2012). Skin care practices for newborns and infants: Review of the clinical evidence for best practices. *Pediatric Dermatology*, 29(1), 1–14.
10. American Diabetes Association. (2011). Standards of medical care in diabetes—2011: Foot care recommendations. *Diabetes Care*, 34(Suppl 1), S11–S61.
11. Reddy, M., Gill, S. S., Rochan, P. A. (2006). Preventing pressure ulcers: A systematic review. *JAMA*, 296(8), 974–984.
12. LeBlanc, K., Baranoski, S. (2009). Prevention and management of skin tears. *Adv Skin Wound Care*, 22(7), 325–332.
13. Hess, C. (2002). *Clinical Guide to Wound Care*. 4th ed. Philadelphia: Lippincott Williams & Wilkins.
14. Carrington, A. L., Abbott, C. A., Griffiths, J. et al. (2008). Peripheral vascular and nerve function associated with lower limb amputation in people with and without diabetes. *Clin Sci,* 101(3), 261–266.
15. Catania, K., Huang, C., James, P., et al. (2007). PUPPI: The pressure ulcer prevention protocol interventions. *Am J Nurs*, 107(4), 44–51.
16. Okan, K., Woo, K., Ayello, E. A. (2007). The role of moisture balance in wound healing. *Adv Skin Wound Care*, 20(1), 39–53.
17. Langemo, D., Hanson, D., Hunter, S. (2011). Incontinence and incontinence-associated dermatitis. *Adv Skin Wound Care*, 4(3), 126–140.
18. Wadland, D. L. (2010). Maintaining skin integrity in the OR. *OR Nurse 2011*, 4(2), 26–32.
19. MayoClinic Staff. (2014). Itchy skin (pruritis) (various pages). Retrieved January 2015 from http://www.mayoclinic.org/diseases-conditions/itchy-skin/basics/causes/con-20028460.
20. Hu, S. (2008). Psychogenic pruritus: A review. Retrieved January 2015 from http://www.vgrd.org/archive/cases/2008/pruritus/pruritus.html.

risk for impaired Skin Integrity

Taxonomy II: Safety/Protection—Class 2 Physical Injury 00247) [**Diagnostic Division:** Safety], 1975; Revised 1998, 2010, 2013

DEFINITION: Vulnerable to alteration in epidermis and/or dermis, which may compromise health.

RISK FACTORS

External

Chemical injury agent (e.g., burn, capsaicin, methylene chloride, mustard agent); radiation therapy
Hypothermia; hyperthermia
Excretions; secretions; humidity; moisture
Extremes of age
Mechanical factors (e.g., shearing forces, pressure, physical immobility; [restraint])

Internal

Alteration in metabolism; inadequate nutrition [e.g., obesity, emaciation]
Alteration in pigmentation, skin turgor, or sensation (resulting from spinal cord injury, diabetes mellitus, etc.)
Hormonal change
Immunodeficiency; impaired circulation; [presence of edema]
Pharmaceutical agent
Pressure over bony prominence
Psychogenic factor [e.g., obsessive compulsive disorder]
Note: A risk diagnosis is not evidenced by signs and symptoms, as the problem has not occurred; rather, nursing interventions are directed at prevention.
Sample Clinical Applications: AIDs; atherosclerosis, anemias; arthritis; coronary artery disease; dementias; amputation; Buerger's disease, burns; CVA; COPD; CHF; diabetes mellitus, obesity; peripheral vascular disease, Raynaud's disease, thrombophlebitis

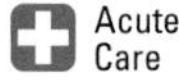

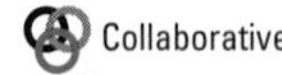

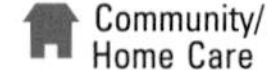

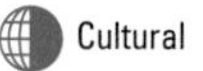

DESIRED OUTCOMES/EVALUATION CRITERIA

Sample NOC linkages:

Risk Control: Personal actions to prevent, eliminate, or reduce modifiable health threats

Immobility Consequences: Physiological: Severity of compromise in physiological functioning due to impaired physical mobility

Tissue Integrity: Skin & Mucous Membranes: Structural intactness and normal physiological function of skin and mucous membranes

Client Will (Include Specific Time Frame)

- Identify individual risk factors.
- Verbalize understanding of treatment or therapy regimen.
- Demonstrate behaviors or techniques to prevent skin breakdown.

ACTIONS/INTERVENTIONS

Sample NIC linkages:

Risk Identification: Analysis of potential risk factors, determination of health risks, and prioritization of risk reduction strategies for an individual or group

Skin Surveillance: Collection and analysis of patient data to maintain skin and mucous membrane integrity

Pressure Management: Minimizing pressure to body parts

NURSING PRIORITY NO. 1 To assess causative/contributing factors:

- Identify client with underlying conditions or problems that have potential for *skin integrity problems, such as (1) disease processes that affect circulation and perfusion of tissues (e.g., arteriosclerosis, venous insufficiency, hypertension, obesity, diabetes, malignant neoplasms), (2) medications (e.g., anticoagulants, corticosteroids, immunosuppressives, antineoplastics) that adversely affect or impair healing, (3) radiation (can break down internal tissues as well as skin), (4) nutrition and hydration (e.g., malnutrition deprives the body of protein and calories required for cell growth and repair, dehydration impairs transport of oxygen and nutrients), and (5) psychological stress and/or psychiatric conditions (e.g., skin excoriation is practiced to avoid increased anxiety or in reaction to a dreaded event, or may be elicited by an obsession). Disruption in skin integrity can be intentional (e.g., surgical incision) or unintentional (e.g., accidental trauma, drug effect, allergic reaction) and closed (e.g., contusion, abrasion, rash) or open (e.g., laceration, skin tears, penetrating wound, ulcerations).*[1–5,14]
- Note general health. *Many factors (e.g., debilitation; immobility; use of restraints; extremes of age; mental and psychiatric status; dehydration or malnutrition; presence of chronic disease; occupational, treatment, and environmental hazards) can affect the ability of the skin to perform its functions (e.g., protection, sensation, movement and growth, chemical synthesis, immunity, thermoregulation, and excretion).*[1,2,14]
- Determine client's age and developmental factors or ability to care for self. *Newborn/infant's skin is thin. Babies and children are prone to skin rashes associated with viral, bacterial, and fungal infections and allergic reactions. In adolescence, hormones stimulate hair growth and sebaceous gland activity. In adults, it takes longer to replenish epidermis cells, resulting in increased risk of skin cancers and infection. In older adults, there is decreased epidermal regeneration, fewer sweat glands, and less subcutaneous fat and elastin and collagen, causing skin to become thinner, drier, and less responsive to pain sensations.*[1,3,4,6–8]
- Evaluate client's skin care practices and hygiene issues. *Individual's skin may be sensitive or oily, dry, and scaly, and it is affected by bathing frequency (or lack of bathing), temperature of water, and types of soap and other cleansing agents. Incontinence (urinary or bowel) and ineffective hygiene can result in serious skin impairment and discomfort.*
- Note presence of compromised vision, sensation, hearing, or speech *that may impact client's self-care as relates to skin care (e.g., diabetic with impaired vision probably cannot satisfactorily examine own feet).*[9]

- Ascertain allergy history. *Individual may be sensitive or allergic to substances (e.g., insects, grasses, medications, lotions, soaps, foods) that can adversely affect the skin.*
- Assess blood supply (e.g., capillary return time, color, warmth) and sensation of skin surfaces or affected area on a regular basis *to provide comparative baseline and opportunity for timely intervention when problems are noted.*
- Calculate ankle-brachial index *to evaluate actual or potential for impairment of circulation to lower extremities. Result less than 0.9 indicates need for close monitoring or more aggressive intervention (e.g., tighter blood glucose and weight control in diabetic client).*[10,11]
- Review lab results (e.g., hemoglobin/hematocrit, blood glucose, albumin, protein) *to evaluate causative factors or ability to heal. Note: Albumin less than 3.5 correlates to decreased wound healing and increased incidence of pressure ulcers.*[12]

NURSING PRIORITY NO. 2 To maintain optimal skin integrity:[1,2,8]

- Perform routine skin inspections, assessing color, temperature, surface changes, texture, and contours. Evaluate color changes in areas of least pigmentation (e.g., sclera, conjunctiva, nailbeds, buccal mucosa, tongue, palms, soles of feet). Report potential problem areas (e.g., reddened/blanched areas, rashes) promptly. *Systematic inspection can identify developing problems and promotes early intervention, thus reducing likelihood of progression to skin breakdown.*[14]
- Handle client gently (particularly infant, young child, elderly frail). *Epidermis of infants and very young children is thin and lacks subcutaneous depth that will develop with age. Skin of the older client is also thin, less elastic, and prone to injury, such as bruising and skin tears.*[2,5]
- Practice and instruct client/caregiver(s) in scrupulous hand hygiene and clean or sterile technique, as appropriate, *to reduce incidence of contamination or infection.*
- Maintain and instruct in overall good skin hygiene (e.g., shower instead of bath, wash thoroughly, pat dry, gently massage with lotion or appropriate cream) *to reduce risk of dermal trauma, improve circulation, and promote comfort.*
- Provide preventative skin care to incontinent client: Change continence pads or diapers frequently, cleanse perineal skin daily and after each incontinence episode, and apply skin protectant ointment *to minimize contact with irritants (urine, stool, excessive moisture).*[13]
- Cleanse skin after diaphoretic episodes *to maintain normal skin pH and flora and limit potential for infection.*
- Develop regularly timed repositioning schedule for client with mobility and sensation impairments, using turn sheet, as needed; encourage or assist with periodic weight shifts for client in chair *to reduce stress on pressure points and to promote circulation to tissues.*
- Use proper turning and transfer techniques. *Avoids movements that cause friction or shearing (e.g., pulling client with parallel force, dragging movements).*
- Pay special attention to bony prominences and other pressure points (e.g., heels, toes, elbows) when positioning client *to prevent pressure trauma and impaired circulation.*
- Provide foam, flotation, alternating pressure, or air mattress *to reduce or relieve pressure on skin, tissues, and lesions, decreasing tissue ischemia.*
- Use appropriate padding or pressure-reducing devices (e.g., egg crate, gel pads, heel rolls, or foam boots), when indicated, *to reduce pressure on sensitive areas and enhance circulation to compromised tissues.*
- Encourage ambulation. *Promotes circulation and reduces risks associated with immobility.*
- Provide for safety measures (e.g., assistive devices or sufficient personnel, grab bars, clear pathways, safe chairs, properly fitting hose and footwear, use of heating pads or lamps, restraints) during ambulation and other interventions *to reduce risk of dermal injury.*
- Avoid or limit use of plastic material (e.g., rubber sheet, plastic-backed linen savers) and remove wet or wrinkled linens promptly. *Moisture potentiates skin breakdown and increases risk for infection.*
- Use paper tape or a nonadherent dressing on frail skin and remove it gently, or use stockinette, tubular or gauze wrap, or other similar product instead of tape to secure dressings and drains *to limit dermal injury.*[5]

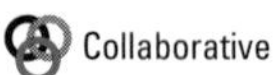

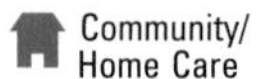

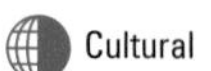

- Avoid use of latex products *when client has known or suspected sensitivity.* Refer to ND Latex Allergy Response.
- Apply hot and cold applications judiciously *to reduce risk of dermal injury in persons with circulatory and neurosensory impairments.*
- Provide adequate clothing or covers; protect from drafts *to prevent vasoconstriction and reduction of circulation to skin.*
- Keep bedclothes dry, use nonirritating materials, and keep bed free of wrinkles, crumbs, etc., *to prevent skin irritation.*
- Try colloidal bath, application of lotions, or careful use of ice pack *to decrease irritable itching.*
- Keep nails cut short, encouraging client *to refrain from scratching,* or suggest use of/obtain order for mittens (considered a restraint), if necessary, *to prevent dermal injury from scratching.*
- Refer to NDs impaired Skin Integrity and risk for Pressure Ulcer for additional interventions, as indicated.

NURSING PRIORITY NO. 3 To promote healthy skin (Teaching/Discharge Considerations):

- Discuss importance of skin and measures to maintain proper skin functioning. *The integumentary system is the largest multifunctional organ of the body and thus merits special care.*
- Encourage regular inspection and monitoring of skin for changes and effective skin care in preventing skin problems. *Early detection and reporting to healthcare providers promotes timely evaluation and intervention.*
- Counsel diabetic and neurologically impaired client regarding the necessity of meticulous skin care, especially of lower extremities. *Healing of lower-extremity injuries tends to be more problematic in this population, resulting in increased incidence of amputation.*
- Avoid products containing perfumes, dyes, preservatives *(may cause dermatitis reactions)* or alcohol, povidone-iodine, and hydrogen peroxide *(may hinder healing).*
- Instruct in care of skin and extremities during cold or hot weather (e.g., wearing gloves, and clean, dry socks; properly fitting shoes or boots; face protection) *to reduce risk of tissue damage, especially in clients with impaired sensation.*
- Recommend elevation of lower extremities when sitting *to enhance venous return and reduce edema formation.*
- Encourage consistent exercise program (active or assistive) *to enhance circulation.*
- Discuss need for adequate nutritional intake (including adequate protein, lipids, calories, trace minerals, multivitamins) *to promote skin health and healing and to maintain general good health.*
- Determine fluid needs and sources for hydration (e.g., oral, tube feeding, ambient room humidity) *to reduce and replenish transepidermal water loss.*
- Encourage restriction or abstinence from smoking, *which can cause vasoconstriction.*
- Discuss importance of limiting lengthy or unnecessary sun exposure and avoiding use of tanning beds. Emphasize necessity of avoiding exposure to sunlight in specific conditions (e.g., systemic lupus, tetracycline or psychotropic drug use, radiation therapy) as well as potential for development of skin cancer.
- Advise use of high sun protection factor (SPF) sunblock or sunscreen, particularly on young child, client with fair skin (prone to burn), client using multiple medications, etc., *to limit skin damage (immediate and over time) associated with sun exposure.*

DOCUMENTATION FOCUS

Assessment/Reassessment

- Individual findings, including individual risk factors.

Planning

- Plan of care and who is involved in planning.
- Teaching plan.

Implementation/Evaluation

- Responses to interventions, teaching, and actions performed.
- Attainment or progress toward desired outcome(s).
- Modifications to plan of care.

Discharge Planning

- Long-term needs and who is responsible for actions to be taken.

References

1. Calianno, C. (2002). Patient hygiene, part 2—Skin care: Keeping the outside healthy. *Nursing*, 32(6), 1–13.
2. Lund, C. H., Osborne, J. W., Kuller, J. (2001). Neonatal skin care: Clinical outcomes of the AWHONN/NANN evidence-based clinical practice guideline. *J Neonatal Nurs*, 30(1), 30–40.
3. Llewellyn, S. (2002). *Skin integrity and wound care (lecture materials).* Chapel Hill, NC: Cape Fear Community College Nursing Program.
4. Colburn, L. (2001). Prevention for chronic wounds. In Krasner, D., Rodeheaver, G., Sibbald, R. G. (eds). *Chronic Wound Care: A Clinical Source Book for Healthcare Professionals.* 2nd ed. Wayne, PA: HMP Communications.
5. LeBlanc, K., Baranoski, S. (2009). Prevention and management of skin tears. *Adv Skin Wound Care*, 22(7), 325–332.
6. McGovern, C. (2003, updated 2014). Skin, hair and nail assessment. Unit 2 (lecture materials). Villanova University College of Nursing. Retrieved January 2015 from http://www10.homepage.villanova.edu/marycarol.mcgovern/2104/SkinHairNail2.htm.
7. Engel, J. (2002). *Pocket Guide to Pediatric Assessment.* 4th ed. St. Louis, MO: Mosby.
8. Wiersema, L. A., Stanley, M. (1999). The aging integumentary system. In Stanley, M., Beare, P. G. (eds). *Gerontological Nursing: A Health Promotion/Protection Approach.* 2nd ed. Philadelphia: F. A. Davis.
9. American Diabetes Association (2011). Standards of medical care in diabetes—2011: Foot care recommendations. *Diabetes Care*, 34(Suppl 1), S11–S61.
10. Murabito, J. M., Evans, J. C., Larson, M. G., et al. (2003). The ankle-brachial index in the elderly and risk of stroke, coronary disease and death. *Arch Intern Med*, 163(16), 1939–1942.
11. Carrington, A. L., Abbott, C. A., Griffiths, J., et al. (2001). Peripheral vascular and nerve function associated with lower limb amputation in people with and without diabetes. *Clin Sci*, 101(3), 261–266.
12. Catania, K., Huang, C., James, P., et al. (2007). PUPPI: The pressure ulcer prevention protocol interventions. *Am J Nurs*, 107(4), 44–51.
13. Gray, M., Bliss, D. Z., Doughty, D. B., et al. (2007). Incontinence-associated dermatitis: A consensus. *J Wound Ostomy Continence Nurs*, 34(1), 45–54.
14. Hu, S. (2008). Psychogenic pruritus: A review. Retrieved January 2015 from http://www.vgrd.org/archive/cases/2008/pruritus/pruritus.html.

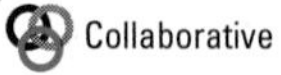

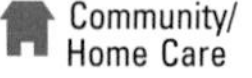

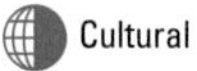

readiness for enhanced Sleep

Taxonomy II: Activity/Rest—Class 1 Sleep/Rest (00165) [**Diagnostic Division:** Activity/Rest], Submitted 2002; Revised 2013

DEFINITION: A pattern of natural, periodic suspension of relative consciousness to provide rest and sustain a desired lifestyle, which can be strengthened.

DEFINING CHARACTERISTICS

Subjective

Expresses desire to enhance sleep

Sample Clinical Applications: Postoperative recovery, chronic pain, pregnancy—prenatal/postpartal period, sleep apnea

DESIRED OUTCOMES/EVALUATION CRITERIA

Sample NOC linkages:

Sleep: Natural periodic suspension of consciousness during which the body is restored

Rest: Quantity and pattern of diminished activity for mental and physical rejuvenation

Comfort Status: Environmental: Environmental ease, comfort, and safety of surroundings

Client Will (Include Specific Time Frame)

- Identify individually appropriate interventions to promote sleep.
- Verbalize feeling rested after sleep.
- Adjust lifestyle to accommodate routines that promote sleep.

ACTIONS/INTERVENTIONS

Sample NIC linkages:

Sleep Enhancement: Facilitation of regular sleep/wake cycles

Relaxation Therapy: Use of techniques to encourage and elicit relaxation for the purpose of decreasing undesirable signs and symptoms such as pain, muscle tension, or anxiety

Environmental Management: Manipulation of the patient's surroundings for therapeutic benefit, sensory appeal, and psychological well-being

NURSING PRIORITY NO. 1 To determine motivation for continued improvement:

- Listen to client's reports of sleep quantity and quality. Determine client's perception of adequate sleep. *Reveals client's experience and expectations regarding sleep. Provides opportunity to address misconceptions or unrealistic expectations and plan for interventions.*
- Observe or obtain feedback from client/significant other(s) regarding usual bedtime, number of hours of sleep, and time of arising *to determine usual sleep pattern and provide comparative baseline for improvements.*
- Ascertain motivation and expectation for change. *Motivation to improve and high expectations can encourage client to make changes that will improve his or her life. However, unrealistic expectations may hamper efforts.*
- Note client report of potential for alteration of habitual sleep time (e.g., change of work pattern or rotating shifts) or change in normal bedtime (e.g., hospitalization). *Helps identify circumstances that are known to interrupt sleep patterns and that could disrupt the person's biological rhythms.*[1,6]

NURSING PRIORITY NO. 2 To assist client to enhance sleep/rest:

- Review client's usual bedtime rituals, routines, and sleep environment needs. *Provides information on client's management of the situation and identifies areas that might be modified when the need arises.*

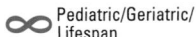

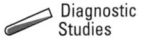

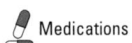

- Discuss or implement effective age-appropriate bedtime rituals for infant/child (e.g., rocking, story reading, cuddling, favorite blanket or toy). *Rituals can enhance ability to fall asleep, reinforce that bed is a place to sleep, and promote sense of security for child.*[2]
- Provide quiet environment and comfort measures (e.g., back rub, washing hands and face, cleaning and straightening sheets) for client in facility. *Promotes relaxation and readiness for sleep.*
- Arrange care *to provide for uninterrupted periods for rest.* Explain necessity of disturbances for monitoring vital signs or other care when client is hospitalized. Do as much care as possible during night without waking client. *Allows for longer periods of uninterrupted sleep, especially during night.*
- Suggest limiting fluid intake in evening if nocturia or bed-wetting is a problem *to reduce need for nighttime elimination.*
- Provide instruction in use of necessary equipment. *Client may use oxygen or continuous positive airway pressure system to improve sleep/rest in presence of hypoxia or sleep apnea.*
- Discuss dietary matters, such as limiting chocolate, heavy meals, caffeine, or alcoholic beverages prior to bedtime, *which are substances known to impair falling or staying asleep. Use of alcohol at bedtime may help individual fall asleep, but ensuing sleep is then fragmented.*[7]
- Explore or implement use of warm bath, intake of light protein snack before bedtime, comfortable room temperature, soothing music, or favorite calming television show. *Nonpharmaceutical aids can enhance falling asleep without the undesired side effects associated with medications.*
- Investigate use of sleep mask, darkening shades or curtains, earplugs, and low-level background (white) noise in situations *where sleep might not come easily or be disturbed by environmental factors.*
- Recommend continuing same schedule for sleep throughout week—including days off. *Maintaining sleep pattern helps sustain biological rhythms.*

NURSING PRIORITY NO. 3 To promote optimum sleep:

- Assure client that occasional sleeplessness should not threaten health. *Knowledge that occasional insomnia is universal and usually not harmful may promote relaxation and relief from worry.*[3]
- Encourage regular exercise during the day *to aid in stress control and release of energy. Note: Exercise at bedtime may stimulate rather than relax client and may actually interfere with sleep.*[5]
- Assist to develop individual program of relaxation (e.g., biofeedback, self-hypnosis, visualization, progressive muscle relaxation). *Reduces sympathetic response and stress to aid in inducing sleep.*[4]
- Address sleep management techniques that may be useful during stressful conditions or lifestyle changes (e.g., pregnancy, new baby, menopause, medical procedures, new job, moving, change in relationship, grief).
- Recommend periodic review of medications. *Many prescription and over-the-counter (OTC) drugs can disrupt sleep.*
- Advise using prescription or OTC sleep medications sparingly. *These medications, while useful for promoting sleep in the short term, can interfere with rapid eye movement sleep.*

DOCUMENTATION FOCUS

Assessment/Reassessment

- Assessment findings, including specifics of sleep pattern and effects on lifestyle/level of functioning.
- Any medications used, interventions tried, previous therapies.
- Motivation and expectations for change.

Planning

- Plan of care and who is involved in planning.
- Teaching plan.

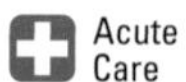

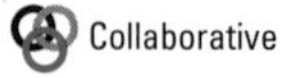

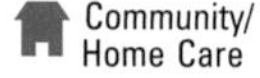

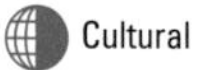

Implementation/Evaluation

- Client's response to interventions, teaching, and actions performed.
- Attainment or progress toward desired outcome(s).
- Modifications to plan of care.

Discharge Planning

- Long-term needs and who is responsible for actions to be taken.
- Specific referrals made.

References

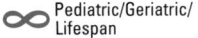

1. Cochran, H. (2003). Diagnose and treat primary insomnia. *Nurse Pract*, 28(9), 13–27.
2. Mindell, J. (1997). *Sleeping Through the Night: How Infants, Toddlers, and Their Parents Can Get a Good Night's Sleep*. New York: HarperCollins.
3. National Institute of Neurological Disorders and Stroke. (Updated 2014). Brain basics: Understanding sleep. Retrieved November 2015 from http://www.ninds.nih.gov/disorders/brain_basics/understanding_sleep.htm.
4. Cox, H. C., Hinz, M. D., Lubno, M. A., et al. (2002). ND: Sleep Pattern, disturbed. *Clinical Applications of Nursing Diagnosis: Adult, Child, Women's, Psychiatric, Gerontic, and Home Health Considerations*. 4th ed. Philadelphia: F. A. Davis.
5. Grandjean, C. K., Gibbons, S. W. (2000). Assessing ambulatory geriatric sleep complaints. *Nurse Pract: Am J Prim Health Care*, 25(9), 25–35.
6. Pronitis-Ruotolo, D. (2001). Surviving the night shift: Making Zeitgeber work for you. *Am J Nurs*, 101(7), 63–68.
7. National Sleep Foundation. (2003). Sleep hygiene. Retrieved November 2015 from http://www.sleepfoundation.org/article/ask-the-expert/sleep-hygiene.

Sleep Deprivation

Taxonomy II: Activity/Rest—Class 1 Sleep/Rest (00096) [**Diagnostic Division:** Activity/Rest], 1998

DEFINITION: Prolonged periods of time without sleep (sustained natural, periodic suspension of relative consciousness).

RELATED FACTORS

Overstimulating environment; environmental barrier; treatment regimen
Average daily physical activity is less than recommended for gender and age; sustained circadian asynchrony; age-related sleep stage shifts
Sustained inadequate sleep hygiene; nonrestorative sleep pattern (i.e., due to caregiver responsibilities, parenting practices, sleep partner)
Prolonged discomfort (e.g., physical, psychological); conditions with periodic limb movement (e.g., restless leg syndrome, nocturnal myoclonus); sleep-related enuresis or painful erections
Nightmares; sleep walking; sleep terror
Sleep apnea
Sundowner's syndrome; dementia
Idiopathic central nervous system hypersomnolence; narcolepsy; familial sleep paralysis

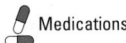

DEFINING CHARACTERISTICS

Subjective

Decrease in functional ability
Malaise; lethargy; fatigue

(continues on page 800)

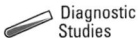

Sleep Deprivation (continued)
Anxiety
Perceptual disorders; heightened sensitivity to pain

Objective
Restlessness; irritability
Alteration in concentration; decrease in reaction time
Drowsiness; listlessness; apathy
Fleeting nystagmus; hand tremors
Confusion; transient paranoia; agitation; combativeness; hallucinations
Sample Clinical Applications: Chronic obstructive pulmonary disease (COPD), heart failure (nocturia), chronic pain, sleep apnea, pregnancy, postpartum, colic, dementia, Alzheimer's disease, anxiety disorders, post-traumatic stress disorder

DESIRED OUTCOMES/EVALUATION CRITERIA

Sample NOC linkages:
Sleep: Natural periodic suspension of consciousness during which the body is restored
Rest: Quantity and pattern of diminished activity for mental and physical rejuvenation
Pain Control: Personal actions to control pain

Client Will (Include Specific Time Frame)
- Identify individually appropriate interventions to promote sleep.
- Verbalize understanding of sleep disorder.
- Adjust lifestyle to accommodate chronobiological rhythms.
- Report improvement in sleep and rest pattern.

Sample NOC linkages:
- **Family Coping:** Family actions to manage stressors that tax family resources

Family Will (Include Specific Time Frame)
- Deal appropriately with parasomnias.

ACTIONS/INTERVENTIONS

Sample NIC linkages:
Sleep Enhancement: Facilitation of regular sleep/wake cycles
Anxiety Reduction: Minimizing apprehension, dread, foreboding, or uneasiness related to an unidentified source or anticipated danger
Environmental Management: Comfort: Manipulation of the patient's surroundings for promotion of optimal comfort

NURSING PRIORITY NO. 1 To assess causative/contributing factors:

- Note client's age and developmental stage. *The average adult requires 7 to 8 hours of sleep, although recent research indicates that the average total hours of sleep have decreased to less than 7 hours per night over the last few decades.[19] Teenagers require about 9 hours, and infants require about 16 hours. Pregnant women and new mothers, while needing more sleep, usually are sleep deprived. Studies show that sleep disorders occur in 35% to 45% of children 2 to 18 years of age,[13,18] and adolescents and young adults don't get enough sleep, have irregular sleep patterns, and are at risk for problem sleepiness.[15] Menopausal women often report interrupted sleep because of hot flashes or hormonal influences, and older people tend to sleep fewer hours and report less restful sleep and need for more sleep.[1–5,12,13]*

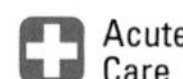

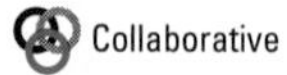

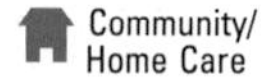

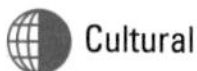

- Determine presence of physical or psychological stressors. *These include multiple, varying factors, such as night-shift work hours or rotating shifts; pain (acute and chronic), current or recent illness, and hospitalization, especially in intensive care unit; death of a spouse or loss of a job; new baby in the home and inadequate sleep-promoting behaviors; etc.*
- Note presence of diagnoses *that are known to affect sleep (e.g., mental confusion or dementias, certain brain infections [e.g., encephalitis], brain injury, narcolepsy; chronic pain; obsessive/compulsive disorder, anxiety, depression, other major psychological disorders; drug or alcohol abuse; restless leg syndrome; sleep-induced respiratory disorders—sleep-disordered breathing, obstructive sleep apnea, childhood snoring with sleep apnea).*[4,5,20]
- Evaluate medication regimen for products affecting sleep. *Diet pills or other stimulants, sedatives, antidepressants, antihypertensives, diuretics, narcotics, agents with anticholinergic effects,* and need for medications requiring nighttime dosing *can inhibit getting to sleep or remaining asleep.*[6,7,17]
- Note environmental factors *affecting sleep (e.g., unfamiliar or uncomfortable sleep environment, excessive noise and light, frequent checking of vital signs, uncomfortable temperature, roommate irritations or actions—snoring, watching television late at night) that impair falling or staying asleep. Note: Clients in critical care units are known to experience lack of sleep or frequent disruptions, often compounding their illness.*[7]
- Determine presence of parasomnias: nightmares or terrors, sleepwalking or talking, or other complex behaviors during sleep. *May occur at any age, with as many as 30% of children (peak age 4 to 8 years) having a sleep disorder at some time.*[17] Note reports of terror, brief periods of paralysis, and sense of body being disconnected from the brain. *Occurrence of sleep paralysis, though not widely recognized in the United States, has been well documented elsewhere and may result in feelings of fear and reluctance to go to sleep. May require more extensive evaluation for serious sleep disorders.*[8,14]

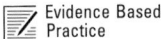

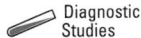

NURSING PRIORITY NO. 2 To assess degree of impairment:

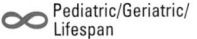

- Assess client's usual sleep patterns and current sleep disturbance, relying on client's/significant other's (SO's) report of problem. Incorporate screening information into in-depth sleep diary or testing if needed. *Usual sleep patterns are individual, but sleep loss has been shown to be the most common complaint reported in primary care settings;*[3,9] *therefore, screening for the problem should be routine. Data collected from a comprehensive assessment is needed to determine etiology of challenging sleep disturbances, including the stage of sleep that is impaired.*[7]
- Ascertain quality of sleep for bed partner/family members. *Loud irregular snoring (sleep apnea), periodic nightmares or sleep terrors, sleep talking, sleepwalking, or involuntary muscle activity can interfere with sleep of bed partner/entire family.*[17]
- Determine client's sleep expectations. *Individual may have faulty beliefs or attitudes about sleep and unrealistic sleep expectations (e.g., "I must get 8 hours of sleep every night, or I can't accomplish anything").*[9]
- Ascertain duration of current problem and effect on life and functional ability. *Client may not get enough sleep and not realize that life functioning is being impaired (e.g., can't concentrate in school, falls asleep when stopped at a light while driving).*[9]
- Listen to subjective reports of sleep quality (e.g., "short, interrupted") and response from lack of good sleep (feeling foggy, sleepy, and woozy; fighting sleep; fatigue). *Helps clarify client's perception of sleep quantity and quality and response to inadequate sleep.*[9]
- Observe for physical signs of fatigue. *Client may display restlessness, irritability, disorientation, frequent yawning, and/or other changes in mood, behavior, or performance (e.g., inability to tolerate stress, problems with concentration or learning). Fatigue, daytime sleepiness, and functional impairment have been reported as significant problems in teens and the elderly.*[2,3,9,12,17,21]
- Determine interventions client has tried to date. *Helps identify appropriate options and may reveal additional interventions that can be attempted.*
- Distinguish client's beneficial bedtime habits from detrimental ones *(e.g., drinking milk in the late evening [instead of coffee], restricting fluid intake, avoiding stimulating exercise, watching TV in bed, eliminating afternoon naps).*

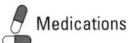

- Instruct client and/or bed partner to keep a sleep-wake log *to document symptoms and identify factors that are interfering with sleep.*
- Obtain a chronological chart *to determine client's peak performance and sleep rhythms.*
- Investigate anxious feelings *to help determine basis and appropriate anxiety-reduction techniques or behavioral therapy needs.*[17,21]

NURSING PRIORITY NO. 3 To assist client to establish optimal sleep pattern :[1,3,6,7,9–11,18,21]

- Review medications being taken and their effect on sleep, suggesting modifications in regimen *if medications are found to be interfering.*
- Encourage client to restrict caffeine and other stimulating substances from late-afternoon and evening intake. Recommend avoidance of bedtime alcohol. *Alcohol and some medications can produce immediate sleep followed by early awakening or difficulty remaining asleep.*
- Avoid eating large evening or late-night meals.
- Recommend light bedtime snack (protein, simple carbohydrate, low fat) and/or glass of warm milk for individuals who feel hungry, ingested 15 to 30 min before retiring. *Sense of fullness and satiety can encourage sleep.*
- Limit evening fluid intake if nocturia is present *to reduce need for nighttime elimination.*
- Promote adequate physical exercise activity during day, finishing workout at least 3 hr before bedtime. *Enhances expenditure of energy and release of tension so that client feels ready for sleep or rest. Note: Rigorous exercise close to bedtime can delay onset of sleep.*
- Suggest abstaining from daytime naps or napping in the morning *to improve ability to fall asleep at night.*
- Recommend quiet relaxing activities prior to bedtime such as reading, listening to soothing music, and meditation to *reduce stimulation and promote relaxation.*
- Discuss or implement effective age-appropriate bedtime rituals (e.g., going to bed at same time each night, brushing teeth, reading, drinking warm milk, rocking, story reading, cuddling, favorite blanket or toy) *to enhance client's ability to fall asleep, reinforce that bed is a place to sleep, and promote sense of security for child.*
- Provide back massage or other therapeutic touching activities, as appropriate. *Touch can be relaxing and emotionally pleasing, given that the client has SO's undivided attention for a few moments.*
- Provide calm, quiet environment for client, *to manage controllable sleep-disrupting factors (e.g., reduce noise and talking, dim lights, shut room door, adjust room temperature as needed, silence or reduce volume on phones, beepers, alarms, television, radios).*
- Administer pain medication first *to make sure client is pain-free* and then sedatives or other sleep medications *(so that hypnotic will be more effective)* when indicated, noting client's response. Time pain medications for peak effect and duration *to reduce need for redosing during prime sleep hours.*
- Discuss appropriate use of benzodiazepines when indicated. *May be useful in some clients for reducing risk of injury associated with sleepwalking or for management of severe sleep terrors. When possible, avoid use of longer-acting benzodiazepines in the elderly, as they are associated with prolonged sedation and increased risk of falls.*[17,21]
- Instruct client to get out of bed, leave bedroom, and engage in relaxing activities *if unable to fall asleep* and not return to bed until feeling sleepy.
- Recommend and instruct client in relaxation techniques (e.g., visualization, breathing, yoga).
- Refer for biofeedback, cognitive therapy, etc., *when measures that are more intensive are needed or desired to cope with stressors and promote relaxation.*
- Collaborate with healthcare team for evaluation and treatment of more serious sleep problems (e.g., obstructive sleep apnea, narcolepsy, sleep paralysis, bed-wetting, nocturnal leg cramps, restless leg syndrome).[13,14,16,17]
- Refer to physician and/or sleep specialist for evaluation and management of obstructive sleep apnea, such as medical or surgical treatment of obesity, medications and/or structural surgery (e.g., alteration of facial

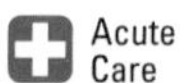
Acute Care
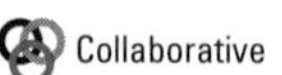
Collaborative
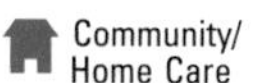
Community/ Home Care
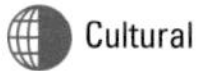
Cultural

structures, removal of tonsils and adenoids in children),[16] or apnea/oxygenation therapy (continuous positive airway pressure, such as Respironics), *when sleep apnea is severe as documented by sleep-disorder studies.*[22]

NURSING PRIORITY NO. 4 To promote wellness (Teaching/Discharge Considerations):

- Review possibility of next-day drowsiness or "rebound" insomnia and temporary memory loss *that may be associated with sleep disorders and prescription sleep medications.*
- Discuss short-term use and appropriateness of over-the-counter sleep medications or herbal supplements. Note possible side effects and drug interactions.
- Identify appropriate safety precautions (e.g., securing doors, windows, and stairways; placing client bedroom on first floor) and attach audible alarm to bedroom door *to alert parents when child is sleepwalking.*[16]
- Refer to support group or counselor *to help deal with psychological stressors (e.g., grief, sorrow, chronic pain).* (Refer to NDs Grieving, chronic Sorrow, and chronic Pain.)
- Encourage family counseling as indicated *to help deal with concerns arising from parasomnias (e.g., sleep talking, sleepwalking, night terrors).*
- Refer to sleep specialist for sleep studies *when problem is unresponsive to customary interventions.*

DOCUMENTATION FOCUS

Assessment/Reassessment
- Assessment findings, including specifics of sleep pattern (current and past) and effects on lifestyle/level of functioning.
- Medications used, interventions tried, previous therapies.
- Family history of similar problem.
- Effects of sleep disturbance on SO/family.

Planning
- Plan of care and who is involved in planning.
- Teaching plan.

Implementation/Evaluation
- Client's response to interventions, teaching, and actions performed.
- Attainment or progress toward desired outcome(s).
- Modifications to plan of care.

Discharge Planning
- Long-term needs and who is responsible for actions to be taken.
- Specific referrals made.

References

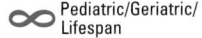

1. Mindell, J. (1997). *Sleeping Through the Night: How Infants, Toddlers, and Their Parents Can Get a Good Night's Sleep.* New York: HarperCollins.
2. National Sleep Foundation. (2000). Adolescent sleep needs and patterns: Research report and resource guide. Retrieved November 2015 from http://sleepfoundation.org/sites/default/files/sleep_and_teens_report1.pdf.
3. National Sleep Foundation. Do women need more sleep than men? Retrieved November 2015 from http://www.sleepfoundation.org/alert/do-women-need-more-sleep-men.
4. Sateia, M. J., Doghramji, K., Hauri, P. J., et al. (2000). Evaluation of chronic insomnia: An American Academy of Sleep Medicine review. *Sleep,* 23(2), 243–308.
5. Subcommittee on Obstructive Sleep Apnea Syndrome, American Academy of Pediatrics Section on Pediatric Pulmonology. (2002). Clinical practice guideline: Diagnosis and management of childhood obstructive sleep apnea syndrome. *Pediatrics,* 109(4), 704–712.
6. Barroso, J. (2002). HIV-related fatigue: Nursing interventions to help patients manage. *Am J Nurs,* 102(5), 83–86.

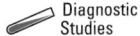

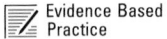

7. Honkus, V. L. (2003). Sleep deprivation in critical care units. *Crit Care Nurs Quart*, 26(3), 179–191.
8. Russo, M. B., Shaikh, S. (Reviewed 2015). Sleep: Understanding the basics. Retrieved November 2015 from http://www.emedicinehealth.com/sleep_understanding_the_basics/article_em.htm.
9. Cochran, H. (2003). Diagnose and treat primary insomnia. *Nurse Pract*, 28(9), 13–27.
10. Pronitis-Ruotolo, D. (2001). Surviving the night shift: Making Zeitgeber work for you. *Am J Nurs*, 101(7), 63–68.
11. Cmiel, C. A. (2004). Noise control: A nursing team's approach to sleep promotion. *Am J Nurs*, 104(2), 40–48.
12. National Agricultural Safety Database. (No date). Sleep deprivation: Cause and consequences. Fact sheet for Nebraska Rural Health and Safety Coalition. Retrieved November 2015 from http://nasdonline.org/document/871/d000705/sleep-deprivation-causes-and-consequences.html.
13. Neuspiel, D. R., Stubbs, E. H. (Updated 2015). Nightmare Disorder. Retrieved November 2015 from http://emedicine.medscape.com/article/914428-overview.
14. Derrer, D. T. (Reviewer). (2014). Sleep disorders and parasomnias. Retrieved November 2015 from http://www.webmd.com/sleep-disorders/guide/parasomnias.
15. National Sleep Foundation Sleep and Teens Task Force. (2000). *Adolescent Sleep Needs and Patterns: Research Report and Resource Guide*. Washington, DC: National Sleep Foundation, 2–4.
16. Garcia, J., Wills, L. (2002). Sleep disorders in children and teens: Helping patients and their families get some sleep. *Postgrad Med*, 107(3), 161–188.
17. Schenck, C. H., Mahowald, M. W. (2002). Parasomnias: Managing bizarre sleep-related behavior disorders. *Postgrad Med*, 107(3), 145–160.
18. Davis, C. P. (Reviewer). (2014). Sleep disorders: A visual guide: Slideshow. Retrieved November 2015 from http://www.medicinenet.com/sleep_disorders_pictures_slideshow/article.htm.
19. Aldabal, L., Bahammam, A. S. (2011). Metabolic, endocrine, and immune consequences of sleep deprivation. *Open Respir Med J*, 5, 31–43.
20. Cole, M. G., Dependukuri, N. (2003). Risk factors for depression among the elderly community subjects: A systematic review and meta-analysis. *Am J Psychiatr*, 160(6), 1147–1156.
21. Townsend-Roccichelli, J., Sandford, J. T., VandelWaa, E. (2010). Managing sleep disorders in the elderly. *Am J Primary Health*, 35(5), 30–37.
22. Barthlen, G. M. (2002). Sleep disorders: Obstructive sleep apnea, restless leg syndrome, and insomnia in geriatric patients. *Geriatrics*, 57(11), 34–39.

disturbed Sleep Pattern

Taxonomy II: Activity/Rest—Class 1 Sleep/Rest (00198) [**Diagnostic Division:** Activity/Rest], Submitted 1980; Revised 1998 2006.

DEFINITION: Time-limited interruptions of sleep amount and quality due to external factors.

RELATED FACTORS

Environmental barrier (e.g., ambient temperature/humidity, daylight/darkness exposure, ambient noise, unfamiliar setting); immobilization
Nonrestorative sleep pattern (i.e., due to caregiver responsibilities, parenting practices, sleep partner)
Insufficient privacy; disruption caused by sleep partner

DEFINING CHARACTERISTICS

Subjective

Difficulty initiating sleep; unintentional awakening
Feeling unrested; dissatisfaction with sleep

Objective

Alteration in sleep pattern
Difficulty in daily functioning
Sample Clinical Applications: Hospitalized or long-term care client, ill family member

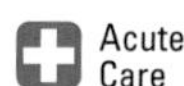

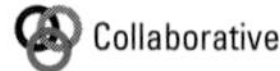

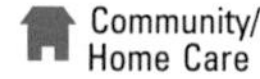

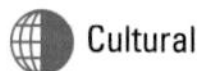

DESIRED OUTCOMES/EVALUATION CRITERIA

Sample NOC linkages:

Sleep: Natural periodic suspension of consciousness during which the body is restored

Comfort Status: Environment: Environmental ease, comfort, and safety of surroundings

Client Will (Include Specific Time Frame)

- Report improved sleep.
- Report increased sense of well-being and feeling rested.
- Identify individually appropriate interventions to promote sleep.

ACTIONS/INTERVENTIONS

Sample NIC linkages:

Sleep Enhancement: Facilitation of regular sleep/wake cycles

Environmental Management: Comfort: Manipulation of the patient's surroundings for promotion of optimal comfort

NURSING PRIORITY NO. 1 To assess causative/contributing factors:

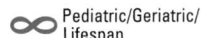

- Identify presence of factors known to interfere with sleep, including current illness or hospitalization, new baby or sick family member in home, etc. *Sleep problems can arise from internal and external factors and may require assessment over time to differentiate specific cause(s). Note: Unresolved long-term disturbances in sleep are thought to be associated with dysfunction of the immune system, interference with wound healing, neurological and behavioral changes, and significant impairment of quality of life.*[1,10] Refer to ND Sleep Deprivation.
- Ascertain presence of short-term alteration in sleep patterns, such as can occur with travel (jet-lag), sharing bed with new sleep partner, fighting with family member, crisis at work, loss of job, or death in family. *Helps identify circumstances that are known to interrupt sleep acutely but do not necessarily represent long-term conditions. These situations may require short-term interventions but are often resolved over time.*[2]
- Note environmental factors, such as unfamiliar or uncomfortable room, excessive noise and light, uncomfortable temperature, frequent medical and monitoring interventions, and roommate actions (e.g., snoring, watching television late at night, wanting to talk). *These factors can reduce client's ability to rest and sleep at a time when more rest is needed. Note: Clients in critical care units are known to experience lack of sleep or frequent disruptions, often compounding their illness.*[3]

NURSING PRIORITY NO. 2 To evaluate sleep and degree of dysfunction:

- Assess client's usual sleep patterns and compare with current sleep disturbance, relying on client's/significant other's report of problem *to ascertain intensity and duration of problems.*
- Listen to reports of sleep quality (e.g., "short, interrupted") and response from lack of good sleep (e.g., feeling foggy, sleepy, and woozy; fighting sleep; fatigue). *Helps clarify client's perception of sleep quantity and quality and response to inadequate sleep.*[4]
- Determine client's sleep expectations. *Individual may have faulty beliefs or attitudes about sleep and/or unrealistic sleep expectations (e.g., "I must get 8 hours of sleep every night, or I can't accomplish anything").*[4]
- Observe for physical signs of fatigue (e.g., restlessness, hand tremors, thick speech, drooping eyes, inattention, lack of interest in activities).
- Incorporate screening information into in-depth sleep diary or testing if needed. *Information collected from a comprehensive assessment may be needed to evaluate the type and etiology of sleep disturbance and identify useful treatment options.*[4,5]

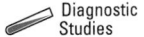

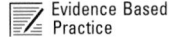

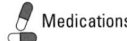

NURSING PRIORITY NO. 3 To assist client to establish optimal sleep/rest patterns:

- Manage environment for hospitalized client:[1,3,6,7]
  Adjust ambient lighting *to maintain daytime light and nighttime dark.*
  Provide privacy as indicated, such as requesting visitors to leave, closing room door, "quiet, patient sleeping" sign, etc.
  Encourage usual bedtime activities such as washing face and hands and brushing teeth.
  Provide bedtime care such as straightening bed sheets, changing damp linens or gown, and back massage *to promote physical comfort.*
  Turn on soft music, calm TV program, or quiet environment, as client prefers, *to enhance relaxation.*
  Minimize sleep-disrupting factors (e.g., shut room door; adjust room temperature as needed; reduce talking and other disturbing noises such as phones, beepers, alarms). *Studies show that use of these interventions can promote readiness for sleep and improve sleep duration and quality.*[8]
  Perform monitoring and care activities without waking client whenever possible. *Allows for longer periods of uninterrupted sleep, especially during night.*
  Avoid or limit use of physical restraints in accordance with client's needs and facility policy.
- Refer to physician or sleep specialist as indicated *for specific interventions and/or therapies, including medications and biofeedback.*
- Refer to NDs Insomnia and Sleep Deprivation for related interventions and rationale.

NURSING PRIORITY NO. 4 To promote optimal sleep (Teaching/Discharge Considerations):

- Assure client that occasional sleeplessness should not threaten health and that resolving time-limited situation can restore healthful sleep. *Knowledge that occasional insomnia is universal and usually not harmful may promote relaxation and relief from worry, which can perpetuate the problem.*[9]
- Problem solve immediate needs. *Short-term solutions (e.g., sleeping in different rooms if partner's illness is keeping client awake, acquiring a fan if sleeping quarters are too warm, getting a substitute to provide care to ill family member so client can get a good night's rest) may be needed until client adjusts to situation or crisis is resolved, with resulting return to more usual sleep pattern.*
- Encourage appropriate indoor light settings during day and night, especially exposure to bright light or sunlight in the morning; avoidance of daytime napping as appropriate for age and situation; and being active during day and more passive in evening. *Helps in promotion of normal sleep-wake patterns.*[6,9]
- Encourage use of aids to block out light and sound, such as sleep mask, room-darkening shades, earplugs, and white noise.[7]
- Discuss use and appropriateness of over-the-counter sleep medications or herbal supplements *to provide assistance in falling and staying asleep.*

DOCUMENTATION FOCUS

Assessment/Reassessment

- Assessment findings, including specifics of sleep pattern (current and past) and effects on lifestyle and level of functioning.
- Specific interventions, medications, or previously tried therapies.

Planning

- Plan of care and who is involved in planning.
- Teaching plan.

Implementation/Evaluation

- Response to interventions, teaching, and actions performed.
- Attainment or progress toward desired outcome(s).
- Modifications to plan of care.

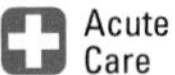

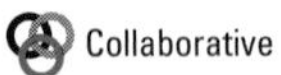

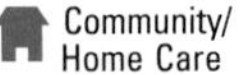

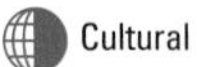

Discharge Planning

- Long-term needs and who is responsible for actions to be taken.
- Available resources, specific referrals made.

References

1. Weinhouse, G. L., Schwab, R. J. (2006). Sleep in the critically ill patient. *Sleep*, 29(5), 707–716.
2. Schutte-Rodin, S., Broch, L., Buysee, D., et al. (2008). Clinical guideline for the evaluation and management of chronic insomnia in adults. *J Clin Sleep Med*, 4(5), 487–504.
3. Patel, M., Chipman, J., Carlin, B. W., et al. (2008). Sleep in the intensive care setting. *Crit Care Nurs Q*, 31(4), 309–318.
4. Cochran, H. (2003). Diagnose and treat primary insomnia. *Nurse Pract*, 28(9), 13–27.
5. Honkus, V. L. (2003). Sleep deprivation in critical care units. *Crit Care Nurs Q*, 26(3), 179–191.
6. Cole, C., Richards, K. (2007). Sleep disruption in older adults. *Am J Nurs*, 107(5), 40–49.
7. Floyd, J. A. (2008). Sleep enhancement. In Ackley, B. J., Ladwig, G. B., Swan, B. A., et al. (eds). *Evidence-Based Nursing Care Guidelines: Medical-Surgical Interventions*. St. Louis, MO: Mosby Elsevier.
8. Olson, D. M., Borel, C. O., Laskowitz, D. T., et al. (2001). Quiet time: A nursing intervention to promote sleep in neurocritical care units. *Am J Crit Care*, 10(2), 74–78.
9. National Institute of Neurological Disorders and Stroke. (Updated 2014). Brain basics. Understanding sleep. Retrieved November 2015 from http://www.ninds.nih.gov/disorders/brain_basics/understanding_sleep.htm.
10. Aldabal, L., Bahammam, A. S. (2011). Metabolic, endocrine, and immune consequences of sleep deprivation. *Open Respir Med J*, 5, 31–43.

impaired Social Interaction

Taxonomy II: Role Relationships—Class 3 Role Performance (00052) [**Diagnostic Division:** Social Interaction], Submitted 1986

DEFINITION: Insufficient or excessive quantity or ineffective quality of social exchange.

RELATED FACTORS

Insufficient knowledge about ways to enhance mutuality
Insufficient skills to enhance mutuality
Communication barrier
Disturbance of self-concept
Absence of significant other
Impaired mobility
Therapeutic isolation
Sociocultural dissonance
Environmental barrier
Disturbance in thought processes

DEFINING CHARACTERISTICS

Subjective

Discomfort in social situations
Dissatisfaction with social engagement (e.g., belonging, caring, interest, shared history)
Family reports change in interaction (e.g., style, pattern)

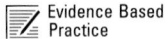

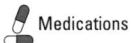

(continues on page 808)

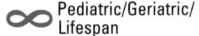

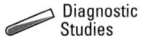

impaired Social Interaction (continued)

Objective

Impaired social functioning

Dysfunctional interaction with others

Sample Clinical Applications: Brain injury, stroke, cancer, neuromuscular disease (e.g., multiple sclerosis [MS]), cerebral palsy, substance abuse, Alzheimer's disease, schizophrenia, autism

DESIRED OUTCOMES/EVALUATION CRITERIA

Sample NOC linkages:

Social Interaction Skills: Personal behaviors that promote effective relationships

Child Development: (specify 6–11 years or 12–17): Milestones of physical, cognitive, and psychosocial progression by [specify] years of age

Social Involvement: Social interactions with persons, groups, or organizations

Client Will (Include Specific Time Frame)

- Verbalize awareness of factors causing or promoting impaired social interactions.
- Identify feelings that lead to poor social interactions.
- Express desire or be involved in achieving positive changes in social behaviors and interpersonal relationships.
- Give self positive reinforcement for changes that are achieved.
- Develop effective social support system; use available resources appropriately.

ACTIONS/INTERVENTIONS

Sample NIC linkages:

Socialization Enhancement: Facilitation of another person's ability to interact with others

Behavior Modification: Social Skills: Assisting the patient to develop or improve interpersonal social skills

Complex Relationship Building: Establishing a therapeutic relationship with a patient to promote insight and behavioral change

NURSING PRIORITY NO. 1 To assess causative/contributing factors:

- Review social history with client/significant others (SO[s]) and go back far enough in time to note when changes in social behavior or patterns of relating occurred or began. *For example, loss or long-term illness of loved one; failed relationships; loss of occupation, financial, or political (power) position; change in status in family hierarchy (job loss, aging, illness); and poor coping or adjustment to developmental stage of life, as with marriage, birth or adoption of child, or children leaving home are situations that may affect quality of social exchange.*[1]
- Ascertain ethnic, cultural, or religious implications for the client. *These factors can dictate choice of behaviors and may even script interactions with others. Client may perceive behaviors as normal because of belief system or may have conflict regarding behaviors that may not be accepted by larger society.*[1,5,6]
- Review medical history, noting stressors of physical or long-term illness (e.g., stroke, cancer, MS, head injury, Alzheimer's disease), mental illness (e.g., schizophrenia), medications, substance use, debilitating accidents, learning disabilities (e.g., sensory integration difficulties, autism spectrum disorder, Asperger's disorder), and emotional disabilities. *Conditions such as these can isolate individual who feels disconnected from others, resulting in difficulty relating in social situations.*[3,4]
- Note presence of visual or hearing impairments. *Individuals with these conditions may find communication barriers are increased, social interaction is affected, and interventions need to be designed to promote involvement with others in positive ways.*[1,3]

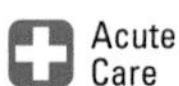

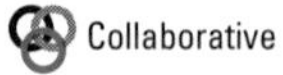

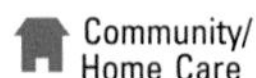

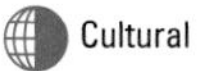

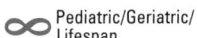

- Determine family patterns of relating and social behaviors. Explore possible family scripting of behavioral expectations in the children and how the client was affected. *Parents are important in teaching their children social skills (e.g., sharing, taking turns, allowing others to talk without interrupting). Family may not have effective patterns of relating to others, and the child learns these skills in this setting. Often child reflects family expectations rather than own desires, which may result in conforming or rebellious behaviors.*[2,6,10]
- Observe client while relating to family/SO(s) and note observations of prevalent patterns. *Identification of patterns will help with plan for change.*[2]
- Encourage client to verbalize feeling of discomfort about social situations. Note any causative factors, recurring precipitating patterns, and barriers to using support systems. *Identifies areas of concern and suggests possible ways to learn new skills.*[2]

NURSING PRIORITY NO. 2 To assess degree of impairment:

- Encourage client to verbalize perceptions of reasons for problems. Active listen, noting indications of hopelessness, powerlessness, fear, anxiety, grief, anger, feeling unloved or unlovable, problems with sexual identity, and hate (directed or not). *These feelings arise from the anxiety that comes with the need to participate with others in social situations and begin to interfere with work, friendships, and life in general.*[5,7]
- Observe and describe social and interpersonal behaviors in objective terms, noting speech patterns and body language (1) in the therapeutic setting and (2) in normal areas of daily functioning (if possible), including family, job, and social or entertainment settings. *Provides information about extent of anxiety client experiences in different settings and suggests possible interventions.*[5,7]
- Determine client's use of coping skills and defense mechanisms. *Symptoms associated with social anxiety affect ability to be involved in social situations, making client's life miserable and seriously interfering with work, friendships, and family life.*[5,7]
- Evaluate possibility of client being the victim of or using destructive behaviors against self or others. (Refer to ND risk for other-directed/self-directed Violence.) *Problems of poor communication lead to frustration and anger, leaving the individual with few coping skills, and may result in destructive behaviors.*[1,2,10]
- Interview family, SO(s), friends, spiritual leaders, coworkers, as appropriate. *Obtaining observations of client's behavioral changes from others associated with the individual provides a broader view of actual problems and how behavior affects client's life/others.*[5]

NURSING PRIORITY NO. 3 To assist client/SO(s) to recognize/make positive changes in impaired social and interpersonal interactions:

- Establish therapeutic relationship using positive regard for the person, active listening, and providing safe environment for self-disclosure. *Client who is having difficulty interacting in social situations needs to feel comfortable and accepted before he or she is willing to talk about self and concerns.*[1,2]
- Have client list behaviors that cause discomfort. *Anxiety usually has physical symptoms (e.g., a racing heart, dry mouth, shaky voice, blushing, sweating, nausea), and once it is recognized, client can choose to begin treatment to change.*[5,7]
- Have family/SO(s) list client's behaviors that are causing discomfort for them. *Anxiety is contagious, and by identifying specific behaviors, all members of the family can begin to deal appropriately with them so they are diminished.*[5,7]
- Review negative behaviors observed previously by caregivers, coworkers, etc. *Others may see behaviors and the problems associated with them, such as unwillingness to participate in necessary activities (eating in a public place, interviewing for a job) and may provide additional information needed to develop an appropriate plan of care.*[1]
- Compare lists and validate reality of perceptions. Help client prioritize those behaviors needing change. *Each individual may have a different view of what constitutes a problem, and by comparing lists, each person hears how others view the problems, enabling the client/family to identify behaviors or concerns to be dealt with.*[1,7]

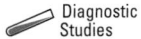

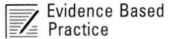

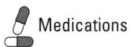

- Explore with client and role-play means of making agreed-on changes in social interactions or behaviors (as determined earlier). *Client needs to learn social skills if he or she has never learned the elements of interacting with others in social settings. Role-playing one-on-one is less threatening and can help individual identify with another and practice new social skills.*[5]
- Role-play random social situations in therapeutically controlled environment with "safe" therapy group. Have group note behaviors, both positive and negative, and discuss these and any changes needed. *Having client participate in a controlled group environment provides opportunities to try out different behaviors in a built-in social setting where members can make friends and provide mutual advice and comfort.*[1,5]
- Role-play changes and discuss impact. Include family/SO(s) as indicated. *Provides opportunity for person to recognize changes in feelings and behavior and enhances comfort with new behaviors.*[4]
- Provide positive reinforcement for improvement in social behaviors and interactions. *Encourages continuation of desired behaviors and efforts for change.*[5]
- Participate in multidisciplinary client-centered conferences *to evaluate progress*. Involve everyone associated with client's care, family members, SO(s), and therapy group. *These conferences have the advantage of providing information from and to each participant in an atmosphere of trust where questions can be asked, decisions can be made, and goals for the future can be agreed on.*[1]
- Work with the client to alleviate underlying negative self-concepts *because they often impede positive social interactions. By replacing negative thoughts with positive messages, client can reduce anxiety and develop a positive sense of self-esteem. While this is not an easy process, the rewards are great when client is willing to practice consistently.*[2]
- Involve neurologically impaired client in individual or group interactions as situation allows. *Individual may not be able to interact appropriately because of disabilities, but involvement in the group provides an opportunity to practice and relearn skills to enable reintegration into social situations.*[1,8]
- Refer for family therapy as indicated. *Social behaviors and interpersonal relationships involve more than the individual, and family may need additional help to resolve ongoing family problems.*[1,2]

NURSING PRIORITY NO. 4 To promote wellness (Teaching/Discharge Considerations):

- Encourage client to keep a daily journal in which social interactions of each day can be reviewed and the comfort or discomfort experienced noted with possible causes or precipitating factors. *Helps client to identify specific problem areas and begin to choose to take responsibility for own behavior(s).*[5,7]
- Assist the client to develop positive social skills through practice of skills in real social situations accompanied by a support person. Provide positive feedback with the use of "I" messages during interactions with client. *Cognitive and behavioral methods can help individuals overcome fears with the help of a trusted person. "I" messages convey a positive message, individual does not feel criticized, and he or she is encouraged to continue new thinking and behaviors.*[1,5]
- Discuss the use of medications when indicated and monitor for effectiveness and side effects. *Several kinds of drugs have been found to be effective in the treatment of social anxiety problems; selective serotonin reuptake inhibitors (SSRIs), such as paroxetine (Paxil) and sertraline (Zoloft), are often the first choice. Antianxiety drugs, such as clonazepam (Klonopin), buspirone (BusPar), and alprazolam (Xanax), can reduce anxiety and may be used alone or in conjunction with SSRIs. Propranolol (Inderal) has been found to be useful for performance anxiety, and when taken an hour before the scheduled event, may suppress the physical symptoms of anxiety.*[5,7]
- Seek community programs for client involvement that promote positive behaviors the client is striving to achieve. *Encouraging reading materials, attending classes, community support groups, and lectures for self-help can help to alleviate negative self-concepts that lead to impaired social interactions.*[2,5]
- Involve in a music-based program, if available (e.g., the Listening Program). *There is a direct correlation between the musical portion of the brain and the language area, and the use of these programs may result in better communication skills. It is theorized that the use of music increases function of the middle ear muscles as a portal to the social engagement system.*[9]

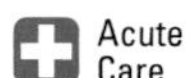

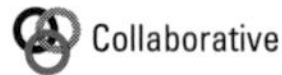

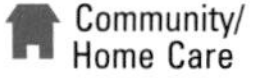

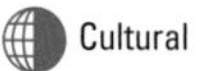

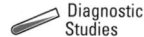

- Encourage ongoing family or individual therapy as long as it is promoting growth and positive change. Be alert to possibility of therapy being used as a crutch. *While therapy groups can be useful, individuals can become dependent on the process and not move on to managing on their own.*[1]
- Provide for occasional follow-up for reinforcement of positive behaviors after professional relationship has ended. *Change is difficult and identifying problems that may arise during these contacts can enhance maintenance and enable client/family to continue to progress.*[2]
- Refer to psychiatric clinical nurse specialist when indicated. *May need additional assistance to promote long-term change.*[1]

DOCUMENTATION FOCUS

Assessment/Reassessment

- Individual findings, including factors affecting interactions, nature of social exchanges, specifics of individual behaviors, and type of learning disability present.
- Cultural or religious beliefs and expectations.
- Perceptions and response of others.

Planning

- Plan of care and who is involved in the planning.
- Teaching plan.

Implementation/Evaluation

- Responses to interventions, teaching, and actions performed.
- Attainment or progress toward desired outcome(s).
- Modifications to plan of care.

Discharge Planning

- Long-term needs and who is responsible for actions to be taken.
- Community resources, specific referrals made.

References

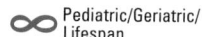

1. Townsend, M. C. (2003). *Psychiatric Mental Health Nursing Concepts of Care*. 4th ed. Philadelphia: F. A. Davis.
2. Doenges, M. E., Townsend, M. C., Moorhouse, M. F. (1998). *Psychiatric Care Plans: Guidelines for Individualizing Care*. 3rd ed. Philadelphia: F. A. Davis.
3. Cox, H., Hinz, M. D., Lubno, M. A., et al. (2002). *Clinical Applications of Nursing Diagnosis: Adult, Child, Women's, Psychiatric, Gerontic, and Home Health Considerations*. 4th ed. Philadelphia: F. A. Davis.
4. Drew, N. (1991). Combating the social isolation of chronic mental illness. *J Psychosoc Nurs*, 29(6), 14–17.
5. No author listed. (2003). Beyond shyness and stage fright: Social anxiety disorder. *Harv Ment Health Lett*, 20(3), 1–4.
6. Purnell, L. D. (2011). *Guide to Culturally Competent Health Care*. 2nd ed. Philadelphia: F. A. Davis.
7. No author listed. (2012). Generalized anxiety disorder. *Encyclopedia of Mental Disorders*. Retrieved November 2015 from http://www.minddisorders.com/Flu-Inv/Generalized-anxiety-disorder.html.
8. Beck, T. J., Bellis, T. J. (2007). (Central) auditory processing disorders: Overview and amplifications. *Hearing J*, 60(5), 44–47.
9. Advanced Brain Technologies. (2012). The listening program. Retrieved November 2015 from http://a.advancedbrain.com/tlp/the_listening_program.jsp.
10. Olsen, G., Fuller, M. L. (Updated 2010). Family interactions patterns: Bullying and victimization in children. Retrieved November 2015 from http://www.education.com/reference/article/family-interaction-patterns-bullying/.

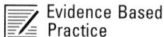

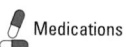

Social Isolation

Taxonomy II: Comfort—Class 3 Social Comfort (00053) [**Diagnostic Division:** Social Interaction], Submitted 1982

DEFINITION: Aloneness experienced by the individual and perceived as imposed by others and as a negative or threatening state.

RELATED FACTORS

Factors impacting satisfying personal relationships (e.g., developmental delay); developmentally inappropriate interests
Alteration in physical appearance, mental status
Alteration in wellness
Social behavior incongruent with norms; values incongruent with cultural norms
Insufficient personal resources (e.g., poor achievement, poor insight, affect unavailable and poorly controlled)
Inability to engage in satisfying personal relationships

DEFINING CHARACTERISTICS

Subjective

Aloneness imposed by others
Insecurity in public; desires to be alone
Inability to meet expectations of others; purposelessness
Developmentally inappropriate interests; values incongruent with cultural norms
Feeling different from others

Objective

Absence of support system; history of rejection
Sad or flat affect; withdrawn; poor eye contact
Disabling condition; illness
Developmental delay
Preoccupation with own thoughts; repetitive or meaningless actions; hostility
Cultural incongruence; member of a subculture;
Sample Clinical Applications: Traumatic injuries, facial scarring/acne, chemotherapy, AIDS, dementia, major depression, conduct disorder, developmental delay, paranoid disorders, schizophrenia

DESIRED OUTCOMES/EVALUATION CRITERIA

Sample NOC linkages:

Social Involvement: Social interactions with persons, groups, or organizations
Loneliness Severity: Severity of emotional, social, or existential isolation response
Social Support: Reliable assistance from others

Client Will (Include Specific Time Frame)

- Identify causes and actions to correct isolation.
- Verbalize willingness to be involved with others.
- Participate in activities or programs at level of ability or desire.
- Express increased sense of self-worth.

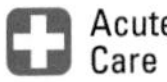
Acute Care
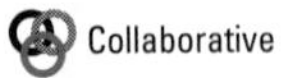
Collaborative
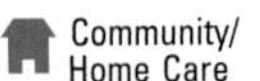
Community/ Home Care
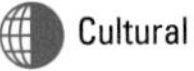
Cultural

ACTIONS/INTERVENTIONS

Sample NIC linkages:
Socialization Enhancement: Facilitation of another person's ability to interact with others
Behavior Management: Social Skills: Assisting the patient to develop or improve interpersonal social skills
Visitation Facilitation: Promoting beneficial visits by family and friends

NURSING PRIORITY NO. 1 To assess causative/contributing factors:

- Determine presence of factors as listed in Related Factors and other concerns (e.g., elderly, female, adolescent, ethnic or racial minority, economically or educationally disadvantaged, hearing or visually impaired). *Identifying individual factors allows for developing an accurate plan of care for the client.*[5]
- Perform physical exam, paying particular attention to any illnesses identified. *Individuals who are isolated appear to be susceptible to health problems, especially coronary heart disease, although little is understood about why that is.*[10]
- Note onset of physical or mental illness and whether recovery is anticipated or condition is chronic or progressive. *Individual may withdraw from activities because of concern about how others view changes that occur due to illness, concern with own thoughts, and alterations in physical appearance or mental status. Anticipated length of illness may dictate choice of interventions.*[1,4]
- Identify blocks to social contacts. *Reluctance to engage in social activities may be the result of problems such as physical immobility, sensory deficits, housebound for any reason, incontinence, financial constraints, and/or transportation difficulties. Individual may be afraid of what others might think of her or him, be concerned with embarrassing self, or not having money or means of transportation for desired activities.*[1]
- Ascertain implications of cultural values or religious beliefs for the client *that may dictate choice of behaviors and may even script interactions with others. Client may perceive behaviors as normal because of belief system or may have conflict regarding behaviors that may not be accepted by larger society.*[1,5,6]
- Assess factors in client's life that may contribute to sense of helplessness. *Losses, such as a spouse, parent, or other, or presence of chronic pain or other disabling conditions may cause individual to withdraw, desire to be alone, and refuse to participate in therapeutic activities.*[1,3]
- Listen to comments of client regarding sense of isolation. Differentiate isolation from solitude and loneliness *that may be acceptable or by choice. Provides clues to what client is thinking and feeling about current situation. Client who chooses to be alone and is satisfied may not need further intervention. Note: Research indicates that perceived social isolation is a risk factor for, and may contribute to, poorer overall cognitive performance, faster cognitive decline, poorer executive functioning, increased negativity, and heightened sensitivity to social threats. These differences impact on emotions, decisions, behaviors, and interpersonal interactions.*[3,5,11,12]
- Assess client's feelings about self, sense of ability to control situation, sense of hope, and coping skills. *If client is isolating self because of negative feelings, lack of hope, etc., measures to promote self-esteem will need to be taken.*[5]
- Identify support systems available to the client, including presence of/relationship with extended family. *People with social anxiety often do not have support systems because of their withdrawal from contact with others. Often the family of origin may be anxious and does not provide the encouragement and support needed by a temperamentally inhibited child or may be too helpful, enabling client to withdraw further. It is difficult for these individuals to ask for help because they are afraid to meet new people and often find support only when they seek help for other conditions, such as depression.*[4,9]
- Identify behavior response of isolation. *Individual may display behaviors such as excessive sleeping or daydreaming, which also may potentiate isolation.*[7,10]
- Note drug use (prescription and illicit). *Individual may begin to use drugs such as alcohol or cocaine to control anxiety in social situations.*[7]

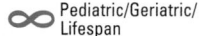

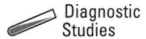

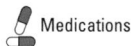

- Review history and elicit information about traumatic events that may have occurred. (Refer to ND Post-Trauma-Syndrome.) *While little is known about the origins of social anxiety disorders, clients who have experienced a traumatic event may withdraw from contact and suffer from anxiety when faced with having to deal with social situations.*[1,5]

NURSING PRIORITY NO. 2 To alleviate conditions that contribute to client's sense of isolation:

- Establish therapeutic nurse-client relationship. *Promotes trust and acceptance, allowing client to feel safe and free to discuss sensitive matters without being judged.*[2]
- Spend time interacting with client and identify other resources available. *Getting to know client and identifying concerns about being involved in activities with others can lead to appropriate interventions. Other people such as volunteers, social workers, and chaplains may be able to spend time with client, enhancing circle of trusted people.*[4]
- Develop plan of action with client. Look at available resources; support risk-taking behaviors, financial planning, appropriate medical and self-care, etc. *Helping client to learn how to manage these issues of daily living can increase self-confidence and help individual to feel more comfortable in social settings.*[5]
- Introduce client to those with similar or shared interests and other supportive people. *Provides role models and encourages getting to know others who share feelings of anxiety, providing an opportunity to develop social skills and learn some ways of problem solving to deal with anxiety.*[2,5]
- Promote participation in recreational or special interest activities in setting that client views as safe. *These activities have the advantage of providing physical and mental stimulation for client who feels isolated and anxious in social settings.*[2,9]
- Provide positive reinforcement when client makes move(s) toward other(s). *Acknowledges and encourages continuation of efforts, helping client toward independence.*[1,7]
- Identify foreign language resources for client who speaks another language. *A professional interpreter is important to ensure accuracy of interpretation; newspapers and radio programming in appropriate foreign language helps client feel connected with own community.*[6,8]
- Assist client to problem solve solutions to short-term or imposed isolation. *Condition may require individual to be isolated from others for his or her and/or others' protection, and working together to decide how to manage loneliness can promote successful outcome.*[1,3]
- Encourage open visitation when possible and/or telephone or computer contacts. *Maintains involvement with others, promoting social involvement, especially when client is unable to go out to activities.*[3]
- Provide environmental stimuli when client is confined. *Open curtains in room, display pictures of family or views of nature, promote television and radio listening, and provide Internet access to help client feel less isolated.*[3]
- Provide for placement in sheltered community when necessary. *The individual who is mentally impaired may be unable to learn to participate in society and display socially acceptable behaviors and will benefit from an environment that offers structure and assistance.*[3]

NURSING PRIORITY NO. 3 To promote wellness (Teaching/Discharge Considerations):

- Assist client to learn social skills as needed. *Enhancing problem solving, communication, social skills, and learning skills to manage activities of daily living will improve sense of self-esteem.*[4]
- Encourage and assist client to enroll in classes as appropriate. *Assertiveness, vocational, and sex education classes may provide skills to improve ability to engage more effectively in social situations.*[5]
- Involve children and adolescents in age-appropriate programs or activities, as indicated. *Promotes socialization skills and peer contact to enable young person to learn by interacting with others.*[5]
- Help client differentiate between isolation and loneliness or aloneness and discuss how to avoid slipping into an undesired state. *Time for the individual to be alone is important to the maintenance of mental health, but the sadness created by isolation and loneliness needs different interventions.*[2,11]
- Involve client in programs directed to correction and prevention of identified causes of problem. *Activities such as senior citizen services, daily telephone contact, house sharing, pets, day-care centers, and church resources can help individual move out of isolation and become involved in life.*[5,10]

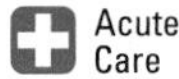

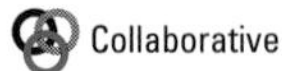

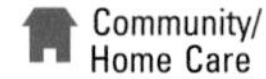

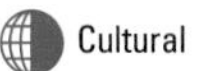

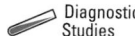

- Discuss use of medications, as indicated. *Prescribed medications, such as selective serotonin reuptake inhibitors, can be very effective in treating social disorders.*[3,7]
- Refer to counselor or therapist, as appropriate. *Facilitates grief work, promotes relationship building, and provides opportunity to work toward improvement of individual issues affecting social interactions.*[1]

DOCUMENTATION FOCUS

Assessment/Reassessment

- Individual findings, including precipitating factors, effect on lifestyle, relationships, and functioning.
- Client's perception of situation.
- Cultural or religious factors.
- Availability and use of resources and support systems.

Planning

- Plan of care and who is involved in planning.
- Teaching plan.

Implementation/Evaluation

- Responses to intervention, teaching, and actions performed.
- Attainment or progress toward desired outcome(s).
- Modifications to plan of care.

Discharge Planning

- Long-term needs and who is responsible for actions to be taken.
- Available resources, specific referrals made.

References

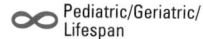

1. Robinson, L., Smith, M., Segal, J., et al. (Updated 2015). Emotional and psychological trauma: Symptoms, treatment and recovery. HelpGuide.org. Retrieved November 2015 from http://www.helpguide.org/articles/ptsd-trauma/emotional-and-psychological-trauma.htm.
2. Doenges, M. E., Townsend, M. C., Moorhouse, M. F. (1998). *Psychiatric Care Plans: Guidelines for Individualizing Care*. 3rd ed. Philadelphia, PA: F. A. Davis.
3. Cox, H., Hinz, M. D., Lubno, M. A., et al. (2002). *Clinical Applications of Nursing Diagnosis: Adult, Child, Women's, Psychiatric, Gerontic, and Home Health Considerations*. 4th ed. Philadelphia: F. A. Davis.
4. Drew, N. (1991). Combating the social isolation of chronic mental illness. *J Psychosoc Nurs*, 29(6), 14–17.
5. No author listed. (2003). Beyond shyness and stage fright: Social anxiety disorder. *HarvMen Health Lett*, 20(4), 1–4.
6. Purnell, L. D. (2011). *Guide to Culturally Competent Health Care*. Philadelphia: F. A. Davis.
7. No author listed. (2012). Generalized anxiety disorder. Encyclopedia of Mental Disorders. Retrieved November 2015 from http://www.minddisorders.com/Flu-Inv/Generalized-anxiety-disorder.html.
8. Andrulis, D. P. (2002). What a Difference an Interpreter Can Make: Health Care Experiences of Uninsured with Limited English Proficiency. *The Access Project*. Boston: Brandeis University.
9. McPherson, M., Smith-Lovin, L., Brashears, M. (2006). Social isolation in U.S.: Changes in core discussion networks over two decades. *Am Sociol Rev*, 71(3), 353–375.
10. House, J. (2001). Social isolation kills, but how and why? *Psychosom Med*, 63(2), 273–274.
11. No author listed. (Updated 2015). Isolation. GoodTherapy.org. Retrieved November 2015 from http://www.goodtherapy.org/therapy-for-isolation.html.
12. Cacioppo, J. T., Hawkley, L. C. (2009). Perceived social isolation and cognition. *Trends Cogn Sci*, 13(10), 447–454.

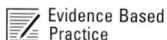

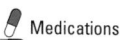

chronic Sorrow

Taxonomy II: Coping/Stress Tolerance—Class 2 Coping Responses (00137) [**Diagnostic Division:** Ego Integrity], Submitted 1998

DEFINITION: Cyclical, recurring, and potentially progressive pattern of pervasive sadness experienced (by a parent, caregiver, individual with chronic illness or disability) in response to continual loss, throughout the trajectory of an illness or disability.

RELATED FACTORS

Death of significant other
Chronic illness or disability (e.g., physical, mental); crises in illness or disability management
Crises related to developmental stage; missed opportunities or milestones
Length of time as a caregiver

DEFINING CHARACTERISTICS

Subjective

Overwhelming negative feelings
Sadness (e.g., periodic, recurrent)
Feelings that interfere with well-being (e.g., personal, social)

Sample Clinical Applications: Cancer, multiple sclerosis (MS), Parkinson's disease, AIDS, amyotrophic lateral sclerosis (ALS), prematurity, genetic or congenital defects, infertility, dementia, Alzheimer's disease, bipolar disorder, schizophrenia, developmental delay

DESIRED OUTCOMES/EVALUATION CRITERIA

Sample NOC linkages:

Depression Level: Severity of level of melancholic mood and loss of interest in life events
Depression Self-Control: Personal actions to minimize melancholy and maintain interest in life events
Hope: Optimism that is personally satisfying and life supporting

Client Will (Include Specific Time Frame)

- Acknowledge presence and impact of sorrow.
- Demonstrate progress in dealing with loss(es) as evidenced by recognizing positive aspects of situation.
- Participate in work and/or self-care activities of daily living (ADLs) as able.
- Verbalize a sense of progress toward resolution of sorrow and hope for the future.

ACTIONS/INTERVENTIONS

Sample NIC linkages:

Mood Management: Providing for safety, stabilization, recovery, and maintenance of a patient who is experiencing dysfunctionally depressed or elevated mood
Grief Work Facilitation: Assistance with the resolution of a significant loss
Hope Inspiration: Enhancing the belief in one's capacity to initiate and sustain actions

NURSING PRIORITY NO. 1 To assess causative/contributing factors and effect on life:

- Determine current or recent events or conditions contributing to client's state of mind, as listed in Related Factors (e.g., death of loved one, chronic physical or mental illness or disability). *Individual information is necessary when formulating a plan of care to address appropriate issues.*[1]

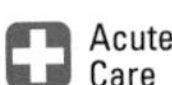

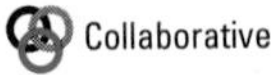

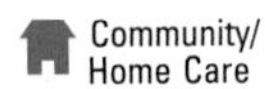

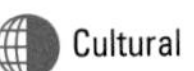

- Note cues of sadness. *Expressions of feelings of loss, such as sighing, faraway looks, unkempt appearance, inattention to conversation, and refusing food, can be indicators of sorrow that is not being dealt with. Note: Chronic sorrow may be cyclical—at times deepening versus times of feeling somewhat better.*[4,5]
- Be aware of use of avoidance behaviors. *Anger, withdrawal, and denial are part of the grieving process and may be used to avoid dealing with the reality of what has happened. However, in a situation that is unchangeable, such as a developmentally disabled child or a child with diabetes, sorrow is seen as a normal response and will continue to be a factor even as the family copes with the condition.*[5,7]
- Identify cultural values or religious beliefs and possible conflicts. *Expressions of sorrow are influenced by these beliefs and may result in conflicts. Or, individual/family may have difficulty living up to the expectations of others (e.g., "God does not give us more than we can handle").*[6]
- Ascertain response of family/SOs to client's situation and support provided. *Parents who have chronically ill children or premature babies, adults who have multiple sclerosis, and elderly caregivers of spouses with dementia may continue to have feelings of sorrow even though they seem to be managing fairly well; due to cyclic nature of sorrow, they will require ongoing support/assistance from others to cope.*[4,7,11]
- Determine level of functioning and ability to care for self/others. Assess needs of family/SO. *Individual who is coping with chronic illness (e.g., Parkinson's disease, MS, HIV/AIDS) may exhibit chronic sorrow related to the illness, fear of death, poverty, and isolation associated with these conditions, which may lead to difficulty managing ADLs for self or meeting needs of family.*[2,3,11]
- Refer to NDs caregiver Role Strain, ineffective Coping, and complicated Grieving, as appropriate.

NURSING PRIORITY NO. 2 To assist client to move through sorrow:

- Encourage verbalization about situation. Active-listen feelings and be available for support and assistance. *Helpful in beginning resolution and acceptance. Individuals involved, client, and caregivers benefit from being able to talk freely about the situation. Active listening conveys a message of acceptance and helps individual come to own resolution.*[1,5]
- Encourage expression of anger, fear, or anxiety. (Refer to appropriate NDs.) *Individual needs to deal with these feelings before she or he can move forward.*[1]
- Acknowledge reality of feelings of guilt or blame, including hostility toward spiritual power. (Refer to ND Spiritual Distress.) *It was believed that grief had an end stage, but research has shown that individuals with chronic conditions, such as diabetes mellitus, MS, and disabling conditions, continue to experience chronic sorrow and lifelong recurring sadness. Understanding this can help individual accept that these feelings are real, and when they are validated, they can be dealt with.*[4,5,10]
- Provide comfort and availability as well as caring for physical needs. *The way healthcare professionals respond to families is important to helping them cope with the situation as physical care is given.*[5,9,11]
- Discuss ways individual has dealt with past losses and reinforce use of previously effective coping skills. *As client begins to look at how they have handled previous situations, effective coping skills can be recalled and applied to current situation.*[2,9]
- Instruct in and encourage use of visualization and relaxation skills. *Learning these stress-management skills can help the individual relax, enhancing ability to deal with feelings of sorrow regarding the long-term situation.*[5,8]
- Discuss use of medication when depression is interfering with ability to manage life. *Client may benefit from the short-term use of an antidepressant medication to help with dealing with situation.*[1]
- Assist SOs to cope with client response. *Family/SO may not be dysfunctional, but may be intolerant and lack understanding of individual responses to long-term illness. Grief is unique to each individual and may not always follow a particular course to resolution that is understood by all.*[4,5,11]
- Include family/SO in setting realistic goals for meeting individual needs. *Inclusion of all family members ensures they all have the same information and are all working toward effective coping strategies.*[4,5]

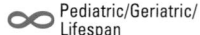

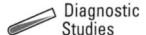

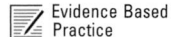

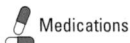

NURSING PRIORITY NO. 3 To promote wellness (Teaching/Discharge Considerations):

- Discuss healthy ways of dealing with difficult situations. *Providing information about effective communication skills, understanding condition they are dealing with, and expectations of the course of the illness or condition can promote personal growth and lead to a positive outcome for the family.*[7,8]
- Have client identify familial, religious, and cultural factors that have meaning for him or her. *May help bring loss or distressing situation into perspective and promote grief or sorrow resolution.*[6]
- Encourage involvement in usual activities, exercise, and socialization within limits of physical and psychological state. *Energy is restored and individuals can go on with their lives when they are willing and able to continue activities.*[5,7]
- Introduce concept of mindfulness (living in the moment) and encourage client to recognize and embrace moments of joy in own life. *Promotes feelings of capability and belief that this moment can be dealt with or enjoyed.*[4,8]
- Refer to other resources (e.g., pastoral care, counseling, psychotherapy, respite care providers, support groups). *Provides additional help when needed to resolve situation, continue grief work, and move on with life.*[11]

DOCUMENTATION FOCUS

Assessment/Reassessment

- Individual findings, including nature of sorrow, effects on participation in treatment regimen.
- Physical and emotional response to conflict, expressions of sadness.
- Cultural or religious issues and conflicts.
- Reactions of family/SO.

Planning

- Plan of care and who is involved in planning.
- Teaching plan.

Implementation/Evaluation

- Response to interventions, teaching, and actions performed.
- Attainment or progress toward desired outcome(s).
- Modifications to plan of care.

Discharge Planning

- Long-term needs and who is responsible for actions to be taken.
- Available resources, specific referrals made.

References

1. Doenges, M. E., Moorhouse, M. F., Murr, A. C. (2010). *Nurse's Pocket Guide Diagnoses: Interventions and Rationales*. 12th ed. Philadelphia: F. A. Davis.
2. Lindgren, C. L. (1996). Chronic sorrow in persons with Parkinson's and their spouse caregivers. *Sch Inq Nurs Pract*, 10(4), 351–366.
3. Lichtensten, B., Laska, M. K., Clair, J. M. (2002). Chronic sorrow in the HIV-positive patient: Issues of race, gender, and social support. *AIDS Patient Care STDs*, 16(1), 27–38.
4. Kearney, P. (2003, updated 2010). Chronic grief (or is it periodic grief?). Lecture materials, Indiana University. Retrieved November 2015 from http://www.indiana.edu/~famlygrf/units/chronic.html.
5. Lowes, L., Lyne, P. (2000). Chronic sorrow in parents of children with newly diagnosed diabetes: A review of the literature and discussion of the implications for nursing practice. *J Adv Nurs*, 32(1), 41–48.
6. Lipson, J. G., Dibble, S. L., Minarik, P. A. (1996). *Culture & Nursing Care: A Pocket Guide*. San Francisco: UCSF Nursing Press.

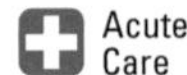

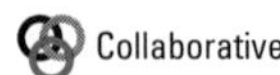

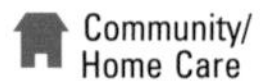

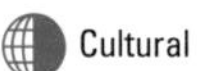

7. Mallow, G. E., Bechtel, G. A. (1999). Chronic sorrow: The experience of parents with children who are developmentally disabled. *J Psychosoc Nurs*, 17(7), 31–43.
8. Kabat-Zinn, J. (1994). *Wherever You Go, There You Are*. New York: Hyperion.
9. Kearney, P. M., Griffin, T. (2001). Between joy and sorrow: Being a parent of a child with a developmental disability. *J Adv Nurs*, 34(5), 582–592.
10. Hobdell, E. (2004). Chronic sorrow and depression in parents of children with neural tube defects. *J Neurosci Nurs*, 36(2), 82–94.
11. Gordon, J. (2009). An evidence-based approach supporting parents dealing with chronic sorrow. *Pediatr Nurs*, 35(2), 115–119.

Spiritual Distress

Taxonomy II: Life Principles—Class 3 Value/Belief/Action Congruence (00066) [**Diagnostic Division:** Ego Integrity], Submitted 1978; Revised 2002, 2013

DEFINITION: A state of suffering related to the impaired ability to experience and integrate meaning in life through connections with self, others, the world, or a superior being.

RELATED FACTORS

Aging; birth of a child
Actively dying; imminent death; death of a significant other; exposure to death
Illness; loss of a body part or function
Increasing dependence on another
Perception of having unfinished business; receiving bad news; life transition; unexpected life event
Loneliness; social alienation; self-alienation; sociocultural deprivation
Treatment regimen
[Challenged belief or value system (e.g., moral or ethical implications of therapy)]

DEFINING CHARACTERISTICS

Subjective

Anxiety, fear
Fatigue; insomnia
Questioning identity; questioning meaning of suffering or life
Connections to self:
Anger; guilt; insufficient courage
Decrease in serenity
Feeling of being unloved; inadequate acceptance
Connections with others:
Alienation
Refuses to interact with significant others or spiritual leader
Separation from support system
Connections with art, music, literature, nature:
Disinterest in nature or reading spiritual literature
Connections with power greater than self:
Anger toward power greater than self
Feeling abandoned; hopelessness; perceived suffering
Inability to pray or participate in religious activities, or to experience the transcendent

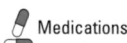

(continues on page 820)

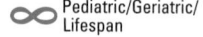

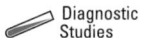

Spiritual Distress (continued)

Objective
Crying
Connections to self:
Ineffective coping strategies; perceived insufficient meaning in life
Connections with art, music, literature, nature:
Decrease in expression of previous pattern of creativity
Connections with power greater than self:
Inability for introspection; sudden changes in spiritual practice; request for a spiritual leader
Sample Clinical Applications: Chronic conditions (e.g., cancer, AIDS, traumatic brain injury vegetative state, infertility); fetal demise, sudden infant death syndrome (SIDS); death of child; traumatic event with fatal outcome or severe disabilities

DESIRED OUTCOMES/EVALUATION CRITERIA

Sample NOC linkages:
Spiritual Health: Connectedness with self, others, higher power, all life, nature, and the universe that transcends and empowers the self
Hope: Optimism that is personally satisfying and life supporting
Psychosocial Adjustment: Life Change: Adaptive psychosocial response of an individual to a significant life change

Client Will (Include Specific Time Frame)
- Verbalize increased sense of connectedness and hope for future.
- Demonstrate ability to help self and participate in care.
- Participate in activities with others, actively seek relationships.
- Discuss beliefs and values about spiritual issues.
- Verbalize acceptance of self as not deserving illness or situation: "No one is to blame."

ACTIONS/INTERVENTIONS

Sample NIC linkages:
Spiritual Support: Assisting the patient to feel balance and connection with a greater power
Hope Inspiration: Enhancing the belief in one's capacity to initiate and sustain actions
Grief Work Facilitation: Assistance with the resolution of a significant loss

NURSING PRIORITY NO. 1 To assess causative/contributing factors:

- Determine client's religious and spiritual orientation, current involvement, and presence of conflicts. *Identification of individual spiritual beliefs and practices that may affect client care, or create conflict between beliefs and treatment, provides for more accurate interventions.*[1]
- Listen to client's/SO's reports or expressions of concern, anger, alienation from God, belief that illness or situation is a punishment for wrongdoing, etc. *Indicates depth of grieving process and possible need for spiritual advisor or other resource to address client's belief system if desired.*[2]
- Assess for influence of cultural beliefs and spiritual values that affect individual in this situation. *Circumstances of illness or situation may conflict with client's view of self, cultural background, and distress over values. For instance, some Catholics may have strong beliefs in the relationship between illness and religious practices.*[5]
- Note recent changes in behavior (e.g., withdrawal from others and creative or religious activities, dependence on alcohol or medications). *Helpful in determining severity and duration of situation and possible need for additional referrals such as substance withdrawal.*[7,11]

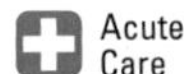

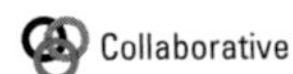

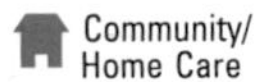

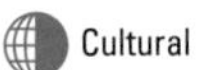

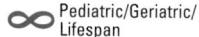

- Assess sense of self-concept and worth and ability to enter into loving relationships. *Lack of connectedness with self or others impairs client's ability to trust others or feel worthy of trust from others, leading to difficulties in relationships with others.*[1,7]
- Observe behavior indicative of poor relationships with others (e.g., manipulative, nontrusting, demanding). *Manipulation is used for management of client's sense of powerlessness because of distrust of others, interfering with relationships with others.*[3,6]
- Determine support systems available to client/SO(s) and how they are used. *Provides insight to client's willingness to pursue outside resources.*[4]
- Determine sense of futility, feelings of hopelessness and helplessness, and lack of motivation to help self. *Indicators that client may see no, or only limited, options, alternatives, or personal choices available; that client lacks energy to deal with situation; and that further evaluation is needed.*
- Note expressions of inability to find meaning in life and/or reason for living. Evaluate suicidal ideation *to refer for mental health evaluation and intervention as indicated. Crisis of the spirit or loss of will to live places client at increased risk for inattention to personal well-being and possible harm to self.*[1,7]

NURSING PRIORITY NO. 2 To assist client/SO(s) to deal with feelings/situation:

- Develop therapeutic nurse-client relationship. Ascertain client's views as to how care provider(s) can be most helpful. Convey acceptance of client's spiritual beliefs and concerns. *Promotes trust and comfort, encouraging client to be open about sensitive matters.*[6]
- Establish environment that promotes free expression of feelings and concerns. *Provides opportunity for client to explore own thoughts and make appropriate decisions regarding spiritual issues.*[4]
- Provide calm, peaceful setting when possible. *Promotes relaxation and enhances opportunity for reflection on situation/discussions with others and meditation.*[3]
- Encourage life review by client. Support client in finding a reason for living. *Promotes sense of hope and willingness to continue efforts to improve situation.*[3]
- Be aware of influence of care provider's own belief system. *It is still possible to be helpful to client while remaining neutral and not espousing own beliefs because client's beliefs and needs are what is important.*[6]
- Identify inappropriate coping behaviors currently being used and associated consequences and discuss with client. *Recognizing negative consequences of actions may enhance desire to change.*[2]
- Set limits on acting-out behavior that is inappropriate/destructive. *Promotes safety for client/others and helps prevent loss of self-esteem.*[2,7]
- Ascertain past successes and coping behaviors. *Helps to determine approaches used previously that may be effective in dealing with current situation, providing encouragement.*[6]
- Problem solve solutions and identify areas for compromise. *May be useful in resolving conflicts that arise from feelings of anxiety regarding questioning of beliefs and current illness or situation.*[3]
- Assist in developing coping skills *to deal with stressors of illness and necessary changes in lifestyle.*[7,9]

NURSING PRIORITY NO. 3 To facilitate setting goals and moving forward:

- Use therapeutic communication skills of reflection and active listening. *Conveys message of competence and helps client find own solutions to concerns.*[7]
- Involve client in refining healthcare goals and therapeutic regimen as appropriate. *Promotes feelings of control over what is happening, enhancing commitment to plan and optimizing outcomes.*[3]
- Encourage client/family to ask questions. *Demonstrates support for individual's willingness to learn.*
- Discuss difference between grief and guilt and help client to identify and deal with each. Point out consequences of actions based on guilt. *Aids client in assuming responsibility for own actions and avoids acting out of false guilt.*[6]
- Identify role models (e.g., individual experiencing similar situation). *Provides opportunities for sharing of experiences and hope and identifying new options to deal with situation.*[7]

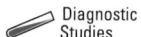

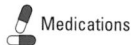

- Assist client to learn use of meditation, mindfulness, and prayer, if desired. *Provides avenue for learning forgiveness to heal past hurts and developing a sense of peace.*[3,8]
- Provide information that anger with God is a normal part of the grieving process. *Realizing these feelings are not unusual can reduce sense of guilt, encourage open expression, and facilitate resolution of grief.*[3,7,11]
- Provide time and privacy to engage in spiritual growth or religious activities as desired (e.g., prayer, meditation, scripture reading, listening to music). *Allows client to focus on self and seek connectedness with spiritual beliefs and values.*[6]
- Encourage and facilitate outings to neighborhood park or nature walks. *Sunshine, fresh air, and activity can stimulate release of endorphins, promoting sense of well-being and encouraging connection with nature.*[6]
- Provide play therapy for child that encompasses spiritual data. *Interactive pleasurable activity promotes open discussion and enhances retention of information. Child will act out feelings in play therapy easier than talking. Provides opportunity for child to practice what has been learned and for therapist to evaluate child's progress.*[3]
- Abide by parents' wishes in discussing and implementing child's spiritual support. *Limits confusion for child and prevents conflict of values and beliefs.*[3]
- Refer to appropriate resources (e.g., pastoral or parish nurse or religious counselor, crisis counselor, hospice; psychotherapy; Alcoholics or Narcotics Anonymous). *Useful in dealing with immediate situation and identifying long-term resources for support to help foster sense of connectedness.*[7,8]
- Refer to NDs ineffective Coping, Powerlessness, Self-Esteem (specify), Social Isolation, and risk for Suicide for additional interventions as indicated.

NURSING PRIORITY NO. 4 To promote spiritual well-being (Teaching/Discharge Considerations):

- Make time for nonjudgmental discussion of philosophical issues or questions about spiritual impact of illness or situation and/or treatment regimen. *Open communication can assist client in reality checks of perceptions and help to identify personal options.*[6]
- Assist client to develop long-term goals for dealing with future and illness situation. *Involvement in planning for desired outcomes enhances commitment to goal, optimizing outcomes.*[7]
- Suggest use of journaling. *Provides opportunity to write feelings and happenings; reviewing them over time can assist in clarifying values and ideas, recognizing and resolving feelings or situation.*[6,10]
- Assist client to identify SO(s)/others who could provide support as needed. *Ongoing support is important to enhance sense of connectedness and continue progress toward goals.*[6]
- Identify spiritual resources that could be helpful (e.g., contact spiritual advisor who has qualifications or experience in dealing with specific problems such as death/dying, relationship problems, substance abuse, suicide). *Provides answers to spiritual questions, assists in the journey of self-discovery, and can help client learn to accept and forgive self.*[6]

DOCUMENTATION FOCUS

Assessment/Reassessment

- Individual findings, including nature of spiritual conflict, and effects of participation in treatment regimen.
- Physical and emotional responses to conflict.

Planning

- Plan of care and who is involved in planning.
- Teaching plan.

Implementation/Evaluation

- Responses to interventions, teaching, and actions performed.
- Attainment or progress toward desired outcome(s).
- Modifications to plan of care.

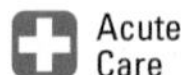

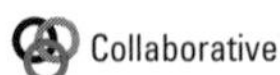

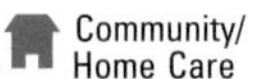

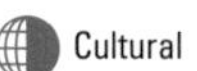

Discharge Planning

- Long-term needs and who is responsible for actions to be taken.
- Available resources, specific referrals made.

References

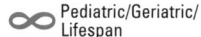

1. Slade, M. (2010). Mental illness and well-being: The central importance of positive psychology and recovery approaches. *BMC Health Serv Res*, 10, 26.
2. Moller, M. D. (1999). Meeting spiritual needs on an inpatient unit. *J Psychosoc Nurs*, 37(11), 5–10.
3. Baldacchino, D., Draper, P. (2001). Spiritual coping strategies: A review of the nursing research literature. *J Adv Nurs*, 34(6), 833–841.
4. Cox, H., Hinz, M. D., Lubno, M. A., et al. (2002). *Clinical Applications of Nursing Diagnosis*. 4th ed. Philadelphia: F. A. Davis.
5. Ludwik, R., Silva, M. C. (2000). Ethics: Nursing around the world: Cultural values and ethical conflicts. *Online J Issues Nurs*. Retrieved March 2015 from http://www.nursingworld.org/MainMenuCategories/ANAMarketplace/ANAPeriodicals/OJIN/Columns/Ethics/CulturalValuesandEthicalConflicts.html.
6. Ross, L. A. (1994). Spiritual aspects of nursing. *J Adv Nurs*, 19(3), 439–447.
7. Townsend, M. C. (2003). *Psychiatric Mental Health Nursing Concepts of Care*. 4th ed. Philadelphia: F. A. Davis.
8. Hospital and Palliative Nurses Association. (Updated 2013). Spiritual distress. Retrieved March 2015 from www.hpna.org/pdf/PatientSheet_SpiritualDistress.pdf.
9. Savrock, J. (2006). Counseling distressed students may be improved by religious/spiritual discussion. Retrieved May 2015 from http://www.ed.psu.edu/news-archive/spiritual.asp.
10. Johnson, C. V., Hayes, J. A. (2003). Troubled spirits: Prevalence and predictors of religious and spiritual concerns among university students and counseling center clients. *J Couns Psychol*, 50(4), 409–419.
11. Hunter, D. (Updated 2014). Grieving the addiction. Retrieved March 2015 from http://www.networktherapy.com/DonnaHunter/default.asp?pid=1534.

risk for Spiritual Distress

Taxonomy II: Life Principles—Class 3 Value/Belief/Action Congruence (00067) [**Diagnostic Division:** Ego Integrity], Submitted 1998; Revised 2013

DEFINITION: Vulnerable to an impaired ability to experience and integrate meaning and purpose in life through connectedness within self, others, literature, nature, and/or a power greater than oneself, which may compromise health.

RISK FACTORS

Physical

Physical or chronic illness; substance abuse

Psychosocial

Anxiety; depression; low self-esteem

Barrier to experiencing love; ineffective relationships

Change in religious ritual or practice; inability to forgive

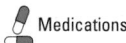

Cultural or racial conflict

Loss; separation from support system; stressors

(continues on page 824)

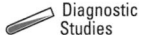

risk for Spiritual Distress (continued)
Developmental
Life transition
Environmental
Environmental change; natural disaster
Note: A risk diagnosis is not evidenced by signs and symptoms, as the problem has not occurred; rather, nursing interventions are directed at prevention.
Sample Clinical Applications: Chronic conditions (e.g., cancer, AIDS, traumatic brain injury vegetative state) infertility; terminal conditions (e.g., end-stage renal disease, lung cancer); fetal demise, sudden infant death syndrome (SIDS); death of spouse or child; traumatic event with fatal outcome or severe disabilities

DESIRED OUTCOMES/EVALUATION CRITERIA

Sample NOC linkages:
Spiritual Health: Connectedness with self, others, higher power, all life, nature, and the universe that transcends and empowers the self
Hope: Optimism that is personally satisfying and life supporting
Psychosocial Adjustment: Life Change: Adaptive psychosocial response of an individual to a significant life change

Client Will (Include Specific Time Frame)
- Identify meaning and purpose in own life that reinforces hope, peace, and contentment.
- Verbalize acceptance of self as being worthy, not deserving of illness or situation, and so forth.
- Identify and use resources appropriately.

ACTIONS/INTERVENTIONS

Sample NIC linkages:
Spiritual Support: Assisting the patient to feel balance and connection with a greater power
Coping Enhancement: Assisting a patient to adapt to perceived stressors, changes, or threats which interfere with meeting life demands and roles
Grief Work Facilitation: Assistance with the resolution of a significant loss

NURSING PRIORITY NO. 1 To assess causative/contributing factors:

- Ascertain current situation (e.g., natural disaster, death of a spouse, personal injustice). *Identification of circumstances that put the individual at risk for loss of connectedness with spiritual beliefs is essential to plan for appropriate interventions.*
- Listen to client's/significant other's (SO's) expressions of anger or concern, belief that illness or situation is a punishment for wrongdoing, etc. *Identifies need for client to talk about and be listened to in regard to concerns about potential loss of control over his or her life.*[3]
- Note reason for living and whether it is directly related to situation. *Tragic occurrences, such as home and business washed away in a flood or lost in a fire, parent whose only child is terminally ill, or loss of a spouse, can cause individual to question previous beliefs.*[1,3]
- Determine client's religious or spiritual orientation, current involvement, and presence of conflicts, especially in current circumstances. *Client may be a member of a religious organization, and whether he or she is active or whether conflicts have risen in relation to current illness or situation will indicate need for assistance from spiritual advisor, pastor, or other resource client would accept.*[1,8,11]

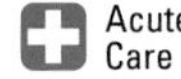

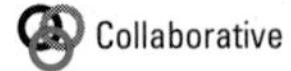

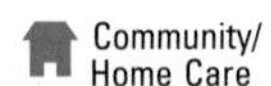

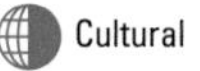

- Assess sense of self-concept, worth, and ability to enter into loving relationships. *Lack of connectedness with self and others impairs client's ability to trust others or feel worthy of trust from others.*[1,7]
- Observe behavior indicative of poor relationships with others. *Client may be manipulative, nontrusting, and demanding because of distrust of self and others, which can interfere with relationships with others, indicating a need for learning positive ways to interact with others.*[2,4]
- Determine support systems available to, and used by, client/SO(s). *Provides insight into individual's willingness to pursue outside resources.*[6,10]
- Ascertain substance use or abuse. *Complicates situation, affects ability to deal with problems in a positive manner, and identifies need for referral to appropriate treatment programs.*[4,9,11]
- Assess for influence of cultural beliefs and spiritual values that affect individual in this situation. *Circumstances of illness or situation may conflict with client's view of self, cultural background, and distress over values. For instance, some Catholics may have strong beliefs in the relationship of illness and religious practices.*[5]

NURSING PRIORITY NO. 2 To assist client/SO(s) to deal with feelings/situation:

- Establish environment that promotes free expression of feelings and concerns. *Provides opportunity for client to explore own thoughts and make appropriate decisions regarding spiritual issues and conflicts.*[7,10,12]
- Use therapeutic communication skills of reflection and active listening. *Communicates confidence in client's ability to find own solutions to concerns.*[7]
- Have client identify and prioritize current or immediate needs. *Helps client focus on what needs to be done and identifies manageable steps to take to achieve goals.*[6]
- Make time for nonjudgmental discussion of philosophical issues or questions about spiritual impact of illness or situation and/or treatment regimen. *Open communication can assist client to make reality checks of perceptions and begin to identify personal options.*[6,12]
- Discuss difference between grief and guilt and help client to identify and deal with each. *Helps client to assume responsibility for own actions, become aware of the consequences of acting out of false guilt.*[6]
- Review coping skills used and their effectiveness in current situation. *Identifies strengths to incorporate into plan and techniques needing revision.*[6]
- Identify role model (e.g., individual experiencing similar situation or disease). *Sharing of experiences and hope provides opportunity for client to look at options as modeled by others and to begin to deal with reality.*[7]
- Provide play therapy for child that encompasses spiritual data. *Interactive pleasurable activity promotes open discussion and enhances retention of information. Child will act out feelings in play therapy easier than talking. Provides opportunity for child to practice what has been learned and for therapist to evaluate child's progress.*[3]
- Abide by parents' wishes in discussing and implementing child's spiritual support. *Limits confusion for child and prevents conflict of values and beliefs.*[3]
- Refer to appropriate resources (e.g., crisis counselor, governmental agencies; pastoral or parish nurse or spiritual advisor who has qualifications or experience dealing with specific problems such as death/dying, relationship problems, substance abuse, suicide; hospice; psychotherapy; Alcoholics or Narcotics Anonymous). *Useful in dealing with immediate situation and identifying long-term resources for support to help foster sense of connectedness.*[7,8,12]

NURSING PRIORITY NO. 3 To promote spiritual well-being (Teaching/Discharge Considerations):

- Role-play new coping techniques. *Provides opportunity to practice and enhances integration of new skills or necessary lifestyle changes.*[4]
- Assist client to learn use of meditation, mindfulness, and prayer, if desired. *Provides avenue for learning forgiveness to heal past hurts and developing a sense of peace.*[3,8]
- Suggest use of journaling. *Provides opportunity to write feelings and happenings; reviewing them over time can assist in clarifying values and ideas and recognizing and resolving feelings or situation.*[6,9]

- Encourage individual to become involved in cultural activities of his or her choosing. *Art, music, plays, and other cultural activities provide a means of connecting with self and others.*
- Discuss possibilities of taking classes and becoming involved in discussion groups or community programs.
- Assist client to identify SO(s) and individuals/support groups who could provide ongoing support. *Having sufficient support can help client maintain spiritual resolve.*[6]
- Discuss benefit of family counseling as appropriate. *Issues of this nature (e.g., situational losses, natural disasters, difficult relationships) affect family dynamics, and family may find it useful to discuss and resolve problems they are experiencing.*[7]

DOCUMENTATION FOCUS

Assessment/Reassessment

- Individual findings, including risk factors, nature of current distress.
- Physical and emotional responses to distress.
- Access to and use of resources.

Planning

- Plan of care and who is involved in planning.
- Teaching plan.

Implementation/Evaluation

- Responses to interventions, teaching, and actions performed.
- Attainment or progress toward desired outcome(s).
- Modifications to plan of care.

Discharge Planning

- Long-term needs and who is responsible for actions to be taken.
- Available resources, specific referrals made.

References

1. Slade, M. (2010). Mental illness and well-being: The central importance of positive psychology and recovery approaches. *BMC Health Serv Res*, 10, 26.
2. Moller, M. D. (1999). Meeting spiritual needs on an inpatient unit. *J Psychosoc Nurs*, 37(11), 5–10.
3. Baldacchino, D., Draper, P. (2001). Spiritual coping strategies: A review of the nursing research literature. *J Adv Nurs*, 34(6), 833–841.
4. Cox, H. C., Hinz, M. D., Lubno, M. A., et al. (2002). *Clinical Applications of Nursing Diagnosis: Adult, Child, Women's, Psychiatric, Gerontic, and Home Health Considerations*. 4th ed. Philadelphia: F. A. Davis.
5. Ludwik, R., Silva, M. C. (2000). Ethics: Nursing around the world: Cultural values and ethical conflicts. Online J Issues Nurs. Retrieved March 2015 from http://www.nursingworld.org/MainMenuCategories/ANAMarketplace/ANAPeriodicals/OJIN/Columns/Ethics/CulturalValuesandEthicalConflicts.html.
6. Ross, L. A. (1994). Spiritual aspects of nursing. *J Adv Nurs*, 19(3), 439–447.
7. Townsend, M. C. (2003). *Psychiatric Mental Health Nursing Concepts of Care*. 4th ed. Philadelphia: F. A. Davis.
8. Hospital and Palliative Nurses Association. (Updated 2013). Spiritual distress-patient/family teaching sheets. Retrieved March 2015 from www.hpna.org/pdf/PatientSheet_SpiritualDistress.pdf.
9. Savrock, J. (2006). Counseling distressed students may be improved by religious discussion. Retrieved March 2015 from http://www.ed.psu.edu/news-archive/spiritual.asp.
10. Johnson, C. V., Hayes, J. A. (2003). Troubled spirits: Prevalence and predictors of religious and spiritual concerns among university students and counseling center clients. *J Couns Psychol*, 50, 409–419.
11. Leigh, J., Bowen, S., Mariatt, G. A. (2005). Spirituality, mindfulness and substance abuse. *Addict Behav*, 30(7), 1335–1341.
12. Smith, A. (2006). Using the Synergy Model to provide spiritual nursing care in critical care settings. *Crit Care Nurs*, 26(4), 41–47.

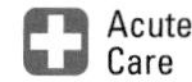

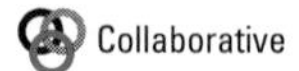

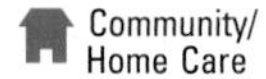

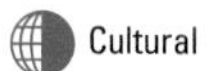

readiness for enhanced Spiritual Well-Being

Taxonomy II: Life Principles—Class 2 Beliefs (00068) [**Diagnostic Division:** Ego Integrity], Submitted 1994; Revised 2002, 2013

DEFINITION: A pattern of experiencing and integrating meaning and purpose in life through connectedness with self, others, art, music, literature, nature, and/or a power greater than oneself, which can be strengthened.

DEFINING CHARACTERISTICS

Subjective

Connections to Self:

Expresses desire to enhance: acceptance, surrender, coping, courage, self-forgiveness, hope, joy, love, serenity (e.g., peace), meaning or purpose in life, satisfaction with philosophy of life

Expresses desire to enhance meditative practice

Connections with Others:

Expresses desire to enhance interaction with significant other/spiritual leaders, service to others

Expresses desire to enhance forgiveness from others

Connections with Art, Music, Literature, and Nature:

Expresses desire to enhance creative energy (e.g., writing, poetry, music), spiritual reading, time outdoors

Connections with Powers Greater than Self:

Expresses desire to enhance participation in religious activity, prayerfulness, reverence, mystical experiences

Sample Clinical Applications: As a health-seeking behavior, the client may be healthy or this diagnosis can occur in any clinical condition

DESIRED OUTCOMES/EVALUATION CRITERIA

Sample NOC linkages:

Spiritual Health: Connectedness with self, others, higher power, all life, nature, and the universe that transcends and empowers the self

Hope: Optimism that is personally satisfying and life supporting

Quality of Life: Extent of positive perception of current life circumstances

Client Will (Include Specific Time Frame)

- Acknowledge the stabilizing and strengthening forces in own life needed for balance and well-being of the whole person.
- Identify meaning and purpose in own life, which reinforces hope, peace, and contentment.
- Verbalize a sense of peace or contentment and comfort of spirit.
- Demonstrate behavior congruent with verbalizations that lend support and strength for daily living.

ACTIONS/INTERVENTIONS

Sample NIC linkages:

Spiritual Growth Facilitation: Facilitation of growth in patients' capacity to identify, connect with, and call upon the source of meaning, purpose, comfort, strength, and hope in their lives

Religious Ritual Enhancement: Facilitating participation in religious practices

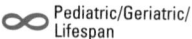

Meditation Facilitation: Facilitating a person to alter his/her level of awareness by focusing specifically on an image or thought

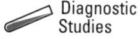

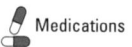

NURSING PRIORITY NO. 1 To determine spiritual state/motivation for growth:

- Ascertain client's perception of current state or degree of connectedness and expectations. *Provides insight as to where client is currently and specific hopes for the future.*[1]
- Ascertain motivation and expectations for change. *Motivation to improve and high expectations can encourage client to make changes that will improve his or her life. However, unrealistic expectations may hamper efforts.*
- Review spiritual or religious history, activities, rituals, and frequency of participation. *Determines basis to build on for growth or change.*[1]
- Determine influence of cultural beliefs or values. *Most individuals are strongly influenced by the spiritual or religious orientation of their family of origin, which can be a major determinate for client's choice of activities and receptiveness to various options.*[5]
- Determine relational values of support systems to client's spiritual centeredness. *The client's family of origin may have differing beliefs from those espoused by the individual, which may be a source of conflict for the client. Comfort can be gained when family and friends share client's beliefs and support the search for spiritual knowledge.*[2]
- Explore meaning or interpretation and relationship of spirituality, life and death, and illness to life's journey. *This information helps client strengthen personal belief system, enabling him or her to move forward and live life to the fullest.*[2,3]
- Clarify the meaning of client's spiritual beliefs or religious practice and rituals to daily living. *Discussing these issues allows client to explore spiritual needs and decide what fits own view of the world to enhance life.*[6]
- Explore ways that spirituality or religious practices have affected client's life and given meaning and value to daily living. Note consequences as well as benefits. *Promotes understanding and appreciation of the difference between spirituality and religion and how each can be used to enhance client's journey of self-discovery.*[3]
- Discuss life's or God's plan (when this is the person's belief) for the individual. *Helpful in determining individual goals and choosing specific options.*[2]

NURSING PRIORITY NO. 2 To assist client to integrate values and beliefs to achieve a sense of wholeness and optimum balance in daily living:

- Explore ways beliefs give meaning and value to daily living. *As client develops understanding of these issues, he or she will provide support for dealing with current and future concerns.*[4]
- Clarify reality and appropriateness of client's self-perceptions and expectations. *Necessary to provide firm foundation for growth. Unrealistic ideas can impede desired improvement.*[2]
- Discuss the importance and value of connections to client's daily life. *The contacts that one has with others sustain the feeling of belonging and connection and promote feelings of wholeness and well-being.*[4,6]
- Identify ways to achieve connectedness or harmony with self, others, nature, and/or a higher power (e.g., meditation, prayer, talking or sharing self with others; being out in nature, gardening, walking; attending religious activities). *This is a highly individual and personal decision, and no action is too trivial to be considered.*[4]

NURSING PRIORITY NO. 3 To enhance optimum spirituality:

- Encourage client to take time to be introspective in the search for peace and harmony. *Finding peace within oneself will carry over to relationships with others and own outlook on life.*[1]
- Discuss use of relaxation or meditative activities (e.g., yoga, tai chi, prayer). *Helpful in promoting general well-being and sense of connectedness with self, nature, and/or spiritual power.*[4,6]
- Suggest attendance or involvement in dream-sharing group *to develop and enhance learning of the characteristics of spiritual awareness and facilitate the individual's growth.*[1]

- Identify ways for spiritual or religious expression. *There are multiple options for enhancing spirituality through connectedness with self/others (e.g., volunteering time to community projects, mentoring, singing in the choir, painting, spiritual writings).*[3,4]
- Encourage participation in desired religious activities and contact with minister or spiritual advisor. *Validating one's beliefs in an external way can provide support and strengthen the inner self.*[1,3]
- Discuss and role-play, as necessary, ways to deal with alternative view or conflict that may occur with family/SO(s)/society or cultural group. *Provides opportunity to try out different behaviors in a safe environment and be prepared for potentialities.*[3]
- Provide bibliotherapy, list of relevant resources (e.g., study groups, parish nurse, poetry society), and reliable Web sites *for later reference, self-paced learning, and ongoing support.*[3]

DOCUMENTATION FOCUS

Assessment/Reassessment

- Assessment findings, including client perception of needs and desire for growth.
- Cultural values or religious beliefs.
- Motivation and expectations for change.

Planning

- Plan for growth and who is involved in planning.

Implementation/Evaluation

- Response to activities, learning, and actions performed.
- Attainment or progress toward desired outcome(s).
- Modifications to plan.

Discharge Planning

- Long-term needs, expectations, and plan of action.
- Specific referrals made.

References

1. Slade, M. (2010). Mental illness and well-being: The central importance of positive psychology and recovery approaches. *BMC Health Serv Res*, 10–26.
2. Moller, M. D. (1999). Meeting spiritual needs on an inpatient unit. *J Psychosoc Nurs*, 37(11), 5–10.
3. Baldacchino, D., Draper, P. (2001). Spiritual coping strategies: A review of the nursing research literature. *J Adv Nurs*, 34(6), 833–841.
4. Cox, H., Hinz, M. D., Lubno, M. A., et al. (2002). *Clinical Applications of Nursing Diagnosis*. 4th ed. Philadelphia: F. A. Davis.
5. Caplan, M. (2011). Psychology and Spirituality: One path or two? Retrieved November 2015 from http://www.huffingtonpost.com/mariana-caplan-phd/spirituality-and-psychology_b_941242.html.
6. Ross, L. A. (1994). Spiritual aspects of nursing. *J Adv Nurs*, 19(3), 439–447.

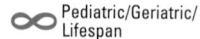

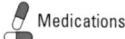

impaired Standing

Taxonomy II: Safety/Protection—Class 2 Activity/Exercise (00238) [**Diagnostic Division:** Safety], Submitted 2013

DEFINITION: Limitation of ability to independently and purposefully attain and/or maintain the body in an upright position from feet to head.

RELATED FACTORS

Circulatory perfusion disorder; impaired metabolic functioning; neurological disorder
Emotional disturbance
Malnutrition; obesity; sarcopenia
Injury to lower extremity
Insufficient endurance or energy
Pain
Prescribed posture; self-imposed relief posture
Surgical procedure

DEFINING CHARACTERISTICS

Objective

Impaired ability to adjust position of one or both lower limbs on uneven surface
Impaired ability to attain or maintain a balanced position of the torso; impaired ability to stress torso with body weight
Impaired ability to flex or extend one or both hips
Inability to or flex or extend one or both knees
Insufficient muscle strength
Sample Clinical Applications: Neuromuscular disorders (e.g., multiple sclerosis [MS], amyotrophic lateral sclerosis [ALS], Parkinson's disease), traumatic injuries (e.g., lower extremity fractures, spinal cord or brain injuries), osteoarthritis, rheumatoid arthritis, hip or knee joint replacement; severe depression, dementia

DESIRED OUTCOMES/EVALUATION CRITERIA

Sample NOC linkages:

Knowledge: Body Mechanics: Extent of understanding conveyed about proper body alignment, balance and coordinated movement
Balance: Ability to maintain body equilibrium
Body Mechanics Performance: Personal actions to maintain proper body alignment and to prevent musculoskeletal strain

Client Will (Include Specific Time Frame)

- Verbalize understanding of individual treatment regimen and safety measures.
- Attain and maintain position of standing function that enables activities and prevents complications.
- Participate in activities of daily living (ADLs) and desired activities.

ACTIONS/INTERVENTIONS

Sample NIC linkages:

Exercise Therapy: Muscle Control: Use of specific activity or exercise protocols to enhance or restore controlled body movement

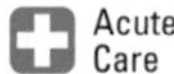

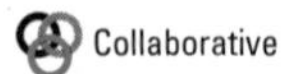

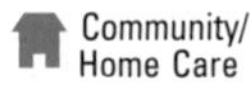

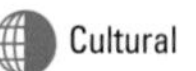

Body Mechanics Promotion: Facilitating the use of position and movement in daily activities to prevent fatigue and musculoskeletal strain or injury

NURSING PRIORITY NO. 1 To identify causative/contributing factors:

- Determine diagnosis that contributes to difficulty with standing balance (e.g., stroke, other neurological disorders [e.g., MS, Parkinson's disease; traumatic brain injury, spinal cord injury with hemi/paraplegia]; vestibular disorders/vertigo; osteoarthritis, rheumatoid arthritis, degenerative joint disease; back pain conditions; lower-limb amputations; psychiatric conditions including severe depression, dementias). *Impaired standing balance has a detrimental effect on a person's functional ability and increases the risk of falling. These conditions can cause postural and balance impairments, muscular weakness, and inadequate range of motion. Sensory deficits may also be involved (e.g., impaired proprioception and/or visual processing, cognitive impairments). For example, sitting and standing balance are major concerns in an amputee's ability to maintain the center of gravity over the base of support. Both balance and coordination are required for weight shifting from one limb to another, thus improving the potential for an optimal gait.*[1] *In persons with chronic neck pain, one study suggested that lack of proprioceptive inhibition of nociceptors at the dorsal horn of the spinal cord would result in subocciptial muscle atrophy and a loss of standing balance.*[2] *Dizziness and/or unsteadiness and episodes of loss of balance are not infrequent complaints of persons with persistent whiplash-associated disorders.*[3]
- Assess client's mental status, noting age, developmental stage, and presence or potential for cognitive dysfunction (e.g., traumatic brain injury, stroke, dementia, extremes of age). *Several studies have suggested that seemingly automatic postural tasks (such as standing balance and walking) require some attention and cognitive processing.*[4,5]
- Determine fall risk, noting factors that may be present. *Fall risk is high in clients with certain conditions (e.g., advanced age or debilitating disease; vision and hearing loss, diminished depth perception; decreased sensation in feet, artificial joints; trauma to lower extremity; amputation, other surgery or immobilizer; presence of severe vertigo with postural sway; generalized or specific leg weakness; reaching upward, forward, or laterally outside of standing balance position).*
- Encourage sitting before attempting standing, when indicated (e.g., supine client with low blood pressure or dehydration, vertigo, first attempt to get up after long period on bedrest). *Longer sitting pause times might improve postural stability after rising from a supine position. One study suggested that longer sitting pause times may also provide improved adaptability to dimly lit environments.*[6]

NURSING PRIORITY NO. 2 To assess functional ability:

- Determine functional status using a 0–4 scale, noting muscle strength and tone, joint mobility, cardiovascular status, balance, and endurance. *Identifies strengths and deficits (e.g., unable to stand without assistance, but can maintain standing position once attained; standing balance improved as vertigo diminishes; standing improves with pain management and nutrition measures, etc.) and may provide information regarding potential for recovery (e.g., client with severe brain injury may have permanent limitations because of impaired cognition affecting memory, judgment, problem solving, and motor planning).*[7,8]
- Determine degree of perceptual or cognitive impairment and ability to follow directions. *Impairments, which may be related to age, chronic or acute disease condition, trauma, surgery, or medications, can necessitate alternative interventions or changes in plan of care.*
- Refer to physician and/or physical therapy specialists, as indicated, *to determine potential for improvement and direction for therapies. May include many different functional and lab tests (e.g., sitting to standing, tolerance, muscle strength and movement, posture and balance monitor, American Spinal Injury Association Impairment Scale, Berger Balance Scale, Functional Independence Measure, electrophysiological and clinical measures of neuropathy).*[9,10]

- Note: Studies have shown that people with the earliest stage of impaired glucose tolerance exhibit deficits in standing balance and trunk position sense, highlighting the importance of early screening for diabetes.[11]

NURSING PRIORITY NO. 3 To promote optimal level of function and prevent complications:

- Assist with treatment of underlying condition(s) *to maximize potential for optimal function.*
- Assist with/refer for rehabilitation therapies and techniques for implementing standing activities. *Various modalities may be used to gain physiological benefits from standing or modified standing therapy. For example, "standing" can be accomplished in a variety of positions with proper support (e.g., a prone-position with blanket under the abdomen), which helps preserve joint range of motion and improves muscle flexibility, weight-bearing ability, and bowel and bladder function even when person is not upright.[12] Note: Research found that a "Standing Strong" program was effective at improving strength, balance, and function, as well as at reducing falls in older adults. This program combines strength training with balance-specific exercises to target the muscular system as well as the three major sensory control systems that control balance.[13]*
- Provide for safety measures as indicated by individual situation, including environmental management and fall prevention. (Refer to ND risk for Falls.)
- Encourage client's participation in self-care activities and in physical or occupational therapies. *Improves body strength and function and enhances self-concept and sense of independence.*
- Administer pain medications before activity as needed *to permit maximal effort and involvement in activity.*
- Collaborate with nutritionist in providing nutritious foods and needed feeding assistance, maximizing client's abilities in ingesting and swallowing (upright position) *to optimize available energy for activities.*
- Demonstrate and assist with use of assitive devices (e.g., side rails, overhead trapeze, roller pads, safety belt, hydraulic lifts, chairs) *for position changes and safe transfers.*
- Refer to NDs Activity Intolerance, impaired bed Mobility, impaired wheelchair Mobility, impaired Transfer Ability, impaired Sitting, and impaired Walking for additional interventions.

NURSING PRIORITY NO. 4 To promote wellness (Teaching/Discharge Considerations):

- Encourage client's/SO's involvement in decision making as much as possible. *Enhances commitment to plan, optimizing outcomes.*
- Demonstrate use of mobility devices (e.g., walkers, strollers, scooters, braces, prosthetics) and have client/caregiver demonstrate knowledge about and safe use of device. Identify appropriate resources for obtaining and maintaining appliances or equipment. *Safe use of mobility aides promotes client's independence and enhances quality of life and safety for client and caregiver.*
- Refer to support and community services as indicated *to provide care, supervision, companionship, respite services, nutritional and ADL assistance, adaptive devices or changes to living environment, financial assistance, etc.*

DOCUMENTATION FOCUS

Assessment/Reassessment

- Individual findings, including level of function and ability to participate in specific or desired activities.

Planning

- Plan of care and who is involved in the planning.
- Teaching plan.

Implementation/Evaluation

- Responses to interventions, teaching, and actions performed.
- Attainment or progress toward desired outcome(s).
- Modifications to plan of care.

Acute Care
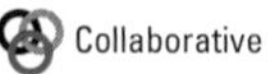
Collaborative
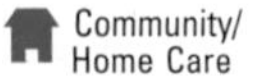
Community/ Home Care
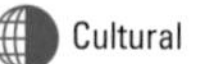
Cultural

Discharge Planning

- Discharge and long-term needs, noting who is responsible for each action to be taken.
- Specific referrals made.
- Sources of and maintenance for assistive devices.

References

1. Gaily, R. S., Clark, C. S. (2002). Physical therapy management of adult lower-limb amputees. Atlas of Limb Prosthetics. Online Orthotics and Prosthetics Virtual Library. Retrieved January 2015 from http://www.oandplibrary.org/alp/.
2. McPartland, J. M., Brodeur, R. R., Hallgren, R. C. (1997). Chronic neck pain, standing balance, and suboccipital muscle atrophy: A pilot study. *J Manipulative Physiol Ther*, 20(1), 24–29.
3. Treleaven, J., Jull, G., LowChoy, N. (2005). Standing balance in persistent whiplash: A comparison between subjects with and without dizziness. *J Rehabil Med*, 37(4), 224–229.
4. Rogers, M. E., Page, P. (2010). Standing Strong: A program to improve strength and balance in older adults. Retrieved January 2015 from http://www.standingstrongprogram.com/wp-content/uploads/2009/05/Standing-Strong-Guide-2010.pdf.
5. Cooper, R., Kuh, P., Hardy, R. (2010). Objectively measured physical capability levels and mortality: Systematic review and meta-analysis. BMJ. Retrieved January 2015 from http://www.bmj.com/content/341/BMJ.c4467.full.
6. Johnson, E. G., Meltzer, J. D. (2012). Effect of sitting pause times on postural stability after supine-to-standing transfer in dimly lit environments. *Geriatr Phys Ther*, 35(1), 15–19.
7. Black, K., Zafonte, R., Millis, S., et al. (2000). Sitting balance following brain injury (does it predict outcome?). *Brain Inj*, 14(2), 141–152.
8. Dworak, P. A., Levy, A. (2005). Strolling along. *Rehabil Manage*, 18(9), 26–31.
9. Gorman, S. L., Rivera, M., McCarthy, L. (2014). Reliability of the function in sitting test (FIST). Rehabilitation Research and Practice. Retrieved January 2015 from http://www.hindawi.com/journals/rerp/2014/593280/.
10. McKinley, W., Kulcarni, U., Pai, A. B. (2013). Functional outcomes per level of spinal cord injury. Retrieved January 2015 from http://emedicine.medscape.com/article/322604-overview#a1.
11. Goldberg, A., Russell, J. W., Alexander, B. B. (2008). Standing balance and trunk position sense in impaired glucose tolerance (IGT)-related peripheral neuropathy. *J Neurol Sci*, 270((1–2)), 165–171.
12. Zwick, D., Dunn, M. (2007). Integrating Iyengar yoga into rehabilitation. *Nursing*, 37((10 Supplement: Therapy Insider)), 10–12.
13. Page, P. (2010). Standing Strong. Bringing evidence to practice for a community-based fall prevention exercise program. *Topics Geriatric Rehabil*, 26(4), 335–352.
14. Gordon, M. (2009). Functional levels code. *Manual of Nursing Diagnosis*. 12th ed. Sudbury, MA: Jones and Bartlett.

Stress Overload

Taxonomy II: Coping/Stress Tolerance—Class 2 Coping Responses (00177) [**Diagnostic Division:** Ego Integrity], Submitted 2006

DEFINITION: Excessive amounts and types of demands that require action.

RELATED FACTORS

Insufficient resources (e.g., financial, social, knowledge)
Excessive stress; stressors; repeated stressors

(continues on page 834)

Stress Overload (continued)
DEFINING CHARACTERISTICS

Subjective
Impaired functioning, decision making
Feeling of pressure; increase in impatience or anger
Negative impact from stress (e.g., physical symptoms, psychological distress, feeling sick)
Excessive stress; tension

Objective
Increase in anger behavior
Sample Clinical Applications: Chronic illness (e.g., multiple sclerosis [MS], diabetes, Parkinson's disease), terminal illness (e.g., ovarian cancer, amyotrophic lateral sclerosis [ALS]), abusive situations, bipolar disorder, depression, social phobia

DESIRED OUTCOMES/EVALUATION CRITERIA

Sample NOC linkages:
Stress Level: Severity of manifested physical or mental tension resulting from factors that alter an existing equilibrium
Anxiety Self-Control: Personal actions to eliminate or reduce feelings of apprehension, tension, or uneasiness from an unidentifiable source
Leisure Participation: Use of relaxing, interesting, and enjoyable activities to promote well-being

Client Will (Include Specific Time Frame)
- Assess current situation accurately.
- Identify ineffective stress-management behaviors and consequences.
- Meet psychological needs as evidenced by appropriate expression of feelings, identification of options, and use of resources.
- Verbalize or demonstrate reduced stress reaction.

ACTIONS/INTERVENTIONS

Sample NIC linkages:
Emotional Support: Provision of reassurance, acceptance, and encouragement during times of stress
Coping Enhancement: Assisting a patient to adapt to perceived stressors, changes, or threats that interfere with meeting life demands and roles
Resiliency Promotion: Assisting individuals, families, and communities in development, use, and strengthening of protective factors to be used in coping with environmental and societal stressors

NURSING PRIORITY NO. 1 To identify causative/precipitating factors and degree of impairment:

- Ascertain what tragic or difficult events have occurred (e.g., family violence, death of loved one; separation from living partner/parent; change in financial status or living conditions; chronic or terminal illness, workplace stress, loss of job or retirement; major trauma; catastrophic natural or man-made event) over remote and recent past *to assist in determining number, duration, and intensity of difficult events causing perception of overwhelming stress.*
- ∞ Ascertain other life events (e.g., job promotion, moving to different home, change in getting married, having a new baby or adding other new family member, child leaving home, adult children returning home, elder parent requiring care, traveling, spending holidays with relatives) that have occurred over recent months. *All such changes, even when desired, can be stressful and can evoke stress reactions.*[2]

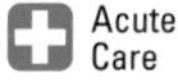

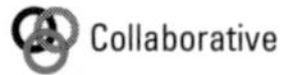

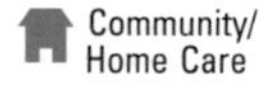

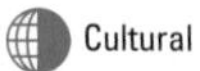

- Evaluate client's report of physical or emotional problems (e.g., fatigue, aches and pains, irritable bowel, skin rashes, frequent colds, sleeplessness, crying spells, anger, feeling overwhelmed or numb, compulsive behaviors) *that can be representing body's response to stress.*[1]
- Determine client's/significant other's (SO's) understanding of events, noting differences in viewpoints.
- Note client's gender, age, and developmental level of functioning. *Although everyone experiences stress and stressors, women, children, young adults, divorced or separated persons, and people in roles or occupations requiring constant multitasking tend to have higher stress-related symptoms. Multiple stressors can weaken immune system and tax physical and emotional coping mechanisms of persons of any age, but particularly the elderly.*[1–3,9]
- Note cultural values or religious beliefs *that may affect client's expectation for self in dealing with situation, ability to ask for help from others, and expectations placed on client by SO/family.*[7]
- Identify client locus of control: internal (expressions of responsibility for self and ability to control outcomes—"I didn't quit smoking") or external (expressions of lack of control over self and environment—"Nothing ever works out"). *Knowing client's locus of control will help in developing a plan of care reflecting client's ability to realistically make changes that will help to manage stress better.*[7]
- Assess emotional responses and coping mechanisms being used.
- Determine stress feelings and self-talk client is engaging in. *Negative self-talk, all-or-nothing or pessimistic thinking, exaggeration, and unrealistic expectations will contribute to stress overload.*[2]
- Assess degree of mastery client has exhibited in life. *Passive individual may have more difficulty being assertive and standing up for rights.*
- Determine presence or absence and nature of resources (e.g., whether family/SO are supportive, lack money, problems with relationship or social functioning).
- Note change in relationships with SO(s). *Conflict in the family, loss of a family member, divorce can result in a change in support client is accustomed to and impair ability to manage situation.*
- Evaluate stress level using appropriate tool (e.g., Stress & Depression, Self-Assessment Tool) to help identify areas of most distress. *While most stress seems to come from disastrous events in individual's life, positive events can also be stressful.*
- Review lab results to identify physiological conditions (e.g., thyroid or other hormone imbalance, anemia, unstable glucose levels, kidney or liver disease) *that may be causing or exacerbating stress.*[1]

NURSING PRIORITY NO. 2 To assist client to deal with current situation:

- Discuss situation or condition in simple, concise manner. *May help client to express emotions, grasp situation, and feel more in control.*
- Active-listen to concerns and provide empathetic presence, using talk and silence as needed.
- Deal with the immediate issues first (e.g., treatment of physical injury, meet safety needs, removal from traumatic or violent environment).
- Collaborate in treatment of underlying conditions (e.g., traumatic injury, chronic or terminal illness, hormone imbalance, depression and other psychiatric disorders).[1]
- Provide or encourage restful environment where possible.
- Assist client in determining whether or not he or she can change stressor or response. *May help client to sort out things over which he or she has control and determine responses that can be modified in order to view life through a more holistic lens.*
- Allow client to react in own way without judgment. Provide support and diversion as indicated.
- Help client to focus on strengths, to set limits on acting-out behaviors, and to learn ways to express emotions in an acceptable manner. *Promotes internal locus of control, enabling client to maintain self-concept and feel more positive about self.*
- Discuss benefits of a "Stop Doing" in place of a "To Do" list. *May help client identify and take action regarding energy drainers (e.g., internalizing others' criticism, fragmented boundaries, power struggles, unprotected personal time) in order to make room for what energizes and brings him/her closer to achieving goals.*[9]

- Address use of ineffective or dangerous coping mechanisms (e.g., substance use or abuse, self-/other-directed violence) and refer for counseling as indicated.

NURSING PRIORITY NO. 3 To promote wellness (Teaching/Discharge Considerations):

- Use client's locus of control to develop individual plan of care *(e.g., for client with internal control, encourage client to take control of own care; for those with external control, begin with small tasks and add as tolerated).*[4]
- Incorporate strengths, assets, and past coping strategies that were successful for client. *Reinforces that client is able to deal with difficult situations.*
- Encourage strengthening of positive SO/family routines and interactions *that support and provide assistance in managing stress.*[5]
- Provide information about stress and exhaustion phase, which occurs when person is experiencing chronic or unresolved stress. *Release of cortisol can contribute to reduction in immune function, resulting in physical illness, mental disability, and life dysfunction.*
- Review stress management and coping skills that client can use:[1,2,4–6]

  Practice behaviors that may help *reduce negative consequences*—change thinking by focusing on positives, reframing thoughts, and changing lifestyle.

  Learn to read own body signs (e.g., shakiness, irritability, sleep disturbances, fatigue).

  Take a step back and reduce obligations, simplify life, and learn to say no *to reduce sense of being overwhelmed.*

  Practice exchanging stresses (i.e., when a new stress comes into play, eliminate or postpone another stress) *to keep total stress level below overstress level.*

  Seek help or assistance in meeting obligations and delegate tasks as appropriate.

  Learn to control and redirect anger.

  Develop and practice positive self-esteem skills.

  Rest, sleep, and exercise on regular schedule or set times *to recuperate and rejuvenate self. Note: A recent study found that physically fit women in their mid-60s had essentially the same response to stress as a group of unfit women in their late 20s.*[8]

  Postpone changes in living situation (e.g., moving, remodeling) if possible.

  Participate in self-help actions (e.g., deep breathing and other relaxation exercises, spend time alone, get involved in recreation or desired activity, plan something fun, develop humor) *to actively relax.*

  Eliminate possible food or environmental allergens and toxins.

  Eat nutritious meals; avoid junk food and excessive sugars.

  Avoid excessive caffeine, alcohol or other drugs, and nicotine *to balance body chemicals and support general health.*

  Take a multivitamin, mineral, and/or trace element preparation.

  Develop spiritual self (e.g., meditate or pray; block negative thoughts; learn to give and take, speak and listen, forgive and move on).

  Interact socially, reach out, and nurture self and others *to reduce loneliness or sense of isolation.*
- Review proper medication use *to manage exacerbating conditions (e.g., depression, mood disorders).*
- Identify community resources (e.g., vocational counseling; educational programs; child or elder care; Women, Infants, and Children program or food stamps; home or respite care) *that can help client manage lifestyle and environmental stress.*
- Refer for therapy, as indicated (e.g., medical treatment, psychological counseling; hypnosis, massage, biofeedback).

DOCUMENTATION FOCUS

Assessment/Reassessment

- Individual findings, noting specific stressors, individual's perception of the situation, locus of control.
- Specific cultural or religious factors.
- Availability and use of support systems and resources.

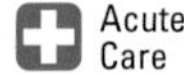

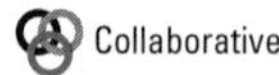

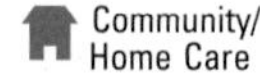

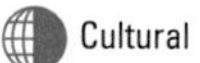

Planning

- Plan of care and who is involved in planning.
- Teaching plan.

Implementation/Evaluation

- Responses to interventions, teaching, and actions performed.
- Attainment or progress toward desired outcome(s).
- Modifications to plan of care.

Discharge Planning

- Long-term needs and who is responsible for actions to be taken.
- Specific referrals made.

References

1. Burns, S. L. (1997–2008). The medical basis of stress, depression, anxiety, sleep problems and drug use. Retrieved November 2015 from http://www.teachhealth.com/.
2. Klimes Institute. (1994–2015). Stress relief. Retrieved November 2015 from http://cecourses.org/preventive-care/stress-relief/.
3. Woolston, C. (Updated 2015). Aging and stress. Retrieved November 2015 from http://consumer.healthday.com/encyclopedia/aging-1/age-health-news-7/aging-and-stress-645997.html.
4. Donatelle, R. (2003). Managing stress: Coping with life's challenges. *Health: The Basics*. 5th ed. San Francisco, CA: Benjamin Cummings.
5. Beckett, C. (2000). Family theory as a framework for assessment. Retrieved November 2015 from http://www2.nau.edu/~nur350-c/class/2_family/theory/lesson2-1-3.html.
6. Harvard Medical School. (2007). *Stress Control: Techniques for Preventing and Easing Stress*. Boston, MA: Harvard Health.
7. Lipson, J. G., Dibble, S. L., Minarik, P. A. (1996). *Culture & Nursing Care: A Pocket Guide*. San Francisco: UCSF Nursing Press.
8. Traustadottir, T., Bosch, P. R., Matt, K., et al. (2005). The HPA axis response to stress in women: Effects of aging and fitness. *Psychoneuroendocrinology*, 30(4), 392–402.
9. Martinuzzi, B. (2007). The breaking point. Retrieved November 2015 from http://www.mindtools.com/pages/article/newTCS_93.htm.

risk for Sudden Infant Death Syndrome

Taxonomy II: Safety/Protection—Class 2 Physical Injury (00156) [**Diagnostic Division:** Safety], Submitted 2002; Revised 2013

DEFINITION: Vulnerable to unpredicted death of an infant.

RISK FACTORS

Modifiable

Delay in or insufficient prenatal care
Infant placed in the prone or side-lying position to sleep
Soft underlayment (e.g., loose items placed near infant)

(continues on page 838)

risk for Sudden Infant Death Syndrome (continued)
Infant overheating or overwrapping
Exposure to smoke
Potentially Modifiable
Young parental age
Low birth weight; prematurity
Nonmodifiable
Male gender
Ethnicity (e.g., African American, Native American)
Season of the year (i.e., winter and fall)
Age 2 to 4 months
Note: A risk diagnosis is not evidenced by signs and symptoms, as the problem has not occurred; rather, nursing interventions are directed at prevention.
Sample Clinical Applications: Any child during first year of life

DESIRED OUTCOMES/EVALUATION CRITERIA

Sample NOC linkages:
Risk Detection: Personal actions taken to identify personal health threats
Risk Control: Actions to eliminate or reduce actual, personal, and modifiable health threats
Knowledge: Infant Care: Extent of understanding conveyed about caring for a baby from birth to first birthday

Parent/Caregiver Will (Include Specific Time Frame)
- Verbalize knowledge of modifiable factors.
- Make changes in environment to prevent death occurring from other factors.
- Follow medically recommended regimen for prenatal and postnatal care.

ACTIONS/INTERVENTIONS

Sample NIC linkages:
Risk Identification: Analysis of potential risk factors, determination of health risks, and prioritization of risk-reduction strategies for an individual or group
Parent Education: Infant: Instruction on nurturing and physical care during the first year of life
Teaching: Infant Safety [specify age 0–12 months]: Instruction on safety during first year of life

NURSING PRIORITY NO. 1 To assess causative/contributing factors:

- Identify individual risk factors pertaining to situation. *Determines modifiable or potentially modifiable factors that can be addressed. Note: SIDS is defined as the sudden death of an infant under 1 year of age, which remains unexplained after a thorough case investigation, including performance of a complete autopsy, examination of the death scene, and review of the clinical history. SIDS is the most common cause of SUIDs between 1 and 6 months, with peak incidence occurring between the second and fourth months. Note: The Centers for Disease Control and Prevention (CDC) statistics published in 2015 state that SIDS is the third leading cause of infant deaths in the United States and the leading cause of death in infants 1 to 12 months old.*[1,7,9–11]
- Determine ethnicity and cultural background of family. *Although the overall rate of SIDS in the United States has declined since 1992, disparities in risk factors and SUIDs rates remain. The CDC reports (2014) that SUID rates for American Indian/Alaska Native and non-Hispanic black infants were more than*

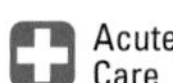
Acute Care
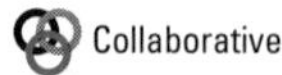
Collaborative
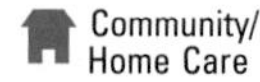
Community/ Home Care
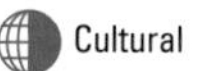
Cultural

twice those of non-Hispanic white infants. SUIDs rates were lowest among Hispanic and Asian/Pacific Islander infants.[7–9,12]

- Note whether mother smoked during pregnancy or is currently smoking. *Many risk factors for SIDS also apply to non-SIDS deaths as well, and smoking is known to negatively affect the fetus prenatally as well as the infant after birth. A large study comparing results of multiple studies concluded there is "substantial evidence to conclude that maternal smoking causes a 3-fold increased risk of SIDS, and possibly 4.7-fold increased risk now that few infants sleep prone."*[1,2,12]
- Assess extent of prenatal care, how early it was begun, and extent to which mother followed recommended care measures. *Prenatal care is important for all pregnancies to afford the optimal opportunity for all infants to have a healthy start to life.*[2–4]
- Determine client's knowledge of premature labor and actions to be taken in the event they occur. *Prompt action can prevent early delivery and the complications of prematurity.*[4]
- Note use of alcohol or other drugs (including prescribed medications) during and after pregnancy. *"Alcohol is one of the most widely abused substances during pregnancy, and its effects on fetal development and infant outcomes have been well studied. Illicit drug use during pregnancy has been associated with a variety of adverse effects, though more research is needed to draw causal connections."*[5,12]

NURSING PRIORITY NO. 2 To promote use of activities to minimize risk of SIDS:

- Emphasize importance of placing infant on his or her back to sleep, both at nighttime and naptime. *Research confirms that fewer babies die of SIDS when they sleep on their backs, not on their tummies or sides.*[6,8]
- Advise all formal child-care providers, as well as grandparents, babysitters, neighbors, or anyone who will have responsibility for the care of the child during sleep, to maintain safe sleeping position in own sleeping place with head and face uncovered. *The recommendation is to always place the infant on the back until he or she can roll over; then repositioning is not required.*[1,2,4,6,7]
- Encourage parents to schedule "tummy time" only while infant is awake. *This activity promotes strengthening of back and neck muscles while parents are close and baby is not sleeping.*[1]
- Encourage well-baby checkups and immunizations. *Keeping babies healthy prevents problems that could put the infant at risk for SIDS. Immunizing infants prevents many illnesses that can be life-threatening.*[1,4,10]
- Encourage breastfeeding, if possible. *Breastfeeding has many advantages (immunological, nutritional, psychosocial), promoting a healthy infant. While this does not preclude the occurrence of SIDS, healthy babies are less prone to many illnesses and health problems. Note: One meta-analysis of 18 studies shows that breastfeeding to any extent and of any duration is protective against SIDS.*[1,4,13]
- Discuss issues of bed-sharing. *Some of the many concerns include* accidental entrapment under a sleeping adult or suffocation by becoming wedged in a couch or cushioned chair. *There are also concerns about accidental death from suffocation when the mother smokes, has recently consumed alcohol, is fatigued, the infant is covered by a blanket or quilt, or there are multiple bed-sharers. Also, studies show that the odds of SIDS is 16 times greater if babies who bed-share are also exposed to secondhand smoke. Research suggests that infants in this setting have more difficulty rousing from sleep, perhaps because smoke exposure changes serotonin pathways of the brain.*[6,13,14]
- Note cultural beliefs about bed-sharing. *Studies show that bed-sharing is growing across all populations in the United States. Bed-sharing is more common among breastfed infants, young unmarried mothers, low-income families where multiple people share a bed. Additional study is needed to better understand bed-sharing practices and associated risks and benefits.*[6,14]

NURSING PRIORITY NO. 3 To promote wellness (Teaching/Discharge Considerations):

- Discuss known facts about SIDS with parents. *SIDS is not preventable, although research indicates that SIDS deaths have reduced since back-sleeping position policy was implemented. The cause is determined only after autopsy and can only be determined after ruling out other causes. SIDS is not the same as suffocation, is not caused by vomiting or choking, is not caused by immunizations, is not contagious, is not the cause of every unexpected infant death, and is not the result of child neglect or abuse.*[1,2,7]

- Recommend attention to factors below that may help in reducing risk:

  Avoid overdressing or overheating infants during sleep. *Baby should be kept warm, but not too warm. Too many layers of clothing or blankets can overheat the infant. Room temperature that is comfortable for an adult will be comfortable for the baby. Note: Infants who were dressed in two or more layers of clothes as they slept had six times the risk of SIDS as those dressed in fewer layers.*[1,4]

  Place infant on a firm mattress in an approved crib. *Avoiding soft mattresses, sofas, cushions, waterbeds, and other soft surfaces, while not known to prevent SIDS, will minimize chance of suffocation.*[1,2]

  Remove fluffy and loose bedding from sleep area, making sure baby's head and face are not covered during sleep. *Using only sleep clothing without a blanket or, if a blanket is used, making sure it is below baby's face and tucked in at the foot of the bed minimizes possibility of suffocation.*[1,2]

  Verify that day-care center/provider(s) are trained in observation and modifying risk factors (e.g., sleeping position) *to reduce risk of death while infant in their care.*

  Discourage excessive checking of the infant. *Since there is nothing that can currently be done (beyond proper sleep positioning) to reduce the occurrence of SIDS, excessive checking only tires the parents and creates an atmosphere of tension and anxiety.*[1,2]

- Discuss the use of apnea monitors, if appropriate. *Apnea monitors are not recommended to prevent SIDS but may be used to monitor other medical problems. Only a small percentage of infants who died of SIDS were known to have prolonged apnea episodes, and monitors are also not medically recommended for subsequent siblings.*[1,2]
- Recommend contacting public health nurse for visit to new mother at least once or twice following discharge. *Researchers found that Native American infants whose mothers received such visits were 80% less likely to die from SIDS than those who were never visited.*[4]
- Refer parents to local SIDS programs and resources for learning (e.g., National SIDS/Infant Death Resource Center and similar Web sites). *Provides reassurance and information for self-paced learning.*[1]
- Encourage consultation with primary care provider if baby shows any signs of illness or behaviors that concern parent. *Promotes timely evaluation and intervention for treatable problems.*[1]

DOCUMENTATION FOCUS

Assessment/Reassessment

- Baseline findings, degree of parental anxiety or concern.
- History of infant deaths within family.

Planning

- Plan of care, specific interventions, and who is involved in planning.
- Teaching plan.

Implementation/Evaluation

- Parent's responses to interventions, teaching, and actions performed.
- Attainment or progress toward desired outcome(s).
- Modifications to plan of care.

Discharge Planning

- Long-term needs and actions to be taken.
- Support systems available, specific referrals made, and who is responsible for actions to be taken.

Acute Care 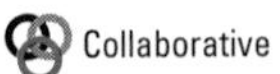 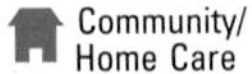 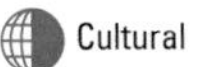

References

1. Angel Eyes (The Colorado SIDS Program). (2013). Infant sleep safety. Retrieved April 2015 from http://www.slideshare.net/425AngelEyes/infant-sleep-safety-understanding-risks-and-exploring-safety-measures.
2. Continuing Education Program on SIDS Risk Reduction. (2005). *U.S. Department of Health and Human Services, National Institutes of Health.*
3. Phillips, C. R. (1996). *Family-Centered Maternity and Newborn Care.* 4th ed. St. Louis, MO: Mosby.
4. London, M. L., Ladewig, P. W., Ball, J. W., et al. (2003). *Maternal & Child Nursing.* 3rd ed. Upper Saddle River, NJ: Prentice Hall.
5. National Institute on Drug Abuse. (Updated 2011). Prenatal exposure to drugs of abuse—May 2011: A research update from the National Institute on Drug Abuse. Retrieved April 2015 from https://www.drugabuse.gov/sites/default/files/prenatal.pdf.
6. SIDS and Kids. (2015). Safe sleeping. Retrieved April 2015 from http://www.sidsandkids.org/safe-sleeping/.
7. Centers for Disease Control and Prevention. (Updated 2015). Sudden unexpected infant deaths and sudden infant death syndrome (various pages). Retrieved April 2015 from hhttp://www.cdc.gov/sids/aboutsuidandsids.htm.
8. American Academy of Pediatrics. (2005). Policy Statement: The changing concept of sudden infant death syndrome: Diagnostic coding shifts, controversies regarding the sleeping environment, and new variations to consider in reducing risk. *Pediatrics,* 116(5), 1245–1255.
9. CDC/NCHS, National Vital Statistics System, Period Linked Birth/Infant Death Data. (2014). Sudden unexpected infant death by race/ethnicity, 2007–2010. Retrieved April 2015 from http://www.cdc.gov/sids/data.htm.
10. Leiter, J. C., Bohm, I. (2007). Mechanisms of pathogenesis in the sudden infant death syndrome. *Resp Physiol Neurobiol,* 159(2), 127–138.
11. Pharoah, P. O., Platt, M. J. (2007). Sudden infant death syndrome in twins and singletons. *Twin Res Hum Gen,* 10(4), 644–648.
12. Mitchell, E. A., Milerad, J. (2006). Smoking and sudden unexpected infant death. Retrieved April 2015 from http://www.who.int/tobacco/media/en/mitchell.pdf.
13. Hauck, F. R., Thompson, J. M., Tanabe, K. O., et. al. (2011). Breastfeeding and reduced risk of sudden infant death syndrome: A meta-analysis. *Pediatrics,* 128(1), 103–110.
14. Horsley, T., Clifford, T., Barrowman, N., et al. (2007). Benefits and harms associated with the practice of bed sharing. *Arch Pediatr Adolesc Med,* 161(3), 237–245.

risk for Suffocation

Taxonomy II: Safety/Protection—Class 2 Physical Injury (00036) [**Diagnostic Division:** Safety], Submitted 1980; Revised 2013

DEFINITION: Vulnerable to inadequate air availability for inhalation.

RISK FACTORS

Internal

Alteration in cognitive or motor functioning; emotional disturbance

Alteration in olfactory function

Face/neck disease or injury

Insufficient knowledge of safety precautions

External

Access to empty refrigerator/freezer; low strung freezer

Eating large mouthfuls [or pieces] of food; small object in airway

(continues on page 842)

risk for Suffocation (continued)
Gas leak; unvented fuel-burning heater; vehicle running in closed garage; smoking in bed
Pacifier around infant's neck; propped bottle in infant's crib
Soft underlayment (e.g., loose items place near infant); playing with plastic bag
Unattended in water
Note: A risk diagnosis is not evidenced by signs and symptoms, as the problem has not occurred; rather, nursing interventions are directed at prevention.
Sample Clinical Applications: Substance use or abuse, spinal cord injury, crushing chest injury, obesity, near-drowning, burn or inhalation injury, sleep apnea, seizure disorder

DESIRED OUTCOMES/EVALUATION CRITERIA

Sample NOC linkages:
Risk Control: Personal actions to prevent, eliminate, or reduce modifiable health threats
Aspiration Prevention: Personal actions to prevent the passage of fluid and solid particles into the lung
Personal Safety Behavior: Personal actions that prevent physical injury to self

Client/Caregiver Will (Include Specific Time Frame)
- Verbalize knowledge of hazards in the environment.
- Identify interventions appropriate to situation.
- Correct hazardous situations to prevent or reduce risk of suffocation.
- Demonstrate cardiopulmonary resuscitation (CPR) skills and how to access emergency assistance.

ACTIONS/INTERVENTIONS

Sample NIC linkages:
Airway Management: Facilitation of patency of air passages
Aspiration Precautions: Prevention or minimization of risk factors in the patient at risk for aspiration
Teaching: Infant Safety: Instruction on safety during first year of life

NURSING PRIORITY NO. 1 To assess causative/contributing factors:
- Determine client's/significant other's (SO's) knowledge of individual safety concerns and environmental hazards present *to identify misconceptions and educational needs. Suffocation can be caused by (1) spasm of airway (e.g., food or water going down wrong way, irritant gases, asthma); (2) airway obstruction (e.g., foreign body, tongue falling back in unconscious person, swelling of tissues from burn injury or allergic reaction); (3) airway compression (e.g., tying rope or band tightly around neck, hanging, throttling, smothering); (4) conditions affecting the respiratory mechanism (e.g., epilepsy, tetanus, rabies, nerve diseases causing paralysis of chest wall or diaphragm); (5) conditions affecting respiratory center in brain (e.g., electric shock; stroke or other brain trauma; medications such as morphine, barbiturates); and (6) compression of the chest (e.g., crushing as might occur with cave-in, motor vehicle crash, pressure in a massive crowd).*[1,5,6]
- Identify level of concern or awareness and motivation of client/SOs to correct safety hazards and improve individual situation. *Lack of commitment may limit willingness to make changes, placing dependent individuals at risk.*
- ∞ Determine age, developmental level, and mentation (e.g., infant/young child, frail elder, person with developmental delay, altered level of consciousness, or cognitive impairments or dementia) *to identify individuals unable to be responsible for or protect self.*
- Assess neurological status and note history of conditions, such as stroke, cerebral palsy, multiple sclerosis, and amyotrophic lateral sclerosis, *that have potential to compromise airway or affect ability to swallow.*

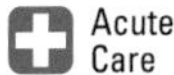

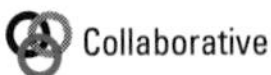

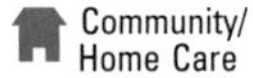

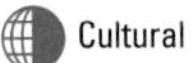

- Determine presence of seizure disorder, noting use of antiepileptics and how well condition is controlled. *Seizure activity (and especially status epileptics) is a major risk factor for respiratory inhibition or arrest, particularly when consciousness is impaired.*[10]
- Note reports of sleep disturbance and daytime fatigue. *May be indicative of sleep apnea (airway obstruction), requiring referral for evaluation.* Refer to NDs Insomnia and Sleep Deprivation.
- Review medication regimen *to note potential for oversedation and respiratory failure (e.g., central nervous system depressants, analgesics, sedatives, antidepressants).*
- Assess for allergies to medications, foods, and environmental factors *that could result in severe reaction or anaphylaxis resulting in respiratory arrest.*
- Be alert to and carefully monitor those individuals who are severely depressed, mentally ill, or aggressive and in restraints. *These individuals could be at risk for suicide by suffocation (e.g., inhaled carbon monoxide or death by strangling or hanging).*[2] Refer to ND risk for Suicide.
- Note signs of respiratory distress (e.g., cough, stridor, wheezing, increased work of breathing) *that could indicate swelling or obstruction of airways.*[3] Refer to NDs ineffective Airway Clearance, risk for Aspiration, ineffective Breathing Pattern, and impaired spontaneous Ventilation, as appropriate, for additional interventions.

NURSING PRIORITY NO. 2 To reverse/correct contributing factors:

- Discuss with client/SO(s) identified environmental or work-related safety hazards and problem solve methods for resolution (e.g., need for smoke and carbon monoxide alarms, vents for household heater, clean chimney, properly strung clothesline, proper venting of machinery exhaust, monitoring of stored chemicals, bracing trench walls when digging).
- Protect airway at all times, especially if client unable to protect self:[2,5,8]

  Use proper positioning, suctioning, and use of airway adjuncts, as indicated, *for comatose or cognitively impaired individual or client with swallowing impairment or obstructive sleep apnea.*

  Provide seizure precautions and antiseizure medication, as indicated.

  Administer medications when client is sitting or standing upright and can swallow without difficulty.

  Emphasize importance of chewing carefully, taking small amounts of food, and using caution *to prevent aspiration when talking or drinking while eating.*

  Provide diet modifications as indicated by specific needs (e.g., developmental level; presence/degree of swallowing disability, impaired cognition) *to reduce risk of aspiration.*

  Avoid physical and mechanical restraints, including vest or waist restraint, side rails, and choke holds. *Can increase client's agitation, causing struggle to escape and resulting in entrapment of head and hanging.*
- Emphasize with client/SO the importance of getting help when beginning to choke or feel respiratory distress (e.g., staying with people instead of leaving table, making gestures across throat, making sure someone recognizes the emergency) *in order to provide timely intervention such as abdominal thrusts and calling 911.*
- Avoid idling automobile (or using fuel-burning heaters) in closed or unvented spaces.
- Emphasize importance of periodic evaluation and repair of gas appliances, furnace, and automobile exhaust system *to prevent exposure to carbon monoxide.*
- Review child protective measures:[2,4,7,8]

  Place infant in supine position for sleep. Refer to ND risk for Sudden Infant Death Syndrome.

  Do not prop baby bottles in infant crib.

  Attach pacifier to clothing—not around neck; remove bib before putting baby in bed.

  Store or dispose of plastic bags (e.g., shopping, garbage, dry cleaning, shipping) out of reach of infants/young children.

  Avoid use of plastic mattress or crib covers.

  Avoid placing infant to sleep on soft surfaces (e.g., beanbag chair, basket with soft sides, soft pillow or comforter, water bed) *that baby can sink into or be unable to free face.*

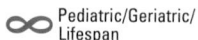

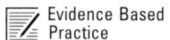

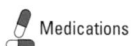

Use a crib with slats that are no more than 2 $^{3}/_{8}$ inches apart *so that baby cannot get head trapped or slip body through slats.*

Refrain from bedsharing with infant/young child *to prevent accidental smothering.*

Provide constant supervision of young children in bathtub or swimming pool.

Make certain that blind and curtain cords, drawstrings on clothing, etc., are out of reach of small children *to prevent accidental hanging.*

Prevent young child/impaired individual from putting objects in mouth (e.g., food such as raw carrots, nuts, seeds, popcorn, hot dogs; toy parts; buttons; balloons; batteries; coins) *that can get lodged in airway and cause choking.*

Lock or remove lid or door of chests, trunks, old refrigerators or freezers *to prevent child from being trapped in airless environment.*

NURSING PRIORITY NO. 3 To promote wellness (Teaching/Discharge Considerations):

- Review safety factors identified in individual situation and methods for remediation.
- Develop plan with client/caregiver for long-range management of situation to avoid risks. *Enhances commitment to plan, optimizing outcomes.*
- Discuss possibility of choking resulting from relaxation of throat muscle and impaired judgment *when combining drinking alcohol with eating.*
- Involve family members in learning and practicing rescue techniques (e.g., treating of choking or breathing problems, CPR) *to deal with emergency situations (especially when at-home client is at risk on a regular basis).*
- Encourage individuals to read package labels and identify and remove safety hazards, such as toys with small parts, and monitor Web sites for product recalls.
- Promote water and swimming pool safety, vigilance, and use of approved flotation equipment, fencing and locked gates, alarm system, etc.
- Discuss fire safety and concerns regarding use of heaters; household gas appliances; and old, discarded appliances. Encourage home fire safety drills yearly.
- Promote public education in techniques for clearing blocked airways (e.g., Heimlich maneuver, CPR).
- Collaborate in community public health education regarding hazards for children (e.g., appropriate toy size for young child; discussing dangers of "huffing" [inhalants] and playing choking or hanging games with preteens; how to spot potential for depression and risk of suicidal gestures in adolescent) *to reduce potential for accidental or intentional suffocation.*[9]

DOCUMENTATION FOCUS

Assessment/Reassessment

- Individual risk factors, including individual's cognitive status and level of knowledge.
- Level of concern and motivation for change.
- Equipment or airway adjunct needs.

Planning

- Plan of care and who is involved in planning.
- Teaching plan.

Implementation/Evaluation

- Responses to interventions, teaching, and actions performed.
- Attainment or progress toward desired outcome(s).
- Modifications to plan of care.

Discharge Planning

- Long-term needs, appropriate preventive measures, and who is responsible for actions to be taken.
- Specific referrals made.

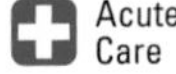

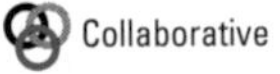

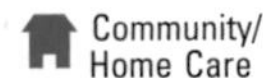

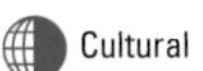

References

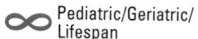

1. Suffocation and artificial respiration. (No date). Fact sheet for WebHealthCentre. Retrieved April 2015 from http://www.webhealthcentre.com/HealthyLiving/first_aid_suffoc.aspx.
2. Masters, K. J., Bellonci, C., Bernet, W., et al. (2001). Summary of the practice parameter for the prevention and management of aggressive behavior in child and adolescent psychiatric institutions with special reference to seclusion and restraint. *J Am Acad Child Adolesc Psychiatry*, 40(11), 1356–1358.
3. Kline, A. (2003). Pinpointing the cause of pediatric respiratory distress. *Nursing*, 33(9), 58–63.
4. Task Force on Infant Sleep Position and Sudden Infant Death Syndrome. (2000). Changing concepts of sudden infant death syndrome: Implications for infant sleeping environment and sleep position. *Pediatrics*, 105(3), 650–656.
5. Green, P. M. (1993). High risk for suffocation. In McFarland, G. K., McFarlane, E. A. (eds). *Nursing Diagnosis and Interventions*. St. Louis, MO: Mosby.
6. Suffocation/choking. Fact Sheet for Manitoba Healthy Schools. Retrieved April 2015 from http://www.gov.mb.ca/healthyschools/topics/safety.html.
7. Centers for Disease Control and Prevention/Kid-Source Online. Preventing choking among infants and young children. Retrieved April 2015 from http://www.kidsource.com/safety/prevent.choke.html.
8. Gavin, M. L. (Reviewed 2013). Household safety: Preventing suffocation. Retrieved April 2015 from http://kidshealth.org/parent/firstaid_safe/home/safety_suffocation.html.
9. Urkin, J., Merrick, J. (2006). The choking game or suffocation roulette in adolescence. *Int J Adolesc Med Health*, 18(2), 207–208.
10. Ko, D. Y. (Updated 2014). Epilepsy and seizures. Retrieved April 2015 from http://emedicine.medscape.com/article/1184846-overview.

risk for Suicide

Taxonomy II: Safety/Protection—Class 3 Violence (00150) [**Diagnostic Division:** Safety], Submitted 2000; Revised 2013

DEFINITION: Vulnerable to self-inflicted, life-threatening injury.

RISK FACTORS

Behavioral
History of suicide attempt
Purchase of a gun; stockpiling medication
Making or changing a will; giving away possessions
Sudden euphoric recovery from major depression
Impulsiveness; marked changes in behavior, attitude, or school performance
Demographic
Age (e.g., elderly people, young adult males, adolescents)
Ethnicity (e.g., white, Native American)
Male gender
Divorced; widowed
Physical
Physical or terminal illness; chronic pain
Psychological
Family history of suicide; history of childhood abuse (e.g., physical, psychological, sexual)
Substance abuse

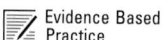

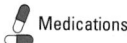

(continues on page 846)

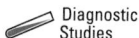

risk for Suicide (continued)
Psychiatric disorder
Guilt
Homosexual youth
Situational
Access to weapon
Living alone; retired; economically disadvantaged; relocation; institutionalization
Loss of autonomy or independence
Adolescents living in nontraditional settings (e.g., juvenile detention center, prison, halfway house, group home)
Social
Loss of important relationship; disruptive family life; insufficient social support; social isolation
Grieving, loneliness
Hopelessness; helplessness
Disciplinary problems; legal difficulty
Cluster suicides
Verbal
Threat of killing self; reports desire to die
Note: A risk diagnosis is not evidenced by signs and symptoms, as the problem has not occurred; rather, nursing interventions are directed at prevention.
Sample Clinical Applications: Acute or chronic brain syndrome, hormonal imbalances (e.g., premenstrual syndrome [PMS], postpartum psychosis), substance use or abuse, chronic or terminal illness (e.g., amyotrophic lateral sclerosis [ALS], cancer), major depression, schizophrenia, bipolar disorder, panic state

DESIRED OUTCOMES/EVALUATION CRITERIA

Sample NOC linkages:
Suicide Self-Restraint: Personal actions to refrain from gestures and attempts at killing self
Coping: Personal actions to manage stressors that tax an individual's resources
Hope: Optimism that is personally satisfying and life supporting

Client Will (Include Specific Time Frame)
- Acknowledge difficulties perceived in current situation.
- Identify current factors that can be dealt with.
- Be involved in planning course of action to correct existing problems.
- Make decision that suicide is not the answer to perceived or real problems.

ACTIONS/INTERVENTIONS

Sample NIC linkages:
Suicide Prevention: Reducing the risk for self-inflicted harm with intent to end life
Behavior Management: Self-Harm: Assisting the patient to decrease or eliminate self-mutilating or self-abusive behaviors
Patient Contracting: Negotiating an agreement with an individual which reinforces a specific behavior change

NURSING PRIORITY NO. 1 To assess causative/contributing factors and degree of risk:

- Note behaviors indicative of intent. *Individual may not make statements of intent, but gestures (e.g., threats, giving away possessions), presence of means (e.g., guns), previous attempts, and presence of hallucinations or delusions may provide clues to intent.*[3,6,11]

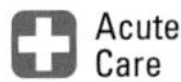

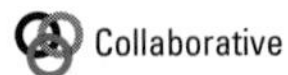

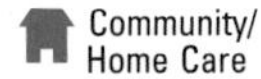

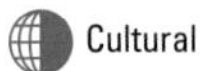

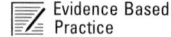

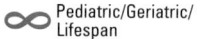

- Ask directly if person is thinking of acting on thoughts or feelings to determine intent. *Most individuals want someone to see what desperate straits they are in, and by bringing the issue into the open, discussion can begin and plans made to keep the person safe.*[3,7]
- Identify degree of risk or potential for suicide and seriousness of threat. Use a risk scale (where available) to prioritize client risk according to severity of threat and availability of means. *Most people who are contemplating suicide send a variety of signals indicating their intent, and recognizing these warning signs allows for immediate intervention. Several risk scales may be used (e.g., Beck's Scale for Suicide Ideation, Linehan's Reasons for Living Inventory, Cole's self-administered adaptation of Linehan's structured interview called the Suicidal Behaviors Questionnaire) to assist in evaluating the severity of risk.*[4,14]
- Note withdrawal from usual activities and lack of social interactions. *These are classic behaviors of the individual who is feeling depressed and sad and may be having negative thoughts of worthlessness.*[6]
- Identify losses client has experienced and meaning of those losses. *Unresolved issues may be contributing to thoughts of hopelessness, feelings of despair, and suicidal ideation.*[3,6]
- Note age and gender. *While women may attempt suicide more frequently, men usually succeed more often. Risk of suicide is greater in teens and the elderly, but there is a rising awareness of risk in early childhood.*[4,8,10]
- Determine cultural or religious beliefs that may be affecting client's thinking about life and death. *Family of origin and culture in which individual grew up influence attitudes toward taking one's own life. Note: A recent study showed that after other factors were controlled, greater moral objections to suicide and lower aggression level in religiously affiliated subjects seemed to function as protective factors against suicide attempts.*[2,4,10]
- Identify conditions such as acute or chronic brain syndrome, epilepsy, panic state, and hormonal imbalance (e.g., PMS, mental illness, postpartum or drug-induced psychosis). *These conditions may interfere with ability to control own behavior leading to impulsive actions that may put client at risk.*[1,4,10,13]
- Review lab results (e.g., blood alcohol, serum glucose, arterial blood gases, electrolytes, renal function tests). *Identifies factors that may affect reasoning ability, interfering with ability to think clearly about issues that are leading to thoughts of suicide.*[1,3,5]
- Assess physical complaints. *Sleeping difficulties and lack of appetite can be indicators of depression and suicidal ideation, requiring further evaluation.*[3,4]
- Review family history for suicidal behavior. *Individual risk is increased when other family members have committed suicide or exhibited symptoms of depression. Studies have shown a possible genetic link toward suicidal behavior.*[12]
- Assess coping behaviors presently used. *Client's current negative thinking may preclude looking at positive behaviors that have been used in the past that would help in the current situation. Client may believe there is no alternative except suicide.*[6,7]
- Ascertain presence of significant others (SOs)/friends available for support. *Individuals who have positive support systems whom they can rely on during a crisis situation are less likely to commit suicide and are more apt to return to a successful life.*[3]
- Determine drug use or "self"-medication. *The use of drugs and alcohol, especially the combination of alcohol and barbiturates, increases the risk of suicide.*[4]
- Note history of disciplinary problems or involvement with judicial system. *Feelings of despair over problems with the legal system and lack of hope about outcome can lead to belief that the only solution is suicide.*[3,10]

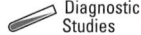

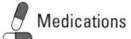

NURSING PRIORITY NO. 2 To assist client to accept responsibility for own behavior and prevent suicide:

- Develop therapeutic nurse-client relationship, providing a consistent care provider. *Promotes sense of trust, allowing individual to discuss feelings openly. Collaborating with the client to better understand the problem affirms the client's ability to solve the current situation.*[3,6]
- Maintain straightforward communication. *By being direct and honest and acknowledging need for attention, care provider can avoid reinforcing manipulative behavior.*[6]

- Explain concern for safety and willingness to help client stay safe. *Clients often believe their concerns will not be taken seriously, and stating clearly that they will be listened to sends a clear message of support and caring.*[6]
- Encourage expression of feelings and make time to listen to concerns. *Acknowledges reality of feelings and that they are okay. Helps individual sort out thinking and begin to develop understanding of situation.*[3,6]
- Give permission to express angry feelings in acceptable ways and let client know someone will be available to assist in maintaining control. *Promotes acceptance and sense of safety while client is regaining own control.*[3,4]
- Acknowledge reality of suicide as an option. Discuss consequences of actions if they follow through on intent. Ask how it will help individual to resolve problems. *Can help client to focus on consequences of actions and begin to discuss the possibility of other options.*[5,7]
- Help client identify more appropriate solutions/behaviors. *Alternative activities, such as exercise, can lessen sense of anxiety and associated physical manifestations.*[3]
- Maintain observation of client and check environment for hazards that could be used to commit suicide. *Increases client safety and reduces risk of impulsive behavior when client is hospitalized.*[11]
- Discuss medication regimen in general and note use of antidepressant medications, especially when there may be a significant organic component to the suicidal ideation. *Certain medications have been shown to increase risk of suicidal ideation or suicide, including (and not limited to) antidepressants, anticonvulsants, pain medications, and smoking-cessation medications. While the use of medications may be helpful in the short term, there are some drawbacks, namely, the length of time it takes for most medications to take effect and the potential for giving a client a means of suicide because of the possibility of a lethal overdose.*[4,6,9,10]
- Reevaluate potential for suicide periodically at key times (e.g., mood changes, increasing withdrawal), as well as when client is feeling better and planning for discharge becomes active. *The highest risk is when the client has both suicidal ideation and sufficient energy with which to act.*[5,6]

NURSING PRIORITY NO. 3 To assist client to plan course of action to correct/deal with existing situation:

- Gear interventions to individual involved. *Age, relationships, and current situation determine what is needed to help client deal with feelings of despair and hopelessness.*[6,10]
- Negotiate contract with client regarding willingness not to do anything lethal for a stated period of time. Specify what care provider will be responsible for and what client responsibilities are. *Making a contract in which the individual agrees to stay alive for a specified period of time, from Day 1 through the entire course of treatment, and which is written and signed by each party may help the client to follow through with therapy to find reason for living. Although there is little research on the effectiveness of these contracts, they are frequently used.*[6]
- Specify alternative actions necessary if client is unwilling to negotiate contract. *Client may be willing to agree to other actions (i.e., calling therapist if feelings are overwhelming) even though he or she is not willing to commit to a contract.*[6]
- Provide directions for actions client can take, avoiding negative statements such as "do nots." *Providing opportunity for client to have control over circumstances can promote a positive attitude and give client some hope for the future.*[3,5]

NURSING PRIORITY NO. 4 To promote wellness (Teaching/Discharge Considerations):

- Promote development of internal control. *Helping the client look at new ways to deal with problems can provide a sense of own ability to solve problems, improve situation, and hope for the future.*[3]
- Assist with learning problem solving, assertiveness training, and social skills. *By learning these new skills, client can begin to feel more confidence in own ability to handle problems that arise and deal with the current situation.*[3,5]
- Engage in physical activity programs. *Promotes release of endorphins and feelings of self-worth, improving sense of well-being and giving client hope.*[3]
- Determine nutritional needs and help client to plan for meeting them. *Enhances general well-being and energy level.*[1,10]

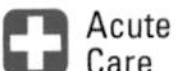

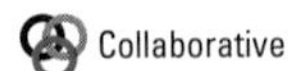

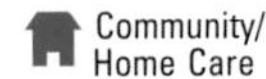

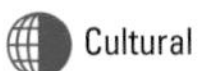

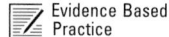

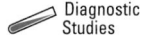

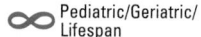

- Review use of antidepressants, noting that it takes 4 to 8 weeks for effects of medication to be observed, and different medications may need to be tried to obtain maximum benefit. Stress importance of continuing medication after symptoms of depression resolve. *Studies of adults age 70 and over reveal significant decrease in relapse when antidepressant continued for 2 years beyond becoming symptom-free.*[10]
- Involve family/SO in planning. *Improves understanding and support when family knows the facts and has a part in planning for rehabilitation efforts for the client.*[1,5]
- Refer to formal resources as indicated. *May need assistance with referrals to individual, group, or marital psychotherapy; substance abuse treatment program; or social services when situation involves mental illness or family disorganization.*[5,10,11]

DOCUMENTATION FOCUS

Assessment/Reassessment

- Individual findings, including nature of concern (e.g., suicidal or behavioral risk factors and level of impulse control, plan of action and means to carry out plan).
- Client's perception of situation, motivation for change.
- Cultural or religious beliefs influencing attitudes about life and suicide.
- Availability of family and other support systems.

Planning

- Plan of care and who is involved in the planning.
- Details of contract regarding suicidal ideation or plans.
- Teaching plan.

Implementation/Evaluation

- Actions taken to promote safety.
- Response to interventions, teaching, and actions performed.
- Attainment or progress toward desired outcome(s).
- Modifications to plan of care.

Discharge Planning

- Long-term needs and who is responsible for actions to be taken.
- Available resources, specific referrals made.

References

1. No author listed. (No date). Suicide. A Different Look at Mental Health. Retrieved April 2015 from http://poetryandinformation.weebly.com/suicide.html.
2. Dervic, K., Oquendo, M. A., Grunebaum, M. F. (2004). Religious affiliation and suicide attempt. *Am J Psychiatry*, 161(12), 2303–2308.
3. Townsend, M. C. (2003). *Psychiatric Mental Health Nursing Concepts of Care*. 4th ed. Philadelphia: F. A. Davis.
4. Soreff, S. (Updated 2015). Suicide. Medscape. Retrieved April 2015 from http://emedicine.medscape.com/article/2013085-overview.
5. Doenges, M., Townsend, M., Moorhouse, M. (1998). *Psychiatric Care Plans: Guidelines for Individualizing Care*. 3rd ed. Philadelphia: F. A. Davis.
6. Jurich, A. P. (2003). The nature of suicide. *Clinical Update (insert in Family Therapy Magazine)*, 3(6), 1–8.
7. Gettinger-Dinner, L. (2007). Suicide risk assessment: What providers need to know. Nurse.com. Retrieved April 2015 from http://news.nurse.com/apps/pbcs.dll/article?AID=200770420001#.VScUNmd0zIU.
8. Whetstone, L., Morrissey, S. (2007). Children at risk: The association between perceived weight status and suicidal thoughts and attempts in middle school youth. *J School Health*, 77(2), 59–66.
9. Sherman, C. (2002). Antisuicidal effect of psychotropics remains uncertain. *Clin Psychiatry News*, 30(8). Retrieved April 2015 from http://www.baumhedlundlaw.com/media/ssri/paxil/FDAHearing/ANTISUICIDAL%20EFFECT%20REMAINS%20UNCERTAIN.pdf.
10. National Institute of Mental Health. (No date). Older adults: Depression & suicide facts. Retrieved April 2015 from http://www.nimh.nih.gov/health/

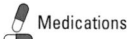

publications/older-adults-depression-and-suicide-facts-fact-sheet/index.shtml.

11. Pearson, J., Stanley, B., King, C., et al. (2001). Issues to consider in intervention research with persons at high risk for suicidality. NIMH. Retrieved April 2015 from http://www.nimh.nih.gov/health/topics/suicide-prevention/issues-to-consider-in-intervention-research-with-persons-at-high-risk-for-suicidality.shtml.
12. Willour, V., Zandii, P. P., DePaulo, J. R., et al. (2007). Study links attempted suicide with genetic evidence identified in previous suicide research. Johns Hopkins Medicine News and Publications. Retrieved April 2015 from http://www.hopkinsmedicine.org/news/media/releases/Study_Links_Attempted_Suicide_with_Genetic_Evidence_Identified_in_Previous_Suicide_Research.
13. Algreeshah, F. S., Benbadis, S. R. (Updated 2013). Psychiatric disorders associated with epilepsy (section on suicidal behaviors). Retrieved April 2015 from http://emedicine.medscape.com/article/1186336-overview#a1.
14. Range, L. M., Knott, E. C. (1997). Twenty suicide assessment instruments: Evaluation and recommendations. *Death Studies*, 21(1), 25–58.

delayed Surgical Recovery

Taxonomy II: Safety/Protection—Class 2 Physical Injury (00100) [**Diagnostic Division:** Safety], Submitted 1998; Revised 2006, 2013

DEFINITION: Extension of the number of postoperative days required to initiate and perform activities that maintain life, health, and well-being.

RELATED FACTORS

American Society of Anesthesiologists (ASA) Physical Status classification score ≥3
Diabetes mellitus
Edema or trauma at surgical site
Extensive or prolonged surgical procedure
Extremes of age; impaired immobility
History of delayed wound healing; perioperative surgical site infection; surgical site contamination
Persistent nausea or vomiting; malnutrition; obesity
Pain
Pharmaceutical agent
Postoperative emotional response; psychological disorder in postoperative period

DEFINING CHARACTERISTICS

Subjective

Discomfort
Loss of appetite
Postpones resumption of work

Objective

Evidence of interrupted healing of surgical area
Excessive time required for recuperation; inability to resume employment
Impaired mobility; requires assistance for self-care

Sample Clinical Applications: Major surgical procedures, traumatic injuries with surgical intervention, chronic conditions (e.g., diabetes mellitus, cancer, HIV/AIDS, chronic obstructive pulmonary disease [COPD])

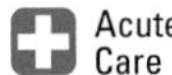

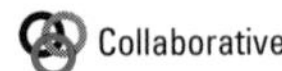

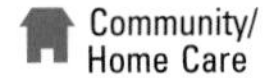

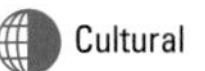

DESIRED OUTCOMES/EVALUATION CRITERIA

Sample NOC linkages:

Wound Healing: Primary Intention: Extent of regeneration of cells and tissues following intentional closure

Self-Care: Activities of Daily Living (ADL): Ability to perform the most basic physical tasks and personal care activities independently with or without assistive device

Endurance: Capacity to sustain activity

Client Will (Include Specific Time Frame)

- Display complete healing of surgical area.
- Perform desired self-care activities.
- Report increased energy and be able to participate in usual (work or employment) activities in a timely manner.

ACTIONS/INTERVENTIONS

Sample NIC linkages:

Self-Care Assistance: Assisting another to perform activities of daily living

Energy Management: Regulating energy use to treat or prevent fatigue and optimize function

Wound Care: Prevention of wound complications and promotion of wound healing

NURSING PRIORITY NO. 1 To assess causative/contributing factors:

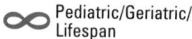

- Identify vulnerable client (e.g., low socioeconomic status or poverty; lack of insurance; inadequate transportation; lack of family or support system; severe trauma or prolonged hospitalization with multiple complicating factors; client with severe anxiety about diagnosis or outcome) *who is at higher risk for adverse outcomes.*[6]
- Determine age, developmental level, and general state of health *to help determine time that may be required for client to resume ADLs and other activities or expectation of time needed for healing. Note: The older adult undergoing surgical treatment is at greater risk for delayed recovery because of age-related changes in numerous systems and protective mechanisms that increase the potential for complications.*[1,7,16]
- Note underlying condition or pathology (e.g., cancer, burns, diabetes, hypothyroidism, obesity, steroid therapy, major trauma, infections, radiation therapy, cardiopulmonary disorders, debilitating illness) *that can adversely affect healing and prolong recuperation time. Note: One study found the incidence of surgical-site infection to be more than five times higher in obese patients and eight times higher in morbidly obese patients than in patients of normal weight. In this population, impaired pulmonary function, hyperglycemia, immobility, and nutritional deficits can compromise wound healing.*[3,8,12]
- Determine the length of operative procedure or time under anesthesia (e.g., typical or lengthy), type and severity of perioperative complications (e.g., trauma, other conditions requiring multiple surgeries; heavy bleeding during procedure), type of surgical wound (e.g., clean; clean-contaminated; grossly contaminated, acutely infected), and development of postoperative complications (e.g., surgical site infection, suture reactions, dehiscence, ventilator-associated pneumonia, deep vein thrombosis) *that can affect the pace of healing or prolong recovery.*[2,3,9]
- Evaluate circulation and sensation in surgical area, noting location of incision. *Lack of blood supply at the wound site can slow healing. Note: Some areas of the body, such as the face and neck, receive the most blood supply and heal the fastest, whereas other areas, such as extremities, take longer to heal. Poor circulation and impaired sensation in extremities, such as in the diabetic person, cause even longer healing times.*[14]
- Determine nutritional status and current intake *to ascertain if nutrition is adequate to support healing. Client may have preexisting nutritional concerns (e.g., elderly person, client with anorexia or morbid obesity) or may have been fasting perioperatively or experienced nausea, vomiting, and loss of appetite postoperatively, depending on the surgical procedure performed and client's reactions to medications (e.g., pain medi-*

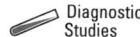

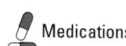

cations, antibiotics). Note: A lack of carbohydrates, proteins, zinc, and vitamins can cause a delay in healing.[2,7,14]

- Review client's preoperative medications/other drug regimen *to ascertain that none could impede healing processes (e.g., aspirin and NSAIDs, chemotherapy agents) or increase bleeding time, (e.g., alcohol and some herbals such as garlic and ginkgo biloba can also be associated with bleeding complications).*[2]
- Perform pain assessment *to ascertain whether pain management is adequate to meet client's needs during recovery.*
- Evaluate client's cognitive and emotional state, noting presence of postoperative changes, including confusion, depression, apathy, and expressions of helplessness, *to determine need for further assessment of possible physical or psychological interferences.*
- Ascertain attitudes and cultural values of individual about condition. *Family beliefs and cultural values, stress and fear related to surgery (and the reason for it), possible stigma about relative condition or disease, or change in body image, as well as motivation to return to usual role and activities, all impact rate and expectations for sick role and recovery.*[5]
- Review results of lab tests (e.g., complete blood count, blood/wound cultures, serum glucose; hormones [e.g., cortisol, glucocorticoid and other hormones associated with inflammation and immune system dysfunction]) *to assess for presence and type of infections, immunosuppression, metabolic or endocrine dysfunction, or other conditions affecting body's ability to heal. Surgical site infections have been found to be tied to hyperglycemia that may impair phagocytosis, negatively affecting the body's normal defense mechanisms. Also, stress-impaired wound healing is mediated primarily through the hypothalamic-pituitary-adrenal hormones, and psychological response–induced unhealthy behaviors.*[11,16]
- Note allergies or history of skin reactions. Evaluate use of plastics (e.g., incontinence pads or moisture barriers), tape/adhesives, or latex materials. *Plastics retain heat and can enhance growth of pathogens in wound. Client sensitivity to adhesives and/or latex can cause skin or tissue reactions that delay primary wound healing and cause additional skin/tissue damage.*[15] Refer to NDs impaired Skin Integrity and Latex Allergy Response.
- Note lifestyle factors (e.g., obesity, cigarette smoking, alcohol abuse, lack of exercise/sedentary lifestyle) *that influence circulation and wound healing and can impede recovery.*[4,17]

NURSING PRIORITY NO. 2 To determine impact of delayed recovery:

- Note length of illness or hospitalization, time of discharge, and progress to date *to compare with general expectations for procedure and situation.*
- Determine client's/significant other's (SO's) expectations for recovery and specific stressors related to delay (e.g., return to work or school, home responsibilities, child care, financial difficulties, limited support system).
- Determine energy level and current participation in ADLs *to compare with usual level of function.*
- Ascertain whether client usually requires assistance in home setting and who provides it, as well as individual's current availability and capability.
- Note client/SO reports of helplessness or inability to cope with situation.
- Obtain psychological assessment of client's emotional status, noting potential problems arising from current situation.

NURSING PRIORITY NO. 3 To promote optimal recovery:

- Inspect incisions or wounds routinely, describing changes (e.g., deepening or healing, wound measurements, presence and type of drainage, development of necrosis).
- Practice and instruct client/caregiver(s) in proper hand hygiene and aseptic technique for incisional care *to reduce incidence of contamination and infection. Note: A recent study showed that while hand-hygiene between patients remains a compliance issue in hospitals, healthcare workers have been found to be more motivated to perform hand hygiene to protect vulnerable patients than they are to protect their own health.*[4,13]

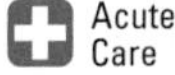

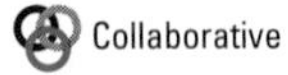

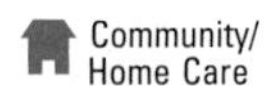

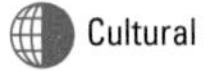

- Administer antibiotics as appropriate and medications to manage postoperative discomforts (e.g., pain, nausea, vomiting) and other concurrent or underlying conditions, such as diabetes, osteoporosis, heart failure, and COPD. *Several types of medications may be needed. For example, client may require antibiotics perioperatively, insulin to support tissue repair, and/or management of chronic pain to improve mobility and tissue recovery.*[10,11]
- Instruct client/SO in necessary self-care of incisions and specific symptom management. *With short hospital stays, client/SO are usually expected to provide a great deal of postoperative care and monitoring at home.*[6]
- Provide wound care expectations and instructions in verbal and written forms *to facilitate self-care and reduce likelihood of misinterpretation of information when client/SO is providing care at home.*[2]
- Instruct client/SO in routine inspection of incision or wound and to report changes in wound indicative of failure to heal (e.g., deepening wound, local or systemic fever, exudates [noting color, amount, and odor], loss of approximation of wound edges) *to establish comparative baseline and allow for early intervention (e.g., antimicrobial therapy, wound irrigation or packing).*
- Avoid or limit use of plastics or latex materials in wound care, as appropriate. *Can delay healing and cause skin breakdown.*
- Collaborate in treatment and assist with wound care, as indicated. *May require barrier dressings, skin-protective agents, wound vac for open or draining wounds, or surgical débridement.* Refer to/include wound care specialist or stomal therapist, as appropriate, *to address treatment interventions to deal with healing difficulties.*
- Provide optimal nutrition with adequate protein *to provide a positive nitrogen balance, which aids in healing and contributes to general good health.*
- Encourage adequate fluid and electrolyte intake *to avoid dehydration of tissues and to promote optimal cellular and organ function.*
- Encourage early ambulation and regular exercise *to promote circulation, improve muscle strength and overall endurance, and reduce risks associated with immobility.*
- Recommend pacing (alternating activity with adequate rest periods) *to reduce fatigue and allow weakened muscles and tissues to recuperate.*
- Employ nonpharmacological healing measures as indicated (e.g., breathing exercises, listening to music, relaxation tapes, biofeedback, hot or cold applications) *to promote relaxation of muscles and tissue healing, as well as improve coping and outlook for positive healing experience.*
- Refer for follow-up care, as indicated (e.g., telephone monitoring, home visit, wound care clinic, pain management program).

NURSING PRIORITY NO. 4 To promote wellness (Teaching/Discharge Considerations):

- Discuss reality of recovery process and client's/SO's expectations. *Individuals are often unrealistic regarding energy and time required for healing and own abilities and responsibilities to facilitate process.*
- Involve client/SO(s) in setting incremental goals. *Enhances commitment to plan and reduces likelihood of frustration, thus blocking progress.*
- Demonstrate self-care skills and provide client/SO with health-related information and psychosocial support *to manage symptoms and pain, thus enhancing well-being.*
- Refer to physical or occupational therapist and/or wound care specialist, as indicated *to address exercise program and home-care needs and identify assistive devices to facilitate independence in ADLs.*
- Identify suppliers for dressings and wound care items or assistive devices as needed.
- Consult nutritionist for individual dietary plan *to meet increased nutritional needs that reflect personal situation and resources.*
- Evaluate home situation (e.g., lives alone, bedroom or bathroom on second floor, availability of assistance) where appropriate, *to evaluate for beneficial adjustments, such as moving bed to first floor, arranging for commode during recovery, and obtaining an in-home emergency call system.*

- Discuss alternative placement (e.g., convalescent or rehabilitation center, as appropriate). *Brief stay with concentrated support and therapy may speed recovery and return to home.*
- Identify community resources (e.g., visiting nurse, home healthcare agency, wound care, Meals on Wheels, respite care). *Facilitates adjustment to home setting.*
- Refer for counseling or support. *May need additional help to overcome feelings of discouragement, deal with changes in life, weight management, and/or smoking cessation.*

DOCUMENTATION FOCUS

Assessment/Reassessment

- Assessment findings, including status of wound healing, individual concerns, family involvement and support factors, availability of resources.
- Cultural expectations.
- Assistive device use or need.

Planning

- Plan of care and who is involved in planning.
- Teaching plan.

Implementation/Evaluation

- Responses of client/SO(s) to plan, interventions, teaching, and actions performed.
- Attainment or progress toward desired outcome(s).
- Modifications to plan of care.

Discharge Planning

- Long-term needs and who is responsible for actions to be taken.
- Specific referrals made.

References

1. Cox, H. C., Hinz, M. D., Lubno, M. A, et al. (2002). ND: Surgical Recovery, delayed. *Clinical Applications of Nursing Diagnosis: Adult, Child, Women's, Psychiatric, Gerontic, and Home Health Considerations*. 4th ed. Philadelphia: F. A. Davis.
2. Semchyshyn, N., Sengelmann, R. D. (2014). Dermatologic surgical complications. Retrieved January 2015 from http://emedicine.medscape.com/article/1128404-overview#a11.
3. Odom-Forren, J. (2006). Preventing surgical site infections. *Nursing*, 36(6), 59–63.
4. Stadelmann, W. K., Degenis, A. G., Tobin, G. R. (1998). Impediments to wound healing. *Am J Surg*, 176(2A suppl), 39S–47S.
5. Purnell, L. D. (2011). *Guide to Culturally Competent Health Care*. 2nd ed. Philadelphia: F. A. Davis.
6. Pieper, B., Sieggreen, M., Freeland, B., et al. (2006). Discharge information needs of patients after surgery. *J Wound Ostomy Continence Nurs*, 33(3), 281–290.
7. Dunn, D. (2006). Age-smart care: Preventing perioperative complications in older adults. *Nursing Made Incredibly Easy!*, 4(3), 30–39.
8. Dunn, D. (2005). Preventing perioperative complications in special populations. *Nursing*, 35(1), 36–43.
9. Gray, M. (2005). Context for WOC practice: Synthesizing the evidence to guide facility wide policies for wound, ostomy and continence care. *J Wound, Ostomy Continence Nurs*, 36(2), 123–125.
10. Sawyer, M., Danielson, D., Degnan, B., et al. (2012, updated 2014). Perioperative Protocol. Institute for Clinical Systems Improvement. Retrieved January 2015 from https://www.icsi.org/_asset/0c2xkr/Periop.pdf.
11. Odom-Forren, J. (2005). Surgical-site infection: Still a reality. *Nurs Manage*, 36(11 Suppl OR Insider), 16–20.
12. Gallagher, S., Langlois, C., Spect, D. W., et al. (2004). Preplanning with protocols for skin and wound care in obese patients. *Adv Skin Wound Care*, 17(8), 442–443.
13. Association for Psychological Science. (2011). Patients' health motivates workers to wash their hands. Retrieved January 2015 from http://www.psychologicalscience.org/index.php/news/releases/

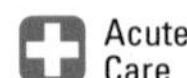
Acute Care
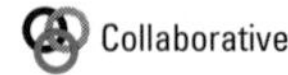
Collaborative
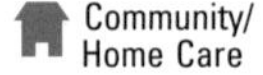
Community/ Home Care
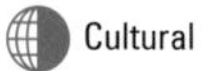
Cultural

patients-health-motivates-workers-to-wash-their-hands.html.
14. Ramsey, C., Koch, F. (2001). The role of sutures in wound healing. Retrieved February 2015 from http://www.infectioncontroltoday.com/articles/2001/09/the-role-of-sutures-in-wound-healing.aspx.
15. Glenn, Y. (2006). When your patient is sensitive to tape. *Nursing*, 36(1), 17–17.
16. Godbout, J. P., Glaser, R. (2006). Stress-induced immune dysregulation: implications for wound healing, infectious disease and cancer. *J Neuroimmune Pharmacol*, 1(4), 421–427.
17. Ahn, C., Mulligan, P., Salcido, R. S. (2008). Smoking—the bane of wound healing: biomedical interventions and social influences. *Adv Skin Wound Care*, 21(5), 227–238.

risk for delayed Surgical Recovery

Taxonomy II: Safety/Protection—Class 2 Physical Injury (00246) [**Diagnostic Division:** Safety], Submitted 2013

DEFINITION: Vulnerable to an extension of the number of postoperative days required to initiate and perform activities that maintain life, health, and well-being, which may compromise health.

RISK FACTORS

American Society of Anesthesiologists (ASA) Physical Status classification score ≥3
Diabetes mellitus
Edema or trauma at surgical site
Extensive or prolonged surgical procedure
Extremes of age; impaired immobility
History of delayed wound healing; perioperative surgical site infection; surgical site contamination
Persistent nausea or vomiting; malnutrition; obesity
Pain
Pharmaceutical agent
Postoperative emotional response; psychological disorder in postoperative period
Note: A risk diagnosis is not evidenced by signs and symptoms, as the problem has not occurred; rather, nursing interventions are directed at prevention
Sample Clinical Applications: Major surgical procedures, traumatic injuries with surgical intervention, chronic conditions (e.g., diabetes mellitus, cancer, HIV/AIDS, chronic obstructive pulmonary disease [COPD])

DESIRED OUTCOMES/EVALUATION CRITERIA

Sample NOC linkages:
Wound Healing: Primary Intention: Extent of regeneration of cells and tissues following intentional closure
Self-Care: Activities of Daily Living (ADL): Ability to perform the most basic physical tasks and personal care activities independently with or without assistive device
Endurance: Capacity to sustain activity

Client Will (Include Specific Time Frame)
- Display complete healing of surgical area.
- Perform desired self-care activities.
- Report increased energy and be able to participate in usual (work or employment) activities in a timely manner.

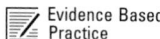

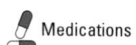

(continues on page 856)

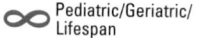

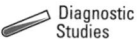

risk for delayed Surgical Recovery (continued)
ACTIONS/INTERVENTIONS

Sample NIC linkages:
Self-Care Assistance: Assisting another to perform activities of daily living
Energy Management: Regulating energy use to treat or prevent fatigue and optimize function
Wound Care: Prevention of wound complications and promotion of wound healing

NURSING PRIORITY NO. 1 To assess causative/contributing risk factors:

- Identify vulnerable client (e.g., low socioeconomic status or poverty, lack of insurance, inadequate transportation, lack of family or support system, severe trauma or prolonged hospitalization with multiple complicating factors, client with severe anxiety about diagnosis or outcome) *who is at higher risk for adverse outcomes.*[1]
- Determine age, developmental level, and general state of health *to help determine time that may be required for client to resume ADLs and other activities or expectation of time needed for healing. Note: The older adult undergoing surgical treatment is at greater risk for delayed recovery because of age-related changes in numerous systems and protective mechanisms that increase the potential for complications.*[2–4]
- Note underlying condition or pathology (e.g., cancer, burns, diabetes, hypothyroidism, obesity, steroid therapy, major trauma, infections, radiation therapy, cardiopulmonary disorders, debilitating illness) *that can adversely affect healing and prolong recuperation time. Note: One study found the incidence of surgical-site infection to be more than five times higher in obese patients and eight times higher in morbidly obese patients than in patients of normal weight. In this population, impaired pulmonary function, hyperglycemia, immobility, and nutritional deficits can compromise wound healing.*[5–7]
- Determine the anticipated length of operative procedure or time under anesthesia (e.g., typical or lengthy), type and severity of perioperative complications (e.g., trauma or other conditions requiring multiple surgeries; heavy bleeding during procedure), and type of surgical wound (e.g., clean; clean-contaminated; grossly contaminated, acutely infected), *which can affect the pace of healing or prolong recovery.*[5,8,9]
- Determine nutritional status and current intake *to ascertain if nutrition is adequate to support healing. Client may have preexisting nutritional concerns (e.g., elderly person, client with anorexia or morbid obesity) or may have been fasting perioperatively or experienced nausea, vomiting, and loss of appetite postoperatively, depending on the surgical procedure performed and client's reactions to medications (e.g., pain medications, antibiotics). Note: A lack of carbohydrates, proteins, zinc, and vitamins can cause a delay in healing.*[3,7,8]
- Review client's preoperative medications/other drug regimen *to ascertain that none could impede healing processes (e.g., aspirin and NSAIDs, chemotherapy agents) or increase bleeding time (e.g., alcohol and some herbals such as garlic and ginkgo biloba can also be associated with bleeding complications).*[8]
- Ascertain attitudes and cultural values of individual about condition. *Family beliefs and cultural values, stress and fear related to surgery (and the reason for it), possible stigma about condition or disease, or change in body image all impact rate and expectations for sick role and recovery.*[10]
- Note allergies or history of skin reactions. Evaluate use of plastics (e.g., incontinence pads or moisture barriers), tape/adhesives, or latex materials. *Plastics retain heat and can enhance growth of pathogens in wound. Client sensitivity to adhesives and/or latex can cause skin or tissue reactions that delay primary wound healing and cause additional skin/tissue damage.*[11] Refer to NDs impaired Skin Integrity and Latex Allergy Response.
- Note lifestyle factors (e.g., obesity, cigarette smoking, alcohol abuse, lack of exercise/sedentary lifestyle) *that influence circulation and wound healing and can impede recovery.*[7,12]

NURSING PRIORITY NO. 2 To promote optimal recovery:

- Inspect incisions or wounds routinely, describing changes (e.g., deepening or healing, wound measurements, presence and type of drainage, development of necrosis).

Acute Care 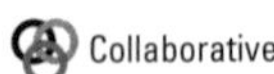 Collaborative 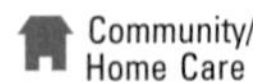 Community/ Home Care 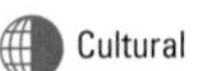 Cultural

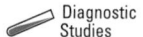

- Practice and instruct client/caregiver(s) in proper hand hygiene and aseptic technique for incisional care *to reduce incidence of contamination and infection. Note: A recent study showed that while hand-hygiene between patients remains a compliance issue in hospitals, healthcare workers have been found to be more motivated to perform hand hygiene to protect vulnerable patients than they are to protect their own health.*[12,13]
- Instruct client/significant other (SO) in necessary self-care of incisions and specific symptom management. *With short hospital stays, client/SO are usually expected to provide a great deal of postoperative care and monitoring at home.*[1]
- Provide wound care expectations and instructions in verbal and written forms *to facilitate self-care and reduce likelihood of misinterpretation of information when client/SO is providing care at home.*[8]
- Instruct client/SO in routine inspection of incision or wound and to report changes in wound indicative of failure to heal (e.g., deepening wound, local or systemic fever, exudates [noting color, amount, odor], loss of approximation of wound edges) *to establish comparative baseline and allow for early intervention.*
- Avoid or limit use of plastics or latex materials in wound care, as appropriate. *Can delay healing and cause skin breakdown.*
- Provide optimal nutrition with adequate protein *to provide a positive nitrogen balance, which aids in healing and contributes to general good health.*
- Encourage adequate fluid and electrolyte intake *to avoid dehydration of tissues and to promote optimal cellular and organ function.*
- Encourage early ambulation and regular exercise *to promote circulation, improve muscle strength and overall endurance, and reduce risks associated with immobility.*
- Recommend pacing (alternating activity with adequate rest periods) *to reduce fatigue and allow weakened muscles and tissues to recuperate.*
- Refer for follow-up care, as indicated (e.g., telephone monitoring, home visit, pain management program).

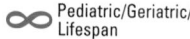

NURSING PRIORITY NO. 3 To promote wellness (Teaching/Discharge Considerations):

- Discuss reality of recovery process and client's/SO's expectations. *Individuals are often unrealistic regarding energy and time required for healing and own abilities and responsibilities to facilitate process.*
- Demonstrate self-care skills and provide client/SO with health-related information and psychosocial support *to manage healing process.*
- Refer to physical or occupational therapist as indicated *to address recovery needs and identify assistive devices to facilitate independence.*
- Consult nutritionist for individual dietary plan *to meet increased nutritional needs that reflect personal situation and resources.*
- Discuss alternative placement (e.g., convalescent or rehabilitation center, as appropriate). *Brief stay with concentrated support and therapy may speed recovery and return to home.*
- Identify community resources (e.g., visiting nurse, home healthcare agency, wound care, Meals on Wheels, respite care). *Facilitates adjustment to home setting.*

DOCUMENTATION FOCUS

Assessment/Reassessment

- Assessment findings, including status of wound healing, individual concerns, family involvement and support factors, availability of resources.
- Cultural expectations.
- Assistive device use or need.

Planning

- Plan of care and who is involved in planning.
- Teaching plan.

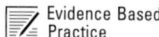

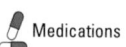

Implementation/Evaluation

- Responses of client/SO(s) to plan, interventions, teaching, and actions performed.
- Attainment or progress toward desired outcome(s).

Discharge Planning

- Long-term needs and who is responsible for actions to be taken.
- Specific referrals made.

References

1. Pieper, B., Sieggreen, M., Freeland, B., et al. (2006). Discharge information needs of patients after surgery. *J Wound Ostomy Continence Nurs*, 33(3), 281–290.
2. Cox, H. C., Hinz, M. D., Lubno, M. A, et al. (2002). ND: Surgical Recovery, delayed. *Clinical Applications of Nursing Diagnosis: Adult, Child, Women's, Psychiatric, Gerontic, and Home Health Considerations*. 4th ed. Philadelphia: F. A. Davis.
3. Dunn, D. (2006). Age-smart care: Preventing perioperative complications in older adults. *Nursing Made Incredibly Easy!*, 4(3), 30–39.
4. Godbout, J. P., Glaser, R. (2006). Stress-induced immune dysregulation: Implications for wound healing, infectious disease and cancer. *J Neuroimmune Pharmacol*, 1(4), 421–427.
5. Odom-Forren, J. (2006). Preventing surgical site infections. *Nursing*, 36(6), 59–63.
6. Dunn, D. (2005). Preventing perioperative complications in special populations. *Nursing*, 35(1), 36–43.
7. Gallagher, S., Langlois, C., Spect, D. W., et al. (2004). Preplanning with protocols for skin and wound care in obese patients. *Adv Skin Wound Care*, 17(8), 442–443.
8. Semchyshyn, N., Sengelmann, R. D. (2014). Dermatologic surgical complications. Retrieved January 2015 from http://emedicine.medscape.com/article/1128404-overview#a11.
9. Gray, M. (2005). Context for WOC practice: Synthesizing the evidence to guide facility wide policies for wound, ostomy and continence care. *J Wound, Ostomy Continence Nurs*, 36(2), 123–125.
10. Purnell, L. D. (2011). *Guide to Culturally Competent Health Care*. 2nd ed. Philadelphia: F. A. Davis.
11. Glenn, Y. (2006). When your patient is sensitive to tape. *Nursing*, 36(1), 17–17.
12. Stadelmann, W. K., Degenis, A. G., Tobin, G. R. (1998). Impediments to wound healing. *Am J Surg*, 176(2A suppl), 39S–47S.
13. Association for Psychological Science. (2011). Patients' health motivates workers to wash their hands. Retrieved January 2015 from http://www.psychologicalscience.org/index.php/news/releases/patients-health-motivates-workers-to-wash-their-hands.html.

impaired Swallowing

Taxonomy II: Nutrition—Class 1 Ingestion (00103) [**Diagnostic Division:** Food/Fluid], Submitted 1986; Nursing Diagnosis Extension and Classification Revision 1998

DEFINITION: Abnormal functioning of the swallowing mechanism associated with deficits in oral, pharyngeal, or esophageal structure or function.

RELATED FACTORS

Congenital Deficits:

Upper airway anomaly; mechanical obstruction [e.g., edema, tracheostomy tube, tumor]; history of enteral feeding

Neuromuscular impairment [e.g., decreased or absent gag reflex, decreased strength or excursion of muscles involved in mastication, perceptual impairment, facial paralysis]; conditions with significant hypotonia

Respiratory condition; congenital heart disease

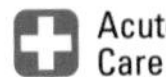
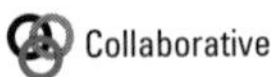
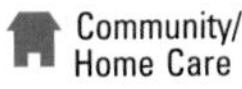
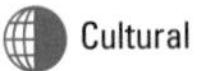

Behavioral feeding problem; self-injurious behavior
Failure to thrive; protein-energy malnutrition
Neurological Problems:
Nasal or nasopharyngeal cavity defect; oropharynx or upper airway abnormality; laryngeal abnormality/defect; tracheal defect
Esophageal reflux disease; achalasia
Trauma; acquired anatomic defects; cranial nerve involvement
Brain injury (e.g., cerebrovascular impairment, neurological illness, trauma, tumor); neurological problems
Prematurity; developmental delay; cerebral palsy

DEFINING CHARACTERISTICS

Subjective
Third Stage: Esophageal
Reports "something stuck"; odynophagia [pain in esophagus on swallowing]
Food refusal; volume limiting
Heartburn; epigastric pain
Nighttime coughing or awakening

Objective
First Stage: Oral
Inefficient suck or nippling
Prolonged bolus formation; tongue action ineffective in forming bolus; premature entry of bolus
Incomplete lip closure; food pushed out of or falls from mouth
Insufficient chewing
Coughing, choking, or gagging before a swallow
Piecemeal deglutition; abnormal oral phase of swallow study
Inability to clear oral cavity; pooling of bolus in lateral sulci; nasal reflux; drooling
Prolonged meal time with insufficient consumption
Second Stage: Pharyngeal
Food refusal
Alteration in head position; delayed or repetitive swallowing
Inadequate laryngeal elevation; abnormal pharyngeal phase of swallow study
Choking; coughing; gagging sensation; nasal reflux; gurgly voice quality
Fevers of unknown etiology; recurrent pulmonary infection
Third Stage: Esophageal
Difficulty swallowing; abnormal esophageal phase of swallow study
Hyperextension of head [e.g., arching during or after meals]
Repetitive swallowing; bruxism
Unexplained irritability surrounding mealtimes
Acidic-smelling breath; regurgitation; vomitus on pillow; vomiting; hematemesis
Sample Clinical Applications:
Brain injury/stroke, neuromuscular conditions (e.g., muscular dystrophy, cerebral palsy, Parkinson's disease, amyotrophic lateral sclerosis [ALS], Guillain-Barré syndrome), facial trauma, head/neck cancer, radical neck surgery/laryngectomy, cleft lip/palate, tracheoesophageal fistula, gastroesophageal reflux disease (GERD), dementia

DESIRED OUTCOMES/EVALUATION CRITERIA

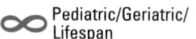

Sample NOC linkages:
Swallowing Status: Safe passage of fluids and solids from the mouth to the stomach
Self-Care: Eating: Ability to prepare and ingest food and fluid independently with or without assistive device

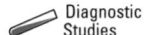

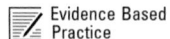

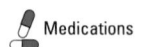

Client Will (Include Specific Time Frame)

- Pass food and fluid from mouth to stomach safely.
- Maintain adequate hydration as evidenced by good skin turgor, moist mucous membranes, and individually appropriate urine output.
- Achieve or maintain desired body weight.

Sample NOC linkage:

Risk Control: Personal actions to prevent, eliminate, or reduce modifiable health threats

Client/Caregiver Will (Include Specific Time Frame)

- Verbalize understanding of causative/contributing factors.
- Identify individually appropriate interventions/actions to promote intake and prevent aspiration.
- Demonstrate feeding methods appropriate to the individual situation.
- Demonstrate emergency measures in the event of choking.

ACTIONS/INTERVENTIONS

Sample NIC linkages:

Swallowing Therapy: Facilitating swallowing and preventing complications of impaired swallowing

Aspiration Precautions: Prevention or minimization of risk factors in the patient at risk for aspiration

Airway Suctioning: Removal of airway secretions by inserting a suction catheter into the patient's oral airway or trachea

NURSING PRIORITY NO. 1 To assess causative/contributing factors and degree of impairment:

- Evaluate client's potential for swallowing problems, noting age and medical conditions (e.g., Parkinson's disease, multiple sclerosis, myasthenia gravis, other neuromuscular conditions). *Swallowing disorders are especially common in the elderly, possibly due to coexistence of variety of neurological, neuromuscular, and/or other conditions. Infants at risk include those born prematurely or born with tracheoesophageal fistula or lip and palate malformation. Persons with traumatic brain injuries often exhibit swallowing impairments regardless of gender or age.*[1,2,13]
- Determine current situation (e.g., intubation, surgery of head, neck, or jaw; cervical spine injury, vocal cord paralysis, problems with saliva production or management; pain with swallowing; mental or anxiety disorder) *that can affect swallowing. Note: Studies show that dysphagia has a significant impact on hospital stay and is a poor prognostic factor. Consequences include problems with nutrition, hydration, quality of life, and social issues.*[7,12]
- Assess client's cognitive and sensory-motor functional status. *Sensory awareness, orientation, concentration, and motor coordination affect desire and ability to swallow safely and effectively.*[4]
- Note voice quality and speech. *Abnormal voice (dysphonia) and abnormal speech patterns (dysarthria) are signs of motor dysfunction of structures involved in oral and pharyngeal swallowing.*[1]
- Note symmetry of facial structures and muscle tone. Assess strength and excursion of muscles involved in chewing and swallowing.
- Note hyperextension of head or arching of neck during or after meals or repetitive swallowing, *which suggests inability to complete swallowing process.*
- Determine infant's ability to initiate and sustain effective suck. *Weak suck results in inefficient nippling, suggesting ineffective movement of tongue and mouth muscles, impairing ability to swallow.*[2] Refer to ND ineffective infant Feeding Pattern.
- Ascertain presence and strength of cough and gag reflex. *Although absence of gag reflex is not necessarily predictive of client's eventual ability to swallow safely, it does increase client's potential for aspiration (overt or silent).*[1] *Coughing, drooling, double swallowing, decreased ability to move food in mouth, and throat clearing with or after swallowing is indicative of swallowing dysfunction and increases risk for aspiration.*[1]

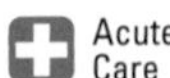

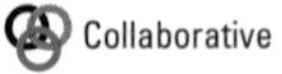

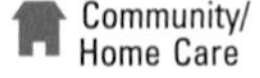

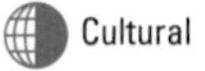

- Auscultate breath sounds *to evaluate the presence of aspiration, especially if client is coughing with intake or has a "gurgly" or "gargly" voice.*
- Inspect oropharyngeal cavity for edema, inflammation, and altered integrity of oral mucosa or structures (e.g., lesions or tumors of the mouth or oral cavity and throat).[1,3]
- Evaluate state of dentition (e.g., poor or missing teeth, ill-fitting dentures) and adequacy of oral hygiene.
- Review medications *that may affect (1) oropharyngeal function (e.g., benzodiazepines, neuroleptics, anticonvulsants, certain sedatives), (2) esophageal function (e.g., NSAIDs, iron preparations, tetracycline, calcium channel blockers), or (3) medications that can cause xerostomia (e.g., anticholinergics, opioids, antidepressants, antineoplastics, diuretics), thus impairing swallowing by means of sedation, pharyngeal weakness, inflammation, dry mouth, etc.*[1]
- Review laboratory test results for underlying problems (e.g., complete blood count) *to screen for infectious or inflammatory conditions* or other metabolic and nutritional studies *that can affect swallowing.*[7]
- Prepare for or assist with diagnostic testing of swallowing activity (e.g., reflex cough test, swallowing electromyography, transnasal or esophageal endoscopy, videofluorographic swallow studies; fiber-optic endoscopic examination of swallowing) *to identify the pathophysiology of swallowing disorder.*[1,3,7]

NURSING PRIORITY NO. 2 To prevent aspiration and maintain airway patency:

- Withhold oral feedings until appropriate diagnostic workup is completed *to determine client's individual factors causing impaired swallowing and identify specific needs.*
- Consult with physician or dietitian regarding meeting current nutritional needs. *May need enteral (preferably by peripheral endoscopic gastrostomy tube) or parenteral feedings in order to obtain nutrition, while reducing risk of aspiration that could accompany nasogastric feedings.*[5]
- Move client to chair for meals, snacks, and drinks when possible; if client must be in bed, raise head of bed as upright as possible with head in anatomic alignment and slightly flexed forward during feeding. Keep client seated upright, or head of bed elevated for 30 to 45 min after feeding, if possible, *to reduce risk of regurgitation and aspiration.*[7,9]
- Instruct client to cough and expectorate *when secretion management is of concern.*
- Have suction equipment available during initial feeding attempts and as indicated. Suction oral cavity if client cannot clear secretions *to prevent aspiration.*
- Instruct client in self-suctioning techniques, when appropriate (e.g., for drooling, frequent choking, structural changes in mouth or throat). *Promotes independence and sense of control.*

NURSING PRIORITY NO. 3 To enhance swallowing ability to meet fluid and caloric body requirements:

- Consult with physician, speech pathologist, dysphagia specialist, gastroenterologist, or rehabilitation team, as indicated. *Therapies may consist of dietary modification, compensatory movements, medical or surgical procedures, etc. For example, medications may help with underlying condition (e.g., swallowing problem associated with Parkinson's disease), surgery (e.g., reconstructive facial surgery following trauma or to correct structural defect in infant), or esophageal dilatation when impaired sphincter function or esophageal strictures impede swallowing. Client/significant other (SO) may learn specific retraining or compensatory techniques (e.g., modifying head and neck posture, strengthening of swallowing muscles, techniques of food placement in mouth).*[1,3,8–10]
- Encourage a rest period before meals *if fatigue is interfering with efforts.*
- Provide analgesics (with caution) before feeding, as indicated, *to enhance comfort, but avoid decreasing awareness or sensory perception.*
- Implement dietary modifications as indicated:[1,3,8–11]

  Provide proper consistency of food and fluids. *Foods that can be formed into a bolus before swallowing, such as gelatin desserts prepared with less water than usual, pudding, and custard; thickened liquids (addition of thickening agent or yogurt, cream soups prepared with less water); thinned purees (hot cereal with water added) or thick drinks, such as nectars or fruit juices that have been frozen into "slush" consistency; and medium-soft boiled or scrambled eggs, canned fruit, and soft-cooked vegetables are most easily swallowed.*

Feed one consistency or texture of food at a time. *Single-textured foods (e.g., pudding, hot cereal, pureed food) should be tolerated well before advancing to soft table foods.*[5]

Avoid milk products and chocolate, *which may thicken oral secretions and impair swallowing,* and sticky foods (e.g., peanut butter, white bread) *that are difficult to swallow or need fluids to completely swallow.*[5]

Ensure temperature (hot or cold versus tepid) of foods and fluids, *which will stimulate sensory receptors.*

Avoid pouring liquid into the mouth or "washing food down" with liquid. *May cause client to lose control of food bolus, increasing risk of aspiration. Note: To avoid posterior head tilting while drinking, some people find drinking from a straw easier than sipping from a cup (if a straw is easier, consider using a flexible one-way straw); if a cup is easier, consider using a "nosey" cup that is double handled and made of durable plastic.*

Feed smaller, more frequent meals *to limit fatigue associated with eating efforts and to promote adequate nutritional intake.*

Determine food preferences of client and present foods in an appealing, attractive manner. *Client may make effort to overcome swallowing problems when food is appealing and desired.*

- Provide or encourage use of proper food placement, chewing, and swallowing techniques:[1,3,8–10]

Provide cognitive cues and specific directions (e.g., remind client to open mouth, chew, or swallow), as indicated, *to enhance concentration and performance of swallowing sequence.*

Focus attention on feeding and swallowing activity by decreasing environmental stimuli, *which may be distracting during feeding. Also, if client is talking or laughing while eating, risk of aspiration is increased.*[6]

Position client on the unaffected side when appropriate, placing food in this side of mouth and having client use the tongue *to assist with managing the food when one side of the mouth is affected (e.g., hemiplegia).*

Manage size of bites—use a small spoon or cut all solid foods into small pieces (e.g., *small bites 1/2 tsp or less are usually easier to swallow*).

Place food midway in oral cavity *to adequately trigger the swallowing reflex.*

Massage the laryngopharyngeal musculature (sides of trachea and neck) gently *to stimulate swallowing.*

Observe oral cavity after each bite and have client check around cheeks with tongue for remaining or unswallowed food *to prevent overloading mouth with food and reduce risk of aspiration.*

Allow ample time for eating (feeding). Incorporate client's eating style and pace when feeding *to avoid fatigue and frustration with process.*

Remain with client during meal *to reduce anxiety and provide assistance if needed.*

Provide positive feedback for client's efforts. *Encourages continuation of efforts and attainment of goals.*

Discontinue feeding and remove any food from mouth if client choking or unable to swallow *to reduce potential for aspiration.*

- Provide oral hygiene following each feeding *to clear mouth of retained food particles and reduce risk of infection and dental carries.*
- Monitor intake, output, and body weight *to evaluate adequacy of fluid and caloric intake and need for changes to therapeutic regimen.*
- Discuss use of tube feedings or parenteral solutions as indicated *for the client unable to achieve adequate nutritional intake.*
- Refer to lactation counselor or support group (e.g., La Leche League) *for breastfeeding guidance and problem solving.* Refer to NDs ineffective Breastfeeding and ineffective infant Feeding Pattern for additional interventions for infants.

NURSING PRIORITY NO. 4 To promote safe swallowing (Teaching/Discharge Considerations):

- Consult with nutritionist *to establish optimum dietary plan considering specific pathology, nutritional needs, and available resources.* (Refer to ND risk for imbalanced Nutrition: less than body requirements.)
- Establish routine schedule for obtaining weight (same time of day and same clothes) and specific weight loss or gain to be reported to primary care provider. *Facilitates timely intervention to change regimen as needed.*
- Consult with pharmacist *to determine if pills may be crushed or if liquids or capsules are available.* Administer medication in gelatin, jelly, or puddings as appropriate.

- Instruct client and/or SO in specific feeding and swallowing techniques. *Enhances client safety and independence.*
- Instruct client/SO in emergency measures in event of choking *to prevent aspiration or more serious complications.*
- Encourage continuation of facial exercise program *to maintain or improve muscle strength.*
- Recommend avoiding food intake within 3 hr of bedtime, eliminating alcohol and caffeine intake, reducing weight if needed, using stress-reduction techniques, and elevating head of bed during sleep *to limit potential for gastric reflux and aspiration.*

DOCUMENTATION FOCUS

Assessment/Reassessment

- Individual findings, including degree and characteristics of impairment, current weight and recent changes, and nutritional status.
- Effects on lifestyle and socialization.

Planning

- Plan of care and who is involved in planning.
- Teaching plan.

Implementation/Evaluation

- Response to interventions, teaching, and actions performed.
- Attainment or progress toward desired outcome(s).
- Modifications to plan of care.

Discharge Planning

- Long-term needs and who is responsible for actions to be taken.
- Available resources and specific referrals made.

References

1. Palmer, J. B., Drennen, J. C., Baba, M. (2000). Evaluation and treatment of swallowing impairments. *Am Fam Physician*, 61(8), 2453–2462.
2. Engel, J. (2002). *Pocket Guide to Pediatric Assessment*. 4th ed. St. Louis: Mosby.
3. Paik, N-J., Dawodu, S. T. (2014). Dysphagia. Retrieved November 2015 from http://emedicine.medscape.com/article/2212409-overview.
4. Poertner, L. C., Coleman, R. F. (1998). Swallowing therapy in adults. *Otolaryngol Clin North Am*, 31(3), 56.
5. Fine, R., Ackley, B. J. (2002). ND: Impaired Swallowing. In Ackley, B. J., Ladwig, G. B. (eds). *Nursing Diagnosis Handbook: A Guide to Planning Care*. 5th ed. St. Louis: Mosby.
6. Galvan, T. J. (2001). Dysphagia: Going down and staying down. *Am J Nurs*, 101(1), 37–42.
7. Stoppler, M. C. (reviewed 2014). Dysphagia (difficulty swallowing). Retrieved November 2015 from http://www.emedicinehealth.com/dysphagia_swallowing_problems/article_em.htm.
8. National Institute for Neurological Disorders and Stroke. (Last modified 2015). Swallowing disorders information page. Retrieved November 2015 from http://www.ninds.nih.gov/disorders/swallowing_disorders/swallowing_disorders.htm.
9. Searle, J. (No date). Eating and swallowing. Retrieved November 2015 from http://huntingtondisease.tripod.com/swallowing/id22.html.
10. McCarron, K. (2006). The shakedown on Parkinson's disease. *Nursing Made Incredibly Easy!*, 4(6), 40–49.
11. Garcia, J. M., Chambers, E. (2010). Managing dysphagia through diet modifications. *Am J Nurs*, 110(11), 26–33.
12. Altman, K. W., Yu, G. P., Schaefer, S. D. (2010). Consequence of dysphagia in the hospitalized patient. *Arch Otolaryngeal Head Neck Surg*, 136(8), 784–789.
13. Morgan, A., Ward, E., Murdoch, B. (2004). Clinical characteristics of acute dysphagia in pediatric patients following traumatic brain injury. *J Head Trauma Rehabil*, 19(3), 226–240.

risk for Thermal Injury

Taxonomy II: Safety/Protection—Class 5 Physical Injury (00220) [**Diagnostic Division:** Safety], Submitted 2010; Revised 2013

DEFINITION: Vulnerable to extreme temperature damage to skin and mucous membranes, which may compromise health.

RISK FACTORS

Alterative in cognitive functioning; neuromuscular impairment, neuropathy
Extremes of age; inadequate supervision
Extremes of environmental temperature; inadequate protective clothing (e.g., flame-retardant sleepwear, gloves, ear coverings)
Fatigue; inattentiveness
Insufficient knowledge of safety precautions (patient, caregiver); unsafe environment
Intoxication (alcohol, drugs); smoking
Treatment regimen
Note: A risk diagnosis is not evidenced by signs and symptoms, as the problem has not occurred; rather, nursing interventions are directed at prevention.
Sample Clinical Applications: Burns, face and head trauma, surgical procedure, radiation therapy, neonatal jaundice, frostbite, dementia/Alzheimer's, attempted suicide

DESIRED OUTCOMES/EVALUATION CRITERIA

Sample NOC linkages:
Tissue Integrity: Skin & Mucous Membrane: Structural intactness and normal physiological function of skin and mucous membranes
Risk Control: Personal actions to prevent, eliminate, or reduce modifiable health threats

Client/Caregivers Will (Include Specific Time Frame)
- Be free of damage to skin or mucous membranes associated with extreme temperatures.
- Demonstrate behaviors and lifestyle changes to reduce risk factors and protect from injury.

ACTIONS/INTERVENTIONS

[This ND is a compilation of a number of situations that can result in injury. Refer to specific NDs, such as Hypothermia, risk for Injury; impaired Skin Integrity; impaired Tissue Integrity; and risk for Trauma, as appropriate, for more specific interventions.]
Sample NIC linkages:
Skin Surveillance: Collection and analysis of patient data to maintain skin and mucous membrane integrity
Risk Identification: Analysis of potential risk factors, determination of health risks, and prioritization of risk reduction strategies for an individual or group

NURSING PRIORITY NO. 1 To identify causative/precipitating factors related to risk:

- Identify client at risk (e.g., chronic illness conditions with weakness, prolonged immobility; acute or chronic confusion, mental illness, dementia, head injury; cultural, familial, and socioeconomic factors adversely affecting lifestyle and home; exposure to environmental chemicals).
- ∞ Note chronological and developmental age of client. *Infants, young children, disabled, and debilitated aged or impaired individuals are not able to protect themselves and may not recognize and/or react appropriately*

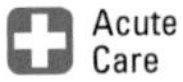

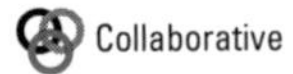

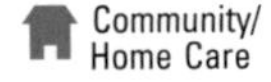

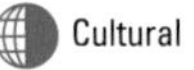

in dangerous situations. A recent study revealed that in the United States, young adults (ages 20–29) were in the highest category for all burn types, while children (5 and under) were most likely to receive scald burns.[1]

- Evaluate client's/significant other's (SO's) level of cognition, competence, decision-making ability, and independence. *Determines ability to attend to safety issues.*
- Ascertain if client is using alcohol/other drugs or medications *that could impair ability to act in best interest of self or others.*
- Evaluate client's lifestyle practices, noting reports of risk-prone behavior (e.g., smoking in bed, failure to use safety equipment when working with chemicals, allowing child to play with matches, unprotected exposure to sun or cold environment) *that can place client or others at high risk for injury.*
- Ascertain knowledge of safety needs and injury prevention, as well as motivation to prevent injury. *Information may reveal areas of misinformation, lack of knowledge, and need for teaching.*

NURSING PRIORITY NO. 2 To assist client/caregiver to reduce or correct individual risk factors:

- Provide client/SO information regarding client's specific situation and consequences of continuing unsafe behaviors *to enhance decision making, clarify expectations and individual needs.*
- Review client's physical and psychological abilities or limitations *to determine adaptations that may be required by current situation.*
- Provide for client's safety while in facility care (e.g., apply hot and cold treatments judiciously, prevent/monitor smoking, supervise bath temperature in confused individuals, young children or elder adults, etc.) *to reduce risk of dermal injury.*
- Ensure client safety when in the operating room:
  - Conduct a fire risk assessment at beginning of each surgical procedure, and continuously monitor for changes in risk during procedure. *The highest risk procedures involve an ignition source (such as electrocautery device), delivery of supplemental oxygen, and the operation of the ignition source near the oxygen (e.g., head, neck, or upper chest surgery).*[2,4]
  - Provide supplemental oxygen safely, using the lowest concentration possible. Use a closed oxygen delivery system (e.g., endotracheal tube) when higher concentrations of oxygen are needed *to reduce amount of oxygen flowing into surgical field.*[2,4]
  - Verify electrical safety of equipment, including intact cords, grounds, and medical engineering verification labels. *Malfunction of equipment can occur during the operative procedure, causing burn injury or death. Note: Ignition sources include, but are not limited to, electrosurgery or electrocautery units and lasers.*[3,4]
  - Place dispersive electrode (electrocautery pad) over largest available muscle mass closest to surgical site, ensuring its contact. *Provides for shortest distance and maximum conductivity to ground to prevent electrical burns.*[4]
  - Ascertain that alcohol-containing skin prep solutions are not pooled under client or in surgical drapes and had sufficient drying time *to prevent sparking with electrocautery equipment activated.*[2,3]
  - Protect surrounding skin and anatomy appropriately when laser equipment is used in surgical procedures, utilizing wet towels, sponges, dams, and cottonoids *to prevent inadvertent skin integrity disruption, hair ignition, and adjacent anatomy injury. Surgical drapes should be configured to minimize the accumulation of oxidizers (oxygen and nitrous oxide) under the drapes and from flowing into the surgical site.*[4]
  - Apply eye protection before laser activation. *Eye protection for specific laser wavelength must be used to prevent injury.*[4]
- Implement skin care protocol for client receiving radiation therapy:
  - Assess skin frequently for side effects of therapy; note breakdown and delayed wound healing. Emphasize importance of reporting open areas to caregiver. *A reddening and/or tanning effect (radiation dermatitis) may develop within the field of radiation.*[5]
  - Avoid rubbing the skin or use of soap, lotions, creams, ointments, powders, or deodorants on area; avoid applying heat or attempting to wash off marks/tattoos placed on skin to pinpoint location for radiation therapy. *These factors can potentiate or otherwise interfere with radiation delivery and may actually increase dermal reaction.*[5]

• ∞ Avoid application of lotion or oils to skin of infants receiving phototherapy for hyperbilirubinemia *to prevent dermal injury,* and cover male groin with small pad *to protect testes from heat-related injury.*[6]
• ∞ Provide or instruct in proper care of skin surfaces during exposure to very cold or hot weather. *Although everyone is at risk for frostbite or sunburn, individuals with impaired sensation or cognition and infants/young children require special attention to deal with extremes in weather (e.g., wearing gloves, boots, a face mask, and goggles when out in very cold weather to avoid frostbite; using sunscreen, limiting time in sun, and wearing light clothing to protect from dermal injury in summer).*[7]
• Discuss importance of self-monitoring of factors that can contribute to occurrence of injury (e.g., fatigue, anger). *Client/significant other (SO) may be able to modify risk through monitoring of actions or postponement of certain actions, especially during times when client is likely to be highly stressed.*
• Perform home assessment, if indicated *to address safety issues. Concerns vary widely and may include evaluation of fire alarms or extinguisher function, safe use of oxygen, checking hot water temperature, or obtaining medical alert device or home health services.*
• Review specific employment concerns or worksite issues and needs (e.g., properly fitting safety equipment, regular use of safety glasses or goggles, safe storage of hazardous substances).
• Discuss need for and refer to sources of supervision (e.g., before- and after-school programs for children, elder day programs, home-care assistance) *when client or care provider is unable or unwilling to attend to safety concerns.*

NURSING PRIORITY NO. 3. To promote wellness (Teaching/Discharge Criteria):

• Identify individual needs and resources for safety education.
• ∞ Prevent burn (flame, scalding, chemical, electrical, sunburn) injuries:[8–12]
Install smoke alarms in kitchen, in every sleeping area, and on every floor of home.
Keep space heaters away from flammable materials and from at-risk persons.
Check all fuel-burning appliances, including fireplaces, for proper functioning.
Store combustibles away from all heat-producing appliances.
Prepare and practice an emergency escape plan.
Avoid smoking in bed. Get rid of used cigarettes carefully. *Fires caused by smoking materials are the leading cause of deaths in house fires.*[9]
Prevent small children from playing with matches or near open flame or stove.
Turn handles of pots and pans toward side of stove or use back burners.
Set the temperature on water heater to 120°F, or use the "low-medium" setting.
Test water temperature before allowing child/impaired person into tub or shower.
Use cool-water humidifiers instead of hot-steam vaporizers.
Store cleaning supplies and other chemicals out of the reach of children *to prevent chemical burns.*
Avoid storing chemicals in food or drink containers; store in original containers with intact labels.
Wear gloves, safety glasses, and other protective clothing when handling chemicals.
Check electrical appliances for proper function and follow manufacturer's safety instructions. Discard frayed or damaged electrical cords *to reduce risk of electrical burn. Note: Most electrical injuries that occur in the home are low-voltage burns and almost exclusively involve either the hands or oral cavity.*[10]
Use child safety plugs in all outlets.
Avoid using electrical appliances while showering or wet.
Stay out of midday sun. Avoid lengthy sun exposure/ultraviolet tanning, especially with specific disease conditions or treatments (e.g., systemic lupus, tetracycline or psychotropic drug use, radiation therapy) *to reduce risk of sunburn.*
Start protecting child from the sun when he or she is a baby, dressing infants in lightweight long pants, long-sleeved shirts, and brimmed hats that shade the neck to prevent sunburn. Sunscreen is often not used in babies under the age of 6 months. *Because children spend a lot of time outdoors playing, they get most of their lifetime sun exposure in their first 18 years.*[11,13]

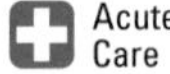

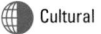
Acute Care
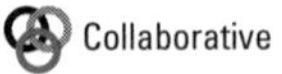
Collaborative
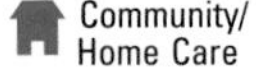
Community/ Home Care

Cultural

- Provide telephone numbers and other contact numbers as individually indicated (e.g., fire, police, physician).
- Refer to resources as indicated (e.g., substance recovery, anger management, or parenting classes) *to address conditions that could exacerbate risk of injury to self or others.*
- Recommend community education programs *to increase awareness of safety measures and available resources.*
- Identify emergency escape plans and routes for home and community *to be prepared in the event of natural or man-made disaster (e.g., fire, toxic chemical release).*

DOCUMENTATION FOCUS

Assessment/Reassessment

- Individual risk factors identified.
- Client concerns or difficulty making and following through with plan.

Planning

- Plan of care and who is involved in planning.
- Teaching plan.

Implementation/Evaluation

- Response to interventions, teaching, and actions performed.
- Attainment or progress toward outcomes.

Discharge Planning

- Referrals to other resources.
- Long-term need and who is responsible for actions.

References

1. American Burn Association, National Burn Repository. (2014). Report of data from 2004–2013. Retrieved April 2015 from http://www.ameriburn.org/2014NBRAnnualReport.pdf.
2. Food and Drug Administration. (2011). Recommendations for healthcare professionals on preventing surgical fires. Retrieved April 2015 from http://www.fda.gov/Drugs/DrugSafety/SafeUseInitiative/PreventingSurgicalFires/ucm270636.htm.
3. Grimes, B. (2007). Essentials of electrosurgical risks. *Perioperative Nursing Clinics*, 2(2), 119–125.
4. Caplan, R. A., Barker, S. J., Connis, R. T., et al. (2008). Practice advisory for the prevention and management of operating room fires. *Anesthesiology*, 108(5), 786–801.
5. Doenges, M. E., Moorhouse, M. F., Murr, A. C. (2010). Cancer. *Nursing Care Plans: Guidelines for Individualizing Client Care Across the Life Span*. 8th ed. Philadelphia: F. A. Davis.
6. No editors listed. (2008). Phototherapy. *Lippincott's Nursing Procedures*. 5th ed. Philadelphia: Williams & Wilkins, 895–897.
7. Geisbrecth, G. G., Wilkerson, J. A. (2006). *Hypothermia, Frostbite and Other Cold Injuries: Prevention, Survival, Rescue and Treatment*. 2nd ed. Seattle, WA: The Mountaineers.
8. Safety for older consumers' home safety checklist. Consumer Product Safety Commission. Retrieved February 2015 from http://www.cpsc.gov//PageFiles/122038/701.pdf.
9. Familydoctor.org editorial staff. (2010). Burns: Preventing burns in your home. Retrieved April 2015 from http://familydoctor.org/familydoctor/en/prevention-wellness/staying-healthy/first-aid/burns-preventing-burns-in-your-home.html.
10. Edlich, R. F., Farinholt, H. M., Winters, K. L., et al. (2005). Modern concepts of treatment and prevention of electrical burns. *J Long Term Eff Med Implants*, 15(5), 511–532.
11. WebMD staff. (Updated 2013). Sunburn-prevention. Retrieved April 2015 from http://www.webmd.com/skin-problems-and-treatments/tc/sunburn-prevention.
12. Heller, J. L. (2011). Chemical burn or reaction. Retrieved April 2015 from http://aspirus.org/AspirusWausauHospital/Health-Information/Chemical-burn-or-reaction-1000059.aspx.
13. Hoeker, J. L. (2013). When is it OK for a baby to wear sunscreen? Mayo Clinic. Retrieved April 2015 from http://www.mayoclinic.org/healthy-lifestyle/infant-and-toddler-health/expert-answers/baby-sunscreen/faq-20058159.

ineffective Thermoregulation

Taxonomy II: Safety/Protection—Class 6 Thermoregulation (00008) [**Diagnostic Division:** Safety], Submitted 1986

DEFINITION: Temperature fluctuation between hypothermia and hyperthermia.

RELATED FACTORS

Trauma; illness
Extremes of age
Fluctuating environmental temperature

DEFINING CHARACTERISTICS

Objective

Fluctuations in body temperature above and below the normal range
Tachycardia; hypertension; increase in respiratory rate
Reduction in body temperature below normal range; skin cool to touch; moderate pallor; mild shivering; piloerection; cyanotic nailbeds; slow capillary refill
Increase in body temperature above normal range; skin warm to touch; flushed skin; seizures

Sample Clinical Applications: Prematurity, brain injury, CVA, intracranial surgery (cerebral edema), infection or sepsis, major surgical procedures

DESIRED OUTCOMES/EVALUATION CRITERIA

Sample NOC linkages:

Thermoregulation: Balance among heat production, heat gain, and heat loss
Thermoregulation: Newborn: Balance among heat production, heat gain, and heat loss during the first 28 days of life

Client/Caregiver Will (Include Specific Time Frame)

- Verbalize understanding of individual factors and appropriate interventions.
- Demonstrate techniques or behaviors to correct underlying condition or situation.
- Maintain body temperature within normal limits.

ACTIONS/INTERVENTIONS

Sample NIC linkages:

Temperature Regulation: Attaining and/or maintaining body temperature within a normal range
Temperature Regulation: Intraoperative: Attaining and/or maintaining desired intraoperative body temperature
Fever Treatment: Management of a patient with hyperpyrexia caused by nonenvironmental factors

NURSING PRIORITY NO. 1 To identify causative/contributing factors:

- ∞ Note client's age (e.g., premature neonate, young child, aging individual), *as it can directly impact ability to maintain or regulate body temperature and respond to changes in environment.*[1,6,9]
- Obtain history concerning present symptoms and correlate with previous episodes or family history and diagnostic studies. *Thermoregulation is a controlled process that maintains the body's core temperature in the range at which most biochemical processes work best (99°F–99.6°F [37.2°C–37.6°C]).*[6] *Exercise, behavioral impulses, and metabolic and hormonal changes influence changes in body temperature, leading to loss or gain of heat.*

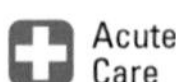

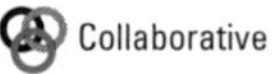

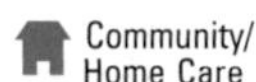

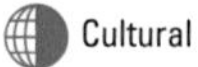

- Determine specific factors involved in current temperature fluctuation (e.g., environmental factors, surgery, infectious process, effects of drugs or toxins, brain or spinal cord injury). *Thermoregulation is affected in two ways: (1) endogenous factors (via diseases or conditions of body/organ systems that affect temperature homeostasis) and (2) exogenous factors (via environmental exposures, medications, and nutrition).*[6] *Understanding the current situation helps to determine the scope of interventions that may be needed (e.g., simple addition of warm blankets during or after surgery, hypothermia therapy following brain trauma).*
- Review lab results (e.g., tests indicative of infection, thyroid or other endocrine tests, drug screens) *to identify potential internal causes of temperature imbalances.*

NURSING PRIORITY NO. 2 To assist with measures to correct/treat underlying cause:

- Monitor temperature by appropriate route (e.g., tympanic, rectal, oral), using the same site and device over time and noting variation from client's usual or normal temperature. *Oral temperature measurement has been shown to be more accurate than tympanic, axillary, or chemical dot thermometers. Rectal and tympanic temperatures most closely approximate core temperature; however, shell temperatures (oral, axillary, touch) are often measured at home and are predictive of fever or subnormal temperatures. Rectal temperature measurement may be the most accurate but is not always expedient (e.g., client declines, is agitated, has rectal lesions or surgery, parent is unskilled or uncomfortable with using rectal thermometer on child). Abdominal temperature monitoring may be done in the premature neonate.*[3,7,8]
- Ensure that cooling and warming equipment and supplies are readily available during childbirth and following procedures or surgery.
- Initiate emergent or immediate interventions, such as cooling or warming measures, fluids, electrolytes, nutrients, and medications (e.g., antipyretics, antibiotics, neoplastics), as indicated, *to restore or maintain body temperature within normal range and optimize organ function.*[1–4]
- Maintain ambient temperature in comfortable range *to prevent or compensate for client's heat production or heat loss (e.g., may need to add or remove clothing or blankets, avoid drafts, reduce or increase room temperature and humidity).*
- Place newborn infant under radiant warmer, cover infant's head with cap, and use layers of lightweight blankets. *Newborns/infants have temperature instability, especially premature or very low-birth-weight infants. Heat loss is greatest through the head and by evaporation and convection.*[5]
- Refer to NDs risk for imbalanced Body Temperature, Hypothermia, or Hyperthermia for additional interventions.

NURSING PRIORITY NO. 3 To promote optimal body temperature (Teaching/Discharge Considerations):

- Review causative or related factors with client/significant others (SOs). *Provides information about what, if any, measures can be implemented to protect client from harm or limit potential for problems associated with ineffective thermoregulation.*
- Discuss appropriate dressing with client/caregivers, such as:
  Wearing layers of clothing that can be removed or added as needed;
  Donning hat and gloves in cold weather;
  Using water-resistant outer gear to protect from wet weather chill; and
  Dressing in light, loose protective clothing in hot weather.
- Review home management of temperature fluctuations in special population (e.g., newborn infant, person with spinal cord injury, frail elder). *Measures could include use of heating pads or ice bags, radiant heaters or fans, adding or removing clothing or blankets, cool or warm liquids and bath water, occlusive wrap in the delivery room, skin-to-skin contact in newborn, etc.*[2–4]
- Provide oral and written information concerning client's disease processes, current therapies, and postdischarge precautions regarding hypothermia or hyperthermia, as appropriate to situation. *Allows for review of instructions for early intervention and implementation of preventive or corrective measures.*
- Refer to teaching section in NDs risk for imbalanced Body Temperature, Hypothermia, or Hyperthermia for related interventions as appropriate.

DOCUMENTATION FOCUS

Assessment/Reassessment

- Individual findings, including nature of problem, degree of impairment, or fluctuations in temperature.

Planning

- Plan of care and who is involved in planning.
- Teaching plan.

Implementation/Evaluation

- Responses to interventions, teaching, and actions performed.
- Attainment or progress toward desired outcome(s).
- Modifications to plan of care.

Discharge Planning

- Long-term needs and who is responsible for actions to be taken.
- Specific referrals made.

References

1. Cox, H. C., Hinz, M. D., Lubno, M. A., et al. (2002). *Clinical Applications of Nursing Diagnosis: Adult, Child, Women's, Psychiatric, Gerontic, and Home Health Considerations*. 4th ed. Philadelphia: F. A. Davis.
2. Helman, R. S., Habal, R. (Updated 2014). Heatstroke. Retrieved March 2015 from http://emedicine.medscape.com/article/166320-overview.htm.
3. Galligan, M. (2006). Proposed guidelines for skin-to-skin treatment of neonatal hypothermia. *Amer J Matern Child Nurs*, 31(5), 298–304.
4. Jones, T. S. (2005). A bolt out of the blue: Dealing with the aftermath of spinal cord injury. *Nursing Made Incredibly Easy!*, 6(3), 14–28.
5. Bissinger, R. L., Annibale, D. J. (2010). Thermoregulation in very low-birth-weight infants during the gold hour results and implications. *Adv Neonatal Care*, 10(5), 230–238.
6. Laberge, M. (2002). Thermoregulation. *Gale Encyclopedia of Nursing and Allied Health*. Farmington Hills, MI: The Gale Group, Inc.
7. O'Grady, N. P., Barie, P. S., Bartlett, J. G., et al. (2008). Guidelines for evaluation of new fever in critically ill adult patients: 2008 update from the American college of Critical Care Medicine and the Infectious Disease Society of America. *Crit Care Med*, 36(4), 1330–1349.
8. Cunha, J. P. (Updated 2014). Fever. Retrieved March 2015 from http://www.medicinenet.com/aches_pain_fever/article.htm.
9. Smith, C. M., Cotter, V. (2008). Age-related changes in health. In Boltz, M., Capezuti, E., Fulmer, T., et al. (eds). *Evidence-Based Geriatric Nursing Protocols for Best Practice*. New York: Springer.

impaired Tissue Integrity

Taxonomy II: Safety/Protection—Physical Injury 00044 [**Diagnostic Division:** Safety], Submitted 1986; Revised 1998, 2013

DEFINITION: Damage to the mucous membrane, cornea, integumentary system, muscular fascia, muscle, tendon, bone cartilage, joint capsule, and/or ligament.

RELATED FACTORS

Alteration in metabolism; imbalanced nutritional state (e.g., obesity, emaciation)
Alteration in sensation; peripheral neuropathy; impaired mobility
Chemical injury agent (e.g., burn, capsaicin, methylene chloride, mustard agent); high voltage power supply; mechanical factor
Excessive fluid volume; impaired circulation; insufficient fluid volume

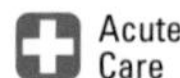

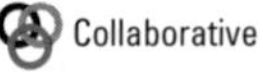

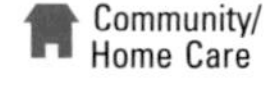

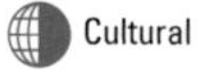

Extremes of age
Extremes of environmental temperature; humidity
Insufficient knowledge about maintaining or protecting tissue integrity
Pharmaceutical agent
Radiation; surgical procedure
[Infection]

DEFINING CHARACTERISTICS

Objective

Damaged or destroyed tissue

Sample Clinical Applications: Abscess, abuse (physical); traumatic injuries, amputation, anemias, burns, cataracts, deep vein thrombsis; diabetes; falls, frostbite; glaucoma, Parkinson's disease, poisoning; substance abuse, malnutrition; vascular occlusive disease

[Note: In reviewing this ND, it is apparent there is much overlap with other diagnoses. We have chosen to present generalized interventions. Although there are commonalities to injury situations, we suggest that the reader refer to other primary diagnoses as indicated, such as risk for Bleeding; risk for Contamination; risk for Falls; ineffective Health Maintenance; impaired Home Maintenance; risk for Infection; risk for Injury; impaired physical Mobility; impaired/risk for impaired Parenting; ineffective Protection; risk for Poisoning; impaired/risk for impaired Skin/Tissue Integrity; delayed/risk for delayed Surgical Recovery; risk for Pressure Ulcer; ineffective Tissue Perfusion; risk for Trauma; risk for self- and other-directed Violence; for additional interventions.]

DESIRED OUTCOMES/EVALUATION CRITERIA

Sample NOC linkages:

Tissue Integrity: Skin & Mucous Membranes: Structural intactness and normal physiological function of skin and mucous membranes

Tissue Perfusion: Peripheral: Adequacy of blood flow through the small vessels of the extremities to maintain tissue function

Client/Caregiver Will (Include Specific Time Frame)

- Verbalize understanding of condition and causative factors.
- Identify interventions appropriate for specific condition.
- Demonstrate behaviors or lifestyle changes to promote healing and prevent complications.

ACTIONS/INTERVENTIONS

Sample NIC linkages:

Wound Care: Prevention of wound complications and promotion of wound healing

Incision Site Care: Cleansing, monitoring, and promotion of healing in a wound that is closed with sutures, clips, or staples

NURSING PRIORITY NO. 1 To identify causative/contributing factors:

- Identify underlying conditions or pathology. Assess for individual factors *that can result in tissue damage or can impede healing, such as (1)* ***trauma that causes internal tissue damage*** *(e.g., burns, high-velocity and penetrating trauma) and fractures (especially long-bone fractures) with hemorrhage, (2)* ***external pressures*** *(e.g., from tight dressings, splints or casting, burn eschar), (3)* ***immobility*** *(e.g., long-term bedrest, traction/cast), (4) presence of* ***conditions affecting peripheral circulation and sensation*** *(e.g., atherosclerosis, diabetes, venous insufficiency), (5)* ***lifestyle factors*** *(e.g., smoking, obesity, sedentary lifestyle), (6)* ***use of***

***medications** (e.g., anticoagulants, corticosteroids, immunosuppressives, antineoplastics) that adversely affect healing, (7) **malnutrition** (deprives the body of protein and calories required for cell growth and repair), and (8) **dehydration** (impairs transport of oxygen and nutrients).*[1–4,11,13,26]

- Note age, developmental stage, and gender. *Children, young adults, elderly persons, and men are at greater risk for injury, which may reflect client's ability or desire to protect self and influences choice of interventions or teaching.*[21,22]
- Determine mechanism of traumatic injury where indicated (e.g., chemical burn affecting skin, mucous membranes; electrical/high voltage injury, car crash, gunshot wound; environmental exposure to toxins or extreme temperatures). *Suggests initial treatment options and potential for tissue damage. Note: Information should include type of injuring agent (e.g., acid or base with route and length of exposure to offending agent; fire; penetration of contaminated object; possibility of coexisting injuries).*[26]
- Assess skin and mucous membranes for color, temperature, and sensation *for adequacy of blood supply and innervation.*
- Evaluate skin and mucous membranes for hydration status; note presence and degree of edema (1+ to 4+) and urine characteristics and output. *Determines presence of circulatory or metabolic imbalances resulting in fluid deficit or overload that can adversely affect cell or tissue health and organ function. Note: Edematous tissues are prone to breakdown.* Refer to NDs risk for imbalanced Fluid Volume, impaired Skin Integrity, and risk for Pressure Ulcer.
- Examine eyes for conjunctivitis, hemorrhage, burns, abrasions, or lacerations as indicated. Note reports of dry, scratchy eye, and vision impairment or pain. *May indicate injury to eye tissues, requiring more intensive evaluation and interventions.*[18] Refer to NDs risk for Dry Eye and risk for Corneal Injury for related interventions.
- Evaluate pulses and calculate ankle-brachial index *to evaluate actual or potential for impairment of circulation to lower extremities. Result less than 0.9 indicates need for close monitoring or more aggressive intervention (e.g., tighter blood glucose and weight control in diabetic client).* Refer to NDs risk for Peripheral Neurovascular Dysfunction and ineffective peripheral Tissue Perfusion.[6,11,13]
- Determine race and ethnic background and family history for genetic factors *that may make individual vulnerable to particular conditions (e.g., sickle cell disease impairs circulation; systemic lupus erythematosis, Marfan syndrome)* and cultural or religious beliefs and practices regarding use of folk remedies or customs *that may damage tissues or impact choice of treatment options.*
- Determine nutritional status and impact of malnutrition on situation (e.g., pressure points on emaciated or elderly client, obesity, lack of activity, slow healing or failure to heal).
- Evaluate client's health and safety practices, noting lack of cleanliness, poor oral care, lack of foot and toenail care, unsafe sexual practices, failure to use safety equipment for occupational or sports-related activities, and unprotected exposure to sun or toxic substances, *that can place client at risk for injury to tissues or impaired function.*
- Note use of prosthetic, diagnostic, or external devices (e.g., artificial limbs, contacts, dentures, endotracheal airways, indwelling catheters, esophageal dilators), *which can cause pressure on/injure delicate tissues or provide entry point for infectious agents.*[10]

NURSING PRIORITY NO. 2 To assess degree of impairment:

- Obtain history of condition (e.g., pressure, venous, or diabetic wound; eye or oral lesions), including whether condition is acute or recurrent, original site and characteristics of wound, and duration of problem and changes that have occurred over time.
- Assess skin and tissues, bony prominences, and pressure areas, noting color, texture, and turgor. Assess areas of least pigmentation for color changes (e.g., sclera, conjunctiva, nailbeds, buccal mucosa, tongue, palms, and soles of feet).
- Assess wound/lesion, documenting (1) location; (2) dimensions and depth in cm; (3) exudates—color, odor, and amount; (4) margins—fixed or unfixed; (5) tunneling/tracts *(full extent of lesions of mucous membranes or subcutaneous tissue may not be visually discernible);* and (6) evidence of necrosis (e.g., color gray to black) or healing (e.g., pink or red granulation tissue) *in order to clarify treatment needs and establish a comparative baseline.*[3,4]

- Classify/stage pressure ulcer(s) using an ulcer classification system, such as the Braden (or similar) scale. (See ND risk for Pressure Ulcer.) *Provides consistent terminology for risk assessment and documentation of pressure ulcers. Note: The National Pressure Ulcer Advisory Panel has updated the definition of a pressure ulcer and the stages of pressure ulcers based on current research and expert opinion. New definitions have been drafted to achieve accuracy, clarity, succinctness, clinical utility, and discrimination between and among the definitions of other pressure ulcer stages and other types of wounds. Deep tissue injury was also added as a distinct pressure ulcer in this updated system.*[5,16,19,20]
- Remeasure and photograph wound(s) periodically *to evaluate progress, development of complications, or delayed healing.*[17]
- Review diagnostic studies (e.g., x-rays, imaging scans, biopsies). *May be necessary to determine cause for and extent of impairment.*
- Obtain specimens of wound exudate or lesions for culture and sensitivity, when appropriate, *to identify effective antimicrobial therapies.*
- Monitor lab studies (e.g., complete blood count, electrolytes, glucose, cultures) *for systemic changes indicative of infection or other systemic complications.*
- Determine psychological effects of condition on the client and family. *Can be devastating for client's body or self-image and esteem—especially if condition is severe, disfiguring, or chronic—as well as costly and burdensome for SO/caregiver.*

NURSING PRIORITY NO. 3 To facilitate healing:

GENERAL[9–11,23–25]

- Modify or eliminate factors contributing to condition, if possible. Assist with treatment of underlying condition(s), as appropriate.
- Provide or encourage optimum nutrition (including protein, lipids, calories, trace minerals, and multivitamins) *to promote tissue health/healing. Nutrients should include adequate protein for tissue/organ maintenance, growth and repair, good immune function, and hormone production. High-quality fats improve energy production and reduction of inflammation. Good-quality carbohydrates provide immediate energy, stable blood sugar and insulin levels.*
- Provide/encourage adequate hydration *to reduce and replenish cellular water loss and enhance circulation. Note: Dehydration can reduce tissue perfusion at a wound site by reducing the blood volume, limiting the supply of oxygen and nutrients.*
- Provide or assist with oral care (e.g., teaching oral and dental hygiene, avoiding extremes of hot or cold, changing position of endotracheal and nasogastric tubes, lubricating lips) *to prevent damage to mucous membranes.* Refer to ND impaired oral Mucous Membranes for related interventions.
- Encourage adequate periods of rest and sleep *to promote healing and meet comfort needs.*
- Promote early and ongoing mobility. Assist with or encourage position changes and active or passive and assistive exercises *to promote circulation and prevent excessive tissue pressure.*

INCISIONS/WOUNDS[9–12,20]

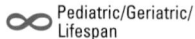

- Inspect lesions or wounds daily for changes (e.g., signs of infection, complications, or healing). *Promotes timely intervention and revision of plan of care.*
- Keep surgical area(s) clean and dry and change dressings or drainage appliances frequently, as indicated, *to prevent accumulation of secretions or excretions that can cause skin and tissue excoriation.*
- Practice aseptic technique for cleansing, dressing, and medicating wounds or lesions. *Reduces risk of infection and/or failure to heal.*
- Protect incision or wound approximation (e.g., use of Steri-Strips, splinting when coughing) and stimulate circulation to surrounding areas *to assist body's natural process of repair.*
- Collaborate with other healthcare providers (e.g., physician, burn specialist, ophthalmologist, infection or wound specialist, ostomy nurse), as indicated, *to assist with developing plan of care for problematic or*

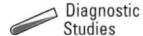

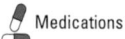

potentially serious wounds. Note: A general surgeon or burn specialist/burn center may be needed for burns (especially burns to hands, face, or perineum. Ophthalmologic consultation is recommended for client with ocular burns from acids or bases if there is any significant degree of corneal or scleral injury. Caustic ingestions may require multiple specialties, including gastroenterology; gastrointestinal surgery; ear, nose, and throat; and surgery.[26]

- Apply appropriate barrier dressings or wound coverings (e.g., semipermeable, occlusive, wet-to-dry, hydrocolloid, hydrogel, polyacrylate moist wound dressing), drainage appliances, and skin-protective agents for open or draining wounds and stomas *to protect the wound and surrounding tissues from excoriating secretions or drainage and to enhance healing. Note: Recent studies are reporting that wet-to-dry dressings are beneficial only for mechanical débridement of wounds, can damage healthy granulation tissue, and can increase risk of infection.*[11,13–15]
- Assist with débridement or enzymatic therapy, as indicated (e.g., burns, severe pressure ulcer).
- Provide appropriate protective and healing devices (e.g., eye pads or goggles; heel protectors, padding, cushions, gel pads; therapeutic beds and mattresses; splints, chronic ulcer dressings, compression wrap).
- Refer to NDs dependent on individual situation (e.g., risk for Peripheral Neurovascular Dysfunction, risk for Perioperative Positioning Injury, risk for Pressure Ulcer, impaired physical/bed Mobility, impaired Skin Integrity, delayed Surgical Recovery; ineffective peripheral Tissue Perfusion, risk for Trauma, risk for Infection) *for related interventions.*

NURSING PRIORITY NO. 4 To correct hazards/minimize impairment:[3–5,7–10]

- Assess IV sites on regular basis for erythema, edema, tenderness, burning, etc., *which indicate infiltration or phlebitis, requiring immediate discontinuation of site use or interventions to heal the area.*
- Use appropriate catheter (e.g., peripheral or central venous) when infusing anticancer or other toxic drugs, and ascertain that IV is patent and infusing well *to prevent infiltration and extravasation with resulting tissue damage.*
- Inspect skin and tissues routinely around incisions and cast edges and traction devices *to ensure proper application and function; note possible development of pressure points.*
- Remove adhesive products with care, removing on horizontal plane and using mineral oil or Vaseline for softening, if needed, *to prevent abrasions or tearing of skin and damage to underlying tissues.*
- Monitor for correct placement of tubes, catheters, and other devices and assess skin tissues around these devices for effects of tape or fasteners or pressure from the devices *to prevent damage to skin and tissues as a result of pressure, friction, or shear forces.*
- Develop regularly timed repositioning schedule for client with mobility and sensation impairments, using adequate personnel and assistive devices as needed; encourage and assist with periodic weight shifts for client in chair *to reduce stress on pressure points and encourage circulation to tissues.*
- Use or demonstrate proper turning and transfer techniques *to avoid movements that cause friction or shearing (e.g., pulling client with parallel force, dragging movements).*
- Provide appropriate mattress (e.g., foam, flotation, alternating-pressure or air mattress) and appropriate padding devices (e.g., foam boots, heel protectors, ankle rolls), when indicated, *to reduce tissue pressure and enhance circulation to compromised tissues.*[13,20]
- Limit use of plastic material (e.g., rubber sheet, plastic-backed linen savers) and remove wet or wrinkled linens promptly. *Moisture potentiates skin and underlying tissues, increasing risk of breakdown and infection.*
- Avoid or restrict use of restraints; use adequate padding and evaluate circulation, movement, and sensation of extremity frequently when restraints are required. *Reduces risk of impaired circulation and tissue ischemia.*
- Elevate linens over affected extremity with bed cradle *to reduce pressure on and irritation of compromised tissues.*
- Encourage physical activity and exercise *to stimulate circulation, enhance organ function, and prevent/limit potential complications of immobility.*

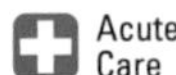

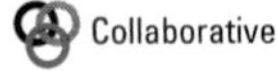

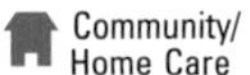

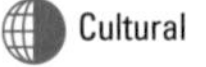

- Provide or assist with oral care (e.g., oral and dental hygiene, avoiding extremes of hot or cold, change position of endotracheal/nasogastric tubes, lubricate lips) *to prevent damage to oral mucous membranes.* Refer to NDs impaired oral Mucous Membrane and risk for Pressure Ulcer for additional interventions.
- Encourage use of adequate clothing or covers; protect from drafts and cold environment *to prevent vasoconstriction that can compromise circulation.*
- Provide or instruct in proper care of extremities during cold or hot weather. *Individuals with impaired sensation or young children/individuals unable to verbalize discomfort require special attention to deal with extremes in weather (e.g., dressing in layers, and wearing gloves clean, dry socks, properly fitting shoes or boots, and a face mask in winter; using sunscreen and wearing light clothing to protect from dermal injury in summer).*
- Advise smoking cessation and refer for resources, if indicated. *Smoking causes vasoconstriction/interferes with healing.*

NURSING PRIORITY NO. 5 To promote wellness (Teaching/Discharge Considerations):

- Encourage verbalizations of feelings and expectations regarding condition and potential for recovery of structure and function.
- Help client and family to identify and implement successful coping skills *to reduce pain or discomforts and to improve quality of life.*
- Discuss importance of follow-up care (e.g., diabetic foot care clinic, wound care specialist, enterostomal therapist) as appropriate, self-monitoring, and reporting of changes in condition or pain characteristics. *Promotes early intervention and reduces potential for complications.*
- Educate the client/caregivers on proper safety precautions regarding hazardous materials, as indicated:[26]
  Inform client/caregivers of various substances in the home that are potentially dangerous.
  Counsel parents on how to keep chemicals out of the reach of children and cognitively impaired persons.
  Consult with local social services agency to evaluate child's home situation.
  Refer client to appropriate agencies for adequate training and protective equipment to protect against hazardous materials/agents in the community or employment setting.
- Review medical regimen (e.g., proper use of topical sprays, creams, ointments, soaks, or irrigations) with client/caregiver *to facilitate tissue healing and prevent complications associated with lack of knowledge about maintaining tissue integrity.*
- Identify required changes in lifestyle, occupation, or environment *necessitated by limitations imposed by condition or to avoid causative factors.*
- Refer to community or governmental resources as indicated (e.g., Public Health Department, Occupational Safety and Health Administration) *for information regarding specific conditions and to report hazards.*

DOCUMENTATION FOCUS

Assessment/Reassessment

- Individual findings, including history of condition, characteristics of wound or lesion, evidence of other organ or tissue involvement.
- Impact on functioning and lifestyle.
- Availability and use of resources.

Planning

- Plan of care and who is involved in planning.
- Teaching plan.

Implementation/Evaluation

- Responses to interventions, teaching, and actions performed.
- Attainment or progress toward desired outcome(s).
- Modifications to plan of care.

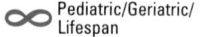

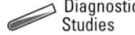

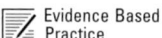

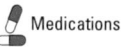

Discharge Planning

- Long-term needs and who is responsible for actions to be taken.
- Specific referrals made.

References

1. Fort, C. W. (2003). How to combat 3 deadly trauma complications. *Nursing*, 33(5), 58–63.
2. Rausal, A. T. (2014). Acute compartment syndrome. Retrieved January 2015 from http://emedicine.medscape.com/article/307668-overview.
3. Llewellyn, S. (2002). *Skin integrity and wound care (lecture materials)*. Chapel Hill, NC: Cape Fear Community College Nursing Program.
4. Colburn, L. (2001). Prevention for chronic wounds. In Krasner, D., Rodeheaver, G., Sibbald, R. G. (eds). *Chronic Wound Care: A Clinical Source Book for Healthcare Professionals*. 2nd ed. Wayne, PA: Health Management.
5. Inouye, S. K., Studenski, S., Tinetti, M. E. (2007). Geriatric syndromes: Clinical, research and policy implications of a core geriatric concept. *J Am Geriatr Soc*, 55(5), 780–791.
6. Murabito, J. M., Evans, J. C., Larson, M. G., et al. (2003). The ankle-brachial index in the elderly and risk of stroke, coronary disease and death. *Arch Intern Med*, 163, 1939–1942.
7. Calianno, C. (2002). Patient hygiene, part 2—Skin care: Keeping the outside healthy. *Nursing*, 32(6). June Clinical suppl.
8. Wiersema, L. A., Stanley, M. (1999). The aging integumentary system. In Stanley, M., Beare, P. G. (eds). *Gerontological Nursing: A Health Promotion/Protection Approach*. 2nd ed. Philadelphia: F. A. Davis, 102–111.
9. McGovern, C. (2014). Skin, hair and nail assessment. Unit 2 (lecture materials). Retrieved January 2015 from http://www10.homepage.villanova.edu/marycarol.mcgovern/2104/SkinHairNail2.htm.
10. Faller, N., Beitz, J. (2001). When a wound isn't a wound: Tubes, drains, fistulas and draining wounds. In Krasner, D., Rodeheaver, G., Sibbald, R. G. (eds). *Chronic Wound Care: A Clinical Source Book for Healthcare Professionals*. 2nd ed. Wayne, PA: Health Management.
11. Bonham, P. A., Flemister, B. G., Goldberg, M., et al. (2009). What's new in lower-extremity arterial disease? WOCN's 2008 Clinical Practice Guideline. *J Wound, Ostomy Continence Nurs*, 36(1), 37–44.
12. Okan, K., Woo, K., Ayello, E. A., et al. (2007). The role of moisture balance in wound healing. *Adv Wound Care*, 20(1), 39–53.
13. Sieggreen, N. Y. (2006). Getting a leg up on managing venous ulcers. *Nursing Made Incredibly Easy!*, 4(6), 52–60.
14. Fleck, C. A. (2009). "Why wet to dry"? *J Am Coll Certified Wound Specialists*, 1(4), 109–113.
15. Cowan, L. G., Stechmiller, J. (2009). Prevalence of wet-to-dry dressings in wound care. *Adv Skin Wound Care*, 22(12), 567–573.
16. Black, J., Baharestani, M. M., Cudigan, J. (2007). From the NPUAP: National Pressure Ulcer Advisory Panel's Updated Pressure Ulcer Staging System. *Adv Skin Wound Care*, 20(5), 269–274.
17. O'Connell-Gifford, E. (2011). The use of photo documentation in wound care. *Medline Healthy Skin Magazine*. Retrieved January 2015 from http://issuu.com/medlineindustries/docs/healthyskinv8i2.
18. Capão, F. J. A., Rocha-Sousa, A., Falcão-Reis, F., et al. (2003). Modern sports eye injuries. *Br J Ophthalmol*, 87(11), 1336–1339.
19. Braden, B. J. (2003). The Braden Scale for predicting pressure sore risk: Reflections after 25 years. *Adv Skin Wound Care*, 25(2), 61.
20. National Pressure Ulcer Advisory Panel. (2014). Prevention and treatment of pressure ulcers: Clinical practice guideline (various pages). Retrieved January 2015 from http://www.npuap.org/resources/educational-and-clinical-resources/prevention-and-treatment-of-pressure-ulcers-clinical-practice-guideline/.
21. Schwebel, D. C., Barton, B. K. (2005). Contributions of multiple risk factors to child injury. *J Pediatr Psychol*, 25, 553–561.
22. Risolainen, L., Heinomen, A., Waller, B., et al. (2009). Gender differences in sport injury risk and types of injuries: A retrospective twelve-month study on cross-country skiers, long distance runners and soccer players. *J Sports Sci Med*, 8, 443–451.
23. Todorovic, V. (2003). Food and wounds: Nutritional factors in wound formation and healing. *Clin Nutr Update*, 8(2), 6–9.
24. Johnston, E. (2007). The role of nutrition in tissue viability. *Wound Essentials*, 2, 10–21.
25. Posthauer, M. (2007). Hydration: An essential nutrient. *Adv Skin Wound Care*, 18(1), 32–33.
26. Cox, R. D. (2013). Chemical burns. Retrieved February 2015 from http://emedicine.medscape.com/article/769336-overview.

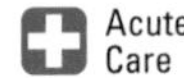

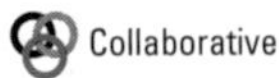

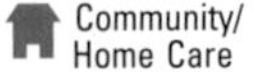

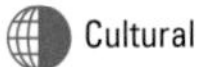

risk for impaired Tissue Integrity

Taxonomy II: Safety/Protection—Physical Injury 000248 [**Diagnostic Division:** Safety], 2013

DEFINITION: Vulnerable to damage to the mucous membrane, cornea, integumentary system, muscular fascia, muscle, tendon, bone cartilage, joint capsule, and/or ligament, which may compromise health.

RISK FACTORS

Alteration in metabolism; imbalanced nutritional state (e.g., obesity, emaciation)
Alteration in sensation; peripheral neuropathy; impaired mobility
Chemical injury agent (e.g., burn, capsaicin, methylene chloride, mustard agent); high voltage power supply; mechanical factor
Excessive fluid volume; impaired circulation; insufficient fluid volume
Extremes of age
Extremes of environmental temperature; humidity
Insufficient knowledge about maintaining or protecting tissue integrity
Pharmaceutical agent
Radiation; surgical procedure
Note: A risk diagnosis is not evidenced by signs and symptoms, as the problem has not occurred; rather, nursing interventions are directed at prevention.
Sample Clinical Applications: Abscess, abuse (physical); traumatic injury, amputation, anemias, burns, cataracts, deep vein thrombosis; diabetes; falls, frostbite; glaucoma, Parkinson's disease, poisoning; substance abuse, malnutrition; vascular occlusive disease
[Note: In reviewing this ND, it is apparent there is much overlap with other diagnoses. We have chosen to present generalized interventions. Although there are commonalities to injury situations, we suggest that the reader refer to other primary diagnoses as indicated, such as risk for Bleeding; risk for Contamination; risk for Falls; ineffective Health Maintenance; impaired Home Maintenance; risk for Infection; risk for Injury; impaired physical Mobility; impaired/risk for impaired Parenting; ineffective Protection; risk for Poisoning; impaired/risk for impaired Skin/Tissue Integrity; delayed/risk for delayed Surgical Recovery; risk for Pressure Ulcer; ineffective Tissue Perfusion; risk for Trauma; risk for self- and other-directed Violence; for additional interventions.]

DESIRED OUTCOMES/EVALUATION CRITERIA

Sample NOC linkages:
Tissue Integrity: Skin & Mucous Membranes: Structural intactness and normal physiological function of skin and mucous membranes
Tissue Perfusion: Peripheral: Adequacy of blood flow through the small vessels of the extremities to maintain tissue function

Client/Caregiver Will (Include Specific Time Frame)
- Verbalize understanding of condition and causative factors.
- Identify interventions appropriate for specific condition.
- Demonstrate behaviors or lifestyle changes to promote healing and prevent complications or recurrence.

Sample NOC linkage:
Wound Healing: Secondary Intention: Extent of regeneration of cells and tissues in an open wound

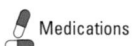

(continues on page 878)

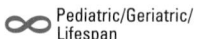

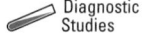

risk for impaired Tissue Integrity (continued)
ACTIONS/INTERVENTIONS

Sample NIC linkages:
Wound Care: Prevention of wound complications and promotion of wound healing
Incision Site Care: Cleansing, monitoring, and promotion of healing in a wound that is closed with sutures, clips, or staples

NURSING PRIORITY NO. 1 To identify risk factors:

- Identify underlying conditions or pathology. Assess for individual factors *that can result in tissue damage or can impede healing, such as (1)* ***trauma that causes internal tissue damage*** *(e.g., burns, high-velocity and penetrating trauma) and fractures (especially long-bone fractures) with hemorrhage, (2)* ***external pressures*** *(e.g., from tight dressings, splints or casting, burn eschar), (3)* ***immobility*** *(e.g., long-term bedrest, traction/cast), (4) presence of* ***conditions affecting peripheral circulation and sensation*** *(e.g., atherosclerosis, diabetes, venous insufficiency), (5)* ***lifestyle factors*** *(e.g., smoking, obesity, sedentary lifestyle), (6)* ***use of medications*** *(e.g., anticoagulants, corticosteroids, immunosuppressives, antineoplastics) that adversely affect healing, (7)* ***malnutrition*** *(deprives the body of protein and calories required for cell growth and repair); and (8)* ***dehydration*** *(impairs transport of oxygen and nutrients).*[1–7]
- Note age, developmental stage, and gender. *Children, young adults, elderly persons, and men are at greater risk for injury, which may reflect client's ability or desire to protect self, and influences choice of interventions or teaching.*[8,9]
- Assess skin and mucous membranes for color, temperature, and sensation *for adequacy of blood supply and innervation.*
- Evaluate skin and mucous membranes for hydration status; note presence and degree of edema (1+ to 4+) and urine characteristics and output. *Determines presence of circulatory or metabolic imbalances resulting in fluid deficit or overload that can adversely affect cell or tissue health and organ function. Note: Edematous tissues are prone to breakdown.* Refer to NDs risk for imbalanced Fluid Volume, impaired Skin Integrity, and risk for Pressure Ulcer.
- Assess skin over bony prominence and pressure areas, noting color, texture, and turgor. Assess areas of least pigmentation for color changes (e.g., nailbeds, buccal mucosa, tongue, palms, soles of feet).
- Evaluate pulses and calculate ankle-brachial index *to evaluate potential for impairment of circulation to lower extremities. Result less than 0.9 indicates need for close monitoring or more aggressive intervention (e.g., tighter blood glucose and weight control in diabetic client).*[5,6,10] Refer to NDs risk for Peripheral Neurovascular Dysfunction and ineffective peripheral Tissue Perfusion.
- Determine nutritional status and potential impact on situation (e.g., pressure points on emaciated or elderly client, obesity, lack of activity, history of slow healing or failure to heal).
- Evaluate client's health and safety practices, noting lack of cleanliness, poor oral care, lack of foot and toenail care, unsafe sexual practices, failure to use safety equipment for occupational or sports-related activities, and unprotected exposure to sun or toxic substances, *that can place client at risk for injury to tissues.*

NURSING PRIORITY NO. 2 To facilitate healing:

GENERAL[5,11–13]

- Assist with treatment of underlying condition(s), as appropriate.
- Provide or encourage optimum nutrition (including protein, lipids, calories, trace minerals, multivitamins) *to promote tissue health/healing* and adequate hydration *to reduce and replenish cellular water loss and enhance circulation.*
- Assess IV sites on regular basis for erythema, edema, tenderness, burning, etc., *which indicate infiltration or phlebitis, requiring immediate discontinuation of site use or interventions to heal the area.*

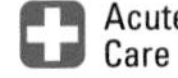

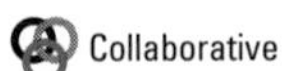

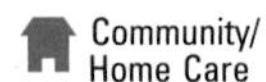

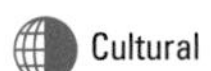

- Use appropriate catheter (e.g., peripheral or central venous) when infusing anticancer or other toxic drugs and ascertain that IV is patent and infusing well *to prevent infiltration and extravasation with resulting tissue damage.*
- Provide or assist with oral care (e.g., teaching oral and dental hygiene, avoiding extremes of hot or cold, changing position of endotracheal and nasogastric tubes, lubricating lips) *to prevent damage to mucous membranes.* Refer to ND impaired oral Mucous Membranes for related interventions.
- Inspect skin and tissues routinely around incisions and cast edges and traction devices *to ensure proper application and function; note possible development of pressure points.*
- Remove adhesive products with care, removing on horizontal plane and using mineral oil or Vaseline for softening, if needed, *to prevent abrasions or tearing of skin and damage to underlying tissues.*
- Monitor for correct placement of tubes, catheters, and other devices and assess skin tissues around these devices for effects of tape or fasteners or pressure from the devices *to prevent damage to skin and tissues as a result of pressure, friction, or shear forces.*
- Develop regularly timed repositioning schedule for client with mobility and sensation impairments, using adequate personnel and assistive devices as needed; encourage and assist with periodic weight shifts for client in chair *to reduce stress on pressure points and encourage circulation to tissues.*
- Use or demonstrate proper turning and transfer techniques *to avoid movements that cause friction or shearing (e.g., pulling client with parallel force, dragging movements).*
- Avoid or restrict use of restraints; use adequate padding and evaluate circulation, movement, and sensation of extremity frequently, when restraints are required. *Reduces risk of impaired circulation and tissue ischemia.*
- Encourage adequate periods of rest and sleep *to promote healing and meet comfort needs.*
- Promote early and ongoing mobility. Assist with or encourage position changes and active or passive and assistive exercises *to promote circulation and prevent excessive tissue pressure.*

INCISIONS/WOUNDS[9–15]

- Inspect lesions or wounds daily for changes (e.g., signs of infection, complications, or healing). *Promotes timely intervention and revision of plan of care.*
- Keep surgical area(s) clean and dry and change dressings or drainage appliances frequently, as indicated, *to prevent accumulation of secretions or excretions that can cause skin and tissue excoriation.*
- Practice aseptic technique for cleansing, dressing, and medicating wounds or lesions. *Reduces risk of infection and/or failure to heal.*
- Protect incision or wound approximation (e.g., use of Steri-Strips, splinting when coughing) and stimulate circulation to surrounding areas *to assist body's natural process of repair.*
- Apply appropriate barrier dressings or wound coverings (e.g., semipermeable, occlusive, wet-to-dry, hydrocolloid, hydrogel, polyacrylate moist wound dressing), drainage appliances, and skin-protective agents for open or draining wounds and stomas *to protect the wound and surrounding tissues from excoriating secretions or drainage and to enhance healing.*
- Refer to NDs dependent on individual situation (e.g., risk for Peripheral Neurovascular Dysfunction, risk for Perioperative Positioning Injury, risk for Pressure Ulcer, impaired physical/bed Mobility, impaired Skin Integrity, delayed Surgical Recovery, ineffective peripheral Tissue Perfusion, risk for Trauma, risk for Infection) *for related interventions.*

NURSING PRIORITY NO. 3 To promote wellness (Teaching/Discharge Considerations):

- Review medical regimen (e.g., proper use of topical sprays, creams, ointments, soaks, or irrigations) with client/caregiver *to prevent complications associated with lack of knowledge about maintaining tissue integrity.*
- Discuss importance of follow-up care (e.g., diabetic foot care clinic, wound care specialist, enterostomal therapist) as appropriate, self-monitoring, and reporting of changes in condition or pain characteristics. *Reduces potential for complications.*
- Advise smoking cessation and refer for resources, if indicated. *Smoking causes vasoconstriction/interferes with healing.*
- Educate client/caregivers on proper safety precautions regarding hazardous materials, as indicated.

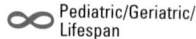

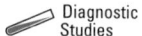

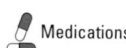

DOCUMENTATION FOCUS

Assessment/Reassessment

- Individual findings, characteristics of wound/incisions, etc.
- Impact on functioning and lifestyle.
- Availability and use of resources.

Planning

- Plan of care and who is involved in planning.
- Teaching plan.

Implementation/Evaluation

- Responses to interventions, teaching, and actions performed.
- Attainment or progress toward desired outcome(s).
- Modifications to plan of care.

Discharge Planning

- Long-term needs and who is responsible for actions to be taken.
- Specific referrals made.

References

1. Fort, C. W. (2003). How to combat 3 deadly trauma complications. *Nursing*, 33(5), 58–63.
2. Rausal, A. T. (2014). Acute compartment syndrome. Retrieved January 2015 from http://emedicine.medscape.com/article/307668-overview.
3. Llewellyn, S. (2002). *Skin integrity and wound care (lecture materials)*. Chapel Hill, NC: Cape Fear Community College Nursing Program.
4. Colburn, L. (2001). Prevention for chronic wounds. In Krasner, D., Rodeheaver, G., Sibbald, R. G. (eds). *Chronic Wound Care: A Clinical Source Book for Healthcare Professionals*. 2nd ed. Wayne, PA: Health Management.
5. Bonham, P. A., Flemister, B. G., Goldberg, M., et al. (2009). What's new in lower-extremity arterial disease? WOCN's 2008 Clinical Practice Guideline. *J Wound, Ostomy Continence Nurs*, 36(1), 37–44.
6. Sieggreen, N. Y. (2006). Getting a leg up on managing venous ulcers. *Nursing Made Incredibly Easy!*, 4(6), 52–60.
7. Cox, R. D. (2013). Chemical burns. Retrieved February 2015 from http://emedicine.medscape.com/article/769336-overview.
8. Schwebel, D. C., Barton, B. K. (2005). Contributions of multiple risk factors to child injury. *J Pediatr Psychol*, 25, 553–561.
9. Risolainen, L., Heinomen, A., Waller, B., et al. (2009). Gender differences in sport injury risk and types of injuries: A retrospective twelve-month study on cross-country skiers, long distance runners and soccer players. *J Sports Sci Med*, 8, 443–451.
10. Murabito, J. M., Evans, J. C., Larson, M. G., et al. (2003). The ankle-brachial index in the elderly and risk of stroke, coronary disease and death. *Arch Intern Med*, 163, 1939–1942.
11. McGovern, C. (2014). Skin, hair and nail assessment. Unit 2 (lecture materials). Retrieved January 2015 from http://www10.homepage.villanova.edu/marycarol.mcgovern/2104/SkinHairNail2.htm.
12. Faller, N., Beitz, J. (2001). When a wound isn't a wound: Tubes, drains, fistulas and draining wounds. In Krasner, D., Rodeheaver, G., Sibbald, R. G. (eds). *Chronic Wound Care: A Clinical Source Book for Healthcare Professionals*. 2nd ed. Wayne, PA: Health Management.
13. Posthauer, M. (2007). Hydration: An essential nutrient. *Adv Skin Wound Care*, 18(1), 32–33.
14. Okan, K., Woo, K., Ayello, E. A., et al. (2007). The role of moisture balance in wound healing. *Adv Wound Care*, 20(1), 39–53.
15. National Pressure Ulcer Advisory Panel. (2014). Prevention and treatment of pressure ulcers: Clinical practice guideline (various pages). Retrieved January 2015 from http://www.npuap.org/resources/educational-and-clinical-resources/prevention-and-treatment-of-pressure-ulcers-clinical-practice-guideline/.

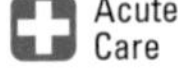

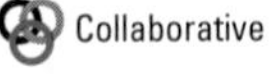

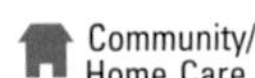

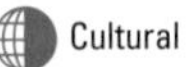

ineffective peripheral Tissue Perfusion

Taxonomy II: Activity/Rest—Class 4 Cardiovascular/Pulmonary Responses (00204) [**Diagnostic Division:** Circulation], Submitted 2008; Revised 2010

DEFINITION: Decrease in blood circulation to the periphery that may compromise health.

RELATED FACTORS

Diabetes mellitus; hypertension
Insufficient knowledge of disease process or aggravating factors (e.g., smoking, sedentary lifestyle, trauma, obesity, salt intake, immobility)
Sedentary lifestyle; smoking

DEFINING CHARACTERISTICS

Subjective

Extremity pain; intermittent claudication
Paresthesia

Objective

Decrease in or absence of peripheral pulses; ankle-brachial index <0.90; decrease in blood pressure in extremities; femoral bruit
Alteration in skin characteristics (e.g., color, elasticity, hair, moisture, nails, sensation, temperature)
Skin color pales with limb elevation; capillary refill time >3 sec; color does not return to lowered limb after 1 min leg elevation
Decrease in pain-free distances achieved in the 6-minute walk test; distance in the 6-minute walk test below normal range (400 m to 700 m in adults)
Edema
Alteration in motor function
Delay in peripheral wound healing; [ulcerations]
Sample Clinical Applications: Atherosclerosis, anemias; arthritis; coronary artery disease; amputation; Buerger's disease, burns; CVA; COPD; CHF; diabetes mellitus, obesity; peripheral vascular disease, Raynaud's disease, thrombophlebitis

DESIRED OUTCOMES/EVALUATION CRITERIA

Sample NOC linkages:

Tissue Perfusion: Peripheral: Adequacy of blood flow through the small vessels of the extremities to maintain tissue function
Knowledge: Disease Process: Extent of understanding conveyed about a specific disease process and prevention of complications

Client Will (Include Specific Time Frame)

- Demonstrate increased perfusion as individually appropriate (e.g., skin warm and dry, peripheral pulses present and strong, absence of edema, free of pain or discomfort).
- Verbalize understanding of condition, therapy regimen, side effects of medications, and when to contact healthcare provider.
- Demonstrate behaviors or lifestyle changes to improve circulation (e.g., engage in regular exercise, cessation of smoking, weight reduction, disease management).

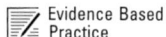

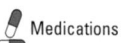

(continues on page 882)

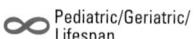

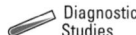

ineffective peripheral Tissue Perfusion (continued)
ACTIONS/INTERVENTIONS

Sample NIC linkages:
Circulatory Care: Arterial Insufficiency: Promotion of arterial circulation
Circulatory Care: Venous Insufficiency: Promotion of venous circulation

NURSING PRIORITY NO. 1 To assess causative/contributing factors:

- Note current situation or presence of conditions that can affect perfusion to all body systems (e.g., congestive heart failure, lung disorders, major trauma, septic or hypovolemic shock, coagulopathies, sickle cell anemia) *affecting systemic circulation and perfusion.*
- Determine history of conditions associated with thrombus or emboli (e.g., problems with coronary or cerebral circulation, stroke; high-velocity trauma with fractures, abdominal or orthopedic surgery, long periods of immobility; inflammatory diseases; chronic lung disease; diabetes with coexisting peripheral vascular disease; estrogen therapy; cancer and cancer therapies; presence of central venous catheters) *to identify client at higher risk for venous stasis, vessel wall injury, and hypercoagulability.*[1,2,14,15]
- Identify presence of high-risk factors or conditions (e.g., smoking, uncontrolled hypertension, obesity, pregnancy, pelvic tumor, paralysis, hypercholesterolemia, varicose veins, arthritis, sepsis). *Places client at greater risk for developing peripheral vascular disease (PVD), including arterial blockage and chronic venous insufficiency, with associated complications.*[3,4,14]
- Note location of restrictive clothing, pressure dressings, circular wraps, and cast or traction device *that may restrict circulation to limb.*
- Ascertain impact on functioning and lifestyle. *For example, leg pain may restrict ambulation or person may develop skin ulceration and healing problems that seriously impact quality of life.*

NURSING PRIORITY NO. 2 To evaluate degree of impairment:

- Assess skin color, temperature, moisture, and whether changes are widespread or localized. *Helps in determining location and type of perfusion problem.*
- Compare skin temperature and color with other limb when assessing extremity circulation. *Helps differentiate type of problem (e.g., deep redness in both hands triggered by vibrating machinery is associated with functional PVD, such as Raynaud's disease; edema, redness, swelling in calf of one leg is associated with localized thrombophlebitis).*[1,5,14–16]
- Assess presence, location, and degree of swelling or edema formation. Measure circumference of extremities, noting differences in size. *Useful in identifying or quantifying edema in involved extremity.*
- Measure capillary refill *to determine adequacy of systemic circulation.*
- Note client's nutritional and fluid status. *Protein-energy malnutrition and weight loss make ischemic tissues more prone to breakdown. Dehydration reduces blood volume and compromises peripheral circulation.*[14]
- Inspect lower extremities for skin texture (e.g., atrophic; shiny appearance; lack of hair; dry, scaly, reddened skin) and skin breaks or ulcerations *that often accompany diminished peripheral circulation.*[2,3,6,14]
- Palpate arterial pulses (bilateral femoral, popliteal, dorsalis pedis, postero-tibial), using handheld Doppler if indicated *to determine level of circulatory problem (e.g., client with intermittent claudication may have palpable pulses that disappear after ambulation).*[2,5]
- Determine pulse equality as well as intensity (e.g., bounding, normal, diminished, absent) and compare with unaffected extremity *to evaluate distribution and quality of blood flow and success or failure of therapy.*[2]
- Evaluate extremity pain reports, noting associated symptoms (e.g., cramping or heaviness, discomfort with walking, progressive temperature or color changes, paresthesia). Determine time (day or night) that symptoms are worse, precipitating or aggravating events (e.g., walking), and relieving factors (e.g., rest, sitting down with legs in dependent position, oral analgesics) *to help isolate and differentiate problems such as intermittent*

Acute Care
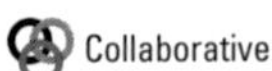
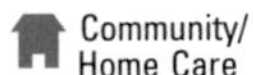
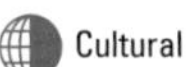

chronic claudication versus loss of function and pain due to acute sustained ischemia related to loss of arterial blood flow.[2,3]

- Assess motor and sensory function. *Problems with ambulation, hypersensitivity or loss of sensation, numbness and tingling are changes that can indicate neurovascular dysfunction or limb ischemia, requiring more evaluation for differentiation of problem.*[2,6]
- Check for calf tenderness or pain on dorsiflexion of foot (Homans' sign) and swelling and redness. *Indicators of deep vein thrombosis (DVT), although DVT is often present without a positive Homans' sign.*[1,15] *Note: While many practitioners continue to use the Homan's sign as part of the physical evaluation for DVT, studies over time have not proven it to be a clinically significant physical assessment tool.*[18]
- Review lab studies (e.g., lipid profile, coagulation studies, hemoglobin/hematocrit, renal/cardiac function tests, inflammatory markers [e.g., D dimer, C-reactive protein]) and diagnostic studies (e.g., Doppler ultrasound, magnetic resonance angiography, venogram, contrast angiography, resting ankle-brachial index, leg segmental arterial pressure measurements) *to determine probability, location, and degree of impairment.*[1–3,6]

NURSING PRIORITY NO. 3 To maximize tissue perfusion:

- Collaborate in treatment of underlying conditions, such as diabetes, hypertension, cardiopulmonary conditions, blood disorders, traumatic injury, hypovolemia, and hypoxemia *to maximize systemic circulation and organ perfusion.*
- Administer medications such as antiplatelet agents, thrombolytics, and antibiotics *to improve tissue perfusion and organ function.*[1,2,4,6,15,16]
- Administer fluids, electrolytes, nutrients, and oxygen as indicated *to promote optimal blood flow, organ perfusion and function.*
- Assist with or prepare for medical procedures such as endovascular stent placement, surgical revascularization procedures, thrombectomy, and sympathectomy *to improve peripheral circulation.*
- Assist with application of elasticized tubular support bandages, adhesive elastic or Velcro wraps (e.g., Circ-Aid), paste bandages (Unna's boot), multilayer bandage regimens, sequential pneumatic compression devices, and custom-fitted compression stockings as indicated *to provide graduated compression of lower extremity in presence of venous stasis ulcer.*[13,15]
- Collaborate with wound care specialist if arterial or venous ulcerations are present. *In-depth wound care may include débridement and various specialized dressings that provide optimal moisture for healing, prevention of infection and further injury.*[14,15]
- Provide interventions to promote peripheral circulation and limit complications:[1–3,7]

  Encourage early ambulation when possible and recommend regular exercise. *Enhances venous return. Studies indicate exercise training may be an effective early treatment for intermittent claudication.*[8]

  Recommend or provide foot and ankle exercises when client unable to ambulate freely *to reduce venous pooling and increase venous return.*[15]

  Provide pressure-relieving devices for immobilized client (e.g., air mattress, foam or sheepskin padding, bed or foot cradle) *to reduce excessive tissue pressure that could lead to skin breakdown.*

  Apply intermittent compression devices or graduated compression stockings to lower extremities *to limit venous stasis, improve venous return, and reduce risk of DVT or tissue ulceration in client who is limited in activity or otherwise at risk.*[9,14–16]

  Assist with or cue client to change position at timed intervals rather than using presence of pain as signal to change positions *because sensation may be impaired.*[6]

  Elevate the legs when sitting, but avoid sharp angulation of the hips or knees *to enhance venous return and minimize edema formation.*

  Avoid massaging the leg in presence of thrombosis *to reduce risk for embolus.*

  Avoid, or carefully monitor, use of heat or cold, such as hot water bottle, heating pad, or ice pack. *Tissues may have decreased sensitivity due to ischemia, increasing risk of dermal injury.*

- Refer to NDs risk for Peripheral Neurovascular Dysfunction, risk for impaired Skin Integrity, impaired Tissue Integrity, and [disturbed Sensory Perception] for additional interventions as appropriate.

NURSING PRIORITY NO. 4 To promote wellness (Teaching/Discharge Considerations):

- Discuss relevant risk factors (e.g., family history, obesity, age, smoking, hypertension, diabetes, clotting disorders) and potential outcomes of atherosclerosis (e.g., systemic and peripheral vascular disease conditions). *Information necessary for client to make informed decisions concerning risk factors and to commit to lifestyle changes necessary to prevent onset of complications or manage symptoms when condition present.*[10,11]
- Identify necessary changes in lifestyle and assist client to incorporate disease management into activities of daily living. *Promotes independence and enhances self-concept regarding ability to deal with change and manage own needs.*
- Emphasize need for regular exercise program *to enhance circulation and promote general well-being.*[12]
- Refer to nutritionist for well-balanced, low-saturated-fat, low-cholesterol diet or other modifications as indicated *to promote weight loss and/or lower cholesterol levels.*
- Discuss care of dependent limbs and foot care as appropriate. *When circulation is impaired, changes in sensation place client at risk for development of lesions or ulcerations that are often slow to heal.*
- Discourage sitting or standing for long periods, wearing constrictive clothing, and crossing legs, *which can restrict circulation and lead to edema.*
- Provide education about relationship between smoking and peripheral vascular circulation, as indicated. *Smoking contributes to development and progression of PVD and is associated with higher rate of amputation in presence of Buerger's disease.*[10,17]
- Educate client/significant other (SO) in reportable symptoms, including any changes in pain level, difficulty walking, and nonhealing wounds, *to provide opportunity for timely evaluation and intervention.*
- Emphasize need for regular medical and laboratory follow-up *to evaluate disease progression and response to therapies, including medications for desired and untoward effects.*
- Review medication regimen with client/SO. *Client may be on various drugs (e.g., antiplatelet agents, blood viscosity–reducing agents, vasodilators, anticoagulants, cholesterol-lowering agents) for treatment of the particular vascular disorder. Any of these medications have harmful side effects and require client teaching and medical monitoring.*[5,14–16]
- Emphasize importance of avoiding use of aspirin, some over-the-counter drugs and supplements, and alcohol when taking anticoagulants.
- Refer to community resources such as smoking-cessation assistance, weight control program, and exercise group *to provide support for lifestyle changes.*

DOCUMENTATION FOCUS

Assessment/Reassessment

- Individual findings, noting nature, extent, and duration of problem, effect on independence and lifestyle.
- Characteristics of pain, precipitators, and what relieves pain.
- Pulses and blood pressure, including above and below suspected lesion as appropriate.

Planning

- Plan of care and who is involved in planning.
- Teaching plan.

Implementation/Evaluation

- Response to interventions/teaching, actions performed.
- Attainment or progress toward desired outcome(s).
- Modifications to plan of care.

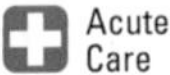

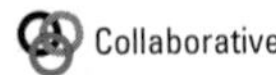

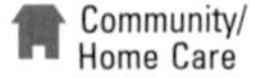

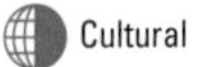

Discharge Planning

- Long-term needs and who is responsible for actions to be taken.
- Available resources, specific referrals made.

References

1. Stockman, J. (2008). In too deep: Understanding deep vein thrombosis. *Nursing Made Incredibly Easy!*, 6(2), 29–38.
2. Sieggreen, M. (2008). Understanding critical limb ischemia. *Nursing*, 38(10), 50–55.
3. Stephens, E. (Updated 2014). Peripheral vascular disease. Retrieved April 2015 from http://emedicine.medscape.com/article/761556-overview.
4. Nieves, J., Capone-Swearer, D. (2006). The clot that changes lives. *Nursing 2006 Critical Care*, 1(3), 18–28.
5. American Heart Association. (Updated 2012). What is peripheral vascular disease? Retrieved April 2015 from http://www.heart.org/idc/groups/heart-public/@wcm/@hcm/documents/downloadable/ucm_300323.pdf.
6. Blach, D. A., Ignatavicius, D. D. (2006). Interventions for clients with vascular problems. In Ignatavicius, D. D., Workman, M. L. (eds). *Medical–Surgical Nursing: Critical Thinking for Collaborative Care*. 5th ed. St. Louis, MO: Elsevier Saunders.
7. Bartley, M. K. (2006). Keep venous thromboembolism at bay. *Nursing*, 36(10), 36–41.
8. Barclay, L. (2009). Hospital-supervised exercise may prevent need for surgery in patients with claudication. Retrieved April 2015 from hhttp://www.medscape.com/viewarticle/588053.
9. Sachdeva, A., Dalton, M., Amaragiri, S. V. (2010). Elastic compression stockings for prevention of deep vein thrombosis. *Cochrane Database Syst Rev*, 7(7).
10. Sieggreen, M. Y. (2006). Getting a leg up on managing venous ulcers. *Nursing Made Incredibly Easy!*, 4(6), 52–60.
11. Baldwin, K. M. (2006). Stroke: It's a knock-out punch. *Nursing Made Incredibly Easy!*, 4(2), 10–23.
12. Frost, K. L., Topp, R. (2006). A physical activity Rx for the hypertensive patient. *Nurse Pract*, 31(4), 29–37.
13. Moses, S. (Updated 2015). Unna's boot. Family practice notebook. Retrieved April 2015 from ht http://www.fpnotebook.com/surgery/Pharm/UnsBt.htm.
14. Calianno, C., Holton, S. J. (2007). Fighting the triple threat of lower extremity ulcers. *Nursing*, 37(3), 57–63.
15. Kehl-Pruett, W. (2006). Deep vein thrombosis in hospitalized patients: A review of evidence-based guidelines for prevention. *Dimens Crit Care Nurs*, 25(2), 53–59.
16. Wipke-Tevis, D. D., Sae-Sia, W. (2004). Caring for vascular leg ulcers. *Home Health Nurse*, 22(4), 237–247.
17. Johns Hopkins Vasculitis Center. (2011). Buerger's disease. Retrieved April 2015 from http://www.hopkinsvasculitis.org/types-vasculitis/buergers-disease/.
18. Grant, B. J. B. (2015). Diagnosis of suspected deep vein thrombosis of the lower extremity. Retrieved April 2015 from http://www.uptodate.com/contents/diagnosis-of-suspected-deep-vein-thrombosis-of-the-lower-extremity.

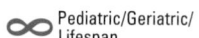

risk for decreased cardiac Tissue Perfusion

Taxonomy II: Activity/Rest—Class 4 Cardiovascular/Pulmonary Responses (00200) [**Diagnostic Division:** Circulation], Submitted 2008; Revised 2013

DEFINITION: Vulnerable to a decrease in cardiac (coronary) perfusion, which may compromise health.

RISK FACTORS

Coronary artery spasm; cardiovascular surgery; cardiac tamponade
Family history of cardiovascular disease
Hypertension; diabetes mellitus; hypovolemia; hypoxemia; hypoxia

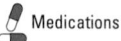

(continues on page 886)

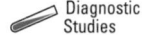

risk for decreased cardiac Tissue Perfusion (continued)

Insufficient knowledge of modifiable risk factors (e.g., smoking, sedentary lifestyle, obesity)
Pharmaceutical agent; substance abuse
Elevated C-reactive protein; hyperlipidemia
Note: A risk diagnosis is not evidenced by signs and symptoms, as the problem has not occurred; rather, nursing interventions are directed at prevention.

Sample Clinical Applications: Angina, coronary artery disease, hypertension, congestive heart failure, diabetes, cardiac surgery, pericarditis, sepsis, anemia, hemorrhagic shock, cocaine use

DESIRED OUTCOMES/EVALUATION CRITERIA

Sample NOC linkages:

Tissue Perfusion: Cardiac: Adequacy of blood flow through the coronary vasculature to maintain heart function

Cardiac Disease Self-Management: Personal actions to manage heart disease, its treatment, and prevent disease progression

Client Will (Include Specific Time Frame)

- Demonstrate adequate coronary perfusion as individually appropriate (e.g., vital signs within client's normal range, free of chest pain or discomfort).
- Identify individual risk factors.
- Verbalize understanding of treatment regimen.
- Demonstrate behaviors or lifestyle changes to maintain or maximize circulation (e.g., cessation of smoking, relaxation techniques, exercise program, dietary plan).

ACTIONS/INTERVENTIONS

Sample NIC linkages:

Cardiac Precautions: Prevention of an acute episode of impaired cardiac function by minimizing myocardial oxygen consumption or increasing myocardial oxygen supply

Hemodynamic Regulation: Optimization of heart rate, preload, afterload, and contractility

NURSING PRIORITY NO. 1 To identify individual risk factors:

- Note presence of conditions such as heart failure, major trauma with blood loss, recent coronary artery bypass graft (CABG) surgery, use of intra-aortic balloon pump, chronic anemia, sepsis, etc. *Conditions such as these can affect systemic circulation, tissue oxygenation, and organ function.*[1,14]
- Note client's age and gender when assessing risk for coronary artery spasm or myocardial infarction. *Risk for heart disorders increases with age, and men are still considered at higher risk for myocardial infarction and experience them earlier in life.*[2] *Although studies show that men have experienced a decline in coronary heart disease mortality in the last 2 decades, due in part to national awareness campaigns, women have not experienced the same recognition and treatment or similar decline in coronary heart disease mortality.*[3]
- Identify lifestyle issues such as obesity, smoking, high cholesterol, excessive alcohol intake, use of drugs such as cocaine, and physical inactivity *that can raise client's risk for coronary artery disease and impaired cardiac tissue perfusion.*[2]
- Determine presence of breathing problems, such as obstructive sleep apnea with oxygen desaturation. *Can produce alveolar hypoventilation, respiratory acidosis, and hypoxia, which can result in cardiac dysrhythmias and cardiac dysfunction.*[8]
- Determine if client is experiencing unusual long-term stress or may have underlying psychiatric disorder (e.g., anxiety or panic) *that may cause or exacerbate coronary artery disease and affect cardiac function.*[5]

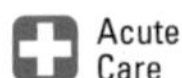

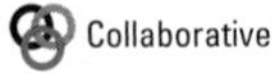

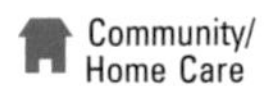

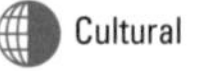

- Review client's medications, noting current use of any vasoactive drugs such as amodirone, dopamine, dobutamine, esmolol, lidocaine, nitroglycerin, and vasopressin. *These medications may be used in emergent situations or to manage blood pressure over time and can exert undesirable and potentially dangerous secondary effects in addition to their intended primary effects. For example, dobutamine given to increase myocardial contractility can also cause tachycardia and hypotension, which increases myocardial workload and oxygen consumption.*[9]
- Review diagnostic studies and lab tests (e.g., electrocardiogram; exercise tolerance tests, myocardial perfusion scan; echocardiogram, bubble echocardiogram; angiography, Doppler ultrasound, chest radiography; oxygen saturation, capnometry, or arterial blood gases; electrolytes, lipid profile; blood urea nitrogen/creatinine, cardiac enzymes) *to identify conditions requiring treatment, and response to therapies.*[7,10,11]

NURSING PRIORITY NO. 2 To determine changes in cardiac status:

- Investigate reports of chest pain, noting changes in characteristics of pain *to evaluate for potential myocardial ischemia or inadequate systemic oxygenation or perfusion of organs. Note: Chest pain is often difficult to diagnose due to variability in symptoms. Leading causes of chest pain (other than heart) include musculoskeletal, gastrointestinal, and pulmonary systems, as well as psychiatric disorders such as panic disorders.*[4–6]
- Monitor vital signs, especially noting blood pressure changes, including hypertension or hypotension, *reflecting systemic vascular resistance problems that alter oxygen consumption and cardiac perfusion.*[1]
- Assess heart sounds and pulses for dysrhythmias. *Can be caused by inadequate myocardial or systemic tissue perfusion, electrolyte or acid-base imbalances.*[13]
- Assess for restlessness, fatigue, changes in level of consciousness; increased capillary refill time; diminished peripheral pulses; and pale, cool skin. *Signs and symptoms of inadequate systemic perfusion, which can cause or affect cardiac function.*[1]
- Inspect for pallor, mottling, cool and clammy skin, and diminished pulses. *Systemic vasoconstriction resulting from reduced cardiac output may be evidenced by poor skin or tissue perfusion and diminished pulses.*[13]
- Investigate reports of difficulty breathing; note respiratory rate outside of acceptable parameters, *which can be indicative of oxygen exchange problems with potential for cardiac dysfunction.*[7]

NURSING PRIORITY NO. 3 To maintain/maximize cardiac perfusion:

- Collaborate in treatment of underlying conditions such as hypovolemia, chronic obstructive pulmonary disease, diabetes, and chronic atrial fibrillation, *to correct or treat disorders that could influence cardiac perfusion or organ function.*
- Maintain hemodynamic stability when client is in postoperative phase of CABG surgery *to keep vital organs adequately perfused. Risk factors in this time frame include dysrhythmias, hypotension or hypertension, cardiac tamponade, and pulmonary dysfunction.*[12]
- Provide supplemental oxygen as indicated *to improve or maintain cardiac and systemic tissue perfusion.*
- Administer fluids and electrolytes as indicated *to maintain systemic circulation and optimal cardiac function.*
- Administer medications (e.g., antihypertensive agents, analgesics, antidysrhythmics, bronchodilators, fibrinolytic agents) *to treat underlying conditions, to prevent thromboembolic phenomena, and to maintain cardiac tissue perfusion and organ function.*[12,13,15]
- Collaborate with dietician or nutritionist to provide easily digestible diet sufficient in nutrients, low in cholesterol and fat, and high in complex carbohydrates *to provide energy and reduce substances harmful to coronary arteries.*[2,16]
- Provide periods of undisturbed rest and calming environment *to reduce myocardial workload.*

NURSING PRIORITY NO. 4 To promote heart health (Teaching/Discharge Considerations):

- Discuss the risk factors (e.g., family history, obesity, age, smoking, hypertension, diabetes, clotting disorders) and potential outcomes of atherosclerosis (e.g., systemic and cardiac disease conditions). *Information necessary for client to make informed decisions concerning risk factors and to commit to lifestyle changes necessary to prevent onset of complications or manage symptoms when condition present.*[2]

- Review difference between modifiable and nonmodifiable risk factors *to assist client/significant other (SO) in understanding those areas in which he/she can take action or make healthy choices*:
  Recommend maintenance of normal weight or weight loss if client is obese *to decrease risk associated with overweight and obesity.*[2]
  Review specific dietary concerns with client, such as reducing animal and dairy fats and increasing plant foods—fruits, vegetables, olive oil, and nuts.[16]
  Encourage smoking cessation, when indicated, offering information about stop-smoking aids and programs. *Smoking causes vasoconstriction compromising perfusion. Smoking cessation is important in the medical management of many contributors to heart attack. These include atherosclerosis (fatty buildups in arteries), thrombosis (blood clots), coronary artery spasm, and cardiac dysrhythmia (heart rhythm problems).*[17]
  Encourage client to engage in regular exercise *to enhance circulation and promote general well-being.*[18]
  Review medications on regular basis *to manage those that affect cardiac function or those given to prevent blood pressure or thromboembolic problems.*
  Discuss drug use where indicated (including cocaine, methamphetamines, alcohol) *to educate client regarding effect of drug on the heart. Note: Studies have found a substantial association between self-reported-cocaine use and physician-diagnosed myocardial infarction. Another study indicates that when methamphetamine is used with alcohol, increased psychological and cardiac effects are observed.*[19–21]
  Discuss coping and stress tolerance. Demonstrate and encourage use of relaxation or stress management techniques *to decrease tension level, thereby improving heart health.*
  Encourage client in high-risk categories (e.g., strong family history, diabetic, prior history of cardiac event) to have regular medical examinations *to provide timely intervention, when needed.*
- Refer to educational or community resources, as indicated. *Client/SO may benefit from instruction and support provided by agencies to engage in healthier heart activities (e.g., weight loss, smoking cessation, exercise).*
- Instruct in blood pressure monitoring at home if indicated; advise purchase of home monitoring equipment; refer to community resources as indicated. *Facilitates management of hypertension, which is a major risk factor for damage to blood vessels or organ function.*[13]

DOCUMENTATION FOCUS

Assessment/Reassessment

- Individual findings, noting specific risk factors.
- Vital signs, cardiac rhythm, presence of dysrhythmias.

Planning

- Plan of care and who is involved in planning.
- Teaching plan.

Implementation/Evaluation

- Response to interventions, teaching, and actions performed.
- Attainment or progress toward desired outcome(s).
- Modifications to plan of care.

Discharge Planning

- Long-term needs and who is responsible for actions to be taken.
- Available resources, specific referrals made.

References

1. Breitenbach, J. E. (2007). Putting an end to perfusion confusion. *Nursing Made Incredibly Easy!*, 5(3), 50–60.
2. American Heart Association. (2013). AHA scientific position: Risk factors and coronary heart disease. Retrieved July 2014 from http://www.ehow.com/facts_5607605_coronary-factors-american-heart-association.html.
3. Yawn, B., Wollan, P. C., Jacobsen, S. J., et al. (2004). Identification of women's coronary heart disease risk factors prior to first myocardial infarction. *J Womens Health*, 13(10), 1087–1096.
4. Fagring, A. J., Gaston-Johansonn, F., Danielseon, E., et al. (2005). Description of unexplained chest pain and its influence on daily life in men and women. *Eur J Cardiovasc Nurs*(4), 337–344.
5. Katerndahl, D. (2004). Panic and plaques: Panic disorder and coronary artery disease in patients with chest pain. *J Am Board Fam Pract*, 17(2), 114–126.
6. Cayley, W. E. (2005). Diagnosing the cause of chest pain. *J Am Fam Physician*, 72(10), 2012–2021.
7. Schulman, C. (2002). End points of resuscitation: Choosing the right parameters to monitor. *Dimens Crit Care Nurs*, 21(1), 2–10.
8. Shahar, E., Whitney, C. W., Redline, S., et al. (2001). Sleep-disordered breathing and cardiovascular disease: Cross sectional results of the sleep heart health study. *Am J Resp Crit Care Med*, 163, 19–25.
9. Miller, J. (2007). Keeping your patient hemodynamically stable. *Nursing*, 37(5), 36–41.
10. Task Force on Pulmonary Embolism, European Society of Cardiology. (Updated 2014). Guidelines on diagnosis and management of acute pulmonary embolism. Retrieved April 2015 from http://www.escardio.org/Guidelines-&-Education/Clinical-Practice-Guidelines/Acute-Pulmonary-Embolism-Diagnosis-and-Management-of.
11. Goldrich, G. (2006). Understanding the 12-lead ECG, part I. *Nursing*, 36(11), 36–41.
12. Mullen-Fortino, M., O'Brien, N. (2008). Caring for the patient after coronary artery bypass graft. *Nursing*, 38(3), 46–52.
13. Bartley, M. K. (2006). Keep venous thromboembolism at bay. *Nursing*, 10(3), 36–41.
14. Eberhardt, R. T., Raffetto, J. D. (2005). Chronic venous insufficiency. *Circulation*, 111(18), 2398–2409.
15. Baldwin, K. M. (2006). Stroke: It's a knock-out punch. *Nursing Made Incredibly Easy!*, 4(2), 10–23.
16. Sacks, F. M., Katan, M. (2002). Randomized clinical trials on the effects of dietary fat and carbohydrate on plasma proteins and cardiovascular disease. *Am J Med*, Suppl 9B, 13–24.
17. Centers for Disease Control and Prevention. (Updated 2012). Smoking and tobacco use: Heart disease and stroke. Retrieved April 2015 from http://www.cdc.gov/tobacco/basic_information/health_effects/heart_disease/.
18. Frost, K. L., Topp, R. (2006). A physical activity Rx for the hypertensive patient. *Nurs Pract*, 31(4), 29–37.
19. Aslibekyan, S., Levitan, E. B., Mittleman, M. A. (2008). Prevalent cocaine use and myocardial infarction. *Am J Cardiol*, 102(8), 966–969.
20. Wright, M. N. J., Martin, M., Goff, T., et al. (2007). Cocaine and thrombosis: A narrative systematic review of clinical and in-vivo studies. *Subst Abuse Treat Prevent Policy*, 27(2).
21. Richards, J. R., Derlet, R. W., Albertson, T. E. (Updated 2014). Methamphetamine toxicity. Retrieved February 2015 from http://emedicine.medscape.com/article/820918-overview.

risk for ineffective cerebral Tissue Perfusion

Taxonomy II: Activity/Rest—Class 4 Cardiovascular/Pulmonary Responses (00201) [**Diagnostic Division:** Circulation], Submitted 2008; Revised 2013

DEFINITION: Vulnerable to a decrease in cerebral tissue circulation, which may compromise health.

RISK FACTORS

Brain injury (e.g., cerebrovascular impairment, neurological illness, trauma, tumor); brain neoplasm
Carotid stenosis; aortic atherosclerosis; arterial dissection
Atrial fibrillation; sick sinus syndrome; atrial myxoma

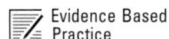

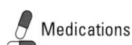

(continues on page 890)

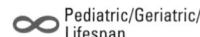

risk for ineffective cerebral Tissue Perfusion (continued)

Recent myocardial infarction; akinetic left ventricular segment; dilated cardiomyopathy; mitral stenosis; mechanical prosthetic valve; infective endocarditis; embolism

Coagulopathy (e.g., sickle cell anemia); disseminated intravascular coagulation; abnormal partial thromboplastin time (PTT); abnormal prothrombin time (PT)

Hypertension; hypercholesterolemia

Substance abuse

Pharmaceutical agent; treatment regime

Note: A risk diagnosis is not evidenced by signs and symptoms, as the problem has not occurred; rather, nursing interventions are directed at prevention.

Sample Clinical Applications: Traumatic brain injury, stroke; atherosclerosis, hypertension, atrial fibrillation, mitral valve stenosis or replacement, transient ischemic attack, sickle cell anemia, cocaine use

DESIRED OUTCOMES/EVALUATION CRITERIA

Sample NOC linkages:

Tissue Perfusion: Cerebral: Adequacy of blood flow through the cerebral vasculature to maintain brain function

Risk Control: Personal actions to prevent, eliminate, or reduce modifiable health threats

Client Will (Include Specific Time Frame)

- Display neurological signs within client's normal range.
- Verbalize understanding of condition, therapy regimen, side effects of medications, and when to contact healthcare provider.
- Demonstrate behaviors or lifestyle changes to improve circulation (e.g., cessation of smoking, relaxation techniques, exercise program, dietary plan).

ACTIONS/INTERVENTIONS

Sample NIC linkages:

Cerebral Perfusion Promotion: Promotion of adequate perfusion and limitation of complications for a patient experiencing or at risk for inadequate cerebral perfusion

Surveillance: Purposeful and ongoing acquisition, interpretation, and synthesis of patient data for clinical decision making

Cerebral Edema Management: Limitation of secondary injury resulting from swelling of brain tissue

NURSING PRIORITY NO. 1 To assess causative/contributing factors:

- Determine history of conditions associated with thrombus or emboli such as stroke, complicated pregnancy, sickle cell disease, fractures (especially long bones or pelvis) *to identify client at higher risk for decreased cerebral perfusion related to bleeding and/or coagulation problems.*
- Note current situation or presence of conditions (e.g., congestive heart failure, major trauma, sepsis, hypertension) *that can affect all body systems and systemic circulation and perfusion.*
- Ascertain potential for presence of acute neurologic conditions, such as traumatic brain injury, tumors, hemorrhage, anoxic brain injury associated with cardiac arrest, and toxic or viral encephalopathies. *These conditions alter the relationship between intracranial volume and pressure, potentially increasing intracranial pressure and decreasing cerebral perfusion.*[1]
- Investigate client reports of headache, particularly when accompanied by loss of coordination, confusion, visual disturbances, difficulty understanding or using language, or a range of progressive neurological deficits. *These symptoms may accompany cerebral perfusion deficits associated with conditions such as stroke, transient ischemic attack, brain trauma, or cerebral arteriovenous malformations.*[2,5]

Acute Care 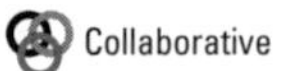 Collaborative 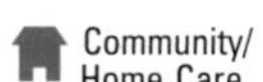 Community/ Home Care 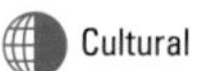 Cultural

- Ascertain if client has history of cardiac problems (e.g., recent myocardial infarction, heart failure, heart valve dysfunction or replacement, chronic atrial fibrillation), *which can impair systemic and cerebral blood flow or cause thromboembolic events to brain.*[3]
- Determine presence of cardiac dysrhythmias. *Can be caused by inadequate myocardial perfusion, electrolyte imbalances, or be associated with brain injury (e.g., bradycardia can accompany traumatic injury; stroke can be precipitated by dysrhythmias).*[3]
- Assess level of consciousness, mental status, speech, and behavior. *Clinical symptoms of decreased cerebral perfusion include fluctuations in consciousness and cognitive functions.*[11]
- Evaluate blood pressure. *Chronic or severe acute hypertension can precipitate cerebrovascular spasm and stroke. Low blood pressure or severe hypotension causes inadequate perfusion of brain, with adverse changes in consciousness/mentation.*[4]
- Verify proper use of antihypertensive medications. *Individuals may stop medication because of lack of symptoms, presence of undesired side effects, and/or cost of drug, potentiating risk of stroke.*
- Review medication regimen noting use of anticoagulants or antiplatelet agents and other drugs *that could cause intracranial bleeding.*
- Review pulse oximetry or arterial blood gases, noting oxygenation level and saturation. *Hypoxia (PaO_2 level less than 60 mg Hg, or O_2 saturation level less than 90%) is associated with reduced cerebral perfusion and increased morbidity and mortality from severe brain injury.*[3,4]
- Review lab studies (e.g., coagulation profiles, complete blood count, electrolytes, lipids, B-type natriuretic peptide) *to identify disorders that increase risk of clotting or bleeding, or other conditions contributing to causing decreased cerebral perfusion.*
- Review results of diagnostic studies (e.g., ultrasound or other imaging scans such as echocardiography, computed tomography, or magnetic resonance angiography; diffusion and perfusion magnetic resonance imaging) *to determine location and severity of disorder that can cause or exacerbate cerebral perfusion problems.*[10]

NURSING PRIORITY NO. 2 To maximize tissue perfusion:

- Collaborate in treatment of underlying conditions (e.g., carotid stent placement, surgical reperfusion procedures, treatment of infections) as indicated *to improve systemic perfusion and organ function.*
- Restore or maintain fluid balance *to maximize cardiac output and prevent decreased cerebral perfusion associated with hypovolemia.*[1,2]
- Manage cardiac dysrhythmias—medication administration, assist with pacemaker insertion. *Reduces risk of diminished cerebral perfusion due to blood clots or low cardiac output.*[1,2]
- Restrict fluids and administer diuretics as indicated *to prevent diminished cerebral perfusion associated with fluid imbalance, hypertension, and cerebral edema.*[1,2]
- Keep head in midline position, when indicated, *to promote venous drainage, preventing or reducing risk of elevated intracranial pressure.*[1,2]
- Maintain optimal head of bed (HOB) placement (e.g., 0, 15, 30 degrees). *Various studies demonstrate different perfusion responses to HOB placement but indicate that cerebral perfusion is reduced when HOB elevated greater than 30 deg. Note: A recent study showed that routine nursing of patients with severe head injury at 30 deg of head elevation within 24 hr after trauma leads to a consistent reduction of intracranial pressure (statistically significant) and an improvement in cerebral perfusion (although not statistically significant) without concomitant deleterious changes in cerebral oxygenation.*[6,12]
- Control fever, monitor hypothermia therapy, and provide supplemental oxygen, as indicated, *to decrease cerebral metabolism and cerebral edema.*[1,2]
- Administer vasoactive medications, as indicated, *to increase cardiac output and/or adequate mean arterial pressure to maintain cerebral perfusion.*[1,2]
- Administer other medications as indicated. *Cortiocosteroids may be used to decrease edema, antihypertensives may be used to manage high blood pressure, and anticoagulants may be used to prevent cerebral embolus.*[1,2]

- Prepare client for surgery as indicated (e.g., carotid endarterectomy, evacuation of hematoma or space-occupying lesion) *to improve cerebral perfusion.*
- Refer to NDs decreased Cardiac Output and decreased Intracranial Adaptive Capacity for additional interventions.

NURSING PRIORITY NO. 3 To promote optimal perfusion (Teaching/Discharge Considerations):

- Review modifiable risk factors, as indicated: *Information can help client make informed choices about remedial actions to reduce risk factors and to commit to lifestyle changes as appropriate.*[2,7]

  Uncontrolled hypertension: *Incidence of stroke increases with systolic blood pressure greater than 140/90 mmHg. Client at risk can learn to self-monitor blood pressure, take prescribed antihypertensive agents consistently, and identify symptoms to report to physician.*

  Smoking: *Smoking causes vasoconstriction and increased arterial wall stiffness, increasing fibrinogen levels and platelet aggregation, and abnormal blood lipids. Numerous recent studies have confirmed a relationship between active and passive smoking, with the maximum risk period being middle life. Smoking cessation immediately lowers risk of stroke.*[8]

  Obesity and unhealthy diet: *Abdominal obesity has been associated with increased risk for ischemic stroke.*[8] *Diet high in cholesterol contributes to development of cerebral atherosclerosis. High intake of sodium can contribute to hypertension.*

  Physical inactivity: *Contributes to obesity and hypertension.*

  Excessive alcohol intake: *Linked to higher risk of stroke because it can cause hypertension, which is a major risk factor. Note: Alcohol intake consumption at higher amounts is associated with increased risk of atrial fibrillation, ventricular fibrillation, dilated cardiomyopathy, hypertension, dyslipidemia, and a systemic anticoagulant effect, all of which increase the risk of stroke.*[7,14]

  Illicit drug use: *Can significantly boost the risk of a deadly or debilitating stroke. Note: Many illicit drugs have been linked to increased stroke risk (i.e., cocaine, amphetamines, opiates, phencyclidine, marijuana).*[9]
- Discuss impact of unmodifiable risk factors such as family history, age, and race. *Understanding effects and interrelationship of all risk factors may encourage client to address what can be changed to improve general well-being and reduce individual risk.*
- Assist client to incorporate disease management into activities of daily living, including regular exercise. *Promotes independence and enhances self-concept regarding ability to deal with change and manage own needs.*
- Emphasize necessity of routine follow-up and laboratory monitoring as indicated. *Important for effective disease management and possible changes in therapeutic regimen.*
- Refer to educational or community resources as indicated. *Client/SO may benefit from instruction and support provided by agencies to engage in healthy activities (e.g., weight loss, smoking cessation, exercise).*

DOCUMENTATION FOCUS

Assessment/Reassessment

- Individual findings, noting specific risk factors.
- Vital signs, blood pressure, cardiac rhythm.
- Medication regimen.
- Diagnostic studies, laboratory results.

Planning

- Plan of care and who is involved in planning.
- Teaching plan.

Implementation/Evaluation

- Response to interventions, teaching, and actions performed.
- Attainment or progress toward desired outcome(s).
- Modifications to plan of care.

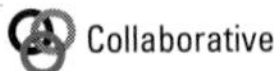

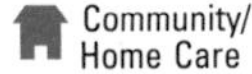

Community/ Home Care
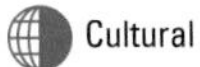

Discharge Planning

- Long-term needs and who is responsible for actions to be taken.
- Available resources, specific referrals made.

References

1. Editorial Staff (2007). Patho puzzler: Don't let your head explode over increased ICP. *Nursing Made Incredibly Easy!*, 5(2), 21–25.
2. Nieves, J., Capone-Swearer, D. (2006). The clot that changes lives. *Nursing 2006 Crit Care*, 1(3), 18–28.
3. Agency for Healthcare Research and Quality. (2003). Pharmacologic management of heart failure and left ventricular systolic dysfunction: Effect in female, black, and diabetic patients, and cost-effectiveness. Retrieved April 2015 from http://archive.ahrq.gov/clinic/tp/hrtfailtp.htm.
4. American Association of Neuroscience Nurses. (Revised 2009). Nursing management of adults with severe traumatic brain injury. Retrieved April 2015 from http://www.aann.org/pdf/cpg/aanntraumaticbraininjury.pdf.
5. Vacca, V. M., Violett, S. (2008). Teamwork integral to treating cerebral arteriovenous malformation. *Nursing*, 3(3), 20–27.
6. McIlvoy, L. H., Meyer, K. (2008). Cerebral perfusion promotion. In Ackley, B. J., et al. (eds). *Evidence-Based-Nursing Care Guidelines: Medical-Surgical Interventions*. St. Louis, MO: Mosby Elsevier.
7. National Stroke Association. (Updated 2014). Lifestyle risk factors (various monographs regarding controllable risk factors). Retrieved April 2015 from http://www.stroke.org/understand-stroke/preventing-stroke/lifestyle-risk-factors.
8. Roger, V. L., Go, A. S., Lloyd-Jones, D. M. (2011). Heart disease and stroke statistics—2011 update: A report from the American Heart Association. *Circulation*, 123, e18–e209.
9. de los Rios, F., Kleindorfer, D. O., Khoury, J., et al. (2012). Trends in substance abuse preceding stroke among young adults: A population-based study. Retrieved April 2015 from http://stroke.ahajournals.org/content/43/12/3179.long.
10. Kochan, J. P., Kanamalla, U. S. (Updated 2013). Cerebral revascularization imaging. Retrieved April 2015 from http://emedicine.medscape.com/article/420186-overview.
11. Sakowitz, O., Unterberg, A. (2006). Detecting and treating microvascular ischemia after subarachnoid hemorrhage. *Curr Opin Crit Car*, 12(2), 103–111.
12. Ng, I. F., Lim, J. B., Wong, H. B. (2004). Effects of head posture on cerebral hemodynamics: Its influences on intracranial pressure, cerebral perfusion pressure, and cerebral oxygenation. *Neurosurgery*, 54(3), 593–599.
13. Girot, M. (2009). Smoking and stroke. *Presse Med*, 38(7–8), 1120–1125.
14. Di Minno, M. N., Franchini, M., Russolillo, A., et al. (2011). Alcohol dosing and the heart: Updating clinical evidence. *Semin Thromb Hemost*, 37(8), 875–884.

risk for ineffective peripheral Tissue Perfusion

Taxonomy II: Activity/Rest—Class 4 Cardiovascular/Pulmonary Responses (00228) [**Diagnostic Division:** Circulation], Submitted 2010; Revised 2013

DEFINITION: Vulnerable to a decrease in blood circulation to the periphery, which may compromise health.

RISK FACTORS

Sedentary lifestyle; smoking
Diabetes; hypertension
Endovascular procedure; trauma
Excessive sodium intake
Insufficient knowledge of disease process, risk factors, or aggravating factors (e.g., smoking, sedentary lifestyle, trauma, obesity, salt intake, immobility)

(continues on page 894)

risk for ineffective peripheral Tissue Perfusion (continued)

Note: A risk diagnosis is not evidenced by signs and symptoms as the problem has not occurred; rather, nursing interventions are directed at prevention

Sample Clinical Applications: Atherosclerosis, coronary artery disease, Raynaud's disease, peripheral vascular disease, Buerger's disease, thrombophlebitis, diabetes mellitus, sickle cell anemia

DESIRED OUTCOMES/EVALUATION CRITERIA

Sample NOC linkages:

Tissue Perfusion; Peripheral: Adequacy of blood flow through the small vessels of the extremities to maintain tissue perfusion

Knowledge: Disease Process: Extent of understanding conveyed about a specific disease process and prevention of complications

Client Will (Include Specific Time Frame)

- Demonstrate adequate perfusion as individually appropriate (e.g., peripheral pulses present and strong, absence of edema, free of pain or discomfort).
- Verbalize understanding of risk factors and when to contact healthcare provider.
- Demonstrate behaviors or lifestyle changes to improve circulation (e.g., engage in regular exercise, cessation of smoking, weight reduction, disease management).

ACTIONS/INTERVENTIONS

Sample NIC linkages:

Circulatory Care: Arterial Insufficiency: Promotion of arterial circulation

Circulatory Care: Venous Insufficiency: Promotion of venous circulation

Teaching: Disease Process: Assisting the patient to understand information related to a specific disease process

NURSING PRIORITY NO. 1 To identify causative/precipitating factors related to risk:

- Note current situation or presence of conditions that can affect perfusion to all body systems (e.g., client admitted for endovascular procedure such as angiography or placement of stent, history or presence of congestive heart failure, lung disorders, major trauma, septic or hypovolemic shock, coagulopathies, sickle cell anemia) *affecting systemic circulation and perfusion.*
- Determine history of conditions associated with thrombus or emboli (e.g., problems with coronary or cerebral circulation, stroke; high-velocity trauma with fractures, abdominal or orthopedic surgery, long periods of immobility; inflammatory diseases; chronic lung disease; diabetes with coexisting peripheral vascular disease (PVD); estrogen therapy; cancer and cancer therapies; presence of central venous catheters) *to identify client at higher risk for venous stasis, vessel wall injury, and hypercoagulability.*[1–4]
- Identify presence of high-risk factors or conditions (e.g., smoking, uncontrolled hypertension, obesity, pregnancy, pelvic tumor, paralysis, hypercholesterolemia, varicose veins, arthritis, sepsis). *Places client at greater risk for developing PVD (including arterial blockage and chronic venous insufficiency) with associated complications.*[3,5,6]

NURSING PRIORITY NO. 2 To assess for and reduce risk of perfusion complications:

- Evaluate reports of extremity pain promptly, noting any associated symptoms (e.g., cramping or heaviness, discomfort with walking, progressive temperature or color changes, paresthesia) *to help isolate and differentiate problems.*
- Note presence and location of restrictive pressure dressings, circular wraps, cast or traction device *that may impede circulation to limb.*

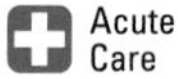

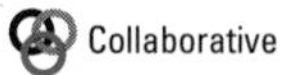

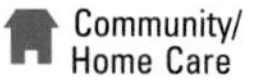

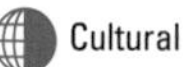

- Assess skin color and temperature in all extremities *for changes that might indicate circulation problem.*
- Compare skin temperature and color with other limb *if developing problem is suspected (e.g., edema, redness, swelling in calf of one leg is associated with localized thrombophlebitis).*[1,3,7]
- Palpate arterial pulses—bilateral radial, femoral, popliteal, dorsalis pedis, and postero-tibial—comparing equality as well as intensity (e.g., bounding, normal, diminished, absent). *Assesses distribution and quality of blood flow.*[2]
- Inspect lower extremities for skin texture (e.g., atrophic; shiny appearance; lack of hair; dry, scaly, reddened skin) and skin breaks or ulcerations *that often accompany diminished peripheral circulation.*[3,5,8]
- Note client's nutritional and fluid status. *Protein-energy malnutrition and weight loss make ischemic tissues more prone to breakdown. Dehydration reduces blood volume and compromises peripheral circulation.*[3,5,8]
- Review lab studies such as lipid profile, coagulation studies, hemoglobin/hematocrit, renal/cardiac function tests, inflammatory markers (e.g., D dimer, C-reactive protein) *to determine potential for circulatory impairment.*

NURSING PRIORITY NO. 3 To maximize tissue perfusion:

- Collaborate in treatment of underlying conditions, such as diabetes, hypertension, cardiopulmonary conditions, blood disorders, traumatic injury, hypovolemia, and hypoxemia *to maximize systemic circulation and organ perfusion.*
- Administer fluids, electrolytes, nutrients, and oxygen as indicated *to promote optimal blood flow and organ and peripheral tissue perfusion and function.*
- Provide interventions to promote peripheral circulation and limit complications:[1,2,4,5,9]

  Encourage early ambulation when possible. *Enhances venous return.*

  Recommend or provide foot and ankle exercises when client unable to ambulate freely *to reduce venous pooling and increase venous return.*

  Provide pressure-relieving/reducing devices for immobilized client (e.g., air mattress, gel or foam padding, bed or foot cradle) *to reduce excessive tissue pressure that could lead to skin breakdown.*

  Apply intermittent compression devices or graduated compression stockings to lower extremities *to limit venous stasis, improve venous return, and reduce risk of deep vein thrombosis or tissue ulceration in client who is limited in activity or otherwise at risk.*[4,10,11]

  Assist with or cue client to change position at timed intervals rather than using presence of pain as signal to change positions, *if sensation is/could be impaired.*

  Elevate the legs when sitting, but avoid sharp angulation of the hips or knees *to enhance venous return and minimize edema formation.*

  Discuss/monitor use of heat or cold, such as hot water bottle, heating pad, or ice pack. *Reduces risk of dermal injury if client has condition associated with decreased sensation or neuropathy.*
- Refer to dietitian or nutritionist to discuss dietary needs such as a well-balanced, low-saturated-fat, low-cholesterol diet or other modifications as indicated *to promote weight loss and/or lower cholesterol levels to improve tissue perfusion.*
- Refer to NDs ineffective peripheral Tissue Perfusion, risk for Peripheral Neurovascular Dysfunction, risk for impaired Skin Integrity, impaired Tissue Integrity, and [disturbed Sensory Perception] for additional interventions as appropriate.

NURSING PRIORITY NO. 4 To promote maintain optimal perfusion (Teaching/discharge Criteria):

- Discuss relevant risk factors (e.g., family history, obesity, age, smoking, hypertension, diabetes, clotting disorders) and potential outcomes of atherosclerosis (e.g., systemic and peripheral vascular disease conditions). *Information necessary for client to make informed choices about risk factors and commit to lifestyle changes as appropriate to prevent onset of complications or manage symptoms when condition is present.*[2,12]
- Identify necessary changes in lifestyle and assist client to incorporate disease management into activities of daily living. *Promotes independence and enhances self-concept regarding ability to deal with change and manage own needs.*

- Emphasize need for regular exercise program *to enhance circulation and promote general well-being.*[13]
- Discourage sitting or standing for long periods, wearing constrictive clothing and crossing legs, *which can restrict circulation and lead to edema.*
- Provide education about relationship between smoking and peripheral vascular circulation, as indicated. *Smoking contributes to development and progression of PVD.*[2,14]
- Educate client/significant other in reportable symptoms, including any changes in pain level, difficulty walking, and nonhealing wounds *to provide opportunity for timely evaluation and intervention.*
- Refer to community resources such as smoking-cessation assistance, weight control program, diabetic educator, and/or exercise group *to provide support for lifestyle changes.*

DOCUMENTATION FOCUS

Assessment/Reassessment

- Individual risk factors identified.
- Client concerns or difficulty making and following through with plan.

Planning

- Plan of care and who is involved in planning.
- Teaching plan.

Implementation/Evaluation

- Response to interventions, teaching, and actions performed.
- Attainment or progress toward outcomes.

Discharge Planning

- Referrals to other resources.
- Long term need and who is responsible for actions.

References

1. Stockman, J. (2008). In too deep: Understanding deep vein thrombosis. *Nursing Made Incredibly Easy!*, 6(2), 29–38.
2. Sieggreen, M. (2008). Understanding critical limb ischemia. *Nursing*, 38(10), 50–55.
3. Calianno, C., Holton, S. J. (2007). Fighting the triple threat of lower extremity ulcers. *Nursing*, 37(3), 57–63.
4. Kehl-Pruett, W. (2006). Deep vein thrombosis in hospitalized patients: A review of evidence-based guidelines for prevention. *Dimens Crit Care Nurs*, 25(2), 53–59.
5. Stephens, E. (Updated 2014). Peripheral vascular disease. Retrieved April 2015 from http://emedicine.medscape.com/article/761556-overview.
6. Nieves, J., Capone-Swearer, D. (2006). The clot that changes lives. *Nursing 2006 Critical Care*, 1(3), 18–28.
7. American Heart Association. (Updated 2012). What is peripheral vascular disease? Retrieved April 2015 from http://www.heart.org/idc/groups/heart-public/@wcm/@hcm/documents/downloadable/ucm_300323.pdf.
8. Sieggreen, M. Y. (2006). Getting a leg up on managing venous ulcers. *Nursing Made Incredibly Easy!*, 4(6), 52–60.
9. Barclay, L. (2009). Hospital-supervised exercise may prevent need for surgery in patients with claudication. Retrieved April 2015 from http://www.medscape.com/viewarticle/588053.
10. Sachdeva, A., Dalton, M., Amaragiri, S. V., et al. (2010). Elastic compression stockings for prevention of deep vein thrombosis. *Cochrane Database Syst Rev*, 7(7), CDOO1484.
11. Wipke-Tevis, D. D., Sae-Sia, W. (2004). Caring for vascular leg ulcers. *Home Healthcare Nurse*, 22(4), 237–247.
12. Baldwin, K. M. (2006). Stroke: It's a knock-out punch. *Nursing Made Incredibly Easy!*, 4(2), 10–23.
13. Frost, K. L., Topp, R. (2006). A physical activity Rx for the hypertensive patient. *Nurse Pract*, 31(4), 29–37.
14. Johns Hopkins Vasculitis Center. (2011). Buerger's disease. Retrieved April 2015 from http://www.hopkinsvasculitis.org/types-vasculitis/buergers-disease/.

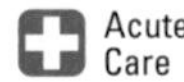

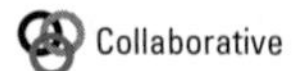

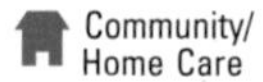

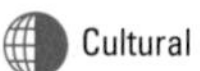

impaired Transfer Ability

Taxonomy II: Activity/Rest—Class 2 Activity/Exercise (00090) [**Diagnostic Division:** Activity/Rest], Submitted 1998; Revised 2006

DEFINITION: Limitation of independent movement between two nearby surfaces.

RELATED FACTORS

Insufficient muscle strength; physical deconditioning; neuromuscular impairment; musculoskeletal impairment
Impaired balance
Pain
Obesity
Impaired vision
Insufficient knowledge of transfer techniques; alteration in cognitive functioning
Environmental barrier (e.g., bed height, inadequate space, wheelchair type, treatment equipment, restraints)

DEFINING CHARACTERISTICS

Subjective or Objective

Impaired ability to transfer between bed and chair, bed and standing position; between chair and car, chair and floor, or chair and standing; on or off a toilet or commode; in or out of bathtub or shower; between uneven levels

Note: Specify level of independence using a standardized functional scale—[refer to ND impaired physical Mobility for suggested functional level classification]

Sample Clinical Applications: Arthritis, fractures, amputation, neuromuscular diseases (e.g., multiple sclerosis [MS], amyotrophic lateral sclerosis [ALS], Guillain-Barré syndrome), paralysis, glaucoma, macular degeneration, dementias

DESIRED OUTCOMES/EVALUATION CRITERIA

Sample NOC linkages:

Transfer Performance: Ability to change body location independently with or without assistive device
Balance: Ability to maintain body equilibrium
Body Positioning: Self-Initiated: Ability to change own body position independently with or without assistive device

Client/Caregiver Will (Include Specific Time Frame)

- Verbalize understanding of situation and appropriate safety measures.
- Master techniques of transfer successfully.
- Make desired transfer safely.

ACTIONS/INTERVENTIONS

Sample NIC linkages:

Self-Care Assistance: Transfer: Assisting a patient with limitation of independent movement to learn to change body location
Body Mechanics Promotion: Facilitating the use of posture and movement in daily activities to prevent fatigue and musculoskeletal strain or injury
Exercise Promotion: Strength Training: Facilitating regular resistive muscle training to maintain or increase muscle strength

NURSING PRIORITY NO. 1 To assess causative/contributing factors:

- Determine presence of conditions that contribute to transfer problems. *Neuromuscular and musculoskeletal problems (such as MS, fractures with splints or casts, back injuries, knee/hip replacement surgery, amputation, quadriplegia or paraplegia, contractures or spastic muscles); agedness (diminished faculties; multiple medications; painful conditions; decreased balance, muscle mass, tone, or strength), and effects of dementias, brain injury, etc., can seriously impact balance and physical and psychological well-being.*[3]
- Evaluate perceptual and cognitive impairments and ability to follow directions. *Plan of care and choice of interventions is dependent upon nature of condition—acute, chronic, or progressive; for example, client with severe brain injury may have permanent limitations because of impaired cognition affecting memory, judgment, problem solving, and motor coordination, requiring more intensive inpatient and long-term care.*
- Note factors complicating current situation. *Recent surgery or traction apparatus, debilitating illness or weakness, and mechanical ventilation or multiple IV/indwelling tubings can restrict movement.*
- Review medication regimen and schedule *to determine possible side effects or drug interactions impairing balance and/or muscle tone.*

NURSING PRIORITY NO. 2 To assess functional ability:

- Perform the "Timed Up and Go" (TUG) test, as indicated, *to assess client's basic ability to transfer and ambulate safely. In this test, the client is asked to get up from a seated position in a chair, stand still momentarily, walk forward 10 feet, turn around, walk back to the chair, turn, and sit down. Factors assessed include sitting balance, ability to transfer from sitting to standing and back to sitting, the pace and stability of ambulation, and the ability to turn without staggering. If the client is not safe with ambulation, assistance may also be required with transfers.*[1] *Note: Client may perform this test adequately and still have difficulty with some transfers, such as in or out of a car or bathtub or from floor to chair.*
- Determine degree of impairment using a 0–4 scale, noting muscle strength and tone, joint mobility, cardiovascular status, balance, and endurance. *Identifies strengths and deficits (e.g., ability to ambulate with assistive devices or problems with balance, failure to attend to one side, inability to bear weight [client is non-weight-bearing or partial weight-bearing]) and may provide information regarding potential for recovery.*[3]
- Observe movement when client is unaware of observations *to note any incongruence with reported abilities.*
- Note emotional and behavioral responses of client/significant other to problems of immobility. *Restrictions or limitations imposed by immobility can cause physical, social, emotional, and financial difficulties for everyone.*

NURSING PRIORITY NO. 3 To promote optimal level of movement:

- Assist with treatment of underlying condition causing dysfunction. *Treatment of condition (e.g., surgery for hip replacement, therapy for unilateral neglect following stroke) can alleviate or improve difficulties with transfer activity.*
- Consult with physical and occupational therapists or rehabilitation team *to develop general and specific muscle strengthening and range-of-motion exercises and transfer training and techniques, as well as recommendations and provision of balance, gait, and mobility aids or adjunctive devices.*[1]
- Position devices (e.g., call light, bed-positioning switch) in easy reach on the bed or chair. *Facilitates transfer and allows client to obtain assistance for transfer as needed.*
- Use appropriate number of people to assist with transfers and correct equipment (e.g., mechanical lift/sling, gait belt, sitting or standing disk pivot) *to safely transfer the client in a particular situation (e.g., chair to bed, chair to car, in or out of shower or tub).*[4–6]
- Demonstrate and assist with use of side rails or stand pole, overhead trapeze, and transfer or sit-to-stand hoist; specialty slings; and/or cane, walker, wheelchair, or crutches, as necessary, *to protect client or care providers from injury during transfers and movements.*[4,5]
- Provide instruction and reinforce information for client and caregivers regarding body and equipment positioning *to improve or maintain balance during transfers.*

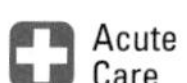
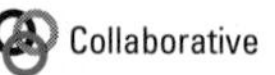
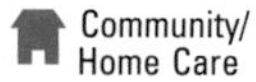
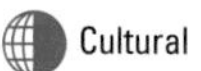

- Monitor body alignment, posture, and balance and encourage wide base of support *when standing to transfer.*
- Use full-length mirror, as needed, *to facilitate client's view of own postural alignment.*

NURSING PRIORITY NO. 4 To maintain safety (Teaching/Discharge Considerations):

- Instruct client/caregiver in appropriate safety measures. *Actions (e.g., proper use of transfer board; locking wheels on bed or chair; correct placement of equipment for optimal body mechanics of client and care-givers(s); use of gait belt, supportive nonslip footwear; good lighting; clearing floor of clutter) are important to facilitating transfers and reducing the possibility of fall and subsequent injury to client and caregiver.*[2]
- Discuss need for and sources of care or supervision. *Home-care agency, before- and after-school programs, senior day care, personal companions, etc., may be required to assist with or monitor activity.*
- Refer to appropriate community resources *for evaluation and modification of environment (e.g., roll-in-shower or tub, correction of uneven floor surfaces and steps, installation of ramps, use of standing tables or lifts).*
- Refer also to NDs impaired bed/physical/wheelchair Mobility, Unilateral Neglect, risk for Falls, or impaired Walking for additional interventions.

DOCUMENTATION FOCUS

Assessment/Reassessment

- Individual findings, including level of function and ability to participate in desired transfers.
- Mobility aides and transfer devices used.

Planning

- Plan of care and who is involved in the planning.
- Teaching plan.

Implementation/Evaluation

- Responses to interventions, teaching, and actions performed.
- Attainment or progress toward desired outcome(s).
- Modifications to plan of care.

Discharge Planning

- Discharge and long-term needs, noting who is responsible for each action to be taken.
- Specific referrals made.
- Sources of and maintenance for assistive devices.

References

1. Cruise, C. M., Koval, K. J. (1998). Rehabilitation of the elderly. *Arch Am Acad Orthop Surg*, 2(1), 103–107.
2. Patient safety during transfers. (2000). *Policy/Operations Manual*. Galveston, TX: UTMB Department of Rehabilitation Services.
3. Kourouche, S., Curtis, K., Watson, W. L., et al. (2011). Identifying risk and raising awareness in older person trauma: A trauma center initiative. *J Trauma Nurs*, 18(3), 163–170.
4. Parsons, K. S., Galinsky, T. L., Waters, T. (2006). Suggestions for preventing musculoskeletal disorders in home healthcare workers, Part 1: Lift and transfer assistance for partially weight-bearing home care patients. *Home Healthc Nurse*, 24(3), 158–164.
5. Parsons, K. S., Galinsky, T. L., Waters, T. (2006). Suggestions for preventing musculoskeletal disorders in home healthcare workers, Part 2: Lift and transfer assistance for non-weight-bearing home care patients. *Home Healthc Nurse*, 24(4), 227–233.
6. Patterson, M., Mechan, P., Hughes, N., et al. (2006). Safe vertical transfer of patient with extremity cast or splint. *Orthop Nurs*, 28(2 Suppl), S18–S23.

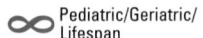

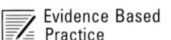

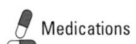

risk for Trauma

Taxonomy II: Safety/Protection—Class 2 Physical Injury (00038) [**Diagnostic Division:** Safety], Submitted 1980; Revised 2013

DEFINITION: Vulnerable to accidental tissue injury (e.g., wound, burn, fracture), which may compromise health.

RISK FACTORS

Internal

Alteration in cognitive functioning; emotional disturbance

Alteration in muscle coordination or sensation (resulting form spinal cord injury, diabetes mellitus, etc); weakness; decrease in eye-hand coordination; impaired balance; insufficient vision

Economically disadvantaged

History of trauma (e.g., physical, psychological, sexual)

Insufficient knowledge or safety precautions

Poor vision; reduced sensation

External [Includes But Is Not Limited To]:

Absent or dysfunctional call-for-aid device; bed in high position; struggling with restraints

Absence of stairway gate or window guard; inadequate stair rails; slippery floor; insufficient anti-slip material in bathroom; use or throw rugs; obstructed passageway; insufficient lighting; unstable chair or ladder

Access to weapon; high crime neighborhood

Children riding in front seat of car; nonuse or misuse of seat restraint; misuse of headgear (e.g., hard hat, motorcycle helmet)

Defective appliance; delay in ignition of gas appliance; grease on stove; electrical hazard (e.g., faulty plug, frayed wire, overloaded outlet/fuse box; unanchored electric wires; gas leak);

Exposure to corrosive product or toxic chemical; inadequately stored corrosive (e.g. lye); exposure to radiation

Extremes of environmental temperature; insufficient protection from heat source; bathing in very hot water; pot handle facing front of stove; use of cracked dishware; flammable object (e.g., clothing, toys); wearing loose clothing around open flame; inadequately stored combustible (e.g., matches, oily rags)

Icicles hanging from roof

Playing with dangerous object or explosive

Proximity to vehicle pathway (e.g., driveway, railroad track); unsafe road or walkway; unsafe operation of heavy equipment (e.g., excessive speed, while intoxicated, without required eyewear)

Smoking in bed or near oxygen

Note: A risk diagnosis is not evidenced by signs and symptoms, as the problem has not occurred; rather, nursing interventions are directed at prevention.

Sample Clinical Applications: Substance intoxication or abuse, peripheral neuropathy, cataracts, glaucoma, macular degeneration, Parkinson's disease, seizure disorder, dementia, major depression, developmental delay

DESIRED OUTCOMES/EVALUATION CRITERIA

Sample NOC linkages:

Physical Injury Severity: Severity of injuries from accidents and trauma

Personal Safety Behavior: Personal actions that prevent physical injury to self

Knowledge: Personal Safety: Extent of understanding conveyed about prevention of unintentional injuries

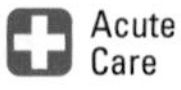

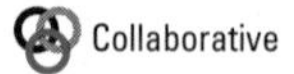

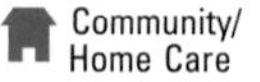

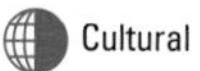

Client/Caregiver Will (Include Specific Time Frame)

- Identify and correct potential risk factors in the environment.
- Demonstrate appropriate lifestyle changes to reduce risk of injury.
- Identify resources to assist in promoting a safe environment.
- Recognize need for and seek assistance to prevent accidents/injuries.

ACTIONS/INTERVENTIONS

[This ND is a compilation of a number of situations that can result in injury. Refer to specific NDs, such as risk for imbalanced Body Temperature; risk for Contamination; risk for Falls; impaired Home Maintenance; Hyperthermia; Hypothermia; risk for Injury; impaired physical Mobility; risk for impaired Parenting; risk for Poisoning; risk for Thermal Injury, [disturbed Sensory Perception]; impaired Skin Integrity; risk for Suffocation; impaired Tissue Integrity; risk for self-/other-directed Violence; impaired Walking, as appropriate, for more specific interventions.]

Sample NIC linkages:

Environmental Management: Safety: Monitoring and manipulation of the physical environment to promote safety

Environmental Management: Worker Safety: Monitoring and manipulation of the worksite environment to promote safety and health of workers

Teaching: Infant [or] Toddler Safety [specify age]: Instruction on safety during first, second, and third years of life

Surveillance: Safety: Purposeful and ongoing collection and analysis of information about the patient and the environment for use in promoting and maintaining patient safety

NURSING PRIORITY NO. 1 To assess causative/contributing factors:

- Determine factors related to individual situation and extent of risk for trauma. *Influences scope and intensity of interventions to manage threats to safety, which are dynamic and constants in every life and situation. Clients interfacing with the healthcare system are at higher risk for trauma for any number of reasons (e.g., illness state, cognitive function, family structure, information and training) and require protection in numerous ways.*[1]
- Note client's age, gender, developmental stage, decision-making ability, level of cognition and competence *to determine client's ability to recognize danger and to protect self. Note: Children, young adults, older persons, and men are at greater risk for injury, which may reflect client's ability or desire to protect self, and influences choice of interventions or teaching.*[12,13]
- Ascertain client's/significant other's (SO's) knowledge of safety needs, injury prevention, and ways of looking at and improving own environment. *Lack of appreciation of significance of individual hazards increases risk of traumatic injury.*[1]
- Assess influence of stressors (e.g., physical, mental, peer related, work related, financial) *that can impair judgment and greatly increase client's potential for injury.*
- Assess mood, coping abilities, and personality styles (i.e., temperament, aggression, impulsive behavior, level of self-esteem). *May result in carelessness or increased risk-taking without consideration of consequences.*[10,11]
- Evaluate individual's emotional and behavioral response to violence in surroundings (e.g., neighborhood, television, peer group). *May affect client's view of and regard for own/others' safety.*[10–12]
- Evaluate environment (home, work, transportation) *for obvious safety hazards, as well as situations that can exacerbate injury or adversely affect client's well-being. Unsafe factors include a vast array of possibilities (e.g., unsafe heating appliances, smoking materials, toxic substances and chemicals, open flames, knives, improperly stored guns, overloaded electrical outlets, dangerous neighborhoods, unsupervised children).*[1]

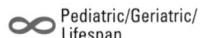

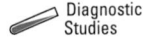

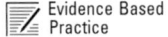

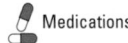

- Review potential occupational risk factors (e.g., works with dangerous tools and machinery, electricity, explosives; police, fire, emergency medical service officers; working with hazardous chemicals, various inhalants, or radiation).
- Note history of accidents during specific period of time, noting circumstances of the accident (e.g., time of day that falls occur, activities going on, who was present). *Investigation of such events can provide clues for client's risk for subsequent events and potential for enhanced safety by a change in the people or environment involved (e.g., client may need assistance when getting up at night, increased playground supervision may be required).*
- Determine potential for abusive behavior by family members/SO(s)/peers. *Anyone, but especially child/frail elder, may require placement if incurring repeated injuries in family/community setting.*
- Note socioeconomic status and availability and use of resources. *Lack of resources, including financial, may limit ability to meet safety needs (e.g., proper child safety seat, appliance repairs, window grates).*
- Review diagnostic studies and laboratory results, noting impairments or imbalances *that may result in or exacerbate conditions, such as confusion, tetany, pathological fractures, etc.*

NURSING PRIORITY NO. 2 To enhance safety in healthcare environment:

- Screen client for safety concerns (e.g., risk for falls, cognitive, developmental, vision/other sensory impairments upon admission and during stay in healthcare facility. Assess for and report changes in client's functional status. Perform thorough assessments regarding safety issues when planning for client discharge. *Failure to accurately assess and intervene or refer regarding these issues can place the client at needless risk and creates negligence issues for the healthcare practitioner.*[8,9,14]
- Monitor client's therapeutic regimen on a continual basis (e.g., client's vital signs, medications, treatment modalities, infusions, nutrition, physical environment) *to prevent healthcare-related injuries.*[9,14]
- Collaborate in treatment of underlying medical, surgical, or psychiatric conditions *to improve cognition and thinking processes, musculoskeletal function, awareness of own safety needs, and general well-being.*
- Refer to physical or occupational therapist as appropriate *to identify high-risk tasks, conduct site visits, select, create, or modify equipment; and provide education about body mechanics and musculoskeletal injuries, as well as provide needed therapies.*[2]
- Emphasize with client importance of obtaining assistance when weak or sedated and when problems of balance, coordination, or postural hypotension are present *to reduce risk of syncope and falls.*
- Provide quiet environment and reduced stimulation as indicated. *Helps limit confusion or overstimulation for clients at risk for such conditions as seizures, tetany, and autonomic hyperreflexia.*
- Demonstrate and encourage use of techniques to reduce or manage stress and vent emotions such as anger and hostility *to reduce risk of violence to self/others.*
- Provide for routine safety needs:[2–7]

  Provide adequate supervision and frequent observation.

  Place young children and confused client/person with dementia near nurses' station.

  Provide for appropriate communication tools (e.g., call light, writing implements and paper; alphabet picture board).

  Demonstrate use and place call bell/light or phone within client's reach.

  Orient or reorient client to environment as needed.

  Encourage client's use of corrective vision and hearing aids.

  Keep bed in low position or place mattress on floor as appropriate.

  Maintain correct body alignment and mechanics.

  Provide positioning as required by situation (e.g., immobilization of fractures).

  Implement appropriate measures to maintain skin and tissue health.

  Protect client (with sensory impairments) from injury due to heat and cold.

  Provide seizure precautions when indicated.

  Lock wheels on bed, wheelchair, and movable furniture.

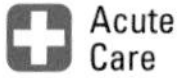

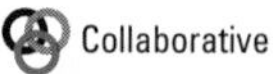

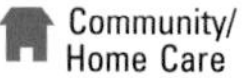

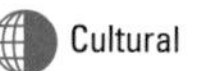

Assist with activities and transfers as needed.
Provide well-fitting, nonskid footwear.
Demonstrate and monitor use of assistive devices, such as cane, walker, crutches, wheelchair, and safety bars.
Clear travel paths, pick up small items from floor; keep furniture in one place and door in one position (completely open or closed).
Provide adequate area lighting.
Follow facility protocol and closely monitor use of restraints when required (e.g., vest, limb, belt, mitten).

- Administer treatments, medications, and therapies in a therapeutic manner.
- Dispose of sharp implements in appropriate container.

NURSING PRIORITY NO. 3 To enhance safety for client in community care setting:

- Provide information to caregivers regarding client's specific disease or condition(s) and associated risks. *For example, postural hypotension, muscle weakness (e.g., multiple sclerosis), dementia, osteoporosis, and head injury can impair function or cognition, impacting client's ability to protect self.*
- Identify interventions and safety devices to promote safe physical environment and individual safety:[5,6,8–11]

Recommend wearing visual or hearing aids *to maximize sensory input.*
Ensure availability of communication devices (e.g., telephone, computer, alarm system, or medical emergency alert device).
Install and maintain electrical and fire safety devices, extinguishers, and alarms.
Review oxygen safety rules.
Identify environmental needs (e.g., decals on glass doors *to show when they are closed;* adequate lighting of stairways, handrails, ramps, bathtub safety tapes *to reduce risk of falls;* lowering temperature on hot water heater *to prevent accidental burns;* creation of ergonomic workstation).
Obtain seat raisers for chairs; ergonomic beds or chairs.
Encourage participation in back-safety classes, injury-prevention exercises, and/or mobility or transfer device training.
Install locked cabinets for medications and toxic household substances and use tamper-proof medication containers.
Review proper storage and disposal of volatile liquids, installation of proper ventilation for use when mixing or using toxic substances, and use of safety glasses or goggles.
Emphasize importance of appropriate use of car restraints and bicycle, skating, or skiing helmets.
Discuss swimming pool fencing and supervision; attending first-aid and cardiopulmonary resuscitation classes.
Obtain trigger locks or gun safes for firearms.

- Initiate appropriate teaching and referrals, *if reckless behavior is occurring or likely to occur (e.g., smoking in bed, driving without safety belts, working with chemicals without safety goggles).*
- Encourage participation in self-help programs *to address individual risks (e.g., assertiveness training, positive self-image to enhance self-esteem, smoking cessation, weight management).*
- Refer to counseling or psychotherapy, as needed, *especially when individual is "accident-prone" or self-destructive behavior is noted.* Refer to ND risk for self-directed Violence.

NURSING PRIORITY NO. 4 To promote optimal safety (Teaching/Discharge Considerations):

- Discuss importance of self-monitoring of conditions or emotions that can contribute to occurrence of injury to self/others (e.g., fatigue, anger, irritability). *Client/SO may be able to modify risk through monitoring of actions or postponement of certain actions, especially during times when client is likely to be highly stressed.*
- Review expectations caregivers have of children, cognitively impaired, or older family members *to identify needed information, required assistance with care, and follow-up that may be needed to provide safe environment for client.*
- Problem solve with client/parent *to provide adequate child supervision after school, during working hours, and on school holidays.*

- ∞ Discuss need for and sources of adult supervision (e.g., senior day care, home health aide, or companion).
- Encourage client's family to identify neighbors or friends willing *to assist elderly/individuals with disabilities in providing such things as checking on client who lives alone, removing snow and ice from walks and steps, assisting with structural maintenance, etc.*
- Explore behaviors related to use of alcohol, tobacco, and recreational drugs and other substances. *Provides opportunity to review consequences of previously determined risk factors (e.g., increase in oral cancer among teenagers using smokeless tobacco, potential consequences of illegal activities, effects of smoking on health of family members as well as fire danger; occurrence of spontaneous abortion, fetal alcohol syndrome or neonatal addiction in prenatal women using tobacco, alcohol, and other drugs).*[10–12]
- Encourage development of fire safety program. *Participation in family fire drills, use of smoke detectors, yearly chimney cleaning, purchase of fire-retardant clothing (especially children's nightwear), fireworks safety, safe use of in-home oxygen or propane sources, etc., enhances home safety.*
- Recommend use of seat belts and approved infant seat in appropriate position in vehicle; fitted helmets for cyclists, motorcyclists, and skateboarders; wearing necessary visual aids; driver training course for new and mature drivers; avoidance of hitchhiking; and substance-abuse program as indicated *to promote transportation safety.*
- Identify community resources (e.g., financial, volunteer) *to assist with necessary home improvements or equipment purchases.*
- Refer to other resources as indicated (e.g., counseling/psychotherapy, parenting classes, budget counseling).
- Provide client/caregiver with emergency contact numbers as individually indicated (e.g., doctor, 911, poison control, police).
- Provide client/caregiver with bibliotherapy and written resources *for later review and self-paced learning.*
- Encourage involvement in community awareness programs and problem solving of identified community needs:

  Participate in self-help programs (e.g., Neighborhood Watch, Helping Hand, after-school activities). *Programs based on identified needs enhance support of community members and potential funding sources.*

  Promote educational opportunities *geared toward increasing awareness of safety measures (e.g., firearms safety) and resources available to the individual.*

  Seek out and involve businesses in volunteer outreach activities such as building safe playgrounds, community or street cleanup, home repair or improvement for frail elders, etc.

  Advocate for and promote solutions for problems of design of buildings, equipment, transportation, and workplace practices *that contribute to accidents.*

DOCUMENTATION FOCUS

Assessment/Reassessment
- Individual risk factors, past and recent history of injuries, awareness of safety needs.

Planning
- Plan of care and who is involved in the planning.
- Teaching plan.

Implementation/Evaluation
- Responses to interventions, teaching, and actions performed.
- Attainment or progress toward desired outcome(s).
- Modifications to plan of care.

Discharge Planning
- Long-term needs and who is responsible for actions to be taken.
- Available resources, specific referrals made.

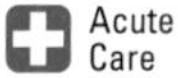

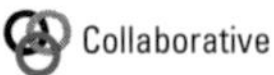

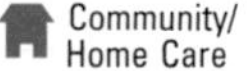

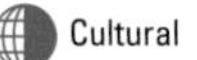

References

1. Ebright, P. R., Patterson, E. S., Render, M. L. (2002). The "New Look" approach to patient safety: A guide for clinical specialist leadership. *Clin Nurs Spec*, 16(5), 247–253.
2. Nelson, A. (ed.) (2006). *Safe Patient Handling and Movement: A Practical Guide for Health Care Professionals*. New York, NY: Springer.
3. Walton, J. (2001). Helping high-risk surgical patients beat the odds. *Nursing*, 31(3), 54–59.
4. Wright, A. (1998). Nursing interventions with advanced osteoporosis. *Home Healthc Nurse*, 16(3), 144–151.
5. Munche, J. A., McCarty, S. M. (2015). Geriatric Rehabilitation. Retrieved April 2015 from http://emedicine.medscape.com/article/318521-overview.
6. Consumer Product Safety Commission. (No date). Safety for older consumers' home safety checklist. Retrieved February 2015 from http://www.cpsc.gov//PageFiles/122038/701.pdf.
7. Daus, C. (1999). Maintaining mobility: Assistive equipment helps the geriatric population stay active and independent. *Rehabil Manage*, 12(5), 58–61.
8. Horn, L. B. (2000). Reducing the risk of falls in the elderly. *Rehabil Manage*, 13(3), 36–38.
9. Kizer, K. W., Blum, L. N. (2005). Safe practices for better health care. Abstract for a portion of the Consensus Report. *Agency for Healthcare Research and Quality*. Retrieved April 2015 from http://www.ncbi.nlm.nih.gov/books/NBK20613/.
10. Gorman-Smith, D., Henry, D. B., Tolan, P. H. (2004). Exposure to community violence and violence perpetration: The protective effects of family functioning. *J Clin Child Psychol*, 33(3), 439–449.
11. Centers for Disease Control and Prevention. (2015). School violence: Risk and protective factors.)Injury Center: Violence prevention. Retrieved April 2015 from http://www.cdc.gov/violenceprevention/youthviolence/riskprotectivefactors.html#RiskFactors.
12. Schwebel, D. C., Barton, B. K. (2005). Contributions of multiple risk factors to child injury. *J Pediatr Psychol*, 30(7), 553–561.
13. Ristolainen, L., Heinonen, A., Waller, B., et al. (2009). Gender differences in sport injury risk and types of injuries: A retrospective twelve-month study on cross-country skiers, long distance runners and soccer players. *J Sports Sci Med*, 8, 443–451.
14. Austin, S. (2008). Seven legal tips for safe nursing practice. *Nursing*, 38(3), 34–39.

Unilateral Neglect

Taxonomy II: Perception/Cognition—Class 1 Attention (00123) [**Diagnostic Division:** Neurosensory], Submitted 1986; Revised 2006

DEFINITION: Impairment in sensory and motor response, mental representation, and spatial attention to the body and the corresponding environment, characterized by inattention to one side and overattention to the opposite side. Left-side neglect is more severe and persistent than right-side neglect.

RELATED FACTORS

Brain injury (e.g., cerebrovascular impairment, neurological illness, trauma, tumor)

DEFINING CHARACTERISTICS

Objective

Hemianopsia; marked deviation of the eyes or trunk to stimuli on the non-neglected side

Failure to move eyes, head, limbs, or trunk in the neglected hemisphere; failure to notice people approaching from the neglected side

Disturbance of sound lateralization

Unaware of positioning of neglected limb

Alteration in safety behavior on neglected side

(continues on page 906)

Unilateral Neglect (continued)

Failure to: eat food from portion of plate on neglected side; dress or groom neglected side

Use of vertical half of page only when writing; impaired performance on line cancellation, line bisection, and target cancellation tests; substitution of letters to form alternative words when reading

Omission of drawing on the neglected side; representational neglect (e.g., distortion of drawing on the neglected side

Perseveration

Transfer of pain sensation to the non-neglected side

Sample Clinical Applications: Traumatic brain injury, CVA/ruptured cerebral aneurysm, brain tumor, glaucoma

DESIRED OUTCOMES/EVALUATION CRITERIA

Sample NOC linkages:

Heedfulness of Affected Side: Personal actions to acknowledge, protect, and cognitively integrate affected body part(s) into self

Self-Care: Activities of Daily Living (ADL): Ability to perform the most basic physical tasks and personal care activities independently with or without assistive device

Client/Caregiver Will (Include Specific Time Frame)

- Acknowledge presence of sensory-perceptual impairment.
- Identify adaptive and protective measures for individual situation.
- Demonstrate behaviors and lifestyle changes necessary to promote physical safety.

Client Will (Include Specific Time Frame)

- Verbalize positive realistic perception of self, incorporating the current dysfunction.
- Perform self-care within level of ability.

ACTIONS/INTERVENTIONS

Sample NIC linkages:

Unilateral Neglect Management: Protecting and safely reintegrating the affected part of the body while helping the patient adapt to disturbed perceptual abilities

Positioning: Deliberative placement of the patient or a body part to promote physiological and/or psychological well-being

Environmental Management: Safety: Monitoring and manipulation of the physical environment to promote safety

NURSING PRIORITY NO. 1 To assess the extent of altered perception and the related degree of disability:

- Identify underlying condition or reason for alterations in sensory/motor/behavioral perceptions as noted in Related Factors. *The client with injury to either side of the brain may experience spatial neglect, but more commonly, it occurs when brain injury affects the right cortical hemisphere, causing left hemiparesis.*[10]
- Observe client's behaviors (as noted in Defining Characteristics) *to determine the extent of impairment (e.g., failure to respond to stimuli, objects, or people on the contralesional side).*
- Ascertain client's/significant other's (SO's) perception of problem and changes and impact on life and future, noting differences in perceptions. *Client is often not aware of, or able to express, spatial perception problems or understand potential effect on future expectations.*
- Assist with/review results of early screening tests. *Tests (often performed at the bedside) may include (and are not limited to) observation to determine if client shows evidence of body neglect such as asymmetric*

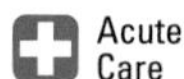
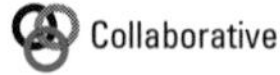
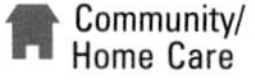
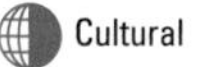

shaving/grooming. Reading test might reveal that client begins reading in the middle of the page. Client may not be able to count fingers on both hands or perceive finger snapping at both ears. Paper and pencil testing may reveal hemispatial neglect through line dissection.[1,9]

- Assess ability to distinguish between right and left. *Unilateral spatial neglect is observed in stroke, brain tumor, or accident victims with damage to the right parietal or parietal-occipital lobe, resulting in misperceptions of space opposite to brain damage. The individual with this condition has information from the left hemispace but no conscious awareness of the information; thus, he/she will pay no attention to the left space.*[1–4]
- Assess sensory awareness (e.g., response to stimulus of hot and cold, dull or sharp); note problems with awareness of motion and proprioception. *Disturbances in these areas may be result of spinal cord injury (where loss of sensation affects body awareness) or brain lesion (where sensation may be intact but awareness is impaired).*
- Note physical signs of neglect (e.g., inability to maintain normal posture; disregard for position of affected limb[s], bumping into objects or walls on the left when ambulating, skin irritation/damage on the left side, indicating lack of awareness of injury).
- Observe ability to function within limits of impairment. Compare with client's perception of own abilities. *Client may or may not be able to learn from mistakes or from observing others depending on the location and severity of the brain lesion.*[5]
- Explore and encourage verbalization of feelings *to identify meaning of loss, dysfunction, or change to the client and impact it may have on assuming ADLs. Note: Expression of loss may be difficult for the client for a variety of reasons. For example, some emotional disturbances and personality changes are caused by the physical effects of brain damage, or the client may be hyperemotional or depressed or be unable to express feelings in the same manner as prior to brain injury.*[5]
- Review results of testing (e.g., computed tomography or magnetic resonance imaging scanning, complete neuropsychological tests) *done to determine cause or type of neglect syndrome (e.g., sensory, motor, representational, personal, spatial, behavioral inattention).*[6–9]

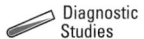

NURSING PRIORITY NO. 2 To promote optimal comfort and safety for the client in the environment:

- Engage in treatment strategies *focused on training of attention to the neglected hemispace:*[1–5,8,9]

  Encourage use of vision and hearing aids if condition requires or client usually wears them *to improve sensory input and interpretation.*

  Remove excess stimuli from the environment *to decrease confusion and reactive stress.*

  Orient or reorient to physical environment and persons interacting with client. *Client with unilateral neglect can also have numerous other cognitive defects affecting ability to think, remember, speak or understand language, and/or interpret environment.*[5]

  Approach client and instruct others to approach client from the unaffected side (e.g., right side, side where vision is not impaired) *to enhance client's awareness and potential for communication.*

  Encourage client to turn head and eyes in full rotation and "scan" the environment *to compensate for visual field loss or when neglect therapies include scanning.*

  Position bedside table and objects (e.g., telephone, call bell, tissues) *within functional field of vision or awareness to facilitate self-care. Note: Therapies may include orienting the client's environment leftward in attempt to help client perceive the neglected space.*

  Place nonessential items (e.g., television, pictures, hairbrush) on affected side during postacute phase once client begins to cross midline *to encourage continuation of retraining behaviors.*

  Discuss affected side while touching, manipulating, and stroking affected side *to focus client's attention on area* and provide objects of various weight, texture, and size for the client to handle *to provide tactile stimuli.*

  Describe where affected areas of body are *when moving or repositioning client.*

  Use descriptive terms to identify body parts rather than "left" and "right"; for example, "Lift this leg" (point to leg) or "Lift your affected leg."

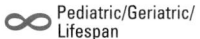

Encourage client to accept affected limb or side as part of self even when it no longer feels like it belongs.
Have client look at and handle affected side *to stimulate awareness* and bring the affected limb across the midline *for client to visualize during care.*
Provide visual cues and assist client to position the affected extremity carefully and teach to routinely visualize placement of the extremity.
Use a mirror to help client adjust position *by visualizing both sides of the body.*

- Provide assistance with ADLs (e.g., feeding, bathing, dressing, grooming, toileting), *which helps client tend to affected side or compensate for client's impairments. Note: Studies show that unilateral neglect is a major factor limiting ADLs and in client being at increased risk for falls.*[11]
- Monitor neglected body part(s) for positioning and anatomic alignment, pressure points, skin irritation or injury, and dependent edema. *Increased risk of injury and pressure ulcer formation necessitates close observation and timely intervention.* (Refer to NDs risk for Peripheral Neurovascular Dysfunction and impaired Tissue Integrity.)
- Assist with ambulation or movement, using appropriate mobility and assistive devices *to promote safety of client and caregiver.*
- Protect from falls and/or collision with objects:
  Position furniture and equipment *so travel path is unobstructed.*
  Remove articles that may create a safety hazard (e.g., footstool, throw rug).
  Ensure adequate lighting in the environment.
  Keep doors wide open or completely closed.
- Refer to NDs impaired Environmental Interpretation Syndrome, risk for Falls/Injury, and Self-Care Deficit (specify) for additional interventions regarding comfort and safety.
- Collaborate with rehabilitation team in strategies (e.g., sensory stimulation techniques such as tapping or stroking, patching one half of each eye, auditory stimulation, wedge prism adaptation techniques, virtual reality technology) *to assist client to overcome or compensate for deficits.*[5,12,13]

NURSING PRIORITY NO. 3 To promote optimal functioning (Teaching/Discharge Considerations):

- Acknowledge and accept feelings of despondency, grief, and anger. *When feelings are openly expressed, client can deal with them and move forward.* (Refer to ND Grieving as appropriate.)
- Encourage family members/SO(s) to treat client normally, to urge client to perform own care as able, and to include client in family activities and outings. *Promotes sense of self-worth and encourages participation in life activities to limit withdrawal and depression.*
- Reinforce to client the reality of the dysfunction and need to compensate. Avoid participating in the client's use of denial. *Delays dealing with reality of situation and limits progress toward goals.*
- Encourage client to continue rehabilitative services *to maximize recovery and enhance independence. Note: Research indicates that most clients with neglect show early recovery, particularly within the first month, and marked improvement within 3 months. In approximately 5% of clients, classic (more severe) symptoms of spatial neglect persist after 6 months or longer. In these individuals, the deficit may be regarded as chronic neglect.*[9]
- Discuss and prepare for ongoing safety issues. *Client may continue to have some functional problems after apparent recovery of spatial neglect, including difficulty with navigating in familiar and unfamiliar environments or safe driving.*[9]
- Identify additional resources to meet individual needs (e.g., Meals on Wheels, home-care rehabilitation services) *to maximize independence and allow client to return to and succeed in community setting.*

DOCUMENTATION FOCUS

Assessment/Reassessment

- Individual findings, including extent of altered perception, degree of disability, effect on independence and participation in ADLs.

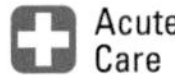

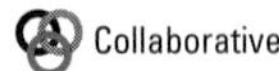

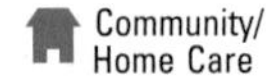

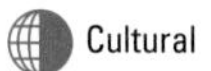

Planning

- Plan of care and who is involved in the planning.
- Teaching plan.

Implementation/Evaluation

- Responses to intervention, teaching, and actions performed.
- Attainment or progress toward desired outcome(s).
- Modifications to plan of care.

Discharge Planning

- Long-term needs and who is responsible for actions to be taken.
- Available resources, specific referrals made.

References

1. Walker, R. (1994). Unilateral neglect: Clinical and experimental studies. *Review for Psyche: An Interdisciplinary Journal of Research on Consciousness*. Archived book review may be accessed at Association for the Scientific Study of Consciousness at http://www.theassc.org/vol_1_1994.
2. Mansoori, L. (2010). Hemispatial neglect syndrome. Student lecture for Brain, Thought and Action (MCDB 3650). University of Colorado. Boulder, CO.
3. Ricci, R., Calhoun, J., Chatterjee, A. (2000). Orientation bias in unilateral neglect: Representational contributions. *Cortex*, 36(5), 671–677.
4. Sinclair, C. (2001). Brain organization as seen in unilateral spatial neglect. Retrieved November 2015 from http://serendip.brynmawr.edu/bb/neuro/neuro01/web2/Sinclair.html.
5. National Institute for Neurological Disorders and Stroke. (2014). Post-stroke rehabilitation fact sheet. Retrieved November 2015 from http://stroke.nih.gov/materials/rehabilitation.htm.
6. Bates, B., Choi, J. Y., Duncan, P. W. (2005). Veterans Affairs/Department of Defense clinical practice guidelines for the management of adult stroke rehabilitation care: An executive summary. *Stroke*, 36(9), 2049–2056.
7. Plummer, P., Morris, M. E., Dunai, J. (2003). Assessment of unilateral neglect. *Phys Ther*, 83(8), 732–740.
8. Swan, L. (2001). Unilateral spatial neglect. *Phys Ther*, 81(9), 1572–1580.
9. Barrett, A. M., John, S. T. (2007, update 2014). Spatial neglect. Retrieved November 2015 from http://emedicine.medscape.com/article/1136474-overview.
10. Vocat, R., Staub, F., Stroppini, T., et al. (2010). Anosognosia for hemiplegia: A clinical-anatomical prospective study. *Brain*, 133, 3578–3597.
11. Czernuszenko, A. (2007). Risk factors for falls in post-stroke patients treated in a neurorehabilitation ward. *Neurol Neurochir Pol*, 41(1), 28–35.
12. Tsirlin, I., Dupierrix, E., Chokron, S., et al. (2009). Uses of virtual reality for diagnosis, rehabilitation and study of unilateral spacial neglect: Review and analysis. *Cyberpsychol Behav*, 12(2), 175–181.
13. Mizuno, K., Tsugi, T., Takebayashi, T., et al. (2011). Prism adaptation therapy enhances rehabilitation of stroke patients with unilateral spatial neglect: A randomized controlled trial. *Neurorehabil Neural Repair*, 25(8), 711–720.

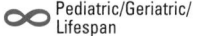

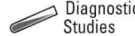

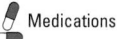

[acute/chronic] Urinary Retention

Taxonomy II: Elimination and Exchange—Class 1 Urinary Function (00023) [**Diagnostic Division:** Elimination], Submitted 1986

DEFINITION: Incomplete emptying of the bladder.

RELATED FACTORS

High urethral pressure
Reflex arc inhibition
Strong sphincter; blockage in urinary tract [e.g., benign prostatic hypertrophy (BPH), perineal swelling]
[Infections; neurological diseases/trauma]
[Pharmaceutical agents (e.g., opiates, atropine, belladonna, psychotropics, antihistamines)]

DEFINING CHARACTERISTICS

Subjective

Sensation of bladder fullness
Dribbling of urine
Dysuria

Objective

Bladder distention
Small or frequent voiding; absent urinary output
Residual urine
Overflow incontinence

Sample Clinical Applications: BPH, prostatitis, cancer, perineal surgery, birth trauma, urethral calculi, multiple sclerosis (MS), spinal cord compression, urinary tract infection (UTI), genital herpes

DESIRED OUTCOMES/EVALUATION CRITERIA

Sample NOC linkages:

Urinary Elimination: Collection and discharge of urine
Symptom Control: Personal actions to minimize perceived adverse changes in physical and emotional functioning
Knowledge: Disease Process: Extent of understanding conveyed about a specific disease process and prevention of complications

Client Will (Include Specific Time Frame)

- Verbalize understanding of causative factors and appropriate interventions for individual situation.
- Demonstrate techniques or behaviors to alleviate or prevent retention.
- Void in sufficient amounts with no palpable bladder distention, experience no postvoid residuals greater than 50 mL, and have no dribbling or overflow.

ACTIONS/INTERVENTIONS

Acute Retention

Sample NIC linkages:

Urinary Catheterization: Insertion of a catheter into the bladder for temporary or permanent drainage of urine
Urinary Retention Care: Assistance in relieving bladder distention
Fluid Monitoring: Collection and analysis of patient data to regulate fluid balance

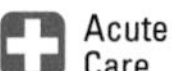

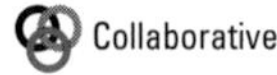

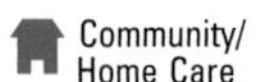

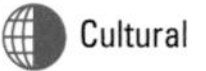

NURSING PRIORITY NO. 1 To assess causative/contributing factors:

- Note presence of pathological conditions, such as neurological injury or disease; kidney or bladder infection or stone formation; and reaction to medications, diagnostic dye, or anesthesia, *that can cause mechanical obstruction, nerve dysfunction, ineffective contraction, or decompensation of detrusor musculature, resulting in ineffective emptying of the bladder and urine retention.*[2]
- Note client's gender and age. *Retention is most common among men (young men due to renal calculi) and older men (where prostate abnormalities or urethral strictures cause outlet obstruction). In either sex, retention may be due to medications (particularly those with anticholinergic effects, including many over-the-counter drugs); severe fecal impaction (which increases pressure on the bladder); or neurogenic bladder in patients with diabetes, multiple sclerosis, Parkinson's disease, or prior pelvic surgery resulting in bladder denervation.*[7,10]
- Investigate reports of sudden loss of ability to pass urine, great difficulty passing urine, pain with urination, blood in urine. *May indicate urinary retention due to UTI or outlet obstruction.*[2]
- Review results of lab tests, such as urinalysis for presence of red and white blood cells, nitrates, glucose, bacteria, and cultures, as indicated. Blood may be tested for infection, electrolyte imbalance, and (in men) prostate-specific antigen *to determine presence of treatable conditions.*
- Review medication regimen *for drugs that can cause or exacerbate retention (e.g., psychotropics, opiates, sedatives, alpha- and beta-blockers, anticholinergics, antihistamines, neuroleptics, anesthesia).*[2]
- Determine anxiety level. *Client may be too embarrassed to void in presence of others or talk about problem with care providers.*
- Examine for fecal impaction, pelvic or perineal surgical site swelling, postpartal edema, vaginal or rectal packing, enlarged prostate, or other "mechanical" factors *that may produce a blockage of the urethra.*
- Strain urine for presence of stones or calculi *that may be causing outlet obstruction or to note when treatments are being effective in stone breakup and removal.*[2]

NURSING PRIORITY NO. 2 To determine degree of interference/disability:

- Ascertain if client can empty bladder completely, partially, or not at all, in spite of urge to urinate. *Signs of urinary retention caused by (1) blockage of the urethra or (2) disruption of complex system of nerves that connects the urinary tract with the brain. In men, blockage is most commonly caused by enlargement of the prostate, cancer, stones, and urethral stricture. Causes that can occur in both genders include scar tissue, injury (as in car crash or fall), blood clots, infection, tumors, and stones (rare). Disruption of nerves or nerve transmission or interpretation of signals can be caused by injury (e.g., spinal cord injury [SCI] or tumor, herniated disk, stroke), pelvic infections, surgery, and certain medications.*[1,2]
- Determine if there has been any significant urine output in the previous 6 to 8 hr. *Small amount of urine may leak out of bladder but generally not enough to relieve symptoms.*
- Note recent amount and type of fluid intake. *Adequate fluid intake is necessary for production of healthy output. If client is not voiding in spite of adequate fluid intake, fluids may be restricted temporarily to prevent bladder overdistention until adequate urine flow is established.*
- Palpate height of the bladder. Ascertain whether client has sensation of bladder fullness and his or her level of discomfort. *Sensation and discomfort can vary depending on underlying cause of retention. Most people with acute retention also feel pain in lower abdomen (pelvis). Back pain, fever, and painful urination may be present with retention if the cause is urinary tract infection.*
- Catheterize, or perform a bladder scan or ultrasound, for bladder residual after voiding *to determine presence and degree of urine retention.*[3]
- Review results of diagnostic tests. *Urine flow rate, bladder capacity, and postvoid residual scanning may be done. Ultrasound, computed tomography (CT) scan, intravenous pyelogram, and cystoscopy can help locate the source of obstruction (e.g., lower or upper tract). Lumbar spine radiographs, CT scan, or magnetic resonance imaging may be done when retention is thought to be due to an acute spinal problem (e.g., herniated disk, spinal cord disruption, infection).*[2,3]

NURSING PRIORITY NO. 3 To assist in treating/preventing retention:

- Assist in treatment to relieve mechanical obstruction (e.g., removal of blockage—vaginal packing, bowel impaction) or apply ice *to reduce perineal swelling.*
- Administer medications as indicated (e.g., antibiotics, stool softeners, pain relievers) *to treat underlying cause.*
- Provide privacy *to reduce retention caused by embarrassment or anxiety.*
- Assist client to sit upright on toilet or commode or stand *to provide functional position of voiding.*
- Encourage warm sitz bath or shower, voiding in tub or shower if need be. *Warm water stimulates bladder to relax and may facilitate voiding.*
- Use ice techniques or spirits of wintergreen, stroke inner thigh, and run water in sink or warm water over perineum if indicated *to stimulate reflex arc.*
- Instruct client with mild or moderate obstructive symptoms to "double void" by urinating, resting on toilet for 3 to 5 min, and then making a second attempt to urinate. *Promotes more efficient bladder evacuation by allowing the detrusor to contract initially and then rest and contract again.*[1]
- Drain bladder (using the appropriate catheter material and size) intermittently or catheterize with indwelling catheter *to resolve acute retention. Note: A variety of different kinds of urethral catheters are available. Some have been developed specifically to lower the risk of catheter-associated infection, such as antiseptic or antibiotic impregnated catheters.*[9]
- Prepare for more intensive interventions (e.g., reconstructive surgery, lithotripsy, prostatectomy) as indicated *to remove source of obstruction, reconstruct sphincter, or provide for urinary diversion.*

NURSING PRIORITY NO. 4 To promote optimal elimination (Teaching/Discharge Considerations):

- Emphasize good voiding habits (e.g., four to six times/day). *Postponing or holding urination for prolonged periods can, over time, overstretch and weaken bladder muscles.*
- Encourage client to report problems immediately *so treatment can be instituted promptly.*
- Emphasize need for adequate fluid intake.
- Encourage adequate fluid intake, including use of acidifying fruit juices or ingestion of vitamin C or Mandelamine *to discourage bacterial growth and stone formation.*[8]
- Adjust fluid intake and timing if indicated, *to prevent bladder distention.*

Chronic Retention

Sample NIC linkages:

Urinary Retention Care: Assistance in relieving bladder distention

Urinary Catheterization: Intermittent: Regular periodic use of a catheter to empty the bladder

NURSING PRIORITY NO. 1 To assess causative/contributing factors:

- Review medical history for diagnoses, such as congenital defects, neurological disorders (e.g., MS, polio), prostatic hypertrophy or surgery, birth canal injury or scarring, and SCI with lower motor neuron injury or bladder stones, *that may cause detrusor-sphincter dysynnergia (loss of coordination between bladder contraction and external urinary sphincter relaxation), detrusor muscle atrophy, or chronic overdistention because of outlet obstruction.*[7,10]
- Determine presence of weak or absent sensory or motor impulses (as with cerebrovascular accidents, spinal injury, or diabetes) *that predispose client to compromised enervation or interpretation of sensory signals resulting in impaired urination.*[7]
- Assess client's medication regimen (e.g., psychotropic, antihistamines, atropine, belladonna) *to consult with primary care provider regarding client's continued use of drugs that are known to potentiate urinary retention.*

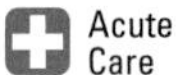
Acute Care
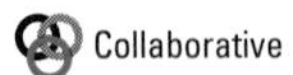
Collaborative
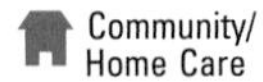
Community/ Home Care
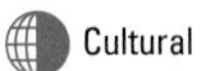
Cultural

NURSING PRIORITY NO. 2 To determine degree of interference/disability:

- Ascertain effect of condition on functioning and lifestyle. *Chronic urinary retention can limit client's desired lifestyle (e.g., daily activities, social functioning) and can lead to chronic incontinence and life-threatening complications (e.g., intractable UTIs, kidney failure).*[4]
- Instruct client/significant other (SO) to maintain voiding log, noting dribbling and frequency and timing of voiding *to determine severity of condition.*[1]
- Determine presence and severity (0–10 scale) of bladder spasms, pelvic pain, and other discomforts.
- Assist with urodynamic testing (e.g., uroflowmetry *to assess urine speed and volume,* cystometrogram *to measure bladder pressure and volume,* bladder scan *to measure retention or postvoid residual, leak point pressure).*[2]

NURSING PRIORITY NO. 3 To assist in treating/preventing retention:

- Collaborate in treatment of underlying conditions (e.g., medications to treat BPH, reducing or eliminating medications responsible for retention, repairing perineal scarring or outlet obstruction), *which may correct or reduce severity of retention and associated overflow or total incontinence.*[10]
- Instruct client/SO in management of voiding problems as indicated:
  Attempt voiding in complete privacy *to reduce embarrassment and distractions.*
  Void on frequent, timed schedule *to maintain low bladder pressure and prevent overdistention of bladder.*
  Maintain consistent fluid intake *to wash out bacteria, avoid infections, and limit bladder stone formation.*[4]
  Adjust fluid amount and timing if indicated *to prevent bladder distention.*
- Establish regular self-catheterization program, as indicated, *to prevent reflux and increased renal pressures and to improve client's quality of life (e.g., ability to participate in desired or needed activities and social interactions). Note: Clean intermittent catheterization is a treatment option for individuals who can urinate but cannot completely empty their bladder.*[4,5,6]
- Perform and instruct client/SO in Credé's method (client or caregiver applies light pressure or tapping on the bladder) or Valsalva's maneuver (client tries to breathe out without letting air escape through the nose or mouth) if appropriate *to stimulate bladder emptying. Note: Client with SCI and spastic bladder may be able to "trigger" the bladder to contract and avoid having to use a catheter.* [7]
- Consult with urologist and prepare for more intensive interventions (e.g., reconstructive surgery, lithotripsy, prostatectomy) as indicated *to remove source of obstruction, reconstruct sphincter, or provide for urinary diversion.*
- Refer for consideration of advanced or research-based therapies (e.g., implanted sacral, tibial, or pelvic electrical stimulating device) *for long-term management of retention.*[4]

NURSING PRIORITY NO. 4 To promote optimum elimination (Teaching/Discharge Considerations):

- Establish regular schedule for bladder emptying whether voiding or using catheter.
- Instruct SO/caregiver(s) in clean intermittent catheterization techniques *so that more than one individual is able to assist the client in care of elimination needs.*[9]
- Instruct client/SO in care when client has indwelling (urethral or suprapubic catheter) or urinary diversion device (e.g., clean technique, emptying and cleaning of leg bag or drainage bag; irrigation and replacement) *to promote self-care, enhance independence, and prevent complications.*[5]
- Emphasize need for adequate fluid intake, including use of acidifying fruit juices or ingestion of vitamin C or Mandelamine. *Maintains renal function, prevents infection and formation of bladder stones, and reduces risk of encrustation around indwelling catheter.*
- Discuss appropriate use of herbal products *such as saw palmetto to improve symptoms of BPH.*
- Review signs/symptoms of complications *to promote timely contact with healthcare provider for evaluation and intervention.*

DOCUMENTATION FOCUS

Assessment/Reassessment

- Individual findings, including nature of problem, degree of impairment, and whether client is incontinent.

Planning

- Plan of care and who is involved in planning.
- Teaching plan.

Implementation/Evaluation

- Response to interventions.
- Attainment or progress toward desired outcome(s).
- Modifications to plan of care.

Discharge Planning

- Long-term needs and who is responsible for actions to be taken.
- Specific referrals made.

References

1. Gray, M. (2000). Urinary retention: Management in the acute care setting (part 2). *Am J Nurs*, 100(8), 36–44.
2. Newman, D. K. (2005). Assessment of the patient with an overactive bladder. *J Wound Ostomy Continence Nurs*, 32(3 suppl), 5–10.
3. National Kidney and Urologic Diseases Information Clearinghouse. (Updated 2014). Urodynamic testing. Fact sheet. Retrieved April 2015 from http://kidney.niddk.nih.gov/KUDISEASES/pubs/urodynamic/index.aspx.
4. Santos, A., Hunt, M. (2005). Managing incontinence: Once a cause of isolation and embarrassment, incontinence does not have to limit quality of life. *Paraplegia News*, 59(11).
5. Herter, R., Kazer, M. W. (2010). Best practices in urinary catheter care. *Home Healthc Nurs*, 28(6), 342–349.
6. Doughty, D., Kisanga, J. (2010). Regulatory guidelines for bladder management in long-term care: Are you in compliance with F-Tag 315? *J Wound, Ostomy Cont Nurs*, 37(4), 399–411.
7. Shenot, P. J. (Updated 2014). Urinary retention (various pages). *The Merck Manual for Health Care Professionals*. Retrieved April 2015 from http://www.merckmanuals.com/professional/genitourinary-disorders/voiding-disorders/urinary-retention.
8. Wyman, J. F. (2003). Treatment of urinary incontinence in men and older women: The evidence shows the efficacy of a variety of techniques. *Am J Nurs*, 103(suppl), 26–35.
9. Smith, J. M. (2003). Indwelling catheter management: From habit-based to evidence-based practice. *J Wound, Ostomy Cont Nurs*, 49(12), 34–45.
10. Policastro, M. A., Sinert, R., Guerrero, P. (Updated 2014). Urinary obstruction. Retrieved April 2015 from http://emedicine.medscape.com/article/778456-overview#showall.

risk for Vascular Trauma

Taxonomy II: Safety/Protection—Class 2 Physical Injury [**Diagnostic Division:** Safety], Submitted 2008; Revised 2013

DEFINITION: Vulnerable to damage to vein and its surrounding tissues related to the presence of a catheter and/or infused solutions, which may compromise health.

RISK FACTORS

Insertion site; difficulty visualizing artery or vein

Inappropriate catheter type or width; inadequate anchoring of catheter

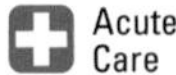

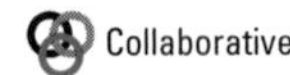

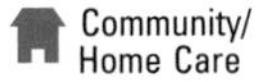

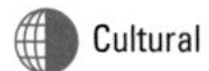

Irritating solution (e.g., concentration, temperature, pH); rapid infusion rate; length of time catheter is in place

Note: A risk diagnosis is not evidenced by signs and symptoms, as the problem has not occurred; rather, nursing interventions are directed at prevention.

Sample Clinical Applications: Surgery, trauma, cancer/chemotherapy, pneumonia, sepsis, dehydration, heat stroke

DESIRED OUTCOMES/EVALUATION CRITERIA

Sample NOC linkages:

Risk Control: Personal actions to prevent, eliminate, or reduce modifiable health threats

Knowledge: Treatment Procedure: Extent of understanding conveyed about a procedure required as part of a treatment regimen

Self-Care: Parenteral Medication: Ability to administer parenteral medications to meet therapeutic goals independently with or without assistive device

Client Will (Include Specific Time Frame)

- Identify sign/symptoms to report to healthcare provider.
- Be free of signs/symptoms associated with venipuncture, infusion solution, or local infection.
- Develop plan for home therapy where indicated and demonstrate appropriate procedures.

ACTIONS/INTERVENTIONS

Sample NIC linkages:

Intravenous (IV) Insertion: Insertion of a needle into a peripheral vein for the purpose of administering fluids, blood, or medications

Intravenous (IV) Therapy: Administration and monitoring of intravenous fluids and medications

Medication Administration: Intravenous: Preparing and giving medications via the intravenous route

NURSING PRIORITY NO. 1 To assess risk factors:

- Determine presence of medical condition(s) requiring IV therapy, such as dehydration, trauma, and surgery; long-term antibiotic treatment of severe infections; cancer therapies; and pain management when oral drugs not effective or practical.
- Note client's age, body size, and weight. *Very young and elderly clients are at risk because of lack of subcutaneous tissue surrounding veins, and veins may be fragile or ropy, causing difficulties with insertion. Forearm veins may be difficult to see in obese, edematous, or dark-skinned individuals.*[3,4]
- Identify particular issues, such as client's emotional state (including fear of needles) and mental or developmental status, *that might interfere with client's ability to cooperate with procedures,* and IV site choices that interfere with client's mobility *to prevent or limit potential for vascular damage.*[3]
- Determine type(s) of solutions being used or planned. *Certain infusates are associated with greater risk of vein irritation and pain (e.g., potassium, contrast media); others are associated with tissue injury, especially upon infiltration into surrounding tissues, including certain antibiotics (e.g., nafcillin, cloxicillin, vancomycin). Hyperosmolar solutions such as total parenteral nutrition can cause tissue damage by altering osmotic pressure. Most cancer chemotherapeutic agents cause direct cellular toxicity after extravasation, and some have potential for causing substantial tissue necrosis (e.g., doxorubicin, vincristine).*[5] *Note: Therapies not appropriate for peripheral short catheters include continuous vesicant therapy, parenteral nutrition, infusates with a pH less than 5 or greater than 9, and solutions with an osmolarity greater than 600 mOsm/L.*[6,7]
- Assess peripheral IV site when one is already in place to determine potential for complications. *Reddened, blanched, tight, translucent, or cool skin; swelling; pain; numbness; streak formation; and a palpable venous cord or purulent drainage are indicative of problem with IV requiring immediate intervention.*[1]

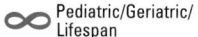

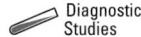

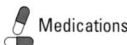

- Assess central venous access device (CVAD), if present, to determine potential for complications. *Inability to aspirate; slowed or absent solution flow; site pain; and engorged veins or swelling in upper arm, chest wall, neck, or jaw on side of catheter insertion may indicate vein or catheter-related thrombus, requiring immediate intervention.*[1,2]

NURSING PRIORITY NO. 2 To reduce potential complications:

- Determine appropriate site choice:
  - Identify extremities and sites that have impaired circulation or injury, such as lymphedema, postoperative swelling, recent trauma, hematoma, axillary lymph node dissection, open wounds, etc.[4] *Leg veins should be avoided in adults due to potential for thrombophlebitis. Antecubital veins should be avoided for peripheral catheters where possible because they limit client's movement and are easily dislodged.*[6]
  - Inspect and palpate chosen veins to determine size and condition. *Vein that is scarred, lumpy, or small and fragile can not only cause problems upon cannulation, but also can impede effectiveness of infusion.*[1,6]
  - Avoid inserting needle in vein valve site. *Damage to this area can cause blood pooling and increase risk of thrombosis.*[3]
- Use a best-practice approach to IV insertion and therapies:
  - Determine best type of access when IV therapy is to be initiated. *Peripheral catheter in forearm is recommended for short-duration, nonirritating solutions of less than 7 days. CVAD placed so that tip is in or near the superior vena cava is appropriate for infusing many kinds of solutions over long periods of time.*[4,8,9]
  - Choose appropriate needle or catheter for situation considering planned length and type of therapy, avoiding steel butterfly needles when possible *to reduce risk of vein injury and infiltration.*[1,2,4] *Over-the-needle catheter for hand or forearm may be ideal for most solutions over a short length of time, while midline catheter may be chosen for chemotherapy or when antibiotic therapy is planned for 1 to 4 weeks; a central venous catheter is used for infusates and other substances that are too irritating to peripheral veins, when client has suffered multiple peripheral sticks, or when one extremity is not available (e.g., amputation, dialysis shunt in one arm).*[4,8]
  - Use appropriate needle gauge. *Size should be smallest diameter possible for chosen vein and solution to be infused to deliver solution at appropriate rate, to promote hemodilution of fluid(s) at the catheter tip, and to reduce mechanical and chemical irritation to vein wall.*[1,3,4]
  - Clean site and inject 1% lidocaine per agency protocol *to reduce risk of infection and pain with needle or cannula insertion. Note: Nursing research is being conducted on the use of lidocaine or normal saline injection for the reduction of the discomfort of venipuncture. One recent small study found intradermal lidocaine superior to bacteriostatic normal saline as an anesthetic pretreatment; however, this study demonstrated that normal saline can provide reasonable pain relief and is thus a practical alternative when intradermal lidocaine is not available or the patient has an allergy to lidocaine.*[10]
  - Stretch and immobilize skin and tissues *to stabilize vein and prevent rolling, requiring multiple sticks.*
  - Insert needle bevel up and hold at a 3- to 10-deg angle *to prevent "blowing" the vein by piercing the back wall.*[2]
  - Release tourniquet immediately when insertion is complete *to prevent intravascular pressure from causing bleeding into surrounding tissues.*[1]
  - Observe for hematoma development and/or reports of pain and discomfort during insertion, *indicating vein damage with bleeding into tissues.*[4]
  - Secure needle or cannula with tape or other securement device *to prevent dislodging and extend catheter dwell time.*[6]
  - Avoid placing tape entirely around arm to anchor catheter. *This may impede venous return and cause venous stasis, pooling of fluid, and infiltration or extravasation into surrounding tissues.*[4]
  - Utilize transparent dressing over insertion site *to protect from external contaminants and to easily observe for potential complications.*

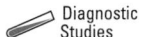

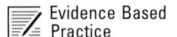

Adhere to recommended infusions, dilutions, and administration rates for medications or irritating substances such as potassium *to reduce incidence of tissue irritation and sloughing.*[2,4,6]

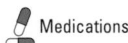

- Consult with IV nurse or other medical provider *to problem solve issues that arise with IVs and/or when different access should be considered (e.g., midline catheter for continuous infusion of irritating solutions, peripheral intravenous central catheter for parenteral nutrition) or for evaluation and interventions for complications such as thrombus development in central catheter tip or in the vein around the catheter.*[4,9]

NURSING PRIORITY NO. 3 To promote optimum therapeutic effect:

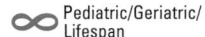

- Observe IV site on a regular basis and instruct client/caregiver to report any discomfort, bruising, redness, swelling, bleeding, or other fluid leaking from site *to allow for prompt intervention and limit serious complications.*
- Replace peripheral catheters every 72 to 96 hr (or per agency policy) *to prevent thrombophlebitis and catheter-related infections.*[4]
- Apply pressure to site when IV is discontinued for sufficient time *to prevent bleeding, especially in client with coagulopathies or on anticoagulants.*[4]
- Adhere to specific protocols related to infection control *to promote safe infusion of solutions or medications and prevent complications.* Refer to ND risk for Infection.
- Identify community resources and suppliers *to support home therapy regimen.*

DOCUMENTATION FOCUS

Assessment/Reassessment

- Assessment findings pre/postinsertion, site choice, use of local anesthetic, type and gauge of needle or cannula inserted, number of sticks required, dressing applied.
- Type, amount, and rate of solution administered, presence of additives.
- Client's response to procedure.

Planning

- Plan of care, specific interventions, and who is involved in the planning.
- Teaching plan as appropriate.

Implementation/Evaluation

- Attainment or progress toward desired outcome(s).
- Modifications to plan of care.

Discharge Planning

- Long-range needs, identifying who is responsible for actions to be taken.
- Community resources for equipment and supplies for home therapy.
- Specific referrals made.

References

1. Hadaway, L. C. (2005). Reopen the pipeline for I.V. therapy. *Nursing*, 35(8), 54–61.
2. Hadaway, L. C., Millam, D. A. (2007). On the road to successful I.V. starts. *Nursing*, 37(8 suppl), 1–14.
3. Rosenthal, K. (2005). Tailor your I.V. insertion techniques for special populations. *Nursing*, 35(5), 36–41.
4. Camp-Sorrell, D., Cope, D. G. (2004). *Access Device Guidelines: Recommendations for Nursing Practice and Education.* 2nd ed. Pittsburgh, PA: Oncology Nursing Society.
5. Dychter, S. S., Gold, D. A., Carson, D. (2012). Intravenous therapy: A review of complications and economic considerations of peripheral access. *J Infus Nurs*, 35(2), 84–91.
6. Infusion Nurses Society. (2006). Infusion nursing standards of practice. *J Infus Nurs*, 29(1 suppl), S1–S92.
7. Gorski, L. A. (2008). Intravenous therapy. In Ackley, B. J., Ladwig, G. B., et al. (eds). *In Evidence-Based Nursing Care Guidelines: Medical-Surgical Interventions.* St. Louis, MO: Mosby Elsevier.

8. Cook, L. S. (2007). Choosing the right intravenous catheter. *Home Healthc Nurse*, 25(8), 523–531.
9. Hadaway, L. C. (2008). Targeting therapy with central venous access devices. *Nursing*, 38(6), 34–40.
10. Burke, S. D., Vercler, S. J., Bye, R. O., et al. (2011). Original research: Local anesthesia before IV catheterization. *Am J Nurs*, 111(2), 40–45.

impaired spontaneous Ventilation

Taxonomy II: Activity/Rest—Class 2 Cardiovascular/Pulmonary Response (00033) [**Diagnostic Division:** Respiration], Submitted 1992

DEFINITION: Decreased energy reserves resulting in an inability to maintain independent breathing that is adequate to support life.

RELATED FACTORS

Alteration in metabolism; [hypermetabolic state (e.g., infection), nutritional deficits or depletion of energy stores]
Respiratory muscle fatigue

DEFINING CHARACTERISTICS

Subjective
Dyspnea
Apprehensiveness

Objective
Alteration in metabolism
Increase in heart rate
Restlessness; decrease in cooperation
Increase in accessory muscle use
Decrease in tidal volume
Decrease in partial pressure of oxygen (Po_2), arterial oxygen saturation (Sao_2); increase in partial pressure of carbon dioxide (Pco_2)

Sample Clinical Applications: Chronic obstructive pulmonary disease (COPD), asthma, pulmonary embolus, acute respiratory distress syndrome, brain injury, chest trauma or surgery, Guillain-Barré syndrome, amyotrophic lateral sclerosis (ALS)

DESIRED OUTCOMES/EVALUATION CRITERIA

Sample NOC linkages:
Mechanical Ventilation Response: Adult: Alveolar exchange and tissue perfusion are effectively supported by mechanical ventilation
Respiratory Status: Ventilation: Movement of air in and out of the lungs
Endurance: Capacity to sustain activity

Client Will (Include Specific Time Frame)
- Reestablish and maintain effective respiratory pattern via ventilator, with absence of retractions or use of accessory muscles, cyanosis, or other signs of hypoxia, and with arterial blood gases (ABGs)/Sao_2 within acceptable range.
- Participate in efforts to wean (as appropriate) within individual's ability.

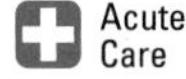

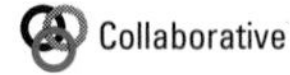

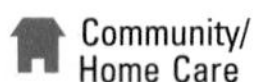

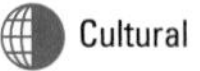

Sample NOC linkage:
Energy Conservation: Personal actions to manage energy for initiating and sustaining activity

Caregiver Will (Include Specific Time Frame)
- Demonstrate behaviors necessary to maintain client's respiratory function.

ACTIONS/INTERVENTIONS

Sample NIC linkages:
Ventilation Assistance: Promotion of an optimal spontaneous breathing pattern that maximizes oxygen and carbon dioxide exchange in the lungs
Mechanical Ventilation Management: Invasive: Assisting the patient receiving artificial breathing support through a device inserted into the trachea
Respiratory Monitoring: Collection and analysis of patient data to ensure airway patency and adequate gas exchange

NURSING PRIORITY NO. 1 To determine degree of impairment:

- Identify client with impending respiratory failure (e.g., developing apnea or slow, shallow breathing; declining mentation or obtunded with need for airway protection).[5]
- Determine presence of conditions that could be associated with hypoventilation. *Causes include (1) central alveolar hypoventilation as a result of congenital defects, drugs, and central nervous system disorders (e.g., stroke, trauma, neoplasms); (2) obesity hypoventilation syndrome is another well-known cause of hypoventilation; (3) chest wall deformities (e.g., kyphoscoliosis, changes after thoracic surgery) can be associated with alveolar hypoventilation, leading to respiratory insufficiency and failure; and (4) neuromuscular diseases that can cause alveolar hypoventilation include myasthenia gravis, ALS, Guillain-Barré, and muscular dystrophy.*[5]
- Assess spontaneous respiratory pattern, noting rate, depth, rhythm, symmetry of chest movement, and use of accessory muscles. *Tachypnea, shallow breathing, and demonstrated or reports of dyspnea (using a numeric or similar scale); increased heart rate and dysrhythmias; pallor or cyanosis; and intercostal retractions and use of accessory muscles indicate increased work of breathing or impaired gas exchange. Note: Studies to date show that no one specific scale has been developed to cover all aspects of breathlessness, but asking the client to rate it some way may be helpful in differentiating this episode from others.*[5,8]
- Auscultate breath sounds, noting presence or absence and equality of breath sounds and adventitious breath sounds (e.g., wheezing) *to evaluate presence and degree of ventilatory impairment.*
- Evaluate ABGs or pulse oximetry and capnography *to determine presence and degree of arterial hypoxemia (PaO_2 less than 55%) and hypercapnia ($PaCO_2$ greater than 45%), resulting in impaired ventilation requiring support.*[6,7]
- Obtain or review results of pulmonary function studies (e.g., lung volumes, inspiratory and expiratory pressures, forced vital capacity), as appropriate, *to assess presence and degree of respiratory insufficiency. Note: Pulmonary function tests revealing (1) vital capacity less than 10 mL/kg; (2) negative inspiratory force less than 25 cm H_2O, and (3) FEV_1 less than 10 mL/kg are standard indicators for intubation and ventilatory management.*[7]
- Investigate etiology of current respiratory failure (e.g., exacerbation of COPD, pneumonia, pulmonary embolus, heart failure, trauma) *to determine client's ventilation needs and most appropriate type of ventilatory support.*
- Review serial chest x-rays and imaging scans (e.g., magnetic resonance imaging, computed tomography) that may be performed *to diagnose underlying disorder and monitor response to treatment.*
- Note response to current measures and respiratory therapy (e.g., bronchodilators, supplemental oxygen, intermittent positive pressure breathing treatments). *Client may already be receiving treatments to maintain airway patency and enhance gas exchange or may have respiratory failure associated with sudden event (e.g., severe trauma, sudden onset respiratory illness, surgery with complications).*
- Ascertain desires of client/significant others (SOs) regarding plan for treatment of respiratory failure, as indicated. *Client may have advance directives and/or prior stated decisions about the level of therapy aggressiveness that*

he or she desires if situation is chronic or long term. Family members may help in decision-making processes if client is a minor or is incapacitated.

NURSING PRIORITY NO. 2 To provide/maintain ventilatory support:

- Collaborate with physician and respiratory care practitioners regarding effective mode of ventilation (e.g., noninvasive oxygenation via continuous positive airway pressure and biphasic positive airway pressure) or intubation and mechanical ventilation (e.g., continuous mandatory, assist control, intermittent mandatory [IMV], pressure support). *Specific mode is determined by client's respiratory requirements, presence of underlying disease process, and the extent to which client can participate in ventilatory efforts. Goals of therapy depend on the reason for mechanical ventilation (e.g., to improve oxygenation, permit sedation, reverse respiratory muscle fatigue).*[9]
- Ensure effective ventilation:[1,7,9]

  Ensure that ventilator settings and parameters are correct as ordered by client situation, including respiratory rate and fraction of inspired oxygen (F_IO_2, expressed as a percentage; tidal volume); peak inspiratory pressure).

  Observe overall breathing pattern, distinguishing between spontaneous respirations and ventilator breaths. *Client may be completely dependent on the ventilator or able to take breaths but have poor oxygen saturation without the ventilator. The client on assist-control ventilation mode can still experience hyper/hypoventilation or "air hunger" and attempt to correct deficiency by overbreathing.*[7]

  Verify that client's respirations are in phase with the ventilator. *Decreases work of breathing, maximizes O_2 delivery when client is not fighting the ventilator.*

  Inflate tracheal or endotracheal tube cuff properly using minimal leak or occlusive technique *to ensure adequate ventilation and delivery of desired tidal volume.*

  Check cuff inflation periodically per facility protocol and whenever cuff is deflated then reinflated *to prevent risks associated with under/overinflation.*

  Check tubings for obstruction (e.g., kinking or accumulation of water) *that can impede flow of oxygen.* Drain tubing, as indicated; refrain from draining toward the client or back into the reservoir, *which can result in contamination and provide medium for growth of bacteria.*

  Check ventilator alarms for proper functioning. Do not turn off alarms, even for suctioning. Verify that alarms can be heard in the nurses' station by care providers *to ensure care provider is alerted to emergent situation or ventilator disconnect.*

  Suction only as needed, using lowest pressure possible, *to clear secretions if client is coughing excessively, has visible secretions, or is tripping high-pressure alarm on ventilator.*

  Remove from ventilator and ventilate manually *if source of ventilator alarm cannot be quickly identified and rectified.*

  Verify that oxygen line is in proper outlet or tank; monitor in-line oxygen analyzer or perform periodic oxygen analysis *to deliver an acceptable oxygen percentage and saturation for client's specific needs.*

  Assess ventilator settings routinely and readjust, as indicated, *according to client's primary disease and results of diagnostic testing.*

  Verify tidal volume set to volume needed for individual situation and proper functioning of spirometer, bellows, or computer readout of delivered volume *to reduce risk of complications associated with alteration in lung compliance or leakage through machine or around tube cuff.*

  Monitor airway pressure for developing complications or equipment problems (e.g., increased airway resistance, retained secretions, decreased lung compliance, client out of phase or off ventilator).

  Promote periodic maximal ventilation of alveoli; check sigh rate intervals (usually 1 1/2 to 2 times tidal volume). *Reduces risk of atelectasis and helps mobilize secretions.*

  Note inspired humidity and temperature; maintain hydration *to prevent excessive drying of mucosa and secretions.*
- Auscultate breath sounds periodically. Note frequent crackles or rhonchi that do not clear with coughing or suctioning. *May indicate developing complications (e.g., atelectasis, pneumonia, acute bronchospasm, pulmonary edema).*

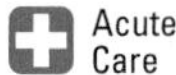
Acute Care
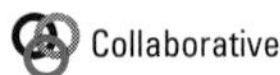
Collaborative
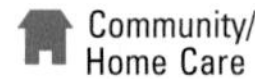
Community/ Home Care
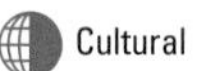
Cultural

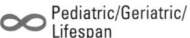

- Note changes in chest symmetry. *May indicate improper placement of endotracheal tube or development of barotrauma.*
- Keep resuscitation bag at bedside *to allow for manual ventilation whenever indicated (e.g., if client is removed from ventilator or troubleshooting equipment problems).*
- Administer and monitor response to medications that promote airway patency and gas exchange *to determine efficacy and need for change.*
- Administer sedation, as required, *to synchronize respirations and reduce work of breathing and energy expenditure.*
- Refer to NDs ineffective Airway Clearance, ineffective Breathing Pattern, and impaired Gas Exchange for related interventions.

NURSING PRIORITY NO. 3 To prepare for/assist with weaning process if appropriate:

- Determine client's physical and psychological readiness to wean soon after intubation, whenever possible, *to limit complications associated with long-term mechanical ventilation. Successful weaning is based on parameters such as (1) evidence for some reversal of the underlying cause of respiratory failure, (2) adequate oxygenation and normal pH, (3) hemodynamic stability, (4) capability and willingness to initiate inspiratory effort, (5) absence of excessive secretions, and (6) nutritional status sufficient to maintain work of breathing.*[1–4,5,7,9]
- Determine mode for weaning. *Recent studies indicate that pressure support mode or multiple daily T-piece trials may be superior to IMV, low-level pressure support may be beneficial for spontaneous breathing trials, and early extubation and institution of noninvasive positive pressure ventilation may have substantial benefits in alert, cooperative client.*[2,4,5]
- Explain to client/SO weaning activities and techniques, individual plan, and expectations. *Reduces fear of unknown, provides opportunities to deal with concerns, clarifies reality of fears, and helps reduce anxiety to a more manageable level.*[3,7]
- Engage client in specialized exercise program *to enhance respiratory muscle strength and general endurance.*
- Maximize weaning effort:

  Elevate head of bed/place in orthopedic chair, if possible, or position *to alleviate dyspnea and to facilitate oxygenation.*

  Coach client in "taking control" of breathing during weaning periods (e.g., to take slower, deeper breaths; practice abdominal or pursed-lip breathing; assume position of comfort) *to maximize respiratory function and reduce anxiety.*

  Instruct in or assist client to perform effective coughing techniques. *Necessary for secretion management after extubation.*

  Provide quiet environment, calm approach, and undivided attention of nurse. *Promotes relaxation, decreasing energy and oxygen requirements.*

  Involve family/SO(s) as appropriate. Provide diversionary activity. *Helps client focus on something other than breathing.*

  Instruct client in use of energy-saving techniques during care activities *to limit oxygen consumption and fatigue associated with work of breathing.*
- Acknowledge and provide ongoing encouragement for client's efforts. Communicate hope for successful weaning response (even partial). *Emotional support can enhance client's commitment to continue weaning activity, maximizing outcomes.*

NURSING PRIORITY NO. 4 To prepare for discharge on ventilator when indicated:

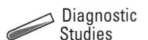

- Ascertain plan for discharge placement (e.g., return home, short-term admission to subacute or rehabilitation center, permanent placement in extended-care facility). *Helps to determine care needs and fiscal impact of home care versus extended-care facility.*

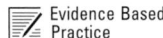

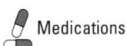

- Review layout of home, noting size of rooms, doorways, placement of furniture, and number and type of electrical outlets *to identify necessary modifications and safety needs.*
- Determine specific equipment needs and resources for equipment and maintenance. Arrange for delivery before client discharge *to allow SO/caregivers to prepare for transfer.*
- Allow sufficient opportunity for SO(s)/family to practice new skills. Role-play potential crisis situations *to enhance confidence in ability to handle client's needs.*
- Demonstrate airway management techniques and proper equipment cleaning practices *to reduce risk of infection.*
- Instruct SO(s)/caregivers in pulmonary physiotherapy measures, as indicated. Refer for home respiratory therapy support, as needed.
- Provide positive feedback and encouragement for efforts of SO(s)/caregivers. *Promotes continuation of desired behaviors.*
- List names and phone numbers for identified contact persons and resources. *Can reduce sense of isolation and enhance likelihood of obtaining assistance and support when needed.*
- Review and provide written or audiovisual materials regarding proper ventilator management, maintenance, and safety for reference in home setting. *Provides information to enhance client's/SO's level of comfort with challenging tasks.*
- Identify signs/symptoms requiring prompt medical evaluation or intervention. *Timely treatment may prevent progression of problem or untoward complications.*
- Obtain no-smoking signs to be posted in home, and remind family members to refrain from smoking *to reduce risk of fire.*
- Have family/SO(s) notify utility company and fire department of presence of ventilator in home. *Client will be placed in high-risk list for follow-up in case of power outage or fire.*

NURSING PRIORITY NO. 5 To promote wellness (Teaching/Discharge Considerations):

- Discuss impact of specific activities on respiratory status and problem-solve solutions *to maximize weaning effort or to reduce incidence of respiratory distress or failure.*
- Monitor health of visitors and persons involved in care *to protect client from sources of infection.*
- Encourage time-out or respite for caregivers *so they may attend to personal needs, wellness, and growth.* Refer to ND risk for caregiver Role Strain.
- Provide opportunities for client/SO(s) to discuss advance directives. *Clarifies parameters for termination of therapy or other end-of-life decisions, as desired.*
- Recommend involvement in support group; introduce to other ventilator-dependent individuals who are successfully managing home ventilation, if desired, *to answer questions, provide role model, assist with problem solving, and offer encouragement and hope for the future.*

DOCUMENTATION FOCUS

Assessment/Reassessment

- Baseline findings, subsequent alterations in respiratory function.
- Results of diagnostic testing.
- Individual risk factors and concerns.

Planning

- Plan of care and who is involved in planning.
- Teaching plan.

Implementation/Evaluation

- Client's/other's responses to interventions, teaching, and actions performed.
- Skill level and assistance needs of SO(s)/family.
- Attainment or progress toward desired outcome(s).
- Modifications to plan of care.

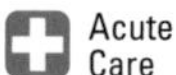

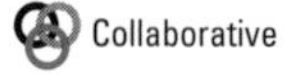

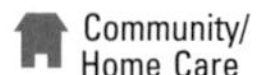

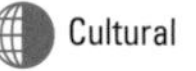

Discharge Planning
- Discharge plan, including appropriate referrals, action taken, and who is responsible for each action.
- Equipment needs and source.
- Resources for support persons or home-care providers.

References

1. Epstein, S. K. (2002). Weaning from mechanical ventilation. *Respir Care*, 47(4), 454–466.
2. MacIntyre, N. R. (2001). Evidence-based guidelines for weaning and discontinuation of ventilatory support. *Chest*, 120(6 suppl), S385–S484.
3. Tasota, F. J., Dobbin, D. (2000). Weaning your patient from mechanical ventilation. *Nursing*, 30(10), 41–46.
4. Stawicki, S. P. (2007). Mechanical ventilation: Weaning and extubation. *OPUS 12 Scientist*, 1(2), 13–16.
5. Fayyaz, J., Lessnau, K.-D. (Updated 2015). Hypoventilation syndromes. Retrieved November 2015 from http://emedicine.medscape.com/article/304381-overview.
6. D'Arcy, Y. (2007). Eye on capnography. *Men Nurs*, 2(2), 25–29.
7. Amitai, A., Sinert, D., Regan, A., et al. (Updated 2013). Ventilator management. Retrieved November 2015 from http://emedicine.medscape.com/article/810126-overview.
8. Bausewein, C., Farquhar, M., Booth, S., et al. (2007). Measurement of breathlessness in advanced disease: A systematic review. *Resp Med*, 101(3), 399–410.
9. Parker, L. C. (2012). Top 10 care essentials for ventilator patients: Evidence-based interventions and teamwork are crucial when caring for patients on mechanical ventilation. Retrieved November 2015 from http://www.medscape.com/viewarticle/761358_2.

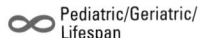

dysfunctional Ventilatory Weaning Response

Taxonomy II: Activity/Rest—Class 4 Cardiovascular/Pulmonary Responses (00034) [**Diagnostic Division:** Respiration], Submitted 1992

DEFINITION: Inability to adjust to lowered levels of mechanical ventilator support that interrupts and prolongs the weaning process.

RELATED FACTORS

Physiological
Ineffective airway clearance
Alteration in sleep pattern
Inadequate nutrition
Pain
[Muscle weakness or fatigue, inability to control respiratory muscles; immobility]
Psychological
Insufficient knowledge of the weaning process
Uncertainty about ability to wean
Decrease in motivation; low self-esteem
Anxiety; fear; insufficient trust in healthcare professionals
Hopelessness; powerlessness
[Unprepared for weaning attempt]

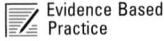

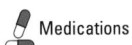

(continues on page 924)

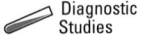

dysfunctional Ventilatory Weaning Response (continued)

Situational

Uncontrolled episodic energy demands
Inappropriate pace of weaning process
Insufficient social support
Environmental barrier (e.g., distractions, low nurse to patient ratio, unfamiliar healthcare staff)
History of ventilator dependence >4 days
History of unsuccessful weaning attempt

DEFINING CHARACTERISTICS

Mild

Subjective

Perceived need for increase in oxygen; breathing discomfort; fatigue, warmth
Fear of machine malfunction

Objective

Restlessness
Mild increase of respiratory rate from baseline
Increase in focus on breathing

Moderate

Subjective

Apprehensiveness

Objective

Increase in blood pressure (<20 mm Hg)/heart rate (<20 beats/min) from baseline
Moderate increase in respiratory rate over baseline; minimal use of respiratory accessory muscles; decrease in air entry on auscultation
Hyperfocused on activities; facial expression of fear
Impaired ability to cooperate or respond to coaching
Diaphoresis
Abnormal skin color (e.g., pale, dusky, cyanosis)

Severe

Objective

Agitation; decrease in level of consciousness
Deterioration in arterial blood gases from baseline
Increase in blood pressure (≥20 mm Hg)/heart rate (≥20 beats/min) from baseline
Significant increase in respiratory rate above baseline; use of significant respiratory accessory muscles; shallow breathing; gasping breaths; paradoxical abdominal breathing
Adventitious breath sounds
Asynchronized breathing with the ventilator
Profuse diaphoresis
Abnormal skin color (e.g., pale, dusky, cyanosis)

Sample Clinical Applications: Traumatic brain injury, stroke, substance overdose, chronic obstructive pulmonary disease (COPD), crushing chest trauma, respiratory or cardiac arrest

DESIRED OUTCOMES/EVALUATION CRITERIA

Sample NOC linkages:

Mechanical Ventilation Weaning Response: Adult: Respiratory and psychological adjustment to progressive removal of mechanical ventilation

Respiratory Status: Ventilation: Movement of air in and out of the lungs
Respiratory Status: Gas Exchange: Alveolar exchange of carbon dioxide and oxygen to maintain arterial blood gas concentrations

---

Client Will (Include Specific Time Frame)

- Actively participate in the weaning process.
- Reestablish independent respiration with arterial blood gases (ABGs) within client's normal range and be free of signs of respiratory failure.
- Demonstrate increased tolerance for activity and participate in self-care within level of ability.

ACTIONS/INTERVENTIONS

Sample NIC linkages:
Mechanical Ventilation Management: Invasive: Assisting the patient receiving artificial breathing support through a device inserted into the trachea
Mechanical Ventilatory Weaning: Assisting the patient to breathe without the aid of a mechanical ventilator
Energy Management: Regulating energy use to treat or prevent fatigue and optimize function

NURSING PRIORITY NO. 1 To identify contributing factors/degree of dysfunction:

- Determine extent and nature of underlying disorders or factors (e.g., preexisting cardiopulmonary diseases, significant trauma, neuromuscular disorders, multisystem organ failure; ventilator-associated pneumonia; complications from surgical procedures) *that contribute to client's reliance on mechanical support, thus affecting weaning efforts.*[7]
- Note length of time client has been on ventilator. Review previous episodes of extubation and reintubation. *Previous unsuccessful weaning attempts (e.g., due to inability to protect airway or clear secretions; oxygen saturation less than 50% on room air) can influence weaning interventions. Although most individuals remain on the ventilator for 7 days or less, some require support for several weeks or more. Weaning is more difficult in those clients and may require multiple attempts.*[1,8]
- Complete Burns Weaning Assessment Program (BWAP) or similar checklist (e.g., stability of vital signs, factors that increase metabolic rate [e.g., sepsis, fever]; hydration status; need for or recent use of analgesia or sedation; nutritional state, muscle strength, and activity level) *to assess systemic parameters that may affect readiness for weaning. Note: A recent study of the use of BWAP score in five adult critical care units found that a score of 50 or higher was linked to successful weaning outcomes.*[1,2,9–11,13]
- Ascertain client's awareness and understanding of weaning process, expectations, and concerns. *Client/significant other (SO) may need specific and repeated instructions during process to allay fears and enhance cooperation. Unrealistic expectations or unvoiced concerns can impair weaning process or willingness to participate.*
- Determine psychological readiness and presence/degree of anxiety. *Weaning provokes anxiety regarding ability to breathe on own and likelihood of ventilator dependence. The client must be highly motivated, be able to actively participate in the weaning process, and be physically comfortable enough to work at weaning.*[3]
- Review lab studies, such as complete blood count, *to determine number and integrity of red blood cells for oxygen transport;* electrolytes; and nutritional markers, such as serum protein and albumin, *to determine if client has sufficient nutritional stores to meet demands of spontaneous breathing and weaning.*[13,10]
- Review chest radiograph, pulse oximetry or ABGs, and/or capnometry. *Before weaning attempts, chest radiograph should show clear lungs or marked improvement in pulmonary congestion. ABGs should document satisfactory oxygenation on an FIO_2 of 40% or less. Capnometry measures end-tidal carbon dioxide values and can be used to confirm correct placement of endotracheal tube and monitor integrity of ventilation equipment.*[3,8]

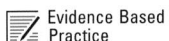

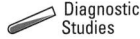

NURSING PRIORITY NO. 2 To support weaning process:

- Discuss with client/SO individual plan and expectations. *May reduce client's anxiety about process and ultimate outcome and support willingness to work at spontaneous breathing trials.*[1]
- Consult with dietitian and nutritional support team for adjustments in composition of diet prior to weaning *to support respiratory muscle strength and work of breathing and to prevent excessive production of* CO_2*, which could alter respiratory drive. Individuals on long-term ventilation may require tube feeding through enteral feedings with high intake of carbohydrates, protein, and calories to improve respiratory muscle function.*[3,8]
- Collaborate in implementing weaning protocols and mode (e.g., spontaneous breathing trials, automatic tube compensation, partial client support by means of synchronized intermittent mandatory ventilation, pressure support ventilation during client's spontaneous breathing) *to optimize the work of breathing and to provide support for spontaneous ventilation.*[4,7,10–12]
- Note response to activity or client care during weaning and limit, as indicated. Provide undisturbed rest or sleep periods. Avoid stressful procedures or situations and nonessential activities *to prevent excessive oxygen consumption or demand with increased possibility of weaning failure.*
- Discuss impact of specific activities on respiratory status, and problem solve solutions to maximize weaning effort.
- Time medications during weaning efforts *to minimize sedative effects.*
- Provide quiet room, calm approach, and undivided attention. *Enhances relaxation, thereby conserving energy.*
- Involve SO(s)/family, as appropriate (e.g., sit at bedside, provide encouragement, help monitor client status).
- Provide diversionary activity (e.g., watching TV, reading aloud) *to focus attention away from breathing when not actively working at breathing exercises.*
- Acknowledge and provide ongoing encouragement for client's efforts.
- Minimize setbacks and focus client attention on gains and progress to date *to reduce frustration that may further impair progress.*

NURSING PRIORITY NO. 3 To prepare for discharge on ventilator when indicated:

- Prepare client/SO for alternative actions when client is unable to resume spontaneous ventilation (e.g., tracheostomy with long-term ventilation support in alternate care setting or home, palliative care or end-of-life procedures). *Customized discharge planning for people new to home ventilation is essential. This must include assessment of the environment, assessment of resources, assessment of caregivers, education and training, and a plan of care.*[5,14]
- Ascertain that all needed equipment is in place, caregivers are trained, and safety concerns have been addressed (e.g., alternative power source, backup equipment, client call or alarm system, established means of client/caregiver communication) *to ease the transfer when client is going home on ventilator.*
- Evaluate caregiver capabilities and burden when client requires long-term ventilator in the home *to determine potential or presence of skill-related problems or emotional issues (e.g., caregiver overload, burnout, or depression). Note: All home caregivers (professionals, family, friends) should receive a comprehensive orientation before caring for someone using a home ventilator. This includes familiarization with the ventilator; alarms and the subsequent actions that must be taken; tracheostomy care; safe transfer of the ventilator user; suctioning techniques; and bag-valve-mask ventilation (use of an Ambu bag) in the case of an emergency, such as accidental disconnection of the ventilator circuit.*[6,14]
- Refer to ND impaired spontaneous Ventilation for additional interventions.

NURSING PRIORITY NO. 4 To promote optimal ventilation (Teaching/Discharge Considerations):

- Encourage client/SO(s) to evaluate impact of ventilatory dependence on their lifestyle and what changes they are willing or unwilling to make when client is discharged on ventilator. *Quality-of-life issues must be examined, including issues of privacy and intimacy, and resolved by the ventilator-dependent client and SO(s). All parties need to understand that ventilatory support is a 24-hr job that ultimately affects everyone.*[14] *Findings may dictate alternative placement such as foster care or extended-care facility.*

Acute Care 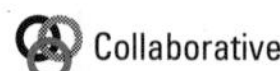 Collaborative 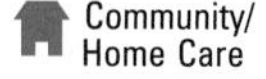 Community/ Home Care 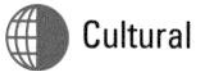 Cultural

- Discuss importance of time for self and identify appropriate sources for respite care. *Initially, caregivers have limited understanding of the magnitude of the demands on their time and energy. Knowing support is available enhances coping abilities.* Refer to ND risk for Caregiver Role Strain.
- Emphasize to client/SO(s) importance of monitoring health of visitors and persons involved in care, avoiding crowds during flu season, obtaining immunizations, etc., *to protect client from sources of infection.*
- Engage in rehabilitation program *to enhance respiratory muscle strength and general endurance or to compensate for deficits.*
- Encourage client/SO(s) to discuss advance directives and ascertain that all care providers are aware of the plan of care. *Clarifies parameters for emergency situations, termination of therapy, or other end-of-life decisions, as desired.*
- Recommend involvement in support group (may be online) and introduce to other ventilator-dependent individuals who are successfully managing home ventilation, if desired, *to answer questions, provide role models, assist with problem solving, and offer encouragement and hope for the future.*
- Identify conditions requiring immediate medical intervention *to treat developing complications and prevent respiratory failure.*

DOCUMENTATION FOCUS

Assessment/Reassessment

- Baseline findings and subsequent alterations.
- Results of diagnostic testing and procedures.
- Individual risk factors.

Planning

- Plan of care, specific interventions, and who is involved in the planning.
- Teaching plan.

Implementation/Evaluation

- Client response to interventions.
- Attainment or progress toward desired outcome(s).
- Modifications to plan of care.

Discharge Planning

- Status at discharge, long-term needs and referrals, indicating who is to be responsible for each action.
- Equipment needs and supplier.

References

1. Tasota, F. J., Dobbin, K. (2000). Weaning your patient from mechanical ventilation. *Nursing*, 30(10), 41.
2. MacIntyre, N. R., Cook, D. J., Ely, E. W., Jr., et al. (2001). Evidence-based guidelines for weaning and discontinuation of ventilatory support. *Chest*, 120(6 suppl), S375–S395.
3. Frakes, M. A. (2001). Measuring end-tidal carbon dioxide: Clinical applications and usefulness. *Crit Care Nurse*, 21(5), 23–35.
4. Henneman, E. A. (2001). Liberating patients from mechanical ventilation: A team approach. *Crit Care Nurse*, 21(3), 25–33.
5. Iregui, M., Malen, J., Tuteur, P., et al. (2002). Determinants of outcome for patients admitted to a long-term-ventilator unit. *South Med J*, 95(3), 310–317.
6. Douglas, S. L., Daly, B. J. (2003). Caregivers of long-term ventilator patients: Physical and psychological outcomes. *Chest*, 123, 1073–1081.
7. Forrette, T. L. (2006). Transitioning from mechanical ventilation. Retrieved April 2012 from http://www.medscape.org/viewarticle/528367.
8. McLean, S. E., Jensen, L. A., Schroeder, D. G., et al. (2006). Improving adherence to a mechanical ventilation weaning protocol for critically ill adults: Outcomes after an implementation program. *Am J Crit Care*, 15(3), 299–309.
9. Burns, S. M. (2005). Mechanical ventilation of clients with acute respiratory distress syndrome and patents requiring weaning: The evidence guiding practice. *Crit Care Nurse*, 25(4), 14–24.

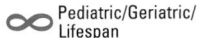

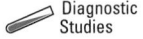

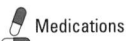

10. Epstein, C. D., Peerless, J. R. (2006). Weaning readiness and fluid balance in older critically ill surgical clients. *Am J Crit Care*, 15(1), 54–64.
11. Stawicki, S. P. (2007). Mechanical ventilation: Weaning and extubation. *OPUS 12 Scientist*, 1(2), 13–16.
12. Unoki, T., Serita, A., Grap, M. J. (2008). Automatic tube compensation during weaning from mechanical ventilation: Evidence and clinical implications. *Crit Care Nurs*, 28(4), 34–42.
13. Burns, S. M., Fisher, C., Tribble, S. S. E. (2010). Multifactor clinical score and outcome of mechanical ventilation weaning trials: Burns Wean Assessment Program. *Am J Crit Care*, 19(431), 439.
14. Stuban, S. L. (2010). Home mechanical ventilation. *Am J Nurs*, 110(5), 63–67.

risk for other-directed Violence

Taxonomy II: Safety/Protection—Class 3 Violence (00138) [**Diagnostic Division:** Safety], Submitted 1980; Revised 1996, 2013

DEFINITION: Vulnerable to behaviors in which an individual demonstrates that he or she can be physically, emotionally, or sexually harmful to others.

RISK FACTORS FOR OTHER-DIRECTED VIOLENCE

Negative body language (e.g., rigid posture, clenching of fists/jaw, hyperactivity, pacing, threatening stances)
Alteration in cognitive functioning
Cruelty to animals; fire-setting
Motor vehicle offense (e.g., traffic violations, use of a motor vehicle to release anger)
Neurological impairment (e.g., positive EEG, head trauma, seizure disorders)
Prenatal or perinatal complications
Pathological intoxication; [toxic reaction to pharmaceutical agent]
Psychotic disorder; [panic states; rage reactions; manic excitement]
Suicidal behavior; impulsiveness; access to weapon
History of childhood abuse (e.g., physical, psychological, sexual), witnessing family violence
Pattern of indirect violence (e.g., tearing objects off walls, urinating/defecating on floor, stamping feet, temper tantrum, throwing objects, breaking a window, slamming doors, sexual advances)
Pattern of other-directed violence (e.g., hitting/kicking/spitting/scratching others, throwing objects/biting someone; attempted rape, rape, sexual molestation; urinating/defecating on a person)
History of substance abuse
Pattern of threatening violence (e.g., verbal threats against property/people, social threats, cursing, threatening notes/letters, threatening gestures, sexual threats)
Pattern of violent antisocial behavior (e.g., stealing, insistent borrowing, insistent demands for privileges, insistent interrupting, refusal to eat/take medication, ignoring instructions)
Sample Clinical Applications: Psychotic conditions (e.g., schizophrenia, paranoia), antisocial personality disorder, dementia, substance abuse (e.g., phencyclidine [PCP], delirium tremens), postpartum psychosis, premenstrual syndrome [PMS], brain injured
[Note: NANDA has separated the diagnosis of Violence with its two elements—other-directed and self-directed. However, the interventions in general address both situations and have been left in one block following the Desired Outcomes section of risk for self-directed Violence.]

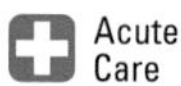

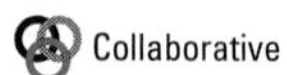

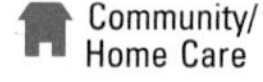

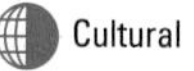

risk for self-directed Violence

Taxonomy II: Safety/Protection—Class 3 Violence (00140) [**Diagnostic Division:** Safety], Submitted 1994; Revised 2013

DEFINITION: Vulnerable to behaviors in which an individual demonstrates that he or she can be physically, emotionally, or sexually harmful to self.

RISK FACTORS FOR SELF-DIRECTED VIOLENCE

Age 15 to 19, ≥45
Marital status (e.g., single, widowed, divorced)
Employment concern (e.g., unemployed, recent job loss/failure); occupation (e.g., executive, administrator/owner of business, professional, semiskilled worker)
Conflict in interpersonal relationship(s)
Pattern of difficulties in family background (e.g., chaotic or conflictual, history of suicide)
Conflict about sexual orientation ; engagement in autoerotic sexual acts
Physical health issue
Mental health issue (e.g., depression, psychosis, severe personality disorder, substance abuse); psychological disorder
History of multiple suicide attempts; suicidal ideation; suicidal plan
Insufficient personal resources (e.g., achievement, insight, affect unavailable and poorly controlled); social isolation
Verbal clues (e.g., talking about death, "better off without me," asking about lethal dosages of medication)
Behavioral clues (e.g., writing forlorn love notes, directing angry messages at a significant other who has rejected the person, giving away personal items, taking out a large life insurance policy)
Note: A risk diagnosis is not evidenced by signs and symptoms, as the problem has not occurred; rather, nursing interventions are directed at prevention.
Sample Clinical Applications: Major depression, postpartum depression/psychosis, Munchausen syndrome, psychosis, substance abuse (e.g., phencyclidine [PCP]), abuse or neglect

DESIRED OUTCOMES/EVALUATION CRITERIA (FOR OTHER-/SELF-DIRECTED VIOLENCE)

Sample NOC linkages:
Aggression Self-Control: Self-restraint of assaultive, combative, or destructive behaviors toward others
Abusive Behavior Self-Restraint: Self-restraint of abusive and neglectful behaviors toward others
Impulse Self-Control: Self-restraint of compulsive or impulsive behaviors
Depression Self-Control: Personal actions to minimize melancholy and maintain interest in life events

Client Will (Include Specific Time Frame)

- Acknowledge realities of the situation.
- Verbalize understanding of why behavior occurs.
- Identify precipitating factors in individual situation.
- Express realistic self-evaluation and increased sense of self-esteem.
- Participate in care and meet own needs in an assertive manner.
- Demonstrate self-control as evidenced by relaxed posture, nonviolent behavior or verbalizations.
- Use resources and support systems in an effective manner.

(continues on page 930)

risk for self-directed Violence (continued)
ACTIONS/INTERVENTIONS (ADDRESSES BOTH OTHER- AND SELF-DIRECTED)

Sample NIC linkages:
Anger Control Assistance: Facilitation of the expression of anger in an adaptive, nonviolent manner
Environmental Management: Violence Prevention: Monitoring and manipulation of the physical environment to decrease the potential for violent behavior directed toward self, others, or environment
Behavior Management: Self-Harm: Assisting the patient to decrease or eliminate self-mutilating or self-abusive behavior

NURSING PRIORITY NO. 1 To assess causative/contributing factors:

- Determine underlying dynamics as listed in Risk Factors.
- Identify conditions, such as acute or chronic brain syndrome, panic state, hormonal imbalance, premenstrual syndrome, postpartum psychosis, drug-induced psychotic states, and postanesthesia or postseizure confusion, *that may interfere with ability to control own behavior and lead to violent episodes.*[1,12]
- Review lab findings (e.g., blood alcohol, drug/tox screen, blood glucose, arterial blood gases, electrolytes, renal function tests). *Provides information about possible treatable sources of behavior.*[2,6]
- Ascertain client's perception of self and situation. Note use of defense mechanisms. *Individuals who are prone to violent behavior may see themselves as victims (denial), may blame others (projection), may not follow social norms, and may be impulsive.*[1]
- Observe and listen for early cues of distress or increasing anxiety. *Behaviors, such as irritability, lack of cooperation, and demanding behavior, and body posture or expression may signal escalating potential for violent behavior and need for immediate intervention.*[1,6]
- Observe for signs of suicidal or homicidal intent. *Perceived morbid or anxious feelings while with the client; warning from the client, "It doesn't matter," "I'd/They'd be better off dead"; mood swings; "accident-prone" or self-destructive behavior; and possession of alcohol or other drug(s) by known substance abuser needs to be noted, taken seriously, and treated appropriately.*[1,6] Refer to ND risk for Suicide.
- Note family history of suicidal or homicidal behavior. *Dynamics in family of origin and current family and parental deprivation or abuse in the early years of an individual's life may contribute to violent behavior in current situation as individual uses violence as a means of solving problems.*[1,10]
- Ask directly if the person is thinking of acting on thoughts or feelings. *Can determine reality and urgency of violent intent and importance of immediate intervention.*[6]
- Determine availability of suicidal or homicidal means. *Identifies urgency of situation and need to intervene by removing lethal means, possibly hospitalizing client, or instituting other measures to ensure safety of client and others.*[1,6,8]
- Assess client coping behaviors. *Client believes there are no alternatives other than violence and has been dealing with frustration and anger in unacceptable ways (yelling, hitting, other violent behaviors) and needs to learn alternative coping skills.*[1,9]
- Identify risk factors and assess for indicators of child abuse or neglect (e.g., unexplained or frequent injuries, failure to thrive). *Visible evidence of physical abuse or neglect makes it more easily recognized; however, behaviors of withdrawal and acting out may also signal the presence of abuse.*[6,9,12]
- Determine presence, extent, and acceptance of violence in the client's culture. *Youth violence has become a national concern with widely publicized school shootings and an increase in arrests of both boys and girls for violent crimes and weapons violations. Young people who are at risk for violence need to be identified, and positive programs aimed at promoting emotional wellness need to be instituted in schools, parent education meetings, churches, and community centers.*[3,7,11]

Acute Care 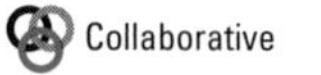 Collaborative 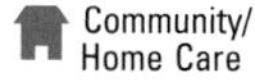 Community/Home Care 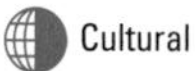 Cultural

NURSING PRIORITY NO. 2 To assist client to accept responsibility for impulsive behavior and potential for violence:

- Develop therapeutic nurse-client relationship. Provide consistent caregiver when possible. *Promotes sense of trust, allowing client to discuss feelings openly and to begin to identify sources of anger and more acceptable ways of dealing with it.*[1,6]
- Maintain straightforward communication. *Avoids reinforcing manipulative behavior. Manipulation is used for management of powerlessness because of distrust of others, fear of loss of power or control, fear of intimacy, and search for approval.*[4,6]
- Discuss motivation for change (e.g., failing relationships, job loss, involvement with judicial system). *Crisis situation can provide impetus for change but requires timely therapeutic intervention to sustain efforts.*[7,8]
- Make time to listen to expressions of feelings. Acknowledge reality of client's feelings and that feelings are okay. (Refer to ND Self-Esteem, specify.) *Promotes understanding of how feelings lead to actions and that individual is responsible for controlling behavior in acceptable ways.*[6]
- Help client recognize that own actions may be in response to own fear (may be afraid of own behavior, loss of control), dependency, and feeling of powerlessness. *Promotes understanding of self and ability to deal with feelings in acceptable ways.*[6,13]
- Confront client's tendency to minimize situation or behavior. *Individuals often want to say that things "are not as bad" as portrayed or "It was just a small argument" and "I didn't think I hit her (or him) that hard." By confronting this minimalization, the reality of the situation can be brought out and discussed, leading to better understanding of the situation and changes in behavior.*[1,6]
- Identify feelings or events (e.g., individual's view of self, hallucinations, individual/family or peer conflict, aggressive behavior) involved in precipitating violent behavior. *By identifying the factors involved in current situation, an appropriate plan can be made to change actions to prevent future violent behavior.*[1,7]
- Discuss impact of behavior on others and consequences of actions. *Discussing these issues openly can help client to develop empathy and understand other person's reactions and begin to change behaviors that can lead to violence.*[5,8]
- Acknowledge reality of suicide or homicide as an option. Discuss consequences of actions if they were to follow through on intent. Ask how it will help client to resolve problems. *Acknowledging the reality of individual's thoughts provides opportunity to look at how actions would affect others, ability to control own behavior, and make choices to live and make a better life for self.*[6,11]
- Accept client's anger without reacting on emotional basis. Give permission to express angry feelings in acceptable ways and let client know that staff will be available to assist in maintaining control. *Promotes acceptance and sense of safety. Client's anger is usually directed at the situation and not at the caregiver, and by remaining separate, the therapist can be more helpful for resolution of the anger.*[6,9]
- Help client identify more appropriate solutions/behaviors. *Motor activities or exercise can lessen sense of anxiety and associated physical manifestations, thus diminishing feelings of anger.*[8]
- Provide directions for actions client can take, avoiding negatives, such as "do nots." *Discussing positive ideas to help client begin to look toward a better future can provide hope that violent behaviors can be changed, promoting feelings of self-worth and belief in control of own self.*[5,13]

NURSING PRIORITY NO. 3 To assist client in controlling behavior:

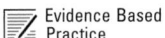

- Contract with client regarding safety of self/others. *Making a contract in which the individual agrees to refrain from any violent behavior for a specified period of time, from Day 1 through the entire course of treatment, and that is written and signed by each party may help the client to follow through with therapy to find more effective ways of resolving conflict. Although there is little research on the effectiveness of these contracts, they are frequently used.*[6,7]
- Give client as much control as possible within constraints of individual situation. *Because control issues are a factor in violent behavior, giving client control in appropriate ways can enhance self-esteem and promote confidence in ability to change behavior.*[7]

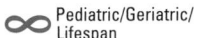

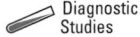

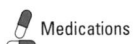

- Be truthful when giving information and dealing with individual. *Builds trust, enhancing therapeutic relationship, and prevents manipulative behavior.*[5]
- Identify current and past successes and strengths. Discuss effectiveness of coping techniques used and possible changes. Refer to ND ineffective Coping. *Client is often not aware of positive aspects of life, and once recognized, they can be used as a basis for change.*[8]
- Give positive reinforcement for client's efforts. *Encourages continuation of desired behaviors.*[1]
- Assist client to distinguish between reality and hallucinations or delusions. *Violent behavior in clients with major mental disorders (schizophrenia, mania) may be in response to command hallucinations and may require more aggressive treatment or hospitalization until behavior is under control.*[1,6]
- Approach in positive manner, acting as if the client has control and is responsible for own behavior. Be aware, though, that the client may not have control, especially if under the influence of drugs (including alcohol). *Individuals will often respond to a positive expectation, reducing threatening actions. Staff needs to be trained in management of this behavior and be prepared to take control of the situation if client is out of control.*[1,6]
- Maintain distance and do not touch client when situation indicates client does not tolerate such closeness. *Individuals who have experienced traumatic events, such as rape, or suffer from posttrauma response may fear close contact even with trusted persons.*[1,6]
- Remain calm and state limits on inappropriate behavior (including consequences) in a firm manner. *Calm manner enables client to de-escalate anger, and knowing what the consequences will be gives an opportunity to choose to change behavior and deal appropriately with situation. Consequences need to be decided beforehand and agreed to by client or they may sound like punishment and be counterproductive.*[1,6,12]
- Direct client to stay in view of staff. *Intervention may be needed to maintain safety of client and others.*[1,6] Refer to ND risk for Suicide.
- Administer prescribed medications (e.g., anti-anxiety or antipsychotic), taking care not to oversedate client. *May be least restrictive way to help client control violent behaviors while learning new coping skills to handle anger and impulsive behavior. The chemistry of the brain is changed by early violence and has been shown to respond to serotonin as well as related neurotransmitter systems, which play a role in restraining aggressive impulses.*[1,6,9]
- Monitor for possible drug interactions and cumulative effects of drug regimen (e.g., anticonvulsants, antidepressants). *May be contributing factor in violent behavior.*[1,6]

NURSING PRIORITY NO. 4 To assist client/SO(s) to correct/deal with existing situation:

- Gear interventions to individual(s) involved based on age, relationship, etc. *Conflict-resolution skills can be learned by all age groups when age-appropriate materials are used.*[5,8]
- Maintain calm, matter-of-fact, nonjudgmental attitude. *Decreases defensive response, allowing individual to think about own responsibility in the conflict and choose positive behaviors instead of usual angry reaction.*[4,5,8]
- Notify potential victims in the presence of serious homicidal threat in accordance with legal and ethical guidelines. *Various Tarasoff statutes exist in many states requiring therapists/healthcare providers to report specific threats to both the individual named and law enforcement when client expresses homicidal intent overtly or covertly in addition to helping the client realize that the proposed action is not wise or in his or her own best interest.*[1]
- Discuss situation with abused or battered person, providing accurate information about choices and effective actions that can be taken. *Promotes understanding of options, giving hope and support for planning for a violence-free future.*[2]
- Assist individual to understand that angry, vengeful feelings are appropriate in the situation and need to be expressed but not acted on. (Refer to ND Post-Trauma Syndrome, as psychological responses may be very similar.) *Helps client accept feelings as natural and begin to learn effective coping skills and promotes sense of control over situation.*[2]
- Identify resources available for assistance (e.g., battered women's shelter, social services, financial). *Helps client to manage immediate needs such as food, shelter, and safety with a long-range goal of attaining or maintaining independence and violence-free life.*[2]

NURSING PRIORITY NO. 5 To promote safety in event of violent behavior:

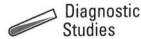

- Provide a safe, quiet environment and remove items from the client's environment that could be used to inflict harm to self/others. *Reducing stimuli can help client to calm down, and removing articles provides for safety of client and staff.*[1,6]
- Maintain distance from client who is striking out or hitting and take evasive or controlling actions, as indicated. *Staff safety is of prime importance, and avoiding physical confrontation until client regains control or take-down team is assembled can prevent injury.*[6]
- Call for additional staff/security personnel. *Having sufficient people available to handle the situation may defuse client's anger, allowing situation to calm down without further action. All personnel need to be trained in take-down techniques.*[6]
- Approach aggressive or attacking client from the front, just out of reach, in a commanding posture with palms down. *Safety is a prime concern, and these actions may defuse the situation.*[6]
- Tell client *"Stop"* in a firm voice. *This may be sufficient to help client control own actions.*[6]
- Maintain direct and constant eye contact when appropriate. *Assists in identifying client's intentions and conveys sense of caring. Eye contact may be perceived as threatening, so it needs to be used cautiously.*[2,6]
- Speak in a low, commanding voice. *Tone of voice conveys message of control and concern and can help to calm the client's anger.*[6]
- Provide client with a sense that caregiver is in control of the situation. *Client is feeling out of control, and seeing that staff are in control provides a feeling of safety.*[6]
- Maintain clear route for staff and client and be prepared to move quickly. *Safety for all is of prime importance, and staff may need to leave the room to regroup while continuing to protect the client. Take-down needs to be done quickly to gain control of the individual.*[6]
- Hold client, using restraints or seclusion when necessary until client regains self-control. *Brief period of physical restraint may be required until client regains control or other therapeutic interventions take effect.*[6]
- Administer medication, as indicated. *Client may require chemical restraint until control is regained.*[1,6]
- Discuss event with client after situation is calmed down and control is regained. *Helping client to understand how feelings of anger had gotten out of control and what can be done to prevent a recurrence can provide a learning opportunity for the individual.*[2,6]

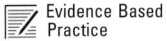

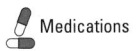

NURSING PRIORITY NO. 6 To promote wellness (Teaching/Discharge Considerations):

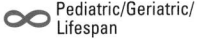

- Promote client involvement in planning care within limits of situation, allowing for meeting own needs for enjoyment. *Individuals often believe they are not entitled to pleasure and good things in their lives and need to learn how to meet these needs in acceptable ways.*[6,13]
- Assist client to learn assertive behaviors. *Manipulative, nonassertive, or aggressive behaviors lead to anger, which can result in violence. Learning assertiveness skills can facilitate change, increase self-esteem, and promote interpersonal relationships.*[1,13]
- Provide information about conflict-resolution skills and help client learn how to use them effectively. *Conflict is always present in human relationships, and learning how to manage conflict is one of the most important tools we can use to solve disagreements and improve relationships.*[4,5,8]
- Discuss reasons for client's behavior with SO(s). Determine desire and commitment of involved parties to sustain current relationships. *Family members may believe individual is purposefully behaving in angry ways, and understanding underlying reasons for behavior can defuse feelings of anger on their part, leading to willingness to resolve problems.*[1,4]
- Develop strategies to help parents learn more effective parenting skills. *Participating in parenting classes and learning appropriate ways of dealing with frustrations can improve family relationships and prevent angry interactions and the possibility of violent behavior.*[4,5]
- Identify support systems. *Presence of family/friends and clergy who can serve as mentors and listen to individual nonjudgmentally can help client defuse angry feelings and learn appropriate ways of dealing with*

them.[1] *Note: Not just the client needs help; those around them also need to learn how to provide positive role models and display a broader array of skills for resolving problems.*

- Refer to formal resources, as indicated. *May need individual or group psychotherapy, substance-abuse treatment program, anger-management class, social services, and/or safe house to facilitate change.*[1]
- Promote violence prevention and emotional literacy programs in the schools and community. *These programs are based on the premise that intelligent management of emotions is critical to successful living. Aggressive youth lack skills in arousal management and nonviolent problem solving, which can be learned in programs and reinforced by the adults in their lives.*[7,11,13]
- Refer to NDs impaired Parenting, family Coping [specify], and Post-Trauma Syndrome.

DOCUMENTATION FOCUS

Assessment/Reassessment

- Individual findings, including nature of concern (e.g., suicidal, homicidal), behavioral risk factors, and level of impulse control, plan of action, and means to carry out plan.
- Client's perception of situation, motivation for change.
- Family history of violence.
- Availability and use of resources.

Planning

- Plan of care and who is involved in the planning.
- Details of contract regarding violence to self/others.
- Teaching plan.

Implementation/Evaluation

- Actions taken to promote safety, including notification of parties at risk.
- Response to interventions, teaching, and actions performed.
- Attainment or progress toward desired outcome(s).
- Modifications to plan of care.

Discharge Planning

- Long-term needs and who is responsible for actions to be taken.
- Available resources, specific referrals made.

References

1. Townsend, M. C. (2003). *Psychiatric Mental Health Nursing Concepts of Care*. 4th ed. Philadelphia, PA: F. A. Davis.
2. Newfield, S. A., Hinz, M. D., Scott-Tilley, D., et al. (2007). *Cox's Clinical Applications of Nursing Diagnosis: Adult, Child, Women's, Psychiatric, Gerontic, and Home Health Considerations*. 5th ed. Philadelphia: F. A. Davis.
3. Zoucha, R. (2006). Considering culture in understanding personal violence. *J Forensic Nurs*, 4(2), 195–196.
4. Doll, L. S., Bonzo, S. E., Mercy, J. A., et al. (eds). (2007). *Handbook of Injury and Violence Prevention*. New York: Springer.
5. Stinnet, W. D. (2011). Turning conflict into cooperation. *Gordon Training Books: Leadership Effectiveness Training*. Solano Beach, CA: Gordon Training International.
6. Doenges, M. E., Townsend, M. C., Moorhouse, M. F. (1998). *Psychiatric Care Plans: Guidelines for Individualizing Care*. 3rd ed. Philadelphia: F. A. Davis.
7. Thomas, S. P. (2003). Identifying and intervening with girls at risk for violence. *J School Nurs*, 19(3), 130–139.
8. Heathfield, S. (2011). Steps in workplace conflict resolution. Avoid these actions in effective conflict resolution. Retrieved April 2015 from http://humanresources.about.com/od/managementtips/a/conflict_solue.htm.
9. Goleman, D. (1995). Early violence leaves its mark on the brain. *New York Times*. Retrieved April 2015 from http://www.nytimes.com/1995/10/03/science/early-violence-leaves-its-mark-on-the-brain.html?pagewanted=1.

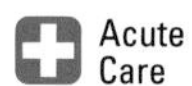
Acute Care
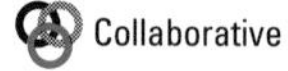
Collaborative
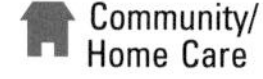
Community/ Home Care
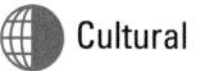
Cultural

10. No author listed. (2013). What is neuroscience? Society for Neuroscience. Retrieved April 2015 from http://www.sfn.org/index.aspx?pagename=whatisneuroscience.
11. Hyman, S. E. (Updated 1999). Thinking about violence in our schools, discussion at the White House. National Institute of Mental Health. Retrieved April 2015 from http://www.namichicago.org/documents/violenceinschools.pdf.
12. Roberts, A. R., Kim, J. H. (2006). Exploring the effects of head injuries among battered women. *J Soc Serv Res*, 32(1), 33–47.
13. Goleman, D. (2006). *Emotional Intelligence: Why It Matters More Than IQ*. 10th Anniversary ed. New York: Bantam.

impaired Walking

Taxonomy II: Activity/Rest—Class 2 Activity/Exercise (00088) [**Diagnostic Division:** Activity/Rest], Submitted 1998; Revised 2006

DEFINITION: Limitation of independent movement within the environment on foot.
[Note: Specify level of independence using a standardized functional scale.]

RELATED FACTORS

Insufficient muscle strength; neuromuscular impairment; musculoskeletal impairment
Decrease in endurance; physical deconditioning
Fear of falling; impaired balance, vision
Pain
Obesity
Alteration in mood; alteration in cognitive functioning
Insufficient knowledge of mobility strategies
Environmental barrier (e.g., stairs, inclines, uneven surfaces, obstacles, distances, lack of assistive device)

DEFINING CHARACTERISTICS

Subjective or Objective

Impaired ability to walk required distance, walk on incline or decline, walk on uneven surface, navigate curbs, climb stairs

Sample Clinical Applications: Arthritis, obesity, amputation, brain injury, stroke, traumatic injury, fractures, chronic pain, peripheral vascular disease (PVD), spinal nerve compression, multiple sclerosis (MS), cerebral palsy, Parkinson's disease, macular degeneration, dementia

DESIRED OUTCOMES/EVALUATION CRITERIA

Sample NOC linkages:

Ambulation: Ability to walk from place to place independently with or without assistive device
Mobility: Ability to move purposefully in own environment independently with or without assistive device
Balance: Ability to maintain body equilibrium

Client Will (Include Specific Time Frame)

- Be able to move about within environment as needed or desired within limits of ability or with appropriate adjuncts.
- Verbalize understanding of situation, risk factors, and safety measures.

(continues on page 936)

impaired Walking (continued)
ACTIONS/INTERVENTIONS

Sample NIC linkages:
Exercise Therapy: Ambulation: Promotion and assistance with walking to maintain or restore autonomic and voluntary body functions during treatment and recovery from illness or injury
Body Mechanics Promotion: Facilitating the use of posture and movement in daily activities to prevent fatigue and musculoskeletal strain or injury
Exercise Therapy: Balance: Use of specific activities, postures, and movements to maintain, enhance, or restore balance

NURSING PRIORITY NO. 1 To assess causative/contributing factors:

- Identify conditions or diagnoses (e.g., advanced age, sensory impairments, pain, obesity, chronic fatigue, cognitive dysfunction, acute illness with weakness, chronic illness [e.g., cardiopulmonary disorders, cancer], musculoskeletal injuries or surgery [e.g., sprains, fractures, tendon or ligament injury; total joint replacement, surgical repair of fractured bone; amputation], balance problems [e.g., inner ear infection, brain injury, stroke], nerve disorders [e.g., MS, Parkinson's disease, cerebral palsy], spinal abnormalities [disease, trauma, degeneration], impaired circulation or neuropathies [e.g., peripheral, diabetic, alcoholic], degenerative bone or muscle disorders [e.g., osteoporosis, muscular dystrophy, myositis], foot conditions [e.g., plantar warts, bunions, ingrown toenails, pressure ulcers]) *that contribute to walking impairment and identify specific needs and appropriate interventions.*[1–6]
- Determine ability to follow directions and presence of emotional or behavioral responses *that may be affecting client's ability or desire to engage in activity.*
- Note client's particular symptoms (e.g., unable to bear weight, can't walk usual distance, limping, staggering, stiff leg, leg pain, shuffling, asymmetric or unsteady gait; can walk on certain surfaces, but not on others). *Influences choice of interventions.*[4–6,8]

NURSING PRIORITY NO. 2 To assess functional ability:

- Perform "Timed Up and Go" (TUG) test, as indicated, to assess client's basic ability to ambulate safely. *Factors assessed include sitting balance, ability to transfer from sitting to standing and back to sitting, the pace and stability of ambulation, and the ability to turn without staggering. Additional testing is indicated for individuals requiring more than 20 sec to complete the test.*[7]
- Evaluate components of walking (e.g., gait, distance covered over time). Determine muscle strength and tone, joint mobility, cardiovascular status, balance, endurance, and use of assistive device. *Identifies strengths and deficits (e.g., ability to ambulate with/without assistive devices) and may provide information regarding potential for recovery (e.g., client with severe brain injury may have permanent limitations because of impaired cognition affecting memory, judgment, problem solving, and motor planning, requiring more intensive inpatient and long-term care).*[6]
- Note whether impairment is temporary or permanent. *Condition may be caused by reversible condition (e.g., weakness associated with acute illness or fractures/surgery with weight-bearing restrictions), or walking impairment can be permanent (e.g., congenital anomalies, amputation, severe rheumatoid arthritis).*[6]
- Assist with or review results of mobility testing (e.g., timing of walking over fixed distance, distance walked over set period of time [endurance], limb movement analysis, leg strength and speed of walking, ambulatory activity monitoring with pedometer) *for differential diagnosis and to guide treatment interventions.*[6,7]
- Note emotional or behavioral responses of client/significant other (SO) to problems of mobility. *Walking impairments can negatively affect self-concept and self-esteem, autonomy, and independence. Social, occupational, and relationship roles can change, leading to isolation, depression, and economic consequences.*

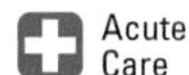

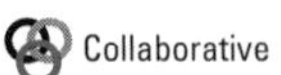

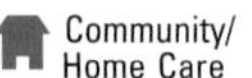

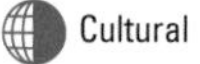

NURSING PRIORITY NO. 3 To promote safe, optimal level of independence in walking:

- Assist with treatment of underlying condition as needed or indicated by individual situation. *Treatment can often reverse or limit dysfunction.*
- Consult with physical therapist, occupational therapist, or rehabilitation team *to develop individual program (e.g., to improve general conditioning, coordination and balance, range-of-motion exercises, specific muscle strengthening), to instruct in specific tasks (e.g., stair climbing or gait training), and to identify and develop appropriate adjunctive devices (e.g., shoe insert, leg brace for proper foot alignment; customized cane, crutches, or walker).*[1]
- Monitor client's cardiopulmonary tolerance for walking. *Increased pulse rate, chest pain, breathlessness, and irregular heartbeat is indicative of need to reduce level of activity.* Refer to ND Activity Intolerance and decreased Cardiac Output for related interventions.
- Encourage adequate rest and gradual increase in walking distance *to reduce fatigue or leg pain associated with walking, and to improve stamina.*[3,4] Refer to NDs Fatigue and risk for peripheral neurovascular Dysfunction.
- Administer medication, as indicated, *to manage pain and maximize level of functioning.* Refer to NDs acute/chronic Pain; chronic Pain Syndrome.
- Implement fall precautions for high-risk clients (e.g., frail or ill elderly, visually or cognitively impaired, person on multiple medications, presence of balance disorders) *to reduce risk of accidental injury.*[3] Refer to NDs risk for Falls and risk for Disuse Syndrome for related interventions.
- Instruct in proper application of prostheses, immobilizers (e.g., walking cast or boot), and braces before walking *to maintain joint stability or immobilization or to maintain alignment during movement.*[2]
- Demonstrate and remind client to properly use assistive devices (e.g., cane, crutches, walker) *individually prescribed and fitted to improve balance, reduce limb pain and dysfunction, and provide support during ambulation.*[1]
- Use adequate personnel and safety devices (e.g., gait belt, properly fitted nonslip shoes, handrail) when ambulating *to prevent injury to client or caregivers.*[1,3,8]
- Limit distractions and provide safe environment. *Allows client to concentrate on walking activities or learning use of assistive devices.*[1]
- Provide cueing as indicated. *Client may need reminders (e.g., lift foot higher, look where going, walk tall) to concentrate on/perform tasks of walking, especially when balance or cognition is impaired.*
- Provide ample time to perform mobility-related tasks *to reduce risk of falling and manage fatigue or pain.*
- Provide positive, constructive feedback *to encourage continuation of efforts and enhance client's self-sufficiency.*[3]
- Assist client to obtain needed information, such as handicapped sticker for close-in parking, sources for mobility scooter, or special public transportation options, when indicated, *to deal with temporary or permanent disability access.*

NURSING PRIORITY NO. 4 To promote wellness (Teaching/Discharge Considerations):

- Evaluate client's home (or work) environment for barriers to walking (e.g., uneven surfaces, many steps, no ramps, long distances between places client needs to walk) *to determine needed changes and make recommendations for client safety.*
- Involve client/SO in problem solving, assisting them to learn ways of managing deficits, *to enhance safety for client with long-term or permanent impairments.*
- Encourage participation in regular active and passive exercise program. Advance levels of exercise, as able, *to improve muscle tone and strength and increase stamina and endurance.*
- Discuss appropriate use of electric scooter, if indicated. *Enhances mobility, especially over distances, to maintain independence and socialization.*
- Identify appropriate resources for obtaining and maintaining appliances, equipment, and environmental modifications *to promote safe mobility.*

- Instruct client/SO in safety measures in home, as individually indicated (e.g., maintaining safe travel pathway, proper lighting, wearing glasses, handrails on stairs, grab bars in bathroom, using walker instead of cane when tired or walking on uneven surface) *to reduce risk of falls.*
- Discuss need for emergency call/support system (e.g., Lifeline, HealthWatch) *to provide immediate assistance for falls and other home emergencies when client lives alone.*

DOCUMENTATION FOCUS

Assessment/Reassessment

- Individual findings, including level of function and ability to participate in specific or desired activities.
- Equipment and assistive device needs.

Planning

- Plan of care and who is involved in the planning.
- Teaching plan.

Implementation/Evaluation

- Responses to interventions, teaching, and actions performed.
- Attainment or progress toward desired outcome(s).
- Modifications to plan of care.

Discharge Planning

- Discharge and long-term needs, noting who is responsible for each action to be taken.
- Specific referrals made.
- Sources of and maintenance for assistive devices.

References

1. Bradley, S. M., Hernandez, C. R. (2011). Geriatric assistive devices. *Am Fam Physician*, 84(4), 405–411.
2. Teplicky, R., Law, M., Russell, D. (2002). The effectiveness of casts, orthotics, and splints for children with neurological disorders. *Infants Young Child*, 15(1), 42–50.
3. Jitramontree, N. (2001). *Evidence-Based Protocol. Exercise Promotion: Walking in Elders [Research Dissemination Core, 53]*. Iowa City, IA: University of Iowa Gerontological Nursing Interventions Research Center.
4. Eberhardt, R. T. (2002). Exercise for intermittent claudication: Walking for life? [Editorial]. *J Cardiopulm Rehabil*, 22(3), 199–200.
5. Walking disorders (various pages). Retrieved November 2015 from http://www.rightdiagnosis.com/sym/walking_disorders.htm.
6. Pearsen, O. R., Busse, M. E., van Deuresn, R. W. M. (2004). Quantification of walking mobility in neurological disorders. *Q J Med*, 97, 463–475.
7. Baer, H. R., Wolf, S. L. (2001). Modified Emory Functional Ambulation Profile: An outcome measure for the rehabilitation of poststroke gait dysfunction. *Stroke*, 32, 973–979.
8. McGuire, J. (2010). Transitional off-loading: An evidence-based approach to pressure redistribution in the diabetic foot. *Adv Skin Wound Care*, 23(4), 175–188.

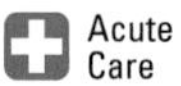

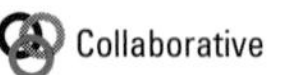

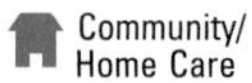

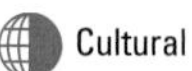

Wandering [specify: sporadic or continual]

Taxonomy II: Activity/Rest—Class 3 Energy Balance (00154) [**Diagnostic Division:** Safety], [Submitted 2000]

DEFINITION: Meandering, aimless, or repetitive locomotion that exposes the individual to harm; frequently incongruent with boundaries, limits, or obstacles.

RELATED FACTORS

Alteration in cognitive functioning; sedation
Cortical atrophy; psychological disorder
Premorbid behavior (e.g., outgoing, sociable personality)
Separation from familiar environment; overstimulating environment
Physiological state (e.g., hunger, thirst, pain, need to urinate)
Time of day

DEFINING CHARACTERISTICS

Objective

Frequent or continuous movement from place to place; pacing
Persistent locomotion in search of something; scanning or searching behavior
Haphazard or fretful locomotion; long periods of locomotion without an apparent destination
Locomotion into unauthorized spaces; trespassing
Locomotion resulting in getting lost; eloping behavior
Impaired ability to locate landmarks in a familiar setting
Locomotion that cannot be easily dissuaded; shadowing a caregiver's locomotion
Hyperactivity
Periods of locomotion interspersed with periods of nonlocomotion (e.g., sitting, standing, sleeping)

Sample Clinical Applications: Brain injury, dementias, developmental delays, major depression, substance abuse, amnesia, fugue

DESIRED OUTCOMES/EVALUATION CRITERIA

Sample NOC linkage:
Physical Injury Severity: Severity of injuries from accidents and trauma

Client Will (Include Specific Time Frame)

- Be free of injury, or unplanned exits.

Sample NOC linkages:
Safe Home Environment: Physical arrangements to minimize environmental factors that might cause physical harm or injury in the home
Safe Wandering: Safe, socially acceptable moving about without apparent purpose in an individual with cognitive impairment

Caregiver(s) Will (Include Specific Time Frame)

- Modify environment, as indicated, to enhance safety.
- Provide for maximal independence of client.

ACTIONS/INTERVENTIONS

Sample NIC linkages:
Elopement Precautions: Minimizing the risk of a patient leaving a treatment setting without authorization when departure presents a threat to the safety of patient or others

(continues on page 940)

Wandering (continued)
Area Restriction: Use of least restrictive limitation of patient mobility to a specified area for purposes of safety or behavior management
Environmental Management: Safety: Monitoring and manipulation of the physical environment to promote safety

NURSING PRIORITY NO. 1 To assess degree of impairment/stage of disease process:

- Ascertain history of client's memory loss and cognitive changes.
- Review responses of collaborative diagnostic examinations (e.g., cognition, functional capacity, behavior, memory impairments, reality orientation, general physical health, and quality of life). *A combination of tests is often needed to complete an evaluation of client's overall condition relating to chronic or irreversible condition. These tests include (but are not limited to) Mini-Mental State Examination, Alzheimer's Disease Assessment Scale cognitive subsection, Functional Assessment Questionnaire, Clinical Global Impression of Change, and Neuropsychiatric Inventory.*[1,2]
- Evaluate client's past history (e.g., individual was very active physically and socially or reacted to stress with physical activity rather than emotional reactions) *to help identify likelihood of wandering. Note: One study showed that a history of prior wandering incidents is a high predictor (72%) for further wandering incidents.*[2,5]
- Note client's age. *Results of a study in selected nursing homes revealed that subjects' age was found to have significant negative correlations with the Revised Algase Wandering Scale—Nursing Home Version overall, suggesting that younger persons with dementia were likely to show more wandering behavior than older ones.*[2,6,7]
- Determine presence of depression. *Research supports the idea that wandering develops more often in depressed client with Alzheimer's disease.*[2]
- Evaluate client's mental status during both daytime and nighttime, noting when client's confusion is most pronounced and when and how long client sleeps. *Information about cognition and behavioral habits can reveal circumstances under which client is likely to wander.*[7]
- Identify client's reason for wandering, if possible. *Client may demonstrate searching behavior (e.g., looking for lost item, pursuing certain unattainable activity), inexhaustible drive to do things and remain busy, or be experiencing sensations (e.g., hunger, thirst, discomfort) without ability to express the actual need.*[2]
- Determine bowel and bladder elimination pattern, timing of incontinence, and presence of constipation *for possible correlation to wandering behavior.*
- Note timing and pattern of wandering behavior. *Client attempting to leave at 5:00 p.m. every day may believe he is going home from work; client may be goal directed (e.g., searching for person or object, escaping from something) or nongoal directed (wandering aimlessly). Knowledge of patterns can prompt caregivers to anticipate need for personal attention.*[2,5]
- Ascertain if client has delusions due to shadows, lights, and noises *to determine necessary changes to environment.*
- Evaluate usual travel patterns. *Activity may be (1) direct (from one location to another without diversion), (2) random (random direction with no obvious stopping point), (3) pacing (back and forth within limited area), or (4) lapping (circling large areas).*[2,5,6]
- Assist with or review results of specific testing (e.g., Revised Algase Wandering Scale, Need-Driven Dementia-Compromised Behavior, similar tool), as indicated. *Researchers are using adjunct tools for clinical assessment that quantify wandering in several domains (as reported by caregivers) to determine individual risks and safety needs.*[2,6]
- Monitor client's need for and use of assistive devices, such as glasses, hearing aids, cane, safe walking shoes, comfortable clothing, etc. *Wandering client is at high risk for falls due to cognitive impairments and the fatigue related to functional decline or forgetting necessary assistive devices or how to properly use them.*

Acute Care
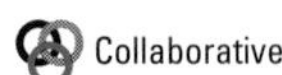
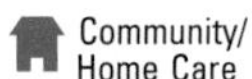
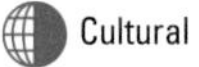

NURSING PRIORITY NO. 2 To assist client/caregiver to deal with wandering:

- Provide a structured daily routine:
  Encourage participation in family activities and familiar routines, such as folding laundry, listening to music, or shared-walking time outdoors. *Activities and exercises may reduce anxiety, depression, and restlessness. Note: Repetitive activity (e.g., rocking, folding laundry, paperwork) may help client with "lapping"—wandering to reduce energy expenditure and fatigue. In addition, studies reveal that wandering may be an adaptive behavior that reflects continuity of premorbid personality traits and lifelong patterns of coping with stress.*[3,7]
  Offer food, fluids, and toileting on a regular schedule when client is unable to verbalize, *as agitation, pacing, or wandering may be associated with these basic needs.*[3]
  Sit with client and talk *when client is socially gregarious, enjoys conversation, or reminiscence is calming.*
  Provide television, radio, or music, *which may be more effective than talking or reading to decrease wandering.*[1]
  Monitor activities, loud conversations, and number of visitors at one time *to prevent overstimulation or increased agitation.*
  Remove items from immediate environment (e.g., coat, hat, keys) *to reduce stimulus for leaving the site.*
- Provide safe place for client to wander:
  Remove environmental safety hazards such as hot water faucets and knobs on kitchen stove, gate or block open stairways, etc.[1,2]
  Keep area free of clutter and place comfortable furniture and other items against the wall or out of travel path *to accommodate safe walking and promote rest periods during times of continual lapping.*[1]
  Install safety locks or latches on doors and windows (*door latches are complex and less accessible*); equip exits with alarms (always turned on; pressure-sensitive doormats that sound an alarm).[1–3]
  Provide for 24-hr supervision, as indicated. *Client can be awake at any time and fail to recognize day or night routines.*
  Consider use of GPS device. Register client with community and national resources such as SafeReturn Program administered by the Alzheimer's Association. *Program registers persons with dementia and operates a 24-hr helpline to facilitate the return of lost persons (800-272-3900).*[2,4,5]
- Ascertain client history of wandering when admitted to facility:
  Place in room near monitoring station; check client location on frequent basis.
  Assign consistent staff as much as possible.
  Create a "wanderer's lounge" or large safe walking area with inaccessible exits or outside gated area.
  Avoid overstimulation from activities or new partner/roommate during rest periods. *Client who is used to wandering in usual living setting may react with increased agitation and emotional outbreaks when admitted to an unfamiliar setting and restricted from wandering. This places both the client and caregivers at risk for injury.*[1–3]
- Use technology to promote safety:
  Provide pressure-sensitive bed or chair alarms *to alert caregivers of movement, especially when client frequently gets up at night or when no one is present.*
  Provide client ID bracelet or necklace with updated photograph, client name, and emergency contact *to assist with identification efforts, particularly when progressive dementia produces marked changes in client's appearance.*[4]
  Obtain electronic locator devices *to find client when there is the potential for client to get lost or go missing.*[4]
  Install verbal door alarm system. *Voice command is more effective at redirecting client and less likely to increase agitation than loud sound.*[1]
- Use universal symbols, large-print signs, portrait-like photographs, pictures, and signs *to assist client in finding way, especially when client has diminished ability or has lost ability to read*
- Avoid using physical or chemical restraints (sedatives) to control wandering behavior. *May increase agitation, sensory deprivation, and falls, and can aggravate wandering behavior.*

NURSING PRIORITY NO. 3 To enhance safety (Teaching/Discharge Considerations):

- Identify problems that are remediable and assist client/significant other (SO) to seek appropriate assistance and access resources. *Encourages problem solving to improve condition rather than accept the status quo.*
- Notify neighbors about client's condition and request that they contact client's family or local police if they see client outside alone. *Community awareness can prevent or reduce risk of client being lost or hurt.*
- Help client/SO and family members develop plan of care when problem is progressive. *Client may initially need part-time assistance at home, progressing to enrollment in day-care program, and then full-time home care or placement in care facility.*
- Refer to community resources, such as day-care programs, support groups, respite care, etc. *Caregiver(s) will require access to multiple kinds of assistance and opportunities to promote problem solving, enhance coping, and obtain necessary respite.*
- Refer to NDs acute/chronic Confusion, risk for Falls, risk for Injury, and [disturbed Sensory Perception (specify)].

DOCUMENTATION FOCUS

Assessment/Reassessment

- Assessment findings, including individual concerns, family involvement, and support factors.
- Availability and use of resources.

Planning

- Plan of care and who is involved in planning.
- Teaching plan.

Implementation/Evaluation

- Responses of client/SO(s) to plan interventions and actions performed.
- Attainment or progress toward desired outcome(s).
- Modifications to plan of care.

Discharge Planning

- Long-term needs and who is responsible for actions to be taken.
- Specific referrals made.

References

1. Health care professionals and Alzheimer's (various pages). (2015). Retrieved November 2015 from http://www.alz.org/health-care-professionals/health-care-clinical-medical-resources.asp.
2. Mayo Clinic Staff. (2015). Alzheimer's: Understand wandering and how to address it. Retrieved November 2015 from http://www.mayoclinic.org/healthy-lifestyle/caregivers/in-depth/alzheimers/art-20046222.
3. Cox, H. C., Hinz, M. D., Lubno, M. A., et al. (2002). ND: Wandering. *Clinical Applications of Nursing Diagnosis: Adult, Child, Women's, Psychiatric, Gerontic, and Home Health Considerations.* 4th ed. Philadelphia: F. A. Davis.
4. Rowe, M. A. (2003). People with dementia who become lost. *Am J Nurs*, 103(7), 32–39.
5. Alzheimer's Disease and Related Disorders SAR Research: Wandering. Retrieved November 2015 from http://www.dbs-sar.com/SAR_Research/wandering.htm.
6. Algase, D. L., Beel-Bates, C., Beattie, E. (2003). Wandering in long term care. *Ann Long Term Care*, 11(1), 33–39.
7. Song, J. A., Algase, D. (2008). Premorbid characteristics and wandering behavior in persons with dementia. *Arch Psychiatr Nurs*, 22(6), 318–327.

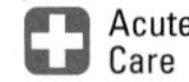
Acute Care
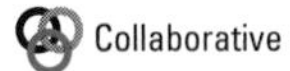
Collaborative
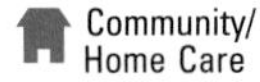
Community/ Home Care
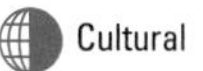
Cultural

CHAPTER 6

Health Conditions and Client Concerns With Associated Nursing Diagnoses

This chapter presents 850 disorders/health conditions and life situations reflecting all specialty areas, with associated nursing diagnoses written as client problem/need statements that include the "related to" and "evidenced by" components.

This section facilitates and helps validate the assessment and diagnosis steps of the nursing process. Because the nursing process is perpetual and ongoing, other nursing diagnoses may be appropriate based on changing individual situations. Therefore, the nurse must continually assess, identify, and validate new client needs and evaluate subsequent care.

To facilitate access to the health conditions/concerns and nursing diagnoses, the conditions are listed alphabetically and coded to identify nursing specialty areas.

MS: Medical-Surgical
PED: Pediatric
OB/GYN: Obstetric/Gynecological
CH: Community/Home
PSY: Psychiatric/Behavioral

There is no separate category for geriatrics because concerns and conditions in this population are subsumed under the other specialty areas and because elderly persons are susceptible to the majority of these problems.

Abdominal hysterectomy MS

Refer to Hysterectomy

Abdominal perineal resection MS

Also refer to Surgery, general

disturbed Body Image may be related to presence of surgical wounds, possibly evidenced by verbalizations of feelings or perceptions, fear of reaction by others, preoccupation with change.

risk for Constipation possibly evidenced by risk factors of decreased physical activity and gastric motility, abdominal muscle weakness, insufficient fluid intake, change in usual foods or eating pattern.

risk for Sexual dysfunction possibly evidenced by risk factors of altered body structure or function, radical resection or treatment procedures, vulnerability, psychological concern about response of significant other(s), and disruption of sexual response pattern (e.g., erection difficulty).

Abortion, elective termination OB

risk for Decisional Conflict possibly evidenced by unclear personal values/beliefs, lack of experience or interference with decision making, information from divergent sources, deficient support system.

deficient Knowledge [Learning Need] regarding reproduction, contraception, self-care, and Rh factor may be related to lack of exposure or recall, misinterpretation of information, possibly evidenced by request for information, statement reflecting misconception, inaccurate follow-through of instructions, development of preventable complications.

risk for Moral Distress may be related to perception of moral or ethical implications of therapeutic procedure, time constraints for decision making.

Anxiety [specify level] may be related to situational or maturational crises, unmet needs, unconscious conflict about essential values or beliefs possibly evidenced by increased tension, apprehension, fear of unspecific consequences, sympathetic stimulation, focus on self.

acute Pain/impaired Comfort may be related to after-effects of procedure, drug effect, possibly evidenced by verbal report, distraction behaviors, changes in muscle tone, changes in vital signs.

risk for maternal Injury possibly evidenced by risk factors of surgical procedure, effects of anesthesia or medications.

Abortion, spontaneous termination **OB**
risk for Bleeding possibly evidenced by risk factor of pregnancy-related complications.

risk for Spiritual distress possibly evidenced by risk factors of challenged beliefs/values, blame for loss directed at self or God.

deficient Knowledge [Learning Need] regarding cause of abortion, self-care, contraception, and future pregnancy may be related to lack of familiarity with new self-healthcare needs, sources for support, possibly evidenced by requests for information and statement of concern or misconceptions, development of preventable complications.

Grieving related to perinatal loss, possibly evidenced by crying, expressions of sorrow, or changes in eating habits or sleep patterns.

risk for Sexual dysfunction possibly evidenced by risk factors of increasing fear of pregnancy or repeat loss, impaired relationship with SO(s), self-doubt regarding own femininity.

Abruptio placentae **OB**
Also refer to Hemorrhage, prenatal

risk for Bleeding possibly evidenced by risk factor of pregnancy-related complication—abruptio placentae.

Fear related to threat of death (perceived or actual) to fetus/self, possibly evidenced by verbalization of apprehension, increased tension, sympathetic stimulation.

acute Pain may be related to collection of blood between uterine wall and placenta, possibly evidenced by verbal reports, abdominal guarding, muscle tension, or alterations in vital signs.

risk for disturbed Maternal-Fetal Dyad possibly evidenced by risk factors of complications of pregnancy, compromised oxygen transport.

Abscess, brain (acute) **MS**
acute Pain may be related to inflammation, edema of tissues, possibly evidenced by reports of headache, restlessness, irritability, and moaning.

risk for Hyperthermia possibly evidenced by risk factors of inflammatory process, hypermetabolic state, and dehydration.

acute Confusion may be related to delirium [cerebral edema, altered perfusion, fever], possibly evidenced by fluctuation in cognition or level of consciousness, increased agitation, restlessness, hallucinations.

risk for Suffocation/Trauma possibly evidenced by risk factors of disease process [seizure activity], cognitive difficulties.

Abscess, gingival **CH**
impaired Dentition may be related to ineffective oral hygiene, access/economic barriers to professional care possibly evidenced by toothache, root caries, purulent drainage.

risk for imbalanced Nutrition: less than body requirements possibly evidenced by risk factor of decreased intake.

Abscess, skin/tissue **CH/MS**
impaired Skin/Tissue Integrity may be related to immunological deficit/infection, possibly evidenced by disruption of skin, destruction of skin layers or tissues, invasion of body structures.

risk for Infection [spread] possibly evidenced by risk factors of broken skin, traumatized tissues, chronic disease, malnutrition, insufficient knowledge.

Abuse, physical **CH/PSY**
Also refer to Battered child syndrome

risk for Trauma possibly evidenced by risk factors of vulnerable client, recipient of verbal threats, history of physical abuse.

Powerlessness may be related to interpersonal interactions, lifestyle of helplessness as evidenced by verbal expressions of having no control, reluctance to express true feelings, apathy, passivity.

chronic low Self-Esteem may be related to continual negative evaluation of self or capabilities, personal vulnerability, willingness to tolerate possible life-threatening domestic violence as evidenced by self-negative verbalization, evaluation of self as unable to deal with events, rejects positive feedback about self.

ineffective Coping may be related to situational or maturational crisis, overwhelming threat to self, personal vulnerability, inadequate support systems, possibly evidenced by verbalized concern about ability to deal with current situation, chronic worry, anxiety, depression, poor self-esteem, inability to problem solve, high illness rate, destructive behavior toward self/others.

Sexual dysfunction may be related to ineffectual or absent role model, vulnerability, physical abuse possibly evidenced by verbalizations, change in sexual behaviors or activities, inability to achieve desired satisfaction.

Abuse, psychological **CH/PSY**
ineffective Coping may be related to situational or maturational crisis, overwhelming threat to self, personal vulnerability, inadequate support systems, possibly evidenced by verbalized concern about ability to deal with current situation, chronic worry, anxiety, depression, poor self-esteem, inability to problem solve, high illness rate, destructive behavior toward self/others.

Powerlessness may be related to abusive relationship, lifestyle of helplessness possibly evidenced by verbal expressions of having no control, reluctance to express true feelings, apathy, passivity.

Sexual dysfunction may be related to ineffectual or absent role model, vulnerability, psychological abuse (harmful relationship), possibly evidenced by reported difficulties, inability to achieve desired satisfaction, conflicts involving values, seeking confirmation of desirability.

Achalasia (cardiospasm) **MS**
impaired Swallowing may be related to neuromuscular impairment, possibly evidenced by observed difficulty in swallowing or regurgitation.

imbalanced Nutrition: less than body requirements may be related to inability or reluctance to ingest adequate nutrients to meet metabolic demands or nutritional needs, possibly evidenced by reported or observed inadequate intake, weight loss, and pale conjunctiva and mucous membranes.

acute Pain may be related to spasm of the lower esophageal sphincter, possibly evidenced by reports of substernal pressure, recurrent heartburn, or gastric fullness (gas pains).

Anxiety [specify level]/Fear may be related to recurrent pain, choking sensation, altered health status, possibly evidenced by verbalizations of distress, apprehension, restlessness, or insomnia.

risk for Aspiration possibly evidenced by risk factor of regurgitation or spillover of esophageal contents.

deficient Knowledge [Learning Need] regarding condition, prognosis, self-care, and treatment needs may be related to lack of familiarity with pathology and treatment of condition, possibly evidenced by requests for information, statement of concern, or development of preventable complications.

Acidosis, metabolic **MS**
Refer to underlying cause/condition, e.g., Diabetic ketoacidosis; Renal failure, Dialysis

Acidosis, respiratory **MS**
(Also refer to underlying cause/condition)

impaired Gas Exchange may be related to ventilation perfusion imbalance (decreased oxygen-carrying capacity of blood, altered oxygen supply, alveolar-capillary membrane changes), possibly evidenced by dyspnea with exertion, tachypnea, changes in mentation, irritability, tachycardia, hypoxia, hypercapnia.

Acne **CH/PED**
impaired Skin Integrity may be related to secretion, infectious process as evidenced by disruptions of skin surface.

disturbed Body Image may be related to change in visual appearance as evidenced by fear of rejection of others, focus on past appearance, negative feelings about body, change in social involvement.

situational low Self-Esteem may be related to adolescence, negative perception of appearance as evidenced by self-negating verbalizations, expressions of helplessness.

Acoustic neuroma **MS**
Also refer to Surgery, general

[disturbed auditory Sensory Perception] may be related to altered sensory reception (compression of eighth cranial nerve), possibly evidenced by unilateral sensorineural hearing loss, tinnitus.

risk for Falls: possibly evidenced by risk factors of hearing difficulties, dizziness, sense of unsteadiness.

Acquired immune deficiency syndrome **CH**
Refer to AIDS

Acromegaly **CH**
chronic Pain may be related to soft tissue swelling, joint degeneration, peripheral nerve compression, possibly evidenced by verbal reports, altered ability to continue previous activities, changes in sleep pattern, fatigue.

disturbed Body Image may be related to biophysical illness and changes, possibly evidenced by verbalization of feelings or concerns, fear of rejection or of reaction of others, negative comments about body, actual change in structure and appearance, change in social involvement.

risk for Sexual dysfunction: possibly evidenced by altered body structure, changes in libido.

Acute respiratory distress syndrome **MS**
Refer to Respiratory distress syndrome, acute

Adams-Stokes syndrome **CH**
Refer to Dysrhythmia, cardiac

ADD **PED**
Refer to Attention deficit disorder

Addiction **CH/PSY**
Refer to specific substance used; Substance dependence/abuse rehabilitation

Addison's disease **MS**
deficient Fluid Volume [hypertonic] may be related to vomiting, diarrhea, increased renal losses, possibly evidenced by delayed capillary refill, poor skin turgor, dry mucous membranes, report of thirst.

risk for Electrolyte Imbalance possibly evidenced by risk factors of vomiting, diarrhea, endocrine dysfunction.

decreased Cardiac Output may be related to hypovolemia and altered electrical conduction (dysrhythmias) or diminished cardiac muscle mass, possibly evidenced by alterations in vital signs, changes in mentation, and irregular pulse or pulse deficit.

CH
Fatigue may be related to decreased metabolic energy production, altered body chemistry (fluid, electrolyte, and glucose imbalance), possibly evidenced by unremitting overwhelming lack of energy, inability to maintain usual routines, decreased performance, impaired ability to concentrate, lethargy, and disinterest in surroundings.

disturbed Body Image may be related to changes in skin pigmentation, mucous membranes, loss of axillary and pubic hair, possibly evidenced by verbalization of negative feelings about body and decreased social involvement.

risk for impaired physical Mobility possibly evidenced by risk factors of neuromuscular impairment (muscle wasting, weakness) and dizziness, syncope.

imbalanced Nutrition: less than body requirements may be related to glucocorticoid deficiency; abnormal fat, protein, and carbohydrate metabolism; nausea, vomiting, anorexia, possibly evidenced by weight loss, muscle wasting, abdominal cramps, diarrhea, and severe hypoglycemia.

risk for impaired Home Maintenance possibly evidenced by risk factors of effects of disease process, impaired cognitive functioning, and inadequate support systems.

Adenoidectomy **PED/MS**
Anxiety [specify level]/Fear may be related to separation from supportive others, unfamiliar surroundings, and perceived threat of injury or abandonment, possibly evidenced by crying, apprehension, trembling, and sympathetic stimulation (pupil dilation, increased heart rate).

risk for ineffective Airway Clearance possibly evidenced by risk factors of sedation, collection of secretions and blood in oropharynx, and vomiting.

risk for deficient Fluid Volume possibly evidenced by risk factors of operative trauma to highly vascular site, hemorrhage.

acute Pain may be related to physical trauma to oronasopharynx, presence of packing, possibly evidenced by restlessness, crying, and facial mask of pain.

Adjustment disorder **PED/PSY**
Refer to Anxiety disorders

Adoption/loss of child custody **PSY**
risk for complicated Grieving possibly evidenced by risk factors of actual loss of child, expectations for future of child/self, thwarted grieving response to loss.

risk for Powerlessness possibly evidenced by risk factors of perceived lack of options, no input into decision process, no control over outcome.

Adrenal crisis, acute **MS**
Also refer to Addison's disease; Shock

deficient Fluid Volume [hypertonic] may be related to failure of regulatory mechanism (damage to or suppression of adrenal gland), inability to concentrate urine, possibly evidenced by decreased venous filling, pulse volume and pressure; hypotension, dry mucous membranes, changes in mentation, decreased serum sodium.

acute Pain may be related to effects of disease process and metabolic imbalances, decreased tissue perfusion, possibly evidenced by reports of severe pain in abdomen, lower back, or legs.

impaired physical Mobility may be related to neuromuscular impairment, decreased muscle strength and control, possibly evidenced by generalized weakness, inability to perform desired activities or movements.

risk for Hyperthermia possibly evidenced by risk factors of presence of illness or infectious process, dehydration.

risk for ineffective Protection possibly evidenced by risk factors of hormone deficiency, drug therapy, nutritional or metabolic deficiencies.

Adrenalectomy — MS

ineffective Tissue Perfusion (specify) may be related to hypovolemia and vascular pooling of blood (vasodilation), possibly evidenced by diminished pulse, pallor or cyanosis, hypotension, and changes in mentation.

risk for Infection possibly evidenced by risk factors of inadequate primary defenses (incision, traumatized tissues), suppressed inflammatory response, invasive procedures.

deficient Knowledge [Learning Need] regarding condition, prognosis, self-care, and treatment needs may be related to unfamiliarity with long-term therapy requirements, possibly evidenced by request for information and statement of concern or misconceptions.

Adrenal insufficiency — CH

Refer to Addison's disease

Affective disorder — PSY

Refer to Bipolar disorder; Depression, major

Affective disorder, seasonal — PSY

Also refer to Depression, major

[intermittent] ineffective Coping may be related to situational crisis (fall-winter season), disturbance in pattern of tension release, and inadequate resources available, possibly evidenced by verbalizations of inability to cope, changes in sleep pattern (too little or too much), reports of lack of energy or fatigue, lack of resolution of problem, behavioral changes (irritability, discouragement).

Agoraphobia — PSY

Also refer to Phobia

Anxiety [panic] may be related to contact with feared situation (public place, crowds), possibly evidenced by tachycardia, chest pain, dyspnea, gastrointestinal distress, faintness, sense of impending doom.

Agranulocytosis — MS

risk for Infection possibly evidenced by risk factor of suppressed inflammatory response.

risk for impaired oral Mucous Membrane possibly evidenced by risk factor of infection.

risk for imbalanced Nutrition: less than body requirements possibly evidenced by risk factor of inability to ingest food or fluids.

AIDS (acquired immunodeficiency syndrome) — MS

Also refer to HIV infection

risk for Infection [progression to sepsis/onset of new opportunistic infection] possibly evidenced by risk factors of depressed immune system, use of antimicrobial agents, inadequate primary defenses, broken skin, traumatized tissue, malnutrition, environmental exposure, invasive procedures, and chronic disease processes.

risk for deficient Fluid Volume possibly evidenced by risk factors of excessive losses—copious diarrhea, profuse sweating, vomiting, hypermetabolic state or fever; and restricted intake—nausea, anorexia, lethargy.

acute/chronic Pain may be related to tissue inflammation or destruction: infections, internal or external cutaneous lesions, rectal excoriation, malignancies, necrosis, peripheral neuropathies, myalgias and arthralgias, possibly evidenced by verbal reports, narrowed focus, alteration in muscle tone, paresthesias, paralysis, guarding behaviors, changes in vital signs (acute), autonomic responses, and restlessness.

risk for ineffective Breathing Pattern/impaired Gas Exchange possibly evidenced by risk factors of muscular impairment—wasting of respiratory musculature, decreased energy, fatigue, respiratory muscle fatigue; retained secretions (tracheobronchial obstruction), pain.

CH

imbalanced Nutrition: less than body requirements may be related to altered ability to ingest, digest, or absorb nutrients (nausea, vomiting, hyperactive gag reflex, gastrointestinal disturbances, fatigue); increased metabolic rate and nutritional needs (fever, infection), possibly evidenced by weight loss, decreased subcutaneous fat or muscle mass; lack of interest in food, aversion to eating, altered taste sensation; abdominal cramping, hyperactive bowel sounds, diarrhea, sore and inflamed buccal cavity, abnormal laboratory results—vitamin, mineral, and protein deficiencies; electrolyte imbalances.

Fatigue may be related to decreased metabolic energy production, increased energy requirements (hypermetabolic state), overwhelming psychological or emotional demands, altered body chemistry (side effects of medication, chemotherapy), sleep deprivation, possibly evidenced by unremitting or overwhelming lack of energy, inability to maintain usual routines, decreased performance, impaired ability to concentrate, lethargy, listlessness, and disinterest in surroundings.

ineffective Protection may be related to chronic disease affecting immune and neurological systems, inadequate nutrition, drug therapies, possibly evidenced by deficient immunity, impaired healing, neurosensory alterations, maladaptive stress response, fatigue, anorexia, disorientation.

PSY

Social Isolation may be related to alterations in physical appearance, mental status, state of wellness; perceptions of unacceptable social behavior or values [phobic fear of others (transmission of disease)], possibly evidenced by expressed feelings of aloneness or rejection, absence of supportive SO(s), and withdrawal from usual activities.

chronic Confusion may be related to physiological changes (hypoxemia, central nervous system infection by HIV, brain malignancies, or disseminated systemic opportunistic infection); altered drug metabolism and excretion, accumulation of toxic elements (renal failure, severe electrolyte imbalance, hepatic insufficiency), possibly evidenced by clinical evidence of organic impairment, altered response to stimuli, memory deficit, and altered personality.

AIDS dementia — CH

Also refer to Dementia, HIV

chronic Confusion/impaired Memory related to physiological changes (neuronal degeneration), possibly evidenced by inaccurate interpretation of or response to stimuli, progressive or long-standing cognitive impairment, short-term memory deficit, impaired socialization, altered personality, and clinical evidence of organic impairment.

ineffective Protection may be related to immune disorder, inadequate nutrition, drug therapies, possibly evidenced by deficient immunity, impaired healing, neurosensory alterations, maladaptive stress response, fatigue, anorexia, disorientation.

Alcohol abuse/withdrawal — CH/MS/PSY

Refer to Alcohol intoxication, acute; Delirium tremens; Substance dependence/abuse rehabilitation

Alcohol intoxication, acute — MS

Also refer to Delirium tremens

acute Confusion may be related to substance abuse, hypoxemia, possibly evidenced by hallucinations, exaggerated emotional response, fluctuation in cognition or level of consciousness, increased agitation.

risk for ineffective Breathing Pattern possibly evidenced by risk factors of hypoventilation syndrome, neuromuscular dysfunction, fatigue.

risk for Aspiration possibly evidenced by risk factors of reduced level of consciousness, depressed cough or gag reflexes, delayed gastric emptying.

Alcoholism — CH

Refer to Substance dependence/abuse rehabilitation

Aldosteronism, primary — MS

deficient Fluid Volume may be related to increased urinary losses, possibly evidenced by dry mucous membranes, poor skin turgor, dilute urine, excessive thirst, weight loss.

impaired physical Mobility may be related to neuromuscular impairment, decreased muscle strength, and pain, possibly evidenced by limited range of motion, slowed movement, limited ability to perform gross/fine motor skills.

risk for decreased Cardiac Output possibly evidenced by risk factors of altered preload and altered heart rhythm.

Alkalosis, metabolic — MS

Refer to underlying cause/condition, e.g., Renal failure, Dialysis

Alkalosis, respiratory — MS

(Also refer to underlying cause/condition.)

impaired Gas Exchange may be related to ventilation perfusion imbalance (decreased oxygen-carrying capacity of blood, altered oxygen supply, alveolar-capillary membrane changes), possibly evidenced by dyspnea, tachypnea, changes in mentation, tachycardia, hypoxia, hypocapnia.

Allergies, seasonal — CH

Refer to Hay fever

Alopecia — CH

disturbed Body Image may be related to effects of illness, therapy, or aging process; change in appearance, possibly evidenced by verbalization of feelings or concerns, fear of rejection or reaction of others, focus on past appearance, preoccupation with change, feelings of helplessness.

ALS — CH

Refer to Amyotrophic lateral sclerosis

Alzheimer's disease — CH

Also refer to Dementia, presenile/senile

risk for Injury/Trauma possibly evidenced by risk factors of inability to recognize or identify danger in environment, disorientation, confusion, impaired judgment, weakness, muscular incoordination, balancing difficulties, altered perception, and seizure activity.

chronic Confusion related to physiological changes (neuronal degeneration), possibly evidenced by inaccurate interpretation of or response to stimuli, progressive or long-standing cognitive impairment, short-term memory deficit, impaired socialization, altered personality, and clinical evidence of organic impairment.

[disturbed Sensory Perception (specify)] may be related to altered sensory reception, transmission, or integration (neurological disease, deficit), socially restricted environment (homebound or institutionalized), sleep deprivation, possibly evidenced by changes in usual response to stimuli, change in problem-solving abilities, exaggerated emotional responses (anxiety, paranoia, hallucinations), inability to tell position of body parts, diminished or altered sense of taste.

Sleep deprivation may be related to sensory impairment, changes in activity patterns, psychological stress (neurological impairment), possibly evidenced by wakefulness, disorientation (day/night reversal), increased aimless wandering, inability to identify need or time for sleeping, changes in behavior, lethargy, dark circles under eyes, and frequent yawning.

ineffective Health Maintenance may be related to deterioration affecting ability in all areas, including coordination, communication, and cognition; ineffective individual or family coping, possibly evidenced by reported or observed inability to take responsibility for meeting basic health practices, lack of equipment/financial or other resources, and impairment of personal support system.

PSY

risk for Stress overload possibly evidenced by risk factors of inadequate resources, chronic illness, physical demands, threats of violence.

compromised family Coping/caregiver Role Strain may be related to disruptive behavior of client, family grief about their helplessness watching loved one deteriorate, prolonged disease or disability progression that exhausts the supportive capacity of SO or family, highly ambivalent family relationships, possibly evidenced by verbalizations of frustrations in dealing with day-to-day care, reports of conflict, feelings of depression, expressed anger/guilt directed toward client, and withdrawal from interaction with client or social contacts.

risk for Relocation Stress Syndrome possibly evidenced by risk factors of little or no preparation for transfer to a new setting, changes in daily routine, sensory impairment, physical deterioration, separation from support systems.

Amenorrhea (secondary or pathological) — GYN

Also refer to Anorexia nervosa

imbalanced Nutrition: less than body requirements may be related to inability to ingest or digest food or absorb nutrients, possibly evidenced by verbal reports, aversion to eating, lack of interest in food, weight loss, excessive hair growth or lanugo, pale conjunctiva and mucous membranes, abnormal lab studies.

risk for Sexual dysfunction possibly evidenced by risk factor of altered body function.

Amphetamine abuse — PSY

Refer to Stimulant abuse

Amputation — MS

risk for ineffective peripheral Tissue Perfusion possibly evidenced by risk factors of reduced arterial or venous blood flow, tissue edema, hematoma formation, hypovolemia.

acute Pain may be related to tissue and nerve trauma, psychological impact of loss of body part, possibly evidenced by reports of incisional or phantom pain, guarding or protective behavior, narrowed or self-focus, and autonomic responses.

impaired physical Mobility may be related to loss of limb (primarily lower extremity), altered sense of balance, pain or discomfort, possibly evidenced by reluctance to attempt movement, impaired coordination; decreased muscle strength, control, and mass.

situational low Self-Esteem may be related to loss of a body part, change in functional abilities, possibly evidenced by verbalization of feelings of powerlessness; grief; preoccupation with loss; negative feelings about body; focus on past strength, function, or appearance; change in usual patterns of responsibility or physical capacity to resume role; fear of rejection or reaction by others; and unwillingness to look at or touch residual limb.

Amyotrophic lateral sclerosis (ALS) **MS**

impaired physical Mobility may be related to muscle wasting, weakness, possibly evidenced by impaired coordination, limited range of motion, and impaired purposeful movement.

ineffective Breathing Pattern/impaired spontaneous Ventilation may be related to neuromuscular impairment, decreased energy, fatigue, tracheobronchial obstruction, possibly evidenced by shortness of breath, fremitus, respiratory depth changes, and reduced vital capacity.

impaired Swallowing may be related to muscle wasting and fatigue, possibly evidenced by recurrent coughing, choking, and signs of aspiration.

PSY

Powerlessness may be related to chronic and debilitating nature of illness, lack of control over outcome, possibly evidenced by expressions of frustration about inability to care for self and depression over physical deterioration.

Grieving may be related to perceived potential loss of self and physiopsychosocial well-being, possibly evidenced by sorrow, choked feelings, expression of distress, changes in eating habits/sleeping patterns, altered communication patterns, and changes in libido.

CH

impaired verbal Communication may be related to physical barrier (neuromuscular impairment), possibly evidenced by impaired articulation, inability to speak in sentences, and use of nonverbal cues (changes in facial expression).

risk for caregiver Role Strain possibly evidenced by risk factors of illness severity of care receiver, complexity and amount of home-care needs, duration of caregiving required, caregiver is spouse, family/caregiver isolation, lack of respite or recreation for caregiver.

Anaphylaxis **CH**

Also refer to Shock

ineffective Airway Clearance may be related to airway spasm (bronchial), laryngeal edema, possibly evidenced by diminished or adventitious breath sounds, cough ineffective or absent, difficulty vocalizing, wide-eyed.

decreased Cardiac Output may be related to decreased preload—increased capillary permeability (third spacing) and vasodilation, possibly evidenced by tachycardia/palpitations, changes in blood pressure, anxiety, restlessness.

Anemia **CH**

Activity Intolerance may be related to imbalance between oxygen supply and demand, possibly evidenced by reports of fatigue and weakness, abnormal heart rate or blood pressure response, decreased exercise or activity level, and exertional discomfort or dyspnea.

imbalanced Nutrition: less than body requirements may be related to failure to ingest or inability to digest food or absorb nutrients necessary for formation of normal red blood cells, possibly evidenced by weight loss or weight below normal for age, height, body build; decreased triceps skinfold measurement, changes in gums and oral mucous membranes; decreased tolerance for activity, weakness, and loss of muscle tone.

deficient Knowledge [Learning Need] regarding condition, prognosis, self-care, and treatment needs may be related to inadequate understanding or misinterpretation of dietary or physiological needs, possibly evidenced by inadequate dietary intake, request for information, and development of preventable complications.

Anemia, iron-deficiency **CH**

Also refer to Anemia

Fatigue may be related to anemia, malnutrition, possibly evidenced by feeling tired, inability to maintain usual routines or level of physical activity.

risk for deficient Fluid Volume possibly evidenced by risk factors of active or chronic blood loss.

risk for impaired oral Mucous Membrane possibly evidenced by risk factors of dehydration, malnutrition, vitamin deficiency.

Anemia, pernicious **CH**

Also refer to Anemia

[disturbed kinesthetic/visual Sensory Perception] may be related to changes in reception or perception, possibly evidenced by paresthesia, inability to tell position of extremities (proprioception), loss of vibratory sensation, changes in sensory acuity (yellow-blue color blindness).

risk for Constipation/Diarrhea possibly evidenced by risk factors of muscular weakness, changes in gastrointestinal motility, neurological impairment.

risk for Injury/Falls possibly evidenced by risk factors of generalized weakness, paresthesia of extremities, loss of proprioception, ataxia.

Anemia, sickle cell **MS**

impaired Gas Exchange may be related to decreased oxygen-carrying capacity of blood, reduced red blood cell life span or premature destruction, abnormal red blood cell structure, increased blood viscosity, pulmonary congestion—impairment of surface phagocytosis, predisposition to bacterial pneumonia and pulmonary infarcts, possibly evidenced by dyspnea, use of accessory muscles, signs of hypoxia—cyanosis, tachycardia, changes in mentation, and restlessness.

ineffective Tissue Perfusion (specify) may be related to stasis, vaso-occlusive nature of sickling, inflammatory response, atrioventricular shunts in pulmonary and peripheral circulation, myocardial damage (small infarcts, iron deposits, fibrosis), possibly evidenced by signs and symptoms dependent on system involved; for example, renal—decreased specific gravity and pale urine in face of dehydration; cerebral—paralysis and visual disturbances; peripheral—distal ischemia, tissue infarctions, ulcerations, bone pain; cardiac—angina, palpitations.

CH

acute/chronic Pain may be related to intravascular sickling with localized vascular stasis, occlusion, infarction or necrosis and deprivation of oxygen and nutrients, accumulation of noxious metabolites, possibly evidenced by reports of localized, generalized, or migratory joint or abdominal/back pain; guarding and distraction behaviors (moaning, crying, restlessness); facial grimacing; narrowed focus; and autonomic responses.

deficient Knowledge [Learning Need] regarding disease process, genetic factors, prognosis, self-care, and treatment needs may be related to lack of exposure or recall, misinterpretation of information, unfamiliarity with resources, possibly evidenced by questions, statements of concern or misconceptions, exacerbation of condition, inadequate follow-through of therapy instructions, and development of preventable complications.

risk for sedentary Lifestyle possibly evidenced by risk factors of lack of interest or motivation, resources; lack of training or knowledge of specific exercise needs, safety concerns, fear of injury.

PED

risk for delayed Development possibly evidenced by risk factors of inadequate nutrition, chronic illness.

compromised family Coping may be related to chronic nature of disease and disability, family disorganization, presence of other crises or situations impacting significant person or parent, lifestyle restrictions, possibly evidenced by SO expressing preoccupation with own reaction and displaying protective behavior disproportionate to client's ability or need for autonomy.

Anencephaly **OB**

Also refer to Fetal demise

Anxiety [specify level] may be related to situational crisis, threat of fetal death, interpersonal transmission or contagion, possibly evidenced by increased tension, apprehension, feelings of inadequacy, somatic complaints, difficulty sleeping.

risk for Decisional Conflict possibly evidenced by risk factors of threat to value/belief system, multiple or divergent sources of information, support system deficit, feelings of guilt (particularly regarding ethical issues such as termination of pregnancy, organ donation).

Aneurysm, abdominal aortic **MS**

Refer to Aortic aneurysm, abdominal

Aneurysm, cerebral **MS**

Refer to Cerebrovascular accident

Aneurysm, ventricular **MS**

decreased Cardiac Output may be related to altered stroke volume (decreased contractility, increased systemic vascular resistance), changes in heart rate or rhythm, possibly evidenced by dyspnea, adventitious breath sounds, S_3/S_4 heart sounds, changes in hemodynamic measurements, dysrhythmias.

ineffective Tissue Perfusion (specify) may be related to decreased arterial blood flow, possibly evidenced by blood pressure changes, diminished pulses, edema, dyspnea, dysrhythmias, altered mental status, decreased renal function.

Activity Intolerance may be related to imbalance between oxygen supply and demand, possibly evidenced by weakness, fatigue, abnormal heart rate/blood pressure response to activity, electrocardiogram changes (dysrhythmias, ischemia).

Angina pectoris **MS**

acute Pain may be related to decreased myocardial blood flow, increased cardiac workload and oxygen consumption, possibly evidenced by verbal reports, narrowed focus, distraction behaviors (restlessness, moaning), and autonomic responses (diaphoresis, changes in vital signs).

risk for decreased Cardiac Output possibly evidenced by transient or prolonged myocardial ischemia and effects of medications, alterations in rate, rhythm, and electrical conduction.

Anxiety [specify level] may be related to situational crises, change in health status or threat of death, negative self-talk, possibly evidenced by verbalized apprehension, expressed concerns, association of condition with loss of abilities, facial tension, extraneous movements, and focus on self.

CH

Activity Intolerance may be related to imbalance between oxygen supply and demand, possibly evidenced by exertional dyspnea, abnormal pulse/blood pressure response to activity, and electrocardiogram changes.

deficient Knowledge [Learning Need] regarding condition, prognosis, self-care, and treatment needs may be related to lack of exposure, inaccurate/misinterpretation of information, possibly evidenced by questions, request for information, statement of concern, and inaccurate follow-through of instructions.

risk for sedentary Lifestyle risk factors may include lack of training or knowledge of specific exercise needs, safety concerns, fear of myocardial injury.

risk for risk-prone Health Behavior possibly evidenced by risk factors of condition requiring long-term therapy/change in lifestyle, multiple stressors, assault to self-concept, and altered locus of control.

Anorexia nervosa — MS

imbalanced Nutrition: less than body requirements may be related to psychological restrictions of food intake or excessive activity, laxative abuse, possibly evidenced by weight loss, poor skin turgor and muscle tone, denial of hunger, unusual hoarding or handling of food, amenorrhea, electrolyte imbalance, cardiac irregularities, hypotension.

risk for deficient Fluid Volume risk factors may include inadequate intake of food and liquids, chronic laxative or diuretic use.

PSY

disturbed Body Image may be related to perceptual developmental changes, possibly evidenced by verbalized perceptions reflecting altered view of body appearance, refusal to verify actual change.

chronic low Self-Esteem may be related to lack of approval, repeated negative reinforcement, perceived lack of respect from others possibly evidenced by reports of feelings of shame or guilt; overly conforming, dependent on others' opinions.

impaired Parenting may be related to issues of control in family, situational or maturational crises, history of inadequate coping methods, possibly evidenced by enmeshed family; dissonance among family members; focus on "identified patient"; family developmental tasks not being met; family members acting as enablers; ill-defined family rules, functions, and roles.

Anthrax, cutaneous — MS/CH

impaired Skin/Tissue Integrity may be related to infectious agent, possibly evidenced by disruption of skin surface, damage to tissues.

impaired Comfort may be related to local edema, effects of circulating toxins, possibly evidenced by reports of headache, muscle aches, nausea, malaise.

risk for Infection [spread/sepsis] possibly evidenced by risk factors of broken skin, tissue destruction, lack of immunity, presence of infective agent.

Anthrax, gastrointestinal — MS

Anxiety [moderate to severe]/Fear may be related to situational crisis, change in health status, threat of death, interpersonal transmission or contagion, possibly evidenced by expressed concerns, apprehension, uncertainty, fearful, increased tension, restlessness, blocking of thought.

risk for deficient Fluid Volume possibly evidenced by risk factors of decreased intake (nausea), excessive loss—bloody vomit or diarrhea, hypermetabolic state.

imbalanced Nutrition: less than body requirements may be related to inability to ingest food or absorb nutrients, increased metabolic demands, possibly evidenced by reports of loss of appetite, nausea, abdominal pain, vomiting, diarrhea.

impaired oral Mucous Membrane may be related to effects of infection, dehydration, possibly evidenced by oropharyngeal ulcerations, oral pain, difficulty swallowing.

Anthrax, inhalation (pulmonary) — MS

Also refer to Ventilator assist/dependence

impaired Comfort may be related to effects of inflammatory response, possibly evidenced by fever, malaise, weakness, fatigue, mild chest pain.

Anxiety [moderate to severe]/Fear may be related to situational crisis, change in health status/threat of death, interpersonal transmission or contagion, possibly evidenced by expressed concerns, apprehension, uncertainty, fearfulness, increased tension, restlessness, blocking of thought.

impaired Gas Exchange may be related to alveolar-capillary membrane changes (fluid collection or shifts into interstitial space or alveoli), possibly evidenced by dyspnea, restlessness, irritability, abnormal rate or depth of respirations, cyanosis, hypoxia, lethargy, confusion.

risk for impaired spontaneous Ventilation possibly evidenced by risk factors of problems with secretion management, mechanical compression of lungs (widening of mediastinum), depletion of energy stores.

Antisocial personality disorder PSY

risk for other-directed Violence possibly evidenced by risk factors of contempt for authority or rights of others, inability to tolerate frustration, need for immediate gratification, easy agitation, vulnerable self-concept, inability to verbalize feelings, use of maladjusted coping mechanisms, history of substance abuse.

ineffective Coping may be related to very low tolerance for external stress, lack of experience of internal anxiety (e.g., guilt, shame), personal vulnerability, unmet expectations, multiple life changes, possibly evidenced by choice of aggression and manipulation to handle problems or conflicts, inappropriate use of defense mechanisms (e.g., denial, projection), chronic worry, anxiety, destructive behaviors, high rate of accidents.

chronic low Self-Esteem may be related to lack of positive or repeated negative feedback, unmet dependency needs, retarded ego development, dysfunctional family system, possibly evidenced by acting-out behaviors (e.g., substance abuse, sexual promiscuity, feelings of inadequacy, nonparticipation in therapy).

compromised/disabled family Coping may be related to family disorganization or role changes, highly ambivalent family relationships, client providing little support in turn for the primary person(s), history of abuse or neglect in the home, possibly evidenced by expressions of concern or complaints, preoccupation of primary person with own reactions to situation, display of protective behaviors disproportionate to client's abilities or need for autonomy.

impaired Social Interaction may be related to inadequate personal resources (shallow feelings), immature interests, underdeveloped conscience, unaccepted social values, possibly evidenced by difficulty meeting expectations of others, lack of belief that rules pertain to self, sense of emptiness or inadequacy covered by expressions of self-conceit, arrogance, contempt; behavior unaccepted by dominant cultural group.

Anxiety disorder, generalized PSY

Anxiety [specify level]/Powerlessness may be related to real or perceived threat to physical integrity or self-concept (may or may not be able to identify the threat), unconscious conflict about essential values or beliefs and goals of life, unmet needs, negative self-talk, possibly evidenced by sympathetic stimulation, extraneous movements (foot shuffling, hand or arm fidgeting, rocking movements, restlessness), persistent feelings of apprehension and uneasiness, a general anxious feeling that client has difficulty alleviating, poor eye contact, focus on self, impaired functioning, free-floating anxiety, impaired functioning, and nonparticipation in decision making.

ineffective Coping may be related to level of anxiety being experienced by the client, personal vulnerability; unmet expectations, unrealistic perceptions, inadequate coping methods or support systems, possibly evidenced by verbalization of inability to cope or problem solve, excessive compulsive behaviors (e.g., smoking, drinking), and emotional tension, alteration in societal participation, high rate of accidents.

Insomnia may be related to stress, repetitive thoughts, possibly evidenced by reports of difficulty in falling/staying asleep, dissatisfaction with sleep, nonrestorative sleep, lack of energy.

risk for compromised family Coping possibly evidenced by risk factors of inadequate or incorrect information or understanding by a primary person, temporary family disorganization and role changes, prolonged disability that exhausts the supportive capacity of SO(s).

impaired Social Interaction/Social Isolation may be related to low self-concept, inadequate personal resources, misinterpretation of internal or external stimuli, hypervigilance, possibly evidenced by discomfort in social situations, withdrawal from or reported change in pattern of interactions, dysfunctional interactions; expressed feelings of difference from others; sad, dull affect.

Anxiety disorders **PED/PSY**

Anxiety [severe/panic] may be related to situational or maturational crisis, internal transmission or contagion, threat to physical integrity or self-concept, unmet needs, dysfunctional family system, independence conflicts, possibly evidenced by somatic complaints, nightmares, excessive psychomotor activity, refusal to attend school, persistent worry, fear of catastrophic doom to family/self.

ineffective Coping may be related to maturational crisis, multiple life changes or losses, personal vulnerability, lack of self-confidence, possibly evidenced by inability to problem solve, persistent or overwhelming fears, inability to meet role expectations, social inhibition, panic attacks.

impaired Social Interaction may be related to excessive self-consciousness, inability to interact with unfamiliar people, altered thought processes possibly evidenced by verbalized or observed discomfort in social situations, inability to receive or communicate a satisfying sense of social engagement—belonging, caring, interest; use of unsuccessful social interaction behaviors.

risk for Self-Mutilation/self-directed Violence possibly evidenced by risk factors of panic states, dysfunctional family, history of self-destructive behaviors, emotional disturbance, increasing motor activity.

compromised/disabled family Coping may be related to situational or developmental crisis (e.g., divorce, addition to family, midlife crisis), unrealistic parental expectations, frequent disruptions in living arrangements, high-risk family situations (neglect or abuse, substance abuse), possibly evidenced by SO reports of frustration with clinging behaviors, emotional lability, harsh or punitive response to tyrannical behaviors, disproportionate protective behaviors.

Anxiolytic abuse **PSY**

Refer to Depressant abuse

Aortic aneurysm, abdominal (AAA) **MS**

risk for ineffective Renal Perfusion possibly evidenced by risk factors of hypertension, hypovolemia, hypoxia.

acute Pain may be related to physical agent [vascular enlargement-dissection or rupture], possibly evidenced by verbal coded reports, guarding behavior, facial mask, change in vital signs.

Aortic aneurysm repair, abdominal **MS**

Also refer to Surgery, general

Anxiety related to change in health status, threat of death, surgical intervention, possibly evidenced by expressed concerns, apprehension, increased tension, changes in vital signs.

risk for Bleeding possibly evidenced by risk factors of aneurysm, treatment-related side effects—surgery, failure of vascular repair.

risk for ineffective Renal Perfusion/peripheral Tissue Perfusion possibly evidenced by risk factors of hypertension, treatment-related side effects—surgery, hypovolemia, hypoxia.

Aortic insufficiency **MS/CH**

Refer to Valvular heart disease

Aortic stenosis **MS**

Also refer to Valvular heart disease

decreased Cardiac Output may be related to altered contractility, altered preload or afterload possibly evidenced by fatigue, dyspnea, changes in vital signs, jugular vein distension, increased CVP/PAWP, and syncope.

risk for impaired Gas Exchange possibly evidenced by risk factor of alveolar-capillary membrane changes.

CH

risk for acute Pain possibly evidenced by risk factors of physical agent [e.g, episodic ischemia of myocardial tissues and stretching of left atrium].

Activity Intolerance may be related to imbalance between oxygen supply and demand [decreased or fixed cardiac output], possibly evidenced by exertional dyspnea, reported fatigue, weakness, and abnormal blood pressure or electrocardiogram changes, dysrhythmias in response to activity.

Aplastic anemia **CH**

Also refer to Anemia

risk for ineffective Protection possibly evidenced by risk factors of abnormal blood profile (leukopenia, thrombocytopenia), drug therapies (antineoplastics, antibiotics, NSAIDs, anticonvulsants).

Fatigue may be related to anemia, disease states, malnutrition, possibly evidenced by verbalization of overwhelming lack of energy, inability to maintain usual routines or level of physical activity, tired, compromised libido, lethargy, increase in physical complaints.

Appendectomy **MS**

Also refer to Surgery, general

risk for Infection possibly evidenced by risk factors of release of pathogenic organisms into peritoneal cavity (prior to or at time of surgery).

Appendicitis **MS**

acute Pain may be related to physical agent [distention of intestinal tissues/inflammation], possibly evidenced by verbal reports, guarding behavior, narrowed focus, and autonomic responses (diaphoresis, changes in vital signs).

risk for deficient Fluid Volume possibly evidenced by risk factors of excessive losses through normal routes (vomiting), deviations affecting intake of fluids (nausea, anorexia), and factors influencing fluid needs (hypermetabolic state).

risk for Infection possibly evidenced by risk factors of tissue destruction [release of pathogenic organisms into peritoneal cavity].

ARDS **MS**

Refer to Respiratory distress syndrome, acute

Arrhythmia, cardiac **MS/CH**

Refer to Dysrhythmia, cardiac

Arterial occlusive disease, peripheral **CH**

ineffective peripheral Tissue Perfusion may be related to deficient knowledge of disease process [PAD], hypertension, smoking, sedentary lifestyle, possibly evidenced by skin characteristics, diminished pulses, claudication, delayed peripheral wound healing.

risk for impaired Walking possibly evidenced by limited endurance, pain.

risk for impaired Skin/Tissue Integrity possibly evidenced by risk factors of altered circulation and sensation.

Arthritis, gouty **CH**

Refer to Gout

Arthritis, juvenile rheumatoid **PED/CH**

Also refer to Arthritis, rheumatoid

risk for delayed Development possibly evidenced by risk factors of chronic illness, effects of required therapy.

risk for Social Isolation possibly evidenced by risk factors of delay in accomplishing developmental task, altered state of wellness, and alterations in physical appearance.

Arthritis, rheumatoid **CH**

acute/chronic Pain may be related to accumulation of fluid, inflammatory process, degeneration of joint, and deformity, possibly evidenced by verbal reports, narrowed focus, guarding or protective behaviors, and physical and social withdrawal.

impaired physical Mobility may be related to musculoskeletal deformity, pain or discomfort, decreased muscle strength, possibly evidenced by limited range of motion, impaired coordination, reluctance to attempt movement, and decreased muscle strength, control, and mass.

Self-Care deficit [specify] may be related to musculoskeletal impairment, decreased strength and endurance, limited range of motion, pain on movement, possibly evidenced by inability to manage activities of daily living.

disturbed Body Image/ineffective Role Performance may be related to change in body structure and function, impaired mobility or ability to perform usual tasks, focus on past strength, function, or appearance, possibly evidenced by negative self-talk, feelings of helplessness, change in lifestyle and physical abilities, dependence on others for assistance, decreased social involvement.

Arthritis, septic **CH**

acute Pain may be related to joint inflammation, possibly evidenced by verbal or coded reports, guarding behaviors, restlessness, narrowed focus.

impaired physical Mobility may be related to joint stiffness, pain or discomfort, reluctance to initiate movement, possibly evidenced by limited range of motion, slowed movement.

Self-Care deficit [specify] may be related to musculoskeletal impairment, pain or discomfort, decreased strength, impaired coordination, possibly evidenced by inability to perform desired activities of daily living.

risk for Infection, spread possibly evidenced by risk factors of presence of infectious process, chronic disease states, invasive procedures.

Arthroplasty **MS**

risk for Infection possibly evidenced by risk factors of breach of primary defenses (surgical incision), stasis of body fluids at operative site, and altered inflammatory response.

risk for Bleeding possibly evidenced by risk factors of surgical procedure, trauma to vascular area.

impaired physical Mobility may be related to decreased strength, pain, musculoskeletal changes, possibly evidenced by impaired coordination and reluctance to attempt movement.

acute Pain may be related to tissue trauma, local edema, possibly evidenced by verbal reports, narrowed focus, guarded movement, and autonomic responses (diaphoresis, changes in vital signs).

Arthroscopy, knee — MS

deficient Knowledge [Learning Need] regarding procedure, outcomes, and self-care needs may be related to unfamiliarity with information or resources, misinterpretations, possibly evidenced by questions and requests for information, misconceptions.

risk for impaired Walking possibly evidenced by joint stiffness, discomfort, prescribed movement restrictions, use of assistive device for ambulation.

Asbestosis — CH

impaired Gas Exchange may be related to alveolar-capillary membrane changes, ventilation perfusion imbalance, possibly evidenced by dyspnea, tachypnea, restlessness, clubbing of fingers, abnormal arterial blood gases.

Activity Intolerance may be related to imbalance between oxygen supply and demand, possibly evidenced by exertional dyspnea, decreased exercise tolerance, abnormal cardiopulmonary response to activity.

ineffective Airway Clearance may be related to inflammatory response to inhaled foreign body (asbestos fibers), smoking or secondhand smoke, infection, possibly evidenced by dyspnea, adventitious breath sounds, increased sputum.

risk for Infection possibly evidenced by risk factors of decrease in ciliary action, stasis of body fluids, chronic disease, malnutrition, insufficient knowledge to avoid exposure.

acute Pain may be related to inflammation or irritation of the parietal pleura, possibly evidenced by verbal reports, guarding or distraction behaviors, self-focus, and autonomic responses (changes in vital signs).

Asperger's disorder (now Autism spectrum disorder) — PED/PSY

impaired Social Interaction may be related to skill deficit about ways to enhance mutuality, communication barriers (poor pragmatic language skills), preoccupations, compulsions, repetitive motor mannerisms, possibly evidenced by observed discomfort in social situations, dysfunctional interactions with others, inability to receive or communicate satisfying sense of belonging.

risk for delayed Development possibly evidenced by risk factor of behavior disorder.

risk for Injury possibly evidenced by risk factors of rituals, repetitive motor mannerisms, clumsiness, poor coordination, vulnerability to manipulation or peer pressure.

Aspiration, foreign body — CH

ineffective Airway Clearance may be related to presence of foreign body, possibly evidenced by dyspnea, ineffective cough, diminished or adventitious breath sounds.

Anxiety [specify] may be related to situational crisis, perceived threat of death, possibly evidenced by apprehension, fearfulness, pupil dilation, increased tension.

risk for Suffocation possibly evidenced by risk factors of lack of safety education or precautions, eating large mouthfuls or pieces of food.

Asthma — MS

Also refer to Emphysema

ineffective Airway Clearance may be related to increased production and retained pulmonary secretions, bronchospasm, decreased energy, fatigue, possibly evidenced by wheezing, difficulty breathing, changes in depth and rate of respirations, use of accessory muscles, and persistent ineffective cough with or without sputum production.

impaired Gas Exchange may be related to altered delivery of inspired oxygen, air trapping, possibly evidenced by dyspnea, restlessness, reduced tolerance for activity, cyanosis, and changes in arterial blood gases and vital signs.

Anxiety [specify level] may be related to perceived threat of death, possibly evidenced by apprehension, fearful expression, and extraneous movements.

CH

Activity Intolerance may be related to imbalance between oxygen supply and demand, possibly evidenced by fatigue and exertional dyspnea.

risk for Contamination possibly evidenced by risk factors of presence of atmospheric pollutants, environmental contaminants in the home (e.g., smoking or secondhand tobacco smoke).

Atelectasis — MS

impaired Gas Exchange may be related to inflammatory process, stasis of secretions affecting oxygen exchange across alveolar membrane, and hypoventilation, possibly evidenced by restlessness, changes in mentation, dyspnea, tachycardia, pallor, cyanosis, and arterial blood gases/oximetry evidence of hypoxia.

Atherosclerosis — CH/MS

Refer to Coronary artery disease: Peripheral vascular disease

Athlete's foot CH

impaired Skin Integrity may be related to fungal invasion, humidity, secretions, possibly evidenced by disruption of skin surface, reports of painful itching.

risk for Infection [spread] possibly evidenced by risk factors of multiple breaks in skin, exposure to moist, warm environment.

Atrial fibrillation CH

Also refer to Dysrhythmia, cardiac

Activity Intolerance may be related to imbalance between oxygen supply and demand, possibly evidenced by dyspnea, dizziness, presyncope, or syncopal episodes.

risk for ineffective cerebral Tissue Perfusion possibly evidenced by risk factors of arterial fibrillation, embolism, thrombolytic therapy.

Atrial flutter CH

Also refer to Dysrhythmia, cardiac

Anxiety [specify] may be related to threat to or change in health status, possibly evidenced by expressed concerns, apprehension, awareness of physiological symptoms (palpitations, dizziness, presyncope or syncopal episodes), focus on self.

Atrial tachycardia CH

Refer to Dysrhythmia, cardiac

Attention deficit disorder PED/PSY

ineffective Coping may be related to situational or maturational crisis, retarded ego development, low self-concept, possibly evidenced by easy distraction by extraneous stimuli, shifting between uncompleted activities.

chronic low Self-Esteem may be related to retarded ego development, lack of positive or repeated negative feedback, negative role models, possibly evidenced by lack of eye contact, derogatory self-comments, hesitance to try new tasks, inadequate level of confidence.

deficient Knowledge [Learning Need] regarding condition, prognosis, and therapy may be related to misinformation or misinterpretations, unfamiliarity with resources, possibly evidenced by verbalization of problems or misconceptions, poor school performance, unrealistic expectations of medication regimen.

Autism spectrum disorder PED/PSY

impaired Social Interaction may be related to abnormal response to sensory input, inadequate sensory stimulation, organic brain dysfunction; delayed development of secure attachment or trust, lack of intuitive skills to comprehend and accurately respond to social cues, disturbance in self-concept, possibly evidenced by lack of responsiveness to others, lack of eye contact or facial responsiveness, treating persons as objects, lack of awareness of feelings in others, indifference or aversion to comfort, affection, or physical contact; failure to develop cooperative social play and peer friendships in childhood.

impaired verbal Communication may be related to inability to trust others, withdrawal into self, organic brain dysfunction, abnormal interpretation or response to or inadequate sensory stimulation, possibly evidenced by lack of interactive communication mode, no use of gestures or spoken language, absent or abnormal nonverbal communication; lack of eye contact or facial expression; peculiar patterns of speech (form, content, or speech production), and impaired ability to initiate or sustain conversation despite adequate speech.

risk for Self-Mutilation possibly evidenced by risk factors of organic brain dysfunction, inability to trust others, disturbance in self-concept, inadequate sensory stimulation, or abnormal response to sensory input (sensory overload); history of physical, emotional, or sexual abuse; and response to demands of therapy, realization of severity of condition.

disturbed Personal Identity may be related to organic brain dysfunction, lack of development of trust, fixation at presymbiotic phase of development, possibly evidenced by lack of awareness of the feelings or existence of others, increased anxiety resulting from physical contact with others, absent or impaired imitation of others, repeating what others say, persistent preoccupation with parts of objects, obsessive attachment to objects, marked distress over changes in environment; autoerotic or ritualistic behaviors, self-touching, rocking, swaying.

compromised/disabled family Coping may be related to family members unable to express feelings; excessive guilt, anger, or blaming among family members regarding child's condition; ambivalent or dissonant family relationships, prolonged coping with problem exhausting supportive ability of family members, possibly evidenced by denial of existence or severity of disturbed behaviors, preoccupation with personal emotional reaction to situation, rationalization that problem will be outgrown, attempts to intervene with child are achieving increasingly ineffective results, family withdraws from or becomes overly protective of child.

Bacteremia **MS**
Refer to Sepsis

Barbiturate abuse **CH/PSY**
Refer to Depressant abuse

Battered child syndrome **PED/CH**
Also refer to Abuse, physical

risk for Trauma possibly evidenced by risk factors of dependent position in relationship(s), vulnerability (e.g., congenital problems/chronic illness), history of previous abuse or neglect, lack or nonuse of support systems by caregiver(s).

risk for disproportionate Growth and/or delayed Development possibly evidenced by risk factors of presence of abuse, exposure to violence, inadequate nutrition/malnutrition; caregiver mental health issue, substance abuse, unplanned/unwanted pregnancy.

interrupted Family Processes/impaired Parenting may be related to poor role model, unrealistic expectations, presence of stressors, and lack of support, possibly evidenced by verbalization of negative feelings, inappropriate caretaking behaviors, and evidence of physical or psychological trauma to child.

PSY

chronic low Self-Esteem may be related to deprivation and negative feedback of family members, personal vulnerability, feelings of abandonment, possibly evidenced by lack of eye contact, withdrawal from social contacts, discounting own needs, nonassertive or passive, indecisive, or overly conforming behaviors.

Post-Trauma Syndrome may be related to sustained or recurrent physical or emotional abuse; possibly evidenced by acting-out behavior, development of phobias, poor impulse control, and emotional numbness.

Bedsores **CH/MS**
Refer to Ulcer, pressure

Bed-wetting **PED**
Refer to Enuresis

Benign prostatic hyperplasia **CH/MS**
[acute/chronic] Urinary Retention/overflow urinary Incontinence may be related to mechanical obstruction (enlarged prostate), decompensation of detrusor musculature, inability of bladder to contract adequately, possibly evidenced by frequency, hesitancy, inability to empty bladder completely, incontinence or dribbling, nocturia, bladder distention, residual urine.

acute Pain may be related to mucosal irritation, bladder distention, colic, urinary infection, and radiation therapy, possibly evidenced by verbal reports of bladder or rectal spasm, narrowed focus, altered muscle tone, grimacing, distraction behaviors, restlessness, and autonomic responses.

risk for deficient Fluid Volume/Electrolyte Imbalance possibly evidenced by risk factors of active fluid volume loss—postobstructive diuresis, endocrine or renal dysfunction.

Fear/Anxiety [specify level] may be related to change in health status (possibility of surgical procedure, malignancy); embarrassment, loss of dignity associated with genital exposure before, during, and after treatment, and concern about sexual ability, possibly evidenced by increased tension, apprehension, worry, expressed concerns regarding perceived changes, and fear of unspecific consequences.

Besnier-Boeck disease **CH**
Refer to Sarcoidosis

Biliary calculus **CH/MS**
Refer to Cholelithiasis

Biliary cancer **MS**
Also refer to Cancer

imbalanced Nutrition: less than body requirements may be related to inability to ingest or absorb nutrients (anorexia, nausea, indigestion), abdominal discomfort, possibly evidenced by aversion to eating, observed lack of intake, muscle wasting, weight loss, and imbalances in nutritional studies.

risk for impaired Skin Integrity possibly evidenced by risk factors of accumulation of bile salts in skin, poor skin turgor, skeletal prominence.

Death Anxiety may be related to lack of successful treatment options, poor prognosis, possibly evidenced by fear of the process of dying, leaving SO/family alone after death, negative death images, concern of overworking caregiver, deep sadness.

Binge-eating disorder **PSY**
Refer to Bulimia nervosa

Bipolar disorder **PSY**
risk for other-directed Violence possibly evidenced by risk factors of irritability, impulsive behavior; delu-

sional thinking; angry response when ideas are refuted or wishes denied; manic excitement, with possible indicators of threatening body language or verbalizations, increased motor activity, overt and aggressive acts, hostility.

imbalanced Nutrition: less than body requirements may be related to inadequate intake in relation to metabolic expenditures, possibly evidenced by body weight 20% or more below ideal weight, observed inadequate intake, inattention to mealtimes, and distraction from task of eating; laboratory evidence of nutritional deficits or imbalances.

risk for Poisoning [lithium toxicity] possibly evidenced by risk factors of narrow therapeutic range of drug, client's ability (or lack of) to follow through with medication regimen and monitoring, and denial of need for information or therapy.

Insomnia may be related to psychological stress, lack of recognition of fatigue/need to sleep, hyperactivity, possibly evidenced by denial of need to sleep, interrupted nighttime sleep, one or more nights without sleep, changes in behavior and performance, increasing irritability, restlessness, and dark circles under eyes.

[disturbed Sensory Perception (specify)]/Stress overload may be related to decrease in sensory threshold, endogenous chemical alteration, psychological stress, sleep deprivation, possibly evidenced by increased distractibility and agitation, anxiety, disorientation, poor concentration, auditory or visual hallucination, bizarre thinking, and motor incoordination.

interrupted Family Processes may be related to situational crises (illness, economics, change in roles); euphoric mood and grandiose ideas or actions of client, manipulative behavior and limit-testing, client's refusal to accept responsibility for own actions, possibly evidenced by statements of difficulty coping with situation, lack of adaptation to change, or not dealing constructively with illness; ineffective family decision-making process, failure to send and receive clear messages, and inappropriate boundary maintenance.

Bladder cancer — MS

Also refer to Cancer; Urinary diversion

impaired urinary Elimination may be related to presence of tumor, possibly evidenced by frequency, burning, dysuria.

acute/chronic Urinary Retention may be related to blockage of urethra, possibly evidenced by sensation of fullness, bladder distention, residual urine, dysuria.

Body dysmorphic disorder — PSY

Refer to Hypochondriasis

Bone cancer — MS/CH

Also refer to Myeloma, multiple; Amputation

acute Pain may be related to bone destruction, pressure on nerves, possibly evidenced by verbal or coded report, protective behavior, autonomic responses.

risk for Trauma possibly evidenced by risk factors of increased bone fragility, general weakness, balancing difficulties.

Bone marrow transplantation — MS/CH

Also refer to Transplantation, recipient

risk for Injury possibly evidenced by risk factors of immune dysfunction or suppression, abnormal blood profile, action of donor T cells.

deficient Diversional Activity may be related to hospitalization or length of treatment, restriction of visitors, limitation of activities, possibly evidenced by expressions of boredom, restlessness, withdrawal, and requests for something to do.

risk for imbalanced Nutrition: less than body requirements possibly evidenced by risk factors of increased metabolic needs for healing, altered ability to ingest nutrients—nausea, vomiting, loss of appetite, taste changes, oral lesions.

Borderline personality disorder — PSY

risk for self-/other-directed Violence/Self-Mutilation possibly evidenced by risk factors of use of projection as a major defense mechanism, pervasive problems with negative transference, feelings of guilt or need to "punish" self, distorted sense of self, inability to cope with increased psychological or physiological tension in a healthy manner.

Anxiety [severe to panic] may be related to unconscious conflicts (experience of extreme stress), perceived threat to self-concept, unmet needs, possibly evidenced by easy frustration and feelings of hurt, abuse of alcohol or other drugs, transient psychotic symptoms, and performance of self-mutilating acts.

chronic low Self-Esteem/disturbed Personal Identity may be related to lack of positive feedback, unmet dependency needs, retarded ego development—fixation at an earlier level of development, possibly evidenced by difficulty identifying self or defining self-boundaries, feelings of depersonalization, extreme mood changes, lack of tolerance of rejection or of being alone, unhappiness with self, striking out at others, performance of ritualistic self-damaging acts, and belief that punishing self is necessary.

Social Isolation may be related to immature interests, unaccepted social behavior, inadequate personal resources, and inability to engage in satisfying personal relationships, possibly evidenced by alternating clinging and distancing behaviors, difficulty meeting expectations of others, experiencing feelings of difference from others, expressing interests inappropriate to developmental age, and exhibiting behavior unaccepted by dominant cultural group.

Botulism (food-borne) **MS**

deficient Fluid Volume may be related to active losses (vomiting, diarrhea, decreased intake), nausea, dysphagia, possibly evidenced by reports of thirst; dry skin or mucous membranes, decreased blood pressure and urine output, change in mental state, increased hematocrit.

impaired physical Mobility may be related to neuromuscular impairment, possibly evidenced by limited ability to perform gross or fine motor skills.

Anxiety [specify level]/Fear may be related to threat of death, interpersonal transmission, possibly evidenced by expressed concerns, apprehension, awareness of physiological symptoms, focus on self.

risk for impaired spontaneous Ventilation possibly evidenced by risk factors of neuromuscular impairment, presence of infectious process.

CH

Contamination may be related to lack of proper precautions in food storage or preparation as evidenced by gastrointestinal and neurological effects of exposure to biological agent.

Bowel obstruction **MS**

Refer to Ileus

Bowel resection **CH**

Refer to Intestinal surgery (without diversion)

BPH **CH/MS**

Refer to Benign prostatic hyperplasia

Brachytherapy (radioactive implants) **MS**

risk for Injury possibly evidenced by risk factors of radiation emitted by client (depending on type of procedure), accidental dislodgement or removal of radiation source.

risk for impaired physical Mobility possibly evidenced by risk factors of prescribed restrictions (48 hours for low-dose implants), reluctance to move (fear of dislodging implants), decreased strength or endurance, depressed mood.

Bradycardia **CH**

Refer to Dysrhythmia, cardiac

Brain attack **MS**

Refer to Cerebrovascular accident

Brain tumor **MS**

Also refer to Cancer

acute Pain may be related to pressure on brain tissues, possibly evidenced by reports of headache, facial mask of pain, narrowed focus, and autonomic responses (changes in vital signs).

impaired Memory may be related to neurological disturbances possibly evidenced by reports of experience of forgetting, inability to recall events/factual information.

[disturbed Sensory Perception (specify)] may be related to altered sensory reception/integration, possibly evidenced by changes in sensory acuity, change in behavior pattern, poor concentration/problem-solving abilities, disorientation.

risk for deficient Fluid Volume possibly evidenced by risk factors of recurrent vomiting from irritation of vagal center in medulla and decreased intake.

Self-Care deficit [specify] may be related to sensory or neuromuscular impairment interfering with ability to perform tasks, possibly evidenced by unkempt or disheveled appearance, body odor, and verbalization or observation of inability to perform activities of daily living.

Breast cancer **MS/CH**

Also refer to Cancer

Anxiety [specify level] may be related to change in health status, threat of death, stress, interpersonal transmission, possibly evidenced by expressed concerns, apprehension, uncertainty, focus on self, diminished productivity.

deficient Knowledge [Learning Need] regarding diagnosis, prognosis, and treatment options may be related to lack of exposure or unfamiliarity with information resources, information misinterpretation, cognitive limitation, anxiety, possibly evidenced by verbalizations, statements of misconceptions, inappropriate behaviors.

risk for disturbed Body Image possibly evidenced by risk factor of surgical procedure, alteration in self-perception.

risk for Sexual dysfunction possibly evidenced by risk factors of health-related changes, medical treatments, concern about relationship with SO.

Bronchitis CH

ineffective Airway Clearance may be related to excessive, thickened mucous secretions, possibly evidenced by presence of rhonchi, tachypnea, and ineffective cough.

Activity Intolerance [specify level] may be related to imbalance between oxygen supply and demand, general weakness, exhaustion—interruption in usual sleep pattern due to cough, discomfort, dyspnea, possibly evidenced by reports of fatigue, dyspnea, and abnormal vital sign response to activity.

acute Pain may be related to inflammation of lung parenchyma, persistent cough, cellular reactions to circulating toxins, possibly evidenced by reports of pleuritic chest pain, guarding affected area, distraction behaviors, and restlessness.

Bronchogenic carcinoma MS/CH

Also refer to Cancer

impaired Gas Exchange may be related to ventilation perfusion imbalance (bronchial narrowing with air trapping, atelectasis), presence of inflammatory exudate possibly evidenced by dyspnea, diminished or adventitious breath sounds, decreased chest expansion (depth of breathing), abnormal arterial blood gases.

risk for ineffective Airway Clearance possibly evidenced by risk factors of retained secretions, inflammatory exudate, bronchial narrowing, pain, smoking or secondhand smoke, infection.

risk for Infection possibly evidenced by risk factors of stasis of body fluids, tissue destruction, chronic disease, malnutrition.

Bronchopneumonia MS/CH

Also refer to Bronchitis

ineffective Airway Clearance may be related to tracheal bronchial inflammation, edema formation, increased sputum production, pleuritic pain, decreased energy, fatigue, possibly evidenced by changes in rate and depth of respirations, abnormal breath sounds, use of accessory muscles, dyspnea, cyanosis, cough with or without sputum production.

impaired Gas Exchange may be related to inflammatory alveolar-capillary membrane changes, ventilation-perfusion mismatch—collection of secretions affecting oxygen exchange across alveolar membrane, hypoventilation, altered release of oxygen at cellular level—fever, shifting oxyhemoglobin curve, possibly evidenced by restlessness, changes in mentation, dyspnea, tachycardia, pallor, cyanosis, and arterial blood gas or oximetry evidence of hypoxia.

risk for Infection [spread] possibly evidenced by risk factors of decreased ciliary action, stasis of secretions, presence of existing infection, immunosuppression, chronic disease, malnutrition.

Brown-Sequard syndrome MS/CH

Also refer to Paraplegia; Quadriplegia

impaired physical Mobility may be related to neuromuscular and sensoriperceptual impairment, possibly evidenced by limited motion, weakness, or paralysis (hemiparaplegia).

[disturbed kinesthetic/tactile Sensory Perception] may be related to altered sensory transmission (e.g., neurological trauma, ischemia, inflammation, infection), possibly evidenced by reported change in sensory acuity—loss of touch, vibration, and position on one side of the body, loss of pain and temperature sensation on opposite side of body (hemianesthesia).

Buck's traction MS

Refer to Traction

Buerger's disease CH

Refer to Peripheral vascular disease

Bulimia nervosa PSY/MS

Also refer to Anorexia nervosa

impaired Dentition may be related to dietary habits, poor oral hygiene, chronic vomiting, possibly evidenced by erosion of tooth enamel, multiple caries, abraded teeth.

impaired oral Mucous Membrane may be related to malnutrition or vitamin deficiency, poor oral hygiene, chronic vomiting, possibly evidenced by sore, inflamed buccal mucosa; swollen salivary glands; ulcerations of mucosa; reports of constant sore mouth or throat.

risk for deficient Fluid Volume possibly evidenced by risk factors of consistent self-induced vomiting, excessive laxative or diuretic use, esophageal erosion or tear (Mallory-Weiss syndrome).

deficient Knowledge [Learning Need] regarding condition, prognosis, complications, and treatment may be related to lack of exposure or recall, unfamiliarity with information about condition, learned maladaptive coping skills, possibly evidenced by verbalization of misconception of relationship of current situation and bingeing and purging behaviors, distortion of body image, verbalization of the problem.

Bunion CH

impaired Walking may be related to inflammation and degeneration of joint, inappropriate footwear, possibly evidenced by inability to walk required distances.

Bunionectomy MS

Also refer to Surgery, general; Postoperative recovery period

impaired Walking may be related to surgical intervention, restrictive therapy, possibly evidenced by inability to walk required distances, navigate curbs, climb stairs.

Burns (dependent on type, degree, and severity of the injury) MS/CH

risk for deficient Fluid Volume/Bleeding possibly evidenced by risk factors of loss of fluids through wounds, capillary damage and evaporation, hypermetabolic state, insufficient intake, hemorrhagic losses.

risk for ineffective Airway Clearance possibly evidenced by risk factors of tracheobronchial obstruction—mucosal edema and loss of ciliary action with smoke inhalation; circumferential full-thickness burns of the neck, thorax, and chest, with compression of the airway or limited chest excursion, trauma—direct upper airway injury by flame, steam, chemicals or gases; fluid shifts, pulmonary edema, decreased lung compliance.

risk for Infection possibly evidenced by risk factors of loss of protective dermal barrier, traumatized tissue, necrosis, decreased hemoglobin, suppressed inflammatory response, environmental exposure/invasive procedures.

acute/chronic Pain may be related to destruction of skin, tissue, and nerves; edema formation; and manipulation of injured tissues, possibly evidenced by verbal reports, narrowed focus, distraction and guarding behaviors, facial mask of pain, and changes in vital signs.

risk for imbalanced Nutrition: less than body requirements possibly evidenced by risk factors of hypermetabolic state as much as 50% to 60% higher than normal proportional to the severity of injury, protein catabolism, anorexia, restricted oral intake.

Post-Trauma Syndrome may be related to life-threatening event, possibly evidenced by reexperiencing the event, repetitive dreams or nightmares, psychic or emotional numbness, and sleep disturbance.

ineffective Protection may be related to extremes of age, inadequate nutrition, anemia, impaired immune system, possibly evidenced by impaired healing, deficient immunity, fatigue, anorexia.

PED

deficient Diversional Activity may be related to long-term hospitalization, frequent lengthy treatments, and physical limitations, possibly evidenced by expressions of boredom, restlessness, withdrawal, and requests for something to do.

risk for delayed Development possibly evidenced by risk factors of effects of physical disability, separation from SO(s), and environmental deficiencies.

Bursitis CH

acute/chronic Pain may be related to inflammation of affected joint, possibly evidenced by verbal reports, guarding behavior, and narrowed focus.

impaired physical Mobility may be related to inflammation and swelling of joint and pain, possibly evidenced by diminished range of motion, reluctance to attempt movement, and imposed restriction of movement by medical treatment.

CABG MS

Refer to Coronary artery bypass surgery

CAD CH/MS

Refer to Coronary artery disease

Calculi, urinary CH/MS

acute Pain may be related to increased frequency or force of ureteral contractions, tissue trauma, edema formation, cellular ischemia, possibly evidenced by reports of sudden, severe, colicky pains; guarding and distraction behaviors; self-focus; and autonomic responses.

impaired urinary Elimination may be related to stimulation of the bladder by calculi, renal or ureteral irritation, mechanical obstruction of urinary flow, inflammation, possibly evidenced by urgency and frequency, oliguria, hematuria.

risk for deficient Fluid Volume possibly evidenced by risk factors of stimulation of renal-intestinal reflexes causing nausea, vomiting, and diarrhea; changes in urinary output, postobstructive diuresis.

deficient Knowledge [Learning Need] regarding condition, prognosis, self-care, and treatment needs may be related to lack of exposure or recall and information misinterpretation, possibly evidenced by requests for information, statements of concern, and recurrence or development of preventable complications.

Cancer **MS**

Also refer to Chemotherapy; Radiation therapy

Fear/Death Anxiety may be related to situational crises, threat to or change in health, socioeconomic status, role functioning, or interaction patterns; threat of death, separation from family, interpersonal transmission of feelings, possibly evidenced by expressed concerns, feelings of inadequacy/helplessness, insomnia; increased tension, restlessness, focus on self, sympathetic stimulation.

Grieving may be related to potential loss of physiological well-being (body part or function), change in lifestyle, perceived potential death, possibly evidenced by anger, sadness, withdrawal, choked feelings, changes in eating or sleep patterns, activity level, libido, and communication patterns.

acute/chronic Pain may be related to the disease process (compression of nerve tissue, infiltration of nerves or their vascular supply, obstruction of a nerve pathway, inflammation), or side effects of therapeutic agents, possibly evidenced by verbal reports, self-focusing or narrowed focus, alteration in muscle tone, facial mask of pain, distraction or guarding behaviors, autonomic responses, and restlessness.

Fatigue may be related to decreased metabolic energy production, increased energy requirements—hypermetabolic state; overwhelming psychological or emotional demands, and altered body chemistry—side effects of medications, chemotherapy, radiation therapy, biotherapy, possibly evidenced by unremitting or overwhelming lack of energy, inability to maintain usual routines, decreased performance, impaired ability to concentrate, lethargy, listlessness, and disinterest in surroundings.

impaired Home Maintenance may be related to debilitation, lack of resources, or inadequate support systems, possibly evidenced by verbalization of problem, request for assistance, and lack of necessary equipment or aids.

PED

risk for interrupted Family Processes possibly evidenced by risk factors of situational or transitional crises—long-term illness, change in roles or economic status; developmental—anticipated loss of a family member.

readiness for enhanced family Coping possibly evidenced by verbalizations of impact of crisis on own values, priorities, goals, or relationships.

Candidiasis **CH**

Also refer to Thrush

impaired Skin/Tissue Integrity may be related to infectious lesions, possibly evidenced by disruption of skin surfaces and mucous membranes.

acute Pain/impaired Comfort may be related to exposure of irritated skin and mucous membranes to excretions (urine, feces), possibly evidenced by verbal or coded reports, restlessness, guarding behaviors.

risk for Sexual dysfunction risk factors include presence of infectious process, vaginal discomfort.

Cannabis abuse **CH**

Refer to Depressant abuse

Carbon monoxide poisoning **MS**

impaired Gas Exchange may be related to altered oxygen-carrying capacity of blood, possibly evidenced by headache, confusion, somnolence, elevated carbon monoxide levels.

Activity Intolerance may be related to imbalance between oxygen supply and demand, possibly evidenced by fatigue, exertional dyspnea.

risk for Trauma/Suffocation possibly evidenced by risk factors of cognitive limitations, altered consciousness, loss of large- or small-muscle coordination (seizure).

Cardiac catheterization **MS**

Anxiety [specify] may be related to threat to or change in health status, stress, family heredity, possibly evidenced by expressed concerns, apprehension, uncertainty, focus on self.

risk for decreased Cardiac Output possibly evidenced by risk factors of altered heart rate or rhythm (vasovagal response, ventricular dysrhythmias), decreased myocardial contractility (ischemia).

risk for decreased cardiac Tissue Perfusion (specify) may be related to coronary artery spasm, hypovolemia, hypoxia [thrombosis, emboli].

risk for adverse Reaction to Iodinated Contrast Media risk factors may include underlying disease—possibly evidenced by risk factors of heart disease, concurrent use of medications (e.g., beta blockers, metformin), history of allergies.

Cardiac conditions, prenatal **OB**

Also refer to Pregnancy, high-risk

risk for Cardiac Output [decompensation] possibly evidenced by risk factors of increased circulating volume, dysrhythmias, altered myocardial contractility, inotropic changes in the heart.

risk for excess Fluid Volume possibly evidenced by risk factors of increasing circulating volume, changes in renal function, dietary indiscretion.

risk for ineffective uteroplacental Tissue Perfusion possibly evidenced by risk factors of changes in circulating volume, right-to-left shunt.

risk for Activity Intolerance possibly evidenced by risk factors of presence of circulatory problems, previous episodes of intolerance, deconditioned status.

Cardiac inflammatory disease **MS**

Refer to Endocarditis; Myocarditis; Pericarditis

Cardiac surgery **MS/PED**

risk for decreased Cardiac Output possibly evidenced by risk factors of altered myocardial contractility secondary to temporary factors—ventricular wall surgery, recent myocardial infarction, response to certain medications or drug interactions; altered preload—hypovolemia, and afterload—systemic vascular resistance; altered heart rate or rhythm—dysrhythmias.

risk for Bleeding/deficient Fluid Volume possibly evidenced by risk factors of intraoperative bleeding with inadequate blood replacement; bleeding related to insufficient heparin reversal, fibrinolysis, or platelet destruction; or volume depletion effects of intraoperative or postoperative diuretic therapy.

risk for impaired Gas Exchange possibly evidenced by risk factors of alveolar-capillary membrane changes (atelectasis), intestinal edema, inadequate function or premature discontinuation of chest tubes, and diminished oxygen-carrying capacity of the blood.

acute Pain/impaired Comfort may be related to tissue inflammation or trauma, edema formation, intraoperative nerve trauma, and myocardial ischemia, possibly evidenced by reports of incisional discomfort or pain in chest and donor site; paresthesia or pain in hand, arm, shoulder, anxiety, restlessness, irritability; distraction behaviors, and changes in heart rate and blood pressure.

impaired Skin/Tissue Integrity related to mechanical trauma (surgical incisions, puncture wounds) and edema evidenced by disruption of skin surface and tissues.

Cardiogenic shock **MS**

Refer to Shock, cardiogenic

Cardiomyopathy **CH/MS**

decreased Cardiac Output may be related to altered contractility, possibly evidenced by dyspnea, fatigue, chest pain, dizziness, syncope.

Activity Intolerance may be related to imbalance between oxygen supply and demand, possibly evidenced by weakness, fatigue, dyspnea, abnormal heart rate or blood pressure response to activity, electrocardiogram changes.

ineffective Role Performance may be related to changes in physical health, stress, demands of job and life, possibly evidenced by change in usual patterns of responsibility, role strain, change in capacity to resume role.

Carotid endarterectomy **MS**

Also refer to Surgery, general

risk for ineffective cerebral Tissue Perfusion possibly evidenced by risk factors of carotid stenosis, embolism, thrombolytic therapy.

Carpal tunnel syndrome **CH/MS**

acute/chronic Pain may be related to pressure on median nerve, possibly evidenced by verbal reports, reluctance to use affected extremity, guarding behaviors, expressed fear of reinjury, altered ability to continue previous activities.

impaired physical Mobility may be related to neuromuscular impairment and pain, possibly evidenced by decreased hand strength, weakness, limited range of motion, and reluctance to attempt movement.

risk for peripheral neurovascular Dysfunction possibly evidenced by risk factors of mechanical compression (e.g., brace, repetitive tasks or motions), immobilization.

deficient Knowledge [Learning Need] regarding condition, prognosis, and treatment and safety needs may be related to lack of exposure or recall, information misinterpretation, possibly evidenced by questions, statements of concern, request for information, inaccurate follow-through of instructions, development of preventable complications.

Casts **CH/MS**

Also refer to Fractures

risk for peripheral neurovascular Dysfunction possibly evidenced by risk factors of presence of fracture(s), mechanical compression (cast), tissue trauma, immobilization, vascular obstruction.

risk for impaired Skin Integrity possibly evidenced by risk factors of pressure of cast, moisture or debris under cast, objects inserted under cast to relieve itching, or altered sensation or circulation.

Self-Care deficit [specify] may be related to impaired ability to perform self-care tasks, possibly evidenced by statements of need for assistance and observed difficulty in performing activities of daily living.

Cataract **CH**

[disturbed visual Sensory Perception] may be related to altered sensory reception or status of sense organs, possibly evidenced by diminished acuity, visual distortions, and change in usual response to stimuli.

risk for Trauma possibly evidenced by risk factors of poor vision, reduced hand-eye coordination.

Anxiety [specify level]/Fear may be related to alteration in visual acuity, threat of permanent loss of vision and independence, possibly evidenced by expressed concerns, apprehension, and feelings of uncertainty.

deficient Knowledge [Learning Need] regarding ways of coping with altered abilities, therapy choices, and lifestyle changes may be related to lack of exposure or recall, misinterpretation, or cognitive limitations, possibly evidenced by requests for information, statement of concern, inaccurate follow-through of instructions, development of preventable complications.

Cataract extraction (postoperative care) **MS**

risk for Injury possibly evidenced by risk factors of increased intraocular pressure, intraocular hemorrhage, vitreous loss.

risk for Infection possibly evidenced by risk factors of invasive procedure, surgical manipulation, presence of chronic disease.

[disturbed visual Sensory Perception] may be related to altered sensory reception (use of eyedrops, cataract glasses), therapeutically restricted environment (surgical procedure, patching), possibly evidenced by visual distortions or blurring, visual confusion, change in depth perception.

Cat scratch disease **CH**

acute Pain may be related to effects of circulating toxins (fever, headache, and lymphadenitis), possibly evidenced by verbal reports, guarding behavior, and autonomic response (changes in vital signs).

Hyperthermia may be related to inflammatory process, possibly evidenced by increased body temperature, flushed warm skin, tachypnea, and tachycardia.

Celiac disease **CH**

imbalanced Nutrition: less than body requirements may be related to inability to absorb nutrients (mucosal damage, loss of villi, proliferation of crypt cells, shortened transit time through gastrointestinal tract), possibly evidenced by weight loss, abdominal distention, steatorrhea, evidence of anemia, vitamin deficiencies.

Diarrhea may be related to irritation, malabsorption, possibly evidenced by abdominal pain, hyperactive bowel sounds, at least three loose stools per day.

risk for deficient Fluid Volume possibly evidenced by risk factors of mild to massive steatorrhea, diarrhea.

Cellulitis **CH/MS**

risk for Infection [abscess, bacteremia] possibly evidenced by risk factors of broken skin, chronic disease, presence of pathogens, insufficient knowledge to avoid exposure to pathogens.

acute Pain/impaired Comfort may be related to inflammatory process, circulating toxins, possibly evidenced by reports of localized pain, headache, guarding behaviors, restlessness, autonomic responses.

impaired Tissue Integrity may be related to trauma, inflammation, or invasion of tissues by infectious bacterial agent, or altered circulation, possibly evidenced by redness, warmth, edema, tenderness, or pain under the surface of skin or deep in tissues.

Cerebral embolism **MS/CH**

Refer to Cerebrovascular accident

Cerebral palsy **PED/CH**

Refer to Palsy, cerebral

Cerebrovascular accident **MS**

ineffective cerebral Tissue Perfusion may be related to interruption of blood flow (occlusive disorder, hemorrhage, cerebral vasospasm or edema), possibly evidenced by altered level of consciousness, changes in vital signs, changes in motor or sensory responses, restlessness, memory loss; sensory, language, intellectual, and emotional deficits.

impaired physical Mobility may be related to neuromuscular involvement (weakness, paresthesia, flaccid or hypotonic paralysis, spastic paralysis), perceptual or cognitive impairment, possibly evidenced by inability to purposefully move involved body parts, limited range of motion; impaired coordination or decreased muscle strength or control.

impaired verbal [and/or written] Communication may be related to impaired cerebral circulation, neuromuscular impairment, loss of facial or oral muscle tone and control; generalized weakness, fatigue, possibly evidenced by impaired articulation, does not or cannot speak (dysarthria); inability to modulate speech, find or name words, identify objects, or inability to comprehend written/spoken language; inability to produce written communication.

Self-Care deficit [specify] may be related to neuromuscular impairment, decreased strength or endurance, loss of muscle control or coordination, perceptual or cognitive impairment, pain, discomfort, and depression, possibly evidenced by stated or observed inability to perform activities of daily living, requests for assistance, disheveled appearance, and incontinence.

risk for impaired Swallowing possibly evidenced by risk factors of muscle paralysis and perceptual impairment.

risk for Unilateral Neglect possibly evidenced by risk factors of sensory loss of part of visual field with perceptual loss of corresponding body segment.

CH

situational low Self-Esteem/disturbed Body Image may be related to functional impairment, loss, focus on past function/strength, and cognitive or perceptual changes, possibly evidenced by actual change in function, self-negating verbalizations, report of perceptions reflecting altered view of body function.

Grieving may be related to loss of processes of body [neuromuscular impairments]; loss of job, role function, status, or independence, possibly evidenced by psychological distress, despair, anger, disorganization.

impaired Home Maintenance may be related to condition of individual family member, insufficient finances, family organization or planning; unfamiliarity with resources, and inadequate support systems, possibly evidenced by members expressing difficulty in managing home in a comfortable manner, requesting assistance with home maintenance, disorderly surroundings, and overtaxed family members.

Cervix, dysfunctional — OB

Refer to Dilation of Cervix, premature

Cesarean birth — OB

Also refer to Cesarean birth, unplanned/postpartal

deficient Knowledge [Learning Need] regarding surgical procedure, expectation, postoperative routines and therapy, and self-care needs may be related to lack of information or misinterpretation, possibly evidenced by statements of concern, questions, and misconceptions.

risk for deficient Fluid Volume/Bleeding possibly evidenced by risk factors of restrictions of oral intake, blood loss.

risk for impaired Attachment possibly evidenced by risk factors of separation, existing health conditions maternal/infant, lack of privacy.

Cesarean birth, postpartal — OB

Also refer to Postpartum periods

risk for impaired Attachment possibly evidenced by risk factors of developmental transition—gain of a family member, situational crisis (e.g., surgical intervention, physical complications interfering with initial acquaintance or interaction, negative self-appraisal).

acute Pain/impaired Comfort may be related to surgical trauma, effects of anesthesia, hormonal effects, bladder or abdominal distention, possibly evidenced by verbal reports (e.g., incisional pain, cramping, afterpains, spinal headache), guarding or distraction behaviors, irritability, facial mask of pain.

risk for situational low Self-Esteem possibly evidenced by risk factors of perceived "failure" at life event, maturational transition, perceived loss of control in unplanned delivery.

risk for Injury possibly evidenced by risk factors of biochemical or regulatory functions (e.g., orthostatic hypotension, development of gestational hypertension or eclampsia), effects of anesthesia, thromboembolism, abnormal blood profile (anemia, excessive blood loss, rubella sensitivity, Rh incompatibility), tissue trauma.

risk for Infection possibly evidenced by risk factors of tissue trauma, broken skin, decreased hemoglobin, invasive procedures or increased environmental exposure, prolonged rupture of amniotic membranes, malnutrition.

Self-Care deficit (specify) may be related to effects of anesthesia, decreased strength and endurance, physical discomfort, possibly evidenced by verbalization of inability to perform desired activities of daily living.

Cesarean birth, unplanned — OB

Also refer to Cesarean birth, postpartal

deficient Knowledge [Learning Need] regarding underlying procedure, pathophysiology, and self-care needs may be related to incomplete or inadequate information, possibly evidenced by request for information, verbalization of concerns or misconceptions, and inappropriate or exaggerated behavior.

Anxiety [specify level] may be related to actual or perceived threat to mother/fetus, emotional threat to self-esteem, unmet needs, expectations, interpersonal transmission, possibly evidenced by increased tension, apprehension, feelings of inadequacy, sympathetic stimulation, and narrowed focus, restlessness.

Powerlessness may be related to interpersonal interaction, perception of illness-related regimen, lifestyle of helplessness, possibly evidenced by verbalization of lack of control, lack of participation in care or decision making, passivity.

risk for disturbed Maternal-Fetal Dyad possibly evidenced by risk factors of compromised oxygen transport, complication of pregnancy.

risk for labor Pain possibly evidenced by risk factors of increased or prolonged contractions, psychological reaction.

risk for Infection possibly evidenced by risk factors of invasive procedures, rupture of amniotic membranes, break in skin, decreased hemoglobin, exposure to pathogens.

Chemical dependence — PSY/CH

Refer to specific agents; Substance dependence/abuse rehabilitation

Chemotherapy — MS/CH

Also refer to Cancer

risk for deficient Fluid Volume possibly evidenced by risk factors of gastrointestinal losses (vomiting), interference with adequate intake (stomatitis, anorexia), losses through abnormal routes (indwelling tubes, wounds, fistulas), hypermetabolic state.

imbalanced Nutrition: less than body requirements may be related to inability to ingest adequate nutrients (nausea, stomatitis, gastric irritation, taste distortions, and fatigue), hypermetabolic state, poorly controlled pain, possibly evidenced by weight loss (wasting), aversion to eating, reported altered taste sensation, sore, inflamed buccal cavity; diarrhea or constipation.

impaired oral Mucous Membrane may be related to side effects of therapeutic agents or radiation, dehydration, and malnutrition, possibly evidenced by ulcerations, leukoplakia, decreased salivation, and reports of pain.

disturbed Body Image may be related to anatomical or structural changes; loss of hair and weight, possibly evidenced by negative feelings about body, preoccupation with change, feelings of helplessness, hopelessness, and change in social environment.

ineffective Protection may be related to inadequate nutrition, drug therapy, radiation, abnormal blood profile, disease state (cancer), possibly evidenced by impaired healing, deficient immunity, anorexia, fatigue.

readiness for enhanced Hope possibly evidenced by expressed desire to enhance belief in possibilities or sense of meaning to life.

Chickenpox — CH/PED

Refer to Measles

Chlamydia trachomatis infection — CH

Refer to Sexually transmitted infection

Cholecystectomy — MS

acute Pain may be related to interruption in skin and tissue layers with mechanical closure (sutures, staples) and invasive procedures including T-tube/nasogastric tube, possibly evidenced by verbal reports, guarding or distraction behaviors, and autonomic responses—changes in vital signs.

ineffective Breathing Pattern may be related to pain, muscular impairment, decreased energy, fatigue, ineffective cough, possibly evidenced by fremitus, tachypnea, decreased respiratory depth and vital capacity, holding breath, reluctance to cough.

risk for deficient Fluid Volume/Bleeding possibly evidenced by risk factors of losses from vomiting or nasogastric aspiration, medically restricted intake, altered coagulation.

Cholelithiasis — CH

acute Pain may be related to obstruction or ductal spasm, inflammatory process, tissue ischemia, necrosis, possibly evidenced by verbal reports, guarding or distraction behaviors, self or narrowed focus, and changes in vital signs.

risk for imbalanced Nutrition: less than body requirements possibly evidenced by risk factors of self-imposed or prescribed dietary restrictions, nausea and vomiting, dyspepsia, pain; loss of nutrients; impaired fat digestion—obstruction of bile flow.

deficient Knowledge [Learning Need] regarding pathophysiology, therapy choices, and self-care needs may be related to lack of information or recall, misinterpretation, possibly evidenced by verbalization of concerns, questions, and recurrence of condition.

Cholera **CH/MS**

deficient Fluid Volume may be related to active volume loss—profuse watery diarrhea, vomiting, possibly evidenced by intense thirst, marked loss of tissue turgor, decreased urine output (oliguria, anuria), change in mental state, hemoconcentration.

risk for Shock possibly evidenced by risk factors of hypotension, hypovolemia, sepsis.

Christmas disease **CH**

Refer to Hemophilia

Chronic obstructive lung disease **CH/MS**

ineffective Airway Clearance may be related to bronchospasm, increased production of tenacious secretions, retained secretions, and decreased energy, fatigue, possibly evidenced by presence of wheezes, crackles, tachypnea, dyspnea, changes in depth of respirations, use of accessory muscles, persistent cough, and chest radiograph findings.

impaired Gas Exchange may be related to altered oxygen delivery (obstruction of airways by secretions/bronchospasm, air trapping) and alveoli destruction, possibly evidenced by dyspnea, restlessness, confusion, abnormal arterial blood gas values—hypoxia, hypercapnia, changes in vital signs, and reduced tolerance for activity.

Activity Intolerance may be related to imbalance between oxygen supply and demand, and generalized weakness, possibly evidenced by verbal reports of fatigue, exertional dyspnea, and abnormal vital sign response.

imbalanced Nutrition: less than body requirements may be related to inability to ingest adequate nutrients (dyspnea, fatigue, medication side effects, sputum production, anorexia), possibly evidenced by weight loss, reported altered taste sensation, decreased muscle mass and subcutaneous fat, poor muscle tone, and aversion to eating or lack of interest in food.

risk for Infection possibly evidenced by risk factors of decreased ciliary action, stasis of secretions, and debilitated state, malnutrition.

Circumcision **PED**

deficient Knowledge [Learning Need] regarding surgical procedure, prognosis, and treatment may be related to lack of exposure, misinterpretation, unfamiliarity with information resources, possibly evidenced by request for information, verbalization of concern or misconceptions, inaccurate follow-through of instructions.

acute Pain may be related to trauma to and edema of tender tissues, possibly evidenced by crying, changes in sleep pattern, refusal to eat.

impaired urinary Elimination may be related to tissue injury, inflammation, development of urethral fistula, possibly evidenced by edema, difficulty voiding.

risk for Bleeding possibly evidenced by risk factors of circumcision, decreased clotting factors immediately after birth, previously undiagnosed problems with bleeding or clotting.

risk for Infection possibly evidenced by risk factors of mmature immune system, invasive procedure/tissue trauma, environmental exposure.

Cirrhosis **MS**

Also refer to Substance dependence/abuse rehabilitation; Hepatitis, acute viral

risk for impaired Liver Function possibly evidenced by risk factors of viral infection, alcohol abuse.

CH

imbalanced Nutrition: less than body requirements may be related to inability to ingest or absorb nutrients (anorexia, nausea, indigestion, early satiety), abnormal bowel function, impaired storage of vitamins, possibly evidenced by aversion to eating, observed lack of intake, muscle wasting, weight loss, and imbalances in nutritional studies.

excess Fluid Volume may be related to compromised regulatory mechanism (syndrome of inappropriate antidiuretic hormone, decreased plasma proteins, malnutrition) and excess sodium or fluid intake, possibly evidenced by generalized or abdominal edema, weight gain, dyspnea, blood pressure changes, positive hepatojugular reflex, change in mentation, altered electrolytes, changes in urine specific gravity, and pleural effusion.

risk for impaired Skin Integrity possibly evidenced by risk factors of altered circulation or metabolic state, poor skin turgor, skeletal prominence, and presence of edema, ascites, accumulation of bile salts in skin.

risk for Bleeding possibly evidenced by risk factors of abnormal blood profile, altered clotting factors—decreased production of prothrombin, fibrinogen, and factors VIII, IX, and X; impaired vitamin K absorption; release of thromboplastin, portal hypertension, development of esophageal varices.

risk for acute Confusion possibly evidenced by risk factors of alcohol abuse, increased serum ammonia level, and inability of liver to detoxify certain enzymes and drugs.

Self-Esteem (specify)/disturbed Body Image may be related to biophysical changes, altered physical appearance, uncertainty of prognosis, changes in role function, personal vulnerability, self-destructive behavior (alcohol-induced disease), possibly evidenced by verbalization of changes in lifestyle, fear of rejection or reaction of others, negative feelings about body or abilities, and feelings of helplessness, hopelessness, powerlessness.

Cleft lip/palate — PED/MS

Also refer to Newborn, special needs

ineffective infant Feeding Pattern may be related to anatomical abnormality, possibly evidenced by inability to sustain an effective suck, inability to coordinate sucking, swallowing, and breathing.

risk for Aspiration possibly evidenced by risk factors of impaired swallowing, regurgitation.

risk for impaired verbal Communication possibly evidenced by risk factors of anatomic defect, developmental delay.

risk for disturbed Body Image/Social Isolation possibly evidenced by risk factors of altered appearance, anatomic deficit, significance of body part (face).

Cocaine hydrochloride poisoning, acute — MS

Also refer to Stimulant abuse; Substance dependence/abuse rehabilitation

ineffective Breathing Pattern may be related to pharmacological effects on respiratory center of the brain, possibly evidenced by tachypnea, altered depth of respiration, shortness of breath, and abnormal arterial blood gases.

risk for decreased Cardiac Output possibly evidenced by risk factors of drug effect on myocardium (degree dependent on drug purity/quality used); alterations in electrical rate, rhythm, or conduction; preexisting myocardiopathy.

CH

risk for impaired Liver Function possibly evidenced by risk factors of cocaine abuse, effect of drug on liver.

Coccidioidomycosis (San Joaquin Valley/Valley Fever) — CH

acute Pain may be related to inflammation, possibly evidenced by verbal reports, distraction behaviors, and narrowed focus.

Fatigue may be related to decreased energy production, states of discomfort, possibly evidenced by reports of overwhelming lack of energy, inability to maintain usual routine, emotional lability, irritability, impaired ability to concentrate, and decreased endurance, decreased libido.

deficient Knowledge [Learning Need] regarding nature and course of disease, therapy, and self-care needs may be related to lack of information, possibly evidenced by statements of concern and questions.

Colectomy — MS

Refer to Intestinal surgery (without diversion)

Colitis, ulcerative — MS

Diarrhea may be related to inflammation or malabsorption of the bowel, presence of toxins or segmental narrowing of the lumen, possibly evidenced by increased bowel sounds and peristalsis; urgency; frequent, watery stools (acute phase); abdominal pain; urgency; cramping.

acute/chronic Pain may be related to inflammation of the intestines, hyperperistalsis, prolonged diarrhea, and anal or rectal irritation, fissures, fistulas, possibly evidenced by verbal reports, guarding or distraction behaviors—restlessness, self-focusing.

risk for deficient Fluid Volume possibly evidenced by risk factors of continued gastrointestinal losses—severe diarrhea, vomiting; capillary plasma loss, restricted intake—nausea, anorexia, hypermetabolic state (inflammation, fever).

CH

imbalanced Nutrition: less than body requirements may be related to altered intake or absorption of nutrients (medically restricted intake, fear that eating may cause diarrhea) and hypermetabolic state, possibly evidenced by weight loss, decreased subcutaneous fat or muscle mass, poor muscle tone, hyperactive bowel sounds, steatorrhea, pale conjunctiva and mucous membranes, and aversion to eating.

ineffective Coping may be related to chronic nature and indefinite outcome of disease, multiple stressors (repeated over time), personal vulnerability, severe pain, inadequate sleep, lack of or ineffective support systems, possibly evidenced by verbalization of inability to cope, discouragement, anxiety; preoccupation with physical self, chronic worry, emotional tension; depression and recurrent exacerbation of symptoms.

risk for Powerlessness possibly evidenced by risk factors of unresolved dependency conflicts, feelings of insecurity, resentment, repression of anger and aggressive feelings; lacking a sense of control in stressful situations, sacrificing own wishes for others, and retreating from aggression or frustration.

Collagen disorders **CH**

Refer to Arthritis, rheumatoid/juvenile rheumatoid; Lupus erythematosus, systemic; Polyarteritis nodosa; Temporal arteritis

Colorectal cancer **MS**

Refer to Cancer; Colostomy

Colostomy **MS**

risk for impaired Skin Integrity possibly evidenced by risk factors of absence of sphincter at stoma, character and flow of effluent and flatus from stoma, reaction to product or removal of adhesive, and improperly fitting appliance.

risk for Diarrhea/Constipation possibly evidenced by risk factors of interruption or alteration of normal bowel function (placement of ostomy), changes in dietary or fluid intake, and effects of medication.

CH

deficient Knowledge [Learning Need] regarding changes in physiological function and self-care/treatment needs may be related to lack of exposure or recall, information misinterpretation, possibly evidenced by questions, statement of concern, inaccurate follow-through of instruction or performance of ostomy care, development of preventable complications.

disturbed Body Image may be related to biophysical changes (presence of stoma, loss of control of bowel elimination) and psychosocial factors (altered body structure, disease process/associated treatment regimen), possibly evidenced by verbalization of change in perception of self, negative feelings about body, fear of rejection or reaction of others, not touching or looking at stoma, and refusal to participate in care.

impaired Social Interaction may be related to fear of embarrassing situation secondary to altered bowel control with loss of contents, odor, possibly evidenced by reduced participation and verbalized or observed discomfort in social situations.

risk for Sexual dysfunction possibly evidenced by altered body structure and function, radical resection and treatment procedures, vulnerability, psychological concern about response of SO(s), and disruption of sexual response pattern (e.g., erection difficulty).

Coma **MS**

risk for Suffocation possibly evidenced by risk factors of cognitive impairment, loss of protective reflexes and purposeful movement.

risk for deficient Fluid Volume/imbalanced Nutrition: less than body requirements possibly evidenced by risk factors of inability to ingest food or fluids, increased needs—hypermetabolic state.

[total] Self-Care deficit may be related to cognitive impairment and absence of purposeful activity, evidenced by inability to perform activities of daily living.

risk for ineffective cerebral Tissue Perfusion possibly evidenced by risk factors of head trauma, substance abuse, embolism, cerebral aneurysm, brain tumor/neoplasm.

risk for Infection possibly evidenced by risk factors of stasis of body fluids (oral, pulmonary, urinary), invasive procedures, and nutritional deficits.

Coma, diabetic **MS**

Refer to Diabetic ketoacidosis

Compartment syndrome, abdominal **MS**

acute Pain may be related to increasing abdominal distention and edema formation, inflammation, possibly evidenced by reports of pain, guarding behaviors, restlessness, narrowed focus.

risk for ineffective Gastrointestinal Perfusion possibly evidenced by risk factors of trauma, abdominal aortic aneurysm, liver dysfunction, sepsis, increasing abdominal pressure.

ineffective Breathing Pattern may be related to abdominal distention, pain possibly evidenced by dyspnea, tachypnea, altered chest excursion.

risk for Shock possibly evidenced by risk factors of hypotension, hypovolemia.

Compartment syndrome, extremity **MS**

acute Pain may be related to increasing pressure within muscle, possibly evidenced by reports of progressing pain distal to injury unrelieved by routine analgesics.

ineffective peripheral Tissue Perfusion may be related to interruption of arterial blood flow, elevated tissue pressures, possibly evidenced by absent or diminished distal pulses, erythema, pain.

risk for peripheral neurovascular Dysfunction possibly evidenced by risk factors of reduction or interruption of blood flow (direct vascular injury, tissue trauma, excessive edema, elevated tissue pressures, hypovolemia).

Complex regional pain syndrome **CH**

acute/chronic Pain may be related to continued nerve stimulation, possibly evidenced by verbal reports, distraction or guarding behaviors, narrowed focus, changes in sleep pattern, and altered ability to continue previous activities.

ineffective peripheral Tissue Perfusion may be related to reduction of arterial blood flow (arteriole vasoconstriction), possibly evidenced by extremity pain, altered skin characteristics, diminished pulses, and edema.

[disturbed tactile Sensory Perception] may be related to altered sensory reception (neurological deficit, pain), possibly evidenced by change in usual response to stimuli—abnormal sensitivity of touch, physiological anxiety, and irritability.

risk for ineffective Role Performance possibly evidenced by risk factors of situational crisis, chronic disability, debilitating pain.

risk for compromised family Coping possibly evidenced by risk factors of temporary family disorganization or role changes, and prolonged disability that exhausts the supportive capacity of SO(s).

Concussion, brain **CH**

Also refer to Postconcussion syndrome

acute Pain may be related to trauma to/edema of cerebral tissue, possibly evidenced by reports of headache, guarding or distraction behaviors, and narrowed focus.

risk for deficient Fluid Volume possibly evidenced by risk factors of vomiting, decreased intake, and hypermetabolic state (fever).

risk for impaired Memory possibly evidenced by risk factor of neurological disturbances.

deficient Knowledge [Learning Need] regarding condition, treatment, safety needs, and potential complications may be related to lack of recall, misinterpretation, cognitive limitation, possibly evidenced by questions, statement of concerns, development of preventable complications.

Conduct disorder (childhood, adolescence) **PSY/PED**

risk for self-/other-directed Violence: possibly evidenced by risk factors of retarded ego development, antisocial character, poor impulse control, dysfunctional family system, loss of significant relationships, history of suicidal or acting-out behaviors.

defensive Coping may be related to inadequate coping strategies, maturational crisis, multiple life changes/losses, lack of control of impulsive actions, and personal vulnerability, possibly evidenced by inappropriate use of defense mechanisms; inability to meet role expectations; poor self-esteem; failure to assume responsibility for own actions; hypersensitivity to slight or criticism; and excessive smoking, drinking, or drug use.

ineffective Impulse Control may be related to chronic low self-esteem, anger, disorder of development, mood, personality possibly evidenced by acting without thinking, irritability, temper outbursts.

chronic low Self-Esteem may be related to life choices perpetuating failure, personal vulnerability, possibly evidenced by self-negating verbalizations, anger, rejection of positive feedback, frequent lack of success in life events.

CH

compromised/disabled family Coping may be related to excessive guilt, anger, or blaming among family members regarding child's behavior; parental inconsistencies; disagreements regarding discipline, limit setting, and approaches; and exhaustion of parental resources (prolonged coping with disruptive child), possibly evidenced by unrealistic parental expectations; rejection or overprotection of child; and exaggerated expressions of anger, disappointment, or despair regarding child's behavior or ability to improve or change.

impaired Social Interaction may be related to retarded ego development, developmental state (adolescence), lack of social skills, low self-concept, dysfunctional family system, and neurological impairment, possibly evidenced by dysfunctional interaction with others (difficulty waiting turn in games or group situations, not seeming to listen to what is being said), difficulty playing quietly and maintaining attention to task or play activity, often shifting from one activity to another and interrupting or intruding on others.

Congestive heart failure **MS**

Refer to Heart failure, chronic

Conjunctivitis, bacterial **CH**

acute Pain/impaired Comfort may be related to inflammation, ocular irritation, edema, possibly evidenced by verbal reports, irritability, guarding behavior.

risk for Infection [spread] possibly evidenced by risk factors of purulent discharge, insufficient knowledge to avoid spread.

risk for ineffective Health Management possibly evidenced by risk factors of length of therapy, perceived benefit.

Connective tissue disease **CH**
Refer to Arthritis, rheumatoid/juvenile rheumatoid; Lupus erythematosus, systemic; Polyarteritis nodosa; Temporal arteritis

Conn's syndrome **MS/CH**
Refer to Aldosteronism, primary

Constipation **CH**
Constipation may be related to weak abdominal musculature, gastrointestinal obstructive lesions, pain on defecation, medications, diagnostic procedures, pregnancy, possibly evidenced by change in character and frequency of stools, feeling of abdominal or rectal fullness or pressure, changes in bowel sounds, abdominal distention.

acute Pain may be related to abdominal fullness or pressure, straining to defecate, and trauma to delicate tissues, possibly evidenced by verbal reports, reluctance to defecate, and distraction behaviors.

deficient Knowledge [Learning Need] regarding dietary needs, bowel function, and medication effect may be related to lack of information, misconceptions, possibly evidenced by development of problem and verbalization of concerns, questions.

Conversion disorder **PSY**
Refer to Somatoform disorders

Convulsions **CH**
Refer to Seizure disorder

COPD **CH**
Refer to Chronic obstructive lung disease

Corneal transplantation **MS**
risk for Injury possibly evidenced by risk factors of intraocular hemorrhage, edema/swelling, changes in visual acuity, increased intraocular pressure, glaucoma.

risk for Infection possibly evidenced by risk factors of surgical manipulation, use of corticosteroids, presence of chronic disease.

[disturbed visual Sensory Perception] may be related to altered sensory reception (use of eyedrops, edema, swelling), therapeutically restricted environment (patching), possibly evidenced by visual distortions, blurring, change in acuity.

Coronary artery bypass surgery **MS**
risk for decreased Cardiac Output possibly evidenced by risk factors of decreased myocardial contractility, diminished circulating volume (preload), alterations in electrical conduction, and increased systemic vascular resistance (afterload).

acute Pain may be related to direct chest tissue and bone trauma, invasive tubes and lines, donor site incision, tissue inflammation, edema formation, intraoperative nerve trauma, possibly evidenced by verbal reports, changes in vital signs, distraction behaviors, restlessness, irritability.

[disturbed Sensory Perception (specify)] may be related to restricted environment (postoperative), sleep deprivation, effects of medications, continuous environmental sounds and activities, and psychological stress of procedure, possibly evidenced by disorientation, alterations in behavior, exaggerated emotional responses, and visual or auditory distortions.

CH
ineffective Role Performance may be related to situational crises (dependent role), recuperative process, uncertainty about future, possibly evidenced by delay or alteration in physical capacity to resume role, change in usual role or responsibility, change in self-/others' perception of role.

Coronary artery disease **CH**
Activity Intolerance may be related to imbalance between oxygen supply and demand, sedentary lifestyle, possibly evidenced by exertional discomfort, pain, fatigue, abnormal heart rate response, electrocardiogram changes—dysrhythmias, ischemia.

risk for decreased Cardiac Output possibly evidenced by risk factors of altered heart rate or rhythm, altered contractility, increased peripheral vascular resistance.

Cor pulmonale **CH/MS**
Also refer to Heart failure, chronic; Chronic obstructive lung disease

Activity Intolerance may be related to imbalance between oxygen supply and demand, generalized weakness, chest pain, possibly evidenced by exertional dyspnea, fatigue, cyanosis.

excess Fluid Volume may be related to compromised regulatory mechanism, possibly evidenced by shortness of breath, dependent edema, jugular vein distention, positive hepatojugular reflux, abnormal breath sounds, change in mental status.

impaired Gas Exchange may be related to ventilation perfusion imbalance (heart failure), possibly evidenced by dyspnea, restlessness, lethargy, cyanosis, abnormal arterial blood gas values (hypoxemia, hypercapnia, acidosis), polycythemia.

Cradle cap CH

Refer to Dermatitis, seborrheic

Craniotomy MS

Also refer to Surgery, general

risk for decreased intracranial Adaptive Capacity possibly evidenced by risk factors of brain injuries, systemic hypotension with intracranial hypertension.

[disturbed Sensory Perception (specify)] may be related to altered sensory reception, transmission or integration (neurological deficit), possibly evidenced by disorientation to time, place, person; motor incoordination, altered communication patterns, restlessness, irritability, change in behavior pattern.

risk for Infection possibly evidenced by risk factors of traumatized tissues, broken skin, invasive procedures, nutritional deficits, altered integrity of closed system (cerebrospinal fluid leak).

Creutzfeldt-Jakob disease CH

impaired Memory may be related to neurological deficits, possibly evidenced by observed experiences of forgetting, inability to perform previously learned skills, inability to recall factual information or recent or past events.

Fear may be related to decreases in functional abilities, progressive deterioration, lack of treatment options, possibly evidenced by apprehension, irritability, defensiveness, suspiciousness, aggressive behavior, social isolation.

impaired Walking may be related to changes in muscle coordination and balance, visual changes, impaired judgment, myoclonic seizures, possibly evidenced by inability to walk desired distances, climb stairs, navigate uneven surfaces.

[disturbed visual Sensory Perception] may be related to altered sensory reception or integration (neurological disease), possibly evidenced by change in sensory acuity (visual field defects, diplopia, dimness, blurring, visual agnosia), change in usual response to stimuli.

[total] Self-Care deficit may be related to cognitive decline, physical limitations, frustration over loss of independence, depression, possibly evidenced by impaired ability to perform activities of daily living, unkempt appearance, poor hygiene, apathy.

risk for caregiver Role Strain possibly evidenced by risk factors of illness severity of care receiver, duration of caregiving required, care receiver exhibiting deviant or bizarre behavior; family/caregiver isolation, lack of respite or recreation, spouse is caregiver.

Crohn's disease MS/CH

Also refer to Colitis, ulcerative

imbalanced Nutrition: less than body requirements may be related to intestinal pain after eating, decreased transit time through bowel, fear that eating may cause diarrhea, possibly evidenced by weight loss, decreased subcutaneous fat and muscle mass, poor muscle tone, aversion to eating, and observed lack of intake.

Diarrhea may be related to inflammation of small intestines, presence of toxins, irritation—particular dietary intake, malabsorption of the bowel, segmental narrowing of the lumen, possibly evidenced by hyperactive bowel sounds, increased peristalsis, cramping, and frequent loose liquid stools.

deficient Knowledge [Learning Need] regarding condition, nutritional needs, and prevention of recurrence may be related to misinterpretation of information, lack of recall, unfamiliarity with resources, possibly evidenced by statements of concern, questions, inaccurate follow-through of instructions, and development of preventable complications or exacerbation of condition.

Croup PED/CH

ineffective Airway Clearance may be related to presence of thick, tenacious mucus and swelling or spasms of the epiglottis, possibly evidenced by harsh, brassy cough; tachypnea; use of accessory breathing muscles; and presence of wheezes.

deficient Fluid Volume may be related to decreased ability or aversion to swallowing, presence of fever, and increased respiratory losses, possibly evidenced by dry mucous membranes; poor skin turgor; and scanty, concentrated urine.

Croup, membranous PED/CH

Also refer to Croup

risk for Suffocation possibly evidenced by risk factors of inflammation of larynx with formation of false membrane.

Anxiety [specify level]/Fear may be related to change in environment, perceived threat to self (difficulty breathing), and transmission of anxiety of adults, possibly evidenced by restlessness, facial tension, glancing about, and sympathetic stimulation.

C-section **OB**
Refer to Cesarean birth, unplanned

Cubital tunnel syndrome **CH**
acute/chronic Pain may be related to pressure on ulnar nerve at elbow, possibly evidenced by verbal reports, reluctance to use affected extremity, guarding behaviors, expressed fear of reinjury, altered ability to continue previous activities.

impaired physical Mobility may be related to neuromuscular impairment and pain, possibly evidenced by decreased pinch or grasp strength, hand fatigue, and reluctance to attempt movement.

risk for peripheral neurovascular Dysfunction possibly evidenced by risk factors of mechanical compression (e.g., brace, repetitive tasks or motions), immobilization.

Cushing's syndrome **CH/MS**
risk for excess Fluid Volume possibly evidenced by risk factor of compromised regulatory mechanism (fluid and sodium retention).

risk for Infection possibly evidenced by risk factors of immunosuppressed inflammatory response, skin and capillary fragility, and negative nitrogen balance.

imbalanced Nutrition: less than body requirements may be related to inability to utilize nutrients (disturbance of carbohydrate metabolism), possibly evidenced by decreased muscle mass and increased resistance to insulin.

Self-Care deficit [specify] may be related to muscle wasting, generalized weakness, fatigue, and demineralization of bones, possibly evidenced by statements of or observed inability to complete or perform activities of daily living.

disturbed Body Image may be related to change in structure or appearance (effects of disease process, drug therapy), possibly evidenced by negative feelings about body, feelings of helplessness, and changes in social involvement.

Sexual dysfunction may be related to loss of libido, impotence, and cessation of menses, possibly evidenced by verbalization of concerns or dissatisfaction with and alteration in relationship with SO.

risk for Trauma [fractures] possibly evidenced by risk factors of increased protein breakdown, negative protein balance, demineralization of bones.

CVA **MS/CH**
Refer to Cerebrovascular accident

Cyclothymic disorder **PSY**
Refer to Bipolar disorder

Cystic fibrosis **CH/PED**
ineffective Airway Clearance may be related to excessive production of thick mucus and decreased ciliary action, possibly evidenced by abnormal breath sounds, ineffective cough, cyanosis, and altered respiratory rate and depth.

risk for Infection possibly evidenced by risk factors of stasis of respiratory secretions and development of atelectasis.

imbalanced Nutrition: less than body requirements may be related to impaired digestive process and absorption of nutrients, possibly evidenced by failure to gain weight, muscle wasting, and retarded physical growth.

deficient Knowledge [Learning Need] regarding pathophysiology of condition, medical management, and available community resources may be related to insufficient information, misconceptions, possibly evidenced by statements of concern, questions; inaccurate follow-through of instructions, development of preventable complications.

compromised family Coping may be related to chronic nature of disease and disability, inadequate or incorrect information or understanding by a primary person, and possibly evidenced by SO attempting assistive or supportive behaviors with less than satisfactory results, protective behavior disproportionate to client's abilities or need for autonomy.

Cystitis **CH**
acute Pain may be related to inflammation and bladder spasms, possibly evidenced by verbal reports, distraction behaviors, and narrowed focus.

impaired urinary Elimination may be related to inflammation or irritation of bladder, possibly evidenced by frequency, nocturia, and dysuria.

deficient Knowledge [Learning Need] regarding condition, treatment, and prevention of recurrence may be related to inadequate information, misconceptions, possibly evidenced by statements of concern and questions; recurrent infections.

Cytomegalic inclusion disease CH
Refer to Cytomegalovirus infection

Cytomegalovirus (CMV) infection CH
[risk for disturbed visual Sensory Perception] possibly evidenced by risk factor of inflammation of the retina.

risk for fetal Infection possibly evidenced by risk factors of transplacental exposure, contact with blood or body fluids.

D&C OB/GYN
Refer to Dilation and curettage

Deep vein thrombosis CH/MS
Refer to Thrombophlebitis

Degenerative disc disease CH/MS
Refer to Herniated nucleus pulposus

Degenerative joint disease CH
Refer to Arthritis, rheumatoid

(Although this is a degenerative process versus the inflammatory process of rheumatoid arthritis, nursing concerns are the same.)

Dehiscence, abdominal wound MS
impaired Skin Integrity may be related to altered circulation, altered nutritional state (obesity, malnutrition), and physical stress on incision, possibly evidenced by poor or delayed wound healing and disruption of skin surface or wound closure.

risk for Infection possibly evidenced by risk factors of inadequate primary defenses (separation of incision, traumatized intestines, environmental exposure).

Fear/Anxiety [severe] may be related to crises, perceived threat of death, possibly evidenced by fearfulness, restless behaviors, and sympathetic stimulation.

deficient Knowledge [Learning Need] regarding condition, prognosis, and treatment needs may be related to lack of information or recall and misinterpretation of information, possibly evidenced by development of preventable complications, requests for information, and statement of concern.

Dehydration PED/CH
deficient Fluid Volume [specify] may be related to etiology as defined by specific situation, possibly evidenced by dry mucous membranes, poor skin turgor, decreased pulse volume and pressure, and thirst.

risk for impaired oral Mucous Membrane possibly evidenced by risk factors of dehydration and decreased salivation.

deficient Knowledge [Learning Need] regarding fluid needs may be related to lack of information/misinterpretation, possibly evidenced by questions, statement of concern, and inadequate follow-through of instructions, development of preventable complications.

Delirium tremens MS/PSY
Also refer to Alcohol intoxication, acute

Anxiety [severe/panic]/Fear may be related to cessation of alcohol intake, physiological withdrawal, threat to self-concept, perceived threat of death, possibly evidenced by increased tension; apprehension; feelings of inadequacy, shame, self-disgust, or remorse; fear of unspecified consequences; identifies object of fear.

[disturbed Sensory Perception (specify)] may be related to exogenous (alcohol consumption and sudden cessation) or endogenous factors (electrolyte imbalance, elevated ammonia and blood urea nitrogen), chemical alterations, sleep deprivation, and psychological stress, possibly evidenced by disorientation, restlessness, irritability, exaggerated emotional responses, bizarre thinking, and visual and auditory distortions or hallucinations.

risk for decreased Cardiac Output possibly evidenced by risk factors of direct effect of alcohol on heart muscle, altered systemic vascular resistance, presence of dysrhythmias.

risk for Trauma possibly evidenced by risk factors of alterations in balance, reduced muscle coordination, cognitive impairment, and involuntary clonic/tonic muscle activity.

imbalanced Nutrition: less than body requirements may be related to poor dietary intake, effects of alcohol on organs involved in digestion, interference with absorption or metabolism of nutrients and amino acids, possibly evidenced by reports of inadequate food intake, altered taste sensation, lack of interest in food, debilitated state, decreased subcutaneous fat or muscle mass, signs of mineral or electrolyte deficiency, including abnormal laboratory findings.

Delivery, precipitous/out of hospital OB
Also refer to Labor, precipitous; Labor stages I–IV

risk for deficient Fluid Volume possibly evidenced by risk factors of presence of nausea/vomiting, lack of intake, excessive vascular loss.

risk for Infection possibly evidenced by risk factors of broken or traumatized tissue, increased environmental exposure, rupture of amniotic membranes.

risk for fetal Injury possibly evidenced by risk factors of rapid descent, pressure changes, compromised circulation, environmental exposure.

Delusional disorder **PSY**

risk for self-/other-directed Violence possibly evidenced by risk factors of perceived threats of danger, increased feelings of anxiety, acting out in an irrational manner.

[severe] Anxiety may be related to inability to trust, possibly evidenced by rigid delusional system, frightened of other people and own hostility.

Powerlessness may be related to lifestyle of helplessness, feelings of inadequacy, interpersonal interaction, possibly evidenced by verbal expressions of no control or influence over situation(s), use of paranoid delusions, aggressive behavior to compensate for lack of control.

impaired Social Interaction may be related to mistrust of others, delusional thinking, lack of knowledge or skills to enhance mutuality, possibly evidenced by discomfort in social situations, difficulty in establishing relationships with others, expression of feelings of rejection, no sense of belonging.

Dementia, HIV **CH/PSY**

Also refer to Dementia, presenile/senile

acute/chronic Confusion may be related to direct central nervous system infection with HIV, disseminated systemic opportunistic infection, hypoxemia, brain malignancies, cerebrovascular accident, vasculitis, altered drug metabolism and excretion, electrolyte imbalance, sleep deprivation, possibly evidenced by fluctuation of cognition, progressive cognitive impairment, increased agitation, restlessness, altered interpretation or response to stimuli, clinical evidence of organic impairment.

[mild to severe] Anxiety may be related to threat to self-concept, unmet needs, perceived threat to or change in health status, interpersonal transmission or contagion, possibly evidenced by reports of feeling scared, shaky, increased tension, loss of control—"going crazy," apprehension, increased wariness, extraneous movements, tremors, increased somatic complaints.

compromised family Coping may be related to prolonged disease progression that exhausts the supportive capacity of SOs, highly ambivalent family relationship, sense of shame or guilt related to diagnosis, other crises SOs may be facing, possibly evidenced by intolerance, rejection, abandonment, neglectful relationships with other family members, SO preoccupied with personal reaction, distortion of reality of health problem.

Dementia, presenile/senile **CH/PSY**

Also refer to Alzheimer's disease

impaired Memory may be related to neurological disturbances, possibly evidenced by observed experiences of forgetting, inability to determine if a behavior was performed, inability to perform previously learned skills, inability to recall factual information or recent or past events.

Fear may be related to decreases in functional abilities, public disclosure of disabilities, further mental or physical deterioration, possibly evidenced by social isolation, apprehension, irritability, defensiveness, suspiciousness, aggressive behavior.

Self-Care deficit [specify] may be related to cognitive decline, physical limitations, frustration over loss of independence, depression, possibly evidenced by impaired ability to perform activities of daily living.

risk for Trauma possibly evidenced by risk factors of changes in muscle coordination/balance, impaired judgment, seizure activity.

risk for caregiver Role Strain possibly evidenced by risk factors of illness severity of care receiver, duration of caregiving required, complexity or amount of caregiving tasks, care receiver exhibiting deviant or bizarre behavior; family/caregiver isolation, lack of respite or recreation, spouse is caregiver.

Grieving may be related to awareness of something "being wrong," predisposition for anxiety and feelings of inadequacy, family perception of potential loss of loved one, possibly evidenced by expressions of distress, anger at potential loss, choked feelings, crying, alteration in activity level, communication patterns, eating habits, and sleep patterns.

Dementia, vascular **CH/PSY**

Refer to Alzheimer's disease

Depersonalization disorder **PSY**

Refer to Dissociative disorders

Depressant abuse **CH/PSY**

Also refer to Drug overdose, acute (depressants)

ineffective Denial may be related to weak underdeveloped ego, unmet self-needs, possibly evidenced by inability to admit impact of condition on life, minimizes symptoms or problem, refuses healthcare attention.

ineffective Coping may be related to weak ego, possibly evidenced by abuse of chemical agents, lack of goal-directed behavior, inadequate problem solving, destructive behavior toward self.

imbalanced Nutrition: less than body requirements may be related to use of substance in place of nutritional food, possibly evidenced by loss of weight, pale conjunctiva and mucous membranes, electrolyte imbalances, anemias.

risk for Injury possibly evidenced by risk factors of changes in sleep, decreased concentration, loss of inhibitions.

Depression, major PSY

risk for self-directed Violence possibly evidenced by risk factors of depressed mood and feelings of worthlessness and hopelessness.

[moderate to severe] Anxiety may be related to stress, unconscious conflict about essential values or goals of life, unmet needs, threat to self-concept, interpersonal transmission or contagion, possibly evidenced by reports of feelings of inadequacy, sleep disturbances, fatigue, difficulty concentrating, diminished productivity/ability to problem solve, rumination.

Insomnia may be related to biochemical alterations (decreased serotonin), unresolved fears and anxieties, and inactivity, possibly evidenced by difficulty in falling or remaining asleep, early morning awakening or awakening later than desired, reports of not feeling rested, physical signs (e.g., dark circles under eyes, excessive yawning); hypersomnia (using sleep as an escape).

Social Isolation/impaired Social Interaction may be related to alterations in mental status or thought processes (depressed mood), inadequate personal resources, decreased energy, inertia, difficulty engaging in satisfying personal relationships, feelings of worthlessness or low self-concept, inadequacy in or absence of significant purpose in life, and knowledge or skill deficit about social interactions, possibly evidenced by decreased involvement with others, expressed feelings of difference from others, remaining in home or bed, refusing invitations of social involvement, and dysfunctional interaction with peers, family, or others.

interrupted Family Processes may be related to situational crises of illness of family member with change in roles or responsibilities, developmental crises (e.g., loss of family member or relationship), possibly evidenced by statements of difficulty coping with situation, family system not meeting needs of its members, difficulty accepting or receiving help appropriately, ineffective family decision-making process, and failure to send and to receive clear messages.

Depression, postpartum OB/PSY

Also refer to Depressive disorders

risk for impaired Attachment possibly evidenced by risk factors of anxiety associated with the parent role, inability to meet personal needs, perceived guilt regarding relationship with infant.

Fatigue may be related to stress, sleep deprivation, depression as evidenced by reports of overwhelming lack of energy, inability to maintain usual routines, increase in physical complaints.

situational low Self-Esteem may be related to developmental changes, disturbed body image, possibly evidenced by evaluation of self as unable to deal with situation, self-negating verbalizations, reports of helplessness.

risk for other-directed Violence possibly evidenced by risk factors of hopelessness, increased anxiety, mood swings, despondency, severe depression, psychosis.

Depressive disorders PSY

Refer to Depression, major; Bipolar disorder; Premenstrual dysphoric disorder

de Quervain's syndrome CH

acute/chronic Pain may be related to inflammation of tendon sheath at base of thumb, swelling, possibly evidenced by verbal reports, reluctance to use affected hand, guarding behaviors, expressed fear of reinjury, altered ability to continue previous activities.

impaired physical Mobility may be related to musculoskeletal impairment, swelling, pain, numbness of thumb and index finger, possibly evidenced by decreased grasp or pinch strength, weakness, limited range of motion of thumb, and reluctance to attempt movement.

Dermatitis, contact CH

acute Pain/impaired Comfort may be related to cutaneous inflammation and irritation, possibly evidenced by verbal reports, irritability, and scratching.

impaired Skin Integrity may be related to exposure to chemicals or environmental allergens, pruritus, possibly evidenced by inflammation, epidermal edema, development of vesicles or bullae.

risk for Infection possibly evidenced by risk factors of broken skin and tissue trauma.

Social Isolation may be related to alterations in physical appearance, possibly evidenced by expressed feelings of rejection and decreased interaction with peers.

Dermatitis, seborrheic — CH

impaired Skin Integrity may be related to chronic inflammatory condition of the skin, possibly evidenced by disruption of skin surface with dry or moist scales, yellowish crusts, erythema, and fissures.

Developmental disorders, pervasive — PED/PSY

Refer to Autism spectrum disorder; Rett's syndrome; Asperger's disorder

Diabetes, gestational — OB

Also refer to Diabetes mellitus

risk for unstable Blood Glucose Level possibly evidenced by risk factors of pregnancy, dietary intake, lack of diabetes management, inadequate blood glucose monitoring.

risk for disturbed Maternal-Fetal Dyad possibly evidenced by risk factors of impaired glucose metabolism, compromised oxygen transport—changes in circulation; treatment-related side effects.

deficient Knowledge [Learning Need] regarding diabetic condition, prognosis, and self-care treatment needs may be related to lack of resources or exposure to information, misinformation, lack of recall, possibly evidenced by questions, statements of misconception, inaccurate follow-through of instructions, development of preventable complications.

Diabetes insipidus — MS/CH

deficient Fluid Volume [hypertonic] may be related to failure of regulatory mechanisms and hormone imbalance (e.g., brain injury, medication, sickle cell anemia, hypothyroidism), possibly evidenced by urinary frequency, thirst, polydipsia, dilute urine, dry skin and mucous membranes, decreased skin turgor, nocturia, increased serum sodium.

risk for ineffective Health Management possibly evidenced by risk factors of complexity of medication regimen, presence of side effects, economic difficulties, inadequate knowledge, perceived seriousness and benefits.

Diabetes, juvenile — PED

Also refer to Diabetes mellitus

risk-prone Health Behavior may be related to inadequate comprehension, negative attitude toward healthcare, multiple stressors and life changes, possibly evidenced by failure to take action that prevents health problems, minimizes health status change, failure to achieve optimal sense of control.

risk for Injury possibly evidenced by risk factors of ineffective control or swings in serum glucose level, changes in mentation, developmental age, risk-taking behaviors.

ineffective Coping may be related to maturational crisis (desire to be like peers), inadequate level of perception of control, gender differences in coping strategies, possibly evidenced by use of forms of coping that impede adaptive behavior, inadequate problem solving, risk taking, destructive behavior toward self (loss of or inadequate diabetic control).

compromised family Coping may be related to inadequate or incorrect information or understanding by primary person(s), other situational or developmental crises or situations the SO(s) may be facing, lifelong condition requiring behavioral changes impacting family, possibly evidenced by family expressions of confusion about what to do, verbalizations that they are having difficulty coping with situation; family does not meet physical or emotional needs of its members; SO(s) preoccupied with personal reaction (e.g., guilt, fear), display protective behavior disproportionate (too little or too much) to client's abilities or need for autonomy.

Diabetes mellitus — CH/PED

deficient Knowledge [Learning Need] regarding disease process/treatment and individual care needs may be related to unfamiliarity with information, lack of recall, misinterpretation, possibly evidenced by requests for information, statements of concern, misconceptions, inadequate follow-through of instructions, and development of preventable complications.

risk for unstable Blood Glucose Level possibly evidenced by risk factors of lack of adherence to diabetes management, medication management, inadequate blood glucose monitoring, physical activity level, health status, stress, rapid growth periods.

risk for ineffective Health Management possibly evidenced by risk factors of complexity and duration of treatment, perceived excessive demands made on individual, powerlessness, perceived susceptibility to complications.

risk for Infection possibly evidenced by risk factors of decreased leukocyte function, circulatory changes, and delayed healing.

[risk for disturbed Sensory Perception (specify)] possibly evidenced by risk factors of endogenous chemical alteration (glucose, insulin, or electrolyte imbalance).

Diabetes mellitus, intrapartum OB

Also refer to Diabetes mellitus

risk for Trauma/impaired fetal Gas Exchange possibly evidenced by risk factors of inadequate maternal diabetic control, presence of macrosomia, or intrauterine growth retardation.

risk for maternal Injury possibly evidenced by risk factors of inadequate diabetic control (hypertension, severe edema, ketoacidosis, uterine atony or overdistention, dystocia).

[mild to moderate] Anxiety may be related to situational "crisis," threat to health status (maternal/fetus), possibly evidenced by increased tension, apprehension, fear of unspecific consequences, sympathetic stimulation.

Diabetes mellitus, postpartum OB

risk for unstable Blood Glucose Level possibly evidenced by risk factors of deficient knowledge of diabetes, medication management, dietary intake, increased metabolic demands (recuperation, lactation).

risk for Injury possibly evidenced by risk factors of biochemical or regulatory complications—uterine atony/hemorrhage, gestational hypertension, hyperglycemia).

risk for impaired Attachment possibly evidenced by risk factors of interruption in bonding process, physical illness, changes in physical abilities.

Diabetic ketoacidosis CH/MS

deficient Fluid Volume [specify] may be related to hyperosmolar urinary losses, gastric losses, and inadequate intake, possibly evidenced by increased urinary output, dilute urine; reports of weakness, thirst; sudden weight loss; hypotension; tachycardia; delayed capillary refill; dry mucous membranes; poor skin turgor.

unstable Blood Glucose Level may be related to medication management, lack of diabetes management, inadequate blood glucose monitoring, presence of infection, possibly evidenced by elevated serum glucose level, presence of ketones in urine, nausea, weight loss, blurred vision, irritability.

Fatigue may be related to decreased metabolic energy production, altered body chemistry (insufficient insulin), increased energy demands (hypermetabolic state, infection), possibly evidenced by overwhelming lack of energy, inability to maintain usual routines, decreased performance, impaired ability to concentrate, listlessness.

risk for Infection possibly evidenced by risk factors of high glucose levels, decreased leukocyte function, stasis of body fluids, invasive procedures, alteration in circulation, and perfusion.

Dialysis, general CH

Also refer to Dialysis, peritoneal; Hemodialysis

imbalanced Nutrition: less than body requirements may be related to inadequate ingestion of nutrients—dietary restrictions, anorexia, nausea, vomiting, stomatitis, sensation of feeling full with continuous ambulatory peritoneal dialysis; loss of peptides and amino acids (building blocks for proteins) during dialysis, possibly evidenced by reported inadequate intake, aversion to eating, altered taste sensation, poor muscle tone, weakness, sore and inflamed buccal cavity, pale conjunctiva and mucous membranes.

Grieving may be related to actual or perceived loss, chronic or fatal illness, and thwarted grieving response to a loss, possibly evidenced by verbal expression of distress or unresolved issues, denial of loss; altered eating habits, sleep and dream patterns, activity levels, libido; crying, labile affect; feelings of sorrow, guilt, and anger.

disturbed Body Image/situational low Self-Esteem may be related to situational crisis and chronic illness with changes in usual roles and body image, possibly evidenced by verbalization of changes in lifestyle, focus on past function, negative feelings about body, feelings of helplessness, powerlessness, extension of body boundary to incorporate environmental objects (e.g., dialysis setup), change in social involvement, overdependence on others for care, not taking responsibility for self-care, lack of follow-through, and self-destructive behavior.

Self-Care deficit [specify] may be related to perceptual or cognitive impairment (accumulated toxins); intolerance to activity, decreased strength and endurance; pain, discomfort, possibly evidenced by reported inability to perform activities of daily living, disheveled, unkempt appearance, strong body odor.

Powerlessness may be related to illness-related regimen and healthcare environment, possibly evidenced by verbal expression of having no control, depression over physical deterioration, nonparticipation in care, anger, and passivity.

compromised/disabled family Coping may be related to inadequate or incorrect information or understanding by a primary person, temporary family disorganization and role changes, client providing little support in turn for the primary person, and prolonged disease or disability progression that exhausts the supportive capacity of significant persons, possibly evidenced by expressions of concern or reports about response of SO(s)/family to client's health problem, preoccupation of SO(s) with personal reactions, display of intolerance or rejection, and protective behavior disproportionate (too little or too much) to client's abilities or need for autonomy.

Dialysis, peritoneal **MS/CH**

Also refer to Dialysis, general

risk for excess Fluid Volume possibly evidenced by risk factors of inadequate osmotic gradient of dialysate, fluid retention—malpositioned, kinked, or clotted catheter; bowel distention, peritonitis, scarring of peritoneum; excessive PO/IV intake.

risk for Trauma possibly evidenced by risk factors of improper placement during insertion or manipulation of catheter.

acute Pain/impaired Comfort may be related to catheter irritation, improper catheter placement, presence of edema, abdominal distention, inflammation, or infection; rapid infusion or infusion of cold or acidic dialysate, possibly evidenced by verbal reports, guarding or distraction behaviors, and self-focus.

risk for Infection [peritonitis] possibly evidenced by risk factors of contamination of catheter or infusion system, skin contaminants, sterile peritonitis—response to composition of dialysate.

risk for ineffective Breathing Pattern possibly evidenced by risk factors of increased abdominal pressure restricting diaphragmatic excursion, rapid infusion of dialysate, pain or discomfort, inflammatory process (e.g., atelectasis/pneumonia).

Diaper rash **PED**

Refer to Candidiasis

Diaphragmatic hernia **CH/MS**

Refer to Hernia, hiatal

Diarrhea **PED/CH**

deficient Knowledge [Learning Need] regarding causative or contributing factors and therapeutic needs may be related to lack of information, misconceptions, possibly evidenced by statements of concern, questions, and development of preventable complications.

risk for deficient Fluid Volume possibly evidenced by risk factors of excessive losses through gastrointestinal tract, altered intake.

acute Pain may be related to abdominal cramping and irritation or excoriation of skin, possibly evidenced by verbal reports, facial grimacing, and autonomic responses.

impaired Skin Integrity may be related to effects of excretions on delicate tissues, possibly evidenced by reports of discomfort and disruption of skin surface, destruction of skin layers.

DIC **MS**

Refer to Disseminated intravascular coagulation

Diffuse axonal (brain) injury **MS**

Refer to Traumatic brain injury; Cerebrovascular accident

Digitalis toxicity **MS/CH**

decreased Cardiac Output may be related to altered myocardial contractility and electrical conduction, properties of digitalis (long half-life and narrow therapeutic range), concurrent medications, age and general health status, and electrolyte/acid-base balance, possibly evidenced by changes in rate, rhythm, and conduction (development or worsening of dysrhythmias), changes in mentation, worsening of heart failure, elevated serum drug levels.

risk for imbalanced Fluid Volume possibly evidenced by risk factors of excessive losses from vomiting or diarrhea, decreased intake, nausea, decreased plasma proteins, malnutrition, continued use of diuretics; excess sodium and fluid retention.

deficient Knowledge [Learning Need] regarding condition, therapy, and self-care needs may be related to information misinterpretation and lack of recall, possibly evidenced by inaccurate follow-through of instructions and development of preventable complications.

Dilation and curettage **OB/GYN**

Also refer to Abortion, elective or spontaneous termination

deficient Knowledge [Learning Need] regarding surgical procedure, possible postprocedural complications, and therapeutic needs may be related to lack of exposure or unfamiliarity with information, possibly evidenced by requests for information and statements of concern, misconceptions.

Dilation of cervix, premature OB

Also refer to Preterm labor

Anxiety [specify level] may be related to situational crisis, threat of death or fetal loss, possibly evidenced by increased tension, apprehension, feelings of inadequacy, sympathetic stimulation, and repetitive questioning.

risk for disturbed Maternal-Fetal Dyad possibly evidenced by risk factors of surgical intervention, use of tocolytic drugs.

Grieving may be related to perceived potential fetal loss, possibly evidenced by expression of distress, guilt, anger, choked feelings.

Dislocation/subluxation of joint CH

acute Pain may be related to lack of continuity of bone/joint, muscle spasms, edema, possibly evidenced by verbal or coded reports, guarded or protective behaviors, narrowed focus, autonomic responses.

risk for Injury possibly evidenced by risk factors of nerve impingement, improper fitting of splint device.

impaired physical Mobility may be related to immobilization device, activity restrictions, pain, edema, decreased muscle strength, possibly evidenced by limited range of motion, limited ability to perform motor skills, gait changes.

Disruptive behavior disorder PED/PSY

Refer to Oppositional defiant disorder

Disseminated intravascular coagulation MS

risk for Shock possibly evidenced by risk factors of failure of regulatory mechanism (coagulation process) and active loss, hemorrhage.

ineffective Tissue Perfusion (specify) may be related to alteration of arterial or venous flow (microemboli throughout circulatory system, and hypovolemia), possibly evidenced by changes in respiratory rate and depth, changes in mentation, decreased urinary output, and development of acral cyanosis and focal gangrene.

Anxiety [specify level]/Fear may be related to sudden change in health status/threat of death, interpersonal transmission/contagion, possibly evidenced by sympathetic stimulation, restlessness, focus on self, and apprehension.

risk for impaired Gas Exchange possibly evidenced by risk factors of reduced oxygen-carrying capacity, development of acidosis, fibrin deposition in microcirculation, and ischemic damage of lung parenchyma.

acute Pain may be related to bleeding into joints/muscles, with hematoma formation, and ischemic tissues with areas of acral cyanosis and focal gangrene, possibly evidenced by verbal reports, narrowed focus, alteration in muscle tone, guarding or distraction behaviors, restlessness, autonomic responses.

Dissociative disorders PSY

[severe/panic] Anxiety/Fear may be related to a maladaptation or ineffective coping continuing from early life, unconscious conflict(s), threat to self-concept, unmet needs, or phobic stimulus, possibly evidenced by maladaptive response to stress (e.g., dissociating self, fragmentation of the personality), increased tension, feelings of inadequacy, and focus on self, projection of personal perceptions onto the environment.

risk for self-/other-directed Violence possibly evidenced by risk factors of dissociative state, conflicting personalities, depressed mood, panic states, and suicidal or homicidal behaviors.

disturbed Personal Identity may be related to psychological conflicts (dissociative state), childhood trauma or abuse, threat to physical integrity and self-concept, and underdeveloped ego, possibly evidenced by alteration in perception or experience of the self, loss of one's own sense of reality and the external world, poorly differentiated ego boundaries, confusion about sense of self, purpose, or direction in life; memory loss, presence of more than one personality within the individual.

compromised family Coping may be related to multiple stressors repeated over time, prolonged progression of disorder that exhausts the supportive capacity of significant person(s), family disorganization and role changes, high-risk family situation, possibly evidenced by family/SO(s) describing inadequate understanding or knowledge that interferes with assistive or supportive behaviors; relationship and marital conflict.

Diverticulitis CH

acute Pain may be related to inflammation of intestinal mucosa, abdominal cramping, and presence of fever and chills, possibly evidenced by verbal reports, guarding or distraction behaviors, autonomic responses, and narrowed focus.

Diarrhea/Constipation may be related to altered structure and function, and presence of inflammation, possibly evidenced by signs and symptoms dependent on specific problem (e.g., increase or decrease in frequency of stools and change in consistency).

deficient Knowledge [Learning Need] regarding disease process, potential complications, therapy, and self-care needs may be related to lack of information, misconceptions, possibly evidenced by statements of concern, request for information, and development of preventable complications.

risk for Powerlessness possibly evidenced by risk factors of chronic nature of disease process and recurrent episodes despite cooperation with medical regimen.

Down syndrome PED/CH

Also refer to Mental delay (formerly retardation)

riek for disproportionate Growth and/or delayed Development possibly evidenced by risk factor of genetic disorder.

risk for Trauma possibly evidenced by risk factors of cognitive difficulties and poor muscle tone or coordination, weakness.

imbalanced Nutrition: less than body requirements may be related to poor muscle tone and protruding tongue, possibly evidenced by weak and ineffective sucking or swallowing and observed lack of adequate intake with weight loss or failure to gain.

interrupted Family Processes may be related to situational or maturational crises requiring incorporation of new skills into family dynamics, possibly evidenced by confusion about what to do, verbalized difficulty coping with situation, unexamined family myths.

risk for complicated Grieving possibly evidenced by risk factors of loss of "the perfect child," chronic condition requiring long-term care, and unresolved feelings.

risk for impaired Attachment possibly evidenced by risk factors of ill infant/child who is unable to effectively initiate parental contact due to altered behavioral organization, inability of parents to meet the personal needs.

risk for Social Isolation possibly evidenced by risk factors of withdrawal from usual social interactions and activities, assumption of total child care, and becoming overindulgent or overprotective.

Dressler's syndrome CH

acute Pain may be related to tissue inflammation and presence of effusion, possibly evidenced by verbal reports of chest pain affected by movement or position and deep breathing, guarding or distraction behaviors, self-focus, and changes in vital signs.

Anxiety [specify level] may be related to threat to or change in health status, possibly evidenced by increased tension, apprehension, restlessness, and expressed concerns.

risk for ineffective Breathing Pattern possibly evidenced by risk factor of pain on inspiration.

risk for impaired Gas Exchange possibly evidenced by risk factor of ventilation perfusion imbalance—pleural effusion, pulmonary infiltrates.

Drug overdose, acute (depressants) MS/PSY

Also refer to Substance dependence/abuse rehabilitation

ineffective Breathing Pattern/impaired Gas Exchange may be related to neuromuscular impairment, central nervous system depression, decreased lung expansion, possibly evidenced by changes in respirations, cyanosis, and abnormal arterial blood gases.

risk for Trauma/Suffocation/Poisoning possibly evidenced by risk factors of central nervous system depression, agitation, hypersensitivity to the drug(s), psychological stress.

risk for self-/other-directed Violence possibly evidenced by suicidal behaviors, toxic reactions to drug(s).

risk for Infection possibly evidenced by risk factors of drug injection techniques, impurities in injected drugs, localized trauma; malnutrition, altered immune state.

Drug withdrawal CH/MS

[disturbed Sensory Perception (specify)] may be related to biochemical imbalance, altered sensory integration possibly evidenced by sensory distortions, poor concentration, irritability, hallucinations.

risk for Injury possibly evidenced by risk factor of central nervous system agitation (depressants).

risk for Suicide possibly evidenced by risk factors of alcohol or substance abuse, legal or disciplinary problems, depressed mood (stimulants).

acute Pain/impaired Comfort may be related to biochemical changes associated with cessation of drug use, possibly evidenced by reports of muscle aches, fever, diaphoresis, rhinorrhea, lacrimation, malaise.

Self-Care deficit (specify) may be related to perceptual or cognitive impairment, therapeutic management (restraints), possibly evidenced by inability to meet own physical needs.

Insomnia may be related to cessation of substance use, fatigue, possibly evidenced by reports of insomnia or hypersomnia, decreased ability to function, increased irritability.

Fatigue may be related to altered body chemistry (drug withdrawal), sleep deprivation, malnutrition, poor physical condition, possibly evidenced by verbal reports of overwhelming lack of energy, inability to maintain usual level of physical activity, inability to restore energy after sleep, compromised concentration.

DTs **MS/PSY**

Refer to Delirium tremens

Duchenne's muscular dystrophy **PED/CH**

Refer to Muscular dystrophy (Duchenne's)

Duodenal ulcer **MS/CH**

Refer to Ulcer, peptic

DVT **CH/MS**

Refer to Thrombophlebitis

Dysmenorrhea **GYN**

acute Pain may be related to exaggerated uterine contractibility, possibly evidenced by verbal reports, guarding or distraction behaviors, narrowed focus, and changes in vital signs.

ineffective Coping may be related to chronic, recurrent nature of problem; anticipatory anxiety, and inadequate coping methods, possibly evidenced by muscular tension, headaches, general irritability, chronic depression, and verbalization of inability to cope, report of poor self-concept.

Dyspareunia **GYN/PSY**

Sexual dysfunction may be related to physical or psychological alteration in function (menopausal involution, allergy to contraceptive, abnormalities of genital tract, guilt, control issues), possibly evidenced by verbalization of problem, inability to achieve desired satisfaction, sexual aversion, alteration in relationship with SO.

Anxiety [specify] may be related to situational crisis, stress, unconscious conflict about essential values, unmet needs, possibly evidenced by expressed concerns, distressed, feelings of inadequacy.

Dysrhythmia, cardiac **CH/MS**

risk for decreased Cardiac Output possibly evidenced by risk factors of altered electrical conduction and reduced myocardial contractility.

deficient Knowledge [Learning Need] regarding medical condition and therapy needs may be related to lack of information, misinterpretation, and unfamiliarity with information resources, possibly evidenced by questions, statement of misconception, failure to improve on previous regimen, and development of preventable complications.

risk for Activity Intolerance possibly evidenced by risk factors of imbalance between myocardial oxygen supply and demand, and cardiac depressant effects of certain drugs (beta blockers, antidysrhythmics).

risk for Poisoning [digitalis toxicity] possibly evidenced by risk factors of limited range of therapeutic effectiveness, lack of education or proper precautions, reduced vision, cognitive limitations.

Dysthymic disorder **PSY/CH**

Refer to Depression, major

Dystocia **OB**

Also refer to Labor, stage I [latent/active phases]

risk for maternal Injury possibly evidenced by risk factors of alteration of muscle tone/contractile pattern, mechanical obstruction to fetal descent, maternal fatigue.

risk for fetal Injury possibly evidenced by risk factors of prolonged labor, fetal malpresentations, tissue hypoxia and acidosis, abnormalities of the maternal pelvis, cephalopelvic disproportion.

risk for deficient Fluid Volume possibly evidenced by risk factors of hypermetabolic state, vomiting, profuse diaphoresis, restricted oral intake, mild diuresis associated with oxytocin administration.

ineffective Coping may be related to situational crisis, personal vulnerability, unrealistic expectations or perceptions, inadequate or exhausted support systems, possibly evidenced by verbalizations and behavior indicative of inability to cope (loss of control, inability to problem solve, or meet role expectations), irritability, reports of fatigue, increased tension.

Eating disorders **CH/PSY**

Refer to Anorexia nervosa; Bulimia nervosa

Ebola **MS**

Also refer to Disseminated intravascular coagulation; Multiple organ dysfunction syndrome

acute Pain/impaired Comfort may be related to infectious process, possibly evidenced by reports of headache, myalgia, abdominal or chest pain, sore throat, fever.

Hyperthermia may be related to inflammatory process, possibly evidenced by increased body temperature, warm skin, headache.

risk for deficient Fluid Volume possibly evidenced by risk factors of inadequate intake (nausea, painful swallowing, abdominal pain), increased losses (vomiting, diarrhea, hemorrhage/disseminated intravascular coagulation), hypermetabolic state (fever).

risk for Infection [spread of or secondary] possibly evidenced by risk factors of mode of transmission, invasive monitoring and procedures, debilitated state, malnutrition, insufficient knowledge or resources to avoid exposure to pathogens.

acute Confusion may be related to infectious process, hypoxemia, possibly evidenced by fluctuations in cognition, agitation, change in level of consciousness (stupor, coma).

Eclampsia — OB

Also refer to Hypertension, gestational

Anxiety [specify]/Fear may be related to situational crisis, threat of change in health status or death (self/fetus), separation from support system, interpersonal contagion, possibly evidenced by expressed concerns, apprehension, increased tension, decreased self-assurance, difficulty concentrating.

risk for maternal Injury possibly evidenced by risk factors of tissue edema, hypoxia, tonic-clonic convulsions, abnormal blood profile or clotting factors.

impaired physical Mobility may be related to prescribed bedrest, discomfort, anxiety, possibly evidenced by difficulty turning, postural instability.

risk for Self-Care deficit (specify) possibly evidenced by risk factors of weakness, discomfort, physical restrictions.

ECT — PSY

Refer to Electroconvulsive therapy

Ectopic pregnancy (tubal) — OB

Also refer to Abortion, spontaneous termination

acute Pain may be related to distention/rupture of fallopian tube, possibly evidenced by verbal reports, guarding or distraction behaviors, facial mask of pain, diaphoresis, and changes in vital signs.

risk for Bleeding/deficient Fluid Volume possibly evidenced by risk factors of pregnancy-related complication, hemorrhagic losses, and decreased or restricted intake.

Anxiety [specify level]/Fear may be related to threat of death and possible loss of ability to conceive, possibly evidenced by increased tension, apprehension, sympathetic stimulation, restlessness, and focus on self.

Eczema — CH

Refer to Dermatitis, contact/seborrheic

acute Pain/impaired Comfort may be related to cutaneous inflammation and irritation, possibly evidenced by verbal reports, irritability, and scratching.

risk for Infection possibly evidenced by risk factors of broken skin and tissue trauma.

Social Isolation may be related to alterations in physical appearance, possibly evidenced by expressed feelings of rejection and decreased interaction with peers.

Edema, pulmonary — MS

excess Fluid Volume may be related to decreased cardiac functioning, excessive fluid and sodium intake, possibly evidenced by dyspnea, presence of crackles (rales), pulmonary congestion on radiograph, restlessness, anxiety, and increased central venous pressure and pulmonary pressures.

impaired Gas Exchange may be related to altered blood flow and decreased alveolar-capillary exchange (fluid collection or shifts into interstitial space and alveoli), possibly evidenced by hypoxia, restlessness, and confusion.

Anxiety [specify level]/Fear may be related to perceived threat of death (inability to breathe), possibly evidenced by responses ranging from apprehension to panic state, restlessness, and focus on self.

Elder abuse — CH/PSY

Refer to Abuse, physical/psychological

Electrical injury — MS

Also refer to Burns

risk for decreased Cardiac Output possibly evidenced by risk factors of altered heart rate and rhythm (ventricular fibrillation, asystole).

impaired [internal] Tissue Integrity may be related to thermal injury (along path of current), altered circulation (massive edema), possibly evidenced by damaged or destroyed tissue, necrosis.

risk for ineffective peripheral Tissue Perfusion possibly evidenced by risk factors of reduction of venous or arterial blood flow (vein coagulation, muscle edema), increased tissue pressure (compartment syndrome).

risk for Trauma/Suffocation possibly evidenced by risk factors of muscle paralysis (central nervous system damage), loss of large- or small-muscle coordination (seizures).

Electroconvulsive therapy PSY

Decisional Conflict may be related to lack of relevant or multiple and divergent sources of information, mistrust of regimen or healthcare personnel, sense of powerlessness, support system deficit.

acute Confusion may be related to central nervous system effects of electric shock, medications, and anesthesia, possibly evidenced by fluctuation in cognition, agitation.

impaired Memory may be related to neurological disturbance (electrical shock), possibly evidenced by reported or observed experiences of forgetting, difficulty recalling recent events or factual information.

Emphysema CH/MS

impaired Gas Exchange may be related to alveolar capillary membrane changes or destruction, possibly evidenced by dyspnea, restlessness, changes in mentation, abnormal arterial blood gas values.

ineffective Airway Clearance may be related to increased production and retained tenacious secretions, decreased energy level, and muscle wasting, possibly evidenced by abnormal breath sounds (rhonchi), ineffective cough, changes in rate and depth of respirations, and dyspnea.

Activity Intolerance may be related to imbalance between oxygen supply and demand, possibly evidenced by reports of fatigue or weakness, exertional dyspnea, and abnormal vital sign response to activity.

imbalanced Nutrition: less than body requirements may be related to inability to ingest food (shortness of breath, anorexia, generalized weakness, medication side effects), possibly evidenced by lack of interest in food, reported altered taste, loss of muscle mass and tone, fatigue, and weight loss.

risk for Infection possibly evidenced by risk factors of inadequate primary defenses (stasis of body fluids, decreased ciliary action), chronic disease process, and malnutrition.

Powerlessness may be related to illness-related regimen and healthcare environment, possibly evidenced by verbal expression of having no control, depression over physical deterioration, nonparticipation in therapeutic regimen, anger, and passivity.

Encephalitis MS

risk for ineffective cerebral Tissue Perfusion possibly evidenced by risk factors of cerebral edema altering or interrupting cerebral arterial or venous blood flow, hypovolemia, exchange problems at cellular level (acidosis).

Hyperthermia may be related to increased metabolic rate, illness, and dehydration, possibly evidenced by increased body temperature; flushed, warm skin; and increased pulse and respiratory rates.

acute Pain may be related to inflammation or irritation of the brain and cerebral edema, possibly evidenced by verbal reports of headache, photophobia, distraction behaviors, restlessness, and changes in vital signs.

risk for Trauma/Suffocation possibly evidenced by risk factors of restlessness, clonic-tonic activity, altered sensorium, cognitive impairment, generalized weakness, ataxia, vertigo.

Encopresis PSY/PED

bowel Incontinence may be related to situational or maturational crisis, psychogenic factors (predisposing vulnerability, threat to physical integrity—child/sexual abuse), possibly evidenced by involuntary passage of stool at least once monthly, strong odor of feces on client, hiding soiled clothing in inappropriate places.

disturbed Body Image/chronic low Self-Esteem may be related to negative view of self, maturational expectations, social factors, stigma attached to loss of body function in public, family's belief that condition is volitional, shame related to body odor, possibly evidenced by angry outbursts or oppositional behavior, verbalization of powerlessness, reluctance to engage in social activities.

compromised family Coping may be related to inadequate or incorrect information or understanding of condition, belief that behavior is volitional, disagreement regarding treatment or coping strategies, possibly evidenced by increasingly ineffective attempts to intervene with child, significant person describes preoccupation with personal reaction (excessive guilt, anger, blame regarding child's condition or behavior), overprotective behavior.

Endocarditis MS

risk for decreased Cardiac Output possibly evidenced by risk factors of inflammation of lining of heart and structural change in valve leaflets.

Anxiety [specify level] may be related to change in health status and threat of death, possibly evidenced by apprehension, expressed concerns, and focus on self.

acute Pain may be related to generalized inflammatory process and effects of embolic phenomena, possibly evidenced by verbal reports, narrowed focus, distraction behaviors, and autonomic responses (changes in vital signs).

risk for Activity Intolerance possibly evidenced by risk factors of imbalance between oxygen supply and demand, debilitating condition.

risk for ineffective Tissue Perfusion (specify) possibly evidenced by risk factors of embolic interruption of arterial flow (embolization of thrombi or valvular vegetations).

End-of-life care **CH**

Refer to Hospice care

Endometriosis **GYN**

acute/chronic Pain may be related to pressure of concealed bleeding, formation of adhesions, possibly evidenced by verbal reports (pain between and with menstruation), guarding or distraction behaviors, and narrowed focus.

Sexual dysfunction may be related to pain secondary to presence of adhesions, possibly evidenced by verbalization of problem and altered relationship with partner.

deficient Knowledge [Learning Need] regarding pathophysiology of condition and therapy needs may be related to lack of information, misinterpretations, possibly evidenced by statements of concern and misconceptions.

Enteral feeding **MS/CH**

imbalanced Nutrition: less than body requirements may be related to conditions that interfere with nutrient intake or increase nutrient need or metabolic demand—cancer and associated treatments, anorexia, surgical procedures, dysphagia, or decreased level of consciousness, possibly evidenced by body weight 10% or more under ideal, decreased subcutaneous fat or muscle mass, poor muscle tone, changes in gastric motility and stool characteristics.

risk for Infection possibly evidenced by risk factors of invasive procedure, surgical placement of feeding tube, malnutrition, chronic disease.

risk for Aspiration possibly evidenced by risk factors of presence of feeding tube, bolus tube feedings, increased intragastric pressure, delayed gastric emptying, medication administration.

risk for imbalanced Fluid Volume possibly evidenced by risk factors of active loss or failure of regulatory mechanisms (specific to underlying disease process or trauma), inability to obtain or ingest fluids.

Fatigue may be related to decreased metabolic energy production, increased energy requirements (hypermetabolic state, healing process), altered body chemistry (medications, chemotherapy), possibly evidenced by overwhelming lack of energy, inability to maintain usual routines or accomplish routine tasks, lethargy, impaired ability to concentrate.

Enteritis **MS/CH**

Refer to Colitis, ulcerative; Crohn's disease

Enuresis **PSY/PED**

impaired urinary Elimination may be related to situational or maturational crisis, psychogenic factors (predisposing vulnerability, threat to physical integrity—abuse), possibly evidenced by nocturnal or diurnal enuresis, strong odor of urine on client, hiding soiled clothing in inappropriate places.

disturbed Body Image/chronic low Self-Esteem may be related to negative view of self, maturational expectations, social factors, stigma attached to loss of body function in public, family's belief condition is volitional, shame related to body odor, possibly evidenced by angry outbursts or oppositional behavior, verbalization of powerlessness, reluctance to engage in social activities.

compromised family Coping may be related to inadequate or incorrect information or understanding of condition, belief that behavior is volitional, disagreement regarding treatment or coping strategies, possibly evidenced by increasingly ineffective attempts to intervene with child, SO describes preoccupation with personal reaction (excessive guilt, anger, blame regarding child's condition or behavior), overprotective behavior.

Epididymitis **MS**

acute Pain may be related to inflammation, edema formation, and tension on the spermatic cord, possibly evidenced by verbal reports, guarding or distraction behaviors (restlessness), and changes in vital signs.

risk for Infection [spread] possibly evidenced by risk factors of presence of inflammation and infectious process, insufficient knowledge to avoid spread of infection.

deficient Knowledge [Learning Need] regarding pathophysiology, outcome, and self-care needs may be related to lack of information, misinterpretations, possibly evidenced by statements of concern, misconceptions, and questions.

Epilepsy CH
Refer to Seizure disorder

Episiotomy OB
acute Pain may be related to tissue trauma, edema, surgical incision, possibly evidenced by verbalizations, guarding behavior, self-focusing.

risk for Infection possibly evidenced by risk factors of broken skin, traumatized tissue, body excretions, inadequate hygiene.

risk for Sexual dysfunction possibly evidenced by risk factors of recent childbirth, presence of incision.

Epistaxis CH
[mild to moderate] Anxiety may be related to situational crisis, threat to health status, interpersonal transmission, possibly evidenced by expressed concerns, apprehension, anxiety.

risk for Aspiration possibly evidenced by risk factor of uncontrolled nasal bleeding.

Epstein-Barr virus CH
Refer to Mononucleosis, infectious

Erectile dysfunction CH/PSY
Sexual dysfunction may be related to altered body function, side effects of medication, possibly evidenced by reports of disruption of sexual response pattern, inability to achieve desired satisfaction.

situational low Self-Esteem may be related to functional impairment, perceived failure to perform satisfactorily, rejection of other(s), possibly evidenced by self-negating verbalizations, expressions of helplessness, powerlessness.

Esophageal reflux disease CH
Refer to Gastroesophageal reflux disease

Esophageal varices CH/MS
Refer to Varices, esophageal

Esophagitis CH
Refer to Gastroesophageal reflux disease; Achalasia

ETOH withdrawal MS/CH
Refer to Alcohol intoxication, acute; Substance dependence/abuse rehabilitation

Evisceration MS
Refer to Dehiscence, abdominal wound

Facial reconstructive surgery MS/CH
Also refer to Surgery, general; Intermaxillary fixation

risk for ineffective Airway Clearance possibly evidenced by risk factors of soft tissue edema, airway trauma, retained secretions.

impaired Skin Integrity may be related to traumatic injury, surgical procedure (incisions/grafts), edema, altered circulation, possibly evidenced by disruption or destruction of skin layers.

Fear/Anxiety may be related to situational crisis, memory of traumatic event, threat to self-concept (disfigurement), possibly evidenced by expressed concerns, apprehension, uncertainty, decreased self-assurance, restlessness.

disturbed Body Image may be related to traumatic event, disfigurement, possibly evidenced by negative feelings about self, fear of rejection reaction by others, preoccupation with change, change in social involvement.

risk for Social Isolation possibly evidenced by risk factor of change in physical appearance.

Failure to thrive, adult CH/MS
Frail Elderly Syndrome may be related to depression, apathy, aging process, fatigue, degenerative condition, possibly evidenced by expressed lack of appetite, difficulty performing self-care tasks, altered mood state, inadequate intake, weight loss, physical decline.

ineffective Protection may be related to inadequate nutrition, anemia, extremes of age, possibly evidenced by fatigue, weakness, deficient immunity, impaired healing, pressure sores.

Failure to thrive, infant/child PED
imbalanced Nutrition: less than body requirements may be related to inability to ingest, digest, or absorb nutrients (defects in organ function or metabolism, genetic factors); physical deprivation; psychosocial factors, possibly evidenced by lack of appropriate weight gain or weight loss, poor muscle tone, pale conjunctiva, and laboratory tests reflecting nutritional deficiency.

risk for disporportionate Growth and/or delayed Development possibly evidenced by risk factors of maladaptive feeding behavior, economically disadvantaged, caregiver mental health issue, presence of abuse (physical, psychological, sexual).

risk for impaired Parenting possibly evidenced by risk factors of lack of knowledge, inadequate bonding, unrealistic expectations for self/infant, and lack of appropriate response of child to relationship.

deficient Knowledge [Learning Need] regarding pathophysiology of condition, nutritional needs, growth/development expectations, and parenting skills may be related to lack of information, misinformation, or misinterpretation, possibly evidenced by verbalization of concerns, questions, misconceptions; or development of preventable complications.

Fat embolism syndrome **MS**

Refer to Pulmonary embolus; Respiratory distress syndrome, acute

Fatigue syndrome, chronic **CH**

Fatigue may be related to disease state, inadequate sleep, possibly evidenced by verbalization of unremitting or overwhelming lack of energy, inability to maintain usual routines, listlessness, compromised concentration.

chronic Pain may be related to chronic physical disability, possibly evidenced by verbal reports of headache, sore throat, arthralgias, abdominal pain, muscle aches, altered ability to continue previous activities, changes in sleep pattern.

Self-Care deficit [specify] may be related to tiredness, pain, discomfort, possibly evidenced by reports of inability to perform desired activities of daily living.

risk for ineffective Role Performance possibly evidenced by risk factors of health alterations, stress.

Febrile seizure **PED**

Hyperthermia may be related to illness, dehydration, decreased ability to perspire, possibly evidenced by increase in body temperature; flushed, warm skin; seizures.

Fecal diversion **MS/CH**

Refer to Colostomy

Fecal impaction **CH**

Constipation may be related to irregular defecation habits, decreased activity, dehydration, abdominal muscle weakness, neurological impairment, possibly evidenced by inability to pass stool, abdominal distention, tenderness or pain, nausea, vomiting, anorexia.

Femoral popliteal bypass **MS**

Also refer to Surgery, general

risk for ineffective peripheral Tissue Perfusion possibly evidenced by risk factors of interruption of arterial blood flow, hypovolemia.

risk for peripheral neurovascular Dysfunction possibly evidenced by risk factors of vascular obstruction, immobilization, mechanical compression, dressings.

impaired Walking may be related to surgical incisions, dressings, possibly evidenced by inability to walk desired distance, climb stairs, negotiate inclines.

Fetal alcohol syndrome **PED**

risk for Injury [central nervous system damage] possibly evidenced by risk factors of external chemical factors (alcohol intake by mother), placental insufficiency, fetal drug withdrawal in utero or postpartum, and prematurity.

disorganized infant Behavior may be related to prematurity, environmental overstimulation, lack of containment or boundaries, possibly evidenced by change from baseline physiological measures, tremors, startles, twitches, hyperextension of arms and legs, deficient self-regulatory behaviors, deficient response to visual or auditory stimuli.

risk for impaired Parenting possibly evidenced by risk factors of mental or physical illness, inability of mother to assume the overwhelming task of unselfish giving and nurturing, presence of stressors (financial or legal problems), lack of available or ineffective role model, interruption of bonding process, lack of appropriate response of child to relationship.

PSY

ineffective [maternal] Coping may be related to personal vulnerability, low self-esteem, inadequate coping skills, and multiple stressors (repeated over period of time), possibly evidenced by inability to meet basic needs, fulfill role expectations, or problem solve; and excessive use of drug(s).

dysfunctional Family Processes may be related to lack of or insufficient support from others, mother's drug problem and treatment status, together with poor coping skills, lack of family stability, overinvolvement of parents with children and multigenerational addictive behaviors, possibly evidenced by abandonment, rejection, neglectful relationships with family members, and decisions and actions by family that are detrimental.

Fetal demise **OB**

Refer to Perinatal loss/death of child

Fetal transfusion syndrome **OB**

Refer to Twin-twin transfusion syndrome

Fibrocystic breast disease CH

[mild to moderate] Anxiety may be related to situational crisis, threat to health status, family heredity, interpersonal transmission, possibly evidenced by expressed concerns, apprehension, uncertainty, fearfulness, focus on self, increased tension.

acute/chronic Pain may be related to physical agents (edema formation, nerve irritation), possibly evidenced by verbal reports, guarded or protective behavior, expressive behavior, self-focusing.

risk for ineffective Coping possibly evidenced by risk factors of situational crisis, perceived high degree of threat, inadequate resources or social supports.

Fibroids, uterine GYN

Refer to Uterine myomas

Fibromyalgia syndrome, primary CH

acute/chronic Pain may be related to idiopathic diffuse condition, possibly evidenced by reports of achy pain in fibrous tissues (muscles, tendons, ligaments), muscle stiffness or spasm, disturbed sleep, guarding behaviors, fear of reinjury or exacerbation, restlessness, irritability, self-focusing, reduced interaction with others.

Fatigue may be related to disease state, stress, anxiety, depression, sleep deprivation, possibly evidenced by verbalization of overwhelming lack of energy, inability to maintain usual routines or level of physical activity, tired, feelings of guilt for not keeping up with responsibilities, increase in physical complaints, listlessness.

risk for Hopelessness possibly evidenced by risk factors of chronic debilitating physical condition, prolonged activity restriction (possibly self-induced), creating isolation, lack of specific therapeutic cure, prolonged stress.

Flail chest MS

Refer to Hemothorax; Pneumothorax

Food poisoning CH/MS

Refer to Gastroenteritis

Fractures MS/CH

Also refer to Casts; Traction

risk for Trauma [additional injury] possibly evidenced by risk factors of loss of skeletal integrity, movement of skeletal fragments, use of traction apparatus.

acute Pain may be related to muscle spasms, movement of bone fragments, tissue trauma, edema, traction or immobility device, stress, and anxiety, possibly evidenced by verbal reports, distraction behaviors, self-focusing or narrowed focus, facial mask of pain, guarding or protective behavior, alteration in muscle tone, and changes in vital signs.

risk for peripheral neurovascular Dysfunction possibly evidenced by risk factors of reduction or interruption of blood flow (direct vascular injury, tissue trauma, excessive edema, thrombus formation, hypovolemia).

impaired physical Mobility may be related to neuromuscular or skeletal impairment, pain, discomfort, restrictive therapies (bedrest, extremity immobilization), and psychological immobility, possibly evidenced by inability to purposefully move within the physical environment, imposed restrictions, reluctance to attempt movement, limited range of motion, and decreased muscle strength or control.

risk for impaired Gas Exchange possibly evidenced by risk factors of altered blood flow, blood or fat emboli, alveolar-capillary membrane changes (interstitial or pulmonary edema, congestion).

deficient Knowledge [Learning Need] regarding healing process, therapy requirements, potential complications, and self-care needs may be related to lack of exposure or recall, misinterpretation of information, possibly evidenced by statements of concern, questions, and misconceptions.

Frostbite MS/CH

impaired Tissue Integrity may be related to altered circulation and thermal injury, possibly evidenced by damaged or destroyed tissue.

acute Pain may be related to diminished circulation with tissue ischemia or necrosis and edema formation, possibly evidenced by verbal reports, guarding or distraction behaviors, narrowed focus, and changes in vital signs.

risk for Infection possibly evidenced by risk factors of traumatized tissue, tissue destruction, altered circulation, and compromised immune response in affected area.

Fusion, cervical MS

Refer to Laminectomy, cervical

Fusion, lumbar MS

Refer to Laminectomy, lumbar

Gallstones CH

Refer to Cholelithiasis

Gangrene, dry MS

ineffective peripheral Tissue Perfusion may be related to interruption in arterial flow, possibly evidenced by cool skin temperature, change in color (black), atrophy of affected part, and presence of pain.

acute Pain may be related to tissue hypoxia and necrotic process, possibly evidenced by verbal reports, guarding or distraction behaviors, narrowed focus, and changes in vital signs.

Gangrene, gas MS

impaired Tissue Integrity may be related to trauma, surgery, infection, altered circulation, possibly evidenced by edema, brown or serous exudate, bronze or blackish green skin color, gas bubbles or crepitation, pain.

[severe] Anxiety/Fear may be related to situational crisis, interpersonal transmission, threat of death, possibly evidenced by expressed concerns, distress, apprehension, fearfulness, restlessness, irritability, focus on self.

risk for ineffective Renal Perfusion possibly evidenced by risk factors of effects of circulating toxins, altered circulation, shock.

risk for Injury possibly evidenced by risk factors of therapeutic intervention (hyperbaric oxygen therapy).

Gas, lung irritant MS/CH

ineffective Airway Clearance may be related to irritation or inflammation of airway, possibly evidenced by marked cough, abnormal breath sounds (wheezes), dyspnea, and tachypnea.

risk for impaired Gas Exchange possibly evidenced by risk factors of irritation or inflammation of alveolar membrane (dependent on type of agent and length of exposure).

Anxiety [specify level] may be related to change in health status and threat of death, possibly evidenced by verbalizations, increased tension, apprehension, and sympathetic stimulation.

Gastrectomy, subtotal MS

Also refer to Surgery, general

risk for imbalanced Nutrition: less than body requirements possibly evidenced by risk factors of restricted oral intake, early satiety, change in digestive process, malabsorption of nutrients, fear of complications (e.g., dumping syndrome, reactive hypoglycemia).

risk for Fatigue possibly evidenced by risk factors of malnutrition, anemia.

risk for Diarrhea possibly evidenced by risk factor of malabsorption.

Gastric partitioning MS

Refer to Gastroplasty

Gastric resection MS

Refer to Gastrectomy, subtotal

Gastric ulcer MS/CH

Refer to Ulcer, peptic

Gastrinoma MS/CH

Refer to Zollinger-Ellison syndrome

Gastritis, acute MS

acute Pain may be related to irritation or inflammation of gastric mucosa, possibly evidenced by verbal reports, guarding or distraction behaviors, and changes in vital signs.

risk for deficient Fluid Volume/Bleeding possibly evidenced by risk factors of excessive losses through vomiting and diarrhea, continued bleeding, reluctance to ingest or restrictions of oral intake.

Gastritis, chronic CH

risk for imbalanced Nutrition: less than body requirements possibly evidenced by risk factors of inability to ingest adequate nutrients (prolonged nausea, vomiting, anorexia, epigastric pain).

deficient Knowledge [Learning Need] regarding pathophysiology, psychological factors, therapy needs, and potential complications may be related to lack of information or recall, unfamiliarity with information resources, information misinterpretation, possibly evidenced by verbalization of concerns, questions, and continuation of problem or development of preventable complications.

Gastroenteritis CH/MS

Diarrhea may be related to toxins, contaminants, travel, infectious process, parasites, possibly evidenced by at least three loose liquid stools per day, hyperactive bowel sounds, abdominal pain.

risk for deficient Fluid Volume possibly evidenced by risk factors of excessive losses (diarrhea, vomiting), hypermetabolic state (infection), decreased intake (nausea, anorexia), extremes of age or weight.

risk for Infection [transmission] possibly evidenced by risk factors of insufficient knowledge to prevent contamination (inappropriate hand hygiene and food handling).

Gastroesophageal reflux disease (GERD) CH

acute/chronic Pain may be related to acidic irritation of mucosa, muscle spasm, recurrent vomiting, possibly evidenced by reports of heartburn, distraction behaviors.

impaired Swallowing may be related to GERD, esophageal defects, achalasia, possibly evidenced by reports of heartburn or epigastric pain, "something stuck" when swallowing, food refusal or volume limiting, nighttime coughing or awakening.

risk for imbalanced Nutrition: less than body requirements possibly evidenced by risk factors of limited intake, recurrent vomiting.

risk for Insomnia possibly evidenced by risk factors of nighttime heartburn, regurgitation of stomach contents.

risk for Aspiration possibly evidenced by risk factors of incompetent lower esophageal sphincter, regurgitation of gastric acid.

Gastrointestinal hemorrhage MS

Refer to Gastritis, acute or chronic; Ulcer, peptic; Colitis, ulcerative; Crohn's disease; Varices, esophageal

Gastroplasty MS

Also refer to Surgery, general

ineffective Breathing Pattern may be related to decreased lung expansion, pain, anxiety, decreased energy, fatigue, tracheobronchial obstruction, possibly evidenced by dyspnea, tachypnea, changes in respiratory depth, reduced vital capacity, wheezes, rhonchi, abnormal arterial blood gases.

risk for ineffective peripheral Tissue Perfusion possibly evidenced by risk factors of diminished blood flow, hypovolemia, immobility or bedrest, interruption of venous blood flow (thrombus).

risk for deficient Fluid Volume possibly evidenced by risk factors of excessive gastric losses, nasogastric suction, diarrhea, reduced intake.

risk for imbalanced Nutrition: less than body requirements possibly evidenced by risk factors of decreased intake, dietary restrictions, early satiety, increased metabolic rate (healing), malabsorption of nutrients, impaired absorption of vitamins.

Diarrhea may be related to changes in dietary fiber and bulk, inflammation, irritation, malabsorption of bowel, possibly evidenced by loose or liquid stools, increased frequency, hyperactive bowel sounds.

Gender identity disorder PSY

(For individuals experiencing persistent and marked distress regarding uncertainty about issues relating to personal identity, e.g., sexual orientation and behavior.)

Anxiety [specify level] may be related to unconscious or conscious conflicts about essential values or beliefs (ego-dystonic gender identification), threat to self-concept, unmet needs, possibly evidenced by increased tension, helplessness, hopelessness, feelings of inadequacy, uncertainty, insomnia, and focus on self, and impaired daily functioning.

ineffective Role Performance/disturbed Personal Identity may be related to crisis in development in which person has difficulty knowing or accepting to which sex he or she belongs or is attracted, sense of discomfort and inappropriateness about anatomic sex characteristics, possibly evidenced by confusion about sense of self, purpose, or direction in life, sexual identification or preference, verbalization of desire to be or insistence that person is the opposite sex, change in self-perception of role, and conflict in roles.

ineffective Sexuality Pattern may be related to ineffective or absent role models and conflict with sexual orientation or preferences, lack of or impaired relationship with an SO, possibly evidenced by verbalizations of discomfort with sexual orientation or role, and lack of information about human sexuality.

risk for compromised/disabled family Coping possibly evidenced by risk factors of inadequate or incorrect information or understanding, SO unable to perceive or to act effectively in regard to client's needs, temporary family disorganization and role changes, and client providing little support in turn for primary person.

readiness for enhanced family Coping possibly evidenced by expression of desire to acknowledge growth impact of crisis/situation, to enhance connection with others who have experienced a similar situation.

Genetic disorder CH/OB

Anxiety may be related to presence of specific risk factors (e.g., exposure to teratogens), situational crisis, threat to self-concept, conscious or unconscious conflict about essential values and life goals, possibly evidenced by increased tension, apprehension, uncertainty, feelings of inadequacy, expressed concerns.

deficient Knowledge [Learning Need] regarding purpose and process of genetic counseling may be related to lack of awareness of ramifications of diagnosis, process necessary for analyzing available options, and information misinterpretation, possibly evidenced by verbalization of concerns, statement of misconceptions, request for information.

risk for interrupted Family Processes possibly evidenced by risk factors of situational crisis, individual/family vulnerability, difficulty reaching agreement regarding options.

Grieving may be related to anticipatory or actual loss (e.g., childbearing or reproductive issues), possibly evidenced by suffering, blame, despair, change in usual routines and activities of daily living.

Spiritual distress may be related to intense inner conflict about the outcome, normal grieving for the loss of the perfect child, anger that is often directed at God/greater power, religious beliefs or moral convictions, possibly evidenced by verbalization of inner conflict about beliefs, questioning of the moral and ethical implications of therapeutic choices, viewing situation as punishment, anger, hostility, and crying.

Genital herpes **CH**

Refer to Herpes simplex; Sexually transmitted infection

Genital warts (human papillomavirus) **CH**

Refer to Sexually transmitted infection

GERD **CH**

Refer to Gastroesophageal reflux disease

GI bleeding **MS**

Refer to Gastritis, acute or chronic; Ulcer, peptic

Gigantism **CH**

Refer to Acromegaly

Gingivitis **CH**

impaired oral Mucous Membrane may be related to ineffective oral hygiene, ill-fitting dentures, decreased salivation, hormonal changes, possibly evidenced by edema, gingival bleeding, hyperplasia, oral pain.

Glaucoma **CH**

[disturbed visual Sensory Perception] may be related to altered sensory reception and altered status of sense organ (increased intraocular pressure, atrophy of optic nerve head), possibly evidenced by progressive loss of visual field.

Anxiety [specify level] may be related to change in health status, presence of pain, possibility or reality of loss of vision, unmet needs, and negative self-talk, possibly evidenced by apprehension, uncertainty, and expressed concern regarding changes in life event.

Glomerulonephritis **PED**

excess Fluid Volume may be related to failure of regulatory mechanism (inflammation of glomerular membrane inhibiting filtration), possibly evidenced by weight gain, edema, anasarca, intake greater than output, and blood pressure changes.

acute Pain may be related to effects of circulating toxins and edema or distention of renal capsule, possibly evidenced by verbal reports, guarding or distraction behaviors, and changes in vital signs.

imbalanced Nutrition: less than body requirements may be related to anorexia and dietary restrictions, possibly evidenced by aversion to eating, reported altered taste, weight loss, and decreased intake.

deficient Diversional Activity may be related to treatment modality and restrictions, fatigue, and malaise, possibly evidenced by statements of boredom, restlessness, and irritability.

risk for disproportionate Growth risk factors may include infection, malnutrition, chronic illness.

Gluten sensitive enteropathy **CH**

Refer to Celiac disease

Goiter **CH**

disturbed Body Image may be related to visible swelling in neck, possibly evidenced by verbalization of feelings, fear of reaction of others, actual change in structure, change in social involvement.

Anxiety may be related to change in health status, progressive growth of mass, perceived threat of death.

risk for imbalanced Nutrition: less than body requirements possibly evidenced by risk factors of decreased ability to ingest or difficulty swallowing.

risk for ineffective Airway Clearance possibly evidenced by risk factors of tracheal compression or obstruction.

Gonorrhea **CH**

Also refer to Sexually transmitted infection

risk for Infection [dissemination/bacteremia] possibly evidenced by risk factors of presence of infectious process in highly vascular area and lack of recognition of disease process.

acute Pain may be related to irritation or inflammation of mucosa and effects of circulating toxins, possibly evidenced by verbal reports of genital or pharyngeal irritation, perineal or pelvic pain, guarding or distraction behaviors.

deficient Knowledge [Learning Need] regarding disease cause, transmission, therapy, and self-care needs may be related to lack of information, misinterpretation, denial of exposure, possibly evidenced by statements of concern, questions, misconceptions, and inaccurate follow-through of instructions, development of preventable complications.

Gout — CH

acute Pain may be related to inflammation of joint(s), possibly evidenced by verbal reports, guarding or distraction behaviors, and changes in vital signs.

impaired physical Mobility may be related to joint pain, edema, possibly evidenced by reluctance to attempt movement, limited range of motion, and therapeutic restriction of movement.

deficient Knowledge [Learning Need] regarding cause, treatment, and prevention of condition may be related to lack of information, misinterpretation, possibly evidenced by statements of concern, questions, misconceptions, and inaccurate follow-through of instructions.

Grand mal seizures — CH/PED

Refer to Seizure disorder

Grave's disease — CH

Refer to Hyperthyroidism

Guillain-Barré syndrome (acute polyneuritis) — MS

risk for ineffective Breathing Pattern/Airway Clearance possibly evidenced by risk factors of weakness or paralysis of respiratory muscles, impaired gag or swallow reflexes, decreased energy, fatigue.

[disturbed Sensory Perception (specify)] may be related to altered sensory reception, transmission, or integration (altered status of sense organs, sleep deprivation); therapeutically restricted environment; endogenous chemical alterations (electrolyte imbalance, hypoxia); and psychological stress, possibly evidenced by reported or observed change in usual response to stimuli, altered communication patterns, and measured change in sensory acuity and motor coordination.

impaired physical Mobility may be related to neuromuscular impairment, pain, discomfort, possibly evidenced by impaired coordination, partial or complete paralysis, decreased muscle strength or control.

Anxiety [specify level]/Fear may be related to situational crisis, change in health status, threat of death, possibly evidenced by increased tension, restlessness, helplessness, apprehension, uncertainty, fearfulness, focus on self, and sympathetic stimulation.

risk for Disuse Syndrome possibly evidenced by risk factors of paralysis and pain.

Gulf War syndrome — CH/MS

[chronic] Fatigue may be related to unknown environmental exposure, stress, anxiety, disease state, possibly evidenced by overwhelming lack of energy, inability to maintain usual routines or level of physical activity, lethargic, compromised concentration.

Anxiety [specify] may be related to exposure to toxins, change in health status, threat of death, change in role function or economic status, unmet needs, possibly evidenced by expressed concerns, apprehension, uncertainty, fear of unspecific consequences, sleep disturbance, irritability, preoccupation.

impaired Memory may be related to neurological disturbances, possibly evidenced by reported or observed experiences of forgetting, inability to recall recent events.

chronic Pain may be related to chronic physical condition, possibly evidenced by verbal reports of muscle or joint pain, headaches, altered ability to continue previous activities, fatigue, reduced interaction with others.

Diarrhea may be related to environmental exposure to toxins, high stress levels/anxiety, possibly evidenced by liquid stools, abdominal pain.

[disturbed visual Sensory Perception] may be related to altered sensory reception, possibly evidenced by blurred vision, photosensitivity.

Hallucinogen abuse — CH/PSY

Also refer to Substance dependence/abuse rehabilitation

Anxiety/Fear may be related to situational crisis, threat to or change in health status, perceived threat of death, inexperience or unfamiliarity with effects of drug, possibly evidenced by assumptions of "losing my mind/control," apprehension, preoccupation with feelings of impending doom, sympathetic stimulation.

Self-Neglect may be related to substance use, executive processing ability, possibly evidenced by inadequate personal/environmental hygiene, nonadherence to health activities.

Self-Care deficit (specify) may be related to perceptual or cognitive impairment, therapeutic management (restraints), possibly evidenced by inability to meet own physical needs.

Hand-foot-mouth disease PED/CH

Also refer to Meningitis, acute meningococcal

impaired oral Mucous Membrane may be related to infection, dehydration, possibly evidenced by oral lesions, ulcers, pain, difficulty eating.

risk for Infection [transmission] possibly evidenced by risk factors of insufficient knowledge to avoid exposure to pathogens, inadequate acquired immunity.

risk for deficient Fluid Volume possibly evidenced by risk factors of deviations affecting intake (oral ulcers and pain), increased fluid needs (hypermetabolic state, fever).

Hansen's disease CH

impaired Skin/Tissue integrity may be related to altered circulation, sensation, pigmentation and [invasion of tissues by bacterial infection], possibly evidenced by symmetric skin lesions lighter than normal color, nodules, plaques, thickened dermis with loss of sensation, and frequent involvement of the nasal mucosa resulting in nasal congestion and epistaxis.

risk for Infection [spread/transmission] possibly evidenced by risk factors of inadequate primary or secondary defenses, insufficient knowledge to avoid exposure to/early treatment of infectious bacterial [*Mycobacterium leprae*] agent.

impaired physical Mobility may be related to neuromuscular and sensoriperceptual impairments, possibly evidenced by muscular weakness, or numbness or absence of sensation in hands, arms, legs, feet.

disturbed Body Image may be related to biophysical illness, trauma, possibly evidenced by permanent nerve damage, [cosmetic damage], actual change in structure, missing body part, fear of reaction or rejection by others.

Hantavirus MS

Refer to Hantavirus pulmonary syndrome

Hantavirus pulmonary syndrome MS

Also refer to Disseminated intravascular coagulation

acute Pain/impaired Comfort may be related to inflammatory process, circulating toxins, possibly evidenced by reports of headache, myalgia, gastrointestinal distress, fever.

impaired Gas Exchange may be related to alveolar-capillary membrane changes (fluid collection or shifts into interstitial space or alveoli), possibly evidenced by dyspnea, restlessness, irritability, abnormal rate or depth of respirations, lethargy, confusion.

[moderate to severe] Anxiety may be related to change in health status, threat of death, interpersonal transmission, possibly evidenced by expressed concerns, distressed, apprehension, extraneous movement.

risk for impaired spontaneous Ventilation possibly evidenced by risk factors of respiratory muscle fatigue, problems with secretion management.

Hashimoto's thyroiditis CH

Refer to Hypothyroidism; Goiter

Hay fever CH

impaired Comfort/acute Pain may be related to irritation or inflammation of upper airway mucous membranes and conjunctiva, possibly evidenced by verbal reports, irritability, and restlessness.

deficient Knowledge [Learning Need] regarding underlying cause, appropriate therapy, and required lifestyle changes may be related to lack of information, possibly evidenced by statements of concern, questions, and misconceptions.

Headache CH/MS

Also refer to Temporal arteritis

acute/chronic Pain may be related to stress, tension, nerve irritation or pressure, vasospasm, increased intracranial pressure, possibly evidenced by verbal or coded reports, pallor, facial mask of pain, guarding or distraction behaviors, restlessness, self-focusing, changes in sleep pattern or appetite, preoccupation with pain.

risk for ineffective Coping possibly evidenced by risk factors of situational crisis, personal vulnerability, inadequate support systems, work overload, no vacations, inadequate relaxation, severe pain, overwhelming threat to self.

deficient Knowledge [Learning Need] regarding condition, prognosis, and treatment needs may be related to lack of exposure or recall, unfamiliarity with information or resources, cognitive limitations, possibly evidenced by request for information, statement of misconceptions, inaccurate follow-through of instructions, development of preventable complications.

Head injury MS/CH

Refer to Traumatic brain injury

Heart attack MS

Refer to Myocardial infarction

Heart failure, chronic — MS

decreased Cardiac Output may be related to altered myocardial contractility, inotropic changes; alterations in rate, rhythm, and electrical conduction; and structural changes (valvular defects, ventricular aneurysm), possibly evidenced by tachycardia, dysrhythmias, changes in blood pressure, extra heart sounds, decreased urine output, diminished peripheral pulses, cool and ashen skin, orthopnea, crackles; dependent or generalized edema and chest pain.

excess Fluid Volume may be related to reduced glomerular filtration rate, increased antidiuretic hormone production, and sodium/water retention, possibly evidenced by orthopnea and abnormal breath sounds, S_3 heart sound, jugular vein distention, positive hepatojugular reflex, weight gain, hypertension, oliguria, generalized edema.

risk for impaired Gas Exchange possibly evidenced by risk factors of alveolar-capillary membrane changes—fluid collection or shifts into interstitial space and alveoli.

CH

Activity Intolerance may be related to imbalance between oxygen supply and demand, generalized weakness, and prolonged bedrest or sedentary lifestyle, possibly evidenced by reported or observed weakness, fatigue; changes in vital signs, presence of dysrhythmias; dyspnea, pallor, and diaphoresis.

risk for impaired Skin Integrity possibly evidenced by risk factors of prolonged chair- or bedrest, edema, vascular pooling, decreased tissue perfusion.

deficient Knowledge [Learning Need] regarding cardiac function, disease process, therapy, and self-care needs may be related to lack of information, misinterpretation, possibly evidenced by questions, statements of concern or misconceptions; development of preventable complications or exacerbations of condition.

Heart transplantation — MS/CH

Refer to Cardiac surgery; Transplantation, recipient

Heat exhaustion — CH/MS

deficient Fluid Volume may be related to excessive losses (profuse sweating), hypermetabolic state (core temperature 101°F to 105°F [38.3°C to 40.6°C]), lack of intake, extremes of age, possibly evidenced by weakness, fatigue, slow pulse, decreased blood pressure, changes in mentation.

Heatstroke — MS

Hyperthermia may be related to prolonged exposure to hot environment, vigorous activity with failure of regulating mechanism of the body, possibly evidenced by high body temperature (greater than 105°F [40.6°C]), flushed/hot skin, tachycardia, and seizure activity.

decreased Cardiac Output may be related to functional stress of hypermetabolic state, altered circulating volume and venous return, and direct myocardial damage secondary to hyperthermia, possibly evidenced by decreased peripheral pulses, dysrhythmias, tachycardia, and changes in mentation.

Hematoma, epidural — MS

acute Confusion may be related to head injury, possibly evidenced by fluctuation in cognition or level of consciousness.

risk for decreased intracranial Adaptive Capacity possibly evidenced by risk factors of brain injuries, decreased cerebral perfusion pressure, systemic hypotension with intracranial hypertension.

risk for ineffective Breathing Pattern possibly evidenced by risk factors of neuromuscular dysfunction (injury to respiratory center of brain), perception or cognitive impairment.

risk for deficient Fluid Volume possibly evidenced by risk factors of restricted oral intake, hypermetabolic state, loss of fluid through normal or abnormal routes.

Hematoma, subdural-acute — MS

Refer to Traumatic brain injury

Hematoma, subdural-chronic — CH

acute/chronic Pain may be related to physical agent (space-occupying clot), possibly evidenced by reports of increasing daily headache.

acute/chronic Confusion may be related to head injury, alcohol abuse, possibly evidenced by fluctuations in cognition, increased agitation, restlessness, misperceptions, inappropriate responses.

impaired physical Mobility may be related to neuromuscular impairment (hemiparesis), decreased muscle strength, cognitive impairment, possibly evidenced by limited ability to perform gross or fine motor skills, gait changes, postural instability.

Hemiplegia, spastic — PED/CH

Refer to Palsy, cerebral

Hemodialysis MS/CH

Also refer to Dialysis, general

risk for Injury [loss of vascular access] possibly evidenced by risk factors of clotting or thrombosis, infection, disconnection, hemorrhage.

risk for deficient Fluid Volume possibly evidenced by risk factors of excessive fluid losses or shifts via ultrafiltration, fluid restrictions, altered coagulation, disconnection of shunt.

risk for excess Fluid Volume possibly evidenced by risk factors of rapid or excessive fluid intake—IV, blood, plasma expanders, or saline given to support blood pressure during procedure.

ineffective Protection may be related to chronic disease state, drug therapy, abnormal blood profile, inadequate nutrition, possibly evidenced by altered clotting, impaired healing, deficient immunity, fatigue, anorexia.

Hemophilia PED

risk for Bleeding/deficient Fluid Volume possibly evidenced by risk factors of impaired coagulation, inherent coagulopathies, trauma, hemorrhagic losses.

risk for acute/chronic Pain possibly evidenced by risk factors of nerve compression from hematomas, nerve damage, or hemorrhage into joint space.

risk for impaired physical Mobility possibly evidenced by risk factors of joint hemorrhage, swelling, degenerative changes, and muscle atrophy.

ineffective Protection may be related to abnormal blood profile, possibly evidenced by altered clotting.

compromised family Coping may be related to prolonged nature of condition that exhausts the supportive capacity of significant person(s), possibly evidenced by protective behaviors disproportionate to client's abilities or need for autonomy.

Hemorrhage, postpartum OB

risk for Shock possibly evidenced by risk factors of hypovolemia—postpartum complications, disseminated intravascular coagulation.

risk for Injury possibly evidenced by risk factors of decreased hemoglobin, tissue hypoxia.

[moderate] Anxiety may be related to situational crisis, threat of change in health status or death, interpersonal transmission or contagion, physiological response (catecholamine release), possibly evidenced by increased tension, apprehension, feelings of inadequacy or helplessness, sympathetic stimulation, self-focus.

risk for Infection possibly evidenced by risk factors of traumatized tissue, stasis of body fluids (lochia), decreased hemoglobin, invasive procedures.

risk for impaired Attachment possibly evidenced by risk factors of interruption in bonding process, physical condition, perceived threat to own survival.

Hemorrhage, prenatal OB

risk for Shock possibly evidenced by risk factors of hypovolemia—ectopic or molar pregnancy, abruptio placentae.

risk for disturbed Maternal-Fetal Dyad possibly evidenced by risk factors of compromised oxygen transport—hypovolemia.

Fear may be related to threat of death [perceived or actual] to self/fetus, possibly evidenced by verbalizations of specific concerns, increased tension, sympathetic stimulation.

acute Pain may be related to muscle contractions, cervical dilation, tissue trauma (fallopian tube rupture), possibly evidenced by reports, distraction behaviors, and change in blood pressure/pulse.

risk for imbalanced Fluid Volume possibly evidenced by risk factors of excessive or rapid replacement of fluid losses.

Hemorrhagic fever, viral MS

Refer to Ebola; Hantavirus pulmonary syndrome

Hemorrhoidectomy MS/CH

acute Pain may be related to edema or swelling and tissue trauma, possibly evidenced by verbal reports, guarding or distraction behaviors, focus on self, and changes in vital signs.

risk for Urinary Retention possibly evidenced by perineal trauma, edema or swelling, and pain.

deficient Knowledge [Learning Need] regarding therapeutic treatment and potential complications may be related to lack of information, misconceptions, possibly evidenced by statements of concern and questions.

Hemorrhoids CH/OB

acute Pain may be related to inflammation and edema of prolapsed varices, possibly evidenced by verbal reports and guarding or distraction behaviors.

Constipation may be related to pain on defecation and reluctance to defecate, possibly evidenced by frequency, less than usual pattern, and hard, formed stools.

Hemothorax **MS**

Also refer to Pneumothorax

risk for Trauma/Suffocation possibly evidenced by risk factors of concurrent disease or injury process, dependence on external device (chest drainage system), and lack of safety education or precautions.

Anxiety [specify level] may be related to change in health status and threat of death, possibly evidenced by increased tension, restlessness, expressed concern, sympathetic stimulation, and focus on self.

Hepatitis, acute viral **MS/CH**

impaired Liver Function related to viral infection as evidenced by jaundice, hepatic enlargement, abdominal pain, marked elevations in serum liver function tests.

Fatigue may be related to decreased metabolic energy production, discomfort, altered body chemistry—changes in liver function, effect on target organs, possibly evidenced by reports of lack of energy, inability to maintain usual routines, decreased performance, and increased physical complaints.

imbalanced Nutrition: less than body requirements may be related to inability to ingest adequate nutrients (nausea, vomiting, anorexia); hypermetabolic state, altered absorption and metabolism—reduced peristalsis, bile stasis, possibly evidenced by aversion to eating or lack of interest in food, altered taste sensation, observed lack of intake, and weight loss.

acute Pain/impaired Comfort may be related to inflammation and swelling of the liver, arthralgias, urticarial eruptions, and pruritus, possibly evidenced by verbal reports, guarding or distraction behaviors, focus on self, and changes in vital signs.

risk for Infection possibly evidenced by risk factors of inadequate secondary defenses and immunosuppression, malnutrition, insufficient knowledge to avoid exposure to pathogens or spread to others.

risk for impaired Tissue Integrity possibly evidenced by risk factor of bile salt accumulation in the tissues.

deficient Knowledge [Learning Need] regarding disease process and transmission, treatment needs, and future expectations may be related to lack of information or recall, misinterpretation, unfamiliarity with resources, possibly evidenced by questions, statement of concerns, misconceptions, inaccurate follow-through of instructions, and development of preventable complications.

Hepatorenal syndrome **MS**

Refer to Cirrhosis; Renal failure, acute

Hernia, hiatal **CH**

chronic Pain may be related to regurgitation of acidic gastric contents, possibly evidenced by verbal reports, facial grimacing, and focus on self.

deficient Knowledge [Learning Need] regarding pathophysiology, prevention of complications, and self-care needs may be related to lack of information, misconceptions, possibly evidenced by statements of concern, questions, and recurrence of condition.

Hernia, inguinal **MS**

Refer to Herniorrhaphy

Herniated nucleus pulposus **CH/MS**

acute/chronic Pain may be related to nerve compression or irritation and muscle spasms, possibly evidenced by verbal reports, guarding or distraction behaviors, preoccupation with pain, self-focus, narrowed focus, changes in vital signs when pain is acute, altered muscle tone or function, changes in eating or sleeping patterns and libido, and physical or social withdrawal.

impaired physical Mobility may be related to pain (muscle spasms), therapeutic restrictions (e.g., rest, braces, or traction), muscular impairment, and depressive mood state, possibly evidenced by reports of pain on movement, reluctance to attempt or difficulty with purposeful movement, decreased muscle strength, impaired coordination, and limited range of motion.

deficient Diversional Activity may be related to length of recuperation period and therapy restrictions, physical limitations, pain and depression, possibly evidenced by statements of boredom, disinterest, "nothing to do," and restlessness, irritability, withdrawal.

Herniorrhaphy **MS/PED**

acute Pain may be related to disruption of skin, tissue, and muscle integrity, possibly evidenced by verbal or coded reports, alteration in muscle tone, distraction or guarding behaviors, narrowed focus, and autonomic responses.

risk for Injury possibly evidenced by risk factors of surgical repair, insertion of graft, increased intra-abdominal pressure (straining at stool, heavy lifting, strenuous activity).

Heroin abuse **CH**

risk for Infection possibly evidenced by risk factors of injection, reuse or sharing of needles, malnutrition, environmental exposure, insufficient knowledge or motivation to avoid pathogens.

imbalanced Nutrition: less than body requirements may be related to inadequate intake, possibly evidenced by anorexia, lack of food or methods to prepare food, economic difficulties, weight loss, poor muscle tone, decreased muscle mass.

risk for Trauma possibly evidenced by risk factors of personal vulnerability, cigarette smoking, lack of safety precautions, driving impaired or under the influence, high-crime neighborhood.

risk for ineffective Protection possibly evidenced by risk factors of effects of substance use, malnutrition, chronic disease, lifestyle choices, unhealthy environment.

Heroin withdrawal — CH/MS

acute Pain/impaired Comfort may be related to cessation of drug, muscle tremors or twitching, possibly evidenced by reports of muscle aches, hot and cold flashes, diaphoresis, lacrimation, rhinorrhea, drug cravings.

[severe] Anxiety may be related to central nervous system hyperactivity, possibly evidenced by apprehension, pervasive anxious feelings, jittery, restlessness, weakness, insomnia, anorexia.

risk for ineffective Health Management possibly evidenced by risk factors of protracted withdrawal, economic difficulties, family or social support deficits, perceived barriers or benefits.

Herpes simplex — CH

acute Pain may be related to presence of localized inflammation and open lesions, possibly evidenced by verbal reports, distraction behaviors, and restlessness.

risk for [secondary] Infection possibly evidenced by risk factors of broken or traumatized tissue, altered immune response, and untreated infection or treatment failure.

risk for Sexual dysfunction possibly evidenced by risdk factors of lack of knowledge, values conflict, or fear of transmitting the disease.

Herpes zoster (shingles) — CH

acute Pain may be related to inflammation, local lesions along sensory nerve(s), possibly evidenced by verbal reports, guarding or distraction behaviors, narrowed focus, and changes in vital signs.

deficient Knowledge [Learning Need] regarding pathophysiology, therapeutic needs, and potential complications may be related to lack of information, misinterpretation, possibly evidenced by statements of concern, questions, and misconceptions.

High altitude pulmonary edema (HAPE) — MS

Also refer to Mountain sickness, acute

impaired Gas Exchange may be related to ventilation perfusion imbalance, alveolar-capillary membrane changes, altered oxygen supply, possibly evidenced by dyspnea, confusion, cyanosis, tachycardia, abnormal arterial blood gases.

excess Fluid Volume may be related to compromised regulatory mechanism, possibly evidenced by shortness of breath, anxiety, edema, abnormal breath sounds, pulmonary congestion.

High altitude sickness — MS

Refer to Mountain sickness, acute; High altitude pulmonary edema

High-risk pregnancy — OB

Refer to Pregnancy, high-risk

Hip replacement — MS

Refer to Total joint replacement

HIV infection — CH

Also refer to AIDS

risk-prone Health Behavior may be related to life-threatening, stigmatizing condition or disease; assault to self-esteem; altered locus of control; inadequate support systems; incomplete grieving; medication side effects (fatigue, depression), possibly evidenced by verbalization of nonacceptance or denial of diagnosis, failure to take action that prevents health problems.

deficient Knowledge [Learning Need] regarding disease, prognosis, and treatment needs may be related to lack of exposure or recall, information misinterpretation, unfamiliarity with information resources, or cognitive limitation, possibly evidenced by statement of misconception, request for information, inappropriate or exaggerated behaviors (hostile, agitated, hysterical, apathetic), inaccurate follow-through of instructions, development of preventable complications.

risk for ineffective Health Management possibly evidenced by risk factors of complexity of healthcare system and access to care, economic difficulties; complexity of therapeutic regimen—confusing or difficult dosing schedule, duration of regimen; mistrust of regimen and/or healthcare personnel—client and provider interactions; health beliefs or cultural influences, perceived seriousness, susceptibility, or benefits of therapy; decisional conflicts, powerlessness.

risk for complicated Grieving possibly evidenced by risk factors of preloss psychological symptoms, predisposition for anxiety and feelings of inadequacy, frequency of major life events.

Hodgkin's disease CH/MS

Also refer to Cancer; Chemotherapy

Anxiety [specify level]/Fear may be related to threat to self-concept and threat of death, possibly evidenced by apprehension, insomnia, focus on self, and increased tension.

deficient Knowledge [Learning Need] regarding diagnosis, pathophysiology, treatment, and prognosis may be related to lack of information, misinterpretation, possibly evidenced by statements of concern, questions, and misconceptions.

acute Pain/impaired Comfort may be related to manifestations of inflammatory response (fever, chills, night sweats) and pruritus, possibly evidenced by verbal reports, distraction behaviors, and focus on self.

risk for ineffective Breathing Pattern/Airway Clearance possibly evidenced by risk factors of tracheobronchial obstruction (enlarged mediastinal nodes or airway edema).

Hospice care CH

acute/chronic Pain may be related to biological, physical, psychological agent; chronic physical disability, possibly evidenced by verbal or coded report, preoccupation with pain, changes in appetite, sleep pattern, altered ability to continue desired activities, guarded or protective behavior, restlessness, irritability, narrowed focus—altered time perception, impaired thought processes.

Activity Intolerance/Fatigue may be related to generalized weakness, bedrest or immobility, pain, progressive disease state or debilitating condition, depressive state, imbalance between oxygen supply and demand, possibly evidenced by inability to maintain usual routine, verbalized lack of desire or interest in activity, decreased performance, lethargy.

Grieving/Death Anxiety may be related to anticipated loss of physiological well-being, change in body function, perceived threat of death, or dying process, possibly evidenced by changes in communication pattern, denial of potential loss, choked feelings, anger, fear of loss of physical or mental abilities, negative death images or unpleasant thoughts about any event related to death or dying, anticipated pain related to dying; powerlessness over issues related to dying, worrying about impact of one's own death on SO(s), being the cause of others' grief and suffering, concerns of overworking the caregiver as terminal illness incapacitates.

compromised/disabled family Coping/caregiver Role Strain may be related to prolonged disease or disability progression, temporary family disorganization and role changes, unrealistic expectations, inadequate or incorrect information or understanding by primary person possibly evidenced by client expressing despair about family reactions or lack of involvement, history of poor relationship between caregiver and care receiver; altered caregiver health status; SO attempting assistive or supportive behaviors with less than satisfactory results; apprehension about future regarding caregiver's ability to provide care; SO describing preoccupation about personal reactions; displaying intolerance, abandonment, rejection; family behaviors that are detrimental to well-being.

risk for Spiritual distress possibly evidenced by risk factors of physical or psychological stress, energy-consuming anxiety, situational losses, blocks to self-love, low self-esteem, inability to forgive.

risk for Moral Distress possibly evidenced by risk factors of conflict among decision makers, cultural conflicts, end-of-life decisions, loss of autonomy, physical distance of decision makers.

Huntington's disease CH

Hopelessness may be related to chronic progressive debilitating condition, possibly evidenced by despondent verbalizations, withdrawal from environs, angry outbursts.

impaired Walking may be related to movement disorder (altered gait, ataxia, dystonia), possibly evidenced by inability to walk required distances, navigate curbs or uneven surfaces, climb stairs.

chronic Confusion may be related to dementia, possibly evidenced by altered interpretation, progressive cognitive impairment, altered personality, impaired memory, impaired socialization.

imbalanced Nutrition: less than body requirements may be related to inability to ingest food (difficulty swallowing, cognitive decline), possibly evidenced by aversion to eating, inadequate food intake, weight loss, decreased subcutaneous fat or muscle mass.

[total] Self-Care deficit may be related to neuromuscular impairment, cognitive decline, possibly evidenced by inability to perform desired activities of daily living.

risk for caregiver Role Strain possibly evidenced by risk factors of progressive deterioration (physical and mental) of care receiver, duration of caregiving required, complexity or amount of caregiving tasks, caregiver's competing role commitments, family isolation, lack of respite or recreation for caregiver, bizarre behavior of care receiver.

Hydrocephalus **PED/MS**

ineffective cerebral Tissue Perfusion may be related to decreased arterial or venous blood flow (compression of brain tissue), possibly evidenced by changes in mentation, restlessness, irritability, reports of headache, pupillary changes, and changes in vital signs.

[disturbed visual Sensory Perception] may be related to pressure on sensory or motor nerves, possibly evidenced by reports of double vision, development of strabismus, nystagmus, pupillary changes, and optic atrophy.

risk for impaired physical Mobility possibly evidenced by risk factors of neuromuscular impairment, decreased muscle strength, and impaired coordination.

risk for decreased intracranial Adaptive Capacity possibly evidenced by risk factors of brain injury, changes in perfusion pressure and intracranial pressure.

CH

risk for Infection possibly evidenced by risk factors of invasive procedure, presence of shunt.

deficient Knowledge [Learning Need] regarding condition, prognosis, long-term therapy needs, and medical follow-up may be related to lack of information, misperceptions, possibly evidenced by questions, statement of concern, request for information, and inaccurate follow-through of instructions, development of preventable complications.

Hydrophobia **CH/MS**

Refer to Rabies

Hyperactivity disorder **PED/PSY**

ineffective Impulse Control may be related to compunction, possibly evidenced by acting without thinking, temper outbursts.

defensive Coping may be related to mild neurological deficits, dysfunctional family system, abuse or neglect, possibly evidenced by denial of obvious problems, projection of blame or responsibility, grandiosity, difficulty in reality testing perceptions.

impaired Social Interaction may be related to retarded ego development, negative role models, neurological impairment, possibly evidenced by discomfort in social situations, interrupts or intrudes on others, difficulty waiting turn in games or group activities, difficulty maintaining attention to task.

disabled family Coping may be related to excessive guilt, anger, or blaming among family members, parental inconsistencies, disagreements regarding discipline or limit-setting approaches, exhaustion of parental expectations, possibly evidenced by unrealistic parental expectations, rejection or overprotection of child, exaggerated expression of feelings, despair regarding child's behavior.

Hyperbilirubinemia **PED**

neonatal Jaundice may be related to prematurity, hemolytic disease, asphyxia, acidosis, hyponatremia, hypoglycemia, difficulty transitioning to extra-uterine life, feeding pattern not well established, abnormal weight loss, possibly evidenced by abnormal blood profile (elevated blood urea nitrogen), yellow-orange skin and sclera.

risk for Injury [effects of treatment] possibly evidenced by risk factors of physical properties of phototherapy and effects on body regulatory mechanisms, invasive procedure (exchange transfusion), abnormal blood profile, chemical imbalances.

deficient Knowledge [Learning Need] regarding condition prognosis, treatment, and safety needs may be related to lack of exposure or recall and information misinterpretation, possibly evidenced by questions, statement of concern, and inaccurate follow-through of instructions, development of preventable complications.

Hyperemesis gravidarum **OB**

deficient Fluid Volume may be related to excessive gastric losses and reduced intake, possibly evidenced by dry mucous membranes, decreased and concentrated urine, decreased pulse volume and pressure, thirst, and hemoconcentration.

risk for Electrolyte Imbalance possibly evidenced by risk factors of vomiting, dehydration.

imbalanced Nutrition: less than body requirements may be related to inability to ingest, digest, or absorb nutrients (prolonged vomiting), possibly evidenced by reported inadequate food intake, lack of interest in food or aversion to eating, and weight loss.

risk for ineffective Coping possibly evidenced by risk factors of situational or maturational crisis (pregnancy, change in health status, projected role changes, concern about outcome).

Hyperparathyroidism, primary **MS**

risk for deficient Fluid Volume possibly evidenced by risk factors of excessive losses through normal routes (vomiting, diarrhea, gastric bleed).

risk for Electrolyte Imbalance possibly evidenced by risk factors of impaired regulatory mechanism, vomiting.

impaired urinary Elimination may be related to anatomical obstruction (renal calculi), possibly evidenced by decreased renal function.

risk for Trauma possibly evidenced by risk factors of decreased calcium levels, bone fragility.

Hypertension **CH**

deficient Knowledge [Learning Need] regarding condition, therapeutic regimen, and potential complications may be related to lack of information or recall, misinterpretation, cognitive limitations, or denial of diagnosis, possibly evidenced by statements of concern, questions, and misconceptions, inaccurate follow-through of instructions, and lack of blood pressure control.

risk-prone Health Behavior may be related to condition requiring change in lifestyle, altered locus of control, and absence of feelings or denial of illness, possibly evidenced by verbalization of nonacceptance of health status change and lack of movement toward independence.

risk for Activity Intolerance possibly evidenced by risk factors of generalized weakness, imbalance between oxygen supply and demand.

risk for Sexual dysfunction possibly evidenced by risk factor of side effects of medication.

MS

risk for decreased Cardiac Output possibly evidenced by risk factors of increased afterload (vasoconstriction), fluid shifts, hypovolemia, myocardial ischemia, ventricular hypertrophy and rigidity.

acute Pain may be related to increased cerebrovascular pressure, possibly evidenced by verbal reports (throbbing pain located in suboccipital region, present on awakening and disappearing spontaneously after being up and about), reluctance to move head, avoidance of bright lights and noise, increased muscle tension.

Hypertension, gestational **OB/CH**

Also refer to Eclampsia

deficient Fluid Volume may be related to a plasma protein loss, decreasing plasma colloid osmotic pressure allowing fluid shifts out of vascular compartment, possibly evidenced by edema formation, sudden weight gain, hemoconcentration, nausea, vomiting, epigastric pain, headaches, visual changes, decreased urine output.

decreased Cardiac Output may be related to hypovolemia, decreased venous return, increased systemic vascular resistance, possibly evidenced by variations in blood pressure and hemodynamic readings, edema, shortness of breath, change in mental status.

risk for disturbed Maternal-Fetal Dyad possibly evidenced by risk factors of compromised oxygen transport—vasospasm of spiral arteries and relative hypovolemia.

deficient Knowledge [Learning Need] regarding pathophysiology of condition, therapy, self-care, nutritional needs, and potential complications may be related to lack of information or recall, misinterpretation, possibly evidenced by statements of concern, questions, misconceptions, inaccurate follow-through of instructions, development of preventable complications.

Hypertension, intrapartum **OB**

risk for imbalanced Fluid Volume possibly evidenced by risk factors of compromised regulatory mechanism, fluid shifts, excessive fluid intake, effects of drug therapy (oxytocin infusion).

risk for impaired fetal Gas Exchange possibly evidenced by risk factors of altered blood flow, vasospasms, prolonged uterine contractions.

impaired urinary Elimination may be related to fluid shifts, hormonal changes, effects of medication, possibly evidenced by changes in amount and frequency of voiding, bladder distention, changes in urine specific gravity, presence of albumin.

risk for maternal Injury possibly evidenced by risk factors of tonic-clonic convulsions, altered clotting factors (release of thromboplastin from placenta).

acute Pain may be related to intensification of uterine activity, myometrial hypoxia, anxiety, possibly evidenced by verbalizations, altered muscle tone, distraction behaviors, autonomic responses, facial mask.

Hypertension, prenatal **OB**

Refer to Hypertension, gestational

Hypertension, pulmonary **CH/MS**

Refer to Pulmonary hypertension

Hyperthyroidism **CH**

Also refer to Thyrotoxicosis

Fatigue may be related to hypermetabolic imbalance with increased energy requirements, irritability of central nervous system, and altered body chemistry, possibly evidenced by verbalization of overwhelming lack of energy to maintain usual routine, decreased performance, emotional lability and irritability, and impaired ability to concentrate.

Anxiety [specify level] may be related to increased stimulation of the central nervous system (hypermetabolic state, pseudocatecholamine effect of thyroid hormones), possibly evidenced by increased feelings of apprehension, overexcitement, or distress; irritability; emotional lability; shakiness; restless movements; tremors.

risk for imbalanced Nutrition: less than body requirements possibly evidenced by risk factors of inability to ingest adequate nutrients for hypermetabolic rate, constant activity level, impaired absorption of nutrients (vomiting, diarrhea), hyperglycemia, relative insulin insufficiency.

risk for Dry Eye possibly evidenced by risk factors of autoimmune diseases (thyroid disease), lack of spontaneous blink reflex, ocular surface damage.

Hypervolemia — CH/MS

excess Fluid Volume may be related to excess fluid and sodium intake, compromised regulatory mechanisms (renal failure, increased antidiuretic hormone), decreased plasma proteins, rapid or excessive administration of isotonic parenteral fluids, possibly evidenced by edema, abnormal breath sounds, S_3 heart sound, shortness of breath, positive hepatojugular reflex—elevated central venous pressure, change in mental status.

Hypochondriasis — PSY

Refer to Somatoform disorders

Hypoglycemia — CH

acute Confusion may be related to inadequate glucose for cellular brain function and effects of endogenous hormone activity, possibly evidenced by increased restlessness, misperceptions, fluctuation in cognition/level of consciousness.

risk for unstable Blood Glucose Level possibly evidenced by risk factors of dietary intake, lack of adherence to diabetes management, inadequate blood glucose monitoring, medication management.

deficient Knowledge [Learning Need] regarding pathophysiology of condition, therapy, and self-care needs may be related to lack of information or recall, misinterpretations, possibly evidenced by development of hypoglycemia and statements of questions, misconceptions.

Hypoparathyroidism (acute) — MS

risk for Electrolyte Imbalance possibly evidenced by risk factor of impaired regulatory mechanism.

risk for Injury possibly evidenced by risk factors of neuromuscular excitability—tetany and formation of renal stones.

acute Pain may be related to recurrent muscle spasms and alteration in reflexes, possibly evidenced by verbal reports, distraction behaviors, and narrowed focus.

risk for ineffective Airway Clearance possibly evidenced by risk factor of spasm of the laryngeal muscles.

Anxiety [specify level] may be related to threat to, or change in, health status, physiological responses.

Hypophysectomy — MS

Also refer to Surgery, general; Cancer

Fear/Anxiety may be related to situational crisis (nature of diagnosis and procedure), change in health status, perceived threat of death, separation from support system, possibly evidenced by expressed concerns, apprehension, being scared, increased tension, extraneous movement, difficulty concentrating.

risk for deficient Fluid Volume possibly evidenced by risk factors of failure of regulatory mechanism (decreased antidiuretic hormone).

risk for Infection possibly evidenced by risk factors of traumatized tissue, invasive procedure, cerebrospinal fluid leak.

Sexual dysfunction may be related to altered body function (loss of anterior pituitary), possibly evidenced by sterility, decreased libido, impotence (male), infertility, atrophy of vaginal mucosa (female).

Hypothermia (systemic) — CH

Also refer to Frostbite

Hypothermia may be related to exposure to cold environment, inadequate clothing, age extremes (very young or elderly), damage to hypothalamus, consumption of alcohol or medications causing vasodilation, possibly evidenced by reduction in body temperature below normal range, shivering, cool skin, pallor.

deficient Knowledge [Learning Need] regarding risk factors, treatment needs, and prognosis may be related to lack of information or recall, misinterpretation, possibly evidenced by statement of concerns, misconceptions, occurrence of problem, and development of complications.

Hypothyroidism **CH**

Also refer to Myxedema

Fatigue may be related to decreased metabolic energy production, possibly evidenced by verbalization of unremitting or overwhelming lack of energy, inability to maintain usual routines, impaired ability to concentrate, decreased libido, irritability, listlessness, decreased performance, increase in physical complaints.

Constipation may be related to decreased peristalsis, lack of physical activity, possibly evidenced by frequency less than usual pattern, decreased bowel sounds, hard dry stools, and development of fecal impaction.

impaired physical Mobility may be related to weakness, fatigue, muscle aches, altered reflexes, and mucin deposits in joints and interstitial spaces, possibly evidenced by decreased muscle strength or control and impaired coordination.

[disturbed Sensory Perception (specify)] may be related to mucin deposits and nerve compression, possibly evidenced by paresthesias of hands and feet or decreased hearing.

Hypovolemia **CH/MS**

deficient Fluid Volume may be related to active fluid loss (hemorrhage, vomiting, gastric intubation, diarrhea, burns, wounds, fistulas), regulatory failure (adrenal disease, recovery phase of acute renal fialure, diabetic ketoacidosis, hyperosmolar nonketotic coma, diabetes insipidus, sepsis), possibly evidenced by thirst, weight loss, poor skin turgor, dry mucous membranes, tachycardia, tachypnea, fatigue, decreased central venous pressure.

Hysterectomy **GYN/MS**

Also refer to Surgery, general

acute Pain may be related to tissue trauma, abdominal incision, edema, hematoma formation, possibly evidenced by verbal reports, guarding or distraction behaviors, and changes in vital signs.

risk for perioperative positioning Injury possibly evidenced by risk factors of immobilization, lithotomy position.

impaired urinary Elimination/risk for [acute] Urinary Retention possibly evidenced by risk factors of mechanical trauma, surgical manipulation, presence of localized edema or hematoma, or nerve trauma with temporary bladder atony.

risk for Sexual dysfunction possibly evidenced by risk factors of concerns regarding altered body function and structure, perceived changes in femininity, changes in hormone levels, loss of libido, and changes in sexual response pattern.

Ileal conduit **MS/CH**

Refer to Urinary diversion

Ileocolitis **MS/CH**

Refer to Crohn's disease

Ileostomy **MS/CH**

Refer to Colostomy

Ileus **MS**

acute Pain may be related to distention, edema and ischemia of intestinal tissue, possibly evidenced by verbal reports, guarding/distraction behaviors, narrowed focus, and changes in vital signs.

Diarrhea/Constipation may be related to presence of obstruction, changes in peristalsis, possibly evidenced by changes in frequency and consistency or absence of stool, alterations in bowel sounds, presence of pain, and cramping.

risk for deficient Fluid Volume possibly evidenced by risk factors of increased intestinal losses (vomiting, diarrhea) and decreased intake.

Immersion foot **MS**

impaired Skin/Tissue Integrity may be related to exposure to cold and wet environment (above freezing), altered circulation, presence of infection, possibly evidenced by tissue maceration, pain, soggy edema.

[disturbed peripheral Sensory Perception] may be related to altered sensory reception, possibly evidenced by paresthesia, numbness.

risk for ineffective Health Maintenance possibly evidenced by risk factors of lack of material resources, poor coping skills, inadequate knowledge of safety needs.

Impetigo **PED/CH**

impaired Skin Integrity may be related to presence of infectious process and pruritus, possibly evidenced by open, crusted lesions.

acute Pain may be related to inflammation and pruritus, possibly evidenced by verbal reports, distraction behaviors, and self-focusing.

risk for [secondary] Infection possibly evidenced by risk factors of broken skin, traumatized tissue, altered immune response, and virulence or contagious nature of causative organism.

risk for Infection [transmission] possibly evidenced by risk factors of virulent nature of causative organism, insufficient knowledge to prevent infection of others.

Impotence **CH**
Refer to Erectile dysfunction

Infant (at 4 weeks) **PED**
readiness for enhanced Knowledge regarding infant care, developmental expectations, safety, and well-being may be related to changing needs of infant, possibly evidenced by questions, expressed concerns or desire to learn more, behaviors congruent with expressed knowledge.

risk for imbalanced Nutrition (specify) possibly evidenced by risk factors of failure to ingest, digest, or absorb adequate calories—insufficient intake, malabsorption, congenital problem, neglect or emotional abuse, or failure to thrive; obesity in one or both parents, rapid transition across growth percentiles.

risk for acute Pain possibly evidenced by risk factor of accumulation of gas in confined space with cramping of intestinal musculature.

risk for Infection possibly evidenced by risk factors of immature immunological response, increased environmental exposure.

risk for Sudden Infant Death Syndrome possibly evidenced by risk factors of sleeping position, secondhand smoke exposure, type of bedding used.

risk for disorganized infant Behavior possibly evidenced by risk factors of immature development of sensory organs, inappropriate or inadequate environmental stimuli, effects of prenatal or intrapartal complications, drugs.

Infant of addicted mother **OB/PED**
risk for Injury [central nervous system damage] possibly evidenced by risk factors of prematurity, hypoxia, effects of medications, substance use, or withdrawal; possible exposure to infectious agents (prenatal, intrapartal).

ineffective Airway Clearance/impaired Gas Exchange may be related to excess mucus production, depression of cough reflex and respiratory center, intrauterine asphyxia, possibly evidenced by tachypnea, tachycardia, cyanosis, nasal flaring, grunting respirations, hypoxia, acidosis.

risk for Infection possibly evidenced by risk factors of presence of maternal infections (Guillain-Barré syndrome, sexually transmitted infection).

risk for imbalanced Nutrition: less than body requirements possibly evidenced by risk factors of inability to ingest, digest, or absorb adequate nutrients to meet metabolic needs (e.g., poor or uncoordinated sucking and swallowing, frequent gastrointestinal irritation with vomiting, diarrhea, repeated regurgitation, frequent hyperactivity).

risk for impaired Skin Integrity possibly evidenced by risk factors of mechanical factors (continual rubbing of face or knees against bedding, scratching face with hands), presence of excretions.

impaired Parenting may be related to lack of available or ineffective role model, unmet emotional maturation needs of parent, lack of support between or from SO, interruption in bonding process, lack of appropriate response of infant, possibly evidenced by reports of role inadequacy or inability to care for infant, inattention to infant needs, inappropriate caretaking behaviors, lack of parental attachment behaviors.

disabled family Coping may be related to SO with chronically unexpressed feelings of guilt, anxiety, hostility, despair; dissonant discrepancy of coping styles; high-risk family situations, possibly evidenced by intolerance, rejection, abandonment, or desertion, neglectful relationships between family members, neglectful care of infant, distortion of reality of parent's health problem or substance use.

Infant of HIV-positive mother **OB/PED**
Also refer to AIDS

risk for Infection possibly evidenced by risk factors of immature immune system, inadequate acquired immunity, suppressed inflammatory response, invasive procedures, malnutrition.

risk for imbalanced Nutrition: risk for less than body requirements possibly evidenced by risk factors of inability to ingest, digest, or absorb nutrients (e.g., impaired suck or swallow, gastrointestinal infection, malabsorption, diarrhea).

risk for delayed Development possibly evidenced by risk factors of separation from SO, inadequate caretaking, inconsistent responsiveness, multiple caretakers, environmental and stimulation deficiencies, effects of chronic condition or disabilities.

deficient Knowledge [Learning Need] regarding condition, prognosis, and treatment needs may be related to lack of exposure, misinterpretation, unfamiliarity with resources, lack of recall or interest in learning, possibly evidenced by questions, statements of misconceptions, inaccurate follow-through of instructions, development of preventable complications.

Infection, ear — PED
Refer to Otitis media

Infection, prenatal — OB
Also refer to AIDS

risk for disturbed Maternal-Fetal Dyad possibly evidenced by risk factors of presence of infection, anemia, inadequate acquired immunity, environmental exposure, rupture of amniotic membranes, treatment-related side effects.

deficient Knowledge [Learning Need] regarding treatment, prevention, and prognosis of condition may be related to lack of exposure to information or unfamiliarity with resources, misinterpretation, possibly evidenced by verbalization of problem, inaccurate follow-through of instructions, development of preventable complications, continuation of infectious process.

impaired Comfort may be related to body response to infective agent, properties of infection (e.g., skin or tissue irritation, development of lesions), possibly evidenced by verbal reports, illness-related symptoms, restlessness, withdrawal from social contacts.

Infection, puerperal — OB/CH
risk for Infection [spread/sepsis] possibly evidenced by risk factors of presence of infection, broken skin, traumatized tissues, high vascularity of involved area, invasive procedures/increased environmental exposure, anemia, chronic disease.

acute Pain may be related to body response to infective agent and toxins, possibly evidenced by verbalizations, restlessness, guarding behavior, self-focusing, and changes in vital signs.

imbalanced Nutrition: less than body requirements may be related to insufficient intake to meet metabolic demands (anorexia, nausea, vomiting, medical restrictions), possibly evidenced by aversion to eating, decreased or lack of oral intake, unanticipated weight loss.

risk for impaired Attachment possibly evidenced by risk factors of interruption in bonding process, separation, physical barriers, maternal fatigue or apathy.

Infection, wound — MS/CH
risk for Infection [sepsis] possibly evidenced by risk factors of presence of infection, broken skin, or traumatized tissues, stasis of body fluids, invasive procedures, increased environmental exposure, chronic disease (e.g., diabetes, anemia, malnutrition), altered immune response, and untoward effect of medications (e.g., opportunistic or secondary infection).

impaired Skin/Tissue Integrity may be related to altered circulation, presence of infection, wound drainage, nutritional deficit, possibly evidenced by delayed healing, damaged tissues, invasion of body structures.

risk for delayed Surgical Recovery possibly evidenced by risk factors of presence of infection, activity restrictions or limitations, nutritional deficiency.

Infertility — CH
situational low Self-Esteem may be related to functional impairment (inability to conceive), unrealistic self-expectations, sense of failure, possibly evidenced by self-negating verbalizations, expressions of helplessness, perceived inability to deal with situation.

chronic Sorrow may be related to perceived physical disability (inability to conceive), possibly evidenced by expressions of anger, disappointment, emptiness, self-blame, helplessness, sadness, feelings interfering with client's ability to achieve maximum well-being.

risk for Spiritual distress possibly evidenced by risk factors of energy-consuming anxiety, low self-esteem, deteriorating relationship with SO, viewing situation as deserved or punishment for past behaviors.

Inflammatory bowel disease — CH
Refer to Colitis, ulcerative; Crohn's disease

Influenza — CH
acute Pain/impaired Comfort may be related to inflammation and effects of circulating toxins, possibly evidenced by verbal reports, distraction behaviors, and narrowed focus.

risk for deficient Fluid Volume possibly evidenced by risk factors of excessive gastric losses, hypermetabolic state, and altered intake.

Hyperthermia may be related to effects of circulating toxins and dehydration, possibly evidenced by increased body temperature; warm, flushed skin; and tachycardia.

risk for ineffective Breathing Pattern possibly evidenced by risk factors of response to infectious process, decreased energy, fatigue.

Inhalant intoxication/abuse — CH/PSY
Refer to Stimulant abuse

Insomnia, acute — CH
Insomnia may be related to daytime activity pattern, social or work schedule inconsistent with chronotype, travel across time zones, fatigue, life change, physical

conditions (dyspnea, gastroesophageal reflux, night sweats), possibly evidenced by verbal reports of difficulties, not feeling well-rested, less than age-normed total sleep time, changes in behavior and performance, physical signs (dark circles under eyes, frequent yawning).

Insomnia, chronic **CH**

Sleep deprivation may be related to sustained environmental stimulation, sustained circadian asynchrony, prolonged use of pharmacological or dietary antisoporifics, prolonged pain, sleep apnea, dementia, narcolepsy, possibly evidenced by daytime drowsiness, decreased ability to perform, lethargy, slowed reaction, apathy.

Insulin resistance syndrome **CH**

Refer to Metabolic syndrome

Insulin shock **MS/CH**

Refer to Hypoglycemia

Intermaxillary fixation **MS/CH**

Also refer to Surgery, general

risk for ineffective Airway Clearance possibly evidenced by risk factors of soft tissue trauma, retained secretions.

risk for Aspiration possibly evidenced by risk factors of facial trauma or surgery, wired jaws, difficulty swallowing.

impaired Tissue Integrity may be related to tissue trauma or damage, intraoperative manipulation, mechanical fixation device, altered circulation, nutritional deficit, possibly evidenced by edema, hematoma, ecchymosis, erythema, inflammation, delayed healing.

impaired verbal Communication may be related to wiring of jaws, edema of mouth and surrounding structures, pain, possibly evidenced by inability or reluctance to talk.

risk for imbalanced Nutrition: less than body requirements possibly evidenced by risk factors of facial and tissue edema, inability to chew, difficulty swallowing, decreased appetite, increased metabolic needs.

Intervertebral disc excision **MS**

Refer to Laminectomy, cervical or lumbar

Intestinal obstruction **MS**

Refer to Ileus

Intestinal surgery (without diversion) **MS**

Also refer to Surgery, general

risk for deficient Fluid Volume possibly evidenced by risk factors of excessive losses through normal routes (vomiting, diarrhea), excessive losses through abnormal routes (indwelling drains, nasogastric/intestinal suctioning, hemorrhage), insufficient replacement, fever.

risk for Infection possibly evidenced by risk factors of chronic disease, malnutrition, opening of abdominal cavity and bowel, stasis of body fluids, altered peristalsis.

Constipation/Diarrhea may be related to effects of anesthesia, surgical manipulation, decreased dietary intake or bulk, physical inactivity, irritation, malabsorption, pain, effects of medication, possibly evidenced by change in bowel habits, change in stool characteristics, hyper-/hypoactive bowel sounds, abdominal pain.

Intracranial infections **MS**

Refer to Abscess, brain [acute]; Encephalitis; Meningitis, acute meningococcal

Irritable bowel syndrome **CH**

acute Pain may be related to abnormally strong intestinal contractions, increased sensitivity of intestine to distention, hypersensitivity to hormones gastrin and cholecystokinin, skin or tissue irritation, perirectal excoriation, possibly evidenced by verbal reports, guarding behavior, expressive behavior (restlessness, moaning, irritability).

Constipation may be related to motor abnormalities of longitudinal muscles, changes in frequency and amplitude of contractions, dietary restrictions, stress, possibly evidenced by change in bowel pattern—decreased frequency, sensation of incomplete evacuation, abdominal pain and distention.

Diarrhea may be related to motor abnormalities of longitudinal muscles, changes in frequency and amplitude of contractions, stress, possibly evidenced by precipitous passing of liquid stool on rising or immediately after eating, rectal urgency, incontinence, bloating.

Kanner's syndrome **PED/PSY**

Refer to Autistic spectrum disorder

Kaposi's sarcoma, AIDS-related **CH/MS**

Also refer to Chemotherapy

disturbed Body Image may be related to widely disseminated lesions of varied color in skin and mucous membranes, possibly evidenced by verbalizations, fear of rejection or reaction of others, negative feelings about body, hiding body parts, change in social involvement.

risk for deficient Fluid Volume possibly evidenced by risk factors of extensive bleeding of visceral lesions.

Kawasaki disease **PED**

Hyperthermia may be related to increased metabolic rate and dehydration, possibly evidenced by increased body temperature greater than normal range, flushed skin, increased respiratory rate, and tachycardia.

acute Pain may be related to inflammation and edema or swelling of tissues, possibly evidenced by verbal reports, restlessness, guarding behaviors, and narrowed focus.

impaired Skin Integrity may be related to inflammatory process, altered circulation, and edema formation, possibly evidenced by disruption of skin surface, including macular rash and desquamation.

impaired oral Mucous Membrane may be related to inflammatory process, dehydration, and mouth breathing, possibly evidenced by pain, hyperemia, and fissures of lips.

risk for decreased Cardiac Output possibly evidenced by risk factors of structural changes and inflammation of coronary arteries, and alterations in rate and rhythm or conduction.

Ketoacidosis **CH**

Refer to Diabetic ketoacidosis

Kidney disease, polycystic **CH**

risk for [urinary tract] Infection possibly evidenced by risk factors of inadequate primary defenses (traumatized tissue, stasis of body fluids), inadequate secondary defenses (suppressed inflammatory response), chronic disease.

acute/chronic Pain may be related to injuring agents—presence of cysts in kidneys or other organs, possibly evidenced by verbal report of back or lower side pain, headaches beyond tolerance, guarded or protective behavior, narrowed focus, sleep disturbance, distraction behaviors.

risk for excess Fluid Volume possibly evidenced by risk factors of oliguria, edema, abnormal breath sounds, jugular vein distention, hypertension.

Kidney failure, acute **MS**

Refer to Renal failure, acute

Kidney failure, chronic **CH/MS**

Refer to Renal failure, chronic

Kidney stone(s) **CH**

Refer to Calculi, urinary

Knee replacement **MS**

Refer to Total joint replacement

Kwashiorkor **PED**

imbalanced Nutrition: less than body requirements may be related to financial or resource limitations, possibly evidenced by inadequate food intake less than recommended daily allowances, lack of food, weight loss, poor muscle tone, decreased subcutaneous fat or muscle mass, abnormal laboratory studies.

risk for Infection possibly evidenced by malnutrition.

risk for disproportionate Growth possibly evidenced by malnutrition, caregiver maladaptive feeding behaviors, deprivation, poverty, impaired insulin response, infection.

Labor, breech presentation **OB**

Anxiety [specify level] may be related to situational crisis, threat to self/fetus, interpersonal transmission, possibly evidenced by increased tension, apprehension, fearfulness, restlessness, sympathetic stimulation.

risk for fetal Injury possibly evidenced by risk factors of entrapment of head, stretching of brachial plexus or spinal cord (nerve damage), hypoxia (brain damage).

Labor, dysfunctional **OB**

Refer to Dystocia

Labor, induced/augmented **OB**

deficient Knowledge [Learning Need] regarding procedure, treatment needs, and possible outcomes may be related to lack of exposure or recall, information misinterpretation, and unfamiliarity with information resources, possibly evidenced by questions, statement of concern, misconception, and exaggerated behaviors.

risk for maternal Injury possibly evidenced by risk factors of adverse effects or response to therapeutic interventions.

risk for impaired fetal Gas Exchange possibly evidenced by risk factors of altered placental perfusion, cord prolapse.

labor Pain may be related to altered characteristics of chemically stimulated contractions, cervical dilation, psychological concerns, possibly evidenced by verbal reports, increased muscle tone, distraction or guarding behaviors, and narrowed focus.

Labor, precipitous **OB**

Anxiety [specify level] may be related to situational crisis, threat to self/fetus, interpersonal transmission, possibly evidenced by increased tension; scared, fearful, restless, jittery; sympathetic stimulation.

risk for impaired Skin/Tissue Integrity possibly evidenced by risk factors of mechanical factors (e.g., pressure, shearing forces).

labor Pain may be related to occurrence of rapid, strong uterine contractions, cervical dilation; psychological issues, possibly evidenced by verbalizations of inability to use learned pain-management techniques, sympathetic stimulation, distraction behaviors (e.g., moaning, restlessness).

Labor, preterm **OB/CH**

Activity Intolerance may be related to muscle and cellular hypersensitivity, possibly evidenced by continued uterine contractions or irritability.

risk for Poisoning possibly evidenced by risk factors of dose-related toxic or side effects of tocolytics.

risk for fetal Injury possibly evidenced by risk factors of delivery of premature/immature infant.

Anxiety [specify level] may be related to situational crisis, perceived or actual threats to self/fetus, and inadequate time to prepare for labor, possibly evidenced by increased tension, restlessness, expressions of concern, and autonomic responses (changes in vital signs).

deficient Knowledge [Learning Need] regarding preterm labor treatment needs and prognosis may be related to lack of information and misinterpretation, possibly evidenced by questions, statements of concern, misconceptions, inaccurate follow-through of instruction, and development of preventable complications.

Labor, stage I (active phase) **OB**

labor Pain/impaired Comfort may be related to contraction-related hypoxia, dilation of tissues, and pressure on adjacent structures combined with stimulation of both parasympathetic and sympathetic nerve endings, possibly evidenced by verbal reports, guarding or distraction behaviors (restlessness), muscle tension, and narrowed focus.

impaired urinary Elimination may be related to altered intake, dehydration, fluid shifts, hormonal changes, hemorrhage, severe intrapartal hypertension, mechanical compression of bladder, and effects of regional anesthesia, possibly evidenced by changes in amount and frequency of voiding, urinary retention, slowed progression of labor, and reduced sensation.

risk for ineffective [individual/couple] Coping possibly evidenced by risk factors of situational crises, personal vulnerability, use of ineffective coping mechanisms, inadequate support systems, and pain.

Labor, stage I (latent phase) **OB**

deficient Knowledge [Learning Need] regarding progression of labor and available options may be related to lack of exposure or recall, information misinterpretation, possibly evidenced by questions, statements of misconceptions, inaccurate follow-through of instructions.

risk for [mild] Anxiety possibly evidenced by risk factors of situational crisis, unmet needs, stress.

risk for ineffective Coping possibly evidenced by risk factors of personal vulnerability, inadequate support systems or coping methods.

Labor, stage I (transition phase) **OB**

labor Pain may be related to mechanical pressure of presenting part, tissue dilation or stretching and hypoxia, stimulation of para/sympathetic nerves, possibly evidenced by verbal reports, narrowed focus.

Fatigue may be related to discomfort, pain, overwhelming psychological emotional demands, increased energy requirements, decreased caloric intake, possibly evidenced by verbalizations, impaired ability to concentrate, emotional lability or irritability, lethargy, altered coping ability.

risk for imbalanced Fluid Volume possibly evidenced by risk factors of reduced intake, excess fluid loss, hemorrhage, excess fluid retention, rapid fluid administration.

risk for decreased Cardiac Output possibly evidenced by risk factors of decreased venous return, hypovolemia, changes in systemic vascular resistance.

Labor, stage II (expulsion) **OB**

labor Pain may be related to strong uterine contractions, tissue stretching and dilation, and compression of nerves by presenting part of the fetus, and bladder distention, possibly evidenced by verbalizations, facial grimacing, narrowed focus, and autonomic responses (diaphoresis).

Cardiac Output [fluctuation] may be related to changes in systemic vascular resistance, fluctuations in venous return (repeated or prolonged Valsalva's maneuvers, effects of anesthesia and medications, dorsal recumbent position occluding the inferior vena cava and partially obstructing the aorta), possibly evidenced by decreased venous return, changes in vital signs (blood pressure, pulse), urinary output, fetal bradycardia.

risk for impaired fetal Gas Exchange possibly evidenced by risk factors of mechanical compression of head or cord, maternal position or prolonged labor affecting placental perfusion, and effects of maternal anesthesia, hyperventilation.

risk for impaired Skin/Tissue Integrity possibly evidenced by risk factors of untoward stretching, lacerations of delicate tissues (precipitous labor, hypertonic contractile pattern, adolescence, large fetus) and application of forceps.

risk for Fatigue possibly evidenced by risk factors of pregnancy, stress, anxiety, sleep deprivation, increased physical exertion, anemia, environmental humidity, temperature, and lights.

Labor, stage III (placental expulsion) OB

acute Pain may be related to tissue trauma, psychological response following delivery, possibly evidenced by verbalizations, changes in muscle tone, restlessness.

risk for deficient Fluid Volume/Bleeding possibly evidenced by risk factors of lack or restriction of oral intake, vomiting, diaphoresis, increased insensible water loss, uterine atony, lacerations of the birth canal, retained placental fragments.

risk for maternal Injury possibly evidenced by risk factors of positioning during delivery and transfers, difficulty with placental separation, abnormal blood profile.

risk for impaired Attachment possibly evidenced by risk factors of physical barriers, separation, anxiety associated with the parent role.

Labor, stage IV (first 4 hr following delivery of placenta) OB

Fatigue may be related to increased physical exertion, sleep deprivation, stress, environmental stimuli, hormonal changes, possibly evidenced by verbalization of overwhelming lack of energy, compromised concentration, listlessness.

acute Pain may be related to effects of hormones and medications, mechanical trauma, tissue edema, physical and psychological exhaustion, anxiety, possibly evidenced by reports of cramping (afterpains), muscle tremors, guarding or distraction behaviors, facial mask.

risk for Bleeding possibly evidenced by risk factors of myometrial fatigue/failure of homeostatic mechanisms (e.g., continued uteroplacental circulation, incomplete vasoconstriction, effects of pregnancy-induced hypertension).

risk for impaired Attachment possibly evidenced by risk factors of maternal fatigue, physical barriers, separation, lack of privacy, anxiety associated with the parent role.

Laceration CH

impaired Skin/Tissue Integrity may be related to trauma, possibly evidenced by disruption of skin layers, invasion of body structures.

risk for Infection possibly evidenced by risk factors of trauma, tissue destruction, increased environmental exposure.

Laminectomy, cervical MS

Also refer to Laminectomy, lumbar

risk for perioperative Positioning Injury possibly evidenced by risk factors of immobilization, muscle weakness, obesity, advanced age.

risk for ineffective Airway Clearance possibly evidenced by risk factors of retained secretions, pain, muscular weakness.

risk for impaired Swallowing possibly evidenced by risk factors of operative edema, pain, neuromuscular impairment.

Laminectomy, lumbar MS

Also refer to Surgery, general

risk for ineffective Tissue Perfusion (specify) possibly evidenced by risk factors of diminished or interrupted blood flow—pressure dressing, edema of operative site, hematoma formation; hypovolemia.

risk for [spinal] Trauma possibly evidenced by risk factors of temporary weakness of spinal column, balancing difficulties, changes in muscle tone and coordination.

acute Pain may be related to traumatized tissues—surgical manipulation, harvesting bone graft; localized inflammation, and edema, possibly evidenced by altered muscle tone, verbal reports, distraction or guarding behaviors, autonomic changes—changes in vital signs, diaphoresis, pallor.

impaired physical Mobility may be related to imposed therapeutic restrictions, neuromuscular impairment, and pain, possibly evidenced by limited range of motion, decreased muscle strength and control, impaired coordination, and reluctance to attempt movement.

risk for [acute] Urinary Retention possibly evidenced by risk factors of reduced mobility, restrictions of position.

Laryngectomy **MS**

Also refer to Cancer; Chemotherapy

ineffective Airway Clearance may be related to partial or total removal of the glottis—impairing ability to breathe, cough, or swallow; temporary or permanent change to neck breathing (dependent on patent stoma), edema formation—surgical manipulation, lymphatic accumulation; and copious, thick secretions, possibly evidenced by dyspnea; changes in rate and depth of respiration; use of accessory respiratory muscles; weak, ineffective cough; abnormal breath sounds; and cyanosis.

impaired Skin/Tissue Integrity may be related to surgical removal of tissues and grafting, effects of radiation or chemotherapeutic agents, altered circulation or reduced blood supply, compromised nutritional status, edema formation, and pooling or continuous drainage of secretions, possibly evidenced by disruption and destruction of skin and tissue layers.

impaired oral Mucous Membrane may be related to dehydration or absence of oral intake, decreased saliva production, poor or inadequate oral hygiene, pathological condition (oral cancer), mechanical trauma (oral surgery), decreased saliva production, difficulty swallowing and pooling of secretions or drooling, and nutritional deficits, possibly evidenced by xerostomia (dry mouth), oral discomfort, thick, mucoid saliva; decreased saliva production, dry and crusted or coated tongue, inflamed lips, absent teeth and gums, poor dental health, and halitosis.

CH

impaired verbal Communication may be related to anatomic deficit (removal of vocal cords), physical barrier (tracheostomy tube), and required voice rest, possibly evidenced by inability to speak, change in vocal characteristics, and impaired articulation.

risk for Aspiration possibly evidenced by risk factors of impaired swallowing, facial and neck surgery, presence of tracheostomy, feeding tube.

Laryngitis **CH/PED**

Refer to Croup

Latex allergy **CH**

Latex Allergy Response may be related to hypersensitivity to latex rubber protein, possibly evidenced by contact dermatitis—erythema, blisters; type IV reaction—eczema, irritation; hypersensitivity—generalized edema, wheezing, bronchospasm, hypotension, cardiac arrest.

Anxiety [specify level]/Fear may be related to threat of death, possibly evidenced by expressed concerns, hypervigilance, restlessness, focus on self.

risk for risk-prone Health Behavior possibly evidenced by risk factors of health status requiring change in occupation.

Laxative abuse **CH**

perceived Constipation may be related to health beliefs, faulty appraisal, impaired cognition/thought processes, possibly evidenced by expectation of daily bowel movement, expected passage of stool at same time every day.

Lead poisoning, acute **PED/CH**

Also refer to Lead poisoning, chronic

Contamination may be related to flaking or peeling paint (young children), improperly lead-glazed ceramic pottery, unprotected contact with lead (e.g., battery manufacture or recycling, bronzing, soldering or welding), imported herbal products or medicinals, possibly evidenced by abdominal cramping, headache, irritability, decreased attentiveness, constipation, tremors.

risk for Trauma possibly evidenced by risk factors of loss of coordination, altered level of consciousness, clonic or tonic muscle activity, neurological damage.

risk for deficient Fluid Volume possibly evidenced by risk factors of excessive vomiting, diarrhea, or decreased intake.

deficient Knowledge [Learning Need] regarding sources of lead and prevention of poisoning may be related to lack of information, misinterpretation, possibly evidenced by statements of concern, questions, and misconceptions.

Lead poisoning, chronic **CH**

Also refer to Lead poisoning, acute

Contamination may be related to flaking or peeling paint (young children), improperly lead-glazed ceramic pottery, unprotected contact with lead (e.g., battery manufacture or recycling, bronzing, soldering or welding), imported herbal products or medicinals, possibly evidenced by chronic abdominal cramping, headache, personality changes, cognitive deficits, seizures, neuropathy.

imbalanced Nutrition: less than body requirements may be related to decreased intake (chemically induced changes in the gastrointestinal tract), possibly evidenced by anorexia, abdominal discomfort, reported metallic taste, and weight loss.

chronic Pain may be related to deposition of lead in soft tissues and bone, possibly evidenced by verbal reports, distraction behaviors, and focus on self.

risk for delayed Development/disproportionate Growth possibly evidenced by risk factors of lead poisoning, chronic illness.

Legionnaires' disease **CH/MS**

Hyperthermia may be related to illness and inflammatory process, possibly evidenced by increased body temperature; flushed, warm skin; chills.

acute Pain/impaired Comfort may be related to infectious agent and inflammatory response, effects of circulating toxins, possibly evidenced by reports of headache, myalgia, high fever, diaphoresis.

ineffective Airway Clearance may be related to tracheal bronchial inflammation, edema formation, increased sputum production, pleuritic pain, decreased energy, fatigue, possibly evidenced by changes in rate and depth of respirations, abnormal breath sounds, use of accessory muscles, dyspnea, cyanosis, ineffective cough—with or without sputum production.

impaired Gas Exchange may be related to inflammatory process, collection of secretions affecting oxygen exchange across alveolar membrane, and hypoventilation, possibly evidenced by restlessness, changes in mentation, dyspnea, tachycardia, pallor, cyanosis, and arterial blood gas or oximetry evidence of hypoxia.

Diarrhea may be related to infectious process, possibly evidenced by liquid stools, abdominal cramping.

risk for Infection [spread] possibly evidenced by risk factors of decreased ciliary action, stasis of secretions, presence of existing infection, improper disposal of contaminated materials.

Leprosy **CH**

Refer to Hansen's disease

Leukemia, acute **MS**

Also refer to Chemotherapy

risk for Infection possibly evidenced by risk factors of inadequate secondary defenses (alterations in mature white blood cells, increased number of immature lymphocytes, immunosuppression and bone marrow suppression), invasive procedures, and malnutrition.

Anxiety [specify level]/Fear may be related to change in health status, threat of death, and situational crisis, possibly evidenced by sympathetic stimulation, apprehension, feelings of helplessness, focus on self, and insomnia.

Activity Intolerance [specify level] may be related to reduced energy stores, increased metabolic rate, imbalance between oxygen supply and demand—anemia, hypoxia; therapeutic restrictions (isolation, bedrest), effect of drug therapy, possibly evidenced by generalized weakness, reports of fatigue and exertional dyspnea, abnormal heart rate or blood pressure response.

acute Pain may be related to physical agents—infiltration of tissues, organs, central nervous system, or expanding bone marrow; chemical agents (antileukemic treatments), psychological manifestations—anxiety, fear, possibly evidenced by verbal reports of abdominal discomfort, arthralgia, bone pain, headache; distraction behaviors, narrowed focus, and autonomic responses—changes in vital signs.

risk for deficient Fluid Volume/Bleeding possibly evidenced by risk factors of excessive losses (vomiting, hemorrhage, diarrhea, coagulopathy), decreased intake (nausea, anorexia), increased fluid need (hypermetabolic state/fever), predisposition for kidney stone formation and tumor lysis syndrome.

Leukemia, chronic **CH**

ineffective Protection may be related to abnormal blood profiles, drug therapy (cytotoxic agents, steroids), radiation treatments, possibly evidenced by deficient immunity, impaired healing, altered clotting, weakness.

Fatigue may be related to disease state, anemia, possibly evidenced by verbalizations, inability to maintain usual routines, listlessness.

imbalanced Nutrition: less than body requirements may be related to inability to ingest nutrients, possibly evidenced by lack of interest in food, anorexia, weight loss, abdominal fullness, pain.

Lice, head **PED/CH**

Refer to Pediculosis capitis

Lice, pubic **CH**

Refer to Pediculosis capitis

Lightning injury **MS**

Also refer to Electrical injury

acute Confusion may be related to central nervous system involvement, possibly evidenced by change in level of consciousness.

impaired Memory may be related to acute hypoxia, decreased cardiac output, electrolyte imbalance, neurological disturbance, possibly evidenced by inability to recall recent events, amnesia.

Liver failure **MS/CH**
Refer to Cirrhosis; Hepatitis, acute viral

Liver transplantation **MS/CH**
Refer to Transplantation, recipient

Lockjaw **MS**
Refer to Tetanus

Long-term care **CH**
(Also refer to condition requiring/contributing to need for facility placement.)

Anxiety [specify level]/Fear may be related to change in health status, role functioning, interaction patterns, socioeconomic status, environment; unmet needs; recent life changes; and loss of friends/SO(s), possibly evidenced by apprehension, restlessness, insomnia, repetitive questioning, pacing, purposeless activity, expressed concern regarding changes in life events, and focus on self.

Grieving may be related to perceived, actual, or potential loss of physiopsychosocial well-being, personal possessions, and SO(s), as well as cultural beliefs about aging and debilitation, possibly evidenced by denial of feelings, depression, sorrow, guilt; alterations in activity level, sleep patterns, eating habits, and libido.

risk for Poisoning [drug toxicity] possibly evidenced by risk factors of effects of aging (reduced metabolism, impaired circulation, precarious physiological balance, presence of multiple diseases and organ involvement) and use of multiple prescribed and over-the-counter drugs.

impaired Memory may be related to neurological disturbances, hypoxia, fluid imbalance, possibly evidenced by inability to recall events/factual information, reports experience of forgetting.

Insomnia may be related to internal factors (illness, psychological stress, inactivity) and external factors (environmental changes, facility routines), possibly evidenced by reports of difficulty in falling asleep, not feeling rested, interrupted sleep, awakening earlier than desired, change in behavior or performance, increasing irritability, and listlessness.

risk for Sexual dysfunction possibly evidenced by risk factors of biopsychosocial alteration of sexuality; interference in psychological or physical well-being, self-image, and lack of privacy/SO.

risk for Relocation Stress Syndrome possibly evidenced by risk factors of temporary or permanent move that may be voluntary or involuntary, lack of predeparture counseling, multiple losses, feeling of powerlessness, lack of or inappropriate use of support system, decreased psychosocial or physical health status.

risk for impaired Religiosity possibly evidenced by risk factors of life transition, ineffective support or coping, lack of social interaction, depression.

LSD (lysergic acid diethylamide) intoxication **MS/PSY**
Also refer to Hallucinogen abuse

risk for Trauma possibly evidenced by risk factors of perceptual distortion, impaired judgment, dangerous decision making, changes in mood.

Anxiety [panic attack] may be related to drug side effects, possibly evidenced by severe apprehension, fear of unspecific consequences, central nervous system excitation, central autonomic hyperactivity.

Lung cancer **MS/CH**
Refer to Bronchogenic carcinoma

Lung transplantation **MS/CH**
Also refer to Transplantation, recipient

risk for impaired Gas Exchange possibly evidenced by risk factors of ventilation-perfusion mismatch, poor healing, stenosis of bronchial or tracheal anastomosis.

risk for Infection possibly evidenced by risk factors of medically induced immunosuppression, suppressed inflammatory response, antibiotic therapy, invasive procedures, effects of chronic or debilitating disease.

Lupus erythematosus, systemic (SLE) **CH**
Fatigue may be related to inadequate energy production, increased energy requirements (chronic inflammation), overwhelming psychological or emotional demands, states of discomfort, and altered body chemistry (including effects of drug therapy), possibly evidenced by reports of unremitting and overwhelming lack of energy, inability to maintain usual routines, decreased performance, lethargy, and decreased libido.

acute Pain may be related to widespread inflammatory process affecting connective tissues, blood vessels, serosal surfaces and mucous membranes, possibly evidenced by verbal reports, guarding or distraction behaviors, self-focusing, and changes in vital signs.

impaired Skin/Tissue Integrity may be related to chronic inflammation, edema formation, and altered circulation, possibly evidenced by presence of skin rash or lesions, ulcerations of mucous membranes, and photosensitivity.

disturbed Body Image may be related to presence of chronic condition with rash, lesions, ulcers, purpura, mottled erythema of hands, alopecia, loss of strength, and altered body function, possibly evidenced by hiding body parts, negative feelings about body, feelings of helplessness, and change in social involvement.

Lyme disease **CH/MS**

acute/chronic Pain may be related to systemic effects of toxins, presence of rash, urticaria, and joint swelling and inflammation, possibly evidenced by verbal reports, guarding behaviors, autonomic responses, and narrowed focus.

Fatigue may be related to increased energy requirements, altered body chemistry, and states of discomfort evidenced by reports of overwhelming lack of energy, inability to maintain usual routines, decreased performance, lethargy, and malaise.

risk for decreased Cardiac Output possibly evidenced by risk factors of alteration in cardiac rate, rhythm, or conduction.

Lymphedema **CH**

disturbed Body Image may be related to physical changes (chronic swelling of lower extremity), possibly evidenced by verbalizations, fear of reaction of others, negative feelings about body, hiding body part, change in social involvement.

impaired Walking may be related to chronic or progressive swelling of lower extremity, possibly evidenced by difficulty walking required distances, climbing stairs, navigating uneven surfaces and declines.

risk for impaired Skin Integrity possibly evidenced by risk factors of altered circulation, significant edema, changes in sensation.

Macular degeneration **CH**

[disturbed visual Sensory Perception] may be related to altered sensory reception, possibly evidenced by reported or measured change in sensory acuity, change in usual response to stimuli.

Anxiety [specify level]/Fear may be related to situational crisis, threat to or change in health status and role function, possibly evidenced by expressed concerns, apprehension, feelings of inadequacy, diminished productivity, impaired attention.

risk for impaired Social Interaction possibly evidenced by risk factors of limited physical mobility, environmental barriers.

Malaria **MS/CH**

Hyperthermia may be related to inflammatory process, possibly evidenced by increased body temperature (106°F [41.1°C]); flushed, warm skin; tachycardia; headache; altered consciousness.

acute Pain/impaired Comfort may be related to infectious agent, inflammatory response, possibly evidenced by reports of headache, backache, myalgia, malaise, high fever, shaking chills, abdominal discomfort.

risk for deficient Fluid Volume possibly evidenced by risk factors of decreased intake (nausea, abdominal pain, prostration), excessive losses (vomiting, diarrhea), hypermetabolic state.

Fatigue may be related to disease state, anemia, lack of restful sleep, possibly evidenced by verbalization of unremitting or overwhelming lack of energy, inability to restore energy even after sleep, lethargy.

Mallory-Weiss syndrome **MS**

Also refer to Achalasia (cardiospasm)

risk for deficient Fluid Volume possibly evidenced by risk factors of excessive vascular losses, presence of vomiting, and reduced intake.

deficient Knowledge [Learning Need] regarding causes, treatment, and prevention of condition may be related to lack of information, misinterpretation, possibly evidenced by statements of concern, questions, and recurrence of problem.

Malnutrition **CH**

Also refer to Anorexia nervosa

Frail Elderly Syndrome may be related to depression, apathy, aging process, fatigue, degenerative condition, possibly evidenced by expressed lack of appetite, difficulty performing self-care tasks, altered mood state, inadequate intake, weight loss, physical decline.

ineffective Protection may be related to inadequate nutrition, anemia, extremes of age, possibly evidenced by fatigue, weakness, deficient immunity, impaired healing, pressure sores.

Marburg disease **MS**

Refer to Ebola

Mastectomy — MS

impaired Skin/Tissue Integrity may be related to surgical removal of skin and tissue, altered circulation, presence of edema, drainage, changes in skin elasticity and sensation, and tissue destruction (radiation), possibly evidenced by disruption of skin surface and destruction of skin layers and subcutaneous tissues.

impaired physical Mobility may be related to neuromuscular impairment, pain, and edema formation, possibly evidenced by reluctance to attempt movement, limited range of motion, and decreased muscle mass and strength.

bathing/dressing Self-Care deficit may be related to temporary decreased range of motion of one or both arms, possibly evidenced by statements of inability to perform or complete self-care tasks.

disturbed Body Image/situational low Self-Esteem may be related to loss of body part denoting femininity, fear of rejection or reaction of others, behaviors inconsistent with self-value system possibly evidenced by not looking at or touching area, self-negating verbalizations, preoccupation with loss, and change in social involvement or relationship.

risk for complicated Grieving possibly evidenced by risk factors of preloss psychological symptoms, predisposition for anxiety and feelings of inadequacy, frequency of major life events.

Mastitis — OB/GYN

acute Pain may be related to erythema and edema of breast tissues, possibly evidenced by verbal reports, guarding or distraction behaviors, self-focusing, and changes in vital signs.

risk for Infection [spread/abscess formation] possibly evidenced by risk factors of traumatized tissues, stasis of fluids, and insufficient knowledge to prevent complications.

deficient Knowledge [Learning Need] regarding pathophysiology, treatment, and prevention may be related to lack of information, misinterpretation, possibly evidenced by statements of concern, questions, and misconceptions.

risk for ineffective Breastfeeding possibly evidenced by risk factors of inability to feed on affected side, interruption in breastfeeding.

Mastoidectomy — PED/MS

risk for Infection [spread] possibly evidenced by risk factors of preexisting infection, surgical trauma, and stasis of body fluids. Also refer to Surgery, general.

acute Pain may be related to inflammation, tissue trauma, and edema formation, possibly evidenced by verbal reports, distraction behaviors, restlessness, self-focusing, and changes in vital signs.

[disturbed auditory Sensory Perception] may be related to presence of surgical packing, edema, and surgical disturbance of middle ear structures, possibly evidenced by reported or tested hearing loss in affected ear.

Measles — CH/PED

acute Pain/impaired Comfort may be related to inflammation of mucous membranes, conjunctiva, and presence of extensive skin rash with pruritus, possibly evidenced by verbal/coded reports, distraction behaviors, self-focusing, and changes in vital signs.

Hyperthermia may be related to presence of viral toxins and inflammatory response, possibly evidenced by increased body temperature; flushed, warm skin; and tachycardia.

risk for [secondary] Infection possibly evidenced by risk factors of altered immune response and traumatized dermal tissues.

deficient Knowledge [Learning Need] regarding condition, transmission, and possible complications may be related to lack of information, misinterpretation, possibly evidenced by statements of concern, questions, misconceptions, and development of preventable complications.

Measles, German — PED/CH

Refer to Rubella

Melanoma, malignant — MS/CH

Refer to Cancer; Chemotherapy

Ménière's disease — CH

Also refer to Vertigo

[disturbed auditory Sensory Perception] may be related to altered state of sensory organ or sensory reception, possibly evidenced by change in sensory acuity, tinnitus, vertigo.

Nausea may be related to inner ear disturbance, possibly evidenced by verbal reports, vomiting.

risk for [total] Self-Care deficit possibly evidenced by risk factors of perceptual impairment, recurrent nausea, general weakness.

Meningitis, acute meningococcal — MS

risk for Infection [spread] possibly evidenced by risk factors of hematogenous dissemination of pathogen, stasis of body fluids, suppressed inflammatory response (medication-induced), and exposure of others to pathogens.

risk for ineffective cerebral Tissue Perfusion possibly evidenced by risk factors of cerebral edema altering or interrupting cerebral arterial or venous blood flow, hypovolemia, exchange problems at cellular level (acidosis).

Hyperthermia may be related to infectious process (increased metabolic rate) and dehydration, possibly evidenced by increased body temperature; warm, flushed skin; and tachycardia.

acute Pain may be related to inflammation and irritation of the meninges with spasm of extensor muscles (neck, shoulders, and back), possibly evidenced by verbal reports, guarding or distraction behaviors, narrowed focus, photophobia, and changes in vital signs.

risk for Trauma/Suffocation possibly evidenced by risk factors of alterations in level of consciousness, possible development of clonic-tonic muscle activity (seizures), generalized weakness, prostration, ataxia, vertigo.

Meniscectomy MS/CH

impaired Walking may be related to pain, joint instability, and imposed medical restrictions of movement, possibly evidenced by impaired ability to move about environment as needed or desired.

deficient Knowledge [Learning Need] regarding postoperative expectations, prevention of complications, and self-care needs may be related to lack of information, possibly evidenced by statements of concern, questions, and misconceptions.

Menopause GYN

ineffective Thermoregulation may be related to fluctuation of hormonal levels, possibly evidenced by skin flushed/warm to touch, diaphoresis, night sweats, cold hands and feet.

Fatigue may be related to change in body chemistry, lack of sleep, depression, possibly evidenced by reports of lack of energy, tiredness, inability to maintain usual routines, decreased performance.

risk for Sexual dysfunction possibly evidenced by risk factors of perceived altered body function, changes in physical response, myths or inaccurate information, impaired relationship with SO.

risk for stress urinary Incontinence possibly evidenced by risk factors of changes in pelvic muscles and loss of structural support.

readiness for enhanced Health Management possibly evidenced by expressed desire for increased control of health practice, describes reduction of symptoms.

Mental delay (formerly retardation) CH

Also refer to Down syndrome

impaired verbal Communication may be related to developmental delay or impairment of cognitive and motor abilities, possibly evidenced by impaired articulation, difficulty with phonation, and inability to modulate speech or find appropriate words (dependent on degree of retardation).

risk for Self-Care deficit [specify] possibly evidenced by risk factors of impaired cognitive ability and motor skills.

risk for Overweight or Obesity possibly evidenced by risk factors of decreased metabolic rate coupled with impaired cognitive development, dysfunctional eating patterns, and sedentary activity level.

risk for sedentary Lifestyle possibly evidenced by risk factors of lack of interest or motivation, resources; lack of training or knowledge of specific exercise needs, safety concerns, fear of injury.

impaired Social Interaction may be related to impaired thought processes, communication barriers, and knowledge or skill deficit about ways to enhance mutuality, possibly evidenced by dysfunctional interactions with peers, family, and/or SO(s), and verbalized or observed discomfort in social situation.

compromised family Coping may be related to chronic nature of condition and degree of disability that exhausts supportive capacity of SO(s), other situational or developmental crises or situations SO(s) may be facing, unrealistic expectations of SO(s), possibly evidenced by preoccupation of SO with personal reaction, SO(s) withdraw(s) or enter(s) into limited interaction with individual, protective behavior disproportionate (too much or too little) to client's abilities or need for autonomy.

impaired Home Maintenance may be related to impaired cognitive functioning, insufficient finances/family organization or planning, lack of knowledge, and inadequate support systems, possibly evidenced by requests for assistance, expression of difficulty in maintaining home, disorderly surroundings, and overtaxed family members.

risk for Sexual dysfunction possibly evidenced by risk factors of biopsychosocial alteration of sexuality, ineffectual or absent role models, misinformation, lack of knowledge, lack of SO(s), and lack of appropriate behavior control.

Mesothelioma CH/MS

Also refer to Asbestosis; Cancer

acute Pain may be related to tissue destruction, possibly evidenced by reports of chest pain (initially nonpleuritic), irritability, self-focusing, autonomic responses.

Activity Intolerance may be related to imbalance between oxygen supply and demand, possibly evidenced by dyspnea, fatigue.

Metabolic syndrome CH

risk for unstable Blood Glucose Level possibly evidenced by risk factors of dietary intake, weight gain, sededentary activity level.

sedentary Lifestyle may be related to deficient knowledge of health benefits of physical exercise, lack of interest, motivation, or resources, possibly evidenced by verbalized preference for activities low in physical activity, choosing a daily routine lacking physical exercise.

risk for ineffective Tissue Perfusion (specify) possibly evidenced by risk factors of arterial plaque formation (elevated triglycerides, low levels of high-density lipoprotein), prothrombotic state, proinflammatory state.

Migraine CH/MS

Refer to Headache

Miscarriage OB

Refer to Abortion, spontaneous termination

Mitral insufficiency MS/CH

Refer to Valvular heart disease

Mitral stenosis MS/CH

Activity Intolerance may be related to imbalance between oxygen supply and demand, possibly evidenced by reports of fatigue, weakness, exertional dyspnea, and tachycardia.

impaired Gas Exchange may be related to altered blood flow, possibly evidenced by restlessness, hypoxia, and cyanosis (orthopnea, paroxysmal nocturnal dyspnea).

decreased Cardiac Output may be related to impeded blood flow as evidenced by jugular vein distention, peripheral or dependent edema, orthopnea, paroxysmal nocturnal dyspnea.

deficient Knowledge [Learning Need] regarding pathophysiology, therapeutic needs, and potential complications may be related to lack of information or recall, misinterpretation, possibly evidenced by statements of concern, questions, inaccurate follow-through of instructions, and development of preventable complications.

Mitral valve prolapse (MVP) CH

Refer to Valvular heart disease

Mononucleosis, infectious CH

Fatigue may be related to decreased energy production, states of discomfort, and increased energy requirements (inflammatory process), possibly evidenced by reports of overwhelming lack of energy, inability to maintain usual routines, lethargy, and malaise.

acute Pain/impaired Comfort may be related to inflammation of lymphoid and organ tissues, irritation of oropharyngeal mucous membranes, and effects of circulating toxins, possibly evidenced by verbal reports, distraction behaviors, and self-focusing.

Hyperthermia may be related to inflammatory process, possibly evidenced by increased body temperature; warm, flushed skin; and tachycardia.

deficient Knowledge [Learning Need] regarding disease transmission, self-care needs, medical therapy, and potential complications may be related to lack of information, misinterpretation, possibly evidenced by statements of concern, misconceptions, and inaccurate follow-through of instructions.

Mood disorders PSY

Refer to Depression, major; Bipolar disorder; Premenstrual dysphoric disorder

Mountain sickness, acute (AMS) CH/MS

acute Pain may be related to reduced oxygen tension, possibly evidenced by reports of headache.

Fatigue may be related to stress, increased physical exertion, sleep deprivation, possibly evidenced by overwhelming lack of energy, inability to restore energy even after sleep, compromised concentration, decreased performance.

risk for deficient Fluid Volume possibly evidenced by risk factors of increased water loss (e.g., overbreathing dry air), exertion, inadequate fluid intake (nausea).

Multiple organ dysfunction syndrome MS

Also refer to specific organs involved; Sepsis; Ventilator assist/dependence

ineffective peripheral Tissue/Renal/Gastrointestinal Perfusion may be related to hypovolemia, selective vasoconstriction, microvascular embolization, possibly evidenced by cool skin, diminished pulses, oliguria or anuria, nausea, abdominal tenderness, hypoactive bowel sounds.

impaired Gas Exchange may be related to ventilation perfusion imbalance, alveolar hypoventilation, possibly evidenced by dyspnea, irritability, confusion, abnormal arterial blood gases.

Activity Intolerance may be related to generalized weakness, bedrest, imbalance between oxygen supply and demand, pain, possibly evidenced by abnormal heart rate and blood pressure response to activity, pallor, exertional discomfort, electrocardiogram changes—dysrhythmias, ischemia.

[severe] Anxiety/Fear may be related to situational crisis, change in health status, threat of death, possibly evidenced by expressed concerns, apprehension, increased tension, fearfulness, restlessness, decreased perceptual field.

imbalanced Nutrition: less than body requirements may be related to restricted intake, inability to digest food, increased metabolic demands, possibly evidenced by weight loss, poor muscle tone, decreased subcutaneous fat and muscle mass, abnormal laboratory studies.

risk for Infection possibly evidenced by risk factors of stasis of body fluids, immunosuppression, malnutrition, invasive devices and procedures, environmental exposure.

Multiple personality — PSY

Refer to Dissociative disorders

Multiple sclerosis — CH

Fatigue may be related to decreased energy production, increased energy requirements to perform activities, psychological and emotional demands, pain or discomfort, medication side effects, possibly evidenced by verbalization of overwhelming lack of energy, inability to maintain usual routine, decreased performance, impaired ability to concentrate, increase in physical complaints.

[disturbed visual/kinesthetic/tactile Sensory Perception] may be related to delayed or interrupted neuronal transmission, possibly evidenced by impaired vision, diplopia, disturbance of vibratory or position sense, paresthesias, numbness, and blunting of sensation.

impaired physical Mobility may be related to neuromuscular impairment, discomfort or pain, sensoriperceptual impairments, decreased muscle strength, control, or mass, deconditioning, as evidenced by limited ability to perform motor skills, limited range of motion, gait changes, postural instability.

Powerlessness/Hopelessness may be related to illness-related regimen, unpredictability of disease, and lifestyle of helplessness, possibly evidenced by verbal expressions of having no control or influence over the situation, depression over physical deterioration that occurs despite client compliance with regimen, nonparticipation in care or decision making when opportunities are provided, passivity, decreased verbalization and affect, isolating behaviors.

impaired Home Maintenance may be related to effects of debilitating disease, impaired cognitive or emotional functioning, insufficient finances, and inadequate support systems, possibly evidenced by reported difficulty, observed disorderly surroundings, and poor hygienic conditions.

compromised/disabled family Coping may be related to situational crises, temporary family disorganization, and role changes, client providing little support in turn for SO(s), prolonged disease and disability progression that exhausts the supportive capacity of SO(s), feelings of guilt, anxiety, hostility, despair, and highly ambivalent family relationships, possibly evidenced by client who expresses or confirms concern about SOs' response to client's illness, SO(s) preoccupied with own personal reactions, intolerance, abandonment, neglectful care of the client, and distortion of reality regarding client's illness.

Mumps — PED/CH

acute Pain may be related to presence of inflammation, circulating toxins, and enlargement of salivary glands, possibly evidenced by verbal reports, guarding or distraction behaviors, self-focusing, and autonomic responses (changes in vital signs).

Hyperthermia may be related to inflammatory process (increased metabolic rate) and dehydration, possibly evidenced by increased body temperature; warm, flushed skin; and tachycardia.

risk for deficient Fluid Volume possibly evidenced by risk factors of hypermetabolic state and painful swallowing, with decreased intake.

Muscular dystrophy (Duchenne's) — PED/CH

impaired physical Mobility may be related to musculoskeletal impairment and weakness, possibly evidenced by decreased muscle strength, control, and mass; limited range of motion; and impaired coordination.

risk for delayed Development possibly evidenced by risk factors of genetic disorder/chronic illness, learning disability.altered ability to perform self-care or self-control activities appropriate to age.

risk for Overweight or Obesity possibly evidenced by risk factors of sedentary lifestyle and dysfunctional eating patterns.

compromised family Coping may be related to situational crisis and emotional conflicts around issues about hereditary nature of condition and prolonged disease and disability that exhausts supportive capacity of family members, possibly evidenced by preoccupation with personal reactions regarding disability and displaying protective behavior disproportionate (too little or too much) to client's abilities and need for autonomy.

Myasthenia gravis — MS

ineffective Breathing Pattern/Airway Clearance may be related to neuromuscular weakness and decreased energy, fatigue, possibly evidenced by dyspnea, changes in rate and depth of respiration, ineffective cough, and adventitious breath sounds.

impaired verbal Communication may be related to neuromuscular weakness, fatigue, and physical barrier (intubation), possibly evidenced by facial weakness, impaired articulation, hoarseness, and inability to speak.

impaired Swallowing may be related to neuromuscular impairment of laryngeal and pharyngeal muscles and muscular fatigue, possibly evidenced by reported or observed difficulty swallowing, coughing, choking, and evidence of aspiration.

Anxiety [specify level]/Fear may be related to situational crisis, threat to self-concept, change in health and socioeconomic status or role function, separation from support systems, lack of knowledge, and inability to communicate, possibly evidenced by expressed concerns, increased tension, restlessness, apprehension, sympathetic stimulation, crying, focus on self, uncooperative behavior, withdrawal, anger, and noncommunication.

CH

deficient Knowledge [Learning Need] regarding drug therapy, potential for crisis (myasthenic or cholinergic), and self-care management may be related to inadequate information, misinterpretation, possibly evidenced by statements of concern, questions, and misconceptions; development of preventable complications.

impaired physical Mobility may be related to neuromuscular impairment, possibly evidenced by reports of progressive fatigue with repetitive or prolonged muscle use, impaired coordination, and decreased muscle strength and control.

[disturbed visual Sensory Perception] may be related to neuromuscular impairment, possibly evidenced by visual distortions (diplopia) and motor incoordination.

Myelitis, transverse — MS/CH

Refer to Paraplegia

Myeloma, multiple — MS/CH

Also refer to Cancer

acute/chronic Pain may be related to destruction of tissues and bone, side effects of therapy, possibly evidenced by verbal or coded reports, guarding or protective behaviors, changes in appetite, weight, sleep; reduced interaction with others.

impaired physical Mobility may be related to loss of integrity of bone structure, pain, deconditioning, depressed mood, possibly evidenced by verbalizations, limited range of motion, slowed movement, gait changes.

risk for ineffective Protection possibly evidenced by risk factors of cancer, drug therapies, radiation treatments, inadequate nutrition.

Myocardial infarction — MS

Also refer to Myocarditis

acute Pain may be related to ischemia of myocardial tissue, possibly evidenced by verbal reports, guarding or distraction behaviors (restlessness), facial mask of pain, self-focusing, and autonomic responses (diaphoresis, changes in vital signs).

Anxiety [specify level]/Fear may be related to threat of death, threat of change of health status, role functioning, and lifestyle; interpersonal transmission and contagion, possibly evidenced by increased tension, fearful attitude, apprehension, expressed concerns or uncertainty, restlessness, sympathetic stimulation, and somatic complaints.

risk for decreased Cardiac Output possibly evidenced by risk factors of changes in rate and electrical conduction, reduced preload, increased systemic vascular resistance, altered muscle contractility, depressant effects of some medications, infarcted or dyskinetic muscle, structural defects.

CH

risk for sedentary Lifestyle possibly evidenced by risk factors of lack of resources; lack of training or knowledge of specific exercise needs, safety concerns, fear of injury

Myocarditis MS

Also refer to Myocardial infarction

Activity Intolerance may be related to imbalance in oxygen supply and demand (myocardial inflammation or damage), cardiac depressant effects of certain drugs, and enforced bedrest, possibly evidenced by reports of fatigue, exertional dyspnea, tachycardia, and palpitations in response to activity, electrocardiogram changes, dysrhythmias, and generalized weakness.

risk for decreased Cardiac Output possibly evidenced by risk factors of altered contractility, altered stroke volume.

deficient Knowledge [Learning Need] regarding pathophysiology of condition, prognosis, treatment, self-care needs, and lifestyle changes may be related to lack of information, misinterpretation, possibly evidenced by statements of concern, misconceptions, inaccurate follow-through of instructions, and development of preventable complications.

Myoclonus, nocturnal CH

Sleep deprivation may be related to periodic limb movement, irresistible urge to move legs to relieve uncomfortable sensations, possibly evidenced by decreased quality of sleep, daytime drowsiness, decreased ability to function, inability to concentrate.

Myofascial pain syndrome CH

Also refer to Fibromyalgia

acute/chronic Pain may be related to nocturnal bruxism (clenching or grinding teeth), possibly evidenced by reports of pain (temporomandibular region), headache, muscular tenderness to palpation, limitation in opening mouth.

risk for impaired Dentition possibly evidenced by risk factors of bruxism, ineffective oral hygiene (limitations in opening mouth).

Myringotomy PED/MS

Refer to Mastoidectomy

Myxedema CH

Also refer to Hypothyroidism

disturbed Body Image may be related to change in structure or function (loss of hair, thickening of skin, masklike facial expression, enlarged tongue, menstrual and reproductive disturbances), possibly evidenced by negative feelings about body, feelings of helplessness, and change in social involvement.

Overweight may be related to decreased metabolic rate and activity level, possibly evidenced by weight gain greater than ideal for height and frame.

risk for decreased Cardiac Output possibly evidenced by risk factors of alteration in heart rhythm, altered contractility.

Narcolepsy CH

Insomnia may be related to medical condition, possibly evidenced by hypersomnia, reports of unsatisfying nighttime sleep, vivid visual or auditory illusions or hallucinations at onset of sleep, sleep interrupted by vivid or frightening dreams.

risk for Trauma possibly evidenced by risk factors of sudden loss of muscle tone, momentary paralysis (cataplexy), sudden inappropriate sleep episodes.

risk for chronic low Self-Esteem possibly evidenced by risk factors of negative evaluation of self, personal vulnerability, chronic physical condition, impaired work or school performance, problems with social relationships, reduced quality of life.

Near drowning MS

impaired Gas Exchange may be related to ventilation perfusion imbalance (patchy atelectasis), alveolar-capillary membrane changes, aspiration or acute reflex laryngospasm, possibly evidenced by severe hypoxia, pale or dusky skin, change in mentation (confusion to coma).

risk for Hypothermia possibly evidenced by risk factor of submersion in very cold water.

NEC PED

Refer to Necrotizing enterocolitis

Necrotizing cellulitis/fasciitis MS

Also refer to Cellulitis; Sepsis

Hyperthermia may be related to inflammatory process, response to circulating toxins, possibly evidenced by body temperature above normal range; flushed, warm skin; tachycardia; altered mental status.

impaired Tissue Integrity may be related to inflammation and edema (infection), ischemia, possibly evidenced by damaged or destroyed tissue, dermal gangrene.

Necrotizing enterocolitis PED

Also refer to Sepsis

imbalanced Nutrition: less than body requirements may be related to inability to digest or absorb nutrients (ischemia of bowel), possibly evidenced by abdominal pain and distention, gastric residuals after feedings, failure to gain weight.

risk for deficient Fluid Volume possibly evidenced by risk factors of vomiting, third-space fluid losses (bowel inflammation, peritonitis), lack of oral intake.

Neglect/abuse — CH/PSY

Refer to Abuse·Battered child syndrome

Nephrectomy — MS

acute Pain may be related to surgical tissue trauma with mechanical closure (suture), possibly evidenced by verbal reports, guarding or distraction behaviors, self-focusing, and changes in vital signs.

risk for deficient Fluid Volume possibly evidenced by risk factors of excessive vascular losses and restricted intake.

ineffective Breathing Pattern may be related to incisional pain with decreased lung expansion, possibly evidenced by tachypnea, fremitus, changes in respiratory depth and chest expansion, and changes in arterial blood gases.

Constipation may be related to reduced dietary intake, decreased mobility, gastrointestinal obstruction (paralytic ileus), and incisional pain with defecation, possibly evidenced by decreased bowel sounds; reduced frequency/amount of stool; and hard, formed stool.

Nephrolithiasis — MS/CH

Refer to Calculi, urinary

Nephrotic syndrome — MS/CH

Also refer to Renal failure, acute/chronic

excess Fluid Volume may be related to compromised regulatory mechanism with changes in hydrostatic or oncotic vascular pressure and increased activation of the renin-angiotensin-aldosterone system, possibly evidenced by edema, anasarca, effusions, ascites, weight gain, intake greater than output, and blood pressure changes.

imbalanced Nutrition: less than body requirements may be related to excessive protein losses and inability to ingest adequate nutrients (anorexia), possibly evidenced by weight loss, muscle wasting (may be difficult to assess due to edema), lack of interest in food, and observed inadequate intake.

risk for Infection possibly evidenced by risk factors of chronic disease and steroidal suppression of inflammatory responses.

risk for impaired Skin Integrity possibly evidenced by risk factors of presence of edema and activity restrictions.

Neuralgia, trigeminal — CH

acute Pain may be related to neuromuscular impairment with sudden violent muscle spasm, possibly evidenced by verbal reports, guarding or distraction behaviors, self-focusing, and changes in vital signs.

deficient Knowledge [Learning Need] regarding control of recurrent episodes, medical therapies, and self-care needs may be related to lack of information or recall and misinterpretation, possibly evidenced by statements of concern, questions, and exacerbation of condition.

Neural tube defect — PED

Refer to Spina bifida

Neuritis — CH

acute/chronic Pain may be related to nerve damage usually associated with a degenerative process, possibly evidenced by verbal reports, guarding or distraction behaviors, self-focusing, and changes in vital signs.

deficient Knowledge [Learning Need] regarding underlying causative factors, treatment, and prevention may be related to lack of information, misinterpretation, possibly evidenced by statements of concern, questions, and misconceptions.

Newborn, growth deviations — PED

Also refer to Newborn, premature

disproportionate Growth may be related to maternal nutrition, substance use or abuse, multiple gestation, prematurity, maternal conditions (e.g., pregnancy-induced hypertension, diabetes), possibly evidenced by birth weight at or below 10th percentile or at or above 90th percentile (considering gestational age, ethnicity, etc.).

imbalanced Nutrition: less than body requirements may be related to decreased nutritional stores, hyperplasia of pancreatic beta cells, and increased insulin production, possibly evidenced by weight deviation from expected, decreased muscle mass/fat stores, electrolyte imbalance.

risk for ineffective Tissue Perfusion (specify) possibly evidenced by risk factors of interruption of arterial or venous blood flow (hyperviscosity associated with polycythemia).

risk for Injury possibly evidenced by risk factors of altered growth, delayed central nervous system or neurological development, abnormal blood profile.

risk for disorganized infant Behavior possibly evidenced by risk factors of functional limitations related to growth deviations (restricting neonate's opportunity to seek out, recognize, and interpret stimuli), electrolyte imbalance, psychological stress, low energy reserves, poor organizational ability, limited ability to control environment.

Newborn, normal **PED**

risk for impaired Gas Exchange possibly evidenced by risk factors of prenatal or intrapartal stressors, excess production of mucus, or cold stress.

risk for Hypothermia possibly evidenced by risk factors of large body surface in relation to mass, limited amounts of insulating subcutaneous fat, nonrenewable sources of brown fat and few white fat stores, thin epidermis with close proximity of blood vessels to the skin, inability to shiver, and movement from a warm uterine environment to a much cooler environment.

risk for impaired Attachment possibly evidenced by risk factors of developmental transition or gain of a family member, anxiety associated with the parent role, lack of privacy (healthcare interventions, intrusive family/visitors).

risk for imbalanced Nutrition: less than body requirements possibly evidenced by risk factors of rapid metabolic rate, high-caloric requirement, increased insensible water losses through pulmonary and cutaneous routes, fatigue, and a potential for inadequate or depleted glucose stores.

risk for Infection possibly evidenced by risk factors of inadequate secondary defenses (inadequate acquired immunity, e.g., deficiency of neutrophils and specific immunoglobulins), and inadequate primary defenses (e.g., environmental exposure, broken skin, traumatized tissues, decreased ciliary action).

Newborn at 1 week **PED**

Also refer to Newborn, normal

risk for Injury possibly evidenced by risk factors of physical (hyperbilirubinemia), environmental (inadequate safety precautions), chemical (drugs in breast milk), psychological (inappropriate parental stimulation or interaction).

risk for Constipation/Diarrhea possibly evidenced by risk factors of type and amount of oral intake, medications or dietary intake of lactating mother, presence of allergies, infection.

risk for impaired Skin Integrity possibly evidenced by risk factors of excretions (ammonia formation from urea), chemical irritation from laundry detergent or diapering material, mechanical factors (e.g., long fingernails).

Newborn, postmature **PED**

risk for impaired Gas Exchange possibly evidenced by risk factors of ventilation perfusion imbalances (meconium aspiration, pneumonitis).

Hypothermia may be related to decreased subcutaneous fat stores, poor metabolic reserves, exposure to cool environment, decreased ability to shiver, possibly evidenced by reduction in body temperature, cool skin, pallor.

risk for imbalanced Nutrition: less than body requirements possibly evidenced by risk factors of placental insufficiency, decreased subcutaneous fat stores, decreased glycogen stores at birth (neonatal hypoglycemia).

risk for impaired Skin Integrity possibly evidenced by risk factors of dry, peeling skin; long fingernails, absence of vernix caseous.

Newborn, premature **PED**

impaired Gas Exchange may be related to alveolar-capillary membrane changes (inadequate surfactant levels), altered blood flow (immaturity of pulmonary arteriole musculature), altered oxygen supply (immaturity of central nervous and neuromuscular systems, tracheobronchial obstruction), altered oxygen-carrying capacity of blood (anemia), and cold stress, possibly evidenced by respiratory difficulties, inadequate oxygenation of tissues, and acidemia.

ineffective Breathing Pattern may be related to immaturity of the respiratory center, poor positioning, drug-related depression and metabolic imbalances, decreased energy, fatigue, possibly evidenced by dyspnea, tachypnea, periods of apnea, nasal flaring, use of accessory muscles, cyanosis, abnormal arterial blood gases, and tachycardia.

risk for ineffective Thermoregulation possibly evidenced by risk factors of immature central nervous system development (temperature regulation center), decreased ratio of body mass to surface area, decreased subcutaneous fat, limited brown fat stores, inability to shiver or sweat, poor metabolic reserves, muted response to hypothermia, and frequent medical/nursing manipulations and interventions.

risk for deficient Fluid Volume possibly evidenced by risk factors of extremes of age and weight, excessive fluid losses (thin skin, lack of insulating fat, increased environmental temperature, immature kidney/failure to concentrate urine).

risk for ineffective infant Feeding Pattern possibly evidenced by risk factors of decreased energy, fatigue; poor positioning; drug-related depression; inability to coordinate sucking, swallowing, and breathing.

risk for disorganized infant Behavior possibly evidenced by risk factors of prematurity (immaturity of central nervous system, hypoxia), lack of containment or boundaries, pain, overstimulation, separation from parents.

risk for Injury [central nervous system damage] possibly evidenced by risk factors of tissue hypoxia, altered clotting factors, metabolic imbalances (hypoglycemia, electrolyte shifts, elevated bilirubin).

Newborn, small for gestational age PED

Refer to Newborn, growth deviations

Newborn, special needs PED

(Also refer to specific condition.)

family Grieving may be related to perceived loss of the perfect child, alterations of future expectations, possibly evidenced by expression of distress at loss, sorrow, guilt, anger, choked feelings; interference with life activities, crying.

deficient parental Knowledge [Learning Need] regarding condition and infant care may be related to lack of or unfamiliarity with information resources, misinterpretation, possibly evidenced by questions, concerns, misconceptions, hesitancy, or inadequate performance of activities.

risk for impaired Attachment possibly evidenced by risk factors of delay or interruption in bonding process (separation, physical barriers), perceived threat to infant's survival, stressors (financial, family needs), lack of appropriate response of newborn, lack of support between or from SOs.

risk for ineffective family Coping possibly evidenced by risk factors of situational crises, temporary preoccupation of SO trying to manage emotional conflicts and personal suffering, being unable to perceive or act effectively in regard to infant's needs, temporary family disorganization.

risk for parental Social Isolation possibly evidenced by risk factors of perceived situational crisis, assuming sole or full-time responsibility for infant's care, lack of or inappropriate use of resources.

Nicotine abuse CH

risk-prone Health Behavior may be related to lack of motivation to change behavior, low state of optimism, absence of social/SO support for change, failure to intend to change behavior, possibly evidenced by denial of health problem, failure to take action, failure to achieve optimal sense of control.

risk for Injury possibly evidenced by risk factors of smoking habits (e.g., in bed, while driving, near combustible chemicals or oxygen), children playing with cigarettes or matches.

risk for impaired Gas Exchange possibly evidenced by risk factors of progressive airflow obstruction, decreased oxygen supply (carbon monoxide).

risk for ineffective peripheral Tissue Perfusion possibly evidenced by risk factors of reduction of arterial or venous blood flow.

Nicotine withdrawal CH

readiness for enhanced Health Management (smoking cessation) possibly evidenced by expressed concerns or desire to seek higher level of wellness.

risk for Overweight possibly evidenced by risk factors of eating in response to internal cues (substitution of food for activity of smoking).

risk for ineffective Health Management possibly evidenced by risk factors of economic difficulties, lack of support from SO/friends, continued environmental exposure to secondhand smoke or smoking activity.

Nonketotic hyperosmolar syndrome MS

deficient Fluid Volume may be related to excessive renal losses, inadequate oral intake, extremes of age, presence of infection, possibly evidenced by sudden weight loss, dry skin and mucous membranes, poor skin turgor, hypotension, increased pulse, fever, change in mental status (confusion to coma).

decreased Cardiac Output may be related to decreased preload (hypovolemia), altered heart rhythm (hyper-/hypokalemia), possibly evidenced by decreased hemodynamic pressures (e.g., central venous pressure), electrocardiogram changes, dysrhythmias.

imbalanced Nutrition: less than body requirements may be related to inadequate utilization of nutrients (insulin deficiency), decreased oral intake, hypermetabolic state, possibly evidenced by recent weight loss, imbalance between glucose and insulin levels.

risk for Trauma possibly evidenced by risk factors of weakness, cognitive limitations, altered consciousness, loss of large- or small-muscle coordination (risk for seizure activity).

Obesity CH

Obesity may be related to excessive intake in relation to metabolic needs, possibly evidenced by weight 20% greater than ideal for height and frame, sedentary activity level, reported or observed dysfunctional eating patterns, and excess body fat by triceps skinfold or other measurements.

sedentary Lifestyle may be related to lack of interest or motivation, resources; lack of training or knowledge of specific exercise needs, safety concerns or fear of injury, possibly evidenced by demonstration of physical deconditioning, choice of a daily routine lacking physical exercise.

Activity Intolerance may be related to imbalance between oxygen supply and demand, and sedentary lifestyle, possibly evidenced by fatigue or weakness, exertional discomfort, and abnormal heart rate and blood pressure response.

risk for Sleep deprivation possibly evidenced by risk factor of sleep apnea.

PSY

disturbed Body Image/chronic low Self-Esteem may be related to view of self in contrast to societal values, family, or subcultural encouragement of overeating; control, sex, and love issues, perceived failure at ability to control weight, possibly evidenced by negative feelings about body, fear of rejection or reaction of others, feeling of hopelessness or powerlessness, and lack of follow-through with treatment plan.

impaired Social Interaction may be related to verbalized or observed discomfort in social situations, self-concept disturbance, absence of or ineffective supportive SO(s), limited mobility, possibly evidenced by reluctance to participate in social gatherings, verbalized or observed discomfort in social situations, dysfunctional interactions with others, feelings of rejection.

Obesity-hypoventilation syndrome CH

Refer to Pickwickian syndrome

Obsessive-compulsive disorder PSY

[severe] Anxiety may be related to earlier life conflicts, possibly evidenced by repetitive actions, recurring thoughts, decreased social and role functioning.

risk for impaired Skin/Tissue Integrity possibly evidenced by risk factors of repetitive behaviors related to cleansing (e.g., hand hygiene, brushing teeth, showering).

risk for ineffective Role Performance possibly evidenced by risk factors of psychological stress, health-illness problems.

Opioid abuse CH/PSY

Refer to Depressant abuse; Heroin abuse/withdrawal

Oppositional defiant disorder PED/PSY

ineffective Coping may be related to situational or maturational crisis, mild neurological deficits, retarded ego development, dysfunctional family system, negative role models, possibly evidenced by inability to meet age-appropriate role expectations, hostility toward others, defiant response to requests or rules, inability to delay gratification.

impaired Social Interaction may be related to retarded ego development, dysfunctional family, negative role models, neurological impairment, possibly evidenced by discomfort in social situations, difficulty playing or interacting with others, aggressive behavior, refusal to comply with requests of others.

chronic low Self-Esteem may be related to retarded ego development, lack of positive or repeated negative feedback, mild neurological deficits, negative role models, possibly evidenced by lack of eye contact, lack of self-confidence, physical risk-taking, distraction of others to cover up own failures, projection of blame.

compromised/disabled family Coping may be related to anger, excessive guilt, blaming among family members regarding child's behavior, parental inconsistencies or disagreements regarding discipline and limit-setting, exhaustion of parental resources, possibly evidenced by unrealistic parental expectations, rejection or overprotection of child, exaggerated expressions of anger, disappointment, despair.

Organic brain syndrome CH

Refer to Alzheimer's disease

Osgood-Schlatter disease PED

acute Pain may be related to inflammation and swelling in region of patellar tendon, possibly evidenced by verbal reports, protective behavior, change in muscle tone.

impaired Walking may be related to inflammatory process (knee), possibly evidenced by impaired ability to walk desired distances, climb or descend stairs.

risk for ineffective Health Management possibly evidenced by risk factors of age (adolescence), perceived seriousness or benefit, competitive nature, peer pressure.

Osteitis deformans CH

Refer to Paget's disease, bone

Osteoarthritis (degenerative joint disease) CH

Refer to Arthritis, rheumatoid

(Although this is a degenerative process versus the inflammatory process of rheumatoid arthritis, nursing concerns are the same.)

Osteomalacia CH

Refer to Rickets

Osteomyelitis MS/CH

acute Pain may be related to inflammation and tissue necrosis, possibly evidenced by verbal reports, guarding or distraction behaviors, self-focus, and autonomic responses (changes in vital signs).

Hyperthermia may be related to increased metabolic rate and infectious process, possibly evidenced by increased body temperature and warm, flushed skin.

ineffective bone Tissue Perfusion may be related to inflammatory reaction with thrombosis of vessels, destruction of tissue, edema, and abscess formation, possibly evidenced by bone necrosis, continuation of infectious process, and delayed healing.

risk for impaired Walking possibly evidenced by risk factors of inflammation and tissue necrosis, pain, joint instability.

deficient Knowledge [Learning Need] regarding pathophysiology of condition, long-term therapy needs, activity restriction, and prevention of complications may be related to lack of information, misinterpretation, possibly evidenced by statements of concern, questions, and misconceptions, and inaccurate follow-through of instructions.

Osteoporosis CH

risk for Trauma possibly evidenced by risk factors of loss of bone density and integrity increasing risk of fracture with minimal or no stress.

acute/chronic Pain may be related to vertebral compression on spinal nerve, muscles, or ligaments; spontaneous fractures, possibly evidenced by verbal reports, guarding or distraction behaviors, self-focus, and changes in sleep pattern.

impaired physical Mobility may be related to pain and musculoskeletal impairment, possibly evidenced by limited range of motion, reluctance to attempt movement, expressed fear of reinjury, and imposed restrictions or limitations.

Otitis media PED

acute Pain may be related to inflammation, edema, pressure, possibly evidenced by verbal or coded report, guarding behavior, restlessness, crying.

[disturbed auditory Sensory Perception] may be related to decreased sensory reception, possibly evidenced by reported change in sensory acuity, auditory distortions, change in usual response to stimuli.

risk for delayed Development possibly evidenced by risk factors of auditory impairment, frequent ear infections.

Ovarian cancer MS

Also refer to Cancer

disturbed Body Image may be related to surgical change in reproductive organs, surgical menopause, loss of hair and weight, possibly evidenced by negative feelings about body/sense of mutilation, preoccupation with change, feelings of helplessness, hopelessness, and change in social involvement.

Sexual dysfunction may be related to change in sexual organs, postoperative menopause, vulnerability, possibly evidenced by verbalizations of problem, inability in achieving desired satisfaction, alterations in relationship with SO.

Paget's disease, bone CH

acute Pain may be related to compression/entrapment of nerves, joint degeneration, possibly evidenced by reports of headache, back or joint pain.

Fatigue may be related to disease state and hypermetabolic condition, possibly evidenced by overwhelming lack of energy, inability to maintain usual routines, tired.

disturbed Body Image may be related to physical deformities (enlarged skull, bowing of long bones), possibly evidenced by verbalization of feelings reflecting altered view of body, negative feelings about body, fear of rejection or reaction of others, change in social involvement.

[disturbed auditory Sensory Perception] may be related to altered sensory reception or transmission (nerve compression), possibly evidenced by decreased auditory acuity.

risk for impaired Walking possibly evidenced by risk factors of bowing of long bones, hobbling gait, joint stiffness and pain, paresis or paralysis.

risk for Injury/Falls possibly evidenced by risk factors of bone deformity or fragility, joint stiffness and pain, altered gait.

risk for decreased Cardiac Output possibly evidenced by risk factors of excessive circulatory demands (metabolically active and highly vascular nature of lesions).

Palliative care **CH**

Refer to Hospice care

Palsy, cerebral **PED/CH**

impaired physical Mobility may be related to muscular weakness or hypertonicity, increased deep tendon reflexes, tendency to contractures, and underdevelopment of affected limbs, possibly evidenced by decreased muscle strength, control, mass; limited range of motion, and impaired coordination.

compromised family Coping may be related to permanent nature of condition, situational crisis, emotional conflicts, temporary family disorganization, and incomplete information or understanding of client's needs, possibly evidenced by verbalized anxiety or guilt regarding client's disability, inadequate understanding and knowledge base, and displaying protective behaviors disproportionate (too little or too much) to client's abilities or need for autonomy.

risk for delayed Development possibly evidenced by risk factors of congenital disorder/brain injury, seizure disorder, visual/hearing impairment.

Pancreas transplantation **MS/CH**

Refer to Transplantation, recipient

Pancreatic cancer **MS**

Also refer to Cancer

acute Pain/impaired Comfort may be related to pressure on surrounding organs and nerves, possibly evidenced by verbal reports, guarding or distraction behaviors, focus on self, and autonomic responses (changes in vital signs).

imbalanced Nutrition: less than body requirements may be related to inability to ingest or digest food, absorb nutrients, increased metabolic needs, possibly evidenced by inadequate food intake, anorexia, abdominal pain after eating, weight loss, cachexia.

risk for Infection possibly evidenced by risk factors of stasis of body fluids (biliary obstruction), malnutrition.

risk for impaired Tissue Integrity possibly evidenced by risk factors of poor skin turgor, skeletal prominence, presence of edema, ascites, bile salt accumulation in the tissues.

Pancreatitis **MS**

acute Pain may be related to obstruction of pancreatic and biliary ducts, chemical contamination of peritoneal surfaces by pancreatic exudate, autodigestion of pancreas, extension of inflammation to the retroperitoneal nerve plexus, possibly evidenced by verbal reports, guarding or distraction behaviors, self-focusing, grimacing, changes in vital signs, and alteration in muscle tone.

risk for deficient Fluid Volume/Bleeding possibly evidenced by risk factors of excessive gastric losses (vomiting, nasogastric suctioning), increase in size of vascular bed (vasodilation, effects of kinins), third-space fluid transudation, ascites formation, alteration of clotting process, hemorrhage.

risk for unstable Blood Glucose Level possibly evidenced by risk factors of compromised physical health status, excessive stress, ineffective medication management.

imbalanced Nutrition: less than body requirements may be related to vomiting, decreased oral intake, prescribed dietary restrictions, altered ability to digest nutrients—loss of digestive enzymes, possibly evidenced by reported inadequate food intake, aversion to eating, reported altered taste sensation, weight loss, and reduced muscle mass.

risk for Infection possibly evidenced by risk factors of inadequate primary defenses (stasis of body fluids, altered peristalsis, change in pH secretions), immunosuppression, nutritional deficiencies, tissue destruction, and chronic disease.

Panic disorder **PSY**

Fear may be related to unfounded morbid dread of a seemingly harmless object or situation, possibly evidenced by physiological symptoms, mental or cognitive behaviors indicative of panic, withdrawal from or total avoidance of situations that place client in contact with feared object.

[severe to panic] Anxiety may be related to unidentified stressors, contact with feared object or situation, limitations placed on ritualistic behavior, possibly evidenced by attacks of immobilizing apprehension, physical, mental, or cognitive behaviors indicative of panic; expressed feelings of terror or inability to cope.

Paralysis, infantile **PED**

Refer to Poliomyelitis

Paranoid personality disorder **PSY**

risk for other-/self-directed Violence possibly evidenced by risk factors of perceived threats of danger, paranoid delusions, and increased feelings of anxiety.

[severe] Anxiety may be related to inability to trust (has not mastered tasks of trust versus mistrust), possibly evidenced by rigid delusional system (serves to provide relief from stress that justifies the delusion), frightened of other people and own hostility.

Powerlessness may be related to feelings of inadequacy, lifestyle of helplessness, maladaptive interpersonal interactions (e.g., misuse of power, force; abusive relationships), sense of severely impaired self-concept, and belief that individual has no control over situation(s), possibly evidenced by paranoid delusions, use of aggressive behavior to compensate, and expressions of recognition of damage paranoia has caused self and others.

[disturbed Sensory Perception (specify)] may be related to psychological stress, possibly evidenced by change in behavior pattern/usual response to stimuli.

compromised family Coping may be related to temporary or sustained family disorganization/role changes, prolonged progression of condition that exhausts the supportive capacity of SO(s), possibly evidenced by family system not meeting physical, emotional, or spiritual needs of its members; inability to express or to accept wide range of feelings; inappropriate boundary maintenance; SO(s) describe(s) preoccupation with personal reactions.

Paranoid schizophrenia **PSY**

Refer to Schizophrenia (schizophrenic disorders)

Paraphilias **PSY**

ineffective Sexuality Pattern may be related to conflict with sexual orientation or variant preferences, possibly evidenced by alterations in achieving sexual satisfaction, difficulty achieving desired satisfaction in socially acceptable ways.

chronic low Self-Esteem may be related to psychosocial factors (e.g., achievement of sexual satisfaction in deviant ways), substance use, possibly evidenced by expressions of shame or guilt, self-destructive behaviors, feelings of powerlessness, helplessness.

interrupted Family Processes may be related to situational crisis (e.g., revelation of sexual deviance or dysfunction), possibly evidenced by expressions of confusion about or difficulty dealing with situation, inappropriate boundary maintenance, family system does not meet emotional or security needs, failure to deal with traumatic experience constructively.

Paraplegia **MS/CH**

Also refer to Quadriplegia

impaired Transfer Ability may be related to loss of muscle function and control, injury to upper extremity joints (overuse).

[disturbed kinesthetic/tactile Sensory Perception] may be related to neurological deficit with loss of sensory reception and transmission, psychological stress, possibly evidenced by reported or measured change in sensory acuity, change in usual response to stimuli, anxiety, disorientation, bizarre thinking, exaggerated emotional responses.

reflex urinary Incontinence/impaired urinary Elimination may be related to disruption of bladder innervation, bladder atony, fecal impaction, possibly evidenced by lack of awareness of bladder distention, retention, incontinence, or overflow, urinary tract infections—kidney stone formation, renal dysfunction.

situational low Self-Esteem may be related to situational crisis, loss of body functions, change in physical abilities, perceived loss of self or identity, possibly evidenced by negative feelings about body or self, feelings of helplessness or powerlessness, delay in taking responsibility for self-care or participation in therapy, and change in social involvement.

Sexual dysfunction may be related to loss of sensation, altered function, and vulnerability, possibly evidenced by seeking of confirmation of desirability, verbalization of concern, alteration in relationship with SO, and change in interest in self/others.

Parathyroidectomy **MS**

acute Pain may be related to presence of surgical incision and effects of calcium imbalance (bone pain, tetany), possibly evidenced by verbal reports, guarding or distraction behaviors, self-focus, and changes in vital signs.

risk for excess Fluid Volume possibly evidenced by risk factors of preoperative renal involvement, stress-induced release of antidiuretic hormone, and changing calcium or other electrolyte levels.

risk for ineffective Airway Clearance possibly evidenced by risk factors of edema formation and laryngeal nerve damage.

deficient Knowledge [Learning Need] regarding postoperative care, complications, and long-term needs may be related to lack of information or recall, misinterpretation, possibly evidenced by statements of concern, questions, and misconceptions.

Parent-child relational problem PED/PSY

impaired Parenting may be related to lack of or ineffective role model, lack of support between or from SO, interruption in bonding process, unrealistic expectations for self/child/partner, presence of stressors, lack of appropriate response of child to parent, possibly evidenced by frequent verbalization of disappointment in child, inability to care for or discipline child, lack of parental attachment behaviors, child abuse or abandonment.

chronic low Self-Esteem/ineffective Role Performance may be related to view self as "poor" or ineffective parent, belief that seeking help is an admission of defeat or failure, psychiatric or physical illness of the child, possibly evidenced by change in usual patterns or responsibility, expressions of lack of information, lack of follow-through of therapy, nonparticipation in therapy.

interrupted Family Process may be related to situational crisis of child/adolescent, maturational crisis (e.g., adolescence, midlife), possibly evidenced by expressions of confusion and difficulty coping with situation; family system not meeting physical, emotional, or security needs of members; difficulty accepting help; parents not respecting each other's parenting practices.

compromised/disabled family Coping may be related to individual preoccupation with own emotional conflicts and personal suffering or anxiety about the crisis, temporary family disorganization, exhausted supportive capacity of members, highly ambivalent family relationships, possibly evidenced by detrimental decisions or actions, neglected relationships, intolerance, agitation, depression, hostility, aggression.

readiness for enhanced family Coping possibly evidenced by expressing interest in making contact with another person experiencing a similar situation, moving in direction of health-promoting or enriching lifestyle, auditing or negotiating therapy program.

Parenteral feeding MS/CH

imbalanced Nutrition: less than body requirements may be related to conditions that interfere with nutrient intake or increase nutrient need or metabolic demand—cancer and associated treatments, anorexia, surgical procedures, dysphagia, or decreased level of consciousness, possibly evidenced by body weight 10% or more under ideal, decreased subcutaneous fat or muscle mass, poor muscle tone.

risk for Infection possibly evidenced by risk factors of invasive procedure and surgical placement of feeding tube, malnutrition, chronic disease.

risk for Injury [multifactor] possibly evidenced by risk factors of catheter-related complications (air emboli, septic thrombophlebitis).

risk for imbalanced Fluid Volume possibly evidenced by risk factors of active loss or failure of regulatory mechanisms (specific to underlying disease process or trauma), complications of therapy—high glucose solutions or hyperglycemia (hyperosmolar nonketotic syndrome and severe dehydration), inability to obtain or ingest fluids.

Fatigue may be related to decreased metabolic energy production, increased energy requirements (hypermetabolic state, healing process), altered body chemistry (medications, chemotherapy), possibly evidenced by overwhelming lack of energy, inability to maintain usual routines or accomplish routine tasks, lethargy, impaired ability to concentrate.

Parkinson's disease CH

impaired Walking may be related to neuromuscular impairment (muscle weakness, tremors, bradykinesia) and musculoskeletal impairment (joint rigidity), possibly evidenced by inability to move about the environment as desired, increased occurrence of falls.

impaired Swallowing may be related to neuromuscular impairment, muscle weakness, possibly evidenced by reported or observed difficulty in swallowing, drooling, evidence of aspiration (choking, coughing).

impaired verbal Communication may be related to muscle weakness and incoordination, possibly evidenced by impaired articulation, difficulty with phonation, and changes in rhythm and intonation.

risk for Stress overload possibly evidenced by risk factors of inadequate resources, chronic illness, physical demands.

caregiver Role Strain may be related to illness, severity of care receiver, psychological/cognitive problems in care receiver, caregiver is spouse, duration of caregiving required, lack of respite or recreation for caregiver, possibly evidenced by feeling stressed, depressed, worried; lack of resources or support, family conflict.

Passive-aggressive personality disorder PSY

[moderate to severe] Anxiety may be related to unconscious conflict, unmet needs, threat to self-concept, difficulty in asserting self directly, feelings of resentment toward authority figures, possibly evidenced by difficulty resolving feelings or trusting others, passive resistance to demands made by others, extraneous movements, irritability, argumentativeness.

ineffective Coping may be related to inadequate level of confidence in ability to cope or perception of control, uncertainty, high degree of threat, inadequate social support created by characteristics of relationships, disturbance in pattern of tension release, possibly evidenced by verbalizations or inability to cope or ask for help, lack of goal-directed behavior or resolution of problem, lack of assertive behavior, use of forms of coping that impede adaptive behavior, decreased use of social supports, risk-taking.

chronic low Self-Esteem may be related to retarded ego development, unmet dependency needs, early rejection by SO, lack of positive feedback, possibly evidenced by lack of self-confidence, feelings of inadequacy, fear of asserting self, dependency on others, directing frustrations toward others by using covert aggressive tactics, not accepting responsibility for what happens as a result of maladaptive behaviors, failing to work through negative feelings.

Powerlessness may be related to interpersonal interaction, lifestyle of helplessness, dependency feelings, difficulty connecting own passive-resistent behaviors with hostility or resentment, possibly evidenced by experiencing conscious hostility toward authority figures, releasing anger or hostility through others, getting back at others through aggravation.

PCP (phencyclidine) intoxication MS/PSY

Also refer to Hallucinogen abuse

risk for self-/other-directed Violence possibly evidenced by risk factors of drug abuse, psychotic symptomology, impulsivity.

risk for Trauma/Suffocation/Poisoning possibly evidenced by risk factors of clouded sensorium, increased muscle strength, myoclonic jerks or convulsions, ataxia, decreased pain perception, coma.

risk for ineffective cerebral Tissue Perfusion possibly evidenced by risk factors of alterations in blood flow (hypertensive crisis).

Pediculosis capitis PED/CH

impaired Skin Integrity related to presence of nits, intense itching, and scratching; possibly evidenced by redness, excoriation, disruption of skin surface.

risk for Infection [spread] possibly evidenced by risk factors of insufficient knowledge to avoid exposure or transmission of parasite.

Pediculosis pubis CH

Refer to Pediculosis capitis

Pelvic inflammatory disease OB/GYN/CH

risk for Infection [spread] possibly evidenced by risk factors of presence of infectious process in highly vascular pelvic structures, delay in seeking treatment.

acute Pain may be related to inflammation, edema, and congestion of reproductive and pelvic tissues, possibly evidenced by verbal reports, guarding or distraction behaviors, self-focus, and changes in vital signs.

Hyperthermia may be related to inflammatory process and hypermetabolic state, possibly evidenced by increased body temperature; warm, flushed skin; and tachycardia.

risk for situational low Self-Esteem possibly evidenced by risk factors of perceived stigma of physical condition (infection of reproductive system).

deficient Knowledge [Learning Need] regarding cause/complications of condition, therapy needs, and transmission of disease to others may be related to lack of information, misinterpretation, possibly evidenced by statements of concern, questions, misconceptions, and development of preventable complications.

Periarteritis nodosa MS/CH

Refer to Polyarteritis nodosa

Pericarditis MS

acute Pain may be related to tissue inflammation and presence of effusion, possibly evidenced by verbal reports of pain affected by movement or position, guarding or distraction behaviors, self-focus, and changes in vital signs.

Activity Intolerance may be related to imbalance between oxygen supply and demand (restriction of cardiac filling and ventricular contraction, reduced cardiac output), possibly evidenced by reports of weakness, fatigue, exertional dyspnea, abnormal heart rate or blood pressure response, and signs of heart failure.

risk for decreased Cardiac Output possibly evidenced by risk factors of accumulation of fluid (effusion), restricted cardiac filling, and contractility.

Anxiety [specify level] may be related to change in health status and perceived threat of death, possibly evidenced by increased tension, apprehension, restlessness, and expressed concerns.

Perinatal loss/death of child **OB/CH**

Grieving may be related to death of fetus/infant (wanted or unwanted), inability to meet personal expectations, possibly evidenced by verbal expressions of distress, anger, loss, crying, alteration in eating habits or sleep pattern.

situational low Self-Esteem may be related to perceived "failure" at a life event, possibly evidenced by negative self-appraisal in response to life event in a person with a previous positive self-evaluation, verbalization of negative feelings about the self (helplessness, uselessness), difficulty making decisions.

risk for ineffective Role Performance possibly evidenced by risk factors of stress, family conflict, inadequate support system.

risk for interrupted Family Processes possibly evidenced by risk factors of situational crisis, developmental transition [loss of child], family roles shift.

risk for Spiritual distress possibly evidenced by risk factors of loss of loved one, blame for loss directed at self/God, alienation from SO/support systems, challenged belief and value system (birth is supposed to be the beginning of life, not of death), and intense suffering.

Peripheral arterial occlusive disease **CH**

Refer to Arterial occlusive disease, peripheral

Peripheral vascular disease (atherosclerosis) **CH**

ineffective peripheral Tissue Perfusion may be related to reduction or interruption of arterial or venous blood flow, possibly evidenced by changes in skin temperature and color, lack of hair growth, blood pressure and pulse changes in extremity, presence of bruits, and reports of claudication.

Activity Intolerance may be related to imbalance between oxygen supply and demand, possibly evidenced by reports of muscle fatigue, weakness and exertional discomfort (claudication).

risk for impaired Skin/Tissue Integrity possibly evidenced by risk factors of altered circulation with decreased sensation and impaired healing.

Peritonitis **MS**

risk for Infection [spread/septicemia] possibly evidenced by risk factors of inadequate primary defenses (broken skin, traumatized tissue, altered peristalsis), inadequate secondary defenses (immunosuppression), and invasive procedures.

deficient Fluid Volume [mixed] may be related to fluid shifts from extracellular, intravascular, and interstitial compartments into intestines or peritoneal space, excessive gastric losses (vomiting, diarrhea, nasogastric suction), fever, hypermetabolic state, and restricted intake, possibly evidenced by dry mucous membranes, poor skin turgor, delayed capillary refill, weak peripheral pulses, diminished urinary output, dark, concentrated urine; hypotension, and tachycardia.

acute Pain may be related to chemical irritation of parietal peritoneum, trauma to tissues, abdominal distention—accumulation of fluid in abdominal or peritoneal cavity, possibly evidenced by verbal reports, muscle guarding or rebound tenderness, distraction behaviors, facial mask of pain, self-focus, and changes in vital signs.

risk for imbalanced Nutrition: less than body requirements possibly evidenced by risk factors of nausea, vomiting, intestinal dysfunction, metabolic abnormalities, increased metabolic needs.

Persian Gulf syndrome **CH/MS**

Refer to Gulf War syndrome

Personality disorders **PSY**

Refer to Antisocial; Borderline; Obsessive-compulsive; Passive-aggressive; or Paranoid personality disorders

Pertussis **PED**

ineffective Airway Clearance may be related to retained secretions, excessive thick tenacious mucus, infection, possibly evidenced by dyspnea, adventitious breath sounds, hacking/paroxysmal cough.

deficient Fluid Volume may be related to decreased intake, anorexia, vomiting, increased insensible losses (fever, diaphoresis), possibly evidenced by decreased urine output and increased specific gravity, decreased blood pressure, increased pulse rate, decreased skin and tongue turgor, dry skin and mucous membranes.

risk for Infection [transmission/secondary] possibly evidenced by risk factors of contagious nature of disease, stasis of body fluids, malnutrition, insufficient knowledge to avoid exposure to pathogens.

risk for imbalanced Nutrition: less than body requirements possibly evidenced by risk factors of inability to ingest food or absorb nutrients (anorexia, vomiting), increased metabolic demands.

risk for impaired Gas Exchange possibly evidenced by risk factors of compromised airways (tenacious mucus, inflammation), paroxysms of coughing, ventilation perfusion imbalance (atelectasis).

Pervasive developmental disorders PED/PSY

Refer to Autism spectrum disorder; Rett's syndrome; Asperger's disorder

Pheochromocytoma MS

Anxiety [specify level] may be related to excessive physiological (hormonal) stimulation of the sympathetic nervous system, situational crises, threat to or change in health status, possibly evidenced by apprehension, shakiness, restlessness, focus on self, fearfulness, diaphoresis, and sense of impending doom.

deficient Fluid Volume [mixed] may be related to excessive gastric losses (vomiting, diarrhea), hypermetabolic state, diaphoresis, and hyperosmolar diuresis, possibly evidenced by hemoconcentration, dry mucous membranes, poor skin turgor, thirst, and weight loss.

decreased Cardiac Output/ineffective Tissue Perfusion (specify) may be related to altered preload—decreased blood volume, altered systemic vascular resistance, and increased sympathetic activity (excessive secretion of catecholamines), possibly evidenced by cool, clammy skin, change in blood pressure (hypertension, postural hypotension), visual disturbances, severe headache, and angina.

deficient Knowledge [Learning Need] regarding pathophysiology of condition, outcome, and preoperative and postoperative care needs may be related to lack of information or recall, possibly evidenced by statements of concern, questions, and misconceptions.

Phlebitis CH

Refer to Thrombophlebitis

Phobia PSY

Also refer to Anxiety disorder, generalized

Fear may be related to learned irrational response to natural or innate origins (phobic stimulus), unfounded morbid dread of a seemingly harmless object or situation, possibly evidenced by sympathetic stimulation and reactions ranging from apprehension to panic, withdrawal from or total avoidance of situations that place individual in contact with feared object.

impaired Social Interaction may be related to intense fear of encountering feared object, activity or situation; and anticipated loss of control, possibly evidenced by reported change of style or pattern of interaction, discomfort in social situations, and avoidance of phobic stimulus.

Physical abuse CH/PSY

Refer to Abuse, physical; Battered child syndrome

Pickwickian syndrome CH

ineffective Breathing Pattern may be related to obesity, hypoventilation, possibly evidenced by decreased pulmonary function, hypercapnia, hypoxia, reduced effect of carbon dioxide in stimulating respirations.

PID GYN/OB/CH

Refer to Pelvic inflammatory disease

Pinkeye CH

Refer to Conjunctivitis, bacterial

Placenta previa OB

risk for Bleeding/Shock possibly evidenced by risk factors of pregnancy-related complication; hypovolemia, hypotension.

impaired fetal Gas Exchange may be related to altered blood flow, altered oxygen-carrying capacity of blood (maternal anemia), and decreased surface area of gas exchange at site of placental attachment, possibly evidenced by changes in fetal heart rate and activity, and release of meconium.

Fear may be related to threat of death (perceived or actual) to self or fetus, possibly evidenced by verbalization of specific concerns, increased tension, sympathetic stimulation.

risk for deficient Diversional Activity possibly evidenced by risk factors of imposed activity restrictions, bedrest.

Plague, bubonic MS

Hyperthermia may be related to illness, dehydration, possibly evidenced by increased body temperature, tachycardia, chills, confusion.

acute Pain may be related to inflammatory process, enlarged lymph nodes, possibly evidenced by verbal or coded reports, expressive behavior, autonomic responses.

risk for deficient Fluid Volume possibly evidenced by risk factors of fever, decreased oral intake.

risk for impaired Skin Integrity possibly evidenced by risk factor of infectious process.

Plague, pneumonic **MS**
risk for Infection [spread] possibly evidenced by risk factors of contagious nature of disease, close contact with others.

Hyperthermia may be related to illness, dehydration, possibly evidenced by increased body temperature, tachycardia, chills, severe headache, confusion.

impaired Gas Exchange may be related to alveolar-capillary membrane changes, possibly evidenced by tachypnea, dyspnea, stridor, hemoptysis, cyanosis.

deficient Fluid Volume may be related to fever, hypermetabolic state, decreased intake, bleeding diathesis (disseminated intravascular coagulation), possibly evidenced by weakness, decreased venous filling, decreased blood pressure, decreased skin turgor, dry mucous membranes, change in mental state.

Plantar fasciitis **CH**
acute/chronic Pain may be related to inflammation, possibly evidenced by report of stabbing, burning pain, guarding or protective behavior, change in posture and gait, altered ability to continue previous activities.

impaired Walking may be related to musculoskeletal impairment, impaired balance, pain, possibly evidenced by impaired ability to walk required distances or climb stairs.

Pleural effusion **CH/MS**
Also refer to Hemothorax

acute Pain may be related to inflammation/irritation of the parietal pleura, possibly evidenced by verbal reports, guarding or distraction behaviors, self-focus, and changes in vital signs.

ineffective Breathing Pattern may be related to pain on inspiration, possibly evidenced by decreased respiratory depth, tachypnea, and dyspnea.

risk for impaired Gas Exchange possibly evidenced by risk factors of ventilation perfusion imbalance.

Pleurisy **CH**
acute Pain may be related to inflammation and irritation of the parietal pleura, possibly evidenced by verbal reports, guarding or distraction behaviors, self-focus, and changes in vital signs.

ineffective Breathing Pattern may be related to pain on inspiration, possibly evidenced by decreased respiratory depth, tachypnea, and dyspnea.

risk for Infection [pneumonia] possibly evidenced by risk factors of stasis of pulmonary secretions, decreased lung expansion, and ineffective cough.

PMDD **GYN/PSY**
Refer to Premenstrual dysphoric disorder

PMS **GYN/PSY**
Refer to Premenstrual dysphoric disorder

Pneumoconiosis (black lung) **CH**
Refer to Pulmonary fibrosis

Pneumonia **CH/MS**
Refer to Bronchitis; Bronchopneumonia

Pneumonia, ventilator associated **CH**
Refer to Bronchopneumonia

Pneumothorax **MS**
Also refer to Hemothorax

ineffective Breathing Pattern may be related to decreased lung expansion (air accumulation), musculoskeletal impairment, pain, inflammatory process, possibly evidenced by dyspnea, tachypnea, altered chest excursion, respiratory depth changes, use of accessory muscles, nasal flaring, cough, cyanosis, and abnormal arterial blood gases.

risk for decreased Cardiac Output possibly evidenced by risk factors of compression or displacement of cardiac structures.

acute Pain may be related to irritation of nerve endings within pleural space by foreign object (chest tube), possibly evidenced by verbal reports, guarding or distraction behaviors, self-focus, and changes in vital signs.

Poliomyelitis **CH**
Also refer to Postpolio syndrome

ineffective Breathing Pattern may be related to neuromuscular dysfunction and intercostal muscle impairment, hypoventilation syndrome, possibly evidenced by dyspnea, decreased depth of breathing, altered chest excursion, respiratory failure.

impaired physical Mobility related to neuromuscular dysfunction and musculoskeletal impairment, decreased muscle strength, control or mass; contracture, decreased endurance, pain, prescribed movement restriction or bracing, possibly evidenced by limited ability to move, uncoordinated or jerky movements, gait changes, exaggerated lateral postural sway, postural instability.

Self-Care deficit [specify] may be related to neuromuscular impairment, weakness, pain, fatigue, possibly evidenced by reported or observed inability to perform specified activities.

risk for Infection [transmission] possibly evidenced by risk factors of inadequate acquired immunity, malnutrition, or insufficient knowledge to avoid exposure to or transmission of pathogen.

Polyarteritis nodosa MS/CH

ineffective Tissue Perfusion (specify) may be related to reduction or interruption of blood flow, possibly evidenced by organ tissue infarctions, changes in organ function, and development of organic psychosis.

Hyperthermia may be related to widespread inflammatory process, possibly evidenced by increased body temperature and warm, flushed skin.

acute Pain may be related to inflammation, tissue ischemia, and necrosis of affected area, possibly evidenced by verbal reports, guarding or distraction behaviors, self-focus, and changes in vital signs.

Grieving may be related to perceived loss of self, possibly evidenced by expressions of sorrow and anger, altered sleep or eating patterns, changes in activity level, and libido.

Polycythemia vera CH

Activity Intolerance may be related to imbalance between oxygen supply and demand, possibly evidenced by reports of fatigue, weakness.

ineffective Tissue Perfusion (specify) may be related to reduction or interruption of arterial or venous blood flow (insufficiency, thrombosis, or hemorrhage), possibly evidenced by pain in affected area, impaired mental ability, visual disturbances, and color changes of skin and mucous membranes.

Polyradiculitis, acute inflammatory MS

Refer to Guillain-Barré syndrome

Postconcussion syndrome CH

acute/chronic Pain may be related to neuronal damage, possibly evidenced by reports of headache.

Anxiety [specify level] may be related to situational crisis, change in health status, ongoing nature of disability, stress, unmet needs, possibly evidenced by expressed concerns, apprehension, uncertainty, feelings of inadequacy, focus on self, difficulty concentrating.

risk for impaired Memory may be related to neurological disturbances possibly evidenced by inability to recall events/factual information, reports experience of forgetting.

Postmaturity syndrome PED

Refer to Newborn, postmature

Postmyocardial syndrome CH

Refer to Dressler's syndrome

Postoperative recovery period MS

ineffective Breathing Pattern may be related to neuromuscular and perceptual or cognitive impairment, decreased lung expansion and energy, and tracheobronchial obstruction, possibly evidenced by changes in respiratory rate and depth, reduced vital capacity, apnea, cyanosis, and noisy respirations.

risk for imbalanced Body Temperature possibly evidenced by risk factors of exposure to cool environment, effect of medications and anesthetic agents, extremes of age or weight, and dehydration.

risk for acute Confusion possibly evidenced by risk factors of pharmaceutical agents—anesthesia, pain.

risk for deficit Fluid Volume possibly evidenced by risk factors of restriction of oral intake, loss of fluid through abnormal routes (indwelling tubes, drains) and normal routes (vomiting, loss of vascular integrity, changes in clotting ability), extremes of age and weight.

acute Pain may be related to disruption of skin, tissue, and muscle integrity; musculoskeletal or bone trauma; and presence of tubes and drains, possibly evidenced by verbal reports, alteration in muscle tone, facial mask of pain, distraction or guarding behaviors, narrowed focus, and autonomic responses.

impaired Skin/Tissue Integrity may be related to mechanical interruption of skin or tissues, altered circulation, effects of medication, accumulation of drainage, and altered metabolic state, possibly evidenced by disruption of skin and tissues.

risk for Infection possibly evidenced by risk factors of broken skin, traumatized tissues, stasis of body fluids, presence of pathogens or contaminants, environmental exposure, and invasive procedures.

Postpartum blues OB/PSY

Refer to Depression, postpartum

Postpartum period, 4 to 48 hours OB/CH

acute Pain/impaired Comfort may be related to tissue trauma, edema, muscle contractions, bladder fullness, and physical or psychological exhaustion, possibly evidenced by reports of cramping (afterpains), self-focusing, alteration in muscle tone, distraction behaviors, and changes in vital signs.

Breastfeeding (specify) may be related to level of knowledge, previous experiences, infant gestational age, level of support, physical structure or characteristics of the maternal breasts, possibly evidenced by maternal verbalization regarding level of satisfaction, observations of breastfeeding process, infant response and weight gain.

risk for impaired Attachment possibly evidenced by risk factors of lack of support between or from SO(s), ineffective or no role model, anxiety associated with the parental role, unrealistic expectations, unmet social or emotional maturation needs of client/partner, presence of stressors (e.g., financial, housing, employment).

risk for deficient Fluid Volume/Bleeding possibly evidenced by risk factors of excessive blood loss during delivery, reduced intake or inadequate replacement, nausea, vomiting, increased urine output, and insensible losses.

impaired urinary Elimination may be related to hormonal effects (fluid shifts, continued elevation in renal plasma flow), mechanical trauma, tissue edema, and effects of medication or anesthesia, possibly evidenced by frequency, dysuria, urgency, incontinence, or retention.

Constipation may be related to decreased muscle tone associated with diastasis recti, prenatal effects of progesterone, dehydration, excess analgesia or anesthesia, pain (hemorrhoids, episiotomy, or perineal tenderness), prelabor diarrhea and lack of intake, possibly evidenced by frequency less than usual pattern, hard-formed stool, straining at stool, decreased bowel sounds, and abdominal distention.

Insomnia may be related to pain, discomfort, intense exhilaration or excitement, anxiety, exhausting process of labor and delivery, and needs or demands of family members, possibly evidenced by verbal reports of difficulty in falling asleep or staying asleep, not feeling well-rested, interrupted sleep, lack of energy.

Postpartum period, 4 to 6 weeks OB/CH

readiness for enhanced family Coping possibly evidenced by family member(s) moving in direction of health-promoting and enriching lifestyle.

disturbed Body Image may be related to unrealistic expectations of postpartum recovery, permanency of some changes, possibly evidenced by verbalization of negative feelings about body, feelings of helplessness, preoccupation with change, focus on past appearance, fear of rejection or reaction of others.

risk for Sexual dysfunction possibly evidenced by risk factors of health-related transition, changes in body function (including lactation), lack of privacy, fear of pregnancy.

readiness for enhanced Parenting possibly evidenced by expressed willingness to enhance parenting, physical and emotional needs of infant/children are met, bonding evident.

Postpartum period, postdischarge to 4 weeks OB/CH

risk for Fatigue possibly evidenced by risk factors of physical and emotional demands of infant and other family members, psychological stressors, continued discomfort.

Breastfeeding (specify) may be related to level of knowledge and support, previous experiences, infant gestational age, physical structure or characteristics of maternal breast, demands of home life and employment, possibly evidenced by maternal verbalizations regarding level of satisfaction, observations of feeding process, infant response and weight gain.

risk for imbalanced Nutrition: less than body requirements possibly evidenced by risk factors of intake insufficient to meet metabolic demands or correct existing deficiencies (e.g., lactation, anemia, excessive blood loss, infection, excessive tissue trauma, desire to regain prenatal weight).

risk for Infection possibly evidenced by risk factors of tissue trauma, broken skin, decreased Hb, invasive procedures, increased environmental exposure, malnutrition.

risk for ineffective Coping/compromised family Coping possibly evidenced by risk factors of situational or developmental changes, temporary family disorganization or role changes, little support provided by partner/family members.

risk for impaired Parenting possibly evidenced by risk factors of situational crisis—addition and demands of new family member, changes in responsibilities of family members; sleep disruption, lack of support from SO/family members, young parental age, life stressors—financial, employment, home environment, lack of resources.

Postpartum psychosis **OB/PSY**

Also refer to Depression, postpartum

ineffective Coping may be related to situational/maturational crisis, inadequate level of confidence in ability to cope, inadequate level of perception of control, possibly evidenced by inability to meet basic needs, inability to problem solve, sleep pattern disturbance, poor concentration.

risk for other-directed Violence possibly evidenced by risk factors of mood swings, increased anxiety, despondency, hopelessness, psychotic symptomatology.

Postpolio syndrome **CH**

Anxiety [specify]/Fear may be related to change in health status, progressive and debilitating disease, change in role function and economic status, possibly evidenced by expressed concerns, uncertainty, awareness of physiological symptoms, worrisome, sleep disturbance, forgetfulness.

Fatigue may be related to disease state, stress, anxiety, sleep deprivation, depression, possibly evidenced by overwhelming lack of energy, inability to maintain usual routines or level of physical activity, difficulty concentrating.

chronic Pain may be related to chronic physical disability, joint degeneration, possibly evidenced by reports of deep aching pain, altered ability to continue previous activities, change in sleep patterns, reduced interaction with others.

impaired Walking/physical Mobility may be related to neuromuscular impairment, decreased muscle strength and atrophy, decreased endurance, pain, inability to stand erect (flat back syndrome), possibly evidenced by gait disturbances, joint or postural instability, decreased ability to perform gross motor skills.

Sleep Deprivation may be related to sleep apnea (central and obstructive), chronic pain, possibly evidenced by daytime drowsiness, decreased ability to function, inability to concentrate.

impaired Swallowing may be related to neuromuscular impairment, pharyngeal muscle weakness, possibly evidenced by coughing, choking, recurrent pulmonary infections.

ineffective Airway Clearance may be related to neuromuscular dysfunction (muscle weakness and atrophy), retained secretions, possibly evidenced by diminished or adventitious breath sounds (chronic microatelectasis), poor cough (decreased pulmonary compliance, increased chest wall tightness).

Post-traumatic stress disorder **PSY**

Post-Trauma Syndrome related to having experienced a traumatic life event, possibly evidenced by reexperiencing the event, somatic reactions, psychological or emotional numbness, altered lifestyle, impaired sleep, self-destructive behaviors, difficulty with interpersonal relationships, development of phobia, poor impulse control or irritability, and explosiveness.

risk for other-directed Violence possibly evidenced by risk factors of startled reaction, an intrusive memory causing a sudden acting out of a feeling as if the event were occurring; use of alcohol or other drugs to ward off painful effects and produce psychic numbing, breaking through the rage that has been walled off, response to intense anxiety or panic state, and loss of control.

ineffective Coping may be related to personal vulnerability, inadequate support systems, unrealistic perceptions, unmet expectations, overwhelming threat to self, and multiple stressors repeated over a period of time, possibly evidenced by verbalization of inability to cope or difficulty asking for help, muscular tension, headaches, chronic worry, and emotional tension.

complicated Grieving may be related to actual or perceived object loss (loss of self as seen before the traumatic incident occurred as well as other losses incurred in or after the incident), loss of physiopsychosocial well-being, thwarted grieving response to a loss, and lack of resolution of previous grieving responses, possibly evidenced by verbal expression of distress at loss, anger, sadness, labile affect; alterations in eating habits, sleep or dream patterns, libido; reliving of past experiences, expression of guilt, and alterations in concentration.

interrupted Family Processes may be related to situational crisis, failure to master developmental transitions, possibly evidenced by expressions of confusion about what to do and by family having difficulty coping, family system not meeting physical, emotional, or spiritual needs of its members; not adapting to change or dealing with traumatic experience constructively, and ineffective family decision-making process.

Preeclampsia **OB**

Refer to Hypertension, gestational; Abruptio placentae

Pregnancy, 1st trimester **OB/CH**

risk for imbalanced Nutrition: less than body requirements possibly evidenced by risk factors of changes in appetite, insufficient intake (nausea, vomiting, inadequate financial resources and nutritional knowledge), meeting increased metabolic demands (increased thyroid activity associated with the growth of fetal and maternal tissues).

impaired Comfort may be related to hormonal influences, physical changes, possibly evidenced by verbal reports (nausea, breast changes, leg cramps, hemorrhoids, nasal stuffiness), alteration in muscle tone, inability to relax.

risk for disturbed Maternal-Fetal Dyad possibly evidenced by risk factors of environmental or hereditary factors, problems of maternal well-being (e.g., malnutrition, substance use).

[maximally compensated] Cardiac Output may be related to increased fluid volume, maximal cardiac effort and hormonal effects of progesterone and relaxin (places the client at risk for hypertension and/or circulatory failure), and changes in peripheral resistance (afterload), possibly evidenced by variations in blood pressure and pulse, syncopal episodes, presence of pathological edema.

readiness for enhanced family Coping possibly evidenced by movement toward health-promoting and enriching lifestyle, choosing experiences that optimize pregnancy experience and wellness.

risk for Constipation possibly evidenced by risk factors of changes in dietary or fluid intake, smooth muscle relaxation, decreased peristalsis, and effects of medications (e.g., iron).

Fatigue/Insomnia may be related to increased carbohydrate metabolism, altered body chemistry, increased energy requirements to perform activities of daily living, discomfort, anxiety, inactivity, possibly evidenced by reports of overwhelming lack of energy, inability to maintain usual routines, difficulty falling asleep, dissatisfaction with sleep, decreased quality of life.

risk for ineffective Role Performance possibly evidenced by risk factors of maturational crisis, developmental level, history of maladaptive coping, absence of support systems.

deficient Knowledge [Learning Need] regarding normal physiological/psychological changes and self-care needs may be related to lack of information or recall and misinterpretation of normal physiological or psychological changes and their impact on the client/family, possibly evidenced by questions, statements of concern, misconceptions, inaccurate follow-through of instructions, and development of preventable complications.

Pregnancy, 2nd trimester — OB/CH

Also refer to Pregnancy, 1st trimester

risk for disturbed Body Image possibly evidenced by risk factors of perception of biophysical changes, response of others.

ineffective Breathing Pattern may be related to impingement of the diaphragm by enlarging uterus, possibly evidenced by reports of shortness of breath, dyspnea, and changes in respiratory depth.

risk for [decompensated] Cardiac Output possibly evidenced by risk factors of increased circulatory demand, changes in preload (decreased venous return) and afterload (increased peripheral vascular resistance), and ventricular hypertrophy.

risk for excess Fluid Volume possibly evidenced by risk factors of changes in regulatory mechanisms, sodium and water retention.

Sexual dysfunction may be related to conflict regarding changes in sexual desire and expectations, fear of physical injury to woman/fetus, possibly evidenced by reported difficulties, limitations or changes in sexual behaviors or activities.

Pregnancy, 3rd trimester — OB/CH

Also refer to Pregnancy, 1st and 2nd trimesters

deficient Knowledge [Learning Need] regarding preparation for labor/delivery and infant care may be related to lack of exposure or experience, misinterpretations of information, possibly evidenced by request for information, statement of concerns, misconceptions.

impaired urinary Elimination may be related to uterine enlargement, increased abdominal pressure, fluctuation of renal blood flow, and glomerular filtration rate, possibly evidenced by urinary frequency, urgency, dependent edema.

risk for ineffective Coping/compromised family Coping possibly evidenced by risk factors of situational or maturational crisis, personal vulnerability, unrealistic perceptions, absent or insufficient support systems.

risk for disturbed Maternal-Fetal Dyad possibly evidenced by risk factors of presence of hypertension, infection, substance use or abuse, altered immune system, abnormal blood profile, tissue hypoxia, premature rupture of membranes.

Pregnancy, adolescent — OB/CH

Also refer to Pregnancy, 1st, 2nd, and 3rd trimesters

interrupted Family Processes may be related to situational or developmental transition (economic, change in roles, gain of a family member), possibly evidenced by family expressing confusion about what to do, unable to meet physical, emotional, or spiritual needs of the members; family inability to adapt to change or to deal with traumatic experience constructively; does not demonstrate respect for individuality and autonomy of its members, ineffective family decision-making process, and inappropriate boundary maintenance.

Social Isolation may be related to alterations in physical appearance, perceived unacceptable social behavior, restricted social sphere, stage of adolescence, and interference with accomplishing developmental tasks, possibly evidenced by expressions of feelings of aloneness, rejection, or difference from others; uncommunicative; withdrawn; no eye contact; seeking to be alone; unacceptable behavior; and absence of supportive SO(s).

situational/chronic low Self-Esteem may be related to situational or maturational crisis, biophysical changes, and fear of failure at life events, absence of support systems, possibly evidenced by self-negating verbalizations, expressions of shame or guilt, fear of rejection or reaction of other, hypersensitivity to criticism, and lack of follow-through or nonparticipation in prenatal care.

deficient Knowledge [Learning Need] regarding pregnancy, developmental/individual needs, and future expectations may be related to lack of exposure, information misinterpretation, unfamiliarity with information resources, lack of interest in learning, possibly evidenced by questions, statement of concern, misconception, sense of vulnerability, denial of reality, inaccurate follow-through of instruction, and development of preventable complications.

risk for impaired Parenting possibly evidenced by risk factors of young parental age, insufficient cognitive readiness for parenting; unplanned pregnancy, stressors, low self-esteem, social isolation, insufficient family cohesiveness.

Pregnancy, high-risk OB/CH

Also refer to Pregnancy, 1st, 2nd, and 3rd trimesters

Anxiety [specify level] may be related to situational crisis, threat of maternal/fetal death (perceived or actual), interpersonal transmission or contagion, possibly evidenced by increased tension, apprehension, feelings of inadequacy, somatic complaints, difficulty sleeping.

deficient Knowledge [Learning Need] regarding high-risk situation and preterm labor may be related to lack of exposure to or misinterpretation of information, unfamiliarity with individual risks and own role in risk prevention and management, possibly evidenced by request for information, statement of concerns, misconceptions, inaccurate follow-through of instructions.

risk for disturbed Maternal-Fetal Dyad possibly evidenced by risk factors of maternal health problems, substance use or abuse, exposure to teratogens or infectious agents.

risk for maternal Injury possibly evidenced by risk factors of preexisting medical conditions, complications of pregnancy.

risk for Activity Intolerance possibly evidenced by risk factors of presence of circulatory or respiratory problems, uterine irritability.

risk for interrupted Family Processes possibly evidenced by risk factors of situational crisis, change in health status of family member, family role shift, economic stressors.

risk for ineffective Health Management possibly evidenced by risk factors of client value system, health beliefs, cultural influences, issues of control, presence of anxiety, complexity of therapeutic regimen, economic difficulties, perceived susceptibility.

Pregnancy-induced hypertension OB/CH

Refer to Hypertension, gestational

Pregnancy, postmaturity OB

Anxiety [specify level] may be related to situational crisis, threat to maternal/fetal health status (perceived or actual), interpersonal transmission or contagion, possibly evidenced by increased tension, apprehension, irritability, feelings of inadequacy, somatic complaints.

ineffective [uteroplacental] Tissue Perfusion may be related to placental involution, multiple infarcts, and villous degeneration, possibly evidenced by decrease in fetal motion, meconium staining of amniotic fluid, intrauterine growth restriction, late decelerations on fetal monitor.

risk for maternal Injury possibly evidenced by risk factors of dysfunctional or prolonged labor.

risk for fetal Injury possibly evidenced by risk factors of prolonged labor (tissue hypoxia, acidosis), meconium aspiration.

Premature ejaculation CH

Sexual dysfunction may be related to altered body function, partner-related issues, possibly evidenced by reports of disruption of sexual response pattern, inability to achieve desired satisfaction.

situational low Self-Esteem may be related to functional impairment, perceived failure to perform satisfactorily, rejection of other(s), possibly evidenced by self-negating verbalizations, expressions of helplessness, powerlessness.

Premature infant **OB/PED**

Refer to Newborn, premature

Premenstrual dysphoric disorder **GYN/PSY**

chronic Pain may be related to cyclic changes in female hormones affecting other systems (e.g., vascular congestion, spasms), vitamin deficiency, fluid retention, possibly evidenced by increased tension, apprehension, jitteriness, verbal reports, distraction behaviors, somatic complaints, self-focusing, physical and social withdrawal.

[moderate to panic] Anxiety may be related to cyclic changes in female hormones affecting other systems, possibly evidenced by feelings of inability to cope or loss of control, depersonalization, increased tension, apprehension, jitteriness, somatic complaints, and impaired functioning.

ineffective Coping may be related to personal vulnerability, threat to self-concept, multiple stressors, possibly evidenced by reports of inability to cope, inadequate problem solving, sleep pattern disturbance.

excess Fluid Volume may be related to abnormal alterations of hormonal levels, possibly evidenced by edema formation, weight gain, and periodic changes in emotional status/irritability.

deficient Knowledge [Learning Need] regarding pathophysiology of condition and self-care and treatment needs may be related to lack of information, misinterpretation, possibly evidenced by statements of concern, questions, misconceptions, and continuation of condition, exacerbating symptoms.

Premenstrual tension syndrome **GYN/PSY**

Refer to Premenstrual dysphoric disorder

Prenatal substance abuse **OB**

Refer to Substance dependence/abuse, prenatal

Pressure ulcer or sore **CH**

Also refer to Ulcer, decubitus

ineffective peripheral Tissue Perfusion may be related to reduced or interrupted blood flow, possibly evidenced by presence of inflamed, necrotic lesion.

deficient Knowledge [Learning Need] regarding cause, prevention of condition, and potential complications may be related to lack of information or misinterpretation, possibly evidenced by statements of concern, questions, misconceptions, and inaccurate follow-through of instructions.

Preterm labor **OB/CH**

Refer to Labor, preterm

Prostate cancer **MS**

Also refer to Cancer; Prostatectomy

[acute/chronic] Urinary Retention may be related to blockage of urethra, possibly evidenced by sensation of bladder fullness, dysuria, small and frequent voiding, residual urine, bladder distention.

acute Pain may be related to destruction of tissues, pressure on surrounding structures, bladder distention, possibly evidenced by verbal reports, restlessness, irritability, autonomic responses.

Prostatectomy **MS**

Also refer to Surgery, general

impaired urinary Elimination may be related to mechanical obstruction (blood clots, edema, trauma, surgical procedure, pressure or irritation of catheter and balloon) and loss of bladder tone, possibly evidenced by dysuria, frequency, dribbling, incontinence, retention, bladder fullness, suprapubic discomfort.

risk for Bleeding/deficient Fluid Volume possibly evidenced by risk factors of trauma to highly vascular area with excessive vascular losses, restricted intake, postobstructive diuresis.

acute Pain may be related to irritation of bladder mucosa and tissue trauma/edema, possibly evidenced by verbal reports (bladder spasms), distraction behaviors, self-focus, and autonomic responses (changes in vital signs).

disturbed Body Image may be related to perceived threat of altered body and sexual function, possibly evidenced by preoccupation with change or loss, negative feelings about body, and statements of concern regarding functioning.

CH

risk for Sexual dysfunction possibly evidenced by risk factors of situational crisis (incontinence, leakage of urine after catheter removal, involvement of genital area) and threat to self-concept, change in health status.

Prostatitis, acute CH

Also refer to Cystitis

acute Pain/impaired Comfort may be related to inflammatory response, possibly evidenced by reports of low back and pelvic pain, arthralgia, myalgia.

impaired urinary Elimination may be related to localized swelling, urinary tract infection, possibly evidenced by dysuria or burning on urination, frequency, urgency, nocturia, obstructed voiding.

Hyperthermia may be related to illness, possibly evidenced by high fever; chills; flushed, warm skin.

risk for ineffective Health Management possibly evidenced by risk factors of length of therapy, perceived seriousness or benefits.

Prostatitis, chronic CH

Also refer to Cystitis

impaired Comfort/acute Pain may be related to inflammatory response, possibly evidenced by reports of back, pelvic, or scrotal discomfort; low-grade fever.

impaired urinary Elimination may be related to localized swelling, urinary tract infection, possibly evidenced by dysuria, frequency, urgency.

Pruritus CH

acute Pain may be related to cutaneous hyperesthesia and inflammation, possibly evidenced by verbal reports, distraction behaviors, and self-focus.

risk for impaired Skin Integrity possibly evidenced by risk factors of mechanical trauma (scratching) and development of vesicles or bullae that may rupture.

Psoriasis CH

impaired Skin Integrity may be related to increased epidermal cell proliferation and absence of normal protective skin layers, possibly evidenced by scaling papules and plaques.

disturbed Body Image may be related to cosmetically unsightly skin lesions, possibly evidenced by hiding affected body part, negative feelings about body, feelings of helplessness, and change in social involvement.

Psychological abuse CH/PSY

Refer to Abuse, psychological

PTSD PSY

Refer to Post-traumatic stress disorder

Pulmonary edema MS

impaired Gas Exchange may be related to alveolar-capillary membrane changes (fluid collection or shifts into interstitial space or alveoli), possibly evidenced by dyspnea, restlessness, irritability, abnormal rate and depth of respirations, lethargy, confusion.

[moderate to severe] Anxiety may be related to change in health status, threat of death, interpersonal transmission, possibly evidenced by expressed concerns, distressed, apprehension, extraneous movement.

risk for impaired spontaneous Ventilation possibly evidenced by risk factors of respiratory muscle fatigue, problems with secretion management.

Pulmonary edema, high altitude MS

Refer to High altitude pulmonary edema

Pulmonary embolus MS

ineffective Breathing Pattern may be related to tracheobronchial obstruction (inflammation, copious secretions or active bleeding), decreased lung expansion, inflammatory process, possibly evidenced by changes in depth or rate of respiration, dyspnea, use of accessory muscles, altered chest excursion, abnormal breath sounds (crackles, wheezes), and cough (with or without sputum production).

impaired Gas Exchange may be related to ventilation-perfusion imbalance, alveolar-capillary membrane changes (atelectasis, airway or alveolar collapse, pulmonary edema and effusion, excessive secretions, active bleeding), possibly evidenced by profound dyspnea, restlessness, apprehension, somnolence, cyanosis, and changes in arterial blood gas or pulse oximetry (hypoxemia and hypercapnia).

Fear/Anxiety [specify level] may be related to severe dyspnea, inability to breathe normally, perceived threat of death, threat to or change in health status, physiological response to hypoxemia, acidosis, and concern regarding unknown outcome of situation, possibly evidenced by restlessness, irritability, withdrawal or attack behavior, sympathetic stimulation (cardiovascular excitation, pupil dilation, sweating, vomiting, diarrhea), crying, voice quivering, and impending sense of doom.

Pulmonary fibrosis CH

impaired Gas Exchange may be related to alveolar-capillary membrane changes (inflammation, development of scar tissue), ventilation-perfusion imbalance (retained secretions), possibly evidenced by dyspnea, adventitious breath sounds, nonproductive cough, cyanosis.

Anxiety [specify]/Fear may be related to situational crisis, change in health status, threat of death, interpersonal transmission, possibly evidenced by expressed concerns, apprehension, uncertainty, ruminations, increased tension.

Activity Intolerance may be related to imbalance between oxygen supply and demand, generalized weakness, possibly evidenced by exertional dyspnea, abnormal heart rate and blood pressure response to activity, cyanosis.

risk for Infection possibly evidenced by risk factors of stasis of secretions, chronic disease, drug therapies (corticosteroids, cytotoxins).

Pulmonary hypertension **CH/MS**

impaired Gas Exchange may be related to changes in alveolar membrane, increased pulmonary vascular resistance, possibly evidenced by dyspnea, irritability, decreased mental acuity, somnolence, abnormal arterial blood gases.

decreased Cardiac Output may be related to increased pulmonary vascular resistance, decreased blood return to left side of heart, possibly evidenced by increased heart rate, dyspnea, fatigue.

Activity Intolerance may be related to imbalance between oxygen supply and demand, possibly evidenced by reports of weakness, fatigue, abnormal vital signs with activity.

[mild to moderate] Anxiety may be related to change in health status, stress, threat to self-concept, possibly evidenced by expressed concerns, uncertainty, anxiety, awareness of physiological symptoms, diminished productivity and ability to problem solve.

Pulmonic insufficiency **MS/CH**

Refer to Valvular heart disease

Pulmonic stenosis **MS/CH**

Refer to Valvular heart disease

Purpura, idiopathic thrombocytopenic **CH**

ineffective Protection may be related to abnormal blood profile, drug therapy (corticosteroids or immunosuppressive agents), possibly evidenced by altered clotting, fatigue, deficient immunity.

Activity Intolerance may be related to decreased oxygen-carrying capacity, imbalance between oxygen supply and demand, possibly evidenced by reports of fatigue, weakness.

deficient Knowledge [Learning Need] regarding therapy choices, outcomes, and self-care needs may be related to lack of information, misinterpretation, possibly evidenced by statements of concern, questions, and misconceptions.

Pyelonephritis **MS**

acute Pain may be related to acute inflammation of renal tissues, possibly evidenced by verbal reports, guarding or distraction behaviors, self-focus, and changes in vital signs.

Hyperthermia may be related to inflammatory process and increased metabolic rate, possibly evidenced by increase in body temperature; warm, flushed skin; tachycardia; and chills.

impaired urinary Elimination may be related to inflammation and irritation of bladder mucosa, possibly evidenced by dysuria, urgency, and frequency.

deficient Knowledge [Learning Need] regarding therapy needs and prevention may be related to lack of information, misinterpretation, possibly evidenced by statements of concern, questions, misconceptions, and recurrence of condition.

Pyloric stenosis **PED**

deficient Fluid Volume may be related to excessive projectile vomiting, possibly evidenced by decreased, concentrated urine; poor skin turgor, dry skin and mucous membranes, lethargy.

imbalanced Nutrition: less than body requirements may be related to inability to digest or absorb nutrients, possibly evidenced by weight loss, poor muscle tone, pale conjunctiva and mucous membranes.

Quadriplegia **MS/CH**

Also refer to Paraplegia

ineffective Breathing Pattern may be related to impairment of innervation of diaphragm—lesions at or above C5, complete or mixed loss of intercostal muscle function, reflex abdominal spasms, gastric distention, possibly evidenced by decreased respiratory depth, dyspnea, cyanosis, and abnormal arterial blood gases.

risk for Trauma [additional spinal injury] possibly evidenced by risk factors of temporary weakness, instability of spinal column.

Grieving may be related to perceived loss of self, anticipated alterations in lifestyle and expectations, and limitation of future options and choices, possibly evidenced by expressions of distress, anger, sorrow; choked feelings; and changes in eating habits, sleep, communication patterns.

[total] Self-Care deficit related to neuromuscular impairment, evidenced by inability to perform self-care tasks.

bowel Incontinence/Constipation may be related to disruption of nerve innervation, perceptual impairment, changes in dietary and fluid intake, change in activity level, possibly evidenced by inability to evacuate bowel voluntarily; increased abdominal pressure and distention; dry, hard formed stool; change in bowel sounds.

impaired bed/wheelchair Mobility may be related to loss of muscle function and control.

risk for Autonomic Dysreflexia possibly evidenced by risk factors of altered nerve function (spinal cord injury at T6 or above); bladder, bowel, or skin stimulation (tactile, pain, thermal).

impaired Home Maintenance may be related to permanent effects of injury, inadequate or absent support systems and finances, and lack of familiarity with resources, possibly evidenced by expressions of difficulties, requests for information and assistance, outstanding debts or financial crisis, and lack of necessary aids and equipment.

Rabies CH/MS

Hyperthermia may be related to infection, possibly evidenced by fever, malaise.

risk for ineffective Airway Clearance possibly evidenced by risk factors of excessive salivation, muscle spasms (laryngeal, pharyngeal).

deficient Fluid Volume related to inability to drink (severe painful pharyngeal muscle spasms), excessive salivation, possibly evidenced by extreme thirst, decreased skin turgor, decreased output/concentrated urine.

risk for trauma possibly evidenced by risk factors of progressive restlessness, uncontrollable excitement, inability to utilize physical restraints for safety.

Radiation syndrome/poisoning MS

(Dependent on dose and duration of exposure)

[severe] Anxiety/Fear may be related to situational crisis, threat of death, interpersonal transmission and contagion, unmet needs, possibly evidenced by expressed concerns, fearfulness, hopelessness, restlessness, agitation, anguish, increased tension, awareness of physiological symptoms.

deficient Fluid Volume may be related to intractable nausea, vomiting, diarrhea (gastrointestinal tissue necrosis and atrophy), interference with adequate intake (stomatitis, anorexia), hemorrhagic losses (thrombocytopenia), possibly evidenced by dry skin and mucous membranes, poor skin turgor, decreased venous filling, reduced pulse volume and pressure, hypotension, weakness, change in mentation.

acute Confusion may be related to central nervous system inflammation, decreased circulation/hypotension, effects of circulating toxins, possibly evidenced by fluctuations in cognition or level of consciousness, agitation.

ineffective Protection may be related to effects of radiation, abnormal blood profile (leukopenia, thrombocytopenia, anemia), inadequate nutrition, possibly evidenced by neurosensory alterations, anorexia, deficient immunity, impaired healing, altered clotting, disorientation.

risk for Infection possibly evidenced by risk factors of inadequate primary defenses (traumatized or necrotic tissues, stasis of body fluids, altered peristalsis), inadequate secondary defenses (anemia, leukopenia).

Sexual dysfunction may be related to altered body function, possibly evidenced by amenorrhea, decreased libido, infertility.

Radiation therapy CH

Also refer to Brachytherapy; Cancer

Nausea may be related to therapeutic procedure, irritation to gastrointestinal system, possibly evidenced by verbal reports, vomiting, gastric stasis.

imbalanced Nutrition: less than body requirements may be related to inability to ingest adequate nutrients (nausea, stomatitis, and fatigue), hypermetabolic state, possibly evidenced by weight loss, aversion to eating, reported altered taste sensation, sore, inflamed buccal cavity, diarrhea.

impaired oral Mucous Membrane may be related to side effects of radiation, dehydration, and malnutrition, possibly evidenced by ulcerations, leukoplakia, decreased salivation, and reports of pain.

ineffective Protection may be related to inadequate nutrition, radiation, abnormal blood profile, disease state (cancer), possibly evidenced by impaired healing, deficient immunity, anorexia, fatigue.

Radical neck surgery MS

Refer to Laryngectomy

Rape CH

deficient Knowledge [Learning Need] regarding required medical/legal procedures, prophylactic treatment for individual concerns (sexually transmitted in-

fection, pregnancy), and community resources and supports may be related to lack of information, possibly evidenced by statements of concern, questions, misconceptions, and exacerbation of symptoms.

Rape-Trauma Syndrome related to actual or attempted sexual penetration without consent, possibly evidenced by wide range of emotional reactions, including anxiety, fear, anger, embarrassment, and multisystem physical complaints.

risk for impaired Tissue Integrity possibly evidenced by risk factors of forceful sexual penetration and trauma to fragile tissues.

PSY

ineffective Coping may be related to personal vulnerability, unmet expectations, unrealistic perceptions, inadequate support systems or coping methods, multiple stressors repeated over time, overwhelming threat to self, possibly evidenced by verbalizations of inability to cope or difficulty asking for help, muscular tension/headaches, emotional tension, chronic worry.

Sexual dysfunction may be related to biopsychosocial alteration of sexuality (stress of posttrauma response), vulnerability, loss of sexual desire, impaired relationship with SO, possibly evidenced by alteration in achieving sexual satisfaction, change in interest in self/others, preoccupation with self.

Raynaud's disease — CH

acute/chronic Pain may be related to vasospasm and altered perfusion of affected tissues, and ischemia or destruction of tissues, possibly evidenced by verbal reports, guarding of affected parts, self-focusing, and restlessness.

ineffective peripheral Tissue Perfusion may be related to periodic reduction of arterial blood flow to affected areas, possibly evidenced by pallor, cyanosis, coolness, numbness, paresthesia, slow healing of lesions.

deficient Knowledge [Learning Need] regarding pathophysiology of condition, potential for complications, treatment, and self-care needs may be related to lack of information, misinterpretation, possibly evidenced by statements of concern, questions, and misconceptions; development of preventable complications.

Raynaud's phenomenon — CH

Refer to Raynaud's disease

Reactive attachment disorder — PED/PSY

Refer to Anxiety disorders—PED

Reflex sympathetic dystrophy — CH

Refer to Complex regional pain syndrome

acute/chronic Pain may be related to continued nerve stimulation, possibly evidenced by verbal reports, distraction or guarding behaviors, narrowed focus, changes in sleep patterns, and altered ability to continue previous activities.

ineffective peripheral Tissue Perfusion may be related to reduction of arterial blood flow (arteriole vasoconstriction), possibly evidenced by reports of pain, decreased skin temperature and pallor, diminished arterial pulsations, and tissue swelling.

[disturbed tactile Sensory Perception] may be related to altered sensory reception (neurological deficit, pain), possibly evidenced by change in usual response to stimuli, abnormal sensitivity of touch, physiological anxiety, and irritability.

risk for ineffective Role Performance possibly evidenced by risk factors of situational crisis, chronic disability, debilitating pain.

risk for compromised family Coping possibly evidenced by risk factors of temporary family disorganization and role changes and prolonged disability that exhausts the supportive capacity of SO(s).

Regional enteritis — CH

Refer to Crohn's disease

Renal disease, end-stage — CH/MS

Also refer to Renal failure, chronic

Death Anxiety may be related to progressive debilitating disease, unmet needs, inadequate support system, personal vulnerability, past negative experiences, possibly evidenced by fear of the process of dying or loss of abilities, concerns of unfinished business, powerlessness, loss of control, denial of impending death.

Renal failure, acute (Kidney injury, acute) — MS

excess Fluid Volume may be related to compromised regulatory mechanisms (decreased kidney function), possibly evidenced by weight gain, edema, anasarca, intake greater than output, venous congestion, changes in blood pressure and central venous pressure, altered electrolyte levels, decreased hemoglobin and hematocrit, pulmonary congestion on x-ray.

risk for imbalanced Nutrition: less than body requirements possibly evidenced by risk factors of inability to ingest or digest adequate nutrients—anorexia, nausea, vomiting, ulcerations of oral mucosa, and increased metabolic needs; protein catabolism, therapeutic dietary restrictions.

risk for Infection possibly evidenced by risk factors of depression of immunological defenses, invasive procedures or devices, changes in dietary intake, malnutrition.

risk for acute Confusion possibly evidenced by risk factors of electrolyte imbalance, increased blood urea nitrogen/creatinine, azotemia.

Renal failure, chronic CH/MS

Also refer to Dialysis, general

risk for decreased Cardiac Output possibly evidenced by risk factors of fluid imbalances affecting circulating volume, myocardial workload, and systemic vascular resistance; alterations in rate, rhythm, and cardiac conduction (electrolyte imbalances, hypoxia); accumulation of toxins (urea); soft-calcification.

risk for Bleeding possibly evidenced by risk factors of abnormal blood profile—suppressed erythropoietin production and secretion, decreased red blood cell production and survival, altered clotting factors; increased capillary fragility.

risk for acute Confusion possibly evidenced by risk factors of electrolyte imbalance, increased blood urea nitrogen/creatinine, azotemia, malnutrition, decreased hemoglobin.

risk for impaired Skin Integrity possibly evidenced by risk factors of altered metabolic state, circulation (anemia with tissue ischemia), and sensation (peripheral neuropathy), decreased skin turgor, reduced activity, immobility, accumulation of toxins in the skin.

risk for impaired oral Mucous Membrane possibly evidenced by risk factors of decreased or lack of salivation, fluid restrictions, chemical irritation (conversion of urea in saliva to ammonia).

Renal transplantation MS

Also refer to Transplantation, recipient

risk for excess Fluid Volume possibly evidenced by risk factors of compromised regulatory mechanism (implantation of new kidney requiring adjustment period for optimal functioning).

disturbed Body Image may be related to failure and subsequent replacement of body part and medication-induced changes in appearance, possibly evidenced by preoccupation with loss or change, negative feelings about body, and focus on past strength and function.

Fear may be related to potential for transplant rejection or failure and threat of death, possibly evidenced by increased tension, apprehension, concentration on source, and verbalizations of concern.

risk for Infection possibly evidenced by risk factors of broken skin or traumatized tissue, stasis of body fluids, immunosuppression, invasive procedures, nutritional deficits, and chronic disease.

CH

risk for ineffective Coping/compromised family Coping possibly evidenced by risk factors of situational crises, family disorganization and role changes, prolonged disease exhausting supportive capacity of SO/family, therapeutic restrictions/long-term therapy needs.

Repetitive motion injury CH

Refer to Carpal tunnel syndrome

Respiratory distress syndrome, acute MS

ineffective Airway Clearance may be related to loss of ciliary action, increased amount and viscosity of secretions, and increased airway resistance, possibly evidenced by presence of dyspnea, changes in depth and rate of respiration, use of accessory muscles for breathing, wheezes, crackles, cough with or without sputum production.

impaired Gas Exchange may be related to changes in pulmonary capillary permeability with edema formation, alveolar hypoventilation and collapse, with intrapulmonary shunting, possibly evidenced by tachypnea, use of accessory muscles, cyanosis, hypoxia per arterial blood gases or oximetry, anxiety and changes in mentation.

risk for deficient Fluid Volume possibly evidenced by risk factors of active loss from diuretic use and restricted intake.

risk for decreased Cardiac Output possibly evidenced by risk factors of alteration in preload (hypovolemia, vascular pooling, diuretic therapy, and increased intrathoracic pressure, use of ventilator, and positive end-expiratory pressure [PEEP]).

Anxiety [specify level]/Fear may be related to physiological factors (effects of hypoxemia), situational crisis, change in health status/threat of death, possibly evidenced by increased tension, apprehension, restlessness, focus on self, and sympathetic stimulation.

risk for [pulmonary] Injury possibly evidenced by risk factor of increased airway pressure associated with mechanical ventilation (PEEP).

Respiratory distress syndrome (premature infant) PED

Also refer to Newborn, premature

impaired Gas Exchange may be related to alveolar-capillary membrane changes (inadequate surfactant levels), altered oxygen supply (tracheobronchial obstruction, atelectasis), altered blood flow (immaturity of pulmonary arteriole musculature), altered oxygen-carrying capacity of blood (anemia), and cold stress, possibly evidenced by tachypnea, use of accessory muscles and retractions, expiratory grunting, pallor or cyanosis, abnormal arterial blood gases, and tachycardia.

impaired Spontaneous Ventilation may be related to respiratory muscle fatigue and metabolic factors, possibly evidenced by dyspnea, increased metabolic rate, restlessness, use of accessory muscles, and abnormal arterial blood gases.

risk for Infection possibly evidenced by risk factors of inadequate primary defenses (decreased ciliary action, stasis of body fluids, traumatized tissues), inadequate secondary defenses (deficiency of neutrophils and specific immunoglobulins), invasive procedures, and malnutrition (absence of nutrient stores, increased metabolic demands).

risk for ineffective Gastrointestinal Perfusion possibly evidenced by risk factors of persistent fetal circulation and exchange problems.

risk for impaired Attachment possibly evidenced by risk factors of premature/ill infant who is unable to effectively initiate parental contact (altered behavioral organization), separation, physical barriers, anxiety associated with the parental role and demands of infant.

Respiratory syncytial virus PED

impaired Gas Exchange may be related to inflammation of airways, ventilation perfusion imbalance (areas of consolidation), apnea, possibly evidenced by dyspnea, abnormal arterial blood gases/hypoxia.

ineffective Airway Clearance may be related to infection, retained secretions, exudate in alveoli, inflammation of airways, possibly evidenced by dyspnea, adventitious breath sounds, cough.

risk for deficient Fluid Volume possibly evidenced by risk factors of increased insensible losses (fever, diaphoresis), decreased oral intake.

Restless leg syndrome CH

Refer to Myoclonus, nocturnal

Retinal detachment CH

[disturbed visual Sensory Perception] related to decreased sensory reception, possibly evidenced by visual distortions, decreased visual field, and changes in visual acuity.

[mild to moderate] Anxiety may be related to situational crisis, change in health status and role function, possibly evidenced by expressed concerns, apprehension, uncertainty, focus on self.

deficient Knowledge [Learning Need] regarding therapy, prognosis, and self-care needs may be related to lack of information, misconceptions, possibly evidenced by statements of concern and questions.

risk for impaired Home Maintenance possibly evidenced by risk factors of visual limitations, activity restrictions.

Rett's syndrome PED/PSY

Also refer to Autism spectrum disorder

delayed Development may be related to effects of physical and mental disability, possibly evidenced by delay or inability in performing skills and self-care or self-control activities appropriate for age.

impaired Walking/physical Mobility may be related to neuromuscular impairment, joint stiffness, contractures, disuse, possibly evidenced by limited range of motion, inability to perform gross motor skills, walk, or reposition self.

risk for Trauma possibly evidenced by risk factors of cognitive deficits, lack of muscle tone and coordination, seizure activity.

imbalanced Nutrition: less than body requirements may be related to poor muscle tone, dependence on others and inability to meet own needs, possibly evidenced by weak and ineffective sucking or swallowing and observed lack of adequate intake with weight loss or failure to gain.

risk for complicated Grieving possibly evidenced by risk factors of loss of "the perfect child," chronic condition requiring long-term care, and unresolved feelings.

Reye's syndrome PED

deficient Fluid Volume may be related to failure of regulatory mechanism (diabetes insipidus), excessive gastric losses (pernicious vomiting), and altered intake, possibly evidenced by increased and dilute urine output, sudden weight loss, decreased venous filling, dry mucous membranes, decreased skin turgor, hypotension, and tachycardia.

ineffective cerebral Tissue Perfusion may be related to diminished arterial or venous blood flow and hypovolemia, possibly evidenced by memory loss, altered consciousness, and restlessness, agitation.

risk for Trauma possibly evidenced by risk factors of generalized weakness, reduced coordination, and cognitive deficits.

ineffective Breathing Pattern may be related to decreased energy and fatigue, cognitive impairment, tracheobronchial obstruction, and inflammatory process (aspiration pneumonia), possibly evidenced by tachypnea, abnormal arterial blood gases, cough, and use of accessory muscles.

Rheumatic fever **PED**

acute Pain may be related to migratory inflammation of joints, possibly evidenced by verbal reports, guarding or distraction behaviors, self-focus, and changes in vital signs.

Hyperthermia may be related to inflammatory process, hypermetabolic state, possibly evidenced by increased body temperature; warm, flushed skin; and tachycardia.

Activity Intolerance may be related to generalized weakness, joint pain, and medical restrictions or bedrest, possibly evidenced by reports of fatigue, exertional discomfort, and abnormal heart rate in response to activity.

risk for decreased Cardiac Output possibly evidenced by risk factor of altered contractility.

Rheumatic heart disease **PED/MS**

Also refer to Valvular heart disease

Activity Intolerance may be related to imbalance between oxygen supply and demand, generalized weakness, and prolonged bedrest or sedentary lifestyle, possibly evidenced by reported or observed weakness, fatigue, changes in vital signs, presence of dysrhythmias, dyspnea, pallor.

risk-prone Health Behavior may be related to health status requiring change in lifestyle or restriction of desired activities, unrealistic expectations, negative attitudes, possibly evidenced by denial of situation, demonstration of nonacceptance of health status, failure to achieve optimal sense of control.

risk for ineffective Health Management possibly evidenced by risk factors of complexity and duration of therapeutic regimen, imposed restrictions or limitations, economic difficulties, family patterns of healthcare, perceived seriousness or benefits.

risk for impaired Gas Exchange possibly evidenced by risk factors of alveolar-capillary membrane changes (fluid collection or shifts into interstitial space or alveoli).

Rhinitis, allergic **CH**

Refer to Hay fever

Rickets **PED**

risk for disproportionate Growth /delayed Development possibly evidenced by risk factors of inadequate nutrition, economically disadvantaged, chronic illness, prematurity.

deficient Knowledge [Learning Need] regarding cause, pathophysiology, therapy needs and prevention may be related to lack of information, possibly evidenced by statements of concern, questions, misconceptions, and inaccurate follow-through of instructions.

Ringworm, tinea **CH**

Also refer to Athlete's foot

impaired Skin Integrity may be related to fungal infection of the dermis, possibly evidenced by disruption of skin surfaces and presence of lesions.

deficient Knowledge [Learning Need] regarding infectious nature, therapy, and self-care needs may be related to lack of information, misinformation, possibly evidenced by statements of concern, questions, and recurrence and spread.

Rocky Mountain spotted fever **CH/MS**

Refer to Typhus

RSD **CH**

Refer to Reflex sympathetic dystrophy

RSV **PED**

Refer to Respiratory syncytial virus

Rubella **PED/CH**

acute Pain/impaired Comfort may be related to inflammatory effects of viral infection and presence of desquamating rash, possibly evidenced by verbal reports, distraction behaviors, restlessness.

deficient Knowledge [Learning Need] regarding contagious nature, possible complications, and self-care needs may be related to lack of information, misinterpretations, possibly evidenced by statements of concern, questions, and inaccurate follow-through of instructions.

Rubeola **PED/CH**

Refer to Measles

Ruptured intervertebral disc — CH/MS

Refer to Herniated nucleus pulposus

Sarcoidosis — CH

Also refer to Pulmonary fibrosis

Fatigue may be related to disease state, anemia, possibly evidenced by lack of energy, lethargy, decreased performance, inability to maintain usual routines.

risk for Injury possibly evidenced by risk factors of autoimmune dysfunction, abnormal blood profile—thrombocytopenia, leukopenia, anemia; sensory dysfunction.

SARS (sudden acute respiratory syndrome) — MS

Hyperthermia may be related to inflammatory process, possibly evidenced by high fever, chills, rigors, headache.

acute Pain/impaired Comfort may be related to inflammation and circulating toxins, possibly evidenced by reports of myalgia, headache, malaise.

impaired Gas Exchange may be related to ventilation perfusion imbalance (interstitial infiltrates, areas of consolidation), possibly evidenced by dyspnea, changes in mentation or level of consciousness, restlessness, hypoxemia.

risk for impaired spontaneous Ventilation possibly evidenced by risk factors of hypermetabolic state, infection, depletion of energy stores, respiratory muscle fatigue.

Death Anxiety may be related to uncertainty of prognosis, possibly evidenced by report of apprehension; increased pulse and respiratory rate, muscle tension, pupil dilation.

risk for ineffective Protection possibly evidenced by risk factors of inadequate nutrition, abnormal blood profile (leukopenia, thrombocytopenia).

Scabies — CH

impaired Skin Integrity may be related to presence of invasive parasite and development of pruritus, possibly evidenced by disruption of skin surface and inflammation.

deficient Knowledge [Learning Need] regarding communicable nature, possible complications, therapy, and self-care needs may be related to lack of information, misinterpretation, possibly evidenced by questions and statements of concern about spread to others.

Scarlet fever — PED

Hyperthermia may be related to effects of circulating toxins, possibly evidenced by increased body temperature; warm, flushed skin; and tachycardia.

acute Pain/impaired Comfort may be related to inflammation of mucous membranes and effects of circulating toxins (malaise, fever), possibly evidenced by verbal reports, distraction behaviors, guarding (decreased swallowing), and self-focus.

risk for deficient Fluid Volume possibly evidenced by risk factors of hypermetabolic state (hyperthermia) and reduced intake.

Schizoaffective disorder — PSY

risk for other-/self-directed Violence possibly evidenced by risk factors of depressed mood, feelings of worthlessness, hopelessness, unsatisfactory parent-child relationship, feelings of abandonment by SOs, anger turned inward or directed at the environment, punitive superego, irrational feelings of guilt, numerous failures, misinterpretation of reality.

Social Isolation may be related to developmental regression, depressed mood, feelings of worthlessness, egocentric behaviors (offending others and discouraging relationships), delusional thinking, fear of failure, unresolved grief, possibly evidenced by sad, dull affect; absence of support systems; uncommunicative, withdrawn, or catatonic behavior; absence of eye contact; preoccupation with own thoughts; repetitive or meaningless actions.

imbalanced Nutrition: less than body requirements may be related to energy expenditure in excess of intake, refusal or inability to take time to eat, lack of attention to or recognition of hunger cues, possibly evidenced by lack of interest in food, weight loss, pale conjunctiva and mucous membranes, poor muscle tone and skin turgor, amenorrhea, abnormal laboratory studies.

Schizophrenia (schizophrenic disorders) — PSY

[disturbed Sensory Perception (specify)] may be related to biochemical/electrolyte imbalance, psychological stress, possibly evidenced by disorientation to space/time, hallucinations, change in behavior pattern.

impaired verbal Communication may be related to altered perceptions, alteration in self-concept, psychological barriers, e.g., psychosis possibly evidenced by inappropriate verbalizations, difficulty in comprehending usual communication pattern, difficulty in use of facial expressions.

Social Isolation may be related to alterations in mental status, mistrust of others, delusional thinking, unacceptable social behaviors, inadequate personal resources, and inability to engage in satisfying personal relationships, possibly evidenced by difficulty in establishing relationships with others; dull affect, uncommunicative or withdrawn behavior, seeking to be alone, inadequate or absent significant purpose in life, and expression of feelings of rejection.

risk for self-/other-directed Violence possibly evidenced by risk factors of disturbances of thinking and feeling (depression, paranoia, suicidal ideation), lack of development of trust and appropriate interpersonal relationships, catatonic or manic excitement, toxic reactions to drugs (alcohol).

ineffective Coping may be related to personal vulnerability, inadequate support system(s), unrealistic perceptions, inadequate coping methods, and disintegration of thought processes, possibly evidenced by impaired judgment, cognition, and perception; diminished problem-solving or decision-making capacities, poor self-concept, chronic anxiety, depression, inability to perform role expectations, and alteration in social participation.

CH

interrupted Family Processes/disabled family Coping may be related to ambivalent family system or relationships, change of roles, and difficulty of family member in coping effectively with client's maladaptive behaviors, possibly evidenced by deterioration in family functioning, ineffective family decision-making process, difficulty relating to each other, client's expressions of despair at family's lack of reaction or involvement, neglectful relationships with client, extreme distortion regarding client's health problem, including denial about its existence and severity, or prolonged overconcern.

ineffective Health Maintenance/impaired Home Maintenance may be related to impaired cognitive and emotional functioning, altered ability to make deliberate and thoughtful judgments, altered communication, and lack of or inappropriate use of material resources, possibly evidenced by inability to take responsibility for meeting basic health practices in any or all functional areas and demonstrated lack of adaptive behaviors to internal or external environmental changes, disorderly surroundings, accumulation of dirt, unwashed clothes, repeated hygienic disorders.

Self-Care deficit [specify] may be related to perceptual and cognitive impairment, immobility (withdrawal, isolation, or decreased psychomotor activity), and side effects of psychotropic medications, possibly evidenced by inability or difficulty in areas of feeding self, keeping body clean, dressing appropriately, toileting self, or changes in bowel and bladder elimination.

Sciatica **CH**

acute/chronic Pain may be related to peripheral nerve root compression, possibly evidenced by verbal reports, guarding or distraction behaviors, and self-focus.

impaired physical Mobility may be related to neurological pain and muscular involvement, possibly evidenced by reluctance to attempt movement and decreased muscle strength and mass.

Scleroderma **CH**

Also refer to Lupus erythematosus, systemic (SLE)

impaired physical Mobility may be related to musculoskeletal impairment and associated pain, possibly evidenced by decreased strength, decreased range of motion, and reluctance to attempt movement.

ineffective Tissue Perfusion (specify) may be related to reduced arterial blood flow (arteriolar vasoconstriction), possibly evidenced by changes in skin temperature and color, ulcer formation, and changes in organ function (cardiopulmonary, gastrointestinal, renal).

imbalanced Nutrition: less than body requirements may be related to inability to ingest, digest, or absorb adequate nutrients (sclerosis of the tissues rendering mouth immobile, decreased peristalsis of esophagus and small intestines, atrophy of smooth muscle of colon), possibly evidenced by weight loss, decreased intake, and reported or observed difficulty swallowing.

risk-prone Health Behavior may be related to disability requiring change in lifestyle, inadequate support systems, assault to self-concept, and altered locus of control, possibly evidenced by verbalization of nonacceptance of health status change and lack of movement toward independence or future-oriented thinking.

disturbed Body Image may be related to skin changes with induration, atrophy, and fibrosis, loss of hair, and skin and muscle contractures, possibly evidenced by verbalization of negative feelings about body; focus on past strength, function, or appearance; fear of rejection or reaction by others; hiding body part; and change in social involvement.

Scoliosis **PED**

disturbed Body Image may be related to altered body structure, use of therapeutic device(s), and activity restrictions, possibly evidenced by negative feelings about body, change in social involvement, and preoccupation with situation or refusal to acknowledge problem.

deficient Knowledge [Learning Need] regarding pathophysiology of condition, therapy needs, and possible outcomes may be related to lack of information, misinterpretation, possibly evidenced by statements of concern, questions, misconceptions, and inaccurate follow-through of instructions.

risk-prone Health Behavior may be related to lack of comprehension of long-term consequences of behavior, possibly evidenced by minimizing health status change, failure to take action, and evidence of failure to improve.

Seasonal affective disorder — PSY

Refer to Affective disorder, seasonal

Sedative intoxication/abuse — CH/PSY

Refer to Depressant abuse

Seizure disorder — CH

deficient Knowledge [Learning Need] regarding condition and medication control may be related to lack of information, misinterpretations, scarce financial resources, possibly evidenced by questions, statements of concern, misconceptions, incorrect use of anticonvulsant medication, recurrent episodes, or uncontrolled seizures.

chronic low Self-Esteem/disturbed Personal Identity may be related to stigma associated with condition, perception of being out of control or helpless, possibly evidenced by verbalization about changed lifestyle, fear of rejection, negative feelings about "brain" or self, change in usual pattern of responsibility, denial of problem resulting in lack of follow-through or nonparticipation in therapy.

impaired Social Interaction may be related to unpredictable nature of condition and self-concept disturbance, possibly evidenced by decreased self-assurance, verbalization of concern, discomfort in social situations, inability to receive or communicate a satisfying sense of belonging and caring, and withdrawal from social contacts and activities.

risk for Trauma/Suffocation possibly evidenced by risk factors of weakness, balancing difficulties, cognitive limitations, altered consciousness, loss of large- or small-muscle coordination (during seizure).

Separation anxiety disorder — PED/PSY

Refer to Anxiety disorders—PED

Sepsis — MS

Also refer to Sepsis, puerperal

risk for deficient Fluid Volume possibly evidenced by risk factors of marked increase in vascular compartment—massive vasodilation, vascular shifts to interstitial space, and reduced intake.

risk for decreased Cardiac Output possibly evidenced by risk factors of decreased preload (venous return and circulating volume), altered afterload (increased systemic vascular resistance), negative inotropic effects of hypoxia, complement activation, and lysosomal hydrolase.

risk for Shock possibly evidenced by risk factors of infection/sepsis, hypovolemia—fluid shifts or third spacing; hypotension, hypoxemia.

Sepsis, puerperal — OB

risk for Infection [spread] possibly evidenced by risk factors of presence of infection, broken skin, or traumatized tissues, rupture of amniotic membranes, high vascularity of involved area, stasis of body fluids, invasive procedures, or increased environmental exposure, chronic disease (e.g., diabetes mellitus, anemia, malnutrition), altered immune response, and untoward effect of medications (e.g., opportunistic or secondary infection).

Hyperthermia may be related to inflammatory process, hypermetabolic state, dehydration, effect of circulating endotoxins on the hypothalamus, possibly evidenced by increase in body temperature, warm, flushed skin; increased respiratory rate and tachycardia.

risk for impaired Attachment possibly evidenced by risk factors of interruption in bonding process, physical illness, perceived threat to own survival.

risk for ineffective peripheral Tissue Perfusion possibly evidenced by risk factors of interruption or reduction of blood flow—presence of infectious thrombi.

risk for Shock possibly evidenced by risk factors of infection, hypovolemia, hypotension, hypoxemia.

Septicemia — MS

Refer to Sepsis

Serum sickness — CH

acute Pain may be related to inflammation of the joints and skin eruptions, possibly evidenced by verbal reports, guarding or distraction behaviors, and self-focus.

deficient Knowledge [Learning Need] regarding nature of condition, treatment needs, potential complications, and prevention of recurrence may be related to lack of information, misinterpretation, possibly evidenced by statements of concern, questions, misconceptions, and inaccurate follow-through of instructions.

Severe acute respiratory syndrome **MS**
Refer to SARS

Sexual desire disorder **PSY**
Sexual dysfunction may be related to boredom or conflict in relationship, depression, hormonal imbalance, harmful relationships, traumatic events in childhood, possibly evidenced by loss of sexual desire, disruption of sexual response pattern, alteration in relationship with SO.

Anxiety [specify] may be related to situational crisis, stress, unconscious conflict about essential values, unmet needs, possibly evidenced by expressed concerns, distress, feelings of inadequacy, fear of unspecific consequences.

situational low Self-Esteem may be related to perceived functional impairment, emotional insecurity, rejection by SO, possibly evidenced by expressions of helplessness, self-negating verbalizations, change in involvement with partner.

Sexual dysfunctions **PSY**
Refer to Dyspareunia; Erectile dysfunction; Sexual desire disorder; Vaginismus

Sexually transmitted infection **GYN/CH**
risk for Infection [transmission] possibly evidenced by risk factors of contagious nature of infecting agent and insufficient knowledge to avoid exposure to or transmission of pathogens.

impaired Skin/Tissue Integrity may be related to invasion of and irritation by pathogenic organism(s), possibly evidenced by disruptions of skin and tissue, and inflammation of mucous membranes.

deficient Knowledge [Learning Need] regarding condition, prognosis, potential complications, therapy needs, and transmission may be related to lack of information, misinterpretation, lack of interest in learning, possibly evidenced by statements of concern, questions, misconceptions, inaccurate follow-through of instructions, and development of preventable complications.

Shingles **CH**
Refer to Herpes zoster

Shock **MS**
Also refer to Shock, cardiogenic; Shock, hypovolemic/hemorrhagic; Sepsis

ineffective Tissue Perfusion (specify) may be related to changes in circulating volume or vascular tone, possibly evidenced by changes in skin color and temperature and pulse pressure, reduced blood pressure, changes in mentation, and decreased urinary output.

Anxiety [specify level] may be related to change in health status and threat of death, possibly evidenced by increased tension, apprehension, sympathetic stimulation, restlessness, and expressions of concern.

Shock, cardiogenic **MS**
Also refer to Shock

decreased Cardiac Output may be related to structural damage, decreased myocardial contractility, and presence of dysrhythmias, possibly evidenced by electrocardiogram changes, variations in hemodynamic readings, jugular vein distention, cold and clammy skin, diminished peripheral pulses, and decreased urinary output.

risk for impaired Gas Exchange possibly evidenced by risk factors of ventilation perfusion imbalance, alveolar-capillary membrane changes.

Shock, hypovolemic/hemorrhagic **MS**
Also refer to Shock

deficient Fluid Volume may be related to excessive vascular loss, inadequate intake or replacement, possibly evidenced by hypotension, tachycardia, decreased pulse volume and pressure, change in mentation, and decreased, concentrated urine.

Shock, septic **MS**
Refer to Sepsis

Sicca syndrome **CH**
Refer to Sjögren syndrome

Sick building syndrome **CH**
Contamination may be related to presence of atmospheric or environmental contaminants in building (e.g., volatile organic compounds, carbon monoxide, asbestos, dust, fungi, molds, pollens, tobacco smoke), flooring surface (carpeted surfaces hold contaminant residue more than hard floor surfaces), poorly ventilated areas, lack of effective protection, possibly evidenced by headaches; eye, nose, or throat irritation; dry cough; dry or itchy skin; dizziness; nausea; difficulty in concentrating; fatigue.

Fatigue may be related to occupation or employment in a specific building or zone within a building as evidenced by reports of being tired, lethargic; decreased performance

Sick sinus syndrome **MS**

Also refer to Dysrhythmia, cardiac

decreased Cardiac Output may be related to alterations in rate, rhythm, and electrical conduction, possibly evidenced by electrocardiogram indication of dysrhythmias, reports of palpitations, weakness, changes in mentation or consciousness, and syncope.

risk for Trauma possibly evidenced by risk factors of changes in cerebral perfusion with altered consciousness, loss of balance.

SIDS **PED**

Refer to Sudden infant death syndrome

Sinusitis, chronic **CH**

acute/chronic Pain may be related to inflammatory process, possibly evidenced by reports of headache and facial pain, irritability, change in sleep, fatigue.

risk for Infection [spread] possibly evidenced by risk factors of chronic irritation and inflamed tissues, stasis of body fluids, improper handling of infectious material.

Sjögren syndrome **CH**

impaired oral Mucous Membrane related to decreased salivation, possibly evidenced by xerostomia (dry mouth), oral pain or discomfort, self-report of bad or diminished taste, difficulty eating and swallowing.

risk for impaired Tissue Integrity (cornea, mucous membranes) possibly evidenced by risk factors of impaired production of tears, mucus.

risk for Infection possibly evidenced by risk factors of decreased secretions, tissue dryness and damage.

[risk for disturbed visual Sensory Perception] possibly evidenced by risk factors of altered sensory reception (light sensitivity, blurred vision, corneal ulcers).

Skin cancer **CH**

impaired Skin Integrity may be related to invasive growth, surgical excision may be evidenced by disruption of skin surface, destruction of dermis.

risk for acute Pain possibly evidenced by risk factors of ulceration of skin, surgical incision.

risk for disturbed Body Image possibly evidenced by risk factors of skin lesion, surgical intervention.

deficient Knowledge [Learning Need] regarding condition, prognosis, treatment, and prevention may be related to lack of information, misinterpretation, possibly evidenced by statements of concern, questions, misconceptions, inaccurate follow-through of instructions, development of preventable complications, or recurrence.

SLE **CH**

Refer to Lupus erythematosus, systemic

Sleep apnea **CH**

Sleep deprivation may be related to sleep apnea (recurrent apneic episodes followed by gasping arousal), possibly evidenced by daytime drowsiness, tiredness, decreased ability to perform, slowed mentation.

impaired Gas Exchange may be related to altered oxygen supply (recurrent apneic episodes lasting 10 seconds to 2 minutes), possibly evidenced by morning headache, decreased mental acuity, abnormal arterial blood gases (hypoxemia, hypercapnia), dysrhythmias (e.g., extreme bradycardia, ventricular tachycardia).

risk for ineffective Health Management possibly evidenced by risk factors of duration of therapy, associated discomfort, perceived seriousness or benefit.

Smallpox **MS**

risk of Infection [spread] possibly evidenced by risk factors of contagious nature of organism, inadequate acquired immunity, presence of chronic disease, immunosuppression.

deficient Fluid Volume may be related to hypermetabolic state, decreased intake (pharyngeal lesions, nausea), increased losses (vomiting), fluid shifts from vascular bed, possibly evidenced by reports of thirst; decreased blood pressure, venous filling, and urinary output; dry mucous membranes; decreased skin turgor; change in mental state; elevated hematocrit.

impaired Tissue Integrity may be related to immunological deficit, possibly evidenced by disruption of skin surface, cornea, mucous membranes.

Anxiety [specify level]/Fear may be related to threat of death, interpersonal transmission or contagion, separation from support system, possibly evidenced by expressed concerns, apprehension, restlessness, focus on self.

CH

interrupted Family Processes may be related to temporary family disorganization, situational crisis, change in health status of family member, possibly evidenced by changes in satisfaction with family, stress-reduction behaviors, mutual support, expression of isolation from community resources.

ineffective community Coping may be related to man-made disaster (bioterrorism), inadequate resources for problem solving, possibly evidenced by deficits of community participation, high illness rate, excessive community conflicts, expressed vulnerability or powerlessness.

Snake bite, venomous — MS

[severe] Anxiety/Fear may be related to situational crisis, threat of death, interpersonal transmission, possibly evidenced by expressed concerns, apprehension, irritability, jitteriness, increased tension, tremors.

acute Pain/impaired Comfort may be related to effects of toxins (edema formation, erythema, enlargement of lymph nodes, nausea, fever, diaphoresis, muscle fasciculations), possibly evidenced by reports of pain and paresthesias, guarded behavior, restlessness, autonomic responses.

impaired Skin Integrity may be related to trauma, inflammation, altered circulation, possibly evidenced by disruption and destruction of skin layers (skin tense, discolored, necrosis around bite).

risk for deficient Fluid Volume possibly evidenced by risk factors of excessive losses (vomiting, edema formation, hemorrhage from mucous membranes).

Snow blindness — CH

[disturbed visual Sensory Perception] may be related to altered status of sense organ (irritation of the conjunctiva, hyperemia), possibly evidenced by intolerance to light (photophobia) and decreased or loss of visual acuity.

acute Pain may be related to irritation and vascular congestion of the conjunctiva, possibly evidenced by verbal reports, guarding or distraction behaviors, and self-focus.

Anxiety [specify level] may be related to situational crisis and threat to or change in health status, possibly evidenced by increased tension, apprehension, uncertainty, worry, restlessness, and focus on self.

Somatoform disorders — PSY

ineffective Coping may be related to severe level of anxiety that is repressed, personal vulnerability, unmet dependency needs, fixation in earlier level of development, retarded ego development, and inadequate coping skills, possibly evidenced by verbalized inability to cope or problem solve, high illness rate, multiple somatic complaints of several years' duration, decreased functioning in social and occupational settings, narcissistic tendencies with total focus on self and physical symptoms, demanding behaviors, history of "doctor shopping," and refusal to attend therapeutic activities.

chronic Pain may be related to severe level of repressed anxiety, low self-concept, unmet dependency needs, history of self or loved one having experienced a serious illness, possibly evidenced by verbal reports of severe, prolonged pain; guarded movement or protective behaviors, facial mask of pain, fear of reinjury, altered ability to continue previous activities, social withdrawal, demands for therapy and medication.

[disturbed Sensory Perception (specify)] may be related to psychological stress (narrowed perceptual fields, expression of stress as physical problems or deficits), poor quality of sleep, presence of chronic pain, possibly evidenced by reported change in voluntary motor or sensory function (paralysis, anosmia, aphonia, deafness, blindness, loss of touch or pain sensation), la belle indifférence (lack of concern over functional loss).

impaired Social Interaction may be related to inability to engage in satisfying personal relationships, preoccupation with self and physical symptoms, altered state of wellness, chronic pain, and rejection by others, possibly evidenced by preoccupation with own thoughts, sad, dull affect; absence of supportive SO(s), uncommunicative or withdrawn behavior, lack of eye contact, and seeking to be alone.

Spina bifida — PED

Also refer to Paraplegia; Newborn, special needs

bowel Incontinence/Constipation may be related to disruption of nerve innervation, perceptual impairment, reduced activity level, possibly evidenced by inability to evacuate bowel voluntarily, increased abdominal pressure or distention, dry and hard formed stool, change in bowel sounds.

risk for impaired Walking/physical Mobility possibly evidenced by risk factors of neuromuscular impairment, developmental delay, musculoskeletal impairments—clubfoot, hip dislocation, joint deformities, kyphosis.

risk for decreased intracranial Adaptive Capacity possibly evidenced by risk factors of structural changes (aqueductal stricture, malformation of brain stem).

risk for Infection possibly evidenced by risk factors of increased environmental exposure, invasive procedures, traumatized tissues (cerebrospinal fluid leak).

Spinal cord injury (SCI) MS/CH

Refer to Paraplegia; Quadriplegia

Splenectomy MS/CH

Refer to Surgery, general

risk for Infection possibly evidenced by risk factors of inadequate secondary defenses (decreased antibody synthesis, reduced immunoglobulin M), insufficient knowledge or motivation to avoid exposure to pathogens.

risk for ineffective Health Management possibly evidenced by risk factors of length of therapy, economic difficulties, perceived benefits.

Spongiform encephalopathy CH

Refer to Creutzfeldt-Jakob disease

Sprain of ankle or foot CH

acute Pain may be related to trauma to and swelling in joint, possibly evidenced by verbal reports, guarding or distraction behaviors, self-focusing, and changes in vital signs.

impaired Walking may be related to musculoskeletal injury, pain, and therapeutic restrictions, possibly evidenced by reluctance to attempt movement, inability to move about environment easily.

Sprue, nontropical CH

Refer to Celiac disease

Stapedectomy MS

risk for Trauma possibly evidenced by risk factors of increased middle-ear pressure with displacement of prosthesis and balancing difficulties, dizziness.

risk for Infection possibly evidenced by risk factors of surgically traumatized tissue, invasive procedures, and environmental exposure to upper respiratory infections.

acute Pain may be related to surgical trauma, edema formation, and presence of packing, possibly evidenced by verbal reports, guarding or distraction behaviors, and self-focus.

Stasis dermatitis CH

Also refer to Venous insufficiency

impaired Skin Integrity may be related to altered circulation, presence of edema, extremely fragile epidermis, pigmentation, possibly evidenced by erythema, scaling, brown discoloration, disruption of skin surface.

risk for Infection possibly evidenced by risk factors of circulatory stasis, edema formation (small-vessel vasoconstrictive reflexes) in lower extremities, persistent inflammation, tissue destruction.

STI CH

Refer to Sexually transmitted infection

Stillbirth OB

Refer to Perinatal loss/death of child

Stimulant abuse CH

Also refer to Cocaine hydrochloride poisoning, acute; Substance dependence/abuse rehabilitation

imbalanced Nutrition: less than body requirements may be related to anorexia, insufficient or inappropriate use of financial resources, possibly evidenced by reported inadequate intake, weight loss or less than normal weight gain, lack of interest in food, poor muscle tone, signs and laboratory evidence of vitamin deficiencies.

risk for Infection possibly evidenced by risk factors of injection techniques, impurities of drugs, localized trauma and nasal septum damage, malnutrition, altered immune state.

Insomnia may be related to central nervous system sensory alterations, psychological stress, possibly evidenced by constant alertness, racing thoughts preventing rest, denial of need to sleep, reported inability to stay awake, initial insomnia then hypersomnia.

PSY

Fear/Anxiety [specify] may be related to paranoid delusions associated with stimulant use, possibly evidenced by feelings or beliefs that others are conspiring against or are about to attack or kill client.

ineffective Coping may be related to personal vulnerability, negative role-modeling, inadequate support systems, ineffective or inadequate coping skills with substitution of drug, possibly evidenced by use of harmful substance despite evidence of undesirable consequences.

[disturbed Sensory Perception (specify)] may be related to exogenous chemical, altered sensory reception, transmission, or integration (hallucination), altered status of sense organs, possibly evidenced by responding to internal stimuli from hallucinatory experiences, bizarre thinking, anxiety, panic changes in sensory acuity (sense of smell, taste).

Stomatitis **CH**

impaired oral Mucous Membrane may be related to infection, vitamin deficiency, excessive alcohol or tobacco use, ill-fitting dentures, jagged teeth, orthodontic appliances, mouth breathing, nursing bottles with hard or too long nipples, possibly evidenced by oral pain, lesions, ulcers, white patches or plaques, sensitive tongue.

risk for deficient Fluid Volume possibly evidenced by risk factors of oral pain, difficulty swallowing.

Strep throat **CH**

Hyperthermia may be related to illness and effects of toxins, inability to ingest sufficient fluids, possibly evidenced by body temperature above normal range, flushed dry skin, decreased urine output.

acute Pain may be related to injuring biological agent, possibly evidenced by report of throat, head, and abdominal pain, change in ability to eat, crying.

risk for Infection [transmission] possibly evidenced by risk factors of insufficient knowledge to avoid exposure to or transmission of pathogen.

Stress disorder, acute **PSY**

Refer to Post-traumatic stress disorder

Substance dependence/abuse, prenatal **OB**

imbalanced Nutrition: less than body requirements may be related to insufficient dietary intake to meet metabolic needs, inadequate or improper use of financial resources, possibly low weight gain, decreased subcutaneous fat and muscle mass, reported altered taste sensation, lack of interest in food, protein or vitamin deficiencies.

risk for disturbed Maternal-Fetal Dyad possibly evidenced by risk factors of alcohol or drug use, treatment-related side effects.

ineffective Denial/Coping may be related to personal vulnerability, difficulty handling new situations, use of drugs for coping, inadequate support systems, possibly evidenced by denial, lack of acceptance of consequences of drug use, manipulation to avoid responsibility for self, impaired adaptive behaviors.

Powerlessness may be related to substance addiction, episodic compulsive indulgence, failed attempts at recovery, lifestyle of helplessness, possibly evidenced by statements of inability to stop behavior, continuous thinking about drug, alterations in personal, occupational, and social life.

chronic low Self-Esteem may be related to social stigma attached to substance abuse, social expectation that one controls own behavior, continual negative evaluation of self, personal vulnerabilities, possibly evidenced by not taking responsibility for self, lack of follow-through, self-destructive behavior, denial that substance use is a problem.

compromised/disabled Family Coping may be related to codependency issues, situational crisis of pregnancy and drug abuse, family disorganization, exhausted supportive capacity of family members, possibly evidenced by denial or belief that all problems are due to substance use, financial difficulties, severely dysfunctional family, codependent behaviors.

Substance dependence/abuse rehabilitation **PSY/CH**

(Following acute detoxification)

ineffective Denial may be related to threat of unpleasant reality, lack of emotional support from others, overwhelming stress, possibly evidenced by lack of acceptance that drug use is causing the present situation, delay in seeking or refusal of healthcare attention to the detriment of health, use of manipulation to avoid responsibility for self, projection of blame or responsibility for problems.

Powerlessness may be related to substance addiction with/without periods of abstinence, episodic compulsive indulgence, attempts at recovery, and lifestyle of helplessness, possibly evidenced by ineffective recovery attempts, statements of inability to stop behavior, requests for help, constantly thinking about drug or obtaining drug, alteration in personal, occupational, or social life.

imbalanced Nutrition: less than body requirements may be related to insufficient dietary intake to meet metabolic needs for psychological, physiological, or economical reasons, possibly evidenced by weight less than normal for height and body build, decreased subcutaneous fat and muscle mass, reported altered taste sensation, lack of interest in food, poor muscle tone, sore and inflamed buccal cavity, laboratory evidence of protein or vitamin deficiencies.

Sexual dysfunction may be related to altered body function (neurological damage and debilitating effects of drug use), changes in appearance, possibly evidenced by progressive interference with sexual functioning; a significant degree of testicular atrophy, gynecomastia, impotence and decreased sperm counts in men; and loss of body hair, thin soft skin, spider angiomas, and amenorrhea and increase in miscarriages in women.

dysfunctional Family Processes may be related to abuse, history of alcoholism or drug use, inadequate coping skills, lack of problem-solving skills, genetic predisposition or biochemical influences, possibly evidenced by feelings of anger, frustration, responsibility for alcoholic's behavior, suppressed rage, shame, embarrassment, repressed emotions, guilt, vulnerability, disturbed family dynamics, deterioration in family relationships, family denial or rationalization, closed communication systems, triangulating family relationships, manipulation, blaming, enabling to maintain substance use, inability to accept or receive help.

OB

risk for fetal Injury possibly evidenced by risk factors of drug or alcohol use, exposure to teratogens.

deficient Knowledge [Learning Need] regarding condition, effects on pregnancy, prognosis, and treatment needs may be related to lack or misinterpretation of information, lack of recall, cognitive limitations, interference with learning, possibly evidenced by statements of concern, questions, misconceptions, inaccurate follow-through of instructions, development of preventable complications, continued use in spite of complications.

Sudden infant death syndrome — PED

complicated Grieving may be related to unexpected loss of child, lack of anticipatory grieving, possibly evidenced by expressions of distress, guilt, anger; idealization of child, reliving past with little reduction of intensity of grief, labile affect, crying, prolonged interference with life functioning, withdrawal.

risk for impaired Parenting possibly evidenced by risk factors of recent crisis, change in family unit, maladaptive coping strategies, sleep disruption, depression.

risk for interrupted Family Processes possibly evidenced by risk factors of situational crisis, loss of a family member.

risk for chronic Sorrow possibly evidenced by risk factors of death of a loved one, anniversary dates (birth, death, etc.), trigger events (e.g., infants on TV, at play).

Suicide attempt — MS

Also refer to specific means, e.g., Drug overdose, acute; Wound, gunshot

PSY

Hopelessness may be related to long-term stress, abandonment (actual or perceived), deteriorating physical or mental condition, challenged value or belief system, possibly evidenced by verbal cues, passivity, lack of involvement or withdrawal, angry outbursts.

risk for Suicide possibly evidenced by risk factors of prior or current attempt, marked changes in behavior, attitude, or performance, impulsiveness, sudden euphoric recovery from major depression, living alone, loss of independence, economic instability, substance abuse, has a plan and available means.

chronic/situational low Self-Esteem may be related to losses, functional impairment, developmental changes, failures or rejection, possibly evidenced by evaluating self as unable to deal with events, expressions of helplessness, uselessness, shame, or guilt; self-negating verbalizations.

compromised family Coping may be related to temporary family disorganization, role changes, prolonged disease or disability, situational or developmental crises, possibly evidenced by client expressing concern about SO's response to problems, SO confirms ineffective supportive behaviors, SO withdraws from client at the time of need.

Sunstroke — MS

Refer to Heatstroke

Surgery, general — MS

Also refer to Postoperative recovery period

deficient Knowledge [Learning Need] regarding surgical procedure and expectation, postoperative routines, therapy, and self-care needs may be related to lack of information, misinterpretation, possibly evidenced by statements of concern, questions, and misconceptions.

Anxiety [specify level]/Fear may be related to situational crisis, unfamiliarity with environment, change in health status or threat of death and separation from usual support systems, possibly evidenced by increased tension, apprehension, decreased self-assurance, fear of unspecific consequences, focus on self, sympathetic stimulation, and restlessness.

risk for perioperative Positioning Injury possibly evidenced by risk factors of disorientation, immobilization, muscle weakness, obesity, edema.

risk for Injury possibly evidenced by risk factors of wrong client, procedure, site, implants, equipment or materials; interactive conditions between individual and environment; external environment—physical design, structure of environment, exposure to equipment, instrumentation, positioning, use of pharmaceutical agents; internal environment—tissue hypoxia, abnormal blood profile or altered clotting factors, broken skin.

risk for imbalanced Fluid Volume possibly evidenced by risk factors of preoperative fluid deprivation, blood loss, and excessive gastrointestinal losses—vomiting or gastric suction; inappropriate or rapid replacement.

Syndrome X **CH**

Refer to Metabolic syndrome

Synovitis (knee) **CH**

acute Pain may be related to inflammation of synovial membrane of the joint with effusion, possibly evidenced by verbal reports, guarding or distraction behaviors, self-focus, and changes in vital signs.

impaired Walking may be related to pain and decreased strength of joint, possibly evidenced by reluctance to attempt movement, inability to move about environment as desired.

Syphilis, congenital **PED**

Also refer to Sexually transmitted infection

acute Pain may be related to inflammatory process, edema formation, and development of skin lesions, possibly evidenced by irritability or crying that may be increased with movement of extremities and autonomic responses (changes in vital signs).

impaired Skin/Tissue Integrity may be related to exposure to pathogens during vaginal delivery, possibly evidenced by disruption of skin surfaces and rhinitis.

risk for disproportionate Growth/delayed Development possibly evidenced by risk factors of congenital disorder, malnutrition, seizure disorder.

deficient Knowledge [Learning Need] regarding pathophysiology of condition, transmissibility, therapy needs, expected outcomes, and potential complications may be related to caretaker/parental lack of information, misinterpretation, possibly evidenced by statements of concern, questions, and misconceptions.

Syringomyelia **MS**

[disturbed Sensory Perception (specify)] may be related to altered sensory perception (neurological lesion), possibly evidenced by change in usual response to stimuli and motor incoordination.

Anxiety [specify level]/Fear may be related to change in health status, threat of change in role functioning and socioeconomic status, and threat to self-concept, possibly evidenced by increased tension, apprehension, uncertainty, focus on self, and expressed concerns.

impaired physical Mobility may be related to neuromuscular and sensory impairment, possibly evidenced by decreased muscle strength, control, and mass; and impaired coordination.

Self-Care deficit [specify] may be related to neuromuscular and sensory impairments, possibly evidenced by statement of inability to perform care tasks.

Tarsal tunnel syndrome **CH**

acute/chronic Pain may be related to pressure on posterior tibial nerve at ankle, possibly evidenced by verbal reports, reluctance to use affected extremity, guarding behaviors, expressed fear of reinjury, altered ability to continue previous activities.

impaired Walking may be related to neuromuscular impairment and increased pain with walking, possibly evidenced by inability to walk desired distances, climb stairs, navigate curbs or uneven surfaces.

Tay-Sachs disease **PED**

risk for delayed Development possibly evidenced by risk factors of genetic disorder, seizure disorder, visual/hearing impairment.

[disturbed visual Sensory Perception] may be related to neurological deterioration of optic nerve, possibly evidenced by loss of visual acuity.

CH

family Grieving may be related to expected eventual loss of infant/child, possibly evidenced by expressions of distress, denial, guilt, anger, and sorrow; choked feelings; changes in sleep or eating habits; and altered libido.

family Powerlessness may be related to absence of therapeutic interventions for progressive and fatal disease, possibly evidenced by verbal expressions of having no control over situation or outcome, and depression over physical and mental deterioration.

risk for Spiritual distress possibly evidenced by risk factors of challenged belief and value system by presence of fatal condition with racial or religious connotations and intense suffering.

compromised family Coping may be related to situational crisis; temporary preoccupation with managing emotional conflicts and personal suffering; family disorganization; and prolonged, progressive disease, possibly evidenced by preoccupations with personal reactions, expressed concern about reactions of other family members, inadequate support of one another, and altered communication patterns.

TBI — MS/CH

Refer to Traumatic brain injury

Temporal arteritis — CH

acute Pain may be related to arterial inflammation, possibly evidenced by reports of severe headache, scalp tenderness, pain with chewing, myalgia.

[risk for disturbed visual Sensory Perception]: possibly evidenced by altered reception (arterial inflammation, ischemic optic neuropathy).

risk for ineffective Health Management risk factors may include medication side effects, economic difficulties, perceived seriousness or benefits.

Temporomandibular joint syndrome — CH

chronic Pain may be related to pressure on nerves, possibly evidenced by reports of pain in temporomandibular joint area worsened with chewing, muscle tension headache.

risk for imbalanced Nutrition: less than body requirements possibly evidenced by risk factors of inability to ingest food (pain worsened by chewing, limited movement of joint).

[risk for disturbed auditory Sensory Perception] possibly evidenced by risk factors of altered sensory reception (tinnitus, occasional deafness).

Tendonitis — CH

acute/chronic Pain may be related to inflammation, swelling of tendon, possibly evidenced by verbal reports, guarding or protective behavior, fear of reinjury, altered ability to continue previous activities.

impaired physical Mobility may be related to pain, joint stiffness, musculoskeletal impairment, prescribed movement restrictions, possibly evidenced by limited range of motion, limited ability to perform fine or gross motor skills.

risk for ineffective Role Performance possibly evidenced by risk factors of health alterations, fatigue, pain.

Testicular cancer — MS

Also refer to Cancer

disturbed Body Image may be related to surgical change in reproductive organs, loss of hair and weight, possibly evidenced by negative feelings about body and sense of mutilation, preoccupation with change, feelings of helplessness or hopelessness, and change in social environment.

Sexual dysfunction may be related to change in sexual organs, postoperative impotence, vulnerability, possibly evidenced by verbalizations of problem, inability in achieving desired satisfaction, alterations in relationships.

Tetanus — MS

acute Pain may be related to muscle spasms possibly evidenced by reports pain, narrowed focus, facial mask.

bowel/urinary Incontinence may be related to abnormally high abdominal/intestinal pressure possibly evidenced by urgency, inability to delay elimination.

risk for impaired Swallowing possibly evidenced by risk factors of neuromuscular impairment.

risk for impaired spontaneous Ventilation possibly evidenced by risk factors of respiratory muscle fatigue/muscle spasms.

Tetraplegia — MS/CH

Refer to Quadriplegia

Thoracotomy — MS

Refer to Surgery, general; Hemothorax

Thrombophlebitis — CH/MS/OB

ineffective peripheral Tissue Perfusion may be related to interruption of venous blood flow, venous stasis, possibly evidenced by changes in skin color and temperature over affected area, development of edema, pain, diminished peripheral pulses, slow capillary refill.

acute Pain/impaired Comfort may be related to vascular inflammation and irritation, and edema formation (accumulation of lactic acid), possibly evidenced by verbal reports, guarding or distraction behaviors, restlessness, and self-focus.

Anxiety [specify level] may be related to change in health status, perceived or actual threat to self, situational crisis, interpersonal transmission, possibly evidenced by increased tension, apprehension, restlessness, sympathetic stimulation.

risk for impaired physical Mobility possibly evidenced by risk factors of pain and discomfort, restrictive therapies, and safety precautions.

deficient Knowledge [Learning Need] regarding pathophysiology of condition, therapy, self-care needs, and risk of embolization may be related to lack of information or misinterpretation, possibly evidenced by statements of concern, questions, inaccurate follow-through of instructions, and development of preventable complications.

Thrombosis, venous MS

Refer to Thrombophlebitis

Thrush CH

impaired oral Mucous Membrane may be related to presence of infection as evidenced by white patches or plaques, oral discomfort, mucosal irritation, bleeding.

risk for imbalanced Nutrition: less than body requirements possibly evidenced by risk factors of inability to ingest adequate amount of nutrients (oral pain).

Thyroidectomy MS

Also refer to Hyperthyroidism; Hypoparathyroidism (acute), Hypothyroidism

risk for ineffective Airway Clearance possibly evidenced by risk factors of tracheal obstruction—edema, hematoma formation, laryngeal spasms.

impaired verbal Communication may be related to tissue edema, pain or discomfort, and vocal cord injury or laryngeal nerve damage, possibly evidenced by impaired articulation, does not or cannot speak, and use of nonverbal cues or gestures.

risk for Injury [tetany] possibly evidenced by risk factors of chemical imbalance—hypocalcemia, increased release of thyroid hormones; excessive central nervous system stimulation.

risk for head/neck Trauma possibly evidenced by risk factors of loss of muscle control and support, and position of suture line.

acute Pain may be related to presence of surgical incision, manipulation of tissues and muscles, postoperative edema, possibly evidenced by verbal reports, guarding or distraction behaviors, narrowed focus, and autonomic responses—changes in vital signs.

Thyrotoxicosis MS

Also refer to Hyperthyroidism

risk for decreased Cardiac Output possibly evidenced by risk factors of uncontrolled hypermetabolic state increasing cardiac workload; changes in venous return and systemic vascular resistance; and alterations in rate, rhythm, and electrical conduction.

Anxiety [specific level] may be related to physiological factors and central nervous system stimulation (hypermetabolic state and pseudocatecholamine effect of thyroid hormones), possibly evidenced by increased feelings of apprehension, shakiness, loss of control, panic, changes in cognition, distortion of environmental stimuli, extraneous movements, restlessness, and tremors.

deficient Knowledge [Learning Needs] regarding condition, treatment needs, and potential for complications or crisis situation may be related to lack of information or recall, misinterpretation, possibly evidenced by statements of concern, questions, misconceptions, and inaccurate follow-through of instructions.

TIA CH

Refer to Transient ischemic attack

Tic douloureux CH

Refer to Neuralgia, trigeminal

TMJ syndrome CH

Refer to Temporomandibular joint syndrome

Tonsillectomy PED/MS

Refer to Adenoidectomy

Tonsillitis PED

acute Pain may be related to inflammation of tonsils and effects of circulating toxins, possibly evidenced by verbal reports, guarding or distraction behaviors, reluctance/refusal to swallow, self-focus, and changes in vital signs.

Hyperthermia may be related to presence of inflammatory process, hypermetabolic state and dehydration, possibly evidenced by increased body temperature; warm, flushed skin; and tachycardia.

deficient Knowledge [Learning Need] regarding cause/transmission, treatment needs, and potential complications may be related to lack of information, misinterpretation, possibly evidenced by statements of concern, questions, inaccurate follow-through of instructions, and recurrence of condition.

Total joint replacement MS

risk for Infection possibly evidenced by risk factors of inadequate primary defenses (broken skin, exposure of joint), inadequate secondary defenses or immunosuppression (long-term corticosteroid use), invasive procedures and surgical manipulation, implantation of foreign body, and decreased mobility.

impaired physical Mobility may be related to pain and discomfort, musculoskeletal impairment, and surgery and restrictive therapies, possibly evidenced by reluctance to attempt movement, difficulty with purposefully moving within the physical environment, reports of pain or discomfort on movement, limited range of motion, and decreased muscle strength and control.

risk for ineffective peripheral Tissue Perfusion-possibly evidenced by risk factors of reduced arterial or venous blood flow, direct trauma to blood vessels, tissue edema, improper location or dislocation of prosthesis, and hypovolemia.

acute Pain may be related to physical agents (traumatized tissues, surgical intervention, degeneration of joints, muscle spasms) and psychological factors (anxiety, advanced age), possibly evidenced by verbal reports, guarding or distraction behaviors, self-focus, and changes in vital signs.

risk for Constipation possibly evidenced by risk factors of insufficient physical activity, decreased mobility, weakness, insufficient fiber or fluid intake, dehydration, poor eating habits, decreased gastrointestinal motility, effects of medications—anesthesia, opiate analgesics; environmental changes, inadequate toileting.

Tourette's syndrome **CH**

chronic low Self-Esteem may be related to inherited disorder, continual negative evaluation of self and capabilities, personal vulnerability, possibly evidenced by self-negating verbalizations, expressed shame, exaggerated negative feedback about self, hesitancy to try new situations.

Social Isolation may be related to unaccepted social behaviors, inability to engage in satisfying personal relationships, rejection or ridicule by others.

risk for Injury possibly evidenced by risk factors of adverse side effects of medications, negative response of uneducated individuals.

Toxemia of pregnancy **OB**

Refer to Hypertension, gestational

Toxic enterocolitis **PED/MS**

Also refer to Colostomy

deficient Fluid Volume may be related to fulminating losses into the bowel, diarrhea, lack of intake evidenced by decreased concentrated urine, dry mucous membranes, poor skin turgor, decreased venous filling, change in mentation.

risk for decreased Cardiac Output possibly evidenced by risk factors of decreased venous return, altered heart rate and rhythm.

Toxic megacolon **MS**

Refer to Toxic enterocolitis

Toxic shock syndrome **MS**

Also refer to Sepsis

Hyperthermia may be related to inflammatory process, hypermetabolic state and dehydration, possibly evidenced by increased body temperature; warm, flushed skin; and tachycardia.

deficient Fluid Volume [isotonic] may be related to increased gastric losses (diarrhea, vomiting), fever, hypermetabolic state, and decreased intake, possibly evidenced by dry mucous membranes, increased pulse, hypotension, delayed venous filling, decreased concentrated urine, and hemoconcentration.

acute Pain may be related to inflammatory process, effects of circulating toxins, and skin disruptions, possibly evidenced by verbal reports, guarding or distraction behaviors, self-focus, and changes in vital signs.

impaired Skin/Tissue Integrity may be related to effects of circulating toxins and dehydration, possibly evidenced by development of desquamating rash, hyperemia, and inflammation of mucous membranes.

Traction **MS**

Also refer to Casts; Fractures

acute Pain may be related to direct trauma to tissue and bone, muscle spasms, movement of bone fragments, edema, injury to soft tissue, traction or immobility device, anxiety, possibly evidenced by verbal reports, guarding or distraction behaviors, self-focus, alteration in muscle tone, and changes in vital signs.

impaired physical Mobility may be related to neuromuscular and skeletal impairment, pain, psychological immobility, and therapeutic restrictions of movement, possibly evidenced by limited range of motion, inability to move purposefully in environment, reluctance to attempt movement, and decreased muscle strength and control.

risk for Infection possibly evidenced by risk factors of invasive procedures (including insertion of foreign body through skin and bone), presence of traumatized tissue, and reduced activity with stasis of body fluids.

deficient Diversional Activity may be related to length of hospitalization or therapeutic intervention and environmental lack of usual activity, possibly evidenced by statements of boredom, restlessness, and irritability.

Transfusion reaction, blood **MS**

Also refer to Anaphylaxis

risk for imbalanced Body Temperature possibly evidenced by risk factors of infusion of cold blood products, systemic response to toxins.

Anxiety [specify level] may be related to change in health status and threat of death, exposure to toxins, possibly evidenced by increased tension, apprehension, sympathetic stimulation, restlessness, and expressions of concern.

risk for impaired Skin Integrity possibly evidenced by risk factor of immunological response.

Transient ischemic attack CH

ineffective cerebral Tissue Perfusion may be related to interruption of blood flow (e.g., vasospasm), possibly evidenced by altered mental status, behavioral changes, language deficit, change in motor and sensory response.

Anxiety [specify level]/Fear may be related to change in health status, threat to self-concept, situational crisis, interpersonal contagion, possibly evidenced by expressed concerns, apprehension, restlessness, irritability.

risk for ineffective Denial possibly evidenced by risk factors of change in health status requiring change in lifestyle, fear of consequences, lack of motivation.

Transplant, living donor MS

Also refer to Surgery, general; Nephrectomy

Decisional Conflict may be related to multiple or divergent sources of information, family system (demands, expectations, or responsibilities to others), risk to self, possibly evidenced by verbalized uncertainty about choices, questioning personal values or beliefs, delayed decision making, increased tension.

[moderate to severe] Anxiety/Fear may be related to situational crisis, unconscious conflict about essential beliefs or values, familial association, threat to health status or death, possibly evidenced by expressed concerns, apprehension, uncertainty, increased tension, fear of failing family member (e.g., organ rejection), sympathetic stimulation.

Transplantation, recipient MS

Also refer to Surgery, general; Cardiac surgery

Anxiety [specify level]/Fear may be related to unconscious conflict about essential values/beliefs, situational crisis, interpersonal contagion, threat to self-concept, threat of organ rejection or death, side effects of medication, possibly evidenced by increased tension, apprehension, uncertainty, expressed concerns, somatic complaints, sympathetic stimulation, insomnia.

risk for Infection possibly evidenced by risk factors of medically induced immunosuppression, suppressed inflammatory response, antibiotic therapy, invasive procedures, broken skin and traumatized tissue, effects of chronic and debilitating disease.

(Refer to specific conditions relative to compromise or failure of individual transplanted organ, e.g., Renal failure, acute; Heart failure, chronic; Pancreatitis.)

CH

ineffective Coping/compromised family Coping may be related to situational crisis, high degree of threat, uncertainty, family disorganization or role changes, prolonged disease exhausting supportive capacity of family/SO, possibly evidenced by verbalizations, sleep disturbance, fatigue, poor concentration, protective behaviors disproportionate to client's needs, SO describes preoccupation with personal reaction.

ineffective Protection may be related to treatment regimen/pharmaceutical agents, compromised immune system possibly evidenced by weakness, maladaptive stress response.

readiness for enhanced Health Management possibly evidenced by expressed desire to manage treatment and prevention of sequelae, reduction of risk factors, no unexpected sequelae.

risk for ineffective Health Management possibly evidenced by risk factors of complexity of therapeutic regimen and healthcare system, economic difficulties, family patterns of healthcare.

Transurethral resection of prostate MS

Refer to Prostatectomy

Traumatic brain injury (TBI) MS

ineffective cerebral Tissue Perfusion may be related to interruption of blood flow—hemorrhage, hematoma, cerebral edema (localized or generalized response to injury, metabolic alterations, drug or alcohol overdose), decreased systemic blood pressure—hypovolemia, cardiac dysrhythmias; hypoxia, possibly evidenced by altered level of consciousness, memory loss, changes in motor or sensory responses, restlessness, changes in vital signs.

risk for decreased intracranial Adaptive Capacity possibly evidenced by risk factors of brain injuries, systemic hypotension with intracranial hypertension.

risk for ineffective Breathing Pattern possibly evidenced by risk factors of neuromuscular dysfunction—injury to respiratory center of brain; perception or cognitive impairment, tracheobronchial obstruction.

[disturbed Sensory Perception (specify)] may be related to altered sensory reception, transmission or integration (neurological trauma or deficit), possibly evidenced by disorientation to time, place, person; motor incoordination; altered communication patterns; restlessness or irritability; change in behavior pattern.

risk for Infection possibly evidenced by risk factors of traumatized tissues, broken skin, invasive procedures, decreased ciliary action, stasis of body fluids, nutritional deficits, suppressed inflammatory response—steroid use; altered integrity of closed system—cerebrospinal fluid leak.

risk for imbalanced Nutrition: less than body requirements possibly evidenced by risk factors of altered ability to ingest nutrients—decreased level of consciousness; weakness of muscles for chewing or swallowing, hypermetabolic state.

CH

impaired physical Mobility may be related to perceptual or cognitive impairment, decreased strength or endurance, restrictive therapies, safety precautions, possibly evidenced by inability to purposefully move within physical environment—including bed mobility, transfer, ambulation, impaired coordination, limited range of motion, decreased muscle strength and control.

risk for impaired Memory/chronic Confusion possibly evidenced by risk factors of head injury, neurological disturbances.

interrupted Family Processes may be related to situational transition and crisis, uncertainty about ultimate outcome and expectations, possibly evidenced by difficulty adapting to change, family not meeting needs of all members, difficulty accepting/receiving help, inability to express or to accept feelings of members.

Self-Care deficit (specify) may be related to neuromuscular or musculoskeletal impairment, weakness, pain, perceptual or cognitive impairment, possibly evidenced by inability to perform desired or appropriate activities of daily living.

Trench foot — MS

Refer to Immersion foot

Trichinosis — CH

acute Pain may be related to parasitic invasion of muscle tissues, edema of upper eyelids, small localized hemorrhages, and development of urticaria, possibly evidenced by verbal reports, guarding/distraction behaviors (restlessness), and changes in vital signs.

deficient Fluid Volume may be related to hypermetabolic state (fever, diaphoresis); excessive gastric losses (vomiting, diarrhea); and decreased intake and difficulty swallowing, possibly evidenced by dry mucous membranes, decreased skin turgor, hypotension, decreased venous filling, decreased concentrated urine, and hemoconcentration.

ineffective Breathing Pattern may be related to myositis of the diaphragm and intercostal muscles, possibly evidenced by resulting changes in respiratory depth, tachypnea, dyspnea, and abnormal arterial blood gases.

deficient Knowledge [Learning Need] regarding cause, prevention of condition, therapy needs, and possible complications may be related to lack of information, misinterpretation, possibly evidenced by statements of concern, questions, and misconceptions.

Tricuspid insufficiency — CH

Refer to Valvular heart disease

Tricuspid stenosis — CH

Refer to Valvular heart disease

Tubal pregnancy — OB

Refer to Ectopic pregnancy (tubal)

Tuberculosis (pulmonary) — CH

risk for Infection [spread/reactivation] possibly evidenced by risk factors of inadequate primary defenses (decreased ciliary action, stasis of secretions, tissue destruction, and extension of infection), lowered resistance or suppressed inflammatory response, malnutrition, environmental exposure, insufficient knowledge to avoid exposure to pathogens, or inadequate therapeutic intervention.

ineffective Airway Clearance may be related to thick, viscous, or bloody secretions; fatigue with poor cough effort; and tracheal or pharyngeal edema, possibly evidenced by abnormal respiratory rate, rhythm, and depth; adventitious breath sounds—rhonchi, wheezes; stridor and dyspnea.

risk for impaired Gas Exchange possibly evidenced by risk factors of decrease in effective lung surface; atelectasis; destruction of alveolar-capillary membrane; bronchial edema; thick, viscous secretions.

Activity Intolerance may be related to imbalance between oxygen supply and demand, possibly evidenced by reports of fatigue, weakness, and exertional dyspnea.

imbalanced Nutrition: less than body requirements may be related to inability to ingest adequate nutrients (anorexia, effects of drug therapy, fatigue, insufficient financial resources), possibly evidenced by weight loss, reported lack of interest in food or altered taste sensation, and poor muscle tone.

risk for ineffectiveHealth Management possibly evidenced by risk factors of complexity of therapeutic regimen, economic difficulties, family patterns of healthcare, perceived seriousness or benefits (especially during remission), side effects of therapy.

TURP **MS**

Refer to Prostatectomy

Twin-twin transfusion syndrome **OB**

decreased Cardiac Output may be related to altered preload (hypovolemia, anemia) to donor fetus, possibly evidenced by oliguria, oligohydramnios.

excess Fluid Volume may be related to excess fluid intake (shunting of circulation) to recipient fetus, possibly evidenced by polyuria, polyhydramnios.

risk for disproportionate Growth possibly evidenced by risk factor of multiple gestation with imbalanced circulation and nutrition to both fetuses.

Tympanoplasty **MS**

Refer to Stapedectomy

Typhoid fever **MS**

Also refer to Sepsis

risk for Infection [spread] possibly evidenced by risk factors of presence of bacteria in excretions, inadequate knowledge to avoid exposure to pathogen (food or water, fecally contaminated objects).

risk for deficient Fluid Volume possibly evidenced by risk factors of gastric irritation, ulcers.

imbalanced Nutrition: less than body requirements possibly evidenced by risk factors of inability to ingest, digest, or absorb nutrients; hypermetabolic state, possibly evidenced by anorexia, abdominal pain, weight loss.

Typhus **CH/MS**

Hyperthermia may be related to generalized inflammatory process (vasculitis), possibly evidenced by increased body temperature, warm flushed skin, and tachycardia.

acute Pain may be related to generalized vasculitis and edema formation, possibly evidenced by verbal reports, guarding or distraction behaviors, self-focus, and autonomic responses (changes in vital signs).

ineffective Tissue Perfusion (specify) may be related to reduction or interruption of blood flow—generalized vasculitis or thrombi formation, possibly evidenced by reports of headache, abdominal pain, changes in mentation, and areas of peripheral ulceration or necrosis.

Ulcer, decubitus **CH/MS**

impaired Skin/Tissue Integrity may be related to altered circulation, nutritional deficit, fluid imbalance, impaired physical mobility, irritation of body excretions or secretions, and sensory impairments, evidenced by tissue damage or destruction.

acute Pain may be related to destruction of protective skin layers and exposure of nerves, possibly evidenced by verbal reports, distraction behaviors, and self-focus.

risk for Infection possibly evidenced by risk factors of broken or traumatized tissue, increased environmental exposure, and nutritional deficits.

Ulcer, peptic (acute) **MS/CH**

risk for Shock possibly evidenced by risk factors of hypovolemia, hypotension

Fear/Anxiety [specify level] may be related to change in health status and threat of death, possibly evidenced by increased tension, restlessness, irritability, fearfulness, trembling, tachycardia, diaphoresis, lack of eye contact, focus on self, verbalization of concerns, withdrawal, and panic or attack behavior.

acute Pain may be related to caustic irritation and destruction of gastric tissues, reflex muscle spasms in stomach wall, possibly evidenced by verbal reports, distraction behaviors, self-focus, and changes in vital signs.

deficient Knowledge [Learning Need] regarding condition, therapy, self-care needs, and potential complications may be related to lack of information or recall, misinterpretation, possibly evidenced by statements of concern, questions, misconceptions; inaccurate follow-through of instructions; and development of preventable complications or recurrence of condition.

Ulcer, pressure **CH/MS**

Refer to Ulcer, decubitus

Ulcer, venous stasis **CH**

Also refer to Venous insufficiency

impaired Skin/Tissue Integrity may be related to altered venous circulation, edema formation, inflammation, decreased sensation, possibly evidenced by destruction of skin layers, invasion of body structures.

ineffective peripheral Tissue Perfusion may be related to interruption of venous flow—small-vessel vasoconstrictive reflex, possibly evidenced by skin discoloration, edema formation, altered sensation, delayed healing.

Ulnar neuropathy CH
Refer to Cubital tunnel syndrome

Unconsciousness MS
Refer to Coma

Upper GI bleeding MS
Refer to Gastritis, acute or chronic; Ulcer, peptic

Urinary diversion MS/CH
risk for impaired Skin Integrity possibly evidenced by risk factors of absence of sphincter at stoma, character and flow of urine from stoma, reaction to product or chemicals, and improperly fitting appliance or removal of adhesive.

disturbed Body Image related factors may include biophysical factors—presence of stoma, loss of control of urine flow; and psychosocial factors—altered body structure, disease process and associated treatment regimen, such as cancer, possibly evidenced by verbalization of change in body image, fear of rejection or reaction of others, negative feelings about body, not touching or looking at stoma, refusal to participate in care.

acute Pain may be related to physical factors—disruption of skin and tissues, presence of incisions and drains; biological factors—activity of disease process, such as cancer, trauma; and psychological factors—fear, anxiety, possibly evidenced by verbal reports, self-focusing, guarding or distraction behaviors, restlessness, and autonomic responses—changes in vital signs.

impaired urinary Elimination may be related to surgical diversion, tissue trauma, and postoperative edema, possibly evidenced by loss of continence, changes in amount and character of urine, and urinary retention.

Urinary tract infection CH
Refer to Cystitis

Urolithiasis MS/CH
Refer to Calculi, urinary

Uterine bleeding, dysfunctional GYN/MS
Anxiety [specify level] may be related to perceived change in health status and unknown etiology, possibly evidenced by apprehension, uncertainty, fear of unspecified consequences, expressed concerns, and focus on self.

Activity Intolerance may be related to imbalance between oxygen supply and demand, decreased oxygen-carrying capacity of blood (anemia), possibly evidenced by reports of fatigue, weakness.

Uterine myomas GYN
Also refer to Anemia

acute Pain/impaired Comfort may be related to growth, size, and degeneration or twisting of tumors, possibly evidenced by reports of pressure, cramping, guarding behavior, irritability.

impaired urinary Elimination may be related to uterine pressure on bladder, possibly evidenced by frequency, urgency.

risk for deficient Fluid Volume possibly evidenced by risk factor of excessive or chronic blood loss.

Uterus, rupture of, in pregnancy OB
risk for Shock possibly evidenced by risk factors of hypovolemia, hypotension.

acute Pain may be related to tissue trauma and irritation of accumulating blood, possibly evidenced by verbal reports, guarding or distraction behaviors, self-focus, and autonomic responses—changes in vital signs.

Anxiety [specify level] may be related to threat of death of self/fetus, interpersonal contagion, physiological response—release of catecholamines, possibly evidenced by fearful or scared affect, sympathetic stimulation, stated fear of unspecified consequences, and expressed concerns.

UTI CH
Refer to Cystitis

Vaginal hysterectomy MS
Refer to Hysterectomy

Vaginismus GYN/PSY
acute Pain may be related to muscle spasm and hyperesthesia of the nerve supply to vaginal mucous membrane, possibly evidenced by verbal reports, distraction behaviors, and self-focus.

Sexual dysfunction may be related to physical or psychological alteration in function (severe spasms of vaginal muscles), possibly evidenced by verbalization of problem, inability to achieve desired satisfaction, and alteration in relationship with SO.

Vaginitis GYN/CH

impaired Tissue Integrity may be related to irritation or inflammation and mechanical trauma (scratching) of sensitive tissues, possibly evidenced by damaged or destroyed tissue, presence of lesions.

acute Pain may be related to localized inflammation and tissue trauma, possibly evidenced by verbal reports, distraction behaviors, and self-focus.

deficient Knowledge [Learning Need] regarding hygienic needs, therapy, and sexual behaviors or transmission of organisms may be related to lack of information, misinterpretation, possibly evidenced by statements of concern, questions, and misconceptions.

Vaginosis, bacterial GYN

risk for impaired Tissue Integrity possibly evidenced by risk factors of vulvar or vaginal irritation, itching.

risk for [secondary] Infection possibly evidenced by risk factors of prescribed antibiotic therapy, insufficient knowledge to avoid exposure to pathogens.

Valvular heart disease MS

decreased Cardiac Output may be related to alteration in preload, increased arterial pressure and venous congestion, increased afterload, changes in electrical conduction, possibly evidenced by variations in hemodynamic parameters, dysrhythmias and electrocardiogram changes, dyspnea, adventitious breath sounds, cyanosis or pallor, jugular vein distention, fatigue.

Activity Intolerance may be related to imbalance between oxygen supply and demand (decreased or fixed cardiac output), possibly evidenced by reports of fatigue, weakness, abnormal heart rate and blood pressure in response to activity, exertional discomfort or dyspnea.

Anxiety may be related to threat to or change in health status (chronicity of disease), physiological effects, situational crisis (changes in lifestyle, hospitalization), possibly evidenced by expressed concerns, increased tension, apprehension, uncertainty, sympathetic stimulation, insomnia.

risk for excess Fluid Volume risk factors may include increased sodium and water retention, changes in glomerular filtration.

risk for ineffective Tissue Perfusion (specify) possibly evidenced by risk factors of interruption of arterial-venous flow (systemic emboli), venous thrombosis (venous stasis, decreased activity).

VAP MS/CH

Refer to Ventilator assist/dependence; Bronchopneumonia

Varices, esophageal MS

Also refer to Ulcer, peptic (acute)

risk for Bleeding/deficient Fluid Volume possibly evidenced by risk factors of presence of varices, reduced intake, and gastric losses—vomiting; vascular loss.

Anxiety [specify level]/Fear may be related to change in health status and threat of death, possibly evidenced by increased tension, apprehension, sympathetic stimulation, restlessness, focus on self, and expressed concerns.

Varicose veins CH

chronic Pain may be related to venous insufficiency and stasis, possibly evidenced by verbal reports.

disturbed Body Image may be related to change in structure (presence of enlarged, discolored tortuous superficial leg veins), possibly evidenced by hiding affected parts and negative feelings about body.

risk for impaired Skin/Tissue Integrity may be related to altered circulation, venous stasis, and edema formation.

Varicose veins ligation/stripping MS

risk for ineffective peripheral Tissue Perfusion possibly evidenced by risk factors of localized edema, vascular irritation, inadequate venous return, dressings.

impaired Skin Integrity may be related to surgical procedure, pressure dressings, tissue edema, vascular engorgement, possibly evidenced by incisions, development of complications (e.g., ulcerations).

Varicose veins sclerotherapy MS

risk for impaired Skin Integrity possibly evidenced by risk factors of pressure wraps, extravasation of sclerosing agent.

risk for ineffective Health Management possibly evidenced by risk factors of perceived seriousness or benefit, required lifestyle and activity changes, post-procedure dressings.

Variola MS

Refer to Smallpox

Vasculitis CH

Refer to Polyarteritis nodosa; Temporal arteritis

Vasectomy CH/MS

acute Pain/impaired Comfort may be related to manipulation of delicate tissues, edema/hematoma formation, possibly evidenced by verbal reports, guarding behavior, irritability.

deficient Knowledge [Learning Need] regarding self-care and future expectations (issues of reproduction, safety/sexually transmitted diseases) may be related to information misinterpretation, lack of recall, possibly evidenced by verbalizations, misconceptions, inaccurate follow-through of instructions.

Venereal disease CH

Refer to Sexually transmitted infection

Venous insufficiency CH

Also refer to Stasis dermatitis; Ulcer, venous stasis

chronic Pain/impaired Comfort may be related to altered venous circulation, edema formation, possibly evidenced by reports of aching, fullness, tiredness of lower extremities with activity.

risk for risk-prone Health Behavior possibly evidenced by risk factors of health status requiring change in lifestyle, lack of motivation to change behaviors.

risk for ineffective Health Management possibly evidenced by risk factors of economic difficulties, perceived seriousness or benefit, social support deficit.

Ventilator assist/dependence MS/CH

ineffective Breathing Pattern/impaired spontaneous Ventilation may be related to neuromuscular dysfunction, respiratory muscle fatigue, spinal cord injury, hypoventilation syndrome, possibly evidenced by dyspnea, increased work of breathing/use of accessory muscles, reduced vital capacity and total lung volume, changes in respiratory rate, decreased PO_2/SaO_2, increased PCO_2.

ineffective Airway Clearance may be related to artificial airway in trachea, inability to or ineffective cough, possibly evidenced by changes in rate and depth of respirations, abnormal breath sounds, anxiety, restlessness, cyanosis.

impaired verbal Communication may be related to physical barrier (artificial airway), neuromuscular weakness or paralysis, possibly evidenced by inability to speak.

Fear/Anxiety [specify] may be related to situational crisis, threat to self-concept, threat of death or dependency on machine, change in health status, socioeconomic status, or role functioning; interpersonal transmission, possibly evidenced by increased muscle or facial tension, hypervigilance, restlessness, fearfulness, apprehension, expressed concerns, insomnia, negative self-talk.

risk for impaired oral Mucous Membrane possibly evidenced by risk factors of inability to swallow oral fluids, decreased salivation, ineffective oral hygiene, presence of endotracheal tube in mouth.

risk for imbalanced Nutrition: less than body requirements possibly evidenced by risk factors of inability to ingest nutrients, increased metabolic demands.

risk for dysfunctional Ventilatory Weaning Response possibly evidenced by risk factors of limited or insufficient energy stores, sleep disturbance, pain or discomfort, perceived inability to wean, decreased motivation, inadequate support or adverse environment, history of ventilator dependence greater than 1 week or unsuccessful weaning attempts.

Ventricular fibrillation MS

Also refer to Dysrhythmia, cardiac

decreased Cardiac Output may be related to altered electrical conduction and reduced myocardial contractility, possibly evidenced by absence of measurable cardiac output, loss of consciousness, no palpable pulses.

Ventricular tachycardia MS

Also refer to Dysrhythmia, cardiac

risk for decreased Cardiac Output possibly evidenced by risk factors of alteration in heart rhythm, altered contractility.

Vertigo CH

[disturbed kinesthetic Sensory Perception] may be related to altered status of sensory organ (middle or inner ear), altered sensory integration, possibly evidenced by visual distortions, altered sense of balance, falls.

risk for Falls possibly evidenced by risk factors of presence of postural hypotension, acute illness, medications, substance abuse.

West Nile Fever CH/MS

Hyperthermia may be related to infectious process, possibly evidenced by elevated body temperature, skin flushed and warm to touch, tachycardia, increased respiratory rate.

acute Pain may be related to infectious process, circulating toxins, possibly evidenced by reports of headache, myalgia, eye pain, abdominal discomfort.

risk for deficient Fluid Volume possibly evidenced by risk factors of hypermetabolic state, decreased intake, anorexia, nausea, losses from normal routes (vomiting, diarrhea).

risk for impaired Skin Integrity possibly evidenced by risk factors of hyperthermia, decreased fluid intake, alterations in skin turgor, bedrest, circulating toxins.

Whooping cough **PED**

Refer to Pertussis

Wilms' tumor **PED**

Also refer to Cancer; Chemotherapy

Anxiety [specify level]/Fear may be related to change in environment and interaction patterns with family members and threat of death with family transmission and contagion concerns, possibly evidenced by fearful/scared affect, distress, crying, insomnia, and sympathetic stimulation.

risk for Injury possibly evidenced by risk factors of nature of tumor (vascular, mushy with very thin covering) with increased danger of metastasis when manipulated.

interrupted Family Processes may be related to situational crisis of life-threatening illness, possibly evidenced by a family system that has difficulty meeting physical, emotional, and spiritual needs of its members, and inability to deal with traumatic experience effectively.

deficient Diversional Activity may be related to environmental lack of age-appropriate activity (including activity restrictions) and length of hospitalization or treatment, possibly evidenced by restlessness, crying, lethargy, and acting-out behavior.

Withdrawal, drugs/alcohol **CH/MS**

Refer to Alcohol intoxication, acute; Drug overdose, acute (depressants); Drug withdrawal

Wound, gunshot **MS**

(Depends on site and speed/character of bullet.)

risk for Bleeding/deficient Fluid Volume possibly evidenced by risk factors of rauma, vascular losses, restricted oral intake.

acute Pain may be related to destruction of tissue (including organ and musculoskeletal), surgical repair, and therapeutic interventions, possibly evidenced by verbal reports, guarding or distraction behaviors, self-focus, and changes in vital signs.

impaired Tissue Integrity may be related to mechanical factors—yaw of projectile and muzzle blast, possibly evidenced by damaged or destroyed tissue.

risk for Infection possibly evidenced by risk factors of tissue destruction and increased environmental exposure, invasive procedures, and decreased hemoglobin.

CH

risk for Post-Trauma Syndrome possibly evidenced by risk factors of nature of incident (catastrophic accident, assault, suicide attempt) and possibly injury or death of other(s) involved.

Zollinger-Ellison syndrome **MS/CH**

Also refer to Ulcer, peptic

Diarrhea may be related to intestinal irritation—hypersecretion of gastric acid, possibly evidenced by at least three loose liquid stools per day, abdominal pain, change in bowel sounds.

risk for impaired Skin/Tissue Integrity possibly evidenced by risk factors of frequent bowel movements, hyperacidity of liquid stools, esophageal regurgitation.

acute/chronic Pain may be related to acidic irritation of esophageal mucosa (GERD), muscle spasm, possibly evidenced by reports of heartburn, distraction behaviors.

risk for ineffective Health Management possibly evidenced by risk factors of length of therapy, economic difficulties, perceived susceptibility.

APPENDIX A

NANDA-I's Taxonomy II

The 13 domains and their classes are:

Domain 1 Health Promotion: The awareness of well-being or normality of function and the strategies used to maintain control of and enhance that well-being or normality of function

Class 1 Health Awareness: Recognition of normal function and well-being

Class 2 Health Management: Identifying, controlling, performing, and integrating activities to maintain health and well-being

Domain 2 Nutrition: The activities of taking in, assimilating, and using nutrients for the purposes of tissue maintenance, tissue repair, and the production of energy

Class 1 Ingestion: Taking food or nutrients into the body

Class 2 Digestion: The physical and chemical activities that convert foodstuffs into substances suitable for absorption and assimilation

Class 3 Absorption: The act of taking up nutrients through body tissues

Class 4 Metabolism: The chemical and physical processes occurring in living organisms and cells for the development and use of protoplasm and the production of waste and energy, with the release of energy for all vital processes

Class 5 Hydration: The taking in and absorption of fluids and electrolytes

Domain 3 Elimination and Exchange: Secretion and excretion of waste products from the body

Class 1 Urinary Function: The process of secretion, reabsorption, and excretion of urine

Class 2 Gastrointestinal Function: The process of absorption and excretion of the end products of digestion

Class 3 Integumentary Function: The process of secretion and excretion through the skin

Class 4 Respiratory Function: The process of exchange of gases and removal of the end products of metabolism

Domain 4 Activity/Rest: The production, conservation, expenditure, or balance of energy resources

Class 1 Sleep/Rest: Slumber, repose, ease, relaxation, or inactivity

Class 2 Activity/Exercise: Moving parts of the body (mobility), doing work, or performing actions often (but not always) against resistance

Class 3 Energy Balance: A dynamic state of harmony between intake and expenditure of resources

Class 4 Cardiovascular/Pulmonary Responses: Cardiopulmonary mechanisms that support activity/rest

Class 5 Self-Care: Ability to perform activities to care for one's body and bodily functions

Domain 5 Perception/Cognition: The human information-processing system including attention, orientation, sensation, perception, cognition, and communication

Class 1 Attention: Mental readiness to notice or observe

Class 2 Orientation: Awareness of time, place, and person

Class 3 Sensation/Perception: Receiving information through the senses of touch, taste, smell, vision, hearing, and kinesthesia and the comprehension of sensory data resulting in naming, associating, and/or pattern recognition

Class 4 Cognition: Use of memory, learning, thinking, problem solving, abstraction, judgment, insight, intellectual capacity, calculation, and language

Class 5 Communication: Sending and receiving verbal and nonverbal information

Domain 6 Self-Perception: Awareness about the self

Class 1 Self-Concept: The perception(s) about the total self

Class 2 Self-Esteem: Assessment of one's own worth, capability, significance, and success

Class 3 Body Image: A mental image of one's own body

Domain 7 Role Relationships: The positive and negative connections or associations between people or groups of people and the means by which those connections are demonstrated

Class 1 Caregiving Roles: Socially expected behavior patterns by people providing care who are not healthcare professionals

Class 2 Family Relationships: Associations of people who are biologically related or related by choice

Class 3 Role Performance: Quality of functioning in socially expected behavior patterns

Domain 8 Sexuality: Sexual identity, sexual function, and reproduction

Class 1 Sexual Identity: The state of being a specific person in regard to sexuality and/or gender

Class 2 Sexual Function: The capacity or ability to participate in sexual activities

Class 3 Reproduction: Any process by which human beings are produced

Domain 9 Coping/Stress Tolerance: Contending with life events/life processes

Class 1 Posttrauma Responses: Reactions occurring after physical or psychological trauma

Class 2 Coping Responses: The process of managing environmental stress

Class 3 Neurobehavioral Stress: Behavioral responses reflecting nerve and brain function

Domain 10 Life Principles: Principles underlying conduct, thought, and behavior about acts, customs, or institutions viewed as being true or having intrinsic worth

Class 1 Values: The identification and ranking of preferred modes of conduct or end states

Class 2 Beliefs: Opinions, expectations, or judgments about acts, customs, or institutions viewed as being true or having intrinsic worth

Class 3 Value/Belief/Action Congruence: The correspondence or balance achieved among values, beliefs, and actions

Domain 11 Safety/Protection: Freedom from danger, physical injury, or immune system damage; preservation from loss; and protection of safety and security

Class 1 Infection: Host responses following pathogenic invasion

Class 2 Physical Injury: Bodily harm or hurt

Class 3 Violence: The exertion of excessive force or power so as to cause injury or abuse

Class 4 Environmental Hazards: Sources of danger in the surroundings

Class 5 Defensive Processes: The processes by which the self protects itself from the nonself

Class 6 Thermoregulation: The physiological process of regulating heat and energy within the body for purposes of protecting the organism

Domain 12 Comfort: Sense of mental, physical, or social well-being or ease

Class 1 Physical Comfort: Sense of well-being or ease and/or freedom from pain

Class 2 Environmental Comfort: Sense of well-being or ease in/with one's environment

Class 3 Social Comfort: Sense of well-being or ease with one's social situation

Domain 13 Growth/Development: Age-appropriate increases in physical dimensions, maturation of organ systems, and/or progression through the developmental milestones

Class 1 Growth: Increases in physical dimensions or maturity of organ systems

Class 2 Development: Progression or regression through a sequence of recognized milestones in life

APPENDIX B

Definitions of Taxonomy II Axes

AXIS 1 DIAGNOSTIC FOCUS: The focus of the diagnosis (principal element or the fundamental and essential part, the root, of the diagnostic concept)

AXIS 2 SUBJECT OF THE DIAGNOSIS: The subject of the diagnosis. Values are:

Individual: A single human being distinct from others, a person

Caregiver: A family member or helper who regularly looks after a child or sick, elderly, or disabled person

Family: Two or more people having continuous or sustained relationships, perceiving reciprocal obligations, sensing common meaning, and sharing certain obligations toward others; related by blood and/or choice

Group: A number of people with shared characteristics

Community: A group of people living in the same locale under the same governance; examples include neighborhoods and cities

When the unit of care is not explicitly stated, it becomes the individual by default

AXIS 3 JUDGMENT: A descriptor or modifier that limits or specifies the meaning of the diagnostic focus. Values are:

Complicated: Consisting of many interconnecting parts or elements; involving many different and confusing aspects

Compromised: Made vulnerable, or to function less effectively

Decreased: Smaller or fewer in size, amount, intensity, or degree

Defensive: Used or intended to defend or protect

Deficient/Deficit: Not having enough of a specified quality or ingredient; a deficiency or failing, especially in a neurological or psychological function

Delayed: A period of time by which something is late, slow, or postponed

Disabled: Limited in movements, senses, or activities

Disorganized: Not properly arranged or controlled; scattered or inefficient

Disproportionate: Too large or too small in comparison with something else (norm)

Disturbed: Having had its normal pattern or function disrupted

Dysfunctional: Not operating normally or properly; deviating from the norms of social behavior in a way regarded as bad

Emancipated: Free from legal, social, or political restrictions; liberated

Effective: Successful in producing a desired or intended result

Enhanced: Intensified, increased, or further improved the quality, value, or extent of something

Excess: An amount of something that is more than necessary, permitted, or desirable

Failure: The action or state of not functioning

Frail: Weak and delicate

Functional: Affecting the operation, rather than the structure, of an organ

Imbalanced: Lack of proportion or relation between corresponding things

Impaired: Weakened or damaged (something, especially a faculty or function)

Ineffective: Not producing any significant or desired effect

Insufficient: Not enough, inadequate, incapable, incompetent

Interrupted: A stop in continuous progress of (an activity or process); to break the continuity of something

Labile: Of or characterized by emotions that are easily aroused, freely expressed, and tend to alter quickly and spontaneously

Low: Below average in amount, extent, or intensity; small

Organized: Properly arranged or controlled; efficient

Perceived: Become aware of (something) by the use of one of the senses, especially that of sight; interpreted or looked upon (someone or something) in a particular way; regards as; become aware or conscious of (something); realized or understood

Readiness: Willingness to do something; state of being fully prepared for something

Risk: Situation involving exposure to danger, possibility or vulnerability that something unpleasant or unwelcome will happen

Risk-prone: Likely to or liable to suffer from, do, or experience something, typically something regrettable or unwelcome/dangerous

Unstable: Prone to change, fail, or give way; not stable

AXIS 4 LOCATION: Describes the parts/regions of the body and/or their related functions—all tissues, organs, anatomical sites or structures. Values are:

Bed	*Intracranial*	*Wheelchair*
Bladder	*Neurovascular*	
Bowel	*Peripheral*	
Cardiac	*Renal*	
Cerebral	*Urinary*	
Corneal	*Urinary tract*	
Gastrointestinal	*Vascular*	

AXIS 5 AGE: The age of the person who is the subject of the diagnosis. Values are:

Fetus: An unborn human more than 8 weeks after conception until birth

Neonate: A child <28 days of age

Infant: A child ≥28 days and <1 year of age

Child: Person aged 1 to 9 years, inclusive

Adolescent: Person aged 10 to 19 years, inclusive

Adult: A person older than 19 years of age unless national law defines a person as being an adult at an earlier age

Older adult: A person ≥65 years of age

AXIS 6 TIME: The duration of the nursing diagnosis. Values are:

Acute: Lasting <6 months

Chronic: Lasting ≥3 months

Continuous: Uninterrupted, going on without stopping

Intermittent: Stopping or starting again at intervals, periodic, cyclic

Perioperative: Occurring or performed at or around the time of an operation

Situational: Related to a set of circumstances in which one finds oneself

AXIS 7 STATUS OF THE DIAGNOSIS: The actuality or potentiality of the problem/syndrome or the categorization of the diagnosis as a health promotion diagnosis. Values are:

Problem-Focused: An undesirable human response to health conditions/life processes that exists in the current moment (includes problem-focused syndrome diagnoses)

Health Promotion: Motivation and desire to increase well-being and to actualize human health potential that exists in the current moment (Pender, Murdaugh, & Parsons, 2006)

Risk: Vulnerability for developing in the future an undesirable human response to health conditions/life processes (includes risk syndrome diagnoses)

Pender, N. J., Murdaugh, C. L., & Parsons, M. A. (2006). *Health Principles in Nursing Practice* (5th ed.) Upper Saddle River, NJ: Pearson Prentice-Hall.

Permission from NANDA International. (2012). *NANDA-I Nursing Diagnoses: Definitions & Classification 2012–2014.* Oxford: Wiley-Blackwell.

APPENDIX C

NANDA-I Nursing Diagnoses Organized According to Maslow's Hierarchy of Needs

Self-Actualization

Coping, readiness for enhanced
Coping, readiness for enhanced community
Coping, readiness for enhanced family
Decision-Making, readiness for enhanced
Development, risk for delayed
Emancipated Decision-Making, impaired
Emancipated Decision-Making, readiness for enhanced
Emancipated Decision-Making, risk for impaired
Hope, readiness for enhanced
Knowledge, readiness for enhanced
Power, readiness for enhanced
Religiosity, readiness for enhanced
Self-Concept, readiness for enhanced
Spiritual Well-Being, readiness for enhanced

Self-Esteem

Body Image, disturbed
Coping, defensive
Coping, ineffective
Decisional Conflict
Denial, ineffective
Diversional Activity, deficient
Emotional Control, labile
Human Dignity, risk for compromised
Hopelessness
Impulse Control, ineffective
Moral Distress
Mood Regulation, impaired
Noncompliance [Adherence, ineffective] (specify)
Obesity
Overweight
Overweight, risk for
Personal Identity, disturbed
Post-Trauma Syndrome
Post-Trauma Syndrome, risk for
Powerlessness
Powerlessness, risk for
Rape-Trauma Syndrome
Resilience, impaired
Resilience, risk for impaired
Self-Esteem, chronic low
Self-Esteem, situational low
Self-Esteem, risk for chronic low
Self-Esteem, risk for situational low
Self-Mutilation
Self-Mutilation, risk for
Suicide, risk for
Violence, risk for other-directed
Violence, risk for self-directed

Love and Belonging

Attachment, risk for impaired
Communication, readiness for enhanced
Coping, compromised family
Coping, disabled family
Development, risk for delayed
Family Processes, dysfunctional
Family Processes, interrupted
Family Processes, readiness for enhanced
Loneliness, risk for
Parenting, impaired
Parenting, readiness for enhanced
Parenting, risk for impaired
Religiosity, impaired
Religiosity, risk for impaired
Relocation Stress Syndrome
Relocation Stress Syndrome, risk for
Role Conflict, parental
Role Performance, ineffective
Sexual Dysfunction
Social Interaction, impaired
Social Isolation
Sorrow, chronic
Spiritual Distress
Spiritual Distress, risk for

Safety and Security

Allergy Response, risk for
Anxiety
Autonomic Dysreflexia
Autonomic Dysreflexia, risk for
Behavior, readiness for enhanced organized infant
Role Strain, caregiver
Role Strain, risk for caregiver
Communication, impaired verbal
Confusion, acute
Confusion, chronic
Confusion, risk for acute
Contamination
Contamination, risk for
Coping, ineffective community
Death Anxiety
Disuse Syndrome, risk for
Falls, risk for
Fear
Grieving
Grieving, complicated
Grieving, risk for complicated
Health Behavior, risk-prone
Health Maintenance, ineffective
Health Management, ineffective
Health Management, ineffective family
Health Management, readiness for enhanced
Home Maintenance, impaired
Infection, risk for
Injury, risk for
Injury, risk for corneal
Injury, risk for urinary tract
Jaundice, neonatal
Jaundice, risk for neonatal
Knowledge, deficient [Learning Need] (specify)
Latex Allergy Response
Latex Allergy Response, risk for
Lifestyle, sedentary
Maternal-Fetal Dyad, risk for disturbed
Memory, impaired
Mobility, impaired bed
Mobility, impaired wheelchair
Peripheral Neurovascular Dysfunction, risk for
Positioning Injury, risk for perioperative
Poisoning, risk for
Protection, ineffective
Reaction to Iodinated Contrast Media, risk for adverse
Self-Neglect
Sitting, impaired
Standing, impaired
Stress Overload
Sudden Infant Death Syndrome, risk for
Transfer Ability, impaired
Trauma, risk for
Trauma, risk for vascular
Unilateral Neglect
Walking, impaired
Wandering [specify sporadic or continuous]

Physiological Needs

Activity Intolerance [specify level]
Activity Intolerance, risk for
Adaptive Capacity, decreased intracranial
Airway Clearance, ineffective
Aspiration, risk for
Behavior, disorganized infant
Behavior, risk for disorganized infant
Bleeding, risk for
Blood Glucose Level, risk for unstable
Body Temperature, risk for imbalanced
Breast Milk, insufficient
Breastfeeding, ineffective
Breastfeeding, interrupted
Breastfeeding, readiness for enhanced
Breathing Pattern, ineffective
Cardiac Output, decreased
Cardiac Output, risk for decreased
Cardiovascular Function, risk for impaired
Childbearing Process, ineffective
Childbearing Process, risk for ineffective
Comfort, impaired
Comfort, readiness for enhanced
Constipation
Constipation, chronic functional
Constipation, risk for chronic functional
Constipation, perceived
Constipation, risk for
Dentition, impaired
Diarrhea
Electrolyte Imbalance, risk for
Elimination, impaired urinary
Elimination, readiness for enhanced urinary
Frail Elderly Syndrome
Frail Elderly Syndrome, risk for
Fatigue
Feeding Pattern, ineffective infant
Fluid Balance, readiness for enhanced
Fluid Volume, deficient
Fluid Volume, excess
Fluid Volume, risk for deficient
Fluid Volume, risk for imbalanced
Gas Exchange, impaired
Gastrointestinal Motility, dysfunctional
Gastrointestinal Motility, risk for dysfunctional
Gastrointestinal Perfusion, risk for ineffective
Growth, risk for disproportionate
Hyperthermia
Hypothermia
Hypothermia, risk for
Hypothermia, risk for perioperative
Incontinence, bowel
Incontinence, functional urinary
Incontinence, overflow urinary
Incontinence, reflex urinary
Incontinence, stress urinary
Incontinence, urge urinary
Incontinence, risk for urge urinary
Insomnia
Liver Function, risk for impaired
Mobility, impaired physical
Mucous Membrane, impaired oral
Mucous Membrane, risk for impaired oral
Nausea
Nutrition: less than body requirements, imbalanced
Nutrition, readiness for enhanced
Pain, acute
Pain, chronic
Pain, labor
Pain Syndrome, chronic
Pressure Ulcer, risk for
Renal Perfusion, risk for ineffective
Self-Care, readiness for enhanced
Self-Care Deficit (specify): bathing, dressing, feeding, toileting
[Sensory Perception, disturbed (specify: visual, auditory, kinesthetic, gustatory, tactile, olfactory)]
Sexuality Pattern, ineffective
Skin Integrity, impaired
Skin Integrity, risk for impaired
Sleep, readiness for enhanced
Sleep Deprivation
Sleep Pattern, disturbed
Suffocation, risk for
Surgical Recovery, delayed
Surgical Recovery, risk for delayed
Swallowing, impaired
Thermoregulation, ineffective
Tissue Integrity, impaired
Tissue Integrity, risk for impaired
Tissue Perfusion, ineffective peripheral
Tissue Perfusion, risk for decreased cardiac
Tissue Perfusion, risk for ineffective cerebral
Tissue Perfusion, risk for ineffective peripheral
Urinary Retention [acute/chronic]
Ventilation, impaired spontaneous
Ventilatory Weaning Response, dysfunctional

Doenges & Moorhouse's Diagnostic Division Index

ACTIVITY/REST—*Ability to engage in necessary/desired activities of life (work and leisure) and to obtain adequate sleep/rest*

Activity Intolerance [specify level], 32–36
Activity Intolerance, risk for, 35–38
Activity Planning, ineffective, 39–41
Activity Planning, risk for ineffective, 42–44
Disuse Syndrome, risk for, 264–269
Diversional Activity, deficient, 270–273
Fatigue, 317–322
Insomnia, 485–490
Lifestyle, sedentary, 512–516
Mobility, impaired bed, 532–536
Mobility, impaired wheelchair, 541–544
Sleep Deprivation, 799–804
Sleep Pattern, disturbed, 804–807
Sleep, readiness for enhanced, 797–799
Transfer Ability, impaired, 897–899
Walking, impaired, 935–938

CIRCULATION—*Ability to transport oxygen and nutrients necessary to meet cellular needs*

Adaptive Capacity, decreased intracranial, 45–49
Autonomic Dysreflexia, 70–74
Autonomic Dysreflexia, risk for, 74–77
Bleeding, risk for, 86–90
Cardiac Output, decreased, 126–132
Cardiac Output, risk for decreased, 132–135
Cardiovascular Function, risk for impaired, 135–139
Gastrointestinal Perfusion, risk for ineffective, 373–376
Renal Perfusion, risk for ineffective, 692–695
Shock, risk for, 778–782
Tissue Perfusion, ineffective peripheral, 881–885
Tissue Perfusion, risk for decreased cardiac, 885–889
Tissue Perfusion, risk for ineffective cerebral, 889–893
Tissue Perfusion, risk for ineffective peripheral, 893–896

EGO INTEGRITY—*Ability to develop and use skills and behaviors to integrate and manage life experiences*

Anxiety [specify level], 56–61
Body Image, disturbed, 94–98
Coping, defensive, 215–218
Coping, ineffective, 221–226
Coping, readiness for enhanced, 229–231
Death Anxiety, 237–240
Decisional Conflict, 240–243
Decision-Making, readiness for enhanced, 244–246
Denial, ineffective, 247–249
Emancipated Decision-Making, impaired, 293–295
Emancipated Decision-Making, readiness for enhanced, 295–298
Emancipated Decision-Making, risk for impaired, 298
Emotional Control, labile, 299–301
Fear [specify focus], 323–327
Grieving, 377–381
Grieving, complicated, 381–385
Grieving, risk for complicated, 385–388
Health Behavior, risk-prone, 396–399
Hope, readiness for enhanced, 416–418
Hopelessness, 419–423
Human Dignity, risk for compromised, 423–425
Impulse Control, ineffective, 440–443
Mood Regulation, impaired, 544–546
Moral Distress, 547–550
Personal Identity, disturbed, 616–620
Personal Identity, risk for disturbed, 620–623
Post-Trauma Syndrome, 632–637
Post-Trauma Syndrome, risk for, 638–642
Power, readiness for enhanced, 642–644
Powerlessness, 645–649
Powerlessness, risk for, 649–652
Rape-Trauma Syndrome, 658–663
Relationship, ineffective, 665–668
Relationship, readiness for enhanced, 669–671
Relationship, risk for ineffective, 672–675
Religiosity, impaired, 675–678
Religiosity, readiness for enhanced, 678–680
Religiosity, risk for impaired, 681–684
Relocation Stress Syndrome, 684–688
Relocation Stress Syndrome, risk for, 688–691
Resilience, impaired, 695–698
Resilience, readiness for enhanced, 699–701
Resilience, risk for impaired, 702–705
Self-Concept, readiness for enhanced, 733–736
Self-Esteem, chronic low, 736–740
Self-Esteem, risk for chronic low, 740–744
Self-Esteem, risk for situational low, 748–750
Self-Esteem, situational low, 744–748
Sorrow, chronic, 816–819
Spiritual Distress, 819–823
Spiritual Distress, risk for, 823–826
Spiritual Well-Being, readiness for enhanced, 827–829

ELIMINATION—*Ability to excrete waste products*

Constipation, 185–189
Constipation, perceived, 197–199
Constipation, chronic functional, 189–193
Constipation, risk for, 199–202
Diarrhea, 259–263
Elimination, impaired urinary, 286–290
Elimination, readiness for enhanced urinary, 290–292
Gastrointestinal Motility, dysfunctional, 364–368
Gastrointestinal Motility, risk for dysfunctional, 369–372
Incontinence, bowel, 444–447
Incontinence, functional urinary, 447–450
Incontinence, overflow urinary, 451–453
Incontinence, reflex urinary, 454–457
Incontinence, risk for urge urinary, 464–467
Incontinence, stress urinary, 457–460
Incontinence, urge urinary, 460–464
Urinary Retention [acute/chronic], 910–914

FOOD—*Ability to maintain intake of and utilize nutrients and liquids to meet physiological needs*

Blood Glucose Level, risk for unstable, 90–94
Breast Milk, insufficient, 116–120
Breastfeeding, ineffective, 102–108
Breastfeeding, interrupted, 108–112
Breastfeeding, readiness for enhanced, 113–116
Dentition, impaired, 250–254
Electrolyte Imbalance, risk for, 280–285
Feeding Pattern, ineffective infant, 327–330
Fluid Balance, readiness for enhanced, 330–332
[Fluid Volume, deficient (hyper/hypotonic)], 333–337
Fluid Volume, deficient [isotonic], 337–341
Fluid Volume, excess, 341–345
Fluid Volume, risk for deficient, 345–348
Fluid Volume, risk for imbalanced, 349–352
Liver Function, risk for impaired, 516–519
Mucous Membrane, impaired oral, 550–555
Mucous Membrane, risk for impaired oral, 556–558
Nausea, 559–563
Nutrition: less than body requirements, imbalanced, 567–573
Nutrition, readiness for enhanced, 574–576
Obesity, 576–580
Overweight, 580–586
Overweight, risk for, 587–590
Swallowing, impaired, 858–863

HYGIENE—*Ability to perform activities of daily living*
Self-Care, readiness for enhanced, 730–733
Self-Care Deficit: bathing, dressing, feeding, toileting, 723–730
Self-Neglect, 759–762

NEUROSENSORY—*Ability to perceive, integrate, and respond to internal and external cues*
Behavior, disorganized infant, 77–82
Behavior, readiness for enhanced organized infant, 83–85
Behavior, risk for disorganized infant, 85–86
Confusion, acute, 173–177
Confusion, chronic, 177–181
Confusion, risk for acute, 182–184
Dysfunction, risk for peripheral neurovascular, 276–279
Memory, impaired, 529–532
[Sensory Perception, disturbed (specify: visual, auditory, kinesthetic, gustatory, tactile, olfactory)], 763–769
Stress Overload, 833–837
Unilateral Neglect, 905–909

PAIN/DISCOMFORT—*Ability to control internal/external environment to maintain comfort*
Comfort, impaired, 155–159
Comfort, readiness for enhanced, 159–163
Pain, acute, 591–596
Pain, chronic, 596–602
Pain, labor, 602–606
Pain Syndrome, chronic, 596–602

RESPIRATION—*Ability to provide and use oxygen to meet physiological needs*
Airway Clearance, ineffective, 49–53
Aspiration, risk for, 61–65
Breathing Pattern, ineffective, 121–125
Gas Exchange, impaired, 359–363
Ventilation, impaired spontaneous, 918–923
Ventilatory Weaning Response, dysfunctional, 923–928

SAFETY—*Ability to provide safe, growth-promoting environment*
Allergy Response, risk for, 54–56
Body Temperature, risk for imbalanced, 99–102
Contamination, 202–207
Contamination, risk for, 208–211
Dry Eye, risk for, 273–275
Falls, risk for, 301–306
Frail Elderly Syndrome, 352–356
Frail Elderly Syndrome, risk for, 356–358
Health Maintenance, ineffective, 400–403
Home Maintenance, impaired, 413–416
Hyperthermia, 426–430
Hypothermia, 430–434
Hypothermia, risk for, 435–437
Hypothermia, risk for perioperative, 438–440
Infection, risk for, 467–473
Injury, risk for, 473–478
Injury, risk for corneal, 478–481
Injury, risk for urinary tract, 481–485
Jaundice, neonatal, 490–494
Jaundice, risk for neonatal, 495–497
Latex Allergy Response, 505–509
Latex Allergy Response, risk for, 509–512
Maternal-Fetal Dyad, risk for disturbed, 523–529
Mobility, impaired bed, 532–536
Mobility, impaired physical, 536–540
Poisoning, risk for, 623–628
Positioning Injury, risk for perioperative, 628–632
Pressure Ulcer, risk for, 653–656
Protection, ineffective, 656–657
Reaction to Iodinated Contrast Media, risk for adverse, 663–665
Self-Mutilation, 751–755
Self-Mutilation, risk for, 755–758
Sitting, impaired, 782–786
Skin Integrity, impaired, 786–792
Skin Integrity, risk for impaired, 792–796
Standing, impaired, 830–833
Sudden Infant Death Syndrome, risk for, 837–841
Suffocation, risk for, 841–845
Suicide, risk for, 845–850
Surgical Recovery, delayed, 850–855
Surgical Recovery, risk for delayed, 855–858
Thermal Injury, risk for, 864–867
Thermoregulation, ineffective, 868–870
Tissue Integrity, impaired, 870–876
Tissue Integrity, risk for impaired, 877–880
Trauma, risk for, 900–905
Vascular Trauma, risk for, 914–918
Violence, risk for other-directed, 928
Violence, risk for self-directed, 929–935
Wandering [specify: sporadic or continual], 939–942

SEXUALITY—*[Component of Ego Integrity and Social Interaction] Ability to meet requirements/characteristics of male/female role*
Childbearing Process, ineffective, 139–147
Childbearing Process, readiness for enhanced, 147–154
Childbearing Process, risk for ineffective, 154–155
Sexual Dysfunction, 769–774
Sexuality Pattern, ineffective, 774–778

SOCIAL INTERACTION—*Ability to establish and maintain relationships*
Attachment, risk for impaired, 65–69
Communication, impaired verbal, 163–169
Communication, readiness for enhanced, 169–172
Coping, compromised family, 212–214
Coping, defensive, 215–218
Coping, disabled family, 218–221
Coping, ineffective community, 226–229
Coping, readiness for enhanced community, 232–234
Coping, readiness for enhanced family, 234–236
Family Processes, dysfunctional, 306–310
Family Processes, interrupted, 310–314
Family Processes, readiness for enhanced, 314–317
Loneliness, risk for, 520–523
Parenting, impaired, 607–611
Parenting, readiness for enhanced, 612–614
Parenting, risk for impaired, 615
Role Conflict, parental, 705–708
Role Performance, ineffective, 709–712
Role Strain, caregiver, 713–719
Role Strain, risk for caregiver, 719–723
Social Interaction, impaired, 807–811
Social Isolation, 812–815

TEACHING/LEARNING—*Ability to incorporate and use information to achieve health lifestyle/optimal wellness*
Development, risk for delayed, 254–258
Growth, risk for disproportionate, 388–392
Health, deficient community, 392–395
Health Management, ineffective, 404–407
Health Management, ineffective family, 407–410
Health Management, readiness for enhanced, 410–413
Knowledge, deficient [Learning need (specify)], 498–502
Knowledge [specify], readiness for enhanced, 502–504
Noncompliance [ineffective Adherence] [specify], 563–567

Nursing Diagnoses Index

Activity Intolerance [specify level], 32–36
risk for, 36–38
Activity Planning, ineffective, 39–41
Activity Planning, risk for ineffective, 42–44
Adaptive Capacity, decreased intracranial, 45–49
Airway Clearance, ineffective, 49–53
Allergy Response, risk for, 54–56
Anxiety [specify level], 56–61
Aspiration, risk for, 61–65
Attachment, risk for impaired, 65–69
Autonomic Dysreflexia, 70–74
Autonomic Dysreflexia, risk for, 74–77

Behavior, disorganized infant, 77–82
Behavior, readiness for enhanced organized infant, 83–85
Behavior, risk for disorganized infant, 85–86
Bleeding, risk for, 86–90
Blood Glucose Level, risk for unstable, 90–94
Body Image, disturbed, 94–98
Body Temperature, risk for imbalanced, 99–102
Breastfeeding, ineffective, 102–108
Breastfeeding, interrupted, 108–112
Breastfeeding, readiness for enhanced, 113–116
Breast Milk, insufficient, 116–120
Breathing Pattern, ineffective, 121–125

Cardiac Output, decreased, 126–132
Cardiac Output, risk for decreased, 132–135
Cardiovascular Function, risk for impaired, 135–139
Childbearing Process, ineffective, 139–147
Childbearing Process, readiness for enhanced, 147–154
Childbearing Process, risk for ineffective, 154–155
Comfort, impaired, 155–159
Comfort, readiness for enhanced, 159–163
Communication, impaired verbal, 163–169
Communication, readiness for enhanced, 169–172
Confusion, acute, 173–177
Confusion, chronic, 177–181
Confusion, risk for acute, 182–184
Constipation, 185–189
Constipation, chronic functional, 189–193
Constipation, risk for chronic functional, 194–196
Constipation, perceived, 197–199
Constipation, risk for, 199–202
Contamination, 202–207
Contamination, risk for, 208–211
Coping, compromised family, 212–214
Coping, defensive, 215–218
Coping, disabled family, 218–221
Coping, ineffective, 221–226
Coping, ineffective community, 226–229
Coping, readiness for enhanced, 229–231
Coping, readiness for enhanced community, 232–234
Coping, readiness for enhanced family, 234–236

Death Anxiety, 237–240
Decisional Conflict, 240–243
Decision-Making, readiness for enhanced, 244–246
Denial, ineffective, 247–249
Dentition, impaired, 250–254
Development, risk for delayed, 254–258
Diarrhea, 259–263
Disuse Syndrome, risk for, 264–269
Diversional Activity, deficient, 270–273
Dry Eye, risk for, 273–275
Dysfunction, risk for peripheral neurovascular, 276–279

Electrolyte Imbalance, risk for, 280–285
Elimination, impaired urinary, 286–290
Elimination, readiness for enhanced urinary, 290–292
Emancipated Decision-Making, impaired, 293–295
Emancipated Decision-Making, readiness for enhanced, 295–298
Emancipated Decision-Making, risk for impaired, 298
Emotional Control, labile, 299–301

Falls, risk for, 301–306
Family Processes, dysfunctional, 306–310
Family Processes, interrupted, 310–314
Family Processes, readiness for enhanced, 314–317
Fatigue, 317–322
Fear [specify focus], 323–327
Feeding Pattern, ineffective infant, 327–330
Fluid Balance, readiness for enhanced, 330–332
[Fluid Volume, deficient (hyper/hypotonic)], 333–337
Fluid Volume, deficient [isotonic], 337–341
Fluid Volume, excess, 341–345
Fluid Volume, risk for deficient, 345–348
Fluid Volume, risk for imbalanced, 349–352
Frail Elderly Syndrome, 352–356
Frail Elderly Syndrome, risk for, 356–358

Gas exchange, impaired, 359–363
Gastrointestinal Motility, dysfunctional, 364–368
Gastrointestinal Motility, risk for dysfunctional, 369–372
Gastrointestinal Perfusion, risk for ineffective, 373–376
Grieving, 377–381
Grieving, complicated, 381–385
Grieving, risk for complicated, 385–388
Growth, risk for disproportionate, 388–392

Health, deficient community, 392–395
Health Behavior, risk-prone, 396–399
Health Maintenance, ineffective, 400–403
Health Management, ineffective, 404–407
Health Management, ineffective family, 407–410
Health Management, readiness for enhanced, 410–413
Home Maintenance, impaired, 413–416
Hope, readiness for enhanced, 416–418
Hopelessness, 419–423
Human Dignity, risk for compromised, 423–425
Hyperthermia, 426–430
Hypothermia, 430–434
Hypothermia, risk for, 435–437
Hypothermia, risk for perioperative, 438–440

Impulse Control, ineffective, 440–443
Incontinence, bowel, 444–447
Incontinence, functional urinary, 447–450
Incontinence, overflow urinary, 451–453
Incontinence, reflex urinary, 454–457
Incontinence, risk for urge urinary, 464–467
Incontinence, stress urinary, 457–460
Incontinence, urge urinary, 460–464
Infection, risk for, 467–473
Injury, risk for, 473–478
Injury, risk for corneal, 478–481
Injury, risk for urinary tract, 481–485
Insomnia, 485–490

Jaundice, neonatal, 490–494
Jaundice, risk for neonatal, 495–497

Knowledge, deficient [Learning Need (specify)], 498–502
Knowledge [specify], readiness for enhanced, 502–504

Latex Allergy Response, 505–509
Latex Allergy Response, risk for, 509–512
Lifestyle, sedentary, 512–516
Liver Function, risk for impaired, 516–519
Loneliness, risk for, 520–523

Maternal-Fetal Dyad, risk for disturbed, 523–529
Memory, impaired, 529–532
Mobility, impaired bed, 532–536
Mobility, impaired physical, 536–540
Mobility, impaired wheelchair, 541–544
Mood Regulation, impaired, 544–546
Moral Distress, 547–550
Mucous Membrane, impaired oral, 550–555
Mucous Membrane, risk for impaired oral, 556–558

Nausea, 559–563
Noncompliance [ineffective Adherence] [specify], 563–567
Nutrition: less than body requirements, imbalanced, 567–573
Nutrition, readiness for enhanced, 574–576

Obesity, 576–580
Overweight, 580–586
Overweight, risk for, 587–590

Pain, acute, 591–596
Pain, chronic, 596–602
Pain, labor, 602–606
Pain Syndrome, chronic, 596–602
Parenting, impaired, 607–611
Parenting, readiness for enhanced, 612–614
Parenting, risk for impaired, 615–616
Personal Identity, disturbed, 616–620
Personal Identity, risk for disturbed, 620–623
Poisoning, risk for, 623–628
Positioning Injury, risk for perioperative, 628–632
Post-Trauma Syndrome, 632–637
Post-Trauma Syndrome, risk for, 638–642
Power, readiness for enhanced, 642–644
Powerlessness, 645–649
Powerlessness, risk for, 649–652
Pressure Ulcer, risk for, 653–656
Protection, ineffective, 656–657

Rape-Trauma Syndrome, 658–663
Reaction to Iodinated Contrast Media, risk for adverse, 663–665
Relationship, ineffective, 665–668
Relationship, readiness for enhanced, 669–671
Relationship, risk for ineffective, 672–675
Religiosity, impaired, 675–678
Religiosity, readiness for enhanced, 678–680
Religiosity, risk for impaired, 681–684
Relocation Stress Syndrome, 684–688
Relocation Stress Syndrome, risk for, 688–691
Renal Perfusion, risk for ineffective, 692–695
Resilience, impaired individual, 695–698
Resilience, readiness for enhanced, 699–701
Resilience, risk for impaired, 702–705
Role Conflict, parental, 705–708
Role Performance, ineffective, 709–712
Role Strain, caregiver, 713–719
Role Strain, risk for caregiver, 719–723

Self-Care, readiness for enhanced, 730–733
Self-Care Deficit: bathing, dressing, feeding, toileting, 723–730
Self-Concept, readiness for enhanced, 733–736
Self-Esteem, chronic low, 736–740
Self-Esteem, risk for chronic low, 740–744
Self-Esteem, risk for situational low, 748–750
Self-Esteem, situational low, 744–748
Self-Mutilation, 751–755
Self-Mutilation, risk for, 755–758
Self-Neglect, 759–762
[Sensory Perception, disturbed, (specify: visual, auditory, kinesthetic, gustatory, tactile, olfactory)], 763–769
Sexual Dysfunction, 769–774
Sexuality Pattern, ineffective, 774–778
Shock, risk for, 778–782
Sitting, impaired, 782–786
Skin Integrity, impaired, 786–792
Skin Integrity, risk for impaired, 792–796
Sleep, readiness for enhanced, 797–799
Sleep Deprivation, 799–804
Sleep Pattern, disturbed, 804–807
Social Interaction, impaired, 807–811
Social Isolation, 812–815
Sorrow, chronic, 816–819
Spiritual Distress, 819–823
Spiritual Distress, risk for, 823–826
Spiritual Well-Being, readiness for enhanced, 827–829
Standing, impaired, 830–833
Stress Overload, 833–837
Sudden Infant Death Syndrome, risk for, 837–841
Suffocation, risk for, 841–845
Suicide, risk for, 845–850
Surgical Recovery, delayed, 850–855
Surgical Recovery, risk for delayed, 855–858
Swallowing, impaired, 858–863

Thermal Injury, risk for, 864–867
Thermoregulation, ineffective, 868–870
Tissue Integrity, impaired, 870–876
Tissue Integrity, risk for impaired, 877–880
Tissue Perfusion, ineffective peripheral, 881–885
Tissue Perfusion, risk for decreased cardiac, 885–889
Tissue Perfusion, risk for ineffective cerebral, 889–893
Tissue Perfusion, risk for ineffective peripheral, 893–896
Transfer Ability, impaired, 897–899
Trauma, risk for, 900–905

Unilateral Neglect, 905–909
Urinary Retention [acute/chronic], 910–914

Vascular Trauma, risk for, 914–918
Ventilation, impaired, spontaneous, 918–923
Ventilatory Weaning Response, dysfunctional, 923–928
Violence, risk for other-directed, 928
Violence, risk for self-directed, 929–935

Walking, impaired, 935–938
Wandering [specify: sporadic or continual], 939–942

Index

Abdominal hysterectomy. *See* Hysterectomy
Abdominal perineal resection, 943
Abortion
elective termination, 943–944
spontaneous termination, 944
Abruptio placentae, 944
Abscess
brain, 944
gingival, 944
skin/tissue, 944
Abuse
physical, 944–945
psychological, 945
Achalasia (cardiospasm), 945
Acidosis
metabolic, 945
respiratory, 945
Acne, 945
Acoustic neuroma, 945
Acquired immune deficiency syndrome. *See* AIDS
Acromegaly, 945–946
Activity intolerance [specify level], 32–36
in anemia, 950
in angina pectoris, 952
in aortic stenosis, 954
in asbestosis, 956
in asthma, 956
in atrial fibrillation, 957
in bronchitis, 961
in carbon monoxide poisoning, 963
in cardiomyopathy, 964
in chronic obstructive lung disease, 968
in cor pulmonale, 972
in coronary artery disease, 972
definition of, 32
documentation focus, 35
in dysfunctional uterine bleeding, 1061
in emphysema, 985
in endocarditis, 986
in heart failure, 995
in high-risk pregnancy, 1036
in hospice care, 999
in leukemia, 1011
in mesothelioma, 1016
in mitral stenosis, 1016
in multiple organ dysfunction syndrome, 1017
in myocarditis, 1019
nursing priorities, 33–35
in obesity, 1023
in pericarditis, 1028
in peripheral vascular disease, 1029
in polycythemia vera, 1032
in preterm labor, 1008
in pulmonary fibrosis, 1039
in pulmonary hypertension, 1039
in purpura, 1039
in rheumatic fever, 1044
in rheumatic heart disease, 1044
risk for, 35–38
in cardiac conditions, prenatal, 964
in cardiac dysrhythmia, 983
definition of, 35
documentation focus, 38
in hypertension, 1001
NIC linkages, 37
NOC linkages, 36–37
nursing priorities, 37–38
in tuberculosis, 1059
in valvular heart disease, 1062
in ventricular aneurysm, 951
Activity planning, ineffective, 39–41
definition of, 39
documentation focus, 41
NIC linkages, 39
NOC linkages, 39
nursing priorities, 39–41
risk for, 42–44
definition of, 42
documentation focus, 43–44
NIC linkages, 42
NOC linkages, 42
nursing priorities, 42–43
Acute confusion, 173–177
Adams-Stokes syndrome. *See* Dysrhythmia, cardiac
ADD. *See* Attention deficit disorder
Addiction. *See* Substance dependence/abuse; *specific substances*
Addison's disease, 946
Adenoidectomy, 946
Adjustment disorder. *See* Anxiety disorders
Adoption/loss of child custody, 946
Adrenal crisis, acute, 946–947
Adrenal insufficiency. *See* Addison's disease
Adrenalectomy, 947
Adverse reaction to iodinated contrast media, risk for, in cardiac catheterization, 963
Affective disorder. *See also* Bipolar disorder; Depression, major
seasonal, 947
Agoraphobia, 947
Agranulocytosis, 947
AIDS, 947–948. *See also* HIV infection
AIDS dementia, 948
Airway clearance, ineffective, 49–53
in anaphylaxis, 950
in asbestosis, 956
in asthma, 956
in bronchitis, 961
in bronchopneumonia, 961
in chronic obstructive lung disease, 968
in croup, 973
in cystic fibrosis, 974
definition of, 49
documentation focus, 56
in emphysema, 985
in foreign body aspiration, 956
in gas, lung irritant, 990
in infant of addicted mother, 1004
in laryngectomy, 1010
in Legionnaire's disease, 1011
in myasthenia gravis, 1018
NIC linkages, 50
NOC linkages, 50
nursing priorities, 50–53
in pertussis, 1029
in postpolio syndrome, 1034
in rabies, 1040
in respiratory distress syndrome, acute, 1042
in respiratory syncytial virus, 1043
risk for
in adenoidectomy, 946
in bronchogenic carcinoma, 961
in burns, 962
in cervical laminectomy, 1009
in facial reconstructive surgery, 987
in goiter, 992
in Guillain-Barré syndrome, 993
in Hodgkin's disease, 999
in hypoparathyroidism, 1002
in intermaxillary fixation, 1006
in parathyroidectomy, 1026
in thyroidectomy, 1056
in tuberculosis, 1059
in ventilator assist/dependence, 1063
Alcohol abuse/withdrawal. *See* Alcohol intoxication, acute; Delirium tremens; Substance dependence/abuse
Alcohol intoxication, acute, 948
Alcoholism. *See* Substance dependence/abuse
Aldosteronism, primary, 948
Alkalosis, respiratory, 948
Allergies, seasonal. *See* Hay fever
Allergy response
latex, 505–509
risk for, 54–56
definition of, 54
documentation focus, 56
NIC linkages, 54
NOC linkages, 54
nursing priorities, 54–55
Alopecia, 948–949
ALS. *See* Amyotrophic lateral sclerosis
Alzheimer's disease, 949
Amenorrhea, 949
American Nurses Association (ANA), 1–2
standards of nursing practice of, 5–6
Amphetamine abuse. *See* Stimulant abuse
Amputation, 949–950
Amyotrophic lateral sclerosis, 950
Anaphylaxis, 950. *See* Shock
Anemia, 950–951
aplastic, 954

iron-deficiency, 950
pernicious, 950–951
sickle-cell, 951
Anencephaly, 951. *See also* Perinatal loss/ death of child
Aneurysm
abdominal aortic. *See* Aortic aneurysm, abdominal (AAA)
cerebral. *See* Cerebrovascular accident
ventricular, 951
Angina pectoris, 951–952
Anorexia nervosa, 952
Anthrax
cutaneous, 952
gastrointestinal, 952
inhalation (pulmonary), 952–953
Antisocial personality disorder, 953
Anxiety disorder(s), 754
generalized, 953
Anxiety [specify level], 56–61
in abdominal aortic aneurysm repair, 954
in abortion, 943
in achalasia, 945
in adenoidectomy, 946
in agoraphobia, 947
in anencephaly, 951
in angina pectoris, 952
in anxiety disorder, 953, 954
in asthma, 956
in atrial flutter, 957
in benign prostatic hyperplasia, 958
in borderline personality disorder, 959
in botulism, 960
in breast cancer, 960
in breech labor, 1007
in cardiac catheterization, 963
in cataract, 965
death, 237–240. *See also* Death anxiety
definition of, 56
in dehiscence, 975
in delirium tremens, 975
in delusional disorder, 976
in depression, 977
in diabetes mellitus, intrapartum, 979
in disseminated intravascular coagulation, 981
in dissociative disorders, 981
documentation focus, 60–61
in Dressler's syndrome, 982
in dysfunctional uterine bleeding, 1061
in dyspareunia, 983
in eclampsia, 984
in ectopic pregnancy, 984
in endocarditis, 985–986
in epistaxis, 987
in esophageal varices, 1062
in facial reconstructive surgery, 987
in fibrocystic breast disease, 989
in foreign body aspiration, 956
in gas, lung irritant, 990
in gas gangrene, 990
in gastrointestinal anthrax, 952
in gender identity disorder, 991
in genetic disorder, 991
in glaucoma, 992
in goiter, 992
in Guillain-Barré syndrome, 993
in Gulf War syndrome, 993
in hallucinogen abuse, 993
in hantavirus pulmonary syndrome, 994
in hemothorax, 997
in heroin withdrawal, 998
in high-risk pregnancy, 1036
in HIV dementia, 976
in Hodgkin's disease, 999
in hyperthyroidism, 1002
in hypoparathyroidism, 1002
in hypophysectomy, 1002
in inhalation anthrax, 953
in latex allergy, 1010
in leukemia, 1011
in long-term care, 1012
in LSD intoxication, 1012
in macular degeneration, 1013
in membranous croup, 974
in multiple organ dysfunction syndrome, 1017
in myasthenia gravis, 1018
in myocardial infarction, 1018
NIC linkages, 57
NOC linkages, 57
nursing priorities, 58–60
in obsessive-compulsive disorder, 1023
in panic disorder, 1025
in paranoid personality disorder, 1026
in passive-aggressive personality disorder, 1028
in peptic ulcer, 1060
in pericarditis, 1029
in pheochromocytoma, 1030
in postconcussion syndrome, 1032
in postmaturity pregnancy, 1036
in postpartum hemorrhage, 996
in postpolio syndrome, 1034
in precipitous labor, 1008
in premature dilation of cervix, 981
in premenstrual dysphoric disorder, 1037
in pulmonary edema, 984, 1038
in pulmonary embolus, 1038
in pulmonary fibrosis, 1039
in pulmonary hypertension, 1039
in radiation syndrome/poisoning, 1040
in respiratory distress syndrome, acute, 1042
in retinal detachment, 1043
risk for
in labor, 1008
in preterm labor, 1008
in sexual desire disorder, 1048
in shock, 1048
in smallpox, 1049
in snake bite, 1050
in snow blindness, 1050
in stimulant abuse, 1051
in surgery, 1053
in syringomyelia, 1054
in thrombophlebitis, 1055
in thyrotoxicosis, 1056
in transfusion reaction, 1058
in transient ischemic attack, 1058
in transplant, 1058
in transplantation recipient, 1058
in unplanned cesarean birth, 967
in uterine rupture, 1061
in valvular heart disease, 1062
in ventilator assist/dependence, 1063
in Wilms' tumor, 1064
Anxiolytic abuse. *See* Depressant abuse
Aortic aneurysm, abdominal (AAA), 954
Aortic aneurysm repair, abdominal, 954. *See also* Surgery, general
Aortic insufficiency. *See* Valvular heart disease
Aortic stenosis, 954. *See also* Valvular heart disease
Aplastic anemia, 954
Appendectomy, 954
Appendicitis, 955
ARDS. *See* Respiratory distress syndrome, acute
Arrhythmia, cardiac. *See* Dysrhythmia, cardiac
Arterial occlusive disease, peripheral, 955
Arthritis
gouty, 993
juvenile rheumatoid, 955
rheumatoid, 955
septic, 955
Arthroplasty, 955
Arthroscopy, knee, 956
Asbestosis, 956
Asperger's disorder, 956
Aspiration
foreign body, 956
risk for, 61–65
in achalasia, 945
in alcohol intoxication, 948
in cleft lip/palate, 969
definition of, 61
documentation focus, 64–65
in enteral feeding, 986
in epistaxis, 987
in GERD, 991
in intermaxillary fixation, 1006
in laryngectomy, 1010
NIC linkages, 62
NOC linkages, 62
nursing priorities, 62–64
Assessment, 3
process of, 13–23
client database in, 13
documenting and clustering data on, 11–22
interview in, 13–14
laboratory tests/diagnostic procedures in, 15
physical examination in, 14
reviewing and validating findings in, 22
Assessment tool, 15–22
Asthma, 956
Atelectasis, 956
Atherosclerosis. *See* Coronary artery disease; Peripheral vascular disease (atherosclerosis)
Athlete's foot, 957
Atrial fibrillation, 957
Atrial flutter, 957
Atrial tachycardia. *See* Dysrhythmia
Attachment, risk for impaired, 65–69
in cesarean birth, 966
definition of, 65

documentation focus, 68–69
in Down syndrome, 982
in labor, stage III and IV, 1009
in newborn, 1021
NIC linkages, 66
NOC linkages, 66
nursing priorities, 66–68
in postpartum depression, 977
in postpartum diabetes mellitus, 979
in postpartum hemorrhage, 996
in postpartum period, 1033
in puerperal infection, 1005
in puerperal sepsis, 1047
in respiratory distress syndrome, in premature infant, 1043
in special needs newborn, 1022
Attention deficit disorder, 957
Autism spectrum disorder, 957–958
Autonomic dysreflexia, 70–74
definition of, 70
documentation focus, 73
NIC linkages, 70–71
NOC linkages, 70
nursing priorities, 71–73
risk for, 74–77
definition of, 74
documentation focus, 76–77
NIC linkages, 75
NOC linkages, 75
nursing priorities, 75–76
in quadriplegia, 1040

Bacteremia. *See* Sepsis
Barbiturate abuse. *See* Depressant abuse
Bathing, self-care deficit for, 723–730
Battered child syndrome, 958
Bed-wetting. *See* Enuresis
Bedsores. *See* Ulcer, decubitus
Behavior
disorganized infant, 77–82
definition of, 77
documentation focus, 82
in fetal alcohol syndrome, 988
NIC linkages, 78
NOC linkages, 78
nursing priorities, 79–82
risk for, in newborn with growth deviations, 1021
readiness for enhanced organized infant, 83–85
definition of, 83
documentation focus, 84–85
NIC linkages, 83
NOC linkages, 83
nursing priorities, 83–84
risk for disorganized infant, 85–86
definition of, 85
in infant at 4 weeks, 1004
NOC linkages, 85–86
in premature newborn, 1022
risk-prone health, 396–399. *See also* Health behavior, risk-prone
Benign prostatic hyperplasia, 958
Besnier-Boeck disease. *See* Sarcoidosis
Biliary calculus. *See* Cholelithiasis
Biliary cancer, 958
Binge-eating disorder. *See* Bulimia nervosa
Bipolar disorder, 958–959
Bladder cancer, 959
Bleeding, risk for, 86–90
in abdominal aortic aneurysm repair, 954
in abortion, 944
in abruptio placentae, 944
in arthroplasty, 955
in burns, 962
in cardiac surgery, 964
in cesarean birth, 966
in cholecystectomy, 967
in circumcision, 968
in cirrhosis, 968–969
definition of, 86
documentation focus, 89
in ectopic pregnancy, 984
in esophageal varices, 1062
in gastritis, 990
in gunshot wound, 1064
in hemophilia, 996
in labor, stage III and IV, 1009
in leukemia, 1011
NIC linkages, 87
NOC linkages, 86–87
nursing priorities, 87–89
in pancreatitis, 1025
in placenta previa, 1030
in postpartum period, 1033
in prostatectomy, 1037
in renal failure, 1042
Blood glucose level, risk for unstable, 90–94
definition of, 90
in diabetes mellitus, 978
in diabetic ketoacidosis, 979
documentation focus, 93
in gestational diabetes, 978
in hypoglycemia, 1002
in metabolic syndrome, 1016
NIC linkages, 91
NOC linkages, 90–91
nursing priorities, 91–93
in pancreatitis, 1025
in postpartum diabetes mellitus, 979
Body dysmorphic disorder. *See* Hypochondriasis
Body image, disturbed, 94–98
in abdominal perineal resection, 943
in acne, 945
in acromegaly, 945
in Addison's disease, 946
in alopecia, 948–949
in anorexia nervosa, 952
in cerebrovascular accident, 966
in chemotherapy, 967
in cirrhosis, 969
in colostomy, 970
in Cushing's syndrome, 974
definition of, 94
in dialysis, 979
documentation focus, 98
in encopresis, 985
in enuresis, 986
in facial reconstructive surgery, 987
in goiter, 992
in Hansen's disease, 994
in Kaposi's sarcoma, 1006–1007
in lymphedema, 1013
in mastectomy, 1014
in myxedema, 1019
NIC linkages, 95
NOC linkages, 95
nursing priorities, 95–98
in obesity, 1023
in ovarian cancer, 1024
in Paget's disease, 1024
in postpartum period, 1033
in prostatectomy, 1037
in psoriasis, 1038
in renal transplantation, 1042
in rheumatoid arthritis, 955
risk for
in breast cancer, 961
in cleft lip/palate, 969
in pregnancy, 1035
in skin cancer, 1049
in scleroderma, 1046
in scoliosis, 1046–1047
in systemic lupus erythematosus, 1013
in testicular cancer, 1055
in urinary diversion, 1061
in varicose veins, 1062
Body temperature, risk for imbalanced, 99–102
definition of, 99
documentation focus, 101
NIC linkages, 99
NOC linkages, 99
nursing priorities, 99–101
in postoperative recovery period, 1032
in transfusion reaction, 1057
Bone cancer, 959
Bone marrow transplantation, 959
Borderline personality disorder, 959–960
Botulism, 960
Bowel incontinence. *See* Incontinence, bowel
Bowel obstruction. *See* Ileus
Bowel resection. *See* Intestinal surgery
BPH. *See* Benign prostatic hyperplasia
Brachytherapy (radioactive implants), 960
Bradycardia. *See* Dysrhythmia, cardiac
Brain abscess, 944
Brain attack. *See* Cerebrovascular accident
Brain tumor, 960
Breast cancer, 960–961
Breast milk, insufficient, 116–120
definition of, 116
documentation focus, 119–120
NIC linkages, 117
NOC linkages, 117
nursing priorities, 117–119
Breastfeeding
ineffective, 102–108
definition of, 102
documentation focus, 107
in mastitis, 1014
NIC linkages, 103
NOC linkages, 103
nursing priorities, 103–107
interrupted, 108–112
definition of, 108
documentation focus, 111–112
NIC linkages, 109

NOC linkages, 108–109
nursing priorities, 109–111
in postpartum period, 1033
readiness for enhanced, 113–116
definition of, 113
documentation focus, 115–116
NIC linkages, 113
NOC linkages, 113
nursing priorities, 113–115
Breathing pattern, ineffective, 121–125
in abdominal compartment syndrome, 970
in amyotrophic lateral sclerosis, 950
in cholecystectomy, 967
in cocaine poisoning, 969
definition of, 121
documentation focus, 125
in drug overdose, 982
in gastroplasty, 991
in Guillain-Barré syndrome, 993
in myasthenia gravis, 1018
in nephrectomy, 1020
NIC linkages, 122
NOC linkages, 121
nursing priorities, 122–125
in pickwickian syndrome, 1030
in pleural effusion, 1031
in pleurisy, 1031
in pneumothorax, 1031
in poliomyelitis, 1031
in postoperative recovery period, 1032
in pregnancy, 1035
in premature newborn, 1021
in pulmonary embolus, 1038
in quadriplegia, 1039
in Reye's syndrome, 1044
risk for
in AIDS, 947
in alcohol intoxication, 948
in Dressler's syndrome, 982
in epidural hematoma, 995
in Hodgkin's disease, 999
in influenza, 1005
in peritoneal dialysis, 980
in traumatic brain injury, 1058
in trichinosis, 1059
in ventilator assist/dependence, 1063
Bronchitis, 961
Bronchogenic carcinoma, 916
Bronchopneumonia, 961
Brown-Sequard syndrome, 961
Buck's traction. *See* Traction
Buerger's disease. *See* Peripheral vascular disease (atherosclerosis)
Bulimia nervosa, 961–962
Bunion, 962
Bunionectomy, 962
Burns, 962
Bursitis, 962

C-section. *See* Cesarean birth, unplanned
CABG. *See* Coronary artery bypass surgery
CAD. *See* Coronary artery disease
Calculi, urinary, 962–963
Cancer, 963. *See also specific types*
Candidiasis, 963
Cannabis abuse. *See* Depressant abuse
Carbon monoxide poisoning, 963
Cardiac catheterization, 963
Cardiac conditions, prenatal, 964
Cardiac inflammatory disease. *See* Endocarditis; Myocarditis; Pericarditis
Cardiac output
decreased, 126–132
in Addison's disease, 946
in anaphylaxis, 950
in angina pectoris, 952
in aortic stenosis, 954
in cardiogenic shock, 1048
in cardiomyopathy, 964
definition of, 126
in digitalis toxicity, 980
documentation focus, 131
in gestational hypertension, 1001
in heart failure, 995
in heatstroke, 995
in mitral stenosis, 1016
in myocardial infarction, 1018
in myocarditis, 1019
NIC linkages, 127
NOC linkages, 126–127
in nonketotic hyperglycemic-hyperosmolar coma, 1022
nursing priorities, 127–131
in pheochromocytoma, 1030
in pulmonary hypertension, 1039
in renal failure, 1042
risk for
in aldosteronism, 948
in cardiac catheterization, 963
in cardiac conditions, prenatal, 964
in cardiac dysrhythmia, 983
in cardiac surgery, 964
in cocaine poisoning, 969
in coronary artery bypass surgery, 972
in coronary artery disease, 972
in delirium tremens, 975
in electrical injury, 984
in endocarditis, 985
in hypertension, 1001
in Kawasaki disease, 1007
in labor, 1008
in Lyme disease, 1013
in myxedema, 1019
in Paget's disease, 1025
in pericarditis, 1028
in pneumothorax, 1031
in respiratory distress syndrome, acute, 1042
in rheumatic fever, 1044
in sepsis, 1047
in thyrotoxicosis, 1056
in toxic enterocolitis, 1057
in sick sinus syndrome, 1049
in twin-twin transfusion syndrome, 1060
in valvular heart disease, 1062
in ventricular aneurysm, 951
in ventricular fibrillation, 1063
in ventricular tachycardia, 1063
fluctuations in, in labor, stage II, 1008–1009
[maximally compensated], in pregnancy, 1035
risk for [decompensated], in pregnancy, 1035
risk for decreased, 132–135
definition of, 132
documentation focus, 134
NIC linkages, 133
NOC linkages, 132
nursing priorities, 133–134
Cardiac surgery, 964
Cardiogenic shock. *See* Shock, cardiogenic
Cardiomyopathy, 964
Cardiospasm. *See* Achalasia (cardiospasm)
Cardiovascular function, risk for impaired, 135–139
definition of, 135
documentation focus, 138
NIC linkages, 136
NOC linkages, 135
nursing priorities, 136–138
Care plan, concept mapping, 27–30
Caregiver role strain, 713–719
in Alzheimer's disease, 949
in amyotrophic lateral sclerosis, 950
definition of, 713
in dementia, 976
documentation focus, 718
in hospice care, 999
NIC linkages, 715
NOC linkages, 715
nursing priorities, 715–718
in Parkinson's disease, 1027–1028
risk for, 719–723
in Creutzfeldt-Jakob disease, 973
definition of, 719
documentation focus, 722
in Huntington's disease, 999–1000
NIC linkages, 720
NOC linkages, 720
nursing priorities, 720–722
Carotid endarterectomy, 964
Carpal tunnel syndrome, 964
Casts, 964–965
Cat scratch disease, 965
Cataract, 965
Cataract extraction, 965
Celiac disease, 965
Cellulitis, 965
Cerebral embolism. *See* Cerebrovascular accident
Cerebral palsy. *See* Palsy, cerebral
Cerebrovascular accident, 965–966
Cervix, dysfunctional. *See* Dilation of cervix, premature
Cesarean birth, 966
postpartal, 966
unplanned, 967
Chemotherapy, 967
Chickenpox. *See* Measles
Childbearing process
ineffective, 139–147
definition of, 139
documentation focus, 146
NIC linkages, 140
NOC linkages, 140
nursing priorities, 141–145

risk for, 154–155
definition of, 154
NOC linkages, 154–155
readiness for enhanced, 147–154
definition of, 147
documentation focus, 153
NIC linkages, 148
NOC linkages, 148
nursing priorities, 148–153
Chlamydia trachomatis infection. *See* Sexually transmitted infection
Cholecystectomy, 967
Cholelithiasis, 967–968
Cholera, 968
Christmas disease. *See* Hemophilia
Chronic obstructive lung disease, 968
Circumcision, 968
Cirrhosis, 969
Cleft lip/palate, 969
Client care, concept mapping, 24–26
Client database, 13
Clients, interviewing, 13–14
Clinical Care Classification, 10
Cocaine hydrochloride poisoning, acute, 969
Coccidioidomycosis, 969
Code of Ethics for Nurses, 3
Colectomy. *See* Intestinal surgery
Colitis, ulcerative, 969–970
Collagen disorders. *See* Arthritis; Lupus erythematosus, systemic; Polyarteritis nodosa; Temporal arteritis
Colorectal cancer. *See* Cancer; Colostomy
Colostomy, 905
Coma, 970
Diabetic. *See* Diabetic ketoacidosis
Comfort
impaired, 155–159
in abortion, 943
after cesarean birth, 966
in candidiasis, 963
in cardiac surgery, 964
in cellulitis, 965
in conjunctivitis, 971
in contact dermatitis, 977
in cutaneous anthrax, 952
definition of, 155
documentation focus, 158–159
in drug withdrawal, 982
in ebola, 983
in eczema, 984
in hantavirus pulmonary syndrome, 994
in hay fever, 994
in heroin withdrawal, 998
in Hodgkin's disease, 999
in infectious mononucleosis, 1016
in influenza, 1005
in inhalation anthrax, 952
in labor, 1008
in Legionnaires' disease, 1011
in malaria, 1013
in measles, 1014
NIC linkages, 156
NOC linkages, 155
nursing priorities, 156–158
in pancreatic cancer, 1025
in peritoneal dialysis, 980
in postpartum period, 1033
in pregnancy, 1035
in prenatal infection, 1005
in prostatitis, 1038
in rubella, 1044
in SARS, 1045
in scarlet fever, 1045
in snake bite, 1050
in thrombophlebitis, 1055
in uterine myomas, 1061
in vasectomy, 1063
in venous insufficiency, 1063
in viral hepatitis, 997
readiness for enhanced, 159–163
definition of, 159
documentation focus, 163
NIC linkages, 160
NOC linkages, 160
nursing priorities, 160–162
Communication
impaired verbal, 163–169
in amyotrophic lateral sclerosis, 950
in autism spectrum disorder, 957
in cerebrovascular accident, 966
definition of, 163
documentation focus, 168
in intermaxillary fixation, 1006
in laryngectomy, 1010
in mental delay, 1015
in myasthenia gravis, 1018
NIC linkages, 164–165
NOC linkages, 164
nursing priorities, 165–168
in Parkinson's disease, 1027
risk for, in cleft lip/palate, 969
in schizophrenia, 1045
in thyroidectomy, 1056
in ventilator assist/dependence, 1063
readiness for enhanced, 169–172
definition of, 169
documentation focus, 172
NIC linkages, 170
NOC linkages, 169
nursing priorities, 170–172
Community health, deficient, 392–395
Compartment syndrome, abdominal, 970
Complex regional pain syndrome, 971. *See also* Reflex sympathetic dystrophy
Concept map, components of, 25–26
Concept mapping, 24–31
client care, 24–26
plan of care, 27–30
Concussion, brain, 971
Conduct disorder, 971
Conflict
decisional, 240–243
parental role, 705–708
Confusion
acute, 173–177
in alcohol intoxication, 948
in brain abscess, 944
definition of, 173
documentation focus, 176
in ebola, 984
in electroconvulsive therapy, 985
in epidural hematoma, 995
in HIV dementia, 976
in hypoglycemia, 1002
in lightning injury, 1011
NIC linkages, 173–174
NOC linkages, 173
nursing priorities, 174–176
in radiation syndrome/poisoning, 1040
risk for, 182–184
in cirrhosis, 969
definition of, 182
documentation focus, 184
NIC linkages, 182
NOC linkages, 182
nursing priorities, 182–184
in postoperative recovery period, 1032
in renal failure, 1042
chronic, 177–181
in AIDS, 948
in AIDS dementia, 948
in Alzheimer's disease, 949
definition of, 177
documentation focus, 181
in HIV dementia, 976
in Huntington's disease, 999
NIC linkages, 178
NOC linkages, 178
nursing priorities, 178–180
in subdural-chronic hematoma, 995
in traumatic brain injury, 1059
Congestive heart failure. *See* Heart failure, chronic
Conjunctivitis, bacterial, 971–972
Connective tissue disease. *See* Arthritis; Lupus erythematosus, systemic; Polyarteritis nodosa; Temporal arteritis
Conn's syndrome. *See* Aldosteronism, primary
Constipation, 185–202, 972
chronic functional, 189–193
definition of, 189
documentation focus, 193
NIC linkages, 191
NOC linkages, 190
nursing priorities, 191–192
risk for, 194–196
definition of, 194
documentation focus, 196
NIC linkages, 194
NOC linkages, 194
nursing priorities, 194–196
definition of, 185
in diverticulitis, 981–982
documentation focus, 188–189
in fecal impaction, 988
in hemorrhoids, 996
in hypothyroidism, 1003
in IBS, 1006
in ileus, 1003
in intestinal surgery, 1006
in nephrectomy, 1020
NIC linkages, 186
NOC linkages, 186
nursing priorities, 186–188
perceived, 197–199
definition of, 197
documentation focus, 198
in laxative abuse, 1010
NIC linkages, 197

NOC linkages, 197
nursing priorities, 197–198
in postpartum period, 1033
in quadriplegia, 1040
risk for, 199–202
in abdominal perineal resection, 943
in colostomy, 970
definition of, 199
documentation focus, 201
in newborn at 1 week, 1021
NIC linkages, 200
NOC linkages, 199–200
nursing priorities, 200–201
in pernicious anemia, 950
in pregnancy, 1035
in total joint replacement, 1057
in spina bifida, 1050
Contamination, 202–207
in botulism, 960
definition of, 202
documentation focus, 206–207
in lead poisoning, 1010
NIC linkages, 203–204
NOC linkages, 203
nursing priorities, 204–206
risk for, 208–211
in asthma, 956
definition of, 208
documentation focus, 211
NIC linkages, 209
NOC linkages, 208–209
nursing priorities, 209–211
in sick building syndrome, 1048
Contrast media, iodinated, adverse reaction to, risk for, 663–665
Conversion disorder. *See* Somatoform disorders
Convulsions. *See* Seizure disorders
COPD. *See* Chronic obstructive lung disease
Coping
community
ineffective, 226–229
definition of, 226
documentation focus, 228
NIC linkages, 227
NOC linkages, 227
nursing priorities, 227–228
in smallpox, 1050
readiness for enhanced, 232–234
definition of, 232
documentation focus, 233–234
NIC linkages, 232
NOC linkages, 232
nursing priorities, 232–233
defensive, 215–218
in conduct disorder, 971
definition of, 215
documentation focus, 217
in hyperactivity disorder, 1000
NIC linkages, 215–216
NOC linkages, 215
nursing priorities, 216–217
family
compromised, 212–214
in Alzheimer's disease, 949
in antisocial personality disorder, 953
in anxiety disorder, 953, 954
in autism spectrum disorder, 957–958
in cerebral palsy, 1025
in conduct disorder, 971
in cystic fibrosis, 974
definition of, 212
in dialysis, 980
in dissociative disorders, 981
documentation focus, 214
in encopresis, 985
in enuresis, 986
in gender identity disorder, 991
in hemophilia, 996
in HIV dementia, 976
in hospice care, 999
in juvenile diabetes mellitus, 978
in mental delay, 1015
in multiple sclerosis, 1017
in muscular dystrophy, 1018
NIC linkages, 213
NOC linkages, 212–213
nursing priorities, 213–214
in oppositional defiant disorder, 1023
in paranoid personality disorder, 1026
in parent-child relational problem, 1027
in postpartum period, 1033
in pregnancy, 1035
in renal transplantation, 1042
risk for
in complex regional pain syndrome, 971
in reflex sympathetic dystrophy, 1041
in sickle cell anemia, 951
in substance dependence/abuse, prenatal, 1052
in suicide attempt, 1053
in Tay-Sachs disease, 1054–1055
in transplantation recipient, 1058
disabled, 218–221
in autism spectrum disorder, 957–958
definition of, 218
documentation focus, 220–221
in gender identity disorder, 991
in hospice care, 999
in hyperactivity disorder, 1000
in infant of addicted mother, 1004
in multiple sclerosis, 1017
NIC linkages, 219
NOC linkages, 218–219
nursing priorities, 219–220
in oppositional defiant disorder, 1023
in parent-child relationship problem, 1027
in schizophrenia, 1046
in substance dependence/abuse, prenatal, 1052
ineffective, in special needs newborn, 1022
readiness for enhanced, 234–236
in cancer, 963
definition of, 234
documentation focus, 236
in gender identity disorder, 991
NIC linkages, 235
NOC linkages, 234
nursing priorities, 235–236
in parent-child relational problem, 1027
in postpartum period, 1033
in pregnancy, 1035
ineffective, 221–226
in antisocial personality disorder, 953
in anxiety disorders, 953, 954
in attention deficit disorder, 957
in colitis, ulcerative, 969–970
definition of, 221
in depressant abuse, 977
documentation focus, 225
in dysmenorrhea, 983
in dystocia, 983
in fetal alcohol syndrome, 988
in fibrocystic breast disease, 989
intermittent, in seasonal affective disorder, 947
in juvenile diabetes, 978
in labor, 1008
NIC linkages, 222
NOC linkages, 222
nursing priorities, 223–225
in oppositional defiant disorder, 1023
in passive-aggressive personality disorder, 1028
in physical abuse, 944
in post-traumatic stress disorder, 1034
in postpartum psychosis, 1034
in premenstrual dysphoric disorder, 1037
in psychological abuse, 945
in rape, 1041
risk for
in headache, 994
in hyperemesis gravidarum, 1000
in labor, 1008
in postpartum period, 1033
in pregnancy, 1035
in renal transplantation, 1042
in schizophrenia, 1046
in somatoform disorders, 1050
in stimulant abuse, 1051
in substance dependence/abuse, prenatal, 1052
in transplantation recipient, 993, 1058
readiness for enhanced, 229–231
definition of, 229
documentation focus, 231
NIC linkages, 229–230
NOC linkages, 229
nursing priorities, 230–231
Cor pulmonale, 972–973
Corneal injury, risk for, 478–481
Corneal transplantation, 972
Coronary artery bypass surgery, 972
Coronary artery disease, 972
Cradle cap. *See* Dermatitis, seborrheic
Craniotomy, 973
Creativity, in application of nursing process, 5
Creutzfeldt-Jakob disease, 973
Crohn's disease, 973

Croup, 973
membranous, 973–974
Cubital tunnel syndrome, 974
Cushing's syndrome, 974
CVA. *See* Cerebrovascular accident
Cyclothymic disorder. *See* Bipolar disorder
Cystic fibrosis, 974
Cystitis, 974
Cytomegalic inclusion disease. *See* Cytomegalovirus (CMV) infection
Cytomegalovirus (CMV) infection, 975

Data collection, 13–15
D&C. *See* Dilation and curettage
de Quervain's syndrome, 977
Death anxiety, 237–240
in biliary cancer, 958
in cancer, 963
definition of, 237
documentation focus, 239–240
in end-stage renal disease, 1041
in hospice care, 999
NIC linkages, 237
NOC linkages, 237
nursing priorities, 237–239
in SARS, 1045
Decision-making
emancipated, impaired, 293–295
definition of, 293
documentation focus, 294–295
NIC linkages, 293
NOC linkages, 293
nursing priorities, 294
risk for, 298
readiness for enhanced, 244–246
definition of, 244
documentation focus, 246
NIC linkages, 244
NOC linkages, 244
nursing priorities, 244–246
Decisional conflict, 240–243
in abortion, 943
in anencephaly, 951
definition of, 240
documentation focus, 243
in electroconvulsive therapy, 985
NIC linkages, 241
NOC linkages, 241
nursing priorities, 241–243
in transplant, 1058
Deep vein thrombosis. *See* Thrombophlebitis
Degenerative disc disease. *See* Herniated nucleus pulposus
Degenerative joint disease. *See* Arthritis
Dehiscence, abdominal wound, 975
Dehydration, 975
Delirium tremens, 975
Delivery, precipitous/out of hospital, 975–976
Delusional disorder, 976
Dementia
AIDS, 948
HIV, 976
presenile/senile, 976
vascular. *See* Alzheimer's disease
Denial, ineffective, 247–249
definition of, 247
in depressant abuse, 976–977
documentation focus, 249
NIC linkages, 248
NOC linkages, 247
nursing priorities, 248–249
risk for, in transient ischemic attack, 1058
in substance dependence/abuse, prenatal, 1052
in substance dependence/abuse rehabilitation, 1052
Dentition, impaired, 250–254
in bulimia nervosa, 961
definition of, 250
documentation focus, 253
in gingival abscess, 944
NIC linkages, 250–251
NOC linkages, 250
nursing priorities, 251–253
risk for, in myofascial pain syndrome, 1019
Depersonalization disorder. *See* Dissociative disorders
Depressant abuse, 976–977
Depression
major, 977
postpartum, 977
Depressive disorders. *See* Bipolar disorder; Depression, major; Premenstrual dysmorphic disorder
Dermatitis
contact, 977–978
seborrheic, 978
Development
delayed, in cerebral palsy, 1025
risk for delayed, 254–258. *See also* Growth and development, delayed
in Asperger's syndrome, 956
in burns, 962
definition of, 254
documentation focus, 257–258
in juvenile rheumatoid arthritis, 955
NIC linkages, 255
NOC linkages, 255
nursing priorities, 255–257
in otitis media, 1024
Developmental disorders, pervasive. *See* Asperger's disorder; Autism spectrum disorder; Rett's syndrome
Diabetes
gestational, 978
juvenile, 978
Diabetes insipidus, 978
Diabetes mellitus, 978–979
intrapartum, 979
postpartum, 979
Diabetic ketoacidosis, 979
Diagnosis, 3
Diagnostic procedures, 15
Dialysis
general, 979–980
peritoneal, 980
Diaper rash. *See* Candidiasis
Diaphragmatic hernia. *See* Hernia, hiatal
Diarrhea, 259–263, 980
in celiac disease, 965
in colitis, ulcerative, 969
in Crohn's disease, 973
definition of, 259
in diverticulitis, 981–982
documentation focus, 263
in gastroenteritis, 990
in gastroplasty, 991
in Gulf War syndrome, 993
in IBS, 1006
in ileus, 1003
in intestinal surgery, 1006
in Legionnaire's disease, 1011
NIC linkages, 260
NOC linkages, 259
nursing priorities, 260–262
risk for
in colostomy, 970
in gastrectomy, 990
in newborn at 1 week, 1021
in pernicious anemia, 950
in Zollinger-Ellison syndrome, 1064
DIC. *See* Disseminated intravascular coagulation
Diffuse axonal (brain) injury. *See* Cerebrovascular accident; Traumatic brain injury
Digitalis toxicity, 980
Dignity, risk for compromised human, 423–425
Dilation and curettage, 980–981
Dilation of cervix, premature, 981
Dislocation/subluxation of joint, 981
Disorganized infant behavior. *See* Behavior, disorganized infant
Disruptive behavior disorder. *See* Oppositional defiant disorder
Disseminated intravascular coagulation, 981
Dissociative disorders, 981
Distress. *See* Moral distress; Spiritual distress
Disuse syndrome, risk for, 264–269
definition of, 264
documentation focus, 269
in Guillain-Barré syndrome, 993
NIC linkages, 264–265
NOC linkages, 264
nursing priorities, 265–268
Diversional activity, deficient, 270–273
in bone marrow transplantation, 959
in burns, 962
definition of, 270
documentation focus, 272
in glomerulonephritis, 992
in herniated nucleus pulposus, 997
NIC linkages, 270
NOC linkages, 270
nursing priorities, 270–272
in placenta previa, 1030
in traction, 1057
in Wilms' tumor, 1064
Diverticulitis, 981–982
Documentation, electronic, 9
Down syndrome, 982
Dressing, self-care deficit for, 723–730
Dressler's syndrome, 982
Drowning, near, 1019
Drug overdose, acute, 982

Drug withdrawal, 982–983
Dry eye, risk for, 273–275
  definition of, 273
  documentation focus, 275
  in hyperthyroidism, 1002
  NIC linkages, 274
  NOC linkages, 273
  nursing priorities, 274–275
DTs. *See* Delirium tremens
Duchenne's muscular dystrophy. *See* Muscular dystrophy (Duchenne's)
Duodenal ulcer. *See* Ulcer, peptic
DVT. *See* Thrombophlebitis
Dysmenorrhea, 983
Dyspareunia, 983
Dysrhythmia, cardiac, 983
Dysthymic disorder. *See* Depression, major
Dystocia, 983

Eating disorders. *See* Anorexia nervosa; Bulimia nervosa
Ebola, 983–984
Eclampsia, 984
ECT. *See* Electroconvulsive therapy
Ectopic pregnancy, 984
Eczema, 984. *See* Dermatitis
Edema, pulmonary, 984
Elder abuse. *See* Abuse
Elderly, frail, 352–358. *See also* Frail elderly syndrome
Electrical injury, 984–985
Electroconvulsive therapy, 985
Electrolyte imbalance, risk for, 280–285
  in Addison's disease, 946
  in benign prostatic hyperplasia, 958
  definition of, 280
  documentation focus, 284–285
  in hyperemesis gravidarum, 1000
  in hyperparathyroidism, 1001
  in hypoparathyroidism, 1002
  NIC linkages, 280
  NOC linkages, 280
  nursing priorities, 280–284
Electronic documentation, 9
Emotional control, labile, 299–301
  definition of, 299
  documentation focus, 300–301
  NIC linkages, 299
  NOC linkages, 299
  nursing priorities, 300
Emphysema, 985
Encephalitis, 985
Encopresis, 985
End of life care. *See* Hospice care
Endocarditis, 985–986
Endometriosis, 986
Enteral feeding, 986
Enteritis. *See* Colitis, ulcerative; Crohn's disease
Enuresis, 986
Epididymitis, 986–987
Epilepsy. *See* Seizure disorder
Episiotomy, 987
Epistaxis, 987
Epstein-Barr virus. *See* Mononucleosis, infectious
Erectile dysfunction, 987
Esophageal reflux disease. *See* Gastroesophageal reflux disease (GERD)
Esophageal varices, 1062
Esophagitis. *See* Achalasia (cardiospasm); Gastroesophageal reflux disease (GERD)
Ethical code, 3
ETOH withdrawal. *See* Alcohol intoxication, acute; Substance dependence/abuse
Evaluation, 3–4
Evidence-based practice, 3
Evisceration. *See* Dehiscence, abdominal wound

Facial reconstructive surgery, 987
Failure to thrive
  adult, 987
  infant/child, 987–988
Falls, risk for, 301–306
  in acoustic neuroma, 945
  definition of, 301
  documentation focus, 305
  NIC linkages, 302
  NOC linkages, 302
  nursing priorities, 302–305
  in Paget's disease, 1025
  in pernicious anemia, 951
  in vertigo, 1063
Family health management, ineffective, 407–410
Family processes
  dysfunctional, 306–310
    definition of, 306
    documentation focus, 309–310
    in fetal alcohol syndrome, 988
    NIC linkages, 307–308
    NOC linkages, 307
    nursing priorities, 308–309
    in substance dependence/abuse rehabilitation, 1053
  interrupted, 310–314
    in adolescent pregnancy, 1035–1036
    in battered child syndrome, 958
    in bipolar disorder, 959
    definition of, 310
    in depression, 977
    documentation focus, 313
    in Down syndrome, 982
    NIC linkages, 311
    NOC linkages, 311
    nursing priorities, 311–313
    in paraphilias, 1026
    in parent-child relational problem, 1027
    in post-traumatic stress disorder, 1034
    risk for
      in cancer, 963
      in genetic disorder, 992
      in high-risk pregnancy, 1036
      in perinatal loss/death of child, 1029
      in SIDS, 1053
    in schizophrenia, 1046
    in smallpox, 1049–1050
    in traumatic brain injury, 1059
    in Wilms' tumor, 1064
  readiness for enhanced, 314–317
    definition of, 314
    documentation focus, 316–317
    NIC linkages, 315
    NOC linkages, 315
    nursing priorities, 315–316
Fat embolism syndrome. *See* Pulmonary embolus; Respiratory distress syndrome, acute
Fatigue, 317–322
  in Addison's disease, 946
  in AIDS, 947–948
  in aplastic anemia, 954
  in cancer, 963
  in coccidioidomycosis, 969
  definition of, 317
  in diabetic ketoacidosis, 979
  documentation focus, 322
  in drug withdrawal, 983
  in enteral feeding, 986
  in fibromyalgia, 989
  in Gulf War syndrome, 993
  in hospice care, 999
  in hyperthyroidism, 1001–1002
  in hypothyroidism, 1003
  in infectious mononucleosis, 1016
  in iron-deficiency anemia, 950
  in labor, 1008, 1009
    stage IV, 1009
  in leukemia, 1011
  in Lyme disease, 1013
  in malaria, 1013
  in menopause, 1015
  in mountain sickness, 1016
  in multiple sclerosis, 1017
  NIC linkages, 318
  NOC linkages, 318
  nursing priorities, 318–321
  in Paget's disease, 1024
  in parenteral feeding, 1027
  in postpartum depression, 977
  in postpolio syndrome, 1034
  in pregnancy, 1035
  risk for
    in gastrectomy, 990
    in postpartum period, 1033
  in sarcoidosis, 1045
  in sick building syndrome, 1049
  in systemic lupus erythematosus, 1012
  in viral hepatitis, 997
Fatigue syndrome, chronic, 988
Fear
  in adenoidectomy, 946
  in Hodgkin's disease, 999
  in myocardial infarction, 1018
  in postpolio syndrome, 1034
  in Wilms' tumor, 1064
Fear [specify focus], 323–327
  in abruptio placentae, 944
  in achalasia, 945
  in benign prostatic hyperplasia, 958
  in botulism, 960
  in cancer, 963
  in cataract, 965
  in Creutzfeldt-Jakob disease, 973
  definition of, 323
  in dehiscence, 975

in delirium tremens, 975
in dementia, 976
in dissociative disorders, 981
documentation focus, 326
in eclampsia, 984
in ectopic pregnancy, 984
in esophageal varices, 1062
in facial reconstructive surgery, 987
in gas gangrene, 990
in hallucinogen abuse, 993
in Hodgkin's disease, 999
in hypophysectomy, 1002
in long-term care, 1012
in macular degeneration, 1013
in membranous croup, 974
in multiple organ dysfunction syndrome, 1017
in myasthenia gravis, 1018
NIC linkages, 324
NOC linkages, 323
nursing priorities, 324–326
in panic disorder, 1025
in peptic ulcer, 1060
in phobia, 1030
in placenta previa, 1030
in prenatal hemorrhage, 996
in pulmonary edema, 984
in pulmonary embolus, 1038
in pulmonary fibrosis, 1039
in radiation syndrome/poisoning, 1040
in renal transplantation, 1042
in respiratory distress syndrome, acute, 1042
in smallpox, 1049
in snake bite, 1050
in stimulant abuse, 1051
in transient ischemic attack, 1058
in transplant, 1058
in transplantation recipient, 1058
in ventilator assist/dependence, 1063
Febrile seizure, 988
Fecal diversion. *See* Colostomy
Fecal impaction, 988
Feeding, self-care deficit for, 723–730
Feeding pattern, ineffective infant, 327–330
in cleft lip/palate, 969
definition of, 327
documentation focus, 329
NIC linkages, 328
NOC linkages, 327
nursing priorities, 328–329
risk for, in premature infant, 1022
Femoral popliteal bypass, 988
Fetal alcohol syndrome, 988
Fetal demise. *See* Perinatal loss/death of child
Fetal transfusion syndrome, 1060
Fibrocystic breast disease, 989
Fibroids, uterine. *See* Uterine myomas
Fibromyalgia syndrome, primary, 989
Flail chest. *See* Hemothorax; Pneumothorax
Fluid balance, readiness for enhanced, 330–332
definition of, 330
documentation focus, 332
NIC linkages, 330
NOC linkages, 330
nursing priorities, 330–332
Fluid volume
deficient
in croup, 973
in dehydration, 975
in diabetic ketoacidosis, 979
in esophageal varices, 1062
in gestational hypertension, 1001
in heat exhaustion, 995
hyper/hypotonic, 333–337
in Addison's disease, 946
in adrenal crisis, 946
definition of, 333
documentation focus, 336
NIC linkages, 334
NOC linkages, 333
nursing priorities, 334–336
in hyperemesis gravidarum, 1000
hypertonic, in diabetes insipidus, 978
in hypovolemia, 1003
in hypovolemic/hemorrhagic shock, 1048
isotonic, 337–341
in aldosteronism, 948
in botulism, 960
in cardiac surgery, 964
in cholera, 968
definition of, 337
documentation focus, 340–341
NIC linkages, 338
NOC linkages, 338
nursing priorities, 338–340
in toxic shock syndrome, 1057
mixed
in peritonitis, 1029
in pheochromocytoma, 1030
in nonketotic hyperglycemic-hyperosmolar coma, 1022
in pertussis, 1029
in pneumonic plague, 1031
in pyloric stenosis, 1039
in rabies, 1040
in radiation syndrome/poisoning, 1040
in Reye's syndrome, 1043
risk for, 345–348
in acute mountain sickness, 1016
in adenoidectomy, 946
in AIDS, 947
in anorexia nervosa, 952
in appendicitis, 955
in benign prostatic hyperplasia, 958
in brain concussion, 971
in brain tumor, 960
in bubonic plague, 1030
in bulimia nervosa, 961
in burns, 962
in calculi, urinary, 962
in celiac disease, 965
in cesarean birth, 966
in chemotherapy, 967
in cholecystectomy, 967
in colitis, ulcerative, 969
in coma, 970
definition of, 345
in diarrhea, 980
documentation focus, 348
in dystocia, 983
in ebola, 984
in ectopic pregnancy, 984
in epidural hematoma, 995
in gastritis, 990
in gastroenteritis, 990
in gastrointestinal anthrax, 952
in gastroplasty, 991
in gunshot wound, 1064
in hand-foot-mouth disease, 994
in hemodialysis, 996
in hemophilia, 996
in hyperparathyroidism, 1001
in hypophysectomy, 1002
in ileus, 1003
in influenza, 1005
in intestinal surgery, 1006
in iron-deficiency anemia, 950
in Kaposi's sarcoma, 1007
in labor, stage III, 1009
in lead poisoning, 1010
in leukemia, 1011
in malaria, 1013
in Mallory-Weiss syndrome, 1013
in mumps, 1017
in necrotizing enterocolitis, 1020
in nephrectomy, 1020
NIC linkages, 346
NOC linkages, 346
nursing priorities, 346–348
in pancreatitis, 1025
in postoperative recovery period, 1032
in postpartum period, 1033
in precipitous delivery, 975
in premature newborn, 1021–1022
in prostatectomy, 1037
in respiratory distress syndrome, acute, 1042
in respiratory syncytial virus, 1043
in scarlet fever, 1045
in sepsis, 1047
in snake bite, 1050
in stomatitis, 1052
in typhoid fever, 1060
in uterine myomas, 1061
in West Nile fever, 1064
in smallpox, 1049
in toxic enterocolitis, 1057
in trichinosis, 1059
excess, 341–345
in cirrhosis, 968
in cor pulmonale, 972–973
definition of, 341
documentation focus, 344–345
in glomerulonephritis, 992
in heart failure, 995
in high altitude pulmonary edema, 998
in hypervolemia, 1002
in nephrotic syndrome, 1020
NIC linkages, 342
NOC linkages, 342
nursing priorities, 342–344
in premenstrual dysphoric disorder, 1037
in pulmonary edema, 984
in renal failure, 1041
risk for
in cardiac conditions, prenatal, 964

in Cushing's syndrome, 974
in hemodialysis, 996
in parathyroidectomy, 1026
in peritoneal dialysis, 980
in polycystic kidney disease, 1007
in pregnancy, 1035
in renal transplantation, 1042
in valvular heart disease, 1062
in twin-twin transfusion syndrome, 1060
risk for imbalanced, 349–352
definition of, 349
in digitalis toxicity, 980
documentation focus, 351
in enteral feeding, 986
in intrapartum hypertension, 1001
in labor, 1008
NIC linkages, 349
NOC linkages, 349
nursing priorities, 349–351
in parenteral feeding, 1027
in prenatal hemorrhage, 996
in surgery, 1054
Food poisoning. *See* Gastroenteritis
Fractures, 989. *See also* Casts; Traction
Frail elderly syndrome, 352–356
in adult failure to thrive, 987
definition of, 352
documentation focus, 355
in malnutrition, 1013
NIC linkages, 353
NOC linkages, 353
nursing priorities, 353–355
risk for, 356–358
definition of, 356
documentation focus, 358
NIC linkages, 357
NOC linkages, 357
nursing priorities, 357–358
Frostbite, 989
Fusion
Cervical. *See* Laminectomy, cervical
Lumbar. *See* Laminectomy, lumbar

Gallstones. *See* Cholelithiasis
Gangrene
dry, 990
gas, 990
Gas, lung irritant, 990
Gas exchange
impaired, 359–363
in asbestosis, 956
in asthma, 956
in atelectasis, 956
in bronchogenic carcinoma, 961
in bronchopneumonia, 961
in carbon monoxide poisoning, 963
in chronic obstructive lung disease, 968
in cor pulmonale, 973
definition of, 359
in disseminated intravascular coagulation, 981
documentation focus, 363
in drug overdose, 982
in emphysema, 985
fetal
in intrapartum diabetes mellitus, 979
in placenta previa, 1030
risk for, in labor, stage II, 1009
in gas, lung irritant, 990
in hantavirus pulmonary syndrome, 994
in high altitude pulmonary edema, 998
in infant of addicted mother, 1004
in inhalation anthrax, 953
in Legionnaire's disease, 1011
in mitral stenosis, 1016
in multiple organ dysfunction syndrome, 1017
in near drowning, 1019
NIC linkages, 360
NOC linkages, 359–360
nursing priorities, 360–362
in pleural effusion, 1031
in pneumonic plague, 1031
in postmature newborn, 1021
in premature newborn, 1021
in pulmonary edema, 984, 1038
in pulmonary embolus, 1038
in pulmonary fibrosis, 1038–1039
in pulmonary hypertension, 1039
in respiratory acidosis, 945
in respiratory alkalosis, 948
in respiratory distress syndrome
acute, 1042
in premature infant, 1043
in respiratory syncytial virus, 1043
risk for
in AIDS, 947
in aortic stenosis, 954
in cardiac surgery, 964
in cardiogenic shock, 1048
in Dressler's syndrome, 982
in fractures, 989
in heart failure, 995
in induced labor, 1007
in lung transplantation, 1012
in newborn, 1021
in nicotine abuse, 1022
in pertussis, 1030
in rheumatic heart disease, 1044
in tuberculosis, 1059
in SARS, 1045
in sickle cell anemia, 951
in sleep apnea, 1049
impaired fetal, risk for, in intrapartum hypertension, 1001
Gastrointestinal perfusion, ineffective, in multiple organ dysfunction syndrome, 1016–1017
Gastrectomy, subtotal, 990
Gastric partitioning. *See* Gastroplasty
Gastric resection. *See* Gastrectomy, subtotal
Gastric ulcer. *See* Ulcer, peptic
Gastrinoma. *See* Zollinger-Ellison syndrome
Gastritis
acute, 990
chronic, 990
Gastroenteritis, 990
Gastroesophageal reflux disease (GERD), 991
Gastrointestinal hemorrhage. *See* Colitis, ulcerative; Crohn's disease; Gastritis; Ulcer, peptic; Varices, esophageal
Gastrointestinal motility, dysfunctional, 364–368
definition of, 364
documentation focus, 368
NIC linkages, 365
NOC linkages, 364
nursing priorities, 365–367
risk for, 369–372
definition of, 369
documentation focus, 372
NIC linkages, 369
NOC linkages, 369
nursing priorities, 369–371
Gastrointestinal perfusion, risk for ineffective, 373–376
in compartment syndrome, 970
definition of, 373
documentation focus, 375–376
NIC linkages, 373
NOC linkages, 373
nursing priorities, 374–375
in respiratory distress syndrome in premature infant, 1043
Gastroplasty, 991
Gender identity disorder, 991
Genetic disorder, 991–992
Genital herpes. *See* Herpes simplex; Sexually transmitted infection
Genital warts. *See* Sexually transmitted infection
GERD. *See* Gastroesophageal reflux disease (GERD)
GI bleeding. *See* Gastritis; Ulcer, peptic
Gigantism. *See* Acromegaly
Gingival abscess, 944
Gingivitis, 992
Glaucoma, 992
Glomerulonephritis, 992
Glucose, risk for unstable blood, 90–94
Gluten sensitive enteropathy. *See* Celiac disease
Goiter, 992
Gonorrhea, 992–993. *See also* Sexually transmitted infection
Gout, 993
Grand mal seizures. *See* Seizure disorder
Grave's disease. *See* Hyperthyroidism
Grieving, 377–381
in abortion, 944
in amyotrophic lateral sclerosis, 950
in cancer, 963
in cerebrovascular accident, 966
complicated, 381–385
definition of, 381
documentation focus, 384–385
NIC linkages, 382
NOC linkages, 382
nursing priorities, 382–384
in post-traumatic stress disorder, 1034
risk for, 385–388
in adoption/loss of child custody, 946
definition of, 385
documentation focus, 387–388
in Down syndrome, 982
in HIV infection, 998–999
in mastectomy, 1014

NIC linkages, 386
NOC linkages, 386
nursing priorities, 386–387
in Rett's syndrome, 1043
in SIDS, 1053
definition of, 377
in dementia, 976
in dialysis, 979
documentation focus, 380
family
in special needs newborn, 1022
in Tay-Sachs disease, 1054
in genetic disorder, 992
in hospice care, 999
in long-term care, 1012
NIC linkages, 378
NOC linkages, 377
nursing priorities, 378–380
in perinatal loss/death of child, 1029
in polyarteritis nodosa, 1032
in premature dilation of cervix, 981
in quadriplegia, 1039
Growth, disproportionate
in newborn, 1020
risk for, 388–392
definition of, 388
documentation focus, 391–392
in glomerulonephritis, 992
in kwashiorkor, 1007
in lead poisoning, 1011
NIC linkages, 389
NOC linkages, 389
nursing priorities, 389–391
in twin-twin transfusion syndrome, 1060
Growth and development, delayed
in battered child syndrome, 958
in Down syndrome, 982
in failure to thrive, 987
in infant of HIV-positive mother, 1004
in muscular dystrophy, 1018
in Rett's syndrome, 1043
in rickets, 1044
risk for, in lead poisoning, 1011
in sickle cell anemia, 951
in syphilis, 1054
in Tay-Sachs disease, 1054
Guillain-Barré syndrome (acute polyneuritis), 993
Gulf War syndrome, 993

Hallucinogen abuse, 993
Hand-foot-mouth disease, 994
Hansen's disease, 994
Hantavirus pulmonary syndrome, 994
Hashimoto's thyroiditis. *See* Goiter; Hypothyroidism
Hay fever, 994
Head injury. *See* Traumatic brain injury
Headache, 994
Health, deficient community, 392–395
definition of, 392
documentation focus, 395
NIC linkages, 393
NOC linkages, 393
nursing priorities, 393–395
Health behavior, risk-prone, 396–399
definition of, 396
documentation focus, 399
in HIV infection, 998
in hypertension, 1001
in juvenile diabetes mellitus, 978
NIC linkages, 396
in nicotine abuse, 1022
NOC linkages, 396
nursing priorities, 397–399
in rheumatic heart disease, 1044
risk for
in angina pectoris, 952
in latex allergy, 1010
in scleroderma, 1046
in scoliosis, 1047
in venous insufficiency, 1063
Health maintenance
ineffective, 400–403
in Alzheimer's disease, 949
definition of, 400
documentation focus, 403
NIC linkages, 401
NOC linkages, 400
nursing priorities, 401–402
in schizophrenia, 1046
risk for ineffective, in immersion foot, 1003
Health management
family, ineffective, 407–410
definition of, 407
documentation focus, 409–410
NIC linkages, 408
NOC linkages, 408
nursing priorities, 408–409
ineffective, 404–407
definition of, 404
documentation focus, 406–407
NIC linkages, 404–405
NOC linkages, 404
nursing priorities, 405–406
risk for
in conjunctivitis, 972
in diabetes insipidus, 978
in diabetes mellitus, 978
in heroin withdrawal, 998
in high-risk pregnancy, 1036
in HIV infection, 998
in nicotine withdrawal, 1022
in Osgood-Schlatter disease, 1024
in prostatitis, 1038
in rheumatic heart disease, 1044
in sleep apnea, 1049
in splenectomy, 1051
in temporal arteritis, 1055
in transplantation recipient, 1058
in tuberculosis, 1060
in varicose veins sclerotherapy, 1062
in venous insufficiency, 1063
in Zollinger-Ellison syndrome, 1064
readiness for enhanced, 410–413
definition of, 410
documentation focus, 412
in menopause, 1015
NIC linkages, 411
in nicotine withdrawal, 1022
NOC linkages, 411
nursing priorities, 411–412
in transplantation recipient, 1058
Healthcare information, standardized languages for, 9–12
Heart attack. *See* Myocardial infarction
Heart failure, chronic, 995
Heart transplantation. *See* Cardiac surgery; Transplantation, recipient
Heat exhaustion, 995
Heatstroke, 995
Hematoma
epidural, 995
subdural-acute. *See* Traumatic brain injury
subdural-chronic, 995
Hemiplegia, spastic. *See* Palsy, cerebral
Hemodialysis, 996
Hemophilia, 996
Hemorrhage
postpartum, 996
prenatal, 996
Hemorrhagic fever, viral. *See* Ebola; Hantavirus pulmonary syndrome
Hemorrhoidectomy, 996
Hemorrhoids, 996
Hemothorax, 997
Hepatitis, acute viral, 997
Hepatorenal syndrome. *See* Cirrhosis; Renal failure, acute
Hernia
hiatal, 997
inguinal. *See* Herniorrhaphy
Herniated nucleus pulposus, 997
Herniorrhaphy, 997
Heroin abuse, 997–998
Heroin withdrawal, 998
Herpes simplex, 998
Herpes zoster (shingles), 998
High altitude pulmonary edema (HAPE), 998
High altitude sickness. *See* High altitude pulmonary edema (HAPE); Mountain sickness, acute (AMS)
High-risk pregnancy. *See* Pregnancy, high-risk
Hip replacement. *See* Total joint replacement
HIV infection, 998–999. *See also* AIDS
Hodgkin's disease, 999
Holistic view, 2
Home Health Care Classification, 10
Home maintenance, impaired, 413–416
in cancer, 963
in cerebrovascular accident, 966
definition of, 413
documentation focus, 415–416
in mental delay, 1015
in multiple sclerosis, 1017
NIC linkages, 414
NOC linkages, 414
nursing priorities, 414–415
in quadriplegia, 1040
risk for
in Addison's disease, 946
in retinal detachment, 1043
in schizophrenia, 1046
Hope, readiness for enhanced, 416–418
in chemotherapy, 967

definition of, 416
documentation focus, 418
NIC linkages, 417
NOC linkages, 416
nursing priorities, 417–418
Hopelessness, 419–423
definition of, 419
documentation focus, 422
in Huntington's disease, 999
in multiple sclerosis, 1017
NIC linkages, 419
NOC linkages, 419
nursing priorities, 420–422
risk for, in fibromyalgia, 989
in suicide attempt, 1053
Hospice care, 999
Human dignity, risk for compromised, 423–425
definition of, 423
documentation focus, 425
NIC linkages, 424
NOC linkages, 423–424
nursing priorities, 424–425
Human nature, 2
Huntington's disease, 999–1000
Hydrocephalus, 1000
Hydrophobia. *See* Rabies
Hyperactivity disorder, 1000
Hyperbilirubinemia, 1000
Hyperemesis gravidarum, 1000
Hyperparathyroidism, primary, 1001
Hypertension, 1001
gestational, 1001
intrapartum, 1001
prenatal. *See* Hypertension, gestational
pulmonary. *See* Pulmonary hypertension
Hyperthermia, 426–430
in acute prostatitis, 1038
in bubonic plague, 1030
in cat scratch disease, 965
definition of, 426
documentation focus, 429
in ebola, 984
in encephalitis, 985
in febrile seizure, 988
in heatstroke, 995
in infectious mononucleosis, 1016
in influenza, 1005
in Kawasaki disease, 1007
in Legionnaire's disease, 1011
in malaria, 1013
in measles, 1014
in meningitis, 1015
in mumps, 1017
in necrotizing cellulitis/fasciitis, 1019
NIC linkages, 426
NOC linkages, 426
nursing priorities, 427–429
in osteomyelitis, 1024
in pelvic inflammatory disease, 1028
in pneumonic plague, 1031
in polyarteritis nodosa, 1032
in puerperal sepsis, 1047
in pyelonephritis, 1039
in rabies, 1040
in rheumatic fever, 1044
risk for
in adrenal crisis, 947
in brain abscess, 944
in SARS, 1045
in scarlet fever, 1045
in strep throat, 1052
in tonsillitis, 1056
in toxic shock syndrome, 1057
in typhus, 1060
in West Nile fever, 1063
Hyperthyroidism, 1001–1002
Hypervolemia, 1002
Hypochondriasis. *See* Somatoform disorders
Hypoglycemia, 1002
Hypoparathyroidism (acute), 1002
Hypophysectomy, 1002
Hypothermia, 430–434
definition of, 430
documentation focus, 434
in newborn, postmature, 1021
NIC linkages, 431
NOC linkages, 431
nursing priorities, 432–434
risk for, 435–437
definition of, 435
documentation focus, 437
in near drowning, 1019
in newborn, 1021
NIC linkages, 436
NOC linkages, 436
nursing priorities, 436–437
risk for perioperative, 438–440
definition of, 438
documentation focus, 439–440
NIC linkages, 438
NOC linkages, 438
nursing priorities, 438–439
systemic, 1002
in systemic hypothermia, 1002
Hypothyroidism, 1003
Hypovolemia, 1003
Hysterectomy, 1003

Identity, personal, disturbed, 616–620
Ileal conduit. *See* Urinary diversion
Ileocolitis. *See* Crohn's disease
Ileostomy. *See* Colostomy
Ileus, 1003
Immersion foot, 1003
Impetigo, 1003–1004
Implementation, 3
Impotence. *See* Erectile dysfunction
Impulse control, ineffective, 440–443
in conduct disorder, 971
definition of, 440
documentation focus, 443
in hyperactivity disorder, 1000
NIC linkages, 441
NOC linkages, 441
nursing priorities, 441–443
In integrity, impaired, in postoperative recovery period, 1032
Incontinence
bowel, 444–447
definition of, 444
documentation focus, 446–447
in encopresis, 985
NIC linkages, 445
NOC linkages, 444
nursing priorities, 445–446
in quadriplegia, 1040
in spina bifida, 1050
in tetanus, 1055
urinary
functional, 447–450
definition of, 447
documentation focus, 450
NIC linkages, 448
NOC linkages, 448
nursing priorities, 448–450
overflow, 451–453
in benign prostatic hyperplasia, 958
definition of, 451
documentation focus, 453
NIC linkages, 451
NOC linkages, 451
nursing priorities, 451–453
reflex, 454–457
definition of, 454
documentation focus, 456
NIC linkages, 454
NOC linkages, 454
nursing priorities, 454–456
in paraplegia, 1026
stress, 457–460
definition of, 457
documentation focus, 459
in menopause, 1015
NIC linkages, 457
NOC linkages, 457
nursing priorities, 458–459
in tetanus, 1055
urge, 460–464
definition of, 460
documentation focus, 463
NIC linkages, 461
NOC linkages, 461
nursing priorities, 461–443
risk for, 464–467
definition of, 464
documentation focus, 466
NIC linkages, 465
NOC linkages, 465
nursing priorities, 465–466
Infant
of addicted mother, 1004
at 4 weeks, 1004
of HIV-positive mother, 1004
ineffective feeding pattern, 327–330
Infant behavior, disorganized. *See* Behavior, disorganized infant
Infection
ear. *See* Otitis media
prenatal, 1005
puerperal, 1005
risk for, 467–473
in abscess, 944
in adrenalectomy, 947
in agranulocytosis, 947
in AIDS, 947
in appendectomy, 954
in appendicitis, 955
in arthroplasty, 955

in asbestosis, 956
in athlete's foot, 957
in bacterial vaginosis, 1062
in bronchogenic carcinoma, 961
in bronchopneumonia, 961
in burns, 962
in cataract extraction, 965
in cellulitis, 965
in cesarean birth, 966, 967
in chronic obstructive lung disease, 968
in chronic sinusitis, 1049
in circumcision, 968
in coma, 970
in conjunctivitis, 972
in contact dermatitis, 978
in corneal transplantation, 972
in craniotomy, 973
in Cushing's syndrome, 974
in cutaneous anthrax, 952
in cystic fibrosis, 974
in decubitus ulcer, 1060
definition of, 467
in dehiscence, 975
in diabetes mellitus, 979
in diabetic ketoacidosis, 979
documentation focus, 472
in drug overdose, 982
in ebola, 984
in eczema, 984
in emphysema, 985
in enteral feeding, 986
in epididymitis, 986
in episiotomy, 987
fetal, in CMV infection, 975
in frostbite, 989
in gastroenteritis, 990
in gonorrhea, 992
in gunshot wound, 1064
in hand-foot-mouth disease, 994
in Hansen's disease, 994
in heroin abuse, 997
in herpes simplex, 998
in hydrocephalus, 1000
in hypophysectomy, 1002
in impetigo, 1003
in infant at 4 weeks, 1004
in infant of addicted mother, 1004
in infant of HIV-positive mother, 1004
in intestinal surgery, 1006
in kwashiorkor, 1007
in laceration, 1009
in Legionnaire's disease, 1011
in leukemia, 1011
in lung transplantation, 1012
in mastitis, 1014
in mastoidectomy, 1014
in measles, 1014
in meningitis, 1014–1015
in multiple organ dysfunction syndrome, 1017
in nephrotic syndrome, 1020
in newborn, 1021
NIC linkages, 468
NOC linkages, 468
nursing priorities, 468–472
in pancreatic cancer, 1025
in pancreatitis, 1025
in parenteral feeding, 1027
in pediculosis capitis, 1028
in pelvic inflammatory disease, 1028
in peritoneal dialysis, 980
in peritonitis, 1029
in pertussis, 1029
in pleurisy, 1031
in pneumonic plague, 1031
in poliomyelitis, 1032
in postoperative recovery period, 1032
in postpartum hemorrhage, 996
in postpartum period, 1033
in precipitous delivery, 976
in puerperal infection, 1005
in puerperal sepsis, 1047
in pulmonary fibrosis, 1039
in radiation syndrome/poisoning, 1040
in renal failure, 1042
in renal transplantation, 1042
in respiratory distress syndrome, in premature infant, 1043
in septic arthritis, 955
in sinusitis, 1049
in Sjögren syndrome, 1049
in smallpox, 1049
in spina bifida, 1051
in splenectomy, 1051
in stapedectomy, 1051
in stasis dermatitis, 1051
in stimulant abuse, 1051
in STIs, 1048
in strep throat, 1052
in total joint replacement, 1056
in traction, 1057
in transplantation recipient, 1058
in traumatic brain injury, 1059
in tuberculosis, 1059
in typhoid fever, 1060
urinary tract, in polycystic kidney disease, 1007
in viral hepatitis, 997
in wound infection, 1005
wound, 1005
Infertility, 1005
Inflammatory bowel disease. *See* Colitis, ulcerative; Crohn's disease
Influenza, 1005
Inhalant intoxication/abuse. *See* Stimulant abuse
Injury
corneal, risk for, 478–481
definition of, 478
documentation focus, 480
NIC linkages, 479
NOC linkages, 479
nursing priorities, 479–480
electrical, 984–985
lightning, 1011–1012
perioperative position. *See* Perioperative-positioning injury
risk for, 473–478
in Alzheimer's disease, 949
in Asperger's disorder, 956
in bone marrow transplantation, 959
in brachytherapy, 960
in cataract extraction, 965
in cesarean birth, 966
in corneal transplantation, 972
definition of, 473
in depressant abuse, 977
in diabetes mellitus, postpartum, 979
in dislocation/subluxation of joint, 981
documentation focus, 477
in drug withdrawal, 982
fetal
in breech labor, 1007
in dystocia, 983
in fetal alcohol syndrome, 988
in postmaturity pregnancy, 1036
in precipitous delivery, 976
in preterm labor, 1008
in substance dependence/abuse rehabilitation, 1053
in gas gangrene, 990
in hemodialysis, 996
in herniorrhaphy, 997
in hyperbilirubinemia, 1000
in hypoparathyroidism, 1002
in infant of addicted mother, 1004
in juvenile diabetes, 978
maternal
in abortion, 944
in diabetes mellitus, intrapartum, 979
in dystocia, 983
in eclampsia, 984
in high-risk pregnancy, 1036
in induced labor, 1007
in intrapartum hypertension, 1001
in labor, stage III, 1009
in postmaturity pregnancy, 1036
in newborn, 1020
at 1 week, 1021
NIC linkages, 474
in nicotine abuse, 1022
NOC linkages, 474
nursing priorities, 474–477
in Paget's disease, 1025
in parenteral feeding, 1027
in pernicious anemia, 951
in postpartum hemorrhage, 996
in premature newborn, 1022
pulmonary, in respiratory distress syndrome, acute, 1042
in sarcoidosis, 1045
in surgery, 1053–1054
in thyroidectomy, 1056
in Tourette's syndrome, 1057
in Wilms' tumor, 1064
urinary tract, risk for, 481–485
definition of, 481
documentation focus, 484
NIC linkages, 482
NOC linkages, 481–482
nursing priorities, 482–484
Insomnia, 485–490
acute, 1005–1006
in anxiety disorder, 953
in bipolar disorder, 959
chronic, 1006
definition of, 485
in depression, 977
documentation focus, 489
in drug withdrawal, 983
in long-term care, 1012

in narcolepsy, 954
NIC linkages, 486
NOC linkages, 486
nursing priorities, 486–489
in postpartum period, 1033
in pregnancy, 1035
risk for, in GERD, 991
in stimulant abuse, 1051
Insulin resistance syndrome. *See* Metabolic syndrome
Insulin shock. *See* Hypoglycemia
Intermaxillary fixation, 1006
Intervertebral disc excision. *See* Laminectomy, cervical/lumbar
Interviews, client, 13–14
Intestinal obstruction. *See* Ileus
Intestinal surgery, 1006
Intracranial adaptive capacity, decreased, 45–49
definition of, 45
documentation focus, 48
NIC linkages, 45
NOC linkages, 45
nursing priorities, 45–48
risk for
in craniotomy, 973
in epidural hematoma, 995
in hydrocephalus, 1000
in spina bifida, 1050
in traumatic brain injury, 1058
Intracranial infections. *See* Abscess, brain; Encephalitis; Meningitis, acute meningococcal
Iodinated contrast media, adverse reaction to, risk for, 663–665
Irritable bowel syndrome, 1006
Isolation, social, 812–815. *See also* Social isolation

Jaundice, neonatal, 490–494
definition of, 490
documentation focus, 494
in hyperbilirubinemia, 1000
NIC linkages, 491
NOC linkages, 490–491
nursing priorities, 491–494
risk for, 495–497
definition of, 495
documentation focus, 497
NIC linkages, 495
NOC linkages, 495
nursing priorities, 495–497

Kanner's syndrome. *See* Autism spectrum disorder
Kaposi's sarcoma, AIDS-related, 1006–1007
Kawasaki disease, 1007
Ketoacidosis. *See* Diabetic ketoacidosis
Kidney disease, polycystic, 1007
Kidney failure. *See* Renal failure
Kidney stone(s). *See* Calculi, urinary
Knee replacement. *See* Total joint replacement
Knowledge
deficient [Learning Need], in STIs, 1048
deficient [learning need (specify)], 498–502
in abortion, 943, 944
in achalasia, 945
in adrenalectomy, 947
in anemia, 950
in angina pectoris, 952
in arthroscopy, knee, 956
in attention deficit disorder, 957
in brain concussion, 971
in breast cancer, 960
in bulimia nervosa, 961–962
in calculi, urinary, 963
in cardiac dysrhythmia, 983
in carpal tunnel syndrome, 964
in cataract, 965
in cesarean birth, 966, 967
in cholelithiasis, 968
in circumcision, 968
in coccidioidomycosis, 969
in colostomy, 970
in constipation, 972
in Crohn's disease, 973
in cystic fibrosis, 974
in cystitis, 974
definition of, 498
in dehiscence, 975
in dehydration, 975
in diabetes mellitus, 978
in diarrhea, 980
in digitalis toxicity, 980
in dilation and curettage, 980–981
in diverticulitis, 982
documentation focus, 501
in endometriosis, 986
in epididymitis, 986–987
in failure to thrive, 988
in fractures, 989
in gastritis, 990
in genetic disorder, 991–992
in gestational diabetes, 978
in gestational hypertension, 1001
in gonorrhea, 993
in gout, 993
in hay fever, 994
in headache, 994
in heart failure, 995
in hemorrhoidectomy, 996
in herpes zoster, 998
in hiatal hernia, 997
in high-risk pregnancy, 1036
in HIV infection, 998
in Hodgkin's disease, 999
in hydrocephalus, 1000
in hyperbilirubinemia, 1000
in hypertension, 1001
in hypoglycemia, 1002
in hypothermia, 1002
in induced labor, 1007
in infant of HIV-positive mother, 1004
in infectious mononucleosis, 1016
in labor, 1008
in lead poisoning, 1010
in Mallory-Weiss syndrome, 1013
in mastitis, 1014
in measles, 1014
in meniscectomy, 1015
in mitral stenosis, 1016
in myasthenia gravis, 1018
in myocarditis, 1019
in neuritis, 1020
NIC linkages, 498
NOC linkages, 498
nursing priorities, 499–501
in osteomyelitis, 1024
in parathyroidectomy, 1027
parental, in special needs newborn, 1022
in pelvic inflammatory disease, 1028
in peptic ulcer, 1060
in pheochromocytoma, 1030
in pregnancy, 1035
adolescent, 1036
in premenstrual dysphoric disorder, 1037
in prenatal infection, 1005
in pressure ulcer or sore, 1037
in preterm labor, 1008
in purpura, 1039
in pyelonephritis, 1039
in rape, 1040–1041
in Raynaud's disease, 1041
in retinal detachment, 1043
in rickets, 1044
in ringworm, 1044
in rubella, 1044
in scabies, 1045
in scoliosis, 1047
in seizure disorder, 1047
in serum sickness, 1048
in sickle cell anemia, 951
in skin cancer, 1049
in substance dependence/abuse rehabilitation, 1053
in surgery, 1053
in syphilis, 1054
in thrombophlebitis, 1055–1056
in thyrotoxicosis, 1056
in tonsillitis, 1056
in trichinosis, 1059
in trigeminal neuralgia, 1020
in vaginitis, 1062
in vasectomy, 1063
in viral hepatitis, 997
[specify] readiness for enhanced, 502–504
definition of, 502
documentation focus, 504
in infant at 4 weeks, 1004
NIC linkages, 503
NOC linkages, 502–503
nursing priorities, 503–504
Kwashiorkor, 1007

Labor
breech presentation, 1007
dysfunctional. *See* Dystocia
induced/augmented, 1007
precipitous, 1008
preterm, 1008
stage I (active phase), 1008
stage I (latent phase), 1008

stage I (transition phase), 1008
stage II (expulsion), 1008–1009
stage III (placental expulsion), 1009
stage IV (following delivery), 1009
Labor pain, 602–606
Laboratory tests, 15
Laceration, 1004
Laminectomy
cervical, 1009
lumbar, 1009–1010
Laryngectomy, 1010
Laryngitis. *See* Croup
Latex allergy, 1010
Latex allergy response, 505–509
definition of, 505
documentation focus, 508
NIC linkages, 506
NOC linkages, 505
nursing priorities, 506–508
risk for, 509–512
definition of, 509
documentation focus, 511
NIC linkages, 510
NOC linkages, 510
nursing priorities, 510–511
Laxative abuse, 1010
Lead poisoning
acute, 1010
chronic, 1010–1011
Legionnaire's disease, 1011
Leprosy. *See* Hansen's disease
Leukemia
acute, 1011
chronic, 1011
Lice. *See* Pediculosis capitis
Lifestyle, sedentary, 512–516
definition of, 512
documentation focus, 515
in metabolic syndrome, 1016
NIC linkages, 513
NOC linkages, 513
nursing priorities, 513–515
in obesity, 1023
risk for
in angina pectoris, 952
in mental delay, 1015
in myocardial infarction, 1018–1019
in sickle cell anemia, 951
Lightning injury, 1011–1012
Liver failure. *See* Cirrhosis; Hepatitis, acute viral
Liver function
impaired, in viral hepatitis, 997
risk for impaired, 516–519
definition of, 516
documentation focus, 519
NIC linkages, 516–517
NOC linkages, 516
nursing priorities, 517–519
risk for impairment
in cirrhosis, 968
in cocaine poisoning, 969
Liver transplantation. *See* Transplantation, recipient
Lockjaw. *See* Tetanus
Loneliness, risk for, 520–523
definition of, 520
documentation focus, 522
NIC linkages, 520
NOC linkages, 520
nursing priorities, 520–522
Long-term care, 1012
LSD (lysergic acid diethylamide) intoxication, 1012
Lung cancer. *See* Bronchogenic carcinoma
Lung transplantation, 1012
Lupus erythematosus, systemic (SLE), 1012–1013
Lyme disease, 1013
Lymphedema, 1013

Macular degeneration, 1013
Malaria, 1013
Mallory-Weiss syndrome, 1013
Malnutrition, 1013
Mapping
Concept. *See* Concept mapping
Mind, *See* Mind mapping
Marburg disease. *See* Ebola
Maslow's hierarchy of needs, 2
Mastectomy, 1014
Mastitis, 1014
Mastoidectomy, 1014
Maternal-fetal dyad, risk for disturbed, 523–529
in abruptio placentae, 944
definition of, 523
documentation focus, 527–528
in gestational diabetes, 978
in gestational hypertension, 1001
in high-risk pregnancy, 1036
NIC linkages, 524
NOC linkages, 524
nursing priorities, 524–527
in pregnancy, 1035
in premature dilation of cervix, 981
in prenatal hemorrhage, 996
in prenatal infection, 1005
in substance dependence/abuse, prenatal, 1052
in unplanned cesarean birth, 967
Maternal injury, risk for, in abdominal perineal resection, 944
Measles, 1014
German. *See* Rubella
Megacognitive learning tool, 24
Melanoma, malignant. *See* Cancer; Chemotherapy
Memory, impaired, 529–532
in AIDS dementia, 948
in brain tumor, 960
in Creutzfeldt-Jakob disease, 973
definition of, 529
in dementia, 976
documentation focus, 531
in electroconvulsive therapy, 985
in Gulf War syndrome, 993
in lightning injury, 1012
in long-term care, 1012
NIC linkages, 530
NOC linkages, 529
nursing priorities, 530–531
risk for
in brain concussion, 971
in postconcussion syndrome, 1032
in traumatic brain injury, 1059
Ménière's disease, 1014
Meningitis, acute meningococcal, 1014–1015
Meniscectomy, 1015
Menopause, 1015
Mental delay, 1015–1016
Mesothelioma, 1016
Metabolic syndrome, 1016
Migraine. *See* Headache
Mind-body-spirit connection, 2
Mind mapping, 24–31
client care, 24–26
plan of care, 27–30
Miscarriage. *See* Abortion
Mitral insufficiency. *See* Valvular heart disease
Mitral stenosis, 1016
Mitral valve prolapse (MVP). *See* Valvular heart disease
Mobility
impaired bed, 532–536
definition of, 532
documentation focus, 535
NIC linkages, 533
NOC linkages, 532–533
nursing priorities, 533–535
in quadriplegia, 1040
impaired physical, 536–540
in adrenal crisis, 946–947
in aldosteronism, 948
in amputation, 949
in amyotrophic lateral sclerosis, 950
in arthroplasty, 955
in botulism, 960
in Brown-Sequard syndrome, 961
in bursitis, 962
in carpal tunnel syndrome, 964
in cerebral palsy, 1025
in cerebrovascular accident, 965–966
in cubital tunnel syndrome, 974
in de Quervain's syndrome, 977
definition of, 536
in dislocation/subluxation of joint, 981
documentation focus, 540
in eclampsia, 984
in fractures, 989
in gout, 993
in Guillain-Barré syndrome, 993
in Hansen's disease, 994
in herniated nucleus pulposus, 997
in hypothyroidism, 1003
in lumbar laminectomy, 1009
in mastectomy, 1014
in multiple myeloma, 1018
in multiple sclerosis, 1017
in muscular dystrophy, 1017
in myasthenia gravis, 1018
NIC linkages, 537
NOC linkages, 537
nursing priorities, 537–540
in osteoporosis, 1024
in poliomyelitis, 1031–1032
in postpolio syndrome, 1034

in Rett's syndrome, 1043
in rheumatoid arthritis, 955
risk for
in Addison's disease, 946
in brachytherapy, 960
in hemophilia, 996
in hydrocephalus, 1000
in spina bifida, 1050
in sciatica, 1046
in scleroderma, 1046
in septic arthritis, 955
in subdural-chronic hematoma, 995
in syringomyelia, 1054
in tendonitis, 1055
in thrombophlebitis, 1055
in total joint replacement, 1056–1057
in traction, 1057
in traumatic brain injury, 1059
impaired wheelchair, 541–544
definition of, 541
documentation focus, 543
NIC linkages, 541
NOC linkages, 541
nursing priorities, 542–543
in quadriplegia, 1040
Mononucleosis, infectious, 1016
Mood disorders. *See* Bipolar disorder; Depression; Premenstrual dysphoric disorder
Mood regulation, impaired, 544–546
definition of, 544
documentation focus, 546
NIC linkages, 545
NOC linkages, 545
nursing priorities, 545–546
Moral distress, 547–550
definition of, 547
documentation focus, 549
NIC linkages, 547
NOC linkages, 547
nursing priorities, 547–549
risk for
in abortion, 943
in hospice care, 999
Motility, gastrointestinal, dysfunctional. *See also* Gastrointestinal motility, dysfunctional
Mountain sickness, acute (AMS), 1016
Mucous membrane, oral, impaired, 550–558
Multiple organ dysfunction syndrome, 1016–1017
Multiple personality. *See* Dissociative disorders
Multiple sclerosis, 1017
Mumps, 1017
Muscular dystrophy (Duchenne's), 1017–1018
Myasthenia gravis, 1018
Myelitis, transverse. *See* Paraplegia
Myeloma, multiple, 1018
Myocardial infarction, 1018–1019
Myocarditis, 1019
Myoclonus, nocturnal, 954
Myofascial pain syndrome, 954
Myringotomy. *See* Mastoidectomy
Myxedema, 954
NANDA, NIC, NOC (NNN) Taxonomy of Nursing Practice, 11
NANDA International, 10, 11
Narcolepsy, 1019
Nausea, 559–563
definition of, 559
documentation focus, 562
in Ménière's disease, 1014
NIC linkages, 560
NOC linkages, 559
nursing priorities, 560–562
in radiation therapy, 1040
Near drowning, 1019
NEC. *See* Necrotizing enterocolitis
Necrotizing cellulitis/fasciitis, 1019
Necrotizing enterocolitis, 1019–1020
Need identification, 3
Neglect
self, 759–762
unilateral, 905–909
Neglect/abuse. *See* Abuse
Neonatal jaundice, 490–494. *See also* Jaundice, neonatal
Nephrectomy, 1020
Nephrolithiasis. *See* Calculi, urinary
Nephrotic syndrome, 1020
Neural tube defect. *See* Spina bifida
Neuralgia, trigeminal, 1020
Neuritis, 1020
Newborn
at 1 week, 1021
growth deviations in, 1020–1021
normal, 1021
postmature, 1021
premature, 1021–1022
special needs, 1022
Nicotine abuse, 1022
Nicotine withdrawal, 1022
Nightingale, Florence, 1, 3
Noncompliance [ineffective adherence] [specify], 563–567
definition of, 563
documentation focus, 566
NIC linkages, 564
NOC linkages, 564
nursing priorities, 564–566
Nonketotic hyperglycemic-hyperosmolar coma, 1022–1023
Nursing, language of, 9–12
Nursing care, administering, 3–4
Nursing diagnoses, 10
health conditions and client concerns with, 943–1064
Nursing Interventions Classification (NIC), 10
Nursing Outcomes Classification (NOC), 10, 11
Nursing practice, standards of, 5–6
Nursing process, 1–8
advantages of using, 6–7
application of, 4–5
steps in, 3–4
Nursing profession, defining, 1–3
Nursing's Social Policy Statement, 2
Nutrition
imbalanced
less than body requirements, 567–573
in achalasia, 945
in Addison's disease, 946
in AIDS, 947
in amenorrhea, 949
in anemia, 950
in anorexia nervosa, 952
in biliary cancer, 958
in bipolar disorder, 959
in burns, 962
in celiac disease, 965
in chemotherapy, 967
in cholelithiasis, 967
in chronic obstructive lung disease, 968
in cirrhosis, 968
in colitis, ulcerative, 969
in Crohn's disease, 973
in Cushing's syndrome, 974
in cystic fibrosis, 974
definition of, 567
in delirium tremens, 975
in depressant abuse, 977
in dialysis, 979
documentation focus, 573
in Down syndrome, 982
in emphysema, 985
in enteral feeding, 986
in failure to thrive, 987
in gastrointestinal anthrax, 952
in glomerulonephritis, 992
in heroin abuse, 998
in Huntington's disease, 999
in hyperemesis gravidarum, 1000
in kwashiorkor, 1007
in lead poisoning, 1011
in leukemia, 1011
in multiple organ dysfunction syndrome, 1017
in necrotizing enterocolitis, 1019–1020
in nephrotic syndrome, 1020
in newborn, 1020, 1021
postmature, 1021
NIC linkages, 568
NOC linkages, 568
in nonketotic hyperglycemic-hyperosmolar coma, 1022
nursing priorities, 568–572
in pancreatic cancer, 1025
in pancreatitis, 1025
in parenteral feeding, 1027
in peritonitis, 1029
in pertussis, 1029
in postpartum period, 1033
in pregnancy, 1034–1035
in puerperal infection, 1005
in pyloric stenosis, 1039
in radiation therapy, 1040
in renal failure, 1041
in Rett's syndrome, 1043
risk for
in agranulocytosis, 947
in bone marrow transplantation, 959
in coma, 970
in gastrectomy, 990
in gastritis, 990
in gastroplasty, 991

in GERD, 991
in gingival abscess, 944
in goiter, 992
in hyperthyroidism, 1002
in infant of addicted mother, 1004
in infant of HIV-positive mother, 1004
in intermaxillary fixation, 1006
in temporomandibular joint syndrome, 1055
in traumatic brain injury, 1059
in ventilator assist/dependence, 1063
in schizoaffective disorder, 1045
in scleroderma, 1046
in stimulant abuse, 1051
in substance dependence/abuse, prenatal, 1052
in substance dependence/abuse rehabilitation, 1052
in thrush, 1056
in tuberculosis, 1060
in typhoid fever, 1060
in viral hepatitis, 997
more than body requirements
in mental delay, 1015
in myxedema, 1019
risk for
in muscular dystrophy, 1018
in nicotine withdrawal, 1022
in obesity, 1023
risk for, in infant at 4 weeks, 1004
more than body requirements. *See* Obesity; Overweight
readiness for enhanced, 574–576
definition of, 574
documentation focus, 575–576
NIC linkages, 574
NOC linkages, 574
nursing priorities, 574–575

Obesity, 576–580
definition of, 576
documentation focus, 579
NIC linkages, 577
NOC linkages, 577
nursing priorities, 577–579
Obesity, 1023
risk for
in mental delay, 1015
in muscular dystrophy, 1018
Obesity-hypoventilation syndrome. *See* Pickwickian syndrome
Obsessive-compulsive disorder, 1023
Omaha System-Community Health Classification System (OS), 10, 11
Opioid abuse. *See* Depressant abuse; Heroin abuse/withdrawal
Oppositional defiant disorder, 1023
Oral mucous membrane, impaired, 550–555
in bulimia nervosa, 961
in chemotherapy, 967
definition of, 550
in dehydration, 975
documentation focus, 554
in gastrointestinal anthrax, 952
in gingivitis, 992
in hand-foot-mouth disease, 994
in iron-deficiency anemia, 950
in Kawasaki disease, 1007
in laryngectomy, 1010
NIC linkages, 551
NOC linkages, 551
nursing priorities, 551–554
in radiation therapy, 1040
risk for, 556–558
in agranulocytosis, 947
definition of, 556
documentation focus, 558
NIC linkages, 556
NOC linkages, 556
nursing priorities, 557–558
in renal failure, 1042
in Sjögren syndrome, 1049
in stomatitis, 1052
in thrush, 1056
in ventilator assist/dependence, 1063
Organic brain syndrome. *See* Alzheimer's disease
Osgood-Schlatter disease, 1023–1024
Osteitis deformans. *See* Paget's disease, bone
Osteoarthritis, 1024
Osteoarthritis (degenerative joint disease). *See* Arthritis
Osteomalacia. *See* Rickets
Osteomyelitis, 1024
Osteoporosis, 1024
Otitis media, 1024
Ovarian cancer, 1024
Overweight, 580–586
definition of, 580
documentation focus, 585–586
in myxedema, 1019
NIC linkages, 581
NOC linkages, 581
nursing priorities, 581–585
risk for, 587–590
definition of, 587
documentation focus, 590
in mental delay, 1015
in muscular dystrophy, 1018
NIC linkages, 588
in nicotine withdrawal, 1022
NOC linkages, 587–588
nursing priorities, 588–590

Paget's disease, bone, 1024–1025
Pain
acute, 591–596
in abdominal aortic aneurysm, 954
in abortion, 943
in abruptio placentae, 944
in achalasia, 945
in adenoidectomy, 946
in adrenal crisis, 946
in AIDS, 947
in amputation, 949
in angina pectoris, 951–952
in appendicitis, 955
in arthroplasty, 955
in asbestosis, 956
in benign prostatic hyperplasia, 958
in bone cancer, 959
in brain abscess, 944
in brain concussion, 971
in brain tumor, 960
in bronchitis, 961
in bubonic plague, 1030
in burns, 962
in bursitis, 962
in calculi, urinary, 962
in cancer, 963
in candidiasis, 963
in cardiac surgery, 964
in carpal tunnel syndrome, 964
in cat scratch disease, 965
in cellulitis, 965
in cesarean birth, 966
in cholecystectomy, 967
in cholelithiasis, 967
in circumcision, 968
in coccidioidomycosis, 969
in colitis, ulcerative, 969
in compartment syndrome, 970
in complex regional pain syndrome, 971
in conjunctivitis, 971
in constipation, 972
in contact dermatitis, 977
in coronary artery bypass surgery, 972
in cubital tunnel syndrome, 974
in cystitis, 974
in de Quervain's syndrome, 977
in decubitus ulcer, 1060
definition of, 591
in diarrhea, 980
in dislocation/subluxation of joint, 981
in disseminated intravascular coagulation, 981
in diverticulitis, 981
documentation focus, 595
in Dressler's syndrome, 982
in drug withdrawal, 982
in dry gangrene, 990
in dysmenorrhea, 983
in ebola, 983
in ectopic pregnancy, 984
in eczema, 984
in encephalitis, 985
in endocarditis, 986
in endometriosis, 986
in epididymitis, 986
in episiotomy, 987
in fibrocystic breast disease, 989
in fibromyalgia, 989
in fractures, 989
in frostbite, 989
in gastritis, 990
in GERD, 991
in glomerulonephritis, 992
in gonorrhea, 992
in gout, 993
in gunshot wound, 999
in hantavirus pulmonary syndrome, 994
in hay fever, 994
in headache, 994
in hemophilia, 996
in hemorrhoidectomy, 996
in hemorrhoids, 996

in herniated nucleus pulposus, 997
in herniorrhaphy, 997
in heroin withdrawal, 998
in herpes simplex, 998
in herpes zoster, 998
in Hodgkin's disease, 999
in hospice care, 999
in hypertension, 1001
in hypoparathyroidism, 1002
in hysterectomy, 1003
in IBS, 1006
in ileus, 1003
in impetigo, 1003
in infectious mononucleosis, 1016
in influenza, 1005
in intrapartum hypertension, 1001
in Kawasaki disease, 1007
in labor
stage III, 1009
stage IV, 1009
in Legionnaire's disease, 1011
in leukemia, 1011
in lumbar laminectomy, 1009
in Lyme disease, 1013
in malaria, 1013
in mastitis, 1014
in mastoidectomy, 1014
in measles, 1014
in meningitis, 1015
in mesothelioma, 1016
in mountain sickness, 1016
in multiple myeloma, 1018
in mumps, 1017
in myocardial infarction, 1018
in myofascial pain syndrome, 1019
in nephrectomy, 1020
in neuritis, 1020
NIC linkages, 592
NOC linkages, 591–592
nursing priorities, 592–595
in Osgood-Schlatter disease, 1023
in osteomyelitis, 1024
in osteoporosis, 1024
in otitis media, 1024
in Paget's disease, 1024
in pancreatic cancer, 1025
in pancreatitis, 1025
in parathyroidectomy, 1026
in pelvic inflammatory disease, 1028
in peptic ulcer, 1060
in pericarditis, 1028
in peritoneal dialysis, 980
in peritonitis, 1029
in plantar fasciitis, 1031
in pleural effusion, 1031
in pleurisy, 1031
in pneumothorax, 1031
in polyarteritis nodosa, 1032
in polycystic kidney disease, 1007
in postconcussion syndrome, 1032
in postoperative recovery period, 1032
in postpartum period, 1033
in prenatal hemorrhage, 996
in prostate cancer, 1037
in prostatectomy, 1037
in prostatitis, 1038
in pruritus, 1038
in puerperal infection, 1005
in pyelonephritis, 1039
in Raynaud's disease, 1041
in reflex sympathetic dystrophy, 1041
in rheumatic fever, 1044
in rheumatoid arthritis, 955
risk for
in aortic stenosis, 954
in infant at 4 weeks, 1004
in rubella, 1044
in SARS, 1045
in scarlet fever, 1045
in sciatica, 1046
in septic arthritis, 955
in serum sickness, 1047
in sickle cell anemia, 951
in sinusitis, 1049
in skin cancer, 1049
in snake bite, 1050
in snow blindness, 1050
in sprain, 1051
in stapedectomy, 1051
in strep throat, 1052
in subdural-chronic hematoma, 995
in synovitis, 1054
in syphilis, 1054
in systemic lupus erythematosus, 1012–1013
in tarsal tunnel syndrome, 1054
in temporal arteritis, 1055
in tendonitis, 1055
in tetanus, 1055
in thrombophlebitis, 1055
in thyroidectomy, 1056
in tonsillitis, 1056
in total joint replacement, 1057
in toxic shock syndrome, 1057
in traction, 1057
in trichinosis, 1059
in trigeminal neuralgia, 1020
in typhus, 1060
in urinary diversion, 1061
in uterine myomas, 1061
in uterine rupture, 1061
in vaginismus, 1061
in vaginitis, 1062
in vasectomy, 1063
in viral hepatitis, 997
in West Nile fever, 1063
in Zollinger-Ellison syndrome, 1064
chronic
in acromegaly, 945
in AIDS, 947
in burns, 962
in bursitis, 962
in cancer, 963
in carpal tunnel syndrome, 964
in colitis, ulcerative, 969
in complex regional pain syndrome, 971
in cubital tunnel syndrome, 974
in de Quervain's syndrome, 977
in endometriosis, 986
in fatigue syndrome, chronic, 988
in fibrocystic breast disease, 989
in fibromyalgia, 989
in GERD, 991
in Gulf War syndrome, 993
in headache, 994
in hemophilia, 996
in herniated nucleus pulposus, 997
in hiatal hernia, 997
in hospice care, 999
in lead poisoning, 1011
in Lyme disease, 1013
in multiple myeloma, 1018
in myofascial pain syndrome, 1019
in neuritis, 1020
in osteoporosis, 1024
in plantar fasciitis, 1031
in polycystic kidney disease, 1007
in postconcussion syndrome, 1032
in postpolio syndrome, 1034
in premenstrual dysphoric disorder, 1037
in Raynaud's disease, 1041
in reflex sympathetic dystrophy, 1041
in rheumatoid arthritis, 955
in sciatica, 1046
in sickle cell anemia, 951
in sinusitis, 1049
in somatoform disorders, 1050
in subdural-chronic hematoma, 995
in tarsal tunnel syndrome, 1054
in temporomandibular joint syndrome, 1055
in tendonitis, 1055
in varicose veins, 1062
in venous insufficiency, 1063
in Zollinger-Ellison syndrome, 1064
chronic/chronic pain syndrome (CPS), 596–602
definition of, 596
documentation focus, 601–602
NIC linkages, 598
NOC linkages, 597
nursing priorities, 598–601
labor, 602–606, 1008
definition of, 602
documentation focus, 605–606
in induced labor, 1007
in labor, stage II, 1008
NIC linkages, 603
NOC linkages, 603
nursing priorities, 603–605
in precipitous labor, 1008
risk for, in unplanned cesarean birth, 967
Palliative care. *See* Hospice care
Palsy, cerebral, 1025
Pancreas transplantation. *See* Transplantation, recipient
Pancreatic cancer, 1025
Pancreatitis, 1025
Panic disorder, 1025
Panic state, 59–60
Paralysis, infantile. *See* Poliomyelitis
Paranoid personality disorder, 1026
Paranoid schizophrenia. *See* Schizophrenia
Paraphilias, 1026
Paraplegia, 1026
Parathyroidectomy, 1026–1027
Parent-child relational problem, 1027

Parent-infant attachment. *See* Attachment, risk for impaired
Parental role conflict, 705–708
Parenteral feeding, 1027
Parenting
impaired, 607–611
in anorexia nervosa, 952
in battered child syndrome, 958
definition of, 607
documentation focus, 611
in infant of addicted mother, 1004
NIC linkages, 608–609
NOC linkages, 608
nursing priorities, 609–610
in parent-child relational problem, 1027
risk for, 615–616
in adolescent pregnancy, 1036
definition of, 615
in failure to thrive, 987–988
in fetal alcohol syndrome, 988
NIC linkages, 616
NOC linkages, 616
in postpartum period, 1033
in SIDS, 1053
readiness for enhanced, 612–614
definition of, 612
documentation focus, 614
NIC linkages, 612
NOC linkages, 612
nursing priorities, 612–614
in postpartum period, 1033
Parkinson's disease, 1027–1028
Passive-aggressive personality disorder, 1028
Patient Care Data Set (PCDS), 10
PCP (phencyclidine) intoxication, 1028
Pediculosis capitis, 1028
Pediculosis pubis. *See* Pediculosis capitis
Pelvic inflammatory disease, 1028
Perfusion, tissue, ineffective, 881–885. *See also* Tissue perfusion, ineffective
Periarteritis nodosa. *See* Polyarteritis nodosa
Pericarditis, 1028–1029
Perinatal loss/death of child, 1029
Perioperative Nursing Data Set (PNDS), 10
Perioperative positioning injury, risk for, 628–632
in cervical laminectomy, 1009
definition of, 628
documentation focus, 631
in hysterectomy, 1003
NIC linkages, 629
NOC linkages, 629
nursing priorities, 629–631
in surgery, 1053
Peripheral arterial occlusive disease. *See* Arterial occlusive disease, peripheral
Peripheral neurovascular dysfunction, risk for, 276–279
in carpal tunnel syndrome, 964
in casts, 964–965
in cubital tunnel syndrome, 974
definition of, 276
documentation focus, 279
in extremity compartment syndrome, 971
in femoral popliteal bypass, 988
in fractures, 989
NIC linkages, 276
NOC linkages, 276
nursing priorities, 276–279
Peripheral vascular disease (atherosclerosis), 1029
Peritonitis, 1029
Persian Gulf syndrome. *See* Gulf War syndrome
Personal identity, disturbed, 616–620
in autism spectrum disorder, 957
in borderline personality disorder, 959–960
definition of, 616
in dissociative disorders, 981
documentation focus, 619
in gender identity disorder, 991
NIC linkages, 617
NOC linkages, 617
nursing priorities, 617–619
risk for, 620–623
definition of, 620
documentation focus, 622
NIC linkages, 620–621
NOC linkages, 620
nursing priorities, 621–622
in seizure disorder, 1047
Personality disorders. *See* Antisocial personality disorder; Borderline personality disorder; Obsessive-compulsive disorder; Paranoid personality disorder; Passive-aggressive personality disorder; *specific types*
Pertussis, 1029–1030
Pervasive development disorders. *See* Asperger's disorder; Autism spectrum disorder; Rett's syndrome
Pheochromocytoma, 1030
Philosophical beliefs, 2
Phlebitis. *See* Thrombophlebitis
Phobia, 1030
Physical abuse, 944–945. *See also* Abuse
Physical examination, 14
Pickwickian syndrome, 1030
PID. *See* Pelvic inflammatory disease
Pinkeye. *See* Conjunctivitis, bacterial
Placenta previa, 1030
Plague
bubonic, 1030
pneumonic, 1031
Plan of care, concept mapping, 27–30
Planning, 3
Plantar fasciitis, 1031
Pleural effusion, 1031
Pleurisy, 1031
PMDD. *See* Premenstrual dysphoric disorder
PMS. *See* Premenstrual dysphoric disorder
Pneumoconiosis (black lung). *See* Pulmonary fibrosis
Pneumonia. *See* Bronchitis; Bronchopneumonia
Pneumothorax, 1031
Poisoning
radiation, 1040
risk for, 623–628
in bipolar disorder, 959
in cardiac dysrhythmia, 983
definition of, 623
documentation focus, 627–628
in drug overdose, 982
in long-term care, 1012
NIC linkages, 624
NOC linkages, 624
nursing priorities, 624–627
in PCP intoxication, 1028
in preterm labor, 1008
Poliomyelitis, 1031–1032
Polyarteritis nodosa, 1032
Polycythemia vera, 1032
Polyradiculitis. *See* Guillain-Barré syndrome (acute polyneuritis)
Post-trauma syndrome [specify stage], 632–637
in battered child syndrome, 958
in burns, 962
definition of, 632
documentation focus, 337
NIC linkages, 633
NOC linkages, 633
nursing priorities, 633–637
in post-traumatic stress disorder, 1034
risk for, 638–642
definition of, 638
documentation focus, 641
in gunshot wound, 1064
NIC linkages, 638
NOC linkages, 638
nursing priorities, 638–641
Post-traumatic stress disorder, 1034
Postconcussion syndrome, 1032
Postmaturity syndrome. *See* Newborn, postmature
Postmyocardial syndrome. *See* Dressler's syndrome
Postoperative recovery period, 1032
Postpartum blues. *See* Depression, postpartum
Postpartum depression, 977
Postpartum period, 1033
Postpartum psychosis, 1034
Postpolio syndrome, 1034
Power, readiness for enhanced, 642–644
definition of, 642
documentation focus, 644
NIC linkages, 642
NOC linkages, 642
nursing priorities, 643–644
Powerlessness, 645–649
in adoption/loss of child custody, 946
in amyotrophic lateral sclerosis, 950
in anxiety disorder, 953
definition of, 645
in delusional disorder, 976
in dialysis, 979–980
documentation focus, 648–649
in emphysema, 985
family, in Tay-Sachs disease, 1054
in multiple sclerosis, 1017
NIC linkages, 645
NOC linkages, 645
nursing priorities, 646–648
in paranoid personality disorder, 1026
in passive-aggressive personality disorder, 1028
in physical abuse, 944

in psychological abuse, 945
risk for, 649–652
in colitis, ulcerative, 970
definition of, 649
in diverticulitis, 982
documentation focus, 652
NIC linkages, 650
NOC linkages, 650
nursing priorities, 650–651
in substance dependence/abuse, prenatal, 1052
in substance dependence/abuse rehabilitation, 1052
in unplanned cesarean birth, 967
Preeclampsia. *See* Abruptio placentae; Hypertension, gestational; Hypertension, gestational
Pregnancy
1st trimester, 1034–1035
2nd trimester, 1035
3rd trimester, 1035
adolescent, 1035–1036
ectopic, 984
high-risk, 1036
postmaturity, 1036
Pregnancy-induced hypertension. *See* Hypertension, gestational
Premature ejaculation, 1036–1037
Premature infant. *See* Newborn, premature
Premenstrual dysphoric disorder, 1037
Premenstrual tension syndrome. *See* Premenstrual dysphoric disorder
Prenatal substance abuse. *See* Substance dependence/abuse, prenatal
Pressure ulcer, risk for, 653–656
definition of, 653
documentation focus, 655
NIC linkages, 654
NOC linkages, 653–654
nursing priorities, 654–655
Pressure ulcer or sore, 1037
Preterm labor. *See* Labor, preterm
Prostate cancer, 1037
Prostatectomy, 1037
Prostatic hyperplasia, benign, 958
Prostatitis
acute, 1038
chronic, 1038
Protection, ineffective, 656–657
in adult failure to thrive, 987
in AIDS, 948
in AIDS dementia, 948
in burns, 962
in chemotherapy, 967
definition of, 656
in hemodialysis, 996
in hemophilia, 996
in leukemia, 1011
in malnutrition, 1013
NIC linkages, 657
NOC linkages, 657
in purpura, 1039
in radiation syndrome/poisoning, 1040
in radiation therapy, 1040
risk for
in adrenal crisis, 947
in aplastic anemia, 954
in heroin abuse, 998
in multiple myeloma, 1018
in SARS, 1045
in transplantation recipient, 1058
Pruritus, 1038
Psoriasis, 1038
Psychological abuse, 945. *See also* Abuse
PTSD. *See* Post-traumatic stress disorder
Pulmonary edema, 1038
high altitude. *See* High altitude pulmonary edema (HAPE)
Pulmonary embolus, 1038
Pulmonary fibrosis, 1038–1039
Pulmonary hypertension, 1039
Pulmonic insufficiency. *See* Valvular heart disease
Pulmonic stenosis. *See* Valvular heart disease
Purpura, idiopathic thrombocytopenic, 1039
Pyelonephritis, 1039
Pyloric stenosis, 1039

Quadriplegia, 1039–1040

Rabies, 1040
Radiation syndrome/poisoning, 1040
Radiation therapy, 1040
Radical neck surgery. *See* Laryngectomy
Rape, 1040–1041
Rape-trauma syndrome, 658–663
definition of, 658
documentation focus, 662
NIC linkages, 659
NOC linkages, 658
nursing priorities, 659–662
in rape, 1041
Raynaud's disease, 1041
Raynaud's phenomenon. *See* Raynaud's disease
Reaction to iodinated contrast media, adverse, risk for, 663–665
definition of, 663
documentation focus, 664–665
NIC linkages, 664
NOC linkages, 663
nursing priorities, 664
Reactive attachment disorder. *See* Anxiety disorders
Reflex sympathetic dystrophy, 1041
Regional enteritis. *See* Crohn's disease
Relationship
ineffective, 665–668
definition of, 665
documentation focus, 668
NIC linkages, 666
NOC linkages, 666
nursing priorities, 666–668
risk for, 672–675
definition of, 672
documentation focus, 674
NIC linkages, 672
NOC linkages, 672
nursing priorities, 672–674
readiness for enhanced, 669–671
definition of, 669
documentation focus, 671
NIC linkages, 669
NOC linkages, 669
nursing priorities, 669–671
Religiosity
impaired, 675–678
definition of, 675
documentation focus, 677–678
NIC linkages, 676
NOC linkages, 676
nursing priorities, 676–677
risk for, 681–684
definition of, 681
documentation focus, 683
in long-term care, 1012
NIC linkages, 682
NOC linkages, 681
nursing priorities, 682–683
readiness for enhanced, 678–680
definition of, 678
documentation focus, 680
NIC linkages, 679
NOC linkages, 679
nursing priorities, 679–680
Relocation stress syndrome, 684–688
in Alzheimer's disease, 949
definition of, 684
documentation focus, 687
NIC linkages, 685
NOC linkages, 684–685
nursing priorities, 685–687
risk for, 688–691
definition of, 688
documentation focus, 691
in long-term care, 1012
NIC linkages, 689
NOC linkages, 689
nursing priorities, 689–691
Renal disease, end-stage, 1041
Renal failure
acute, 1041–1042
chronic, 1042
Renal perfusion
ineffective, in multiple organ dysfunction syndrome, 1016–1017
risk for ineffective, 692–695
in abdominal aortic aneurysm repair, 954
definition of, 692
documentation focus, 694
in gas gangrene, 990
NIC linkages, 692
NOC linkages, 692
nursing priorities, 692–694
Renal transplantation, 1042
Repetitive motion injury. *See* Carpal tunnel syndrome
Resilience
impaired, 695–698
definition of, 695
documentation focus, 698
NIC linkages, 696
NOC linkages, 696
nursing priorities, 696–698
risk for, 702–705
definition of, 702
documentation focus, 704

NIC linkages, 651
NOC linkages, 702
nursing priorities, 702–704
readiness for enhanced, 699–701
definition of, 699
documentation focus, 701
NIC linkages, 699
NOC linkages, 699
nursing priorities, 699–70
Respiratory distress syndrome
acute, 1042
in premature infant, 1043
Respiratory syncytial virus, 1043
Restless leg syndrome. *See* Myoclonus, nocturnal
Retinal detachment, 1043
Rett's syndrome, 1043
Reye's syndrome, 104
Rheumatic fever, 1044
Rheumatic heart disease, 1044
Rhinitis, allergic. *See* Hay fever
Rickets, 1044
Ringworm, tinea, 1044
Rocky Mountain spotted fever. *See* Typhus
Role conflict, parental, 705–708
definition of, 705
documentation focus, 708
NIC linkages, 706
NOC linkages, 706
nursing priorities, 706–708
Role performance, ineffective, 709–712
in cardiomyopathy, 964
in coronary artery bypass surgery, 972
definition of, 709
documentation focus, 712
in gender identity disorder, 991
NIC linkages, 710
NOC linkages, 710
nursing priorities, 710–712
in parent-child relational problem, 1027
in rheumatoid arthritis, 955
risk for
in complex regional pain syndrome, 971
in fatigue syndrome, chronic, 988
in obsessive-compulsive disorder, 1023
in perinatal loss/death of child, 1029
in pregnancy, 1035
in reflex sympathetic dystrophy, 1041
in tendonitis, 1055
Role strain, caregiver, 713–719
RSD. *See* Reflex sympathetic dystrophy
RSV. *See* Respiratory syncytial virus
Rubella, 1044
Rubeola. *See* Measles
Ruptured intervertebral disk. *See* Herniated nucleus pulposus

San Joaquin Valley fever. *See* Coccidioidomycosis
Sarcoidosis, 1045
SARS (severe acute respiratory syndrome), 1045
Scabies, 1045
Scarlet fever, 1045
Schizoaffective disorder, 1045
Schizophrenia, 1045–1046
Sciatica, 1046
Science, knowledge of, in application of nursing process, 5
Scleroderma, 1046
Scoliosis, 1046–1047
Seasonal affective disorder. *See* Affective disorder, seasonal
Sedative intoxication/abuse. *See* Depressant abuse
Sedentary lifestyle, 512–516
Seizure disorder, 1047
Self-care, readiness for enhanced, 730–733
definition of, 730
documentation focus, 732–733
NIC linkages, 731
NOC linkages, 731
nursing priorities, 731–732
Self-care deficit: bathing, dressing, feeding, toileting, 723–730
in brain tumor, 960
in casts, 965
in cerebrovascular accident, 966
in cesarean birth, 966
in Creutzfeldt-Jakob disease, 973
in Cushing's syndrome, 974
definition of, 723
in dementia, 976
in dialysis, 979
documentation focus, 729
in drug withdrawal, 982
in fatigue syndrome, chronic, 988
in hallucinogen abuse, 993
in Huntington's disease, 999
in mastectomy, 1014
in Ménière's disease, 1014
NIC linkages, 724
NOC linkages, 724
nursing priorities, 725–729
in poliomyelitis, 1032
in quadriplegia, 1040
in rheumatoid arthritis, 955
risk for
in coma, 970
in eclampsia, 984
in mental delay, 1015
in schizophrenia, 1046
in septic arthritis, 955
in syringomyelia, 1054
in traumatic brain injury, 1059
Self-concept, readiness for enhanced, 733–736
definition of, 733
documentation focus, 735
NIC linkages, 734
NOC linkages, 733
nursing priorities, 734–735
Self-esteem
chronic low, 736–740
in adolescent pregnancy, 1036
in anorexia nervosa, 952
in antisocial personality disorder, 953
in attention deficit disorder, 957
in battered child syndrome, 958
in borderline personality disorder, 959–960
in conduct disorder, 971
definition of, 736
documentation focus, 739
in encopresis, 985
in enuresis, 986
in narcolepsy, 1019
NIC linkages, 737
NOC linkages, 737
nursing priorities, 737–739
in obesity, 1023
in oppositional defiant disorder, 1023
in paraphilias, 1026
in parent-child relational problem, 1027
in passive-aggressive personality disorder, 1028
in physical abuse, 944
risk for, 740–744
definition of, 740
documentation focus, 743
NIC linkages, 741
NOC linkages, 740–741
nursing priorities, 741–743
in seizure disorder, 1047
in substance dependence/abuse, prenatal, 1052
in suicide attempt, 1053
in Tourette's syndrome, 1057
situational low, 744–748
in acne, 945
in adolescent pregnancy, 1036
in amputation, 949
in cerebrovascular accident, 966
in cesarean birth, 966
in cirrhosis, 969
definition of, 744
in dialysis, 979
documentation focus, 747
in erectile dysfunction, 987
in infertility, 1005
in mastectomy, 1014
NIC linkages, 745
NOC linkages, 744–745
nursing priorities, 745–747
in paraplegia, 1026
in perinatal loss/death of child, 1029
in postpartum depression, 977
in premature ejaculation, 1037
risk for, 748–750
definition of, 748
documentation focus, 750
NIC linkages, 748
NOC linkages, 748
nursing priorities, 779–750
in pelvic inflammatory disease, 1028
in sexual desire disorder, 1048
in suicide attempt, 1053
Self-mutilation, 751–755
in autism spectrum disorder, 957
definition of, 751
documentation focus, 754
NIC linkages, 752
NOC linkages, 752
nursing priorities, 752–754
risk for, 755–758
in anxiety disorders, 954
in borderline personality disorder, 959
definition of, 755

documentation focus, 758
NIC linkages, 756
NOC linkages, 755–756
nursing priorities, 756–758
Self-neglect, 759–762
definition of, 759
documentation focus, 761–762
in hallucinogen abuse, 993
NIC linkages, 759
NOC linkages, 759
nursing priorities, 760–761
Sensory perception, disturbed [specify: visual, auditory, kinesthetic, gustatory, tactile, olfactory], 763–769
in acoustic neuroma, 845
in Alzheimer's disease, 949
in bipolar disorder, 959
in brain tumor, 960
in Brown-Sequard syndrome, 961
in cataract, 965
in cataract extraction, 965
in complex regional pain syndrome, 971
in corneal transplantation, 972
in coronary artery bypass surgery, 972
in craniotomy, 973
in Creutzfeldt-Jakob disease, 973
definition of, 763
in delirium tremens, 975
documentation focus, 768
in drug withdrawal, 982
in glaucoma, 992
in Guillain-Barré syndrome, 993
in Gulf War syndrome, 993
in hydrocephalus, 1000
in hypothyroidism, 1003
in immersion foot, 1003
in macular degeneration, 1013
in mastoidectomy, 1014
in Ménière's disease, 1014
in multiple sclerosis, 1017
in myasthenia gravis, 1018
NIC linkages, 764
NOC linkages, 763–764
nursing priorities, 764–768
in otitis media, 1024
in Paget's disease, 1024
in paranoid personality disorder, 1026
in paraplegia, 1026
in pernicious anemia, 950
in reflex sympathetic dystrophy, 1041
in retinal detachment, 1043
risk for
in CMV infection, 975
in diabetes mellitus, 979
in temporal arteritis, 1055
in temporomandibular joint syndrome, 1055
in schizophrenia, 1045
in Sjögren syndrome, 1049
in snow blindness, 1050
in somatoform disorders, 1050
in stimulant abuse, 1051
in syringomyelia, 1054
in Tay-Sachs disease, 1054
in traumatic brain injury, 1059
in vertigo, 1063
Separation anxiety disorder. *See* Anxiety disorders
Sepsis, 1047
puerperal, 1047
Septicemia. *See* Sepsis
Serum sickness, 1047–1048
Severe acute respiratory syndrome. *See* SARS (severe acute respiratory syndrome)
Sexual desire disorder, 1048
Sexual dysfunction, 769–774. *See also* Dyspareunia; Erectile dysfunction; Sexual desire disorder; Vaginismus
in Cushing's syndrome, 974
definition of, 769
documentation focus, 773
in dyspareunia, 983
in endometriosis, 986
in erectile dysfunction, 987
in hypophysectomy, 1002
NIC linkages, 770
NOC linkages, 770
nursing priorities, 770–773
in ovarian cancer, 1024
in paraplegia, 1026
in physical abuse, 944–945
in pregnancy, 1035
in premature ejaculation, 1036–1037
in psychological abuse, 945
in radiation syndrome/poisoning, 1040
in rape, 1041
risk for
in abdominal perineal resection, 943
in abortion, 944
in acromegaly, 945
in amenorrhea, 949
in breast cancer, 961
in candidiasis, 963
in colostomy, 970
in episiotomy, 987
in herpes simplex, 998
in hypertension, 1001
in hysterectomy, 1003
in long-term care, 1012
in menopause, 1015
in mental delay, 1015–1016
in postpartum period, 1033
in prostatectomy, 1037
in sexual desire disorder, 1048
in substance dependence/abuse rehabilitation, 1052
in testicular cancer, 1055
in vaginismus, 1061–1062
Sexuality pattern, ineffective, 774–778
definition of, 774
documentation focus, 777
in gender identity disorder, 991
NIC linkages, 775
NOC linkages, 775
nursing priorities, 775–777
in paraphilias, 1026
Sexually transmitted infection, 1048
Shingles. *See* Herpes zoster (shingles)
Shock, 1048
cardiogenic, 1048
hypovolemic/hemorrhagic, 1048
risk for, 778–782
in abdominal compartment syndrome, 970
in cholera, 968
definition of, 778
in disseminated intravascular coagulation, 981
documentation focus, 781–782
NIC linkages, 779
NOC linkages, 779
nursing priorities, 779–781
in peptic ulcer, 1060
in placenta previa, 1030
in postpartum hemorrhage, 996
in prenatal hemorrhage, 996
in puerperal sepsis, 1047
in sepsis, 1047
in uterine rupture, 1061
septic. *See* Sepsis
Sicca syndrome. *See* Sjögren syndrome
Sick building syndrome, 1048–1049
Sick sinus syndrome, 1049
SIDS. *See* Sudden infant death syndrome
Sinusitis, chronic, 1049
Sitting, impaired, 782–786
definition of, 782
documentation focus, 785
NIC linkages, 783
NOC linkages, 783
nursing priorities, 783–785
Sjögren syndrome, 1049
Skin abscess, 944
Skin cancer, 1049
Skin integrity, impaired, 786–792
in abscess, 944
in acne, 945
in athlete's foot, 957
in candidiasis, 963
in cardiac surgery, 964
in cutaneous anthrax, 952
in decubitus ulcer, 1060
definition of, 786
in dehiscence, 975
in dermatitis, 977–978
in diarrhea, 980
documentation focus, 791
in facial reconstructive surgery, 987
in Hansen's disease, 994
in immersion foot, 1003
in impetigo, 1003
in Kawasaki disease, 1007
in laceration, 1009
in laryngectomy, 1010
in mastectomy, 1014
NIC linkages, 787
NOC linkages, 787
nursing priorities, 787–791
in pediculosis capitis, 1028
in psoriasis, 1038
in ringworm, 1044
risk for, 792–796
in biliary cancer, 958
in casts, 965
in cirrhosis, 968
in colostomy, 970
definition of, 792
documentation focus, 795–796

in heart failure, 995
in infant of addicted mother, 1004
in labor, stage II, 1009
in lymphedema, 1013
in nephrotic syndrome, 1020
in newborn, postmature, 1021
in newborn at 1 week, 1021
NIC linkages, 793
NOC linkages, 793
nursing priorities, 793–795
in obsessive-compulsive disorder, 1023
in peripheral arterial occlusive disease, 955
in peripheral vascular disease, 1029
in plague, bubonic, 1030
in precipitous labor, 1008
in pruritus, 1038
in renal failure, chronic, 1042
in snake bite, 1050
in transfusion reaction, blood, 1058
in urinary diversion, 1061
in varicose veins, 1062
in varicose veins sclerotherapy, 1062
in West Nile fever, 1064
in Zollinger-Ellison syndrome, 1064
in scabies, 1045
in skin cancer, 1049
in stasis dermatitis, 1051
in STIs, 1048
in syphilis, 1054
in systemic lupus erythematosus, 1013
in toxic shock syndrome, 1057
in varicose veins ligation/stripping, 1062
in venous stasis ulcer, 1060–1061
in wound infection, 1005
SLE. *See* Lupus erythematosus, systemic
Sleep, readiness for enhanced, 797–799
definition of, 797
documentation focus, 798–799
NIC linkages, 797
NOC linkages, 797
nursing priorities, 797–798
Sleep apnea, 1049
Sleep deprivation, 799–804
in Alzheimer's disease, 949
definition of, 799
documentation focus, 803
in insomnia, 1006
in myoclonus, 1019
NIC linkages, 800
NOC linkages, 800
nursing priorities, 800–803
in postpolio syndrome, 1034
risk for, in obesity, 1023
in sleep apnea, 1049
Sleep pattern, disturbed, 804–807
definition of, 804
documentation focus, 806–807
NIC linkages, 805
NOC linkages, 805
nursing priorities, 805–806
Smallpox, 1049–1050
Snake bite, venomous, 1050
SNLs. *See* Standardized nursing languages (SNLs)
Snow blindness, 1050
Social interaction, impaired, 807–811
in antisocial personality disorder, 953
in anxiety disorder, 953, 954
in Asperger's disorder, 956
in autism spectrum disorder, 957
in colostomy, 970
in conduct disorder, 971
definition of, 807
in delusional disorder, 976
in depression, 977
documentation focus, 811
in hyperactivity disorder, 1000
in mental delay, 1015
NIC linkages, 808
NOC linkages, 808
nursing priorities, 808–811
in obesity, 1023
in oppositional defiant disorder, 1023
in phobia, 1030
risk for, in macular degeneration, 1013
in seizure disorder, 1047
in somatoform disorders, 1050
Social isolation, 812–815
in adolescent pregnancy, 1036
in AIDS, 948
in anxiety disorder, 953
in borderline personality disorder, 960
in contact dermatitis, 977
definition of, 812
in depression, 977
documentation focus, 815
in eczema, 984
NIC linkages, 813
NOC linkages, 812
nursing priorities, 813–815
parental, risk for, in special needs newborn, 1022
risk for
in cleft lip/palate, 969
in Down syndrome, 982
in facial reconstructive surgery, 987
in juvenile rheumatoid arthritis, 955
in schizoaffective disorder, 1045
in schizophrenia, 1045–1046
in Tourette's syndrome, 1057
Social Policy Statement, 2
Somatoform disorders, 1050
Sorrow, chronic, 816–819
definition of, 816
documentation focus, 818
in infertility, 1005
NIC linkages, 816
NOC linkages, 816
nursing priorities, 816–818
risk for, in SIDS, 1053
Spina bifida, 1050–1051
Spinal cord injury. *See* Paraplegia; Quadriplegia
Spiritual distress, 819–823
definition of, 819
documentation focus, 822–823
in genetic disorder, 992
NIC linkages, 820
NOC linkages, 820
nursing priorities, 820–822
risk for, 823–826
in abortion, 944
definition of, 823
documentation focus, 826
in hospice care, 999
in infertility, 1005
NIC linkages, 824
NOC linkages, 824
nursing priorities, 824–826
in perinatal loss/death of child, 1029
in Tay-Sachs disease, 1054
Spiritual well-being, readiness for enhanced, 827–829
definition of, 827
documentation focus, 829
NIC linkages, 827
NOC linkages, 827
nursing priorities, 828–829
Splenectomy, 1051
Spongiform encephalopathy. *See* Creutzfeldt-Jakob disease
Sprain of ankle or foot, 1051
Sprue, nontropical. *See* Celiac disease
Standardized nursing languages (SNLs), 9–12
NIC labels in, 10
NOC labels in, 11
Standards of nursing practice, 5–6
Standing, impaired, 830–833
definition of, 830
documentation focus, 832–833
NIC linkages, 830–831
NOC linkages, 830
nursing priorities, 831–832
Stapedectomy, 1051
Stasis dermatitis, 1051
Stereotypes, of nursing, 1
STI. *See* Sexually transmitted infection
Stillbirth. *See* Perinatal loss/death of child
Stimulant abuse, 1051
Stomatitis, 1052
Strep throat, 1052
Stress disorder, acute. *See* Post-traumatic stress disorder
Stress overload, 833–837
in bipolar disorder, 959
definition of, 833
documentation focus, 836–837
NIC linkages, 834
NOC linkages, 834
nursing priorities, 834–836
risk for
in Alzheimer's disease, 949
in Parkinson's disease, 1027
Substance dependence/abuse
prenatal, 1052
rehabilitation, 1052–1053
Sudden infant death syndrome, 1053
risk for, 837–841
definition of, 837
documentation focus, 840
in infant at 4 weeks, 1004
NIC linkages, 838
NOC linkages, 838
nursing priorities, 838–840
Suffocation, risk for, 841–845
in brain abscess, 944
in carbon monoxide poisoning, 963
in coma, 970

definition of, 841
documentation focus, 844
in drug overdose, 982
in electrical injury, 985
in encephalitis, 985
in foreign body aspiration, 956
in hemothorax, 997
in membranous croup, 973
in meningitis, 1015
NIC linkages, 842
NOC linkages, 842
nursing priorities, 842–844
in PCP intoxication, 1028
in seizure disorder, 1047
Suicide, risk for, 845–850
definition of, 845
documentation focus, 849
in drug withdrawal, 982
NIC linkages, 846
NOC linkages, 846
nursing priorities, 846–849
in suicide attempt, 1053
Suicide attempt, 1053
Sunstroke. *See* Heatstroke
Surgery, general, 1053–1054
Surgical recovery, delayed, 850–855
definition of, 850
documentation focus, 854
NIC linkages, 851
NOC linkages, 851
nursing priorities, 851–854
risk for, 855–858
definition of, 855
documentation focus, 857–858
NIC linkages, 856
NOC linkages, 855
nursing priorities, 856–857
in wound infection, 1005
Swallowing, impaired, 858–863
in achalasia, 945
in amyotrophic lateral sclerosis, 950
in cerebrovascular accident, 966
definition of, 858
documentation focus, 863
in GERD, 991
in myasthenia gravis, 1018
NIC linkages, 860
NOC linkages, 859–860
nursing priorities, 860–863
in Parkinson's disease, 1027
in postpolio syndrome, 1034
risk for
in cervical laminectomy, 1009
in tetanus, 1055
Syndrome X. *See* Metabolic syndrome
Synovitis (knee), 1054
Syphilis, congenital, 1054
Syringomyelia, 1054
Systemized Nomenclature of Medicine (SNOMED), 11

Tarsal tunnel syndrome, 1054
Tay-Sachs disease, 1054–1055
TBI. *See* Traumatic brain injury (TBI)
Teen pregnancy. *See* Pregnancy, adolescent
Temporal arteritis, 1055
Temporomandibular joint syndrome, 1055
Tendonitis, 1055
Terminology, standardized, 9–12
Testicular cancer, 1055
Tetanus, 1055
Tetraplegia. *See* Quadriplegia
Thermal injury, risk for, 865–867
definition of, 864
documentation focus, 867
NIC linkages, 864
NOC linkages, 864
nursing priorities, 864–867
Thermoregulation, ineffective, 868–870
definition of, 868
documentation focus, 870
in menopause, 1015
NIC linkages, 868
NOC linkages, 868
nursing priorities, 868–869
in premature newborn, 1021
Thoracotomy. *See* Hemothorax; Surgery, general
Thrombophlebitis, 1055–1056
Thrombosis, venous. *See* Thrombophlebitis
Thrush, 1056
Thyroidectomy, 1056
Thyrotoxicosis, 1056
TIA. *See* Transient ischemic attack
Tic douloureux. *See* Neuralgia, trigeminal
Tissue abscess, 944
Tissue integrity, impaired, 870–876
in abscess, 944
in candidiasis, 963
in cardiac surgery, 964
in cellulitis, 965
in cutaneous anthrax, 952
in decubitus ulcer, 1060
definition of, 870
documentation focus, 875–876
in electrical injury, 984
in frostbite, 989
in gas gangrene, 990
in gunshot wound, 1064
in Hansen's disease, 994
in immersion foot, 1003
in intermaxillary fixation, 1006
in laceration, 1009
in laryngectomy, 1010
in mastectomy, 1014
in necrotizing cellulitis/fasciitis, 1019
NIC linkages, 871
NOC linkages, 871
nursing priorities, 871–875
in postoperative recovery period, 1032
risk for, 877–880
in bacterial vaginosis, 1062
definition of, 877
documentation focus, 880
in labor, stage II, 1009
NIC linkages, 877–878
NOC linkages, 877
nursing priorities, 878–879
in obsessive-compulsive disorder, 1023
in pancreatic cancer, 1025
in peripheral arterial occlusive disease, 955
in peripheral vascular disease, 1029
in precipitous labor, 1008
in rape, 1041
in Sjögren syndrome, 1049
in varicose veins, 1062
in viral hepatitis, 997
in Zollinger-Ellison syndrome, 1064
in smallpox, 1049
in STIs, 1048
in syphilis, 1054
in systemic lupus erythematosus, 1013
in toxic shock syndrome, 1057
in vaginitis, 1062
in venous stasis ulcer, 1060–1061
in wound infection, 1005
Tissue perfusion
bone, ineffective, in osteomyelitis, 1024
ineffective
in adrenalectomy, 947
cerebral, risk for, 889–893
in atrial fibrillation, 957
in carotid endarterectomy, 964
in cerebrovascular accident, 965
in coma, 970
definition of, 889
documentation focus, 892–893
in hydrocephalus, 1000
in meningitis, 1015
NIC linkages, 890
NOC linkages, 890
nursing priorities, 890–892
in PCP intoxication, 1028
in Reye's syndrome, 1044
in transient ischemic attack, 1058
in traumatic brain injury, 1058
in disseminated intravascular coagulation, 981
in dry gangrene, 990
in electrical injury, 984
gastrointestinal, 373–376. *See also* Gastrointestinal perfusion, risk for ineffective
in multiple organ dysfunction, 1016–1017
peripheral, 881–885
in arterial occlusive disease, 955
in complex regional pain syndrome, 971
definition of, 881
documentation focus, 884–885
in extremity compartment syndrome, 970
NIC linkages, 882
NOC linkages, 881
nursing priorities, 882–884
in peripheral vascular disease, 1029
in pressure ulcer or sore, 1037
in puerperal sepsis, 1047
in Raynaud's disease, 1041
in reflex sympathetic dystrophy, 1041
risk for, 893–896
in abdominal aortic aneurysm repair, 954
in amputation, 949
definition of, 893
documentation focus, 896
in gastroplasty, 991

NIC linkages, 894
NOC linkages, 894
nursing priorities, 894–896
in total joint replacement, 1057
in varicose veins ligation/stripping, 1062
in thrombophlebitis, 1055
in venous stasis ulcer, 1061
in pheochromocytoma, 1030
in polyarteritis nodosa, 1032
in polycythemia vera, 1032
risk for
in endocarditis, 986
in femoral popliteal bypass, 988
in lumbar laminectomy, 1009
in metabolic syndrome, 1016
in newborn, 1020
in nicotine abuse, 1022
in valvular heart disease, 1062
in scleroderma, 1046
in shock, 1048
in sickle cell anemia, 951
in typhus, 1060
uteroplacental
in postmaturity pregnancy, 1036
risk for, in cardiac conditions, prenatal, 964
in ventricular aneurysm, 951
ineffective cerebral, in encephalitis, 985
risk for decreased cardiac, 885–889
in cardiac catheterization, 963
definition of, 885
documentation focus, 888
NIC linkages, 886
NOC linkages, 886
nursing priorities, 886–888
TMJ syndrome. *See* Temporomandibular joint syndrome
Toileting, self-care deficit for, 723–730
Tonsillectomy. *See* Adenoidectomy
Tonsillitis, 1056
Total joint replacement, 1056–1057
Tourette's syndrome, 1057
Toxemia of pregnancy. *See* Hypertension, gestational
Toxic enterocolitis, 1057
Toxic megacolon. *See* Toxic enterocolitis
Toxic shock syndrome, 1057
Traction, 1057
Transfer ability, impaired, 897–899
definition of, 897
documentation focus, 899
NIC linkages, 897
NOC linkages, 897
nursing priorities, 898–899
in paraplegia, 1026
Transfusion reaction, blood, 1057–1058
Transient ischemic attack, 1058
Transplant, living donor, 1058
Transplantation, recipient, 1058
Transurethral resection of prostate. *See* Prostatectomy
Trauma
head/neck, risk for, in thyroidectomy, 1056
risk for, 900–905
in Alzheimer's disease, 949
in battered child syndrome, 958
in bone cancer, 959
in brain abscess, 944
in carbon monoxide poisoning, 963
in cataract, 965
in Cushing's syndrome, 974
definition of, 900
in delirium tremens, 975
in dementia, 976
documentation focus, 904
in Down syndrome, 982
in drug overdose, 982
in electrical injury, 985
in encephalitis, 985
in fractures, 989
in hemothorax, 997
in heroin abuse, 998
in hyperparathyroidism, 1001
in lead poisoning, 1010
in LSD intoxication, 1012
in lumbar laminectomy, 1009
in meningitis, 1015
in narcolepsy, 1019
NIC linkages, 901
NOC linkages, 900–901
in nonketotic hyperglycemic-hyperosmolar coma, 1022–1023
nursing priorities, 901–904
in osteoporosis, 1024
in PCP intoxication, 1028
in peritoneal dialysis, 980
in physical abuse, 944
in quadriplegia, 1039
in rabies, 1040
in Rett's syndrome, 1043
in Reye's syndrome, 1044
in seizure disorder, 1047
in sick sinus syndrome, 1029
in stapedectomy, 1051
vascular, risk for, 914–918
Traumatic brain injury (TBI), 1058–1059
Trench foot. *See* Immersion foot
Trichinosis, 1059
Tricuspid insufficiency. *See* Valvular heart disease
Tricuspid stenosis. *See* Valvular heart disease
Tubal pregnancy. *See* Ectopic pregnancy
Tuberculosis, 1059–1060
TURP. *See* Prostatectomy
Twin-twin transfusion syndrome, 1060
Tympanoplasty. *See* Stapedectomy
Typhoid fever, 1060
Typhus, 1060

Ulcer
decubitus, 1060
peptic, 1060
pressure. *See* Ulcer, decubitus
risk for, 653–656
venous stasis, 1060–1061
Ulnar neuropathy. *See* Cubital tunnel syndrome
Unconsciousness. *See* Coma
Unified Medical Language System Metathesaurus, 11
Unilateral neglect, 905–909
definition of, 905
documentation focus, 908–909
NIC linkages, 906
NOC linkages, 906
nursing priorities, 906–908
risk for, in cerebrovascular accident, 966
Upper GI bleeding. *See* Gastritis; Ulcer, peptic
Urinary diversion, 1061
Urinary elimination
impaired, 286–290
in bladder cancer, 959
in calculi, urinary, 962
in circumcision, 968
in cystitis, 974
definition of, 286
documentation focus, 289
in enuresis, 986
in hyperparathyroidism, 1001
in hysterectomy, 1003
in intrapartum hypertension, 1001
in labor, 1008
NIC linkages, 286
NOC linkages, 286
nursing priorities, 286–289
in paraplegia, 1026
in postpartum period, 1033
in pregnancy, 1035
in prostatectomy, 1037
in prostatitis, 1038
in pyelonephritis, 1039
in urinary diversion, 1061
in uterine myomas, 1061
readiness for enhanced, 290–292
definition of, 290
documentation focus, 292
NIC linkages, 291
NOC linkages, 290
nursing priorities, 291–292
Urinary retention [acute/chronic], 910–914
in benign prostatic hyperplasia, 958
in bladder cancer, 959
definition of, 910
documentation focus, 914
NIC linkages, 910
NOC linkages, 910
nursing priorities, 911–913
in prostate cancer, 1037
risk for
in hemorrhoidectomy, 996
in hysterectomy, 1003
in lumbar laminectomy, 1010
Urinary tract infection. *See* Cystitis
Urinary tract injury, risk for, 481–485
Urolithiasis. *See* Calculi, urinary
Uterine bleeding, dysfunctional, 1061
Uterine myomas, 1061
Uterus, rupture of, in pregnancy, 1061
UTI. *See* Cystitis

Vaginal hysterectomy. *See* Hysterectomy
Vaginismus, 1061–1062
Vaginitis, 1062
Vaginosis, bacterial, 1062
Valley fever. *See* Coccidioidomycosis
Valvular heart disease, 1062
VAP. *See* Bronchopneumonia; Ventricular assist/dependence
Varices, esophageal, 1062
Varicose veins, 1062
ligation/stripping, 1062
sclerotherapy, 1062
Variola. *See* Smallpox
Vascular trauma, risk for, 914–918
definition of, 914
documentation focus, 917
NIC linkages, 915
NOC linkages, 915
nursing priorities, 915–917
Vasculitis. *See* Polyarteritis nodosa; Temporal arteritis
Vasectomy, 1063
Venereal disease. *See* Sexually transmitted infection
Venous insufficiency, 1063
Ventilation, impaired spontaneous, 918–923
in amyotrophic lateral sclerosis, 950
definition of, 918
documentation focus, 922–923
NIC linkages, 919
NOC linkages, 918
nursing priorities, 919–922
in respiratory distress syndrome in premature infant, 1043
risk for
in botulism, 960
in hantavirus pulmonary syndrome, 994
in inhalation anthrax, 953
in pulmonary edema, 1038
in SARS, 1045
in tetanus, 1055
in ventilator assist/dependence, 1063
Ventilator assist/dependence, 1063
Ventilatory weaning response, dysfunctional, 923–928
definition of, 923
documentation focus, 927
NIC linkages, 925
NOC linkages, 924–925
nursing priorities, 925–927
risk for, in ventilator assist/dependence, 1063
Ventricular fibrillation, 1063
Ventricular tachycardia, 1063
Verbal communication, impaired. *See* Communication, impaired verbal
Vertigo, 1063
Violence
[actual/] risk for other-directed, 928
in antisocial personality disorder, 953
in bipolar disorder, 958–959
in borderline personality disorder, 959
in conduct disorder, 971
definition of, 928
in delusional disorder, 976
in dissociative disorders, 981
in drug overdose, 982
in paranoid personality disorder, 1026
in PCP intoxication, 1028
in post-traumatic stress disorder, 1034
in postpartum depression, 977
in postpartum psychosis, 1034
in schizoaffective disorder, 1045
in schizophrenia, 1046
[actual/] risk for self-directed, 929–935
in anxiety disorders, 954
in borderline personality disorder, 959
in conduct disorder, 971
definition of, 929
in delusional disorder, 976
in depression, 977
in dissociative disorders, 981
documentation focus, 934
in drug overdose, 982
NIC linkages, 930
NOC linkages, 929
nursing priorities, 930–934
in paranoid personality disorder, 1026
in PCP intoxication, 1028
in schizoaffective disorder, 1045
in schizophrenia, 1046
Walking, impaired, 935–938
in bunion, 962
in bunionectomy, 962
in Creutzfeldt-Jakob disease, 973
definition of, 935
documentation focus, 938
in femoral popliteal bypass, 988
in Huntington's disease, 999
in lymphedema, 1013
in meniscectomy, 1015
NIC linkages, 936
NOC linkages, 935
nursing priorities, 936–938
in Osgood-Schlatter disease, 1023
in osteomyelitis, 1024
in Parkinson's disease, 1027
in plantar fasciitis, 1031
in postpolio syndrome, 1034
in Rett's syndrome, 1043
risk for
in arthroscopy, knee, 956
in Paget's disease, 1025
in peripheral arterial occlusive disease, 955
in spina bifida, 1050
in sprain, 1051
in synovitis, 1054
in tarsal tunnel syndrome, 1054
Wandering [specify: sporadic or continual], 939–942
definition of, 939
documentation focus, 942
NIC linkages, 939–940
NOC linkages, 939
nursing priorities, 940–942
West Nile fever, 1063–1064
Wheelchair mobility, impaired, 541–544
Whooping cough. *See* Pertussis
Wilms' tumor, 1064
Withdrawal, drugs/alcohol. *See* Alcohol intoxication, acute; Drug overdose, acute; Drug withdrawal
Wound, gunshot, 1064

Zollinger-Ellison syndrome, 1064

GORDON'S FUNCTIONAL HEALTH PATTERNS*

HEALTH PERCEPTION–HEALTH MANAGEMENT PATTERN

Contamination 202–207
Deficient community health 392–395
Frail elderly syndrome 352–356
Ineffective family health management 407–410
Ineffective health maintenance 400–403
Ineffective health management 404–407
Ineffective protection 656
Noncompliance [ineffective Adherence] [specify] 563–567
Readiness for enhanced health management 410–413
Risk for bleeding 86–90
Risk for contamination 208–211
Risk for falls 301–306
Risk for frail elderly syndrome 356–358
Risk for infection 467–473
Risk for injury 473–478
Risk for perioperative positioning injury 628–632
Risk for poisoning 623–628
Risk for suffocation 841–845
Risk for thermal injury 864–867
Risk for trauma 900–905
Risk for vascular trauma 914–918
Risk-prone health behavior 396–399

NUTRITIONAL–METABOLIC PATTERN

[Deficient fluid volume: hyper/hypotonic] 333–337
Deficient fluid volume [isotonic] 337–341
Excess fluid volume 341–345
Hyperthermia 426–430
Hypothermia 430–434
Imbalanced nutrition: less than body requirements 567–573
Impaired dentition 250–254
Impaired oral mucous membrane 550–555
Impaired skin integrity 786–792
Impaired swallowing 858–863
Impaired tissue integrity 870–876
Ineffective breastfeeding 102–108
Ineffective infant feeding pattern 327–330
Ineffective thermoregulation 868–870
Interrupted breastfeeding 108–112
Insufficient breast milk 116–120
Latex allergy response 505–509
Nausea 559–563
Neonatal jaundice 490–494
Obesity 576–580
Overweight 580–586
Readiness for enhanced breastfeeding 113–116
Readiness for enhanced fluid balance 330–332
Readiness for enhanced nutrition 574–576
Risk for adverse reaction to iodinated contrast media 663–665
Risk for allergy response 54–56
Risk for aspiration 61–65
Risk for deficient fluid volume 345–348
Risk for dry eye 273–275
Risk for electrolyte imbalance 280–285
Risk for hypothermia 435–437
Risk for imbalanced body temperature 99–102
Risk for imbalanced fluid volume 349–352
Risk for impaired liver function 516–519
Risk for impaired oral mucous membrane 556–558
Risk for impaired skin integrity 792–796
Risk for latex allergy response 509–512
Risk for neonatal jaundice 495–497
Risk for overweight 587–590
Risk for perioperative hypothermia 438–440
Risk for pressure ulcer 653–656
Risk for unstable blood glucose level 90–94

ELIMINATION PATTERN

Bowel incontinence 444–447
Chronic functional constipation 189–193
Constipation 185–189
Diarrhea 260–263
Dysfunctional gastrointestinal motility 364–368
Functional urinary incontinence 447–450
Impaired urinary elimination 286–290
Overflow urinary incontinence 451–453
Perceived constipation 197–199
Readiness for enhanced urinary elimination 290–292
Reflex urinary incontinence 454–457
Risk for chronic functional constipation 194–196
Risk for constipation 199–202
Risk for dysfunctional gastrointestinal motility 369–372
Risk for urge urinary incontinence 464–467
Stress urinary incontinence 457–460
Urge urinary incontinence 460–464
Urinary retention [acute/chronic] 910–914

ACTIVITY–EXERCISE PATTERN

Activity intolerance 32–36
Autonomic dysreflexia 70–74
Decreased cardiac output 126–132
Decreased intracranial adaptive capacity 45–49
Deficient diversional activity 270–273
Delayed surgical recovery 850–855
Disorganized infant behavior 77–82
Dysfunctional ventilatory weaning response 923–928
Fatigue 317–322
Impaired bed mobility 532–536
Impaired gas exchange 359–363
Impaired home maintenance 413–416
Impaired physical mobility 536–540
Impaired sitting 782–786
Impaired spontaneous ventilation 918–923
Impaired standing 830–833
Impaired transfer ability 897–899
Impaired walking 935–938
Impaired wheelchair mobility 541–544
Ineffective airway clearance 49–53
Ineffective breathing pattern 121–125
Ineffective peripheral tissue perfusion 881–885
Readiness for enhanced organized infant behavior 83–85
Readiness for enhanced self-care 730–733
Risk for activity intolerance 36–38
Risk for autonomic dysreflexia 74–77
Risk for decreased cardiac output 132–134
Risk for decreased cardiac tissue perfusion 885–889
Risk for delayed development 254–258
Risk for delayed surgical recovery 855–858
Risk for disorganized infant behavior 85–86
Risk for disproportionate growth 388–392
Risk for disuse syndrome 264–269
Risk for impaired cardiovascular function 135–139
Risk for ineffective cerebral tissue perfusion 889–893
Risk for ineffective gastrointestinal perfusion 373–376

*Modified by Marjory Gordon, 2012, with permission.

Risk for ineffective peripheral tissue perfusion 893–896
Risk for ineffective renal perfusion 692–695
Risk for peripheral neurovascular dysfunction 276–279
Risk for shock 778–782
Risk for sudden infant death syndrome 837–841
Sedentary lifestyle 512–516
Self-care deficit: bathing, dressing, feeding, toileting 723–730
Self-neglect 759–762
Wandering [specify sporadic or continual] 939–942

SLEEP-REST PATTERN

Disturbed sleep pattern 804–807
Insomnia 485–490
Readiness for enhanced sleep 797–799
Sleep deprivation 799–804

COGNITIVE-PERCEPTUAL PATTERN

Acute confusion 173–177
Acute pain 591–596
Chronic confusion 177–181
Chronic pain 596–602
Chronic pain syndrome 596–602
Decisional conflict [specify] 240–243
Deficient knowledge [learning need] (specify) 498–502
[Disturbed sensory perception (specify: visual, auditory, kinesthetic, gustatory, tactile, olfactory)] 763–769
Impaired comfort 155–159
Impaired emancipated decision-making 293–295
Impaired memory 529–532
Ineffective activity planning 39–41
Labile emotional control 299–301
Labor pain 602–606
Readiness for enhanced comfort 159–163
Readiness for enhanced decision-making 244–246
Readiness for enhanced emancipated decision-making 295–298
Readiness for enhanced knowledge (specify) 502–504
Risk for acute confusion 182–184
Risk for impaired emancipated decision-making 298
Risk for ineffective activity planning 42–44
Unilateral neglect 905–909

SELF-PERCEPTION-SELFCONCEPT PATTERN

Anxiety [specify level: mild, moderate, severe, panic] 56–61
Chronic low self-esteem 736–740
Death anxiety 237–240
Disturbed body image 94–98
Disturbed personal identity 616–620
Fear 323–327
Hopelessness 419–423
Ineffective impulse control 440–443
Powerlessness 645–649
Readiness for enhanced hope 416–418
Readiness for enhanced power 642–644
Readiness for enhanced self-concept 733–736
Risk for chronic low self-esteem 736–740
Risk for compromised human dignity 423–425
Risk for disturbed personal identity 620–623
Risk for loneliness 520–523
Risk for powerlessness 649–652
Risk for self-directed violence 929–935
Risk for situational low self-esteem 748–750
Situational low self-esteem 744–748

ROLE-RELATIONSHIP PATTERN

Caregiver role strain 713–719
Chronic sorrow 816–819
Complicated grieving 381–385
Dysfunctional family processes 306–310
Grieving 377–381
Impaired parenting 607–611
Impaired social interaction 807–811
Impaired verbal communication 163–169
Ineffective relationship 665–668
Ineffective role performance 709–712
Interrupted family processes 310–314
Parental role conflict 705–708
Readiness for enhanced communication 169–172
Readiness for enhanced family processes 314–317
Readiness for enhanced parenting 612–614
Readiness for enhanced relationship 669–671
Relocation stress syndrome 684–688
Risk for caregiver role strain 719–723
Risk for complicated grieving 385–388
Risk for impaired attachment 65–69
Risk for impaired parenting 615
Risk for ineffective relationship 672–675
Risk for other-directed violence 928
Risk for relocation stress syndrome 688–691
Social isolation 812–815

SEXUALITY-REPRODUCTIVE

Ineffective childbearing process 139–147
Ineffective sexuality pattern 774–778
Rape-trauma syndrome 658–663
Readiness for enhanced childbearing process 147–154
Risk for disturbed maternal-fetal dyad 523–529
Risk for ineffective childbearing process 154
Sexual dysfunction 769–774

COPING-STRESS TOLERANCE PATTERN

Compromised family coping 212–214
Defensive coping 215–218
Disabled family coping 218–221
Impaired mood regulation 544–546
Impaired resilience 695–698
Ineffective community coping 226–229
Ineffective coping 221–226
Ineffective denial 247–249
Post-trauma syndrome [specify stage] 632–637
Readiness for enhanced community coping 232–234
Readiness for enhanced coping 229–231
Readiness for enhanced family coping 234–236
Readiness for enhanced resilience 699–701
Risk for impaired resilience 702–705
Risk for post-trauma syndrome 638–642
Risk for self-mutilation 755–758
Risk for suicide 845–850
Self-mutilation 751–755
Stress overload 833–837

VALUE-BELIEF PATTERN

Impaired religiosity 675–678
Moral distress 547–550
Readiness for enhanced religiosity 678–680
Readiness for enhanced spiritual well-being 827–829
Risk for impaired religiosity 681–684
Risk for spiritual distress 823–826
Spiritual distress 819–823